COMPLETE GUIDE TO PRESCRIPTION & NONPRESCRIPTION

DRUGS

By H. WINTER GRIFFITH, M.D.

Technical consultants:
John D. Palmer, M.D., Ph.D.
William N. Jones, B.S., M.S.
Stephen W. Moore, M.D.

Over 5000 Brand Names
Over 700 Generic Names

THE BODY PRESS/PERIGEE

otice: The information in this book is true and complete to the best of our knowledge.The book is intended only as a guide to drugs used for medical treatment. It is not intended as a replacement for sound medical advice from a doctor. Only a doctor can include the variables of an individual's age, sex and past medical history needed for wise drug prescription. This book does not contain every possible side effect, adverse reaction or interaction with other drugs or substances. Final decision about a drug's safety or effectiveness must be made by the individual and his doctor. All recommendations herein are made without guarantees on the part of the author or the publisher. The author and publisher disclaim all liability in connection with the use of this information.

The Body Press/Perigee Books
are published by
The Berkley Publishing Group
200 Madison Avenue
New York, NY 10016

Published simultaneously in Canada

Library of Congress Cataloging-in-Publication Data

Griffith, H. Winter (Henry Winter).
Complete guide to prescription & nonprescription drugs/
by H. Winter Griffith; technical consultants, John D. Palmer,
William N. Jones.— Rev. for 1996.
p. cm.
Includes index.
ISBN 0-399-52161-5
1. Drugs—Popular works. 2. Drugs, Nonprescription—Popular works.
I. Title. II. Title: Complete guide to prescription and nonprescription drugs.
[DNLM: 1. Drugs—handbooks. 2. Drugs—popular works. 3. Drugs,
Nonprescription—handbooks. 4. Drugs, Nonprescription—popular works.
QV 39 G854c 1996]
RM301.15.G75 1996 93-30019 CIP
615'.1—dc20
DNLM/DLC
for Library of Congress

Printed in the United States of America

1 2 3 4 5 6 7 8 9 10

Contents

About The Author

H. Winter Griffith, M.D., authored 25 medical books, including the *Complete Guide to Symptoms, Illness & Surgery; Complete Guide to Pediatric Symptoms, Illness & Medications*; and *Complete Guide to Sports Injuries*, each now published by The Body Press/Perigee Books. Others include *Instructions for Patients; Drug Information for Patients; Instructions for Dental Patients; Information and Instructions for Pediatric Patients; Vitamins, Minerals and Supplements;* and *Medical Tests—Doctor Ordered and Do-It-Yourself.* Dr. Griffith received his medical degree from Emory University in 1953. After 20 years in private practice, he established and was the first director of a basic medical science program at Florida State University. He then became an associate professor of family and community medicine at the University of Arizona College of Medicine. Until his death in 1993, Dr. Griffith lived in Tucson, Arizona.

Technical Consultants

John D. Palmer, M.D., Ph.D.

Associate professor of pharmacology, University of Arizona College of Medicine

Associate professor of medicine (clinical pharmacology), University of Arizona College of Medicine

William N. Jones, Pharmacist, B.S., M.S.

Clinical pharmacy coordinator, Veterans Administration Medical Center, Tucson, Arizona

Adjunct assistant professor, Department of Pharmacy Practice, College of Pharmacy, University of Arizona

Stephen W. Moore, M.D.

Family physician, Tucson, Arizona

Drugs and You

My first day of pharmacology class in medical school started with a jolt. The professor began by writing on the blackboard, "Drugs are poisons."

I thought the statement was extreme. New drug discoveries promised to solve medical problems that had baffled men for centuries. The medical community was intrigued with new possibilities for drugs.

In the decades since then, many drug "miracles" have lived up to those early expectations. But the years have also shown the damage drugs can cause when they are misused or not fully understood. As a family doctor and teacher, I have developed a healthy respect for what drugs can and can't do. I appreciate my professor's warning more than ever.

A drug cannot "cure." It aids the body's natural defenses to promote recovery. Likewise, a manufacturer or doctor cannot guarantee a drug will be useful for everyone. The complexity of the human body, individual responses in different people and in the same person under different circumstances, past and present health, age and gender influence how well a drug works.

All effective drugs produce desirable changes in the body, but a drug can also cause undesirable adverse reactions or side effects in some people. Despite uncertainties, the drug discoveries of recent years have given us tools to save lives and reduce discomfort. Before you decide whether to take a drug, you or your doctor must ask, "Will the benefits outweigh the risks?"

The purpose of this book is to give you enough information about the most widely used drugs so you can make a wise decision. The information will alert you to potential or preventable problems. You can learn what to do if problems arise.

The information is derived from many authoritative sources and represents the consensus of many experts. Every effort has been made to ensure accuracy and completeness. Where information from different sources conflicts, I have used the majority's opinion, coupled with my clinical judgment and that of my technical consultants. Drug information changes with continuing observations by clinicians and users.

Information in this book applies to generic drugs in both the United States and Canada. Generic names do not vary in these countries, but brand names do.

Be Safe! Tell Your Doctor

Some suggestions for wise drug use apply to all drugs. Always give your doctor or dentist complete information about the drugs you take, including your medical history, your medical plans and your progress while under medication.

MEDICAL HISTORY

Tell the important facts of your medical history including illness and previous experience with drugs. Include allergic or adverse reactions you have had to any medicine in the past. Describe the allergic symptoms you have, such as hay fever, asthma, eye watering and itching, throat irritation and reactions to food. People who have allergies to common substances are more likely to develop drug allergies.

List all drugs you take. Don't forget vitamin and mineral supplements; skin, rectal or vaginal medicines; eyedrops and eardrops; antacids; antihistamines; cold and cough remedies; inhalants and nasal sprays; aspirin, aspirin combinations or other pain relievers;

motion sickness remedies; weight-loss aids; salt and sugar substitutes; caffeine; oral contraceptives; sleeping pills or "tonics."

FUTURE MEDICAL PLANS

Discuss plans for elective surgery, pregnancy and breast-feeding. These conditions may require discontinuing or modifying the dosages of medicines you may be taking.

QUESTIONS

Don't hesitate to ask questions about a drug. Your doctor, nurse or pharmacist will be able to provide more information if they are familiar with you and your medical history.

YOUR ROLE

Learn the generic names and brand names of all your medicines. Write them down to help you remember. If a drug is a mixture, learn the names of its generic ingredients.

TAKING A DRUG

Never take medicine in the dark! Recheck the label before each use. You could be taking the *wrong* drug! Tell your doctor about any unexpected new symptoms you have while taking medicine. You may need to change medicines or have a dose adjustment.

STORAGE

Keep all medicines out of children's reach. Store drugs in a cool, dry place, such as a kitchen cabinet or bedroom. Avoid medicine cabinets in bathrooms. They get too moist and warm at times.

Keep medicine in its original container, tightly closed. Don't remove the label! If directions call for refrigeration, keep the medicine cool, but don't freeze it.

DISCARDING

Don't save leftover medicine to use later. Discard it before the expiration date shown on the container. Dispose safely to protect children and pets.

REFILLS

All refills must be ordered by your doctor or dentist, either in the first prescription or later. Only the pharmacy that originally filled the prescription can refill it without checking with your doctor or previous pharmacy. If you go to a *new* pharmacy, you must have a new prescription, or the new pharmacist must call your doctor or original pharmacy to see if a refill is authorized.

If you need a refill, call your pharmacist and order your refill by number and name.

Use one pharmacy for the whole family if you can. The pharmacist then has a record of all of your drugs and can communicate effectively with your doctor, you and your family.

LEARN ABOUT DRUGS

Study the information in this book's charts regarding your medications. Read each chart completely. Because of space limitations, most information that fits more than one category appears only once. Any time you are prescribed a new medication, read the information on the chart for that drug, then take the time to review the charts on other medications you already take.

Take care of yourself. You are the most important member of your health-care team.

Guide to Drug Charts

The drug information in this book is organized in condensed, easy-to-read charts. Each drug is described in a two-page format, as shown in the sample chart below and opposite. Charts are arranged alphabetically by drug generic names, and in some instances, such as *ADRENOCORTICOIDS, TOPICAL,* by drug class name.

A *generic name* is the official chemical name for a drug. A *brand name* is a drug manufacturer's registered trademark for a generic drug. Brand names listed on the charts include

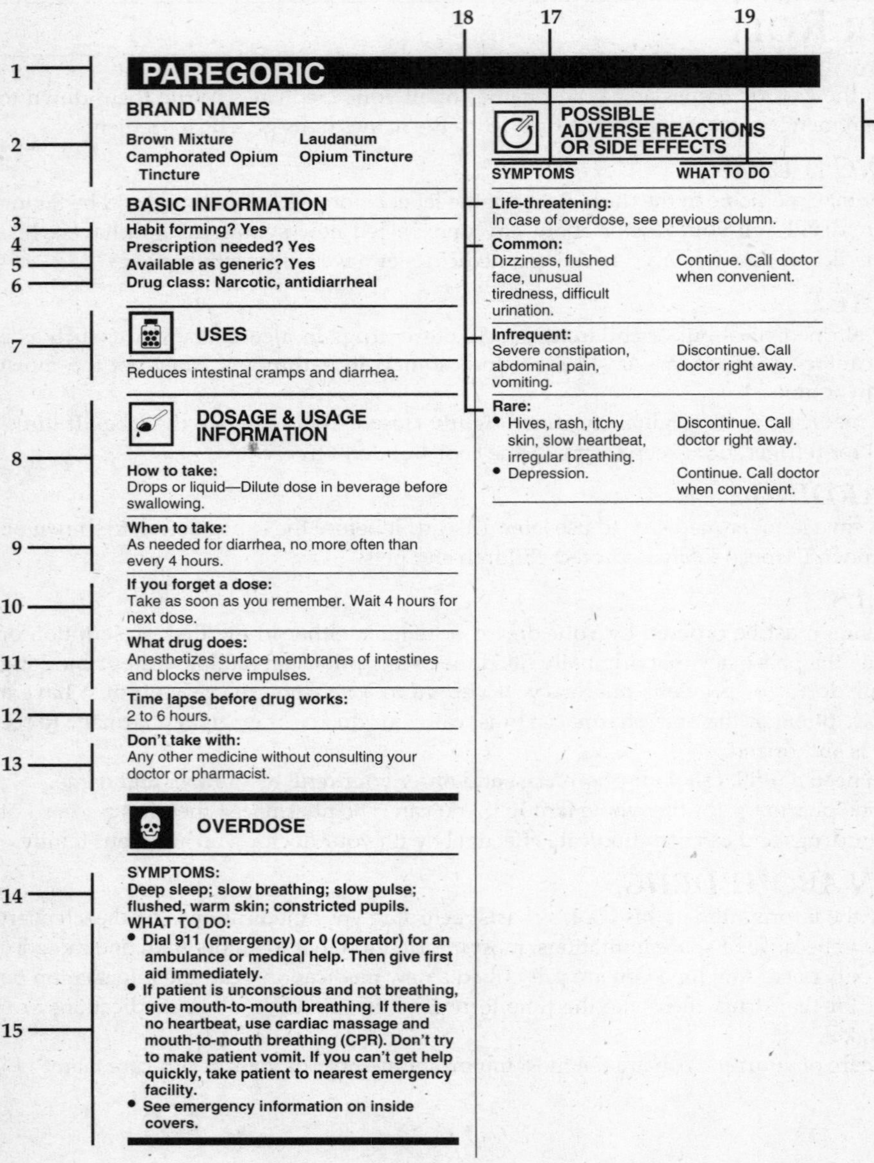

18
17
19
1
PAREGORIC
BRAND NAMES
2
Brown Mixture
Camphorated Opium Tincture
Laudanum
Opium Tincture
BASIC INFORMATION
3 Habit forming? Yes
4 Prescription needed? Yes
5 Available as generic? Yes
6 Drug class: Narcotic, antidiarrheal
7
USES
Reduces intestinal cramps and diarrhea.
8
DOSAGE & USAGE INFORMATION
How to take:
Drops or liquid—Dilute dose in beverage before swallowing.
9
When to take:
As needed for diarrhea, no more often than every 4 hours.
10
If you forget a dose:
Take as soon as you remember. Wait 4 hours for next dose.
11
What drug does:
Anesthetizes surface membranes of intestines and blocks nerve impulses.
12
Time lapse before drug works:
2 to 6 hours.
13
Don't take with:
Any other medicine without consulting your doctor or pharmacist.
OVERDOSE
14
SYMPTOMS:
Deep sleep; slow breathing; slow pulse; flushed, warm skin; constricted pupils.
15
WHAT TO DO:
• Dial 911 (emergency) or 0 (operator) for an ambulance or medical help. Then give first aid immediately.
• If patient is unconscious and not breathing, give mouth-to-mouth breathing. If there is no heartbeat, use cardiac massage and mouth-to-mouth breathing (CPR). Don't try to make patient vomit. If you can't get help quickly, take patient to nearest emergency facility.
• See emergency information on inside covers.
POSSIBLE ADVERSE REACTIONS OR SIDE EFFECTS
16
SYMPTOMS
WHAT TO DO
Life-threatening:
In case of overdose, see previous column.
Common:
Dizziness, flushed face, unusual tiredness, difficult urination.
Continue. Call doctor when convenient.
Infrequent:
Severe constipation, abdominal pain, vomiting.
Discontinue. Call doctor right away.
Rare:
• Hives, rash, itchy skin, slow heartbeat, irregular breathing.
Discontinue. Call doctor right away.
• Depression.
Continue. Call doctor when convenient.

those from the United States and Canada. A generic drug may have one or many brand names.

To find information about a generic drug, look it up in the alphabetical charts. To learn about a brand name, check the index first, where each brand name is followed by the name(s) of its generic ingredients, its drug class name and chart page numbers.

The chart design is the same for every drug. When you are familiar with the chart, you can quickly find information you want to know about a drug.

On the next few pages, each of the numbered chart sections below is explained. This information will guide you in reading and understanding the charts that begin on page 2.

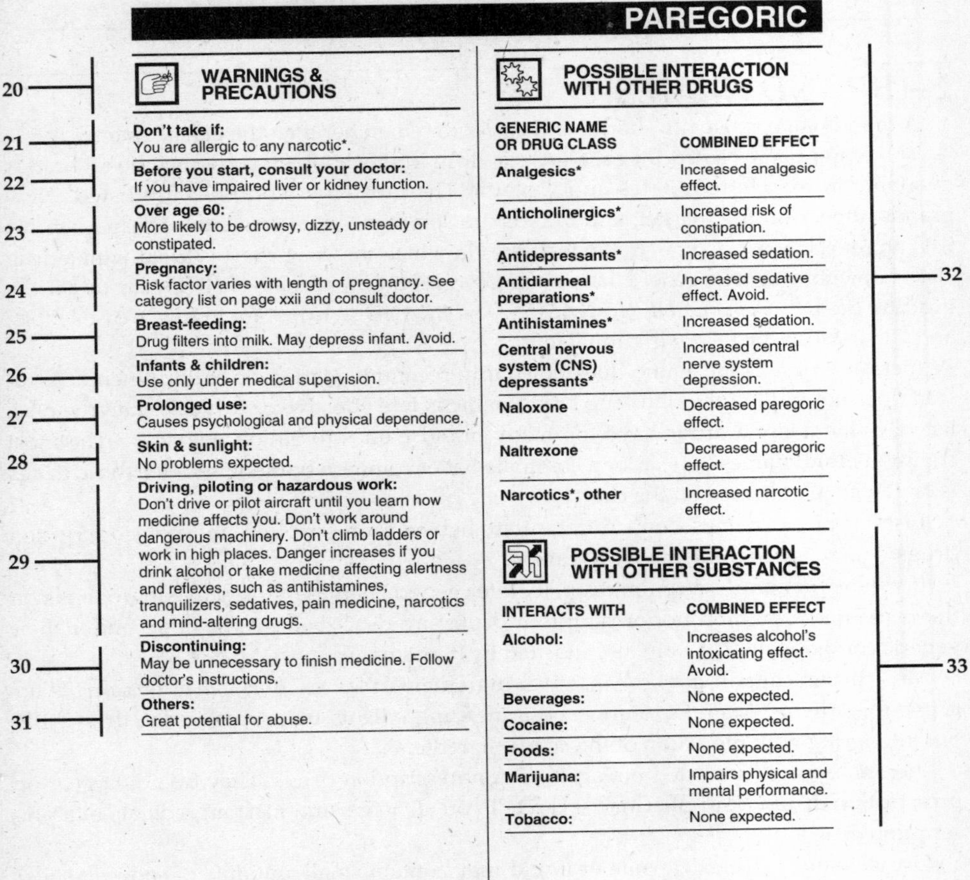

PAREGORIC

WARNINGS & PRECAUTIONS

20 WARNINGS & PRECAUTIONS

21 **Don't take if:**
You are allergic to any narcotic*.

22 **Before you start, consult your doctor:**
If you have impaired liver or kidney function.

23 **Over age 60:**
More likely to be drowsy, dizzy, unsteady or constipated.

24 **Pregnancy:**
Risk factor varies with length of pregnancy. See category list on page xxii and consult doctor.

25 **Breast-feeding:**
Drug filters into milk. May depress infant. Avoid.

26 **Infants & children:**
Use only under medical supervision.

27 **Prolonged use:**
Causes psychological and physical dependence.

28 **Skin & sunlight:**
No problems expected.

29 **Driving, piloting or hazardous work:**
Don't drive or pilot aircraft until you learn how medicine affects you. Don't work around dangerous machinery. Don't climb ladders or work in high places. Danger increases if you drink alcohol or take medicine affecting alertness and reflexes, such as antihistamines, tranquilizers, sedatives, pain medicine, narcotics and mind-altering drugs.

30 **Discontinuing:**
May be unnecessary to finish medicine. Follow doctor's instructions.

31 **Others:**
Great potential for abuse.

POSSIBLE INTERACTION WITH OTHER DRUGS

32

GENERIC NAME OR DRUG CLASS	COMBINED EFFECT
Analgesics*	Increased analgesic effect.
Anticholinergics*	Increased risk of constipation.
Antidepressants*	Increased sedation.
Antidiarrheal preparations*	Increased sedative effect. Avoid.
Antihistamines*	Increased sedation.
Central nervous system (CNS) depressants*	Increased central nerve system depression.
Naloxone	Decreased paregoric effect.
Naltrexone	Decreased paregoric effect.
Narcotics*, other	Increased narcotic effect.

POSSIBLE INTERACTION WITH OTHER SUBSTANCES

33

INTERACTS WITH	COMBINED EFFECT
Alcohol:	Increases alcohol's intoxicating effect. Avoid.
Beverages:	None expected.
Cocaine:	None expected.
Foods:	None expected.
Marijuana:	Impairs physical and mental performance.
Tobacco:	None expected.

***See Glossary**

1—*GENERIC NAME*

Each drug chart is titled by generic name, or in some instances, by the name of the drug class, such as *DIGITALIS PREPARATIONS.*

Sometimes a drug is known by more than one generic name. The chart is titled by the most common one. Less common generic names appear in parentheses following the first. For example, vitamin C is also known as ascorbic acid. Its chart title is *VITAMIN C (Ascorbic Acid)*. The index will include a reference for each name.

Your drug container may show a generic name, a brand name or both. If you have only a brand name, use the index to find the drug's generic name(s), drug class name and chart page numbers.

If your drug container shows no name, ask your doctor or pharmacist for the name and record it on the container.

2—*BRAND NAMES*

A brand name is usually shorter and easier to remember than the generic name.

The brand names listed for each generic drug in this book may not include all brands available in the United States and Canada. The most common ones are listed. New brands appear on the market, and brands are sometimes removed from the market. No list can reflect every change. In the instances in which the drug chart is titled with a drug class name instead of a generic name, the generic and brand names all appear under the heading *BRAND AND GENERIC NAMES*. The *BRAND NAMES* are in lower-case letters, and *GENERIC NAMES* are in capital letters.

Inclusion of a brand name does not imply recommendation or endorsement. Exclusion does not imply that a missing brand name is less effective or less safe than the ones listed. Some generic drugs have too many brand names to list on one chart. The most common brand names appear, or a complete list of common brand names for those drugs is on the page indicated on the chart.

Lists of brand names don't differentiate between prescription and nonprescription drugs. The active ingredients are the same.

If you buy a nonprescription drug, look for generic names of the active ingredients on the container. Common nonprescription drugs are described in this book under their generic components. They are also indexed by brand name.

Most drugs contain *inert*, or inactive, ingredients that are *fillers*, *dyes* or *solvents* for active ingredients. Manufacturers choose inert ingredients that preserve the drug without interfering with the action of the active ingredients.

Inert substances are listed on labels of nonprescription drugs. They do not appear on prescription drugs. Your pharmacist can tell you all active and inert ingredients in a prescription drug.

Occasionally, a tablet, capsule or liquid may contain small amounts of sodium, sugar or potassium. If you are on a diet that severely restricts any of these, ask your pharmacist or doctor to suggest another form.

BASIC INFORMATION

3—*HABIT FORMING*

A drug habit can be physical or psychological. A drug that produces physical dependence leads to addiction. It causes painful and sometimes dangerous effects when withdrawn.

Psychological dependence does not cause dangerous withdrawal effects. It may cause stress and unwanted behavior changes until the habit is broken.

4—PRESCRIPTION NEEDED?

"Yes'' means a doctor must prescribe the drug for you. "No" means you can buy this drug without prescription. Sometimes low strengths of a drug are available without prescription, while high strengths require prescription.

The information about the generic drug applies whether it requires prescription or not. If the generic ingredients are the same, nonprescription drugs have the same dangers, warnings, precautions and interactions as prescribed drugs. The information and warnings on containers for nonprescription drugs may not be as complete as the information in this book. Check both sources.

5—AVAILABLE AS GENERIC?

Some generic drugs have patent restrictions that protect the manufacturer or distributor of that drug. These drugs may be purchased only by brand name.

In recent years, drug manufacturers have marketed more drugs under generic names. Drugs purchased by generic name sometimes are less expensive than brand names.

Some states allow pharmacists to fill prescriptions by brand names or generic names. This allows patients to buy the least expensive form of a drug.

A doctor may specify a brand name because he or she trusts a known source more than an unknown manufacturer of generic drugs. You and your doctor should decide together whether you should buy a medicine by generic or brand name.

Generic drugs manufactured in other countries are not subject to regulation by the U.S. Food and Drug Administration. Drugs manufactured in the United States are subject to regulation.

6—DRUG CLASS

Drugs that possess similar chemical structures and similar therapeutic effects are grouped into classes. Most drugs within a class produce similar benefits, side effects, adverse reactions and interactions with other drugs and substances. For example, all the generic drugs in the narcotic drug class will have similar effects on the body.

Some information on the charts applies to all drugs in a class. For example, a reference may be made to narcotics. The index lists the class—narcotics—and lists drugs in that class.

The names for classes of drugs are not standardized, so classes listed in other references may vary from the classes in this book.

7—USES

This section lists the disease or disorder for which a drug is prescribed.

Most uses listed are approved by the U.S. Food and Drug Administration. Some uses are listed if experiments and clinical trials indicate effectiveness and safety. Still, other uses are included that may not be officially sanctioned, but for which doctors commonly prescribe the drug.

The use for which your doctor prescribes the drug may not appear. You and your doctor should discuss the reason for any prescription medicine you take. You alone will probably decide whether to take a nonprescription drug. This section may help you make a wise decision.

DOSAGE & USAGE INFORMATION

8—HOW TO TAKE

Drugs are available in tablets, capsules, liquids, suppositories, injections, transdermal patches (See Glossary), aerosol inhalants and topical forms such as drops, sprays, creams, ointments and lotions. This section gives general instructions for taking each form.

This information supplements drug label information. If your doctor's instructions differ from the suggestions, follow your *doctor's* instructions.

Instructions are left out for how *much* to take. Dose amounts can't be generalized. Dosages of prescription drugs must be individualized for you by your doctor. Nonprescription drugs have instructions on the labels regarding how much to take.

9—WHEN TO TAKE

Dose schedules vary for medicines and for patients.

Drugs prescribed on a schedule should usually be taken at approximately the same times each day. Some *must* be taken at regular intervals to maintain a steady level of the drug in the body. If the schedule interferes with your sleep, consult with your doctor.

Instructions to take on an empty stomach mean the drug is absorbed best in your body this way. Many drugs must be taken with liquid or food because they irritate the stomach.

Instructions for other dose schedules are usually on the label. Variations in standard dose schedules may apply because some medicines interact with others if you take them at the same time.

10—IF YOU FORGET A DOSE

Suggestions in this section vary from drug to drug. Most tell you when to resume taking the medicine if you forget a scheduled dose.

Establish habits so you won't forget doses. Forgotten doses decrease a drug's therapeutic effect.

11—WHAT DRUG DOES

This is a simple description of the drug's action in the body. The wording is generalized and may not be a complete explanation of the complex chemical process that takes place.

12—TIME LAPSE BEFORE DRUG WORKS

The times given are approximations. Times vary a great deal from person to person, and from time to time in the same person. The figures give you some idea of when to expect improvement or side effects.

13—*DON'T TAKE WITH*

Some drugs create problems when taken in combination with other substances. Most problems are detailed in the Interaction column of each chart. This section mentions substances that don't appear in the Interaction column.

Occasionally, an interaction is singled out if the combination is particularly harmful.

OVERDOSE

14—*SYMPTOMS*

The symptoms listed are most likely to develop with accidental or purposeful overdose. Overdosage may not cause all symptoms listed. Sometimes symptoms are identical to ones listed as side effects. The difference is intensity and severity. You will have to judge. Consult a doctor or poison control center if you have any doubt.

15—*WHAT TO DO*

If you suspect an overdose, whether symptoms are apparent or not, follow instructions in this section. Expanded instructions for emergency treatment for overdose are on the inside back cover.

16—*POSSIBLE ADVERSE REACTIONS OR SIDE EFFECTS*

Adverse reactions or side effects are symptoms that may occur when you take a drug. They are effects on the body other than the desired therapeutic effect.

The term *side effects* implies expected and usually unavoidable effects of a drug. Side effects have nothing to do with the drug's intended use.

For example, the generic drug paregoric reduces intestinal cramps and vomiting. It also often causes a flushed face. The flushing is a side effect that is harmless and does not affect the drug's therapeutic potential. Many side effects disappear in a short time without treatment.

The term *adverse reaction* is more significant. For example, paregoric can cause a serious adverse allergic reaction in some people. This reaction can include hives, rash and severe itch.

Some adverse reactions can be prevented, which is one reason this information is included in the book. Most adverse reactions are minor and last only a short time. With many drugs, adverse reactions that might occur will frequently diminish in intensity as time passes.

The majority of drugs, used properly for valid reasons, offer benefits that outweigh potential hazards.

17—*SYMPTOMS*

Symptoms of commonly known side effects and adverse reactions are listed. Other drug responses may be listed under "Prolonged use," "Skin & sunlight" or "Others." You may experience a symptom that is not listed. It may be a side effect or adverse reaction to the drug, or it may be an additional symptom of the illness. If you are unsure, call your doctor.

18—FREQUENCY

This is an estimation of how often symptoms occur in persons who take the drug. The four most common categories of frequency can be found under the **SYMPTOMS** heading and are as follows. **Life-threatening** means exactly what it says; seek emergency treatment immediately. **Common** means these symptoms are expected and sometimes inevitable. **Infrequent** means the symptoms occur in approximately 1% to 10% of patients. **Rare** means symptoms occur in fewer than 1%.

19—WHAT TO DO

Follow the instructions provided opposite the symptoms that apply to you. If you are concerned or confused, call your doctor.

20—WARNINGS & PRECAUTIONS

Read these entries to determine special information that applies to you.

21—DON'T TAKE IF

This section lists circumstances when drug use is not safe. On some drug labels and in formal medical literature, these circumstances are called *contraindications.*

22—BEFORE YOU START, CONSULT YOUR DOCTOR

This section lists conditions, especially disease conditions, under which a drug should be used only with caution and supervision.

23—OVER AGE 60

As a person ages, physical changes occur that require special considerations. Liver and kidney functions decrease, metabolism slows and the prostate gland enlarges in men.

Most drugs are metabolized or excreted at a rate dependent on kidney and liver functions. Small doses or longer intervals between doses may be necessary to prevent unhealthy concentration of a drug. Toxic effects and adverse reactions occur more frequently and cause more serious problems in older people.

24—PREGNANCY

The best rule to follow during pregnancy is to avoid all drugs, including tobacco and alcohol. Any medicine—prescription or nonprescription—requires medical advice and supervision.

This section will alert you if there is evidence that a drug harms the unborn child. Lack of evidence does not guarantee a drug's safety.

25—BREAST-FEEDING

Many drugs filter into a mother's milk. Some drugs have dangerous or unwanted effects on the nursing infant. This section suggests ways to minimize harm to the child.

26—INFANTS & CHILDREN

Many drugs carry special warnings and precautions for children because of a child's size and immaturity. In medical terminology, *newborns* are babies up to 2 weeks old, *infants* are 2 weeks to 1 year, and *children* are 1 to 12 years.

27—PROLONGED USE

With the exception of immediate allergic reactions, most drugs produce no ill effects during short periods of treatment. However, relatively safe drugs taken for long periods may produce unwanted effects. These are listed. Drugs should be taken in the smallest dose and for the shortest time possible. Nevertheless, some diseases and conditions require an indefinite period of treatment. Your doctor may want to change drugs occasionally or alter your treatment regimen to minimize problems.

The words "functional dependence" sometimes appear in this section. This does not mean *physical* or *psychological addiction*. Sometimes a body function ceases to work naturally because it has been replaced or interfered with by the drug. The body then becomes dependent on the drug to continue the function.

28—SKIN & SUNLIGHT

Many drugs cause *photosensitivity*, which means increased skin sensitivity to ultraviolet rays from sunlight or artificial rays from a sunlamp. This section will alert you to this potential problem.

29—DRIVING, PILOTING OR HAZARDOUS WORK

Any drug that alters moods or that decreases alertness, muscular coordination or reflexes may make these activities particularly hazardous. The effects may not appear in all people, or they may disappear after a short exposure to the drug. If this section contains a warning, use caution until you determine how a new drug affects you.

30—DISCONTINUING

Some patients stop taking a drug when symptoms begin to go away, although complete recovery may require longer treatment.

Other patients continue taking a drug when it is no longer needed. This section gives warnings about prematurely discontinuing. Some drugs cause symptoms days or weeks after they have been discontinued.

31—OTHERS

Warnings and precautions appear here if they don't fit into the other categories. This section includes storage instructions; how to dispose of outdated drugs; changes in blood, urine and other laboratory tests; warnings to persons with chronic illness and other information.

32—POSSIBLE INTERACTION WITH OTHER DRUGS

Drugs interact in your body with other drugs, whether prescription or nonprescription. Interactions affect absorption, elimination or distribution of either drug. The chart lists interactions by generic name, drug class or drug-induced effect. An asterisk (*) beside a drug class name in this column reminds you to "See Glossary" in the back of the book, where that drug class is described and where generic drug names for that class are listed.

If a drug class appears, the generic drug may interact with any drug in that class. Drugs in each class that are included in the book are listed in the index. Occasionally drugs that are not included in this book appear in the Interaction column.

Interactions are sometimes beneficial. You may not be able to determine from the chart which interactions are good and which are bad. Don't guess. Consult your doctor if you take drugs that interact. Some combinations are fatal.

Some drugs have too many interactions to list on one chart. The additional interactions appear on the continuation page indicated at the bottom of the list.

Testing has not been done on all possible drug combinations. It is important to let your doctor or pharmacist know about any drugs you take, both prescription and nonprescription.

33—POSSIBLE INTERACTION WITH OTHER SUBSTANCES

The substances listed here are repeated on every drug chart. All people eat food and drink beverages. Many adults consume alcohol. Many people use cocaine and smoke tobacco or marijuana. This section shows possible interactions between these substances and each drug.

Drugs of Abuse

Each of the drug charts beginning on page 2 contains a section listing the interactions of alcohol, marijuana and cocaine with the therapeutic drug in the bloodstream. These three drugs are singled out because of their widespread use and abuse. The information is factual, not judgmental.

The long-term effects of alcohol and tobacco abuse are numerous. They have been well publicized, and information is provided here as a reminder of the inherent dangers of these drugs.

Drugs of potential abuse include those that are addictive and harmful. They usually produce a temporary, false sense of well-being. The long-term effects, however, are harmful and can be devastating to the body and psyche of the addict.

Refresh your memory frequently about the potential harm from prolonged use of *any* drugs or substances you take. Avoid unwise use of habit-forming drugs.

These are the most common drugs of abuse:

Tobacco (Nicotine)

What it does: Tobacco smoke contains noxious and cancer-producing ingredients. They include nicotine, carbon monoxide, ammonia, and a variety of harmful tars. Carcinogens in smoke probably come from the tars. Most are present in chewing tobacco and snuff as well as smoke from cigarettes, cigars, and pipes. Tobacco smoke interferes with the immune mechanisms of the body.

Short-term effects of average amount: Relaxation of mood if you are a steady smoker. Constriction of blood vessels.

Short-term effects of large amount inhaled: Headache, appetite loss, nausea.

Long-term effects: Greatly enhanced chances of developing lung cancer. Impaired breathing and chronic lung disease (asthma, emphysema, bronchiectasis, lung abscess and others) much more likely. Heart and blood vessel disease more frequent and more severe when they happen. These include myocardial infarction (heart attack), coronary artery disease, heartbeat irregularities, generalized atherosclerosis (hardening of the arteries, making brain, heart, and kidney more vulnerable to disease), peripheral vascular disease such as intermittent claudication, Buerger's disease and others. Tobacco and nicotine lead to an increased incidence of abortion and significantly reduce the birth weight of children brought to term and delivered of women who smoke during pregnancy. Tobacco smoking not only causes higher frequency of lung cancer, but also increases the likelihood of developing cancer of the throat, larynx, mouth, esophagus, bladder, and pancreas.

ALCOHOL

What it does:

•*Central Nervous System*

Depresses, does *not* stimulate, the action of all parts of the central nervous system. It depresses normal mental activity and normal muscle function. Short-term effects of an average amount: relaxation, breakdown of inhibitions, euphoria, decreased alertness. Short-term effects of large amounts: nausea, stupor, hangover, unconsciousness, even death.

•*Gastrointestinal System*

Increases stomach acid, poisons liver function. Chronic alcoholism frequently leads to permanent damage to the liver.

•*Heart and Blood Vessels*

Decreased normal function, leading to heart diseases such as cardiomyopathy and disorders of the blood vessels and kidney, such as high blood pressure. Bleeding from the esophagus and stomach frequently accompany liver disease caused by chronic alcoholism.

•*Unborn Fetus (teratogenicity)*

Alcoholism in the mother carrying a fetus causes *fetal alcohol syndrome (FAS),* which includes the production of mental deficiency, facial abnormalities, slow growth and other major and minor malformations in the newborn.

Signs of Use:

Early signs: Prominent smell of alcohol on the breath, behavior changes (aggressiveness; passivity; lack of sexual inhibition; poor judgment; outbursts of uncontrolled emotion, such as rage or tearfulness).

Intoxication signs: Unsteady gait, slurred speech, poor performance of any brain or muscle function, stupor or coma in *severe* alcoholic intoxication with slow, noisy breathing, cold and clammy skin, heartbeat faster than usual.

Long-term Effects:

Addiction: Compulsive use of alcohol. Persons addicted to alcohol have severe withdrawal symptoms when alcohol is unavailable. Even with successful treatment, addiction to alcohol (and other drugs that cause addiction) has a high tendency to relapse. (Memories of euphoric feelings plus family, social, emotional, psychological, and genetic factors probably are all important factors in producing the addiction.)

Liver disease: Usually cirrhosis; also, deleterious effects on the unborn child of an alcoholic mother.

Loss of sexual function: Impotence, erectile dysfunction, loss of libido.

Increased incidence of cancer: Mouth, pharynx, larynx, esophagus, liver and lung.

Changes in blood: Makes clotting less efficient.

Heart disease: Decreased normal function leading to possible damage and disease.

Stomach and intestinal problems: Increased production of stomach acid.

Interference with expected or normal actions of many medications: Detailed on every chart in this book, drugs such as sedatives, pain killers, narcotics, antihistamines, anticonvulsants, anticoagulants and others.

Marijuana (cannabis, hashish)

What they do: Heighten perception, cause mood swings, relax mind and body.
Signs of use: Red eyes, lethargy, uncoordinated body movements.
Long-term effects: Decreased motivation. Possible brain, heart, lung and reproductive system damage.

Amphetamines

What they do: Speed up physical and mental processes to cause a false sense of energy and excitement. The moods are temporary and unreal.
Signs of use: Dilated pupils, insomnia, trembling.
Long-term effects: Violent behavior, paranoia, possible death from overdose.

Barbiturates

What they do: Produce drowsiness and lethargy.
Signs of use: Confused speech, lack of coordination and balance.
Long-term effects: Disrupt normal sleep pattern. Possible death from overdose, especially in combination with alcohol.

Cocaine

What it does: Stimulates the nervous system, heightens sensations and may produce hallucinations.
Signs of use: Trembling, intoxication, dilated pupils, constant sniffling.
Long-term effects: Ulceration of nasal passages where sniffed. Itching all over body, sometimes with open sores. Possible brain damage or heart rhythm disturbance. Possible death from overdose.

Opiates (codeine, heroin, methadone, morphine, opium)

What they do: Relieve pain, create temporary and false sense of well-being.
Signs of use: Constricted pupils, mood swings, slurred speech, sore eyes, lethargy, weight loss, sweating.
Long-term effects: Malnutrition, extreme susceptibility to infection, the need to increase drug amount to produce the same effects. Possible death from overdose.

Psychedelic Drugs (LSD, Mescaline)

What they do: Produce hallucinations, either pleasant or frightening.
Signs of use: Dilated pupils, sweating, trembling, fever, chills.
Long-term effects: Lack of motivation, unpredictable behavior, narcissism, recurrent hallucinations without drug use ("flashbacks"). Possible death from overdose.

Volatile Substances (Glue, Solvents)

What they do: Produce hallucinations, temporary false sense of well-being and possible unconsciousness.
Signs of use: Dilated pupils, flushed face, confusion.
Long-term effects: Permanent brain, liver, kidney damage. Possible death from overdose.

CHECKLIST FOR SAFER DRUG USE

- Tell your doctor about *any* drug you take (even aspirin, allergy pills, cough and cold preparations, antacids, laxatives, vitamins, etc.) *before* you take *any* new drug.
- Learn all you can about drugs you may take *before* you take them. Information sources are your doctor, your nurse, your pharmacist, this book and other books in your public library.
- Don't take drugs prescribed for someone else—even if your symptoms are the same.
- Keep your prescription drugs to yourself. Your drugs may be harmful to someone else.
- Tell your doctor about any symptoms you believe are caused by a drug—prescription or nonprescription—that you take.
- Take only medicines that are *necessary*. Avoid taking nonprescription drugs while taking prescription drugs for a medical problem.
- Before your doctor prescribes for you, tell him about your previous experiences with any drug—beneficial results, side effects, adverse reactions or allergies.
- Take medicine in good light after you have identified it. If you wear glasses to read, put them on to check drug labels. It is easy to take the wrong drug at the wrong time.
- Don't keep any drugs that change mood, alertness or judgment—such as sedatives, narcotics or tranquilizers—by your bedside. These cause many accidental deaths by overdose. You may unknowingly repeat a dose when you are half asleep or confused.
- Know the names of your medicines. These include the generic name, the brand name and the generic names of all ingredients in a drug mixture. Your doctor, nurse or pharmacist can give you this information.
- Study the labels on all nonprescription drugs. If the information is incomplete or if you have questions, ask the pharmacist for more details.
- If you must deviate from your prescribed dose schedule, tell your doctor.
- Shake liquid medicines before taking (if directed).
- Store all medicines away from moisture and heat. Bathroom medicine cabinets are usually unsuitable.
- If a drug needs refrigeration, don't freeze.
- Obtain a standard measuring spoon from your pharmacy for liquid medicines. Kitchen teaspoons and tablespoons are not accurate enough.
- Follow diet instructions when you take medicines. Some work better on a full stomach, others on an empty stomach. Some drugs are more useful with special diets. For example, medicine for high blood pressure is more effective if accompanied by a sodium-restricted diet.
- Tell your doctor about any allergies you have. A previous allergy to a drug may make it dangerous to prescribe again. People with other allergies, such as eczema, hay fever, asthma, bronchitis and food allergies, are more likely to be allergic to drugs.

- Prior to surgery, tell your doctor, anesthesiologist or dentist about any drug you have taken in the past few weeks. Advise them of any cortisone drugs you have taken within two years.
- If you become pregnant while taking any medicine, including birth control pills, tell your doctor immediately.
- Avoid *all* drugs while you are pregnant, if possible. If you must take drugs during pregnancy, record names, amounts, dates and reasons.
- If you see more than one doctor, tell each one about drugs others have prescribed.
- When you use nonprescription drugs, report it so the information is on your medical record.
- Store all drugs away from the reach of children.
- Note the expiration date on each drug label. Discard outdated ones safely. If no expiration date appears and it has been at least one year since taking the medication, it may be best to discard it.
- Pay attention to the information in the drug charts about safety while driving, piloting or working in dangerous places.
- Alcohol, cocaine, marijuana or other mood-altering drugs, as well as tobacco—mixed with some drugs—can cause a life-threatening interaction, prevent your medicine from being effective or delay your return to health. Common sense dictates that you avoid them during illness.

Cough and Cold Medicines

Coughs and colds are among humans' most common ailments, and the commercial medicines available for treatment are numerous.

There are hundreds of brands of medicines (each with a registered name) designed to relieve symptoms caused by the common cold, influenza and other minor respiratory illnesses. Most of these medications are over-the-counter (OTC) medicines and can be purchased without a prescription.

Although these drugs may be safe when taken alone, interactions between these medicines and other nonprescription or prescription drugs, when taken together, may produce undesirable or unsafe results. So, for your own safety, you should study the information in this book with regard to the ingredients of each brand-name cough or cold medicine you are taking. Follow these steps to learn about the safety of your drug:

1. Determine the brand name of your drug.

2. Look on the label for the generic ingredients that are used in your brand of medicine.

3. For each generic ingredient, consult the index or look up each generic drug in the alphabetized drug charts. Read the information about how to use the drug safely, especially regarding its use (interaction) with other drugs you may be taking simultaneously.

The generic ingredients of cough and cold medicines fall into several drug classes:

Antihistamines control allergy symptoms. All antihistamines may cause drowsiness, decreased reflexes and decreased ability to concentrate. Therefore, don't drive vehicles or pilot aircraft until you learn how this medicine affects you. Don't work around dangerous machinery. Don't climb ladders or work in high places. The danger increases if you drink alcohol or take other medicines that affect alertness and reflexes, such as other antihistamines, tranquilizers, sedatives, pain medicines, narcotics and mind-altering drugs. They all may cause other side effects or adverse reactions.

Decongestants relieve symptoms of nasal or bronchial congestion. All decongestants may cause nervousness, irregular heartbeats in some people, dizziness, confusion and other side effects. Conduct your daily activities with these effects in mind.

Antitussives reduce frequency and severity of cough. These may be either *narcotic* (codeine and hydrocodone) or *non-narcotic* (dextromethorphan). Narcotic cough suppressants are habit-forming and may cause some of the same mental changes that can take place with antihistamines. The most common non-narcotic antitussive medicine, dextromethorphan, is not habit-forming but has other side effects.

Expectorants loosen secretions to make them easier to cough up. The most common expectorant is guaifenesin, which has very few side effects but doesn't loosen secretions very efficiently.

Analgesics relieve aches and pains. The most common analgesics in cough and cold medicines are aspirin, acetaminophen and ibuprofen.

To learn the details about any cough or cold remedy you may take, look up the brand names in the index of this book. Then consult the generic drug charts listed for each brand name.

Pregnancy Risk Category Information

The pregnancy risk category assigned to a medication identifies the potential risk for that particular drug to cause birth defects or death to an unborn child (fetus). These categories are assigned by applying the definitions of the Food and Drug Administration (FDA) to the available clinical information about the drug. Most drugs are tested only on animals and not on humans for safety during pregnancy, because such testing would subject unborn children to unnecessary risks.

It is best to avoid all drugs during pregnancy, but this rating system can help you and your doctor to assess the risk-to-benefit ratio should drug treatment become necessary. You and your doctor should discuss these benefits and risks carefully before any drug treatment is initiated. You should not take any medications (including nonprescription drugs such as laxatives or cold remedies) without your doctor's approval.

Definitions of the drug categories, labeled A, B, C, D, and X, are listed below:

- A: Adequate studies in pregnant women have failed to show a risk to the fetus in the first trimester of pregnancy, and there is no evidence of risk in later trimesters.
- B: Animal studies have not shown an adverse effect on the fetus, but there are no adequate studies in pregnant women; or animal studies have shown an adverse effect on the fetus, but adequate studies in pregnant women have not shown a risk to the fetus.
- C: Animal studies have shown an adverse effect on the fetus, but there are no adequate studies in humans; or there are no studies in animals or women. The drug may be used by pregnant women because of its benefits and despite its potential risks.
- D: There is evidence of risk to the human fetus, but the potential benefits of use by pregnant women may be acceptable despite the potential risks (e.g., a woman might take such a drug in a life-threatening situation or for a serious disease for which safer drugs cannot be used or are ineffective).
- X: Studies in animals and humans show fetal abnormalities, or reports of adverse reactions indicate evidence of fetal risk. The risks involved clearly outweigh potential benefits, and the drug is contraindicated for pregnant women.

Drug Charts

ACETAMINOPHEN

BRAND NAMES

See complete list of brand names in the *Brand Name Directory*, page 890.

BASIC INFORMATION

Habit forming? No
Prescription needed? No
Available as generic? Yes
Drug class: Analgesic, fever reducer

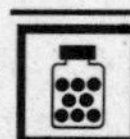

USES

Treatment of mild to moderate pain and fever. Acetaminophen does not relieve redness, stiffness or swelling of joints or tissue inflammation. Use aspirin or other drugs for inflammation.

DOSAGE & USAGE INFORMATION

How to take:

- Tablet or capsule—Swallow with liquid.
- Effervescent granules—Dissolve granules in 4 oz. of cool water. Drink all the water.
- Elixir—Swallow with liquid.
- Suppositories—Remove wrapper and moisten suppository with water. Gently insert larger end into rectum. Push well into rectum with finger.
- Powder—Sprinkle over liquid, then swallow.

When to take:
As needed, no more often than every 3 hours.

If you forget a dose:
Take as soon as you remember. Wait 3 hours for next dose.

What drug does:
May affect hypothalamus—part of brain that helps regulate body heat and receives body's pain messages.

Continued next column

OVERDOSE

SYMPTOMS:
Stomach upset, irritability, sweating, diarrhea, loss of appetite, abdominal cramps, convulsions, coma.
WHAT TO DO:

- **Call your doctor or poison control center for advice if you suspect overdose, even if not sure. Symptoms may not appear until damage has occurred.**
- **See emergency information on inside covers.**

Time lapse before drug works:
15 to 30 minutes. May last 4 hours.

Don't take with:

- Other drugs with acetaminophen. Too much acetaminophen can damage liver and kidneys.
- Any other medicine without consulting your doctor or pharmacist.

POSSIBLE ADVERSE REACTIONS OR SIDE EFFECTS

SYMPTOMS	WHAT TO DO
Life-threatening:	
In case of overdose, see previous column.	
Common:	
Lightheadedness.	Continue. Call doctor when convenient.
Infrequent:	
• Trembling.	Continue. Call doctor when convenient.
• Pain in lower back or side.	Discontinue Call doctor right away.
Rare:	
• Extreme fatigue; rash, itch, hives; sore throat and fever after taking regularly a few days; unexplained bleeding or bruising; blood in urine; painful or frequent urination; jaundice; anemia.	Discontinue. Call doctor right away.
• Decreased volume of urine output.	Continue. Call doctor when convenient.

WARNINGS & PRECAUTIONS

Don't take if:

- You are allergic to acetaminophen.
- Your symptoms don't improve after 2 days' use. Call your doctor.

Before you start, consult your doctor:
If you have kidney disease or liver damage.

Over age 60:
Don't exceed recommended dose. You can't eliminate drug as efficiently as younger persons.

Pregnancy:
No proven harm to unborn child. Avoid if possible. Consult doctor. Risk category B (see page xxii).

Breast-feeding:
No proven harm to nursing infant.

Infants & children:
Use only under medical supervision.

Prolonged use:

- May affect blood system and cause anemia. Limit use to 5 days for children 12 and under, and 10 days for adults.
- Talk to your doctor about the need for follow-up medical examinations or laboratory studies to check liver function, kidney function.

Skin & sunlight:
No problems expected.

Driving, piloting or hazardous work:
Avoid if you feel drowsy. Otherwise, no restrictions.

Discontinuing:
Discontinue in 2 days if symptoms don't improve.

Others:
May interfere with the accuracy of some medical tests.

POSSIBLE INTERACTION WITH OTHER DRUGS

GENERIC NAME OR DRUG CLASS	COMBINED EFFECT
Anticoagulants, oral*	May increase anticoagulant effect. If combined frequently, prothrombin time should be monitored.
Aspirin and other salicylates*	Prolonged use of high doses of both drugs may lead to kidney disease.
Isoniazid	Increased risk of liver damage.
Nicotine	Increased effect of acetaminophen.

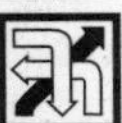

POSSIBLE INTERACTION WITH OTHER SUBSTANCES

INTERACTS WITH	COMBINED EFFECT
Alcohol:	Drowsiness, long-term use may cause toxic effect in liver.
Beverages:	None expected.
Cocaine:	None expected. However, cocaine may slow body's recovery. Avoid.
Foods:	None expected.
Marijuana:	Increased pain relief. However, marijuana may slow body's recovery. Avoid.
Tobacco:	None expected.

*See Glossary

ACETAMINOPHEN & SALICYLATES

BRAND NAMES

See complete list of brand names in the *Brand Name Directory*, page 891.

BASIC INFORMATION

Habit forming? No
Prescription needed? No
High strength: Yes
Low strength: No
Yes, for some combinations
Available as generic? No
Drug class: Analgesic, fever reducer, anti-inflammatory (nonsteroidal)

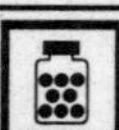

USES

- Treatment of mild pain and fever.
- Salicylates are useful in the treatment of inflammatory conditions such as stiffness, swelling, joint pain of arthritis or rheumatism. For long-term use for inflammatory problems, separate drugs instead of this combination may be safer and more effective.

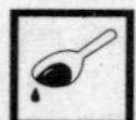

DOSAGE & USAGE INFORMATION

How to take:
- Tablet or capsule—swallow with liquid.
- Effervescent granules—dissolve granules in 4 oz. of cool water.

When to take:
As needed, no more often than every 3 hours or as prescribed by your doctor.

If you forget a dose:
Take as soon as you remember. Wait 3 hours for next dose.

Continued next column

OVERDOSE

SYMPTOMS:
Ringing in ears; nausea; vomiting; diarrhea; dizziness; fever; deep, rapid breathing; hallucinations; coma; unusual sweating; blood in urine; thirst; vision problems; nervousness.
WHAT TO DO:
- **Dial 911 (emergency) or 0 (operator) for an ambulance or medical help. Then give first aid immediately.**
- **See emergency information on inside covers.**

What drug does:
- May affect hypothalamus, the part of the brain that helps regulate body heat and receives body's pain messages.
- May affect production of prostaglandins to reduce inflammation.

Time lapse before drug works:
15 to 30 minutes. May last 4 hours.

Don't take with:
- Other drugs with acetaminophen or aspirin or other salicylates. Too much can cause damage to liver, kidneys and peripheral nerves.
- Any laxative containing cellulose.
- If medicine you take has a buffering agent added, don't take with tetracyclines.
- Any other medicine without consulting your doctor or pharmacist.

POSSIBLE ADVERSE REACTIONS OR SIDE EFFECTS

SYMPTOMS	WHAT TO DO
Life-threatening: In case of overdose, see previous column.	
Common:	
• Jaundice, vomiting blood, black stools, cloudy urine, nausea and vomiting, unexplained tiredness, discomfort on urinating.	Discontinue. Call doctor right away.
• Indigestion or heartburn.	Continue. Call doctor when convenient.
Infrequent:	
Shortness of breath; wheezing (for medicines containing aspirin); decreased urine volume; feet swelling; black or tarry stools; pain on urinating; nausea and vomiting; skin rash, hives; sore throat, fever; easy bruising.	Discontinue. Call doctor right away.
Rare:	
• While taking medicine: Sudden decrease in urine volume.	Discontinue. Call doctor right away.
• After discontinuing medicine: Swelling of feet; rapid weight gain; bloating or puffiness; any urinary problems, such as painful, cloudy or bloody urine.	Check with doctor immediately.

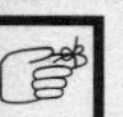

WARNINGS & PRECAUTIONS

Don't take if:
- You are allergic to acetaminophen or any salicylates.*
- Your symptoms don't improve after 3 days use.
- You take a buffered form and need to restrict sodium in your diet.
- You have a peptic ulcer.
- You have a bleeding disorder.

Before you start, consult your doctor:
- If you have ever had peptic ulcers.
- If you have had gout.
- If you have asthma or nasal polyps.
- If you have kidney disease or liver damage.

Over age 60:
Don't exceed recommended dose. More likely to be harmful to kidney and liver or cause hidden bleeding in stomach or intestines. Watch for black stools or decreased urine output.

Pregnancy:
Risk factors vary for drugs in this group. See category list on page xxii and consult doctor.

Breast-feeding:
Drug passes into milk. Avoid drug or discontinue nursing until you finish medicine. Consult doctor on maintaining milk supply.

Infants & children:
Overdose frequent and severe. Keep containers out of children's reach. Consult doctor before giving to persons under age 18 who have fever and discomfort of viral illness, especially chicken pox and influenza. Probably increases risk of Reye's syndrome*.

Prolonged use:
- High doses for severe inflammatory conditions taken for long periods may increase likelihood of kidney damage.
- Talk to your doctor about the need for follow-up medical examinations or laboratory studies to check liver function, kidney function.

Skin & sunlight:
Aspirin combined with sunscreen may decrease sunburn.

Driving, piloting or hazardous work:
No problems expected unless you feel drowsy.

Discontinuing:
No problems expected.

Others:
- Children up to 12 years—Don't take more than 5 doses per day for more than 5 consecutive days.
- Adults—Don't take for more than 10 consecutive days.
- Urine test for sugar may be inaccurate.
- Don't take if container has a strong vinegar-like odor.
- May interfere with the accuracy of some medical tests.

POSSIBLE INTERACTION WITH OTHER DRUGS

GENERIC NAME OR DRUG CLASS	COMBINED EFFECT
Antacids*	Decreased acetaminophen and salicylates effect.
Anticoagulants*	Increased anticoagulant effect. Abnormal bleeding.
Antidiabetic agents*, oral	Low blood sugar.
Anti-inflammatory drugs nonsteroidal (NSAIDs)*	Risk of stomach bleeding and ulcers.
Aspirin and other salicylates*	Likely toxicity.
Barbiturates*	Increased liver toxicity.
Carbamazepine	Increased liver toxicity.
Carteolol	Decreased antihypertensive effect of carteolol.

Continued on page 921

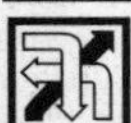

POSSIBLE INTERACTION WITH OTHER SUBSTANCES

INTERACTS WITH	COMBINED EFFECT
Alcohol:	Increased chance of stomach irritation and bleeding.
Beverages:	None expected.
Cocaine:	None expected. However, cocaine may deter body's recovery. Avoid.
Foods:	None expected.
Marijuana:	Possible increased pain relief, but marijuana may deter body's recovery. Avoid.
Tobacco:	None expected.

*See Glossary

ACETOHYDROXAMIC ACID (AHA)

BRAND NAMES

Lithostat

BASIC INFORMATION

Habit forming? No
Prescription needed? Yes
Available as generic? No
Drug class: Antibacterial, antiurolithic

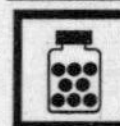

USES

- Treatment for chronic urinary tract infections.
- Prevents formation of urinary tract stones. Will not dissolve stones already present.

DOSAGE & USAGE INFORMATION

How to take:
Tablet—Swallow with liquid. If you can't swallow whole, crumble tablet and take with liquid or food.

When to take:
At the same time each day, according to instructions on prescription label.

If you forget a dose:
Take as soon as you remember up to 2 hours late. If more than 2 hours, wait for next scheduled dose (don't double this dose).

What drug does:
Stops enzyme action that makes urine too alkaline. Alkaline urine favors bacterial growth and stone formation and growth.

Time lapse before drug works:
1 to 3 weeks.

Don't take with:
- Alcohol or iron.
- Any other medicine without consulting your doctor or pharmacist.

OVERDOSE

SYMPTOMS:
Loss of appetite, tremor, nausea, vomiting.
WHAT TO DO:
Overdose unlikely to threaten life. If person takes much larger amount than prescribed, call doctor, poison control center or hospital emergency room for instructions.

POSSIBLE ADVERSE REACTIONS OR SIDE EFFECTS

SYMPTOMS	WHAT TO DO
Life-threatening:	
In case of overdose, see previous column.	
Common:	
Appetite loss, nausea, vomiting, anxiety, depression, mild headache, unusual tiredness.	Continue. Call doctor when convenient.
Infrequent:	
• Loss of coordination, slurred speech, severe headache, sudden change in vision, shortness of breath, clot or pain over a blood vessel, sudden chest pain, leg pain in calf (deep vein blood clot).	Discontinue. Seek emergency treatment.
• Rash on arms and face.	Continue. Call doctor when convenient.
Rare:	
• Sore throat, fever, unusual bleeding, bruising.	Discontinue. Call right away.
• Hair loss.	Continue. Call doctor when convenient.

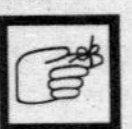

WARNINGS & PRECAUTIONS

Don't take if:
You have severe chronic kidney disease.

Before you start, consult your doctor:
- If you are anemic.
- If you have or have had phlebitis or thrombophlebitis.

Over age 60:
Adverse reactions and side effects may be more frequent and severe than in younger persons.

Pregnancy:
Studies inconclusive on harm to unborn child. Animal studies show fetal abnormalities. Don't use. Risk category X (see page xxii).

Breast-feeding:
Studies inconclusive. May have a potential for adverse reactions in nursing children. Avoid drug or discontinue nursing until you finish medicine. Consult doctor on maintaining milk supply.

Infants & children:
Not recommended. Safety and dosage have not been established.

Prolonged use:
Talk to your doctor about the need for follow-up medical examinations or laboratory studies to check blood pressure, liver function, kidney function, urinary pH.

Skin & sunlight:
No problems expected.

Driving, piloting or hazardous work:
Don't drive or pilot aircraft until you learn how medicine affects you. Don't work around dangerous machinery. Don't climb ladders or work in high places. Danger increases if you drink alcohol or take medicine affecting alertness and reflexes, such as antihistamines, tranquilizers, sedatives, pain medicines, narcotics and mind-altering drugs.

Discontinuing:
Don't discontinue without consulting doctor. Dose may require gradual reduction if you have taken drug for a long time. Doses of other drugs may also require adjustment.

Others:
No problems expected.

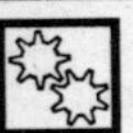

POSSIBLE INTERACTION WITH OTHER DRUGS

GENERIC NAME OR DRUG CLASS	COMBINED EFFECT
Iron	Decreased effects of both drugs.

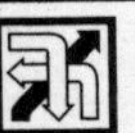

POSSIBLE INTERACTION WITH OTHER SUBSTANCES

INTERACTS WITH	COMBINED EFFECT
Alcohol:	Severe skin rash common in many patients within 30 to 45 minutes after drinking alcohol.
Beverages:	None expected.
Cocaine:	None expected.
Foods:	None expected.
Marijuana:	None expected.
Tobacco:	None expected.

ACYCLOVIR (Oral & Topical)

BRAND NAMES

Zovirax | Zovirax Ointment

BASIC INFORMATION

Habit forming? No
Prescription needed? Yes
Available as generic? No
Drug class: Antiviral

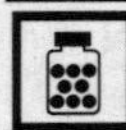

USES

- Treatment and prevention of severe herpes infections of genitals occurring for first time in special cases.
- Treatment of severe herpes infections on mucous membrane of mouth and lips in special cases.
- Used for shingles (herpes zoster) and chicken pox (varicella) in special cases.

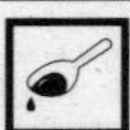

DOSAGE & USAGE INFORMATION

How to take:

- Capsule—Swallow with liquid. If you can't swallow whole, open capsule and take with liquid or food.
- Tablet—Swallow with liquid. If you can't swallow whole, crumble tablet and take with liquid or food.
- Suspension—Swallow with liquid.
- Ointment—Apply to skin and mucous membranes every 3 hours (6 times a day) for 7 days. Use rubber glove when applying. Apply 1/2-inch strip to each sore or blister. Wash before using.

When to use:
As directed on label.

Continued next column

OVERDOSE

SYMPTOMS:
Hallucinations, seizures, kidney shutdown.
WHAT TO DO:

- **Dial 911 (emergency) or 0 (operator) for an ambulance or medical help. Then give first aid immediately.**
- **See emergency information on inside covers.**

If you forget a dose:

- Oral—Take as soon as you remember up to 2 hours late. If more than 2 hours, wait for next scheduled dose (don't double this dose).
- Ointment—Apply as soon as you remember.

What drug does:

- Inhibits reproduction of virus in cells without killing normal cells.
- Does not cure. Herpes may recur.

Time lapse before drug works:
2 hours.

Don't take with:
Any other medicine without consulting your doctor or pharmacist.

POSSIBLE ADVERSE REACTIONS OR SIDE EFFECTS

SYMPTOMS	WHAT TO DO
Life-threatening:	
In case of overdose, see previous column.	
Common:	
Rash, hives, itch, mild pain, burning or stinging of skin, lightheadedness, headache, joint pain, diarrhea.	Continue. Call doctor when convenient.
Infrequent:	
None expected.	
Rare:	
Abdominal pain, decreased appetite, nausea, vomiting.	Continue. Call doctor when convenient.

WARNINGS & PRECAUTIONS

Don't take if:
You are allergic to acyclovir.

Before you start, consult your doctor:
- If pregnant or plan pregnancy.
- If breast-feeding.
- If you have kidney disease.
- If you have any nerve disorder.

Over age 60:
Adverse reactions and side effects may be more frequent and severe than in younger persons.

Pregnancy:
Decide with your doctor whether drug benefits justify risk to unborn child. Risk category C (see page xxii).

Breast-feeding:
- Oral—Drug passes into milk. Avoid drug or discontinue nursing until you finish medicine. Consult doctor for advice on maintaining milk supply.
- Ointment—No special problems expected. Consult doctor.

Infants & children:
Use only under special medical supervision by experienced clinician.

Prolonged use:
- Don't use longer than prescribed time.
- Talk to your doctor about the need for follow-up medical examinations or laboratory studies to check pap smear, kidney function.

Skin & sunlight:
No problems expected.

Driving, piloting or hazardous work:
No problems expected.

Discontinuing:
May be unnecessary to finish medicine. Follow doctor's instructions.

Others:
- Women: Get pap smear every 6 months because those with herpes infections are more likely to develop cancer of the cervix. Avoid sexual activity until all blisters or sores heal.
- Don't get medicine in eyes.
- Protect from freezing.
- Check with doctor if no improvement in 1 week.
- May interfere with the accuracy of some medical tests.

POSSIBLE INTERACTION WITH OTHER DRUGS

GENERIC NAME OR DRUG CLASS	COMBINED EFFECT
Nephrotoxic medications*	Possible increased kidney toxicity.

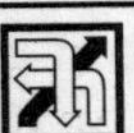

POSSIBLE INTERACTION WITH OTHER SUBSTANCES

INTERACTS WITH	COMBINED EFFECT
Alcohol:	No problems expected.
Beverages:	No problems expected.
Cocaine:	Increased chance of brain and nervous system adverse reaction. Avoid.
Foods:	No problems expected.
Marijuana:	Increased chance of brain and nervous system adverse reaction. Avoid.
Tobacco:	No problems expected.

*See Glossary

ADRENOCORTICOIDS (Nasal Inhalation)

BRAND AND GENERIC NAMES

BECLOMETHASONE (Nasal)
Beconase
Beconase AQ
BUDESONIDE
Decadron Turbinaire
DEXAMETHASONE (Nasal)
FLUTICASONE
Flonase
FLUNISOLIDE (Nasal)
Nasacort
Nasalide
Rhinalar
Rhinocort Aqua
Rhinocort Turbuhaler
TRIAMCINOLONE (Nasal)
Vancenase
Vancenase AQ

BASIC INFORMATION

Habit forming? No
Prescription needed? Yes
Available as generic? Yes, for some
Drug class: Adrenocorticoid (nasal); anti-inflammatory (steroidal), nasal

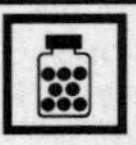

USES

- Treats nasal allergy.
- Treats nasal polyps.
- Treats noninfectious inflammatory nasal conditions.

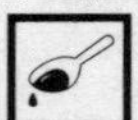

DOSAGE & USAGE INFORMATION

How to take:
- Read patient instruction sheet supplied with your prescription. Usually 1 or 2 sprays into each nostril every 12 hours.
- Save container for possible refills.

When to take:
At the same time each day, according to instructions on prescription label.

If you forget a dose:
Use as soon as you remember up to an hour late. If you remember more than an hour late, skip this dose. Don't double the next dose.

Continued next column

What drug does:
- Subdues inflammation by decreasing secretion of prostaglandins in cells of the lining of the nose and by inhibiting release of histamine.
- Very little, if any, of the nasal adrenocorticoid gets absorbed into the bloodstream.

Time lapse before drug works:
Usually 5 to 7 days, but may be as long as 2 to 3 weeks.

Don't take with:
Any other medicine without consulting your doctor or pharmacist.

OVERDOSE

SYMPTOMS:
None expected.
WHAT TO DO:
Overdose unlikely to threaten life. If person takes much larger amount than prescribed, call doctor, poison control center or hospital emergency room for instructions.

POSSIBLE ADVERSE REACTIONS OR SIDE EFFECTS

SYMPTOMS	WHAT TO DO
Life-threatening: None expected.	
Common: Burning or dryness of nose, sneezing.	Continue. Call doctor when convenient.
Infrequent: Crusting inside the nose, nosebleed, sore throat, ulcers in nose, cough, dizziness, headache, hoarseness, nausea, runny nose, bloody mucus.	Discontinue. Call doctor right away.
Rare:	
• White patches in nose or throat.	Discontinue. Call doctor right away.
• Eye pain, wheezing respiration.	Discontinue. Seek emergency treatment.

ADRENOCORTICOIDS (Nasal Inhalation)

WARNINGS & PRECAUTIONS

Don't take if:
You are allergic to cortisone or any cortisone-like medication.

Before you start, consult your doctor:
If you know you are allergic to any of the propellants in the spray. These include benzalkonium chloride, disodium acetate, phenylethanol, fluorocarbons, propylene glycol.

Over age 60:
No special problems expected.

Pregnancy:
Risk factors vary for drugs in this group. See category list on page xxii and consult doctor.

Breast-feeding:
Drug may pass into milk. Avoid drug or discontinue nursing until you finish medicine. Consult doctor on maintaining milk supply.

Infants & children:
Use only under medical supervision.

Prolonged use:
Not recommended.

Skin & sunlight:
No special problems expected.

Driving, piloting or hazardous work:
Don't drive or pilot aircraft until you learn how medicine affects you. Don't work around dangerous machinery. Don't climb ladders or work in high places. Danger increases if you drink alcohol or take medicine affecting alertness and reflexes.

Discontinuing:
No special problems expected.

Others:
No special problems expected.

POSSIBLE INTERACTION WITH OTHER DRUGS

GENERIC NAME OR DRUG CLASS	COMBINED EFFECT
None expected.	

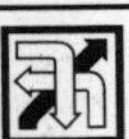

POSSIBLE INTERACTION WITH OTHER SUBSTANCES

INTERACTS WITH	COMBINED EFFECT
Alcohol:	None expected.
Beverages:	None expected.
Cocaine:	None expected.
Foods:	None expected.
Marijuana:	None expected.
Tobacco:	None expected.

***See Glossary**

ADRENOCORTICOIDS (Oral Inhalation)

BRAND AND GENERIC NAMES

AeroBid
AeroBid-M
Azmacort
Beclodisk
Becloforte
BECLOMETHASONE
Beclovent
Beclovent Rotacaps
Bronalide
Budesonide
Decadron Respihaler
DEXAMETHASONE
FLUNISOLIDE
Pulmicort Nebuamp
Pulmicort Turbuhaler
TRIAMCINOLONE
Vanceril

BASIC INFORMATION

Habit forming? No
Prescription needed? Yes
Available as generic? No
Drug class: Anti-inflammatory (inhalation), antiasthmatic

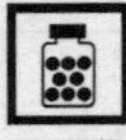

USES

Treatment for prevention of symptoms in patients with chronic bronchial asthma. Does not relieve the symptoms of an acute asthma attack.

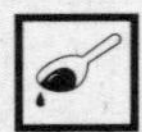

DOSAGE & USAGE INFORMATION

How to take:
Oral inhaler—Follow instructions that come with your prescription or take as directed by your doctor. If you don't understand the instructions or have any questions, consult your doctor or pharmacist. Most effective if taken regularly.

When to take:
Your doctor will determine the dosage amount and schedule that will help control the asthma symptoms and lessen risks of side effects. Usually 1 to 2 inhaled puffs 3 to 4 times a day is sufficient.

If you forget a dose:
Take as soon as you remember. Then spread out the remaining doses for that day at regularly spaced intervals.

Continued next column

OVERDOSE

SYMPTOMS:
None expected.
WHAT TO DO:
Overdose unlikely to threaten life. If person takes much larger amount than prescribed, call doctor, poison control center or hospital emergency room for instructions.

What drug does:
Helps prevent inflammation in the lungs and breathing passages. May decrease progression of severe disease.

Time lapse before drug works:
1 to 4 weeks for the initial response and up to several months for full benefits.

Don't take with:
Any other medicine without consulting your doctor or pharmacist.

POSSIBLE ADVERSE REACTIONS OR SIDE EFFECTS

SYMPTOMS	WHAT TO DO
Life-threatening:	
None expected.	
Common:	
Dry mouth, cough, throat irritation, hoarseness or other voice changes.	Continue. Call doctor when convenient.
Infrequent:	
• Dry throat, headache, nausea, skin bruising, unpleasant taste.	Continue. Call doctor when convenient.
• White curd-like patches in mouth or throat, pain when eating or swallowing (thrush).	Continue, but call doctor right away.
Rare:	
Increased wheezing; difficulty in breathing; pain, tightness or burning in chest; behavior changes (restlessness, nervousness, depression) with budesonide .	Continue, but call doctor right away

WARNINGS & PRECAUTIONS

Don't use if:
You are allergic to any corticosteroids*.

Before you start, consult your doctor:
- If you have osteoporosis.
- If you have or have had tuberculosis.
- If you are taking oral corticosteroid drugs.

Over age 60:
No special problems expected.

Pregnancy:
Risk category C (see page xxii). Decide with your doctor if drug benefits justify any possible risk to unborn child.

Breast-feeding:
Unknown effect. Decide with your doctor if you should continue breast-feeding while using this drug.

Infants & children:
- Should be safe with regular low-dosage regimen. There have been a few reports that long-term use or higher doses may decrease growth rate or cause reduced adrenal gland function. Be sure you and your child's doctor discuss all benefits and risks of the drug.
- Children using large doses of this drug are more susceptible to infectious disease (chicken pox, measles). Avoid exposure to infected people and keep all immunizations up to date.

Prolonged use:
- Talk to your doctor about the need for follow-up medical examinations or laboratory studies to check adrenal function, growth and development in children, pulmonary function, and inhalation technique.
- The drug may lose its effectiveness. If this occurs, consult your doctor.

Skin & sunlight:
No special problems expected.

Driving, piloting or hazardous work:
No special problems expected.

Discontinuing:
Don't discontinue this drug after prolonged use without consulting doctor. Dosage may require a gradual reduction before stopping to avoid any withdrawal symptoms.

Others:
- Advise any doctor or dentist whom you consult that you use this medicine.
- Carry or wear identification to state that you use this medicine.
- Call your doctor if you have any injury, infection or other stress to your body.
- Take medicine only as directed. Do not increase or reduce dosage without doctor's approval.

POSSIBLE INTERACTION WITH OTHER DRUGS

GENERIC NAME OR DRUG CLASS	COMBINED EFFECT
None significant.	

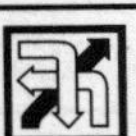

POSSIBLE INTERACTION WITH OTHER SUBSTANCES

INTERACTS WITH	COMBINED EFFECT
Alcohol:	None expected.
Beverages:	None expected.
Cocaine:	Effects not known. Best to avoid.
Foods:	None expected.
Marijuana:	Effects not known. Best to avoid.
Tobacco:	Asthma patients should avoid.

*See Glossary

ADRENOCORTICOIDS (Topical)

BRAND AND GENERIC NAMES

See complete list of brand and generic names in the *Brand Name Directory*, page 891.

BASIC INFORMATION

Habit forming? No
Prescription needed? For some
Available as generic? Yes
Drug class: Adrenocorticoid (topical)

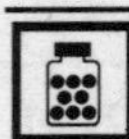

USES

Relieves redness, swelling, itching, skin discomfort of hemorrhoids; insect bites; poison ivy, oak, sumac; soaps, cosmetics; jewelry; burns; sunburn; numerous skin rashes; eczema; discoid lupus erythematosus; swimmers' ear; sun poisoning; hair loss; scars; penphigus; psoriasis; pityriasis rosea.

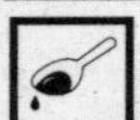

DOSAGE & USAGE INFORMATION

How to use:
- Cream, lotion, ointment, gel—Apply small amount and rub in gently.
- Topical aerosol—Follow directions on container. Don't breathe vapors.
- Other forms—Follow directions on container.

When to use:
When needed or as directed. Don't use more often than directions allow.

If you forget an application:
Use as soon as you remember.

What drug does:
Reduces inflammation by affecting enzymes that produce inflammation.

Time lapse before drug works:
15 to 20 minutes.

Don't use with:
Any other medicine without consulting your doctor or pharmacist.

OVERDOSE

SYMPTOMS:
None expected.
WHAT TO DO:
If person swallows or inhales drug, call doctor, poison control center or hospital emergency room for instructions.

POSSIBLE ADVERSE REACTIONS OR SIDE EFFECTS

SYMPTOMS	WHAT TO DO
Life-threatening: None expected.	
Common: None expected.	
Infrequent: Infection on skin with pain, redness, blisters, pus; skin irritation with burning, itching, blistering or peeling; acne-like skin eruptions.	Continue. Call doctor when convenient.
Rare: None expected.	

Note: Side effects are unlikely if topical adrenocorticoids are used in low doses for short periods of time. High doses for long periods can possibly cause the adverse reactions of cortisone (see CORTISONE).

WARNINGS & PRECAUTIONS

Don't take if:
You are allergic to any topical adrenocorticoid (cortisone) preparation.

Before you start, consult your doctor:
- If you plan pregnancy within medication period.
- If you have diabetes.
- If you have infection at treatment site.
- If you have stomach ulcer.
- If you have tuberculosis.

Over age 60:
Adverse reactions and side effects may be more frequent and severe than in younger persons, especially thinning of the skin.

Pregnancy:
Decide with your doctor whether drug benefits justify risk to unborn child. Risk category C (see page xxii).

Breast-feeding:
No problems expected.

Infants & children:
- Use only under medical supervision. Too much for too long can be absorbed into blood stream through skin and retard growth.
- For infants in diapers, avoid plastic pants or tight diapers.

Prolonged use:
- Increases chance of absorption into blood stream to cause side effects of oral cortisone drugs.
- May thin skin where used.
- Talk to your doctor about the need for follow-up medical examinations or laboratory studies to check complete blood counts (white blood cell count, platelet count, red blood cell count, hemoglobin, hematocrit), adrenal function.

Skin & sunlight:
No problems expected.

Driving, piloting or hazardous work:
No problems expected.

Discontinuing:
May be unnecessary to finish medicine. Follow doctor's instructions.

Others:
- Don't use a plastic dressing longer than 2 weeks.
- Aerosol spray—Store in cool place. Don't use near heat or open flame or while smoking. Don't puncture, break or burn container.
- Don't use for acne or gingivitis.

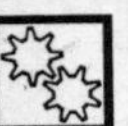

POSSIBLE INTERACTION WITH OTHER DRUGS

GENERIC NAME OR DRUG CLASS	COMBINED EFFECT
Antibacterials* (topical)	Decreased antibiotic effects.
Antifungals* (topical)	Decreased antifungal effect.

POSSIBLE INTERACTION WITH OTHER SUBSTANCES

INTERACTS WITH	COMBINED EFFECT
Alcohol:	None expected.
Beverages:	None expected.
Cocaine:	None expected.
Foods:	None expected.
Marijuana:	None expected.
Tobacco:	None expected.

*See Glossary

ALLOPURINOL

BRAND NAMES

Alloprin
Apo-Allopurinol
Lopurin
Novopural
Purinol
Zyloprim

BASIC INFORMATION

Habit forming? No
Prescription needed? Yes
Available as generic? Yes
Drug class: Antigout

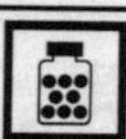

USES

- Treatment for chronic gout.
- Prevention of kidney stones caused by uric acid.

DOSAGE & USAGE INFORMATION

How to take:
Tablet—Swallow with liquid or food to lessen stomach irritation.

When to take:
At the same times each day.

If you forget a dose:
- 1 dose per day—Take as soon as you remember up to 6 hours late. If more than 6 hours, wait for next scheduled dose (don't double this dose).
- More than 1 dose per day—Take as soon as you remember up to 3 hours late. If more than 3 hours, wait for next scheduled dose (don't double this dose).

What drug does:
Slows formation of uric acid by inhibiting enzyme (xanthine oxidase) activity.

Time lapse before drug works:
Reduces blood uric acid in 1 to 3 weeks. May require 6 months to prevent acute gout attacks.

Don't take with:
Any other medicine without consulting your doctor or pharmacist.

OVERDOSE

SYMPTOMS:
None expected.
WHAT TO DO:
Overdose unlikely to threaten life. If person takes much larger amount than prescribed, call doctor, poison control center or hospital emergency room for instructions.

POSSIBLE ADVERSE REACTIONS OR SIDE EFFECTS

SYMPTOMS	WHAT TO DO
Life-threatening: None expected.	
Common: Rash, hives, itch.	Discontinue. Call doctor right away.
Infrequent: • Jaundice (yellow skin or eyes.)	Discontinue. Call doctor right away.
• Drowsiness, diarrhea, stomach pain, nausea or vomiting without other symptoms, headache.	Continue. Call doctor when convenient.
Rare: • Sore throat, fever, unusual bleeding or bruising.	Discontinue. Call doctor right away.
• Numbness, tingling, pain in hands or feet.	Continue. Call doctor when convenient.

WARNINGS & PRECAUTIONS

Don't take if:
You are allergic to allopurinol.

Before you start, consult your doctor:
If you have had liver or kidney problems.

Over age 60:
Adverse reactions and side effects may be more frequent and severe than in younger persons.

Pregnancy:
Decide with your doctor whether drug benefits justify risk to unborn child. Risk category C (see page xxii).

Breast-feeding:
Drug passes into milk. Avoid drug or discontinue nursing. Consult doctor for advice on maintaining milk supply.

Infants & children:
Not recommended.

Prolonged use:
Talk to your doctor about the need for follow-up medical examinations or laboratory studies to check liver function, kidney function, complete blood counts (white blood cell count, platelet count, red blood cell count, hemoglobin, hematocrit), and serum uric-acid determinations.

Skin & sunlight:
No problems expected.

Driving, piloting or hazardous work:
Avoid if you feel drowsy. Use may disqualify you for piloting aircraft.

Discontinuing:
Don't discontinue without doctor's advice until you complete prescribed dose, even though symptoms diminish or disappear.

Others:
Acute gout attacks may increase during first weeks of use. If so, consult doctor about additional medicine.

POSSIBLE INTERACTION WITH OTHER DRUGS

GENERIC NAME OR DRUG CLASS	COMBINED EFFECT
Amoxicillin	Likely skin rash.
Ampicillin	Likely skin rash.
Anticoagulants, oral*	May increase anticoagulant effect.
Antidiabetics, oral*	Increased uric acid elimination.
Azathioprine	Greatly increased azathioprine effect.
Chlorpropamide	May increase chlorpropamide effect.
Chlorthalidone	Decreased allopurinol effect.
Cyclophosphamide	Increased cyclophosphamide toxicity.
Diuretics, thiazide*	Decreased allopurinol effect.
Ethacrynic acid	Decreased allopurinol effect.
Furosemide	Decreased allopurinol effect.
Indapamide	Decreased allopurinol effect.
Iron supplements*	Excessive accumulation of iron in tissues.
Mercaptopurine	Increased mercaptopurine effect.
Metolazone	Decreased allopurinol effect.
Probenecid	Increased allopurinol effect.
Theophylline	May increase theophylline effect.

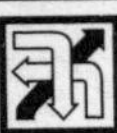

POSSIBLE INTERACTION WITH OTHER SUBSTANCES

INTERACTS WITH	COMBINED EFFECT
Alcohol:	None expected, but may impair management of gout.
Beverages:	Caffeine drinks. Decreased allopurinol effect.
Cocaine:	Decreased allopurinol effect. Avoid.
Foods:	None expected. Low-purine diet* recommended.
Marijuana:	Occasional use—None expected. Daily use—Possible increase in uric acid level.
Tobacco:	None expected.

*See Glossary

AMBENONIUM

BRAND NAMES

Mytelase

BASIC INFORMATION

Habit forming? No
Prescription needed? Yes
Available as generic? No
Drug class: Cholinergic, antimyasthenic

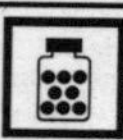

USES

- Diagnosis and treatment of myasthenia gravis.
- Treatment of urinary retention and abdominal distention.

DOSAGE & USAGE INFORMATION

How to take:

- Tablet—Swallow with liquid or food to lessen stomach irritation.
- Extended-release capsules and tablets—Swallow each dose whole with liquid; do not crush.

When to take:
As directed, usually 3 or 4 times a day.

If you forget a dose:
Take as soon as you remember up to 2 hours late. If more than 2 hours, wait for next scheduled dose (don't double this dose).

What drug does:
Inhibits the chemical activity of an enzyme (cholinesterase) so nerve impulses can cross the junction of nerves and muscles.

Continued next column

OVERDOSE

SYMPTOMS:
Muscle weakness or paralysis, cramps, twitching or clumsiness; severe diarrhea, nausea, vomiting, stomach cramps or pain; breathing difficulty; confusion, irritability, nervousness, restlessness, fear; unusually slow heartbeat; seizures, blurred vision, extreme fatigue.
WHAT TO DO:

- **Dial 911 (emergency) or 0 (operator) for an ambulance or medical help. Then give first aid immediately.**
- **See emergency information on inside covers.**

Time lapse before drug works:
3 hours.

Don't take with:
Any other medicine without consulting your doctor or pharmacist.

POSSIBLE ADVERSE REACTIONS OR SIDE EFFECTS

SYMPTOMS	WHAT TO DO
Life-threatening: In case of overdose, see previous column.	
Common:	
• Mild diarrhea, nausea, vomiting, stomach cramps or pain.	Discontinue. Call doctor right away.
• Excess saliva, unusual sweating.	Continue. Call doctor when convenient.
Infrequent:	
• Confusion, irritability.	Discontinue. Seek emergency treatment.
• Constricted pupils, watery eyes, lung congestion, urgent or frequent urination.	Continue. Call doctor when convenient.
Rare: None expected.	

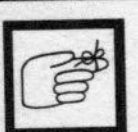

WARNINGS & PRECAUTIONS

Don't take if:
- You are allergic to any cholinergic or bromide.
- You take mecamylamine.

Before you start, consult your doctor:
- If you plan to become pregnant within medication period.
- If you have bronchial asthma.
- If you have heartbeat irregularities.
- If you have urinary obstruction or urinary tract infection.

Over age 60:
Adverse reactions and side effects may be more frequent and severe than in younger persons.

Pregnancy:
Decide with your doctor if benefits justify risk to unborn child. When given intravenously, may increase contractions of the womb close to time of delivery. Risk category C (see page xxii).

Breast-feeding:
No problems expected, but consult doctor.

Infants & children:
Use only under medical supervision.

Prolonged use:
Medication may lose effectiveness. Discontinuing for a few days may restore effect.

Skin & sunlight:
No problems expected.

Driving, piloting or hazardous work:
Don't drive or pilot aircraft until you learn how medicine affects you. Don't work around dangerous machinery. Don't climb ladders or work in high places. Danger increases if you drink alcohol or take medicine affecting alertness and reflexes, such as antihistamines, tranquilizers, sedatives, pain medicine, narcotics and mind-altering drugs.

Discontinuing:
Don't discontinue without doctor's advice until you complete prescribed dose, even though symptoms diminish or disappear.

Others:
No problems expected.

POSSIBLE INTERACTION WITH OTHER DRUGS

GENERIC NAME OR DRUG CLASS	COMBINED EFFECT
Anesthetics, local or general*	Decreased ambenonium effect.
Antiarrhythmics*	Decreased ambenonium effect.
Antibiotics*	Decreased ambenonium effect.
Anticholinergics*	Decreased ambenonium effect. May mask severe side effects.
Cholinergics, other*	Reduced intestinal tract function. Possible brain and nervous-system toxicity.
Guanadrel	Decreased ambenonium effect.
Guanethidine	Decreased ambenonium effect.
Mecamylamine	Decreased ambenonium effect.
Nitrates*	Decreased ambenonium effect.
Procainamide	Decreased ambenonium effect.
Quinidine	Decreased ambenonium effect.
Trimethaphan	Decreased ambenonium effect.

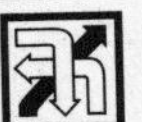

POSSIBLE INTERACTION WITH OTHER SUBSTANCES

INTERACTS WITH	COMBINED EFFECT
Alcohol:	No proven problems with small doses.
Beverages:	None expected.
Cocaine:	Decreased ambenonium effect. Avoid.
Foods:	None expected.
Marijuana:	No proven problems.
Tobacco:	No proven problems.

***See Glossary**

AMILORIDE

BRAND NAMES

Midamor

BASIC INFORMATION

Habit forming? No
Prescription needed? Yes
Available as generic? Yes
Drug class: Diuretic

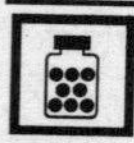

USES

Treatment for high blood pressure and congestive heart failure. Decreases fluid retention and prevents potassium loss.

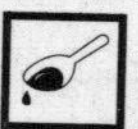

DOSAGE & USAGE INFORMATION

How to take:

- Tablet—Swallow with liquid.
- Capsule—Swallow with liquid. If you can't swallow whole, open capsule and take with liquid or food. Instructions to take on empty stomach mean 1 hour before or 2 hours after eating.

When to take:
At the same time each day, preferably in the morning. May interfere with sleep if taken after 6 p.m.

If you forget a dose:
Take as soon as you remember up to 8 hours late. If more than 8 hours, wait for next scheduled dose (don't double this dose).

Continued next column

OVERDOSE

SYMPTOMS:
Rapid, irregular heartbeat; confusion; shortness of breath; nervousness; extreme weakness.

WHAT TO DO:

- **Dial 911 (emergency) or 0 (operator) for an ambulance or medical help. Then give first aid immediately.**
- **If patient is unconscious and not breathing, give mouth-to-mouth breathing. If there is no heartbeat, use cardiac massage and mouth-to-mouth breathing (CPR). Don't try to make patient vomit. If you can't get help quickly, take patient to nearest emergency facility.**
- **See emergency information on inside covers.**

What drug does:
Blocks exchange of certain chemicals in the kidney so sodium is excreted. Conserves potassium.

Time lapse before drug works:
2 hours.

Don't take with:
Any other medicine without consulting your doctor or pharmacist.

POSSIBLE ADVERSE REACTIONS OR SIDE EFFECTS

SYMPTOMS	WHAT TO DO
Life-threatening:	
In case of overdose, see previous column.	
Common:	
Headache, nausea, appetite loss, vomiting, mild diarrhea constipation, decreased interest in sex.	Continue. Call doctor when convenient.
Infrequent:	
• Shortness of breath, fever, chills, unusual tiredness or weakness confusion.	Discontinue. Call doctor right away.
• Dizziness, bloating, muscle cramps, dry mouth.	Continue. Call doctor when convenient.
Rare:	
None expected.	

WARNINGS & PRECAUTIONS

Don't take if:

- You are allergic to amiloride.
- Your serum potassium level is high.

Before you start, consult your doctor:

- If you plan to become pregnant within medication period.
- If you have diabetes.
- If you have heart disease.
- If you have kidney or liver disease.

Over age 60:
Adverse reactions and side effects may be more frequent and severe than in younger persons. More likely to exceed safe potassium blood levels.

Pregnancy:
No proven harm to unborn child. Avoid if possible. Consult doctor. Risk category B (see page xxii).

Breast-feeding:
No problems expected, but consult doctor.

Infants & children:
Not recommended.

Prolonged use:
Talk to your doctor about the need for follow-up medical examinations or laboratory studies to check blood pressure, kidney function, ECG* and serum electrolytes.

Skin & sunlight:
Increased sensitivity to sunlight.

Driving, piloting or hazardous work:
Don't drive or pilot aircraft until you learn how medicine affects you. Don't work around dangerous machinery. Don't climb ladders or work in high places. Danger increases if you drink alcohol or take medicine affecting alertness and reflexes, such as antihistamines, tranquilizers, sedatives, pain medicine, narcotics and mind-altering drugs.

Discontinuing:
Don't discontinue without doctor's advice until you complete prescribed dose, even though symptoms diminish or disappear.

Others:
Periodic physical checkups and potassium-level tests recommended.

POSSIBLE INTERACTION WITH OTHER DRUGS

GENERIC NAME OR DRUG CLASS	COMBINED EFFECT
Acebutolol	Increased antihypertensive effect. Dosages may require adjustment.
Angiotensin-converting enzyme (ACE) inhibitors*	Possible excessive potassium in blood.
Amiodarone	Increased risk of heartbeat irregularity due to low potassium.
Antihypertensives*	Increased effect of both drugs.
Blood bank blood	Increased potassium levels.
Calcium supplements*	Increased calcium in blood.
Cyclosporine	Increased potassium levels.
Diuretics, other*	Increased effect of both drugs.
Lithium	Possible lithium toxicity.
Nicardipine	Dangerous blood pressure drop. Dosages may require adjustment.
Nimodipine	Dangerous blood pressure drop.
Nitrates*	Excessive blood pressure drop.
Potassium supplements*	Increased potassium levels.
Sodium bicarbonate	Decreased potassium levels.

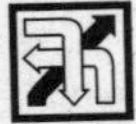

POSSIBLE INTERACTION WITH OTHER SUBSTANCES

INTERACTS WITH	COMBINED EFFECT
Alcohol:	Increased blood pressure drop. Avoid.
Beverages: Low-salt milk.	Possible excess potassium levels. Low-salt milk has extra potassium.
Cocaine:	Blood pressure rise. Avoid.
Foods: Salt substitutes.	Possible excess potassium levels.
Marijuana:	None expected.
Tobacco:	None expected.

*See Glossary

AMILORIDE & HYDROCHLOROTHIAZIDE

BRAND NAMES

Moduret

Moduretic

BASIC INFORMATION

Habit forming? No
Prescription needed? Yes
Available as generic? Yes
Drug class: Diuretic (thiazide), antihypertensive

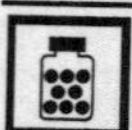

USES

- Controls, but doesn't cure, high blood pressure.
- Reduces fluid retention (edema), decreasing likelihood of congestive heart failure.

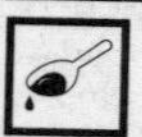

DOSAGE & USAGE INFORMATION

How to take:
Tablet—Swallow with liquid. If you can't swallow whole, crumble tablet and take with liquid or food.

When to take:
At the same time each day, no later than 6 p.m.

If you forget a dose:
Take as soon as you remember up to 2 hours late. If more than 2 hours, wait for next scheduled dose (don't double this dose).

What drug does:
- Forces sodium and water excretion, conserves potassium, reducing body fluid.
- Relaxes muscle cells of small arteries.
- Reduced body fluid and relaxed arteries lower blood pressure.

Time lapse before drug works:
2-6 hours. May require several weeks to lower blood pressure.

Don't take with:
- Any other medicine without consulting your doctor or pharmacist.
- Nonprescription drugs without consulting doctor.

OVERDOSE

SYMPTOMS:
Cramps, weakness, drowsiness, weak pulse, coma, rapid, irregular heartbeat.
WHAT TO DO:
- **Dial 911 (emergency) or 0 (operator) for an ambulance or medical help. Then give first aid immediately.**
- **See emergency information on inside covers.**

POSSIBLE ADVERSE REACTIONS OR SIDE EFFECTS

SYMPTOMS	WHAT TO DO
Life-threatening:	
In case of overdose, see previous column.	
Common:	
• Increased thirst, irregular heartbeat, cramps in muscles, numbness and tingling in hands and feet, thready pulse, shortness of breath.	Discontinue. Call doctor right away.
• Tiredness, weakness, diarrhea, headache, appetite loss, nausea constipation, decreased interest in sex.	Continue. Call doctor when convenient.
Infrequent:	
• Mood changes, dizziness, lightheadedness.	Continue. Call doctor when convenient.
• Fever and chills, red tongue, cracked mouth corners, black stools, dry mouth.	Discontinue. Call doctor right away.
Rare:	
Jaundice; unusual bleeding or bruising; abdominal pain with vomiting; sore throat, sores in mouth; hives, skin rash; joint pain.	Discontinue. Seek emergency treatment.

AMILORIDE & HYDROCHLOROTHIAZIDE

WARNINGS & PRECAUTIONS

Don't take if:
You are allergic to amiloride or any thiazide diuretic drug.

Before you start, consult your doctor:
- If you are allergic to any sulfa drug.
- If you have gout, diabetes, heart disease.
- If you have liver, pancreas or kidney disorder.

Over age 60:
Adverse reactions and side effects may be more frequent and severe than in younger persons, especially dizziness and excessive potassium loss.

Pregnancy:
Consult doctor. Risk category B (see page xxii).

Breast-feeding:
Drug passes into milk. Avoid drug or discontinue nursing until you finish medicine.

Infants & children:
Not recommended unless closely supervised.

Prolonged use:
- You may need medicine to treat high blood pressure for the rest of your life.
- Talk to your doctor about the need for follow-up medical examinations or laboratory studies to check blood pressure, kidney function, electrocardiogram and serum electrolytes.

Skin & sunlight:
May cause rash or intensify sunburn in areas exposed to sun or sunlamp. Avoid overexposure.

Driving, piloting or hazardous work:
Don't drive or pilot aircraft until you learn how medicine affects you. Don't work around dangerous machinery. Don't climb ladders or work in high places. Danger increases if you drink alcohol or take medicine affecting alertness and reflexes, such as antihistamines, tranquilizers, sedatives, pain medicine, narcotics and mind-altering drugs.

Discontinuing:
Don't discontinue without medical advice.

Others:
- Hot weather and fever may cause dehydration and drop in blood pressure. Dose may require temporary adjustment. Weigh daily and report any unexpected weight decreases to your doctor.
- May cause rise in uric acid, leading to gout.
- May cause blood-sugar rise in diabetics.
- Get periodic check-ups and potassium-level laboratory tests.

POSSIBLE INTERACTION WITH OTHER DRUGS

GENERIC NAME OR DRUG CLASS	COMBINED EFFECT
Allopurinol	Decreased allopurinol effect.
Antidepressants, tricyclic*	Dangerous drop in blood pressure. Avoid combination unless under medical supervision.
Antihypertensives, other*	Increased effect of both drugs.
Barbiturates*	Increased hydrochlorothiazide effect.
Beta-adrenergic blocking agents*	Increased antihypertensive effect. Dosages of both drugs may require adjustments.
Blood bank blood	Increased potassium levels.
Carteolol	Increased antihypertensive effect.
Cortisone drugs*	Excessive potassium loss that causes dangerous heart rhythms.

Continued on page 921

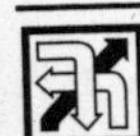

POSSIBLE INTERACTION WITH OTHER SUBSTANCES

INTERACTS WITH	COMBINED EFFECT
Alcohol:	Dangerous blood pressure drop.
Beverages: Low-salt milk.	Possible excess potassium levels. Low-salt milk has extra potassium.
Cocaine:	Increased risk of heart block and high blood pressure.
Foods: Salt substitutes.	Possible excess potassium levels.
Marijuana:	May increase blood pressure.
Tobacco:	None expected.

***See Glossary**

AMINOBENZOATE POTASSIUM

BRAND NAMES

KPAB
Potaba
Potassium Aminobenzoate
Potassium Para-aminobenzoate

BASIC INFORMATION

Habit forming? No
Prescription needed? Yes
Available as generic? No
Drug class: Antifibrosis

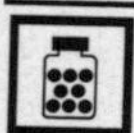

USES

Reduces inflammation and relieves contractions in tissues lying under the skin that have become tight from such disorders as dermatomyositis, Peyronie's disease, scleroderma, pemphigus, morphea.

DOSAGE & USAGE INFORMATION

How to take:

- Tablets—Dissolve in liquid or take with food to prevent stomach upset.
- Capsules—Take with full glass of liquid.
- Oral solution—Swallow with liquid to lessen stomach upset.
- Powder—Mix with liquid.

When to take:
At the same times each day, according to instructions on prescription label. Usually taken with meals and at bedtime with a snack.

If you forget a dose:
Take as soon as you remember up to 2 hours late. If more than 2 hours, wait for next scheduled dose (don't double this dose).

What drug does:
May increase ability of diseased tissues to use oxygen.

Continued next column

OVERDOSE

SYMPTOMS:
Nausea, vomiting.
WHAT TO DO:
Overdose unlikely to threaten life. If person takes much larger amount than prescribed, call doctor, poison control center or hospital emergency room for instructions.

Time lapse before drug works:
May require 3 to 10 months for improvement to begin.

Don't take with:
Any other medicine without consulting your doctor or pharmacist.

POSSIBLE ADVERSE REACTIONS OR SIDE EFFECTS

SYMPTOMS	WHAT TO DO
Life-threatening: None expected.	
Common: Appetite loss, nausea, rash, fever.	Continue. Call doctor when convenient.
Infrequent:	
• Low blood sugar (hunger, anxiety, cold sweats, rapid pulse).	Discontinue. Seek emergency treatment. (Note: Take sugar or honey on the way to emergency room.)
• Sore throat.	Discontinue. Call doctor right away.
Rare: None expected.	

WARNINGS & PRECAUTIONS

Don't take if:
You are allergic to aminobenzoate potassium or para-aminobenzoic acid (PABA).

Before you start, consult your doctor:
- If you have low blood sugar.
- If you have diabetes mellitus.
- If you have kidney disease.

Over age 60:
Adverse reactions and side effects may be more frequent and severe than in younger persons, particularly low blood sugar.

Pregnancy:
Risk factor not designated. See category list on page xxii and consult doctor.

Breast-feeding:
Unknown effect. Consult doctor.

Infants & children:
Not recommended. Safety and dosage have not been established.

Prolonged use:
Talk to your doctor about the need for follow-up medical examinations or laboratory studies to check complete blood counts (white blood cell count, platelet count, red blood cell count, hemoglobin, hematocrit).

Skin & sunlight:
No problems expected.

Driving, piloting or hazardous work:
No problems expected.

Discontinuing:
No problems expected.

Others:
If you become acutely ill and cannot eat well for even a short while, tell your doctor. These circumstances can lead to low blood sugar, and dosage may need adjustment.

POSSIBLE INTERACTION WITH OTHER DRUGS

GENERIC NAME OR DRUG CLASS	COMBINED EFFECT
Dapsone	Decreased dapsone effect.
Methotrexate	Increased methotrexate effect and toxicity.
Salicylates*	May increase salicylate blood level.
Sulfa drugs* (sulfonamides)	Decreased sulfa effect.

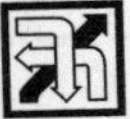

POSSIBLE INTERACTION WITH OTHER SUBSTANCES

INTERACTS WITH	COMBINED EFFECT
Alcohol:	None expected.
Beverages:	None expected.
Cocaine:	None expected.
Foods:	None expected.
Marijuana:	None expected.
Tobacco:	None expected.

*See Glossary

AMINOGLUTETHIMIDE

BRAND NAMES

Cytadren

BASIC INFORMATION

Habit forming? No
Prescription needed? Yes
Available as generic? No
Drug class: Antiadrenal, antineoplastic

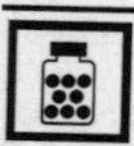

USES

- Treats Cushing's syndrome.
- Treats breast malignancies.

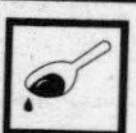

DOSAGE & USAGE INFORMATION

How to take:
Tablets—Swallow with liquid. If you can't swallow whole, crumble tablet and take with liquid or food. Instructions to take on empty stomach mean 1 hour before or 2 hours after eating.

When to take:
Follow doctor's instructions exactly.

If you forget a dose:
Take as soon as you remember up to 2 hours late. If more than 2 hours, wait for next scheduled dose (don't double this dose).

What drug does:
Suppresses adrenal cortex.

Time lapse before drug works:
1 to 2 hours.

Don't take with:
Any other medicines (including over-the-counter drugs such as cough and cold medicines, laxatives, antacids, diet pills, caffeine, nose drops or vitamins) without consulting your doctor.

OVERDOSE

SYMPTOMS:
None expected.
WHAT TO DO:
Overdose unlikely to threaten life. If person takes much larger amount than prescribed, call doctor, poison control center or hospital emergency room for instructions.

POSSIBLE ADVERSE REACTIONS OR SIDE EFFECTS

SYMPTOMS	WHAT TO DO
Life-threatening: None expected.	
Common: Skin rash on face and hands.	Continue. Tell doctor at next visit.
Infrequent:	
• Dizziness, drowsiness, unexplained fatigue, low back pain, pain on urinating, clumsiness, unusual eye movements, appetite loss.	Discontinue. Call doctor right away.
• Vomiting, skin darkening, depression, headache, muscle pain.	Continue. Call doctor when convenient.
Rare: Unusual bleeding or bruising	Discontinue. Call doctor right away.

WARNINGS & PRECAUTIONS

Don't take if:
- You have recently been exposed to chicken pox.
- You have shingles (herpes zoster).

Before you start, consult your doctor:
- If you have decreased thyroid function (hypothyroidism).
- If you have any form of infection.

Over age 60:
Adverse reactions and side effects may be more frequent and severe than in younger persons. You may need smaller doses for shorter periods of time.

Pregnancy:
Risk category D (see page xxii).

Breast-feeding:
Effect not documented. Consult your doctor.

Infants & children:
Effect not documented. Consult your doctor.

Prolonged use:
Talk to your doctor about the need for follow-up medical examinations or laboratory studies to check thyroid function, liver function, serum electrolytes (sodium potassium, chloride) and blood pressure.

Skin & sunlight:
No problems expected.

Driving, piloting or hazardous work:
No problems expected.

Discontinuing:
No special problems expected.

Others:
- Advise any doctor or dentist whom you consult that you take this medicine.
- May affect results in some medical tests.
- May cause decreased thyroid function.

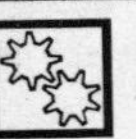

POSSIBLE INTERACTION WITH OTHER DRUGS

GENERIC NAME OR DRUG CLASS	COMBINED EFFECT
Anticoagulants*	Decreased anticoagulant effect.
Clozapine	Toxic effect on the central nervous system.
Cortisone-like drugs*	Decreased cortisone effects.
Dexamethasone	Dexamethasone effect decreased by half.
Trilostane	Too much decrease in adrenal function.

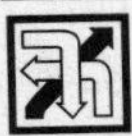

POSSIBLE INTERACTION WITH OTHER SUBSTANCES

INTERACTS WITH	COMBINED EFFECT
Alcohol:	Increased stomach irritation.
Beverages: Coffee, tea, cocoa.	Increased stomach irritation.
Cocaine:	No proven problems.
Foods:	No proven problems.
Marijuana:	No proven problems.
Tobacco:	No proven problems.

***See Glossary**

AMINOSALICYLATE SODIUM

BRAND NAMES

Nemasol-Sodium
P.A.S.
Tubasal

BASIC INFORMATION

Habit forming? No
Prescription needed? Yes
Available as generic? No
Drug class: Antitubercular

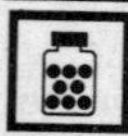

USES

Treatment for tuberculosis (TB).

DOSAGE & USAGE INFORMATION

How to take:
Tablet—Swallow with liquid or food to lessen stomach irritation.

When to take:
At the same times each day.

If you forget a dose:
Take as soon as you remember up to 2 hours late. If more than 2 hours, wait for next scheduled dose (don't double this dose).

What drug does:
- Prevents growth of TB germs.
- Makes TB germs more susceptible to other antituberculosis drugs.

Time lapse before drug works:
6 months.

Don't take with:
Any other medicine without consulting your doctor or pharmacist.

OVERDOSE

SYMPTOMS:
Nausea, vomiting, diarrhea; rapid breathing; convulsions.
WHAT TO DO:
- **Dial 911 (emergency) or 0 (operator) for an ambulance or medical help. Then give first aid immediately.**
- **See emergency information on inside covers.**

POSSIBLE ADVERSE REACTIONS OR SIDE EFFECTS

SYMPTOMS	WHAT TO DO
Life-threatening: In case of overdose, see previous column.	
Common:	
• Painful urination, chills, low back pain, nausea, vomiting.	Discontinue. Call doctor right away.
• Diarrhea or abdominal pain.	Continue. Call doctor when convenient.
Infrequent:	
• Confusion, blood in urine.	Discontinue. Call doctor right away.
• Headache; itchy, dry, puffy skin; rash; light sensitivity; sore throat; fever; swelling in front of neck; decreased sex drive in men; fatigue; weakness.	Continue. Call doctor when convenient.
• Menstrual irregularities, weight gain.	Continue. Tell doctor at next visit.
Rare:	
Jaundice.	Discontinue. Call doctor right away.

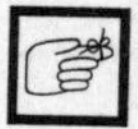

WARNINGS & PRECAUTIONS

Don't take if:
- You are allergic to aminosalicylate sodium, aspirin or other salicylates*.
- Tablets have turned brownish or purplish.

Before you start, consult your doctor:
- If you have ulcers in stomach or duodenum.
- If you have liver or kidney disease.
- If you have epilepsy.
- If you have adrenal insufficiency.
- If you have heart disease or congestive heart failure.
- If you have cancer.
- If you have overactive thyroid.

AMINOSALICYLATE SODIUM

Over age 60:
Adverse reactions and side effects may be more frequent and severe than in younger persons.

Pregnancy:
Decide with your doctor if drug benefits justify risk to unborn child. Risk category C (see page xxii).

Breast-feeding:
No proven problems. Consult doctor.

Infants & children:
Use only under medical supervision.

Prolonged use:
- Enlarged thyroid gland and decreased function.
- Talk to your doctor about the need for follow-up medical examinations or laboratory studies to check liver function, kidney function.

Skin & sunlight:
Increased sensitivity to light.

Driving, piloting or hazardous work:
No problems expected.

Discontinuing:
No problems expected.

Others:
- Treatment may need to continue for several years or indefinitely.
- Periodic blood tests and liver and kidney function studies recommended.

POSSIBLE INTERACTION WITH OTHER DRUGS

GENERIC NAME OR DRUG CLASS	COMBINED EFFECT
Aminobenzoic acid (PABA)	Decreased effect of aminosalicylate sodium.
Anticoagulants*, oral	Increased anticoagulant effect.
Anticonvulsants*, hydantoin	Increased anticonvulsant effect.
Aspirin	Stomach irritation.
Barbiturates*	Oversedation.
Folic acid	Decreased effect of folic acid.
Probenecid	Increased amino-salicylate sodium effect. Possible toxicity.
Rifampin	Decreased rifampin effect.
Sulfa drugs*	Decreased effect of sulfa drugs.
Sulfinpyrazone	Increased amino-salicylate sodium effect. Possible toxicity.
Tetracyclines*	Reduced absorption of aminosalicylate sodium. Space doses 3 hours apart.
Vitamin B-12	Decreased absorption of vitamin B-12.

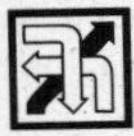

POSSIBLE INTERACTION WITH OTHER SUBSTANCES

INTERACTS WITH	COMBINED EFFECT
Alcohol:	Possible liver disease.
Beverages:	None expected
Cocaine:	None expected.
Foods:	None expected.
Marijuana:	None expected.
Tobacco:	None expected, but tobacco smoking may slow recovery. Avoid.

*See Glossary

AMIODARONE

BRAND NAMES

Cordarone

BASIC INFORMATION

Habit forming? No
Prescription needed? Yes
Available as generic? No
Drug class: Antiarrhythmic

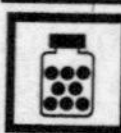

USES

Prevents and treats life-threatening heartbeat irregularities involving both the large chambers of the heart (auricles and ventricles).

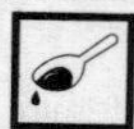

DOSAGE & USAGE INFORMATION

How to take:
Tablets—Swallow whole with liquid or food to lessen stomach irritation. If you can't swallow whole, crumble tablet and take with liquid or food.

When to take:
According to prescription instructions.

If you forget a dose:
Skip this dose and resume regular schedule. Do not double the next dose. If you forget 2 doses or more, consult your doctor.

What drug does:
- Slows nerve impulses in the heart.
- Makes heart muscle fibers less responsive to abnormal electrical impulses arising in the electrical regulatory system of the heart.

Continued next column

OVERDOSE

SYMPTOMS:
Irregular heartbeat, loss of consciousness, seizures.
WHAT TO DO:
- **Dial 911 (emergency) or 0 (operator) for an ambulance or medical help. Then give first aid immediately.**
- **If patient is unconscious and not breathing, give mouth-to-mouth breathing. If there is no heartbeat, use cardiac massage and mouth-to-mouth breathing (CPR). Don't try to make patient vomit. If you can't get help quickly, take patient to nearest emergency facility.**
- **See emergency information on inside covers.**

Time lapse before drug works:
2 to 3 days to 2 to 3 months.

Don't take with:
Any other medicine without consulting your doctor or pharmacist.

POSSIBLE ADVERSE REACTIONS OR SIDE EFFECTS

SYMPTOMS	WHAT TO DO
Life-threatening:	
Shortness of breath, difficulty breathing, cough.	Discontinue. Seek emergency treatment.
Common:	
• Walking difficulty, fever, numbness or tingling in hands or feet, shakiness, weakness in arms and legs.	Discontinue. Call doctor right away.
• Constipation, headache, appetite loss, nausea, vomiting.	Continue. Call doctor when convenient.
Infrequent:	
• Skin color change to blue-gray, blurred vision, cold feeling, dry eyes, nervousness, scrotum swelling or pain, insomnia, swollen feet and ankles, fast or slow heartbeat, eyes hurt in light, weight gain or loss, sweating.	Discontinue. Call doctor right away.
• Bitter or metallic taste, diminished sex drive, dizziness, flushed face, coldness and unusual tiredness.	Continue. Call doctor when convenient.
Rare:	
Jaundice, skin rash.	Discontinue. Call doctor right away.

WARNINGS & PRECAUTIONS

Don't take if:
You are allergic to amiodarone.

Before you start, consult your doctor:
- If you have liver, kidney or thyroid disease.
- If you have heart disease other than coronary artery disease.

Over age 60:
- Adverse reactions and side effects may be more frequent and severe than in younger persons. Ask about smaller doses.
- Pain in legs (while walking) considerably more likely.

Pregnancy:
Risk category D (see page xxii).

Breast-feeding:
Drug passes into milk. Avoid drug or discontinue nursing until you finish medicine. Consult doctor for advice on maintaining milk supply.

Infants & children:
Safety not established. Use only under close medical supervision.

Prolonged use:
- Blue-gray discoloration of skin may appear.
- Don't discontinue without consulting doctor. Dose may require gradual reduction if you have taken drug for a long time. Doses of other drugs may also require adjustment.
- Talk to your doctor about the need for follow-up medical examinations or laboratory studies to check ECG*, SGPT*, serum alkaline phosphatase, SGOT*, thyroid function.

Skin & sunlight:
May cause rash or intensify sunburn in areas exposed to sun or sunlamp. Avoid undue exposure, use sunscreens.

Driving, piloting or hazardous work:
Avoid if you feel dizzy or lightheaded. Otherwise, no problems expected.

Discontinuing:
- Don't discontinue without consulting doctor. Dose may require gradual reduction if you have taken drug for a long time. Doses of other drugs may also require adjustment.
- Notify doctor if cough, fever, breathing difficulty or shortness of breath occur after discontinuing medicine.

Others:
- Learn to check your own pulse. If it drops to lower than 50 or rises to higher than 100 beats per minute, don't take amiodarone until you consult your doctor.
- May interfere with the accuracy of some medical tests.

POSSIBLE INTERACTION WITH OTHER DRUGS

GENERIC NAME OR DRUG CLASS	COMBINED EFFECT
Antiarrhythmics, other*	Increased likelihood of heartbeat irregularity.
Anticoagulants*	Increased anticoagulant effect.
Beta-adrenergic blocking agents*	Increased likelihood of slow heartbeat.
Calcium channel blockers*	Possible heart block.
Cholestyramine	May decrease amiodarone blood levels.
Digitalis	Increased digitalis effect.
Diltiazam	Increased likelihood of slow heartbeat.
Diuretics*	Increased risk of heartbeat irregularity due to low potassium level.
Encainide	Increased effect of toxicity on the heart muscle.
Flecainide	Increased flecainide effect.
Isoniazid	Increased risk of liver damage.
Nicardipine	Possible increased effect and toxicity of each drug.
Nifedipine	Increased likelihood of slow heartbeat.
Phenytoin	Increased effect of phenytoin.
Procainamide	Increased procainamide effect.
Propafenone	Increased effect of both drugs and increased risk of toxicity.
Quinidine	Increased quinidine effect.
Verapamil	Increased likelihood of slow heartbeat.

POSSIBLE INTERACTION WITH OTHER SUBSTANCES

INTERACTS WITH	COMBINED EFFECT
Alcohol:	Increased risk of heartbeat irregularity. Avoid.
Beverages:	None expected.
Cocaine:	Increased risk of heartbeat irregularity. Avoid.
Foods:	None expected.
Marijuana:	Possible irregular heartbeat. Avoid.
Tobacco:	Possible irregular heartbeat. Avoid.

*See Glossary

AMPHETAMINES

BRAND AND GENERIC NAMES

Amfetamine	Dexedrine
AMPHETAMINE	Dexedrine Spansule
AMPHETAMINE SULFATE	DEXTRO-AMPHETAMINE
Biphetamine 12½	METHAMPHETMINE
Biphetamine 20	Oxydess
Desoxyn	Spancap
Desoxyn Gradumet	

BASIC INFORMATION

Habit forming? Yes
Prescription needed? Yes
Available as generic? Yes
Drug class: Central nervous system stimulant

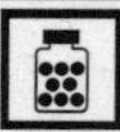

USES

- Prevents narcolepsy (attacks of uncontrollable sleepiness).
- Controls hyperactivity in children under special circumstances.

DOSAGE & USAGE INFORMATION

How to take:
- Tablet—Swallow with liquid.
- Extended-release capsules and tablets—Swallow each dose whole with liquid; do not crush.

When to take:
- At the same times each day.
- Short-acting form—Don't take later than 6 hours before bedtime.
- Long-acting form—Take on awakening.

If you forget a dose:
- Short-acting form—Take up to 2 hours late. If more than 2 hours, wait for next dose (don't double this dose).
- Long-acting form—Take as soon as you remember. Wait 20 hours for next dose.

Continued next column

OVERDOSE

SYMPTOMS:
Rapid heartbeat, hyperactivity, high fever, hallucinations, suicidal or homicidal feelings, convulsions, coma.
WHAT TO DO:
- **Dial 911 (emergency) or 0 (operator) for an ambulance or medical help. Then give first aid immediately.**
- **See emergency information on inside covers.**

What drug does:
- Hyperactivity—Decreases motor restlessness and increases ability to pay attendion.
- Narcolepsy—Increases motor activity and mental alertness; diminishes drowsiness.

Time lapse before drug works:
15 to 30 minutes.

Don't take with:
Any other medicine without consulting your doctor or pharmacist.

POSSIBLE ADVERSE REACTIONS OR SIDE EFFECTS

SYMPTOMS	WHAT TO DO
Life-threatening: In case of overdose, see previous column.	
Common:	
• Irritability, nervousness, insomnia, euphoria.	Continue. Call doctor when convenient.
• Dry mouth.	Continue. Tell doctor at next visit.
• Fast, pounding heartbeat.	Discontinue. Call doctor right away.
Infrequent:	
• Dizziness, reduced alertness, blurred vision, unusual sweating.	Discontinue. Call doctor right away.
• Headache.	Continue. Call doctor when convenient.
• Diarrhea or constipation, appetite loss, stomach pain, nausea, vomiting, weight loss, diminished sex drive, impotence.	Continue. Tell doctor at next visit.
Rare:	
• Rash; hives; chest pain or irregular heartbeat; uncontrollable movements of head, neck, arms, legs.	Discontinue. Call doctor right away.
• Mood changes, swollen breasts.	Continue. Call doctor when convenient.

WARNINGS & PRECAUTIONS

Don't take if:
- You are allergic to any amphetamine.
- You will have surgery within 2 months, including dental surgery, requiring general or spinal anesthesia.

Before you start, consult your doctor:
- If you plan to become pregnant within medication period.
- If you have glaucoma.
- If you have heart or blood vessel disease or high blood pressure.
- If you have overactive thyroid, anxiety or tension.
- If you have a severe mental illness (especially children).

Over age 60:
Adverse reactions and side effects may be more frequent and severe than in younger persons.

Pregnancy:
Decide with your doctor if drug benefits justify risk to unborn child. Consult doctor. Risk category C (see page xxii).

Breast-feeding:
Drug passes into milk.

Infants & children:
Not recommended for children under 12.

Prolonged use:
- Habit forming.
- Talk to your doctor about the need for follow-up medical examinations or laboratory studies to check blood pressure, growth charts in children, reassessment of need for continued treatment.

Skin & sunlight:
No problems expected.

Driving, piloting or hazardous work:
Don't drive or pilot aircraft until you learn how medicine affects you. Don't work around dangerous machinery. Don't climb ladders or work in high places. Danger increases if you drink alcohol or take medicine affecting alertness and reflexes.

Discontinuing:
May be unnecessary to finish medicine. Follow doctor's instructions.

Others:
- This is a dangerous drug and must be closely supervised. Don't use for appetite control or depression. Potential for damage and abuse.
- During withdrawal phase, may cause prolonged sleep of several days.
- Don't use for fatigue or to replace rest.

POSSIBLE INTERACTION WITH OTHER DRUGS

GENERIC NAME OR DRUG CLASS	COMBINED EFFECT
Anesthesias, general*	Irregular heartbeat.
Antidepressants, tricyclic*	Decreased amphetamine effect.
Antihypertensives*	Decreased anti-hypertensive effect.
Beta-adrenergic blocking agents*	High blood pressure, slow heartbeat.
Carbonic anhydrase inhibitors*	Increased amphetamine effect.
Central nervous system (CNS) stimulants,* other	Excessive CNS stimulation.
Doxazosin	Decreased doxazosin effect.
Furazolidine	Sudden and severe high blood pressure.
Haloperidol	Decreased amphetamine effect.
Monoamine oxidase (MAO) inhibitors*	May severely increase blood pressure.
Nabilone	Greater depression of the central nervous system.
Phenothiazines*	Decreased amphetamine effect.
Prazosin	Decreased prazosin effect.
Sodium bicarbonate	Increased amphetamine effect.
Sympathomimetics*	Seizures.
Thyroid hormones*	Heartbeat irregularities.

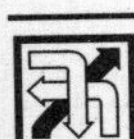

POSSIBLE INTERACTION WITH OTHER SUBSTANCES

INTERACTS WITH	COMBINED EFFECT
Alcohol:	Decreased amphetamine effect. Avoid.
Beverages: Caffeine drinks.	Overstimulation. Avoid.
Cocaine:	Dangerous stimulation of nervous system. Avoid.
Foods:	None expected.
Marijuana:	Frequent use—Severely impaired mental function.
Tobacco:	None expected.

*See Glossary

AMYL NITRITE INHALANT

BRAND NAMES

Amyl Nitrate Inhalant

BASIC INFORMATION

Habit forming? No
Prescription needed? Yes
Available as generic? Yes
Drug class: Coronary vasodilator

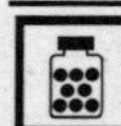

USES

Treats angina pectoris attacks. Note: Don't use amyl nitrite expecting a "high" or as an aphrodisiac. Serious, harmful side effects may occur when amyl nitrate is abused.

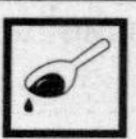

DOSAGE & USAGE INFORMATION

How to take:
Cover the glass capsule with a protective cloth and then crush between your fingers. Inhale 1 to 6 times. Remain seated while you inhale. Repeat dose in 5 minutes if needed.

When to take:
Only when chest pain occurs. If relief doesn't occur with first capsule within 5 minutes, crush another. If inhaling 2 capsules in 10 minutes doesn't bring relief, go to emergency room.

If you forget a dose:
No set dosage schedule. Use only when needed.

What drug does:
Relaxes coronary arteries that supply blood to the heart muscle.

Time lapse before drug works:
1 to 5 minutes.

Don't take with:
Any other medicine without consulting your doctor or pharmacist.

OVERDOSE

SYMPTOMS:
Blue lips, fingernails; dizziness, fainting, head pressure, shortness of breath, fast heartbeat.
WHAT TO DO:

- **Dial 911 (emergency) or 0 (operator) for an ambulance or medical help. Then give first aid immediately.**
- **See emergency information on inside covers.**

POSSIBLE ADVERSE REACTIONS OR SIDE EFFECTS

SYMPTOMS	WHAT TO DO
Life-threatening: In case of overdose, see previous column.	
Common: Continuing fast heartbeat, rapid pulse, headache, flushed face, restlessness.	Discontinue. Call doctor right away.
Infrequent: Dizziness, lightheadedness.	Discontinue. Call doctor right away.
Rare: Continuing dizziness, skin rash.	Discontinue. Call doctor right away.

WARNINGS & PRECAUTIONS

Don't take if:
You have had a recent head injury.

Before you start, consult your doctor:
- If you are anemic.
- If you have glaucoma.
- If you have overactive thyroid.
- If you have had a recent myocardial infarction.

Over age 60:
Adverse reactions and side effects may be more frequent and severe than in younger persons. You may need smaller doses for shorter periods of time.

Pregnancy:
Risk to unborn child outweighs drug benefits. Don't use. Risk category X (see page xxii).

Breast-feeding:
No documented problems. Best to avoid.

Infants & children:
Effect not documented. Consult your pediatrician.

Prolonged use:
Request follow-up studies to check liver function, kidney function, blood counts, platelet counts, heart function and blood pressure.

Skin & sunlight:
No problems expected.

Driving, piloting or hazardous work:
Avoid if you feel confused, drowsy or dizzy.

Discontinuing:
None expected.

Others:
- Advise any doctor or dentist whom you consult that you take this medicine.
- May affect results in some medical tests.

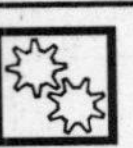

POSSIBLE INTERACTION WITH OTHER DRUGS

GENERIC NAME OR DRUG CLASS	COMBINED EFFECT
Antihypertensives*	Increased side effects of fainting and dizziness.
Sympathomimetics*	Reduces amyl nitrite effects.

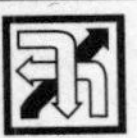

POSSIBLE INTERACTION WITH OTHER SUBSTANCES

INTERACTS WITH	COMBINED EFFECT
Alcohol:	Excess lightheadedness.
Beverages: Coffee, tea, cocoa.	Reduces amyl nitrite effects.
Cocaine:	Central nervous system toxicity. Avoid.
Foods:	None expected.
Marijuana:	Excess central nervous system stimulation. Avoid.
Tobacco:	No special problems expected.

***See Glossary**

ANALGESICS (Topical-Otic)

BRAND AND GENERIC NAMES

ANTIPYRINE AND BENZOCAINE
Aurafair
Auralgan
Aurodex
Auromid
Oto

BASIC INFORMATION

Habit forming? No
Prescription needed? Yes
Available as generic? Yes
Drug class: Analgesic (otic), anesthetic

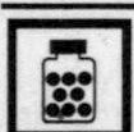

USES

Relieves pain of middle ear infections (otitis media). It does not treat the infection itself.

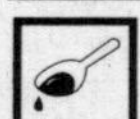

DOSAGE & USAGE INFORMATION

How to use:

- Warm ear drops under running water around the unopened bottle.
- Lie down with affected ear up.
- Adults—Pull ear lobe back and up.
- Children—Pull ear lobe down and back.
- Drop medicine into ear canal until canal is full.
- Stay lying down for 2 minutes.
- Gently insert cotton plug into ear to prevent leaking.

When to use:
Every 1 to 2 hours for 4 hours, then 4 times a day when needed for pain.

If you forget a dose:
Use as soon as you remember.

What drug does:
Functions as a topical anesthetic/analgesic on the eardrum.

Time lapse before drug works:
10 minutes.

Don't use with:
Any other medicine without consulting your doctor or pharmacist.

OVERDOSE

SYMPTOMS:
None expected.
WHAT TO DO:
Not intended for internal use. If child accidentally swallows, call poison control center.

POSSIBLE ADVERSE REACTIONS OR SIDE EFFECTS

SYMPTOMS	WHAT TO DO
Life-threatening: None expected.	
Common: None expected.	
Infrequent: Itching or burning in ear (probably represents allergic reaction).	Discontinue. Call doctor right away.
Rare: None expected.	

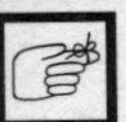

WARNINGS & PRECAUTIONS

Don't use if:
You are allergic to any local anesthetic (name usually ends with "caine").

Before you start, consult your doctor:
If eardrum is ruptured.

Over age 60:
No problems expected.

Pregnancy:
Consult doctor. Risk category C (see page xxii).

Breast-feeding:
No problems expected. Consult doctor.

Infants & children:
No problems expected.

Prolonged use:
Not intended for prolonged use.

Skin & sunlight:
No problems expected.

Driving, piloting or hazardous work:
No problems expected.

Discontinuing:
No problems expected.

Others:
- Keep cool, but don't freeze.
- Don't touch tip of dropper to any other surface.
- Don't rinse the dropper. Wipe with clean cloth and close tightly.

POSSIBLE INTERACTION WITH OTHER DRUGS

GENERIC NAME OR DRUG CLASS	COMBINED EFFECT
None expected.	

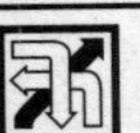

POSSIBLE INTERACTION WITH OTHER SUBSTANCES

INTERACTS WITH	COMBINED EFFECT
Alcohol:	None expected.
Beverages:	None expected.
Cocaine:	None expected.
Foods:	None expected.
Marijuana:	None expected.
Tobacco:	None expected.

*See Glossary

ANDROGENS

BRAND AND GENERIC NAMES

See complete list of brand and generic names in the *Brand Name Directory*, page 892.

BASIC INFORMATION

Habit forming? No
Prescription needed? Yes
Available as generic? Yes
Drug class: Androgen

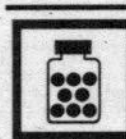

USES

- Corrects male hormone deficiency.
- Reduces "male menopause" symptoms (loss of sex drive, depression, anxiety).
- Decreases calcium loss of osteoporosis (softened bones).
- Blocks growth of breast cancer cells in females.
- Corrects undescended testicles in male children.
- Reduces breast pain and fullness following childbirth.
- Augments treatment of a plastic anemia.
- Stimulates weight gain after illness, injury or for chronically underweight persons.
- Stimulates growth in treatment of dwarfism.

DOSAGE & USAGE INFORMATION

How to take:
- Tablets or capsules—With food to lessen stomach irritation.
- Injection—Once or twice a month.

When to take:
At the same time each day.

If you forget a dose:
Take as soon as you remember up to 2 hours late. If more than 2 hours, wait for next scheduled dose (don't double this dose).

Continued next column

OVERDOSE

SYMPTOMS:
None expected.
WHAT TO DO:
Overdose unlikely to threaten life. If person takes much larger amount than prescribed, call doctor, poison control center or hospital emergency room for instructions.

What drug does:
- Stimulates cells that produce male sex characteristics.
- Replaces hormone deficiencies.
- Stimulates red-blood-cell production.
- Suppresses production of estrogen (female sex hormone).

Time lapse before drug works:
Varies with problems treated. May require 2 or 3 months of regular use for desired effects.

Don't take with:
Any other medicine without consulting your doctor or pharmacist.

POSSIBLE ADVERSE REACTIONS OR SIDE EFFECTS

SYMPTOMS	WHAT TO DO
Life-threatening: Intense itching, weakness, loss of consciousness.	Seek emergency treatment immediately.
Common:	
• Acne or oily skin, deep voice, enlarged clitoris in females; frequent erections, swollen breasts in men.	Continue. Call doctor when convenient.
• Sore mouth; higher sex drive, decreased testicle size, impotence in men.	Continue. Tell doctor at next visit.
Infrequent:	
• Yellow skin or eyes.	Discontinue. Seek emergency treatment.
• Depression or confusion, flushed face, rash or itch, nausea, vomiting, diarrhea, swollen feet or legs, headache, shortness of breath, rapid weight gain, chills, difficult urination; vaginal bleeding in women; scrotum pain in men.	Discontinue. Call doctor right away.
Rare:	
• Hives, black stool.	Discontinue. Seek emergency treatment.
• Sore throat, fever, abdominal pain.	Discontinue. Call doctor right away.
• Appetite loss, halitosis.	Continue. Call doctor when convenient.

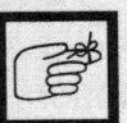

WARNINGS & PRECAUTIONS

Don't take if:
You are allergic to any male hormone.

Before you start, consult your doctor:
- If you might be pregnant.
- If you have cancer of prostate.
- If you have heart disease or arteriosclerosis.
- If you have kidney or liver disease.
- If you have breast cancer (males).
- If you have high blood pressure.
- If you have migraine attacks.
- If you have high level of blood calcium.
- If you have epilepsy.

Over age 60:
- May stimulate sexual activity.
- Can make high blood pressure or heart disease worse.
- Can enlarge prostate and cause urinary retention.

Pregnancy:
Risk to unborn child outweighs drug benefits. Don't use. Risk category X (see page xxii).

Breast-feeding:
Drug passes into milk. Avoid drug or discontinue nursing until you finish medicine. Consult doctor for advice on maintaining milk supply.

Infants & children:
Don't give to children younger than 2. Use with older children only under medical supervision.

Prolonged use:
- Reduces sperm count and volume of semen.
- Possible kidney stones.
- Unnatural hair growth and deep voice in women.
- Talk to your doctor about the need for follow-up medical examinations or laboratory studies to check complete blood counts (white blood cell count, platelet count, red blood cell count, hemoglobin, hematocrit).

Skin & sunlight:
No problems expected.

Driving, piloting or hazardous work:
No problems expected.

Discontinuing:
No problems expected.

Others:
- May cause atrophy of testicles.
- Will not increase strength in athletes.
- May cause liver cancer.
- In women, may cause male-like changes such as deepened voice, increased hair growth.

POSSIBLE INTERACTION WITH OTHER DRUGS

GENERIC NAME OR DRUG CLASS	COMBINED EFFECT
Anticoagulants*	Increased anti-coagulant effect.
Antidiabetic agents*	Increased antidiabetic effect.
Chlorzoxazone	Decreased androgen effect.
Cyclosporine	Increased cyclosporine effect.
Hepatotoxic drugs* (other)	Increased liver toxicity.
Insulin	Increased antidiabetic effect.
Oxyphenbutazone	Decreased androgen effect.
Phenobarbital	Decreased androgen effect.
Phenylbutazone	Decreased androgen effect.

POSSIBLE INTERACTION WITH OTHER SUBSTANCES

INTERACTS WITH	COMBINED EFFECT
Alcohol:	None expected.
Beverages:	None expected.
Cocaine:	No proven problems.
Foods: Salt.	Excessive fluid retention (edema). Decrease salt intake while taking male hormones.
Marijuana:	Decreased blood levels of androgens.
Tobacco:	No proven problems.

***See Glossary**

ANESTHETICS (Ophthalmic)

BRAND AND GENERIC NAMES

Ak-Taine	**Ophthetic**
Alcaine	**Pontocaine**
I-Paracaine	**PROPARACAINE**
Kainaire	**Spectro-Caine**
Ocu-Caine	**TETRACAINE**
Ophthaine	

BASIC INFORMATION

Habit forming? No
Prescription needed? Yes
Available as generic? Yes
Drug class: Anesthetic, local (ophthalmic)

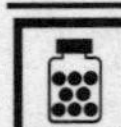

USES

Eliminates pain in eye temporarily to measure pressure in eye to check for glaucoma, remove foreign bodies and stitches and corneal scraping for diagnostic procedures.

DOSAGE & USAGE INFORMATION

How to use:

Eye drops
- Wash hands.
- Apply pressure to inside corner of eye with middle finger.
- Continue pressure for 1 minute after placing medicine in eye.
- Tilt head backward. Pull lower lid away from eye with index finger of the same hand.
- Drop eye drops into pouch and close eye. Don't blink.
- Keep eyes closed for 1 to 2 minutes.

Continued next column

Eye ointment
- Wash hands.
- Pull lower lid down from eye to form a pouch.
- Squeeze tube to apply thin strip of ointment into pouch.
- Close eye for 1 to 2 minutes.
- Don't touch applicator tip to any surface (including the eye). If you accidentally touch tip, clean with warm soap and water.
- Keep container tightly closed.
- Keep cool, but don't freeze.
- Wash hands immediately after using.

When to use:
As directed on label.

If you forget a dose:
Use as soon as you remember.

What drug does:
Blocks conduction of pain impulses.

Time lapse before drug works:
13-15 seconds.

Don't use with:
Other drops in eyes such as antiglaucoma eye drops.

OVERDOSE

SYMPTOMS:
None expected.
WHAT TO DO:
Not intended for internal use. If child accidentally swallows, call poison control center.

POSSIBLE ADVERSE REACTIONS OR SIDE EFFECTS

SYMPTOMS	WHAT TO DO
Life-threatening:	
Anaphylaxis (severe itching, hives, wheezing, runny nose, paleness, cold sweats, coma).	See inside covers.
Common:	
Mild stinging and burning.	Continue. Tell doctor at next visit.
Infrequent:	
Allergic reaction symptoms—itching, pain, redness, swelling, watery eyes.	Discontinue. Call doctor right away.
Rare (extremely):	
Symptoms of excess medicine absorbed by body—Weakness, increased sweating, nervousness, difficult breathing, vomiting, nausea, muscle spasms, irregular heartbeat, dizziness, drowsiness.	Discontinue. Call doctor right away.

WARNINGS & PRECAUTIONS

Don't use if:
You are allergic to any eye anesthetic.

Before you start, consult your doctor:
- If you have ever had an allergic reaction to any local anesthetic applied to skin, ears, mucous membranes or injected, such as benzocaine, butacaine, butamben, chloroprocaine, procaine, propoxycaine.
- If you have had an allergic reaction to sunscreens.

Over age 60:
No problems expected.

Pregnancy:
Studies have not been done. Consult doctor. Risk category C (see page xxii).

Breast-feeding:
No problems expected, but check with doctor.

Infants & children:
Use only under close medical supervision.

Prolonged use:
May retard healing. Avoid if possible.

Skin & sunlight:
No problems expected.

Driving, piloting or hazardous work:
No problems expected.

Discontinuing:
No problems expected.

Others:
- Don't rub or wipe eye until anesthetic has worn off (usually about 20 minutes) or until normal feeling in eye returns.
- Keep cool, but don't freeze.

POSSIBLE INTERACTION WITH OTHER DRUGS

GENERIC NAME OR DRUG CLASS	COMBINED EFFECT

Clinically significant interactions with oral or injected medicines unlikely.

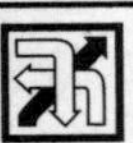

POSSIBLE INTERACTION WITH OTHER SUBSTANCES

INTERACTS WITH	COMBINED EFFECT
Alcohol:	None expected.
Beverages:	None expected.
Cocaine:	None expected.
Foods:	None expected.
Marijuana:	None expected.
Tobacco:	None expected.

ANESTHETICS (Rectal)

BRAND AND GENERIC NAMES

Americaine-Hemorrhoidal
BENZOCAINE
DIBUCAINE
Ethyl Aminobenzoate
Fleet Relief
Nupercainal
Pontocaine Cream
Pontocaine Ointment
PRAMOXINE
Preparation"H"
Proctofoam
TETRACAINE
TETRACAINE AND MENTHOL
Tronolane
Tronothane

BASIC INFORMATION

Habit forming? No
Prescription needed? Yes, for some.
Available as generic? Yes, Dibucaine. No others, but most brands are available without prescription.
Drug class: Anesthetic (rectal)

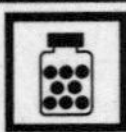

USES

- Relieves pain, itching and swelling of hemorrhoids (piles).
- Relieves pain of rectal fissures (breaks in lining membrane of the anus).

DOSAGE & USAGE INFORMATION

How to use:

- Rectal cream or ointment—Apply to surface of rectum with fingers. Insert applicator into rectum no farther than 1/2 and apply inside. Wash applicator with warm soapy water or discard.
- Aerosol foam—Read patient instructions. Don't insert into rectum. Use the special applicator and wash carefully after using.
- Suppository—Remove wrapper and moisten with water. Lie on side. Push blunt end of suppository into rectum with finger. If suppository is too soft, run cold water over wrapper or put in refrigerator for 15 to 45 minutes before using.

When to use:
As directed.

Continued next column

OVERDOSE

SYMPTOMS:
None expected.
WHAT TO DO:
Not intended for internal use. If child accidentally swallows, call poison control center.

If you forget a dose:
Use as soon as you remember.

What drug does:
Deadens nerve endings to pain and touch.

Time lapse before drug works:
5 to 15 minutes.

Don't use with:
Any other medicine without consulting your doctor or pharmacist.

POSSIBLE ADVERSE REACTIONS OR SIDE EFFECTS

SYMPTOMS	WHAT TO DO
Life-threatening: None expected.	
Common: None expected.	
Infrequent:	
• Nervousness, trembling, hives, rash, itch, inflammation or tenderness not present before application, slow heartbeat.	Discontinue. Call doctor right away.
• Dizziness, blurred vision, swollen feet.	Continue. Call doctor when convenient.
Rare:	
• Blood in urine.	Discontinue. Call doctor right away.
• Increased or painful urination.	Continue. Call doctor when convenient.

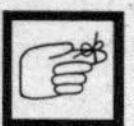

WARNINGS & PRECAUTIONS

Don't use if:
You are allergic to any topical anesthetic.

Before you start, consult your doctor:
- If you have skin infection at site of treatment.
- If you have had severe or extensive skin disorders such as eczema or psoriasis.
- If you have bleeding hemorrhoids.

Over age 60:
Adverse reactions and side effects may be more frequent and severe than in younger persons.

Pregnancy:
Risk factors vary for drugs in this group. See category list on page xxii and consult doctor.

Breast-feeding:
No problems expected. Consult doctor.

Infants & children:
Use caution. More likely to be absorbed through skin and cause adverse reactions.

Prolonged use:
Possible excess absorption. Don't use longer than 3 days for any one problem.

Skin & sunlight:
No problems expected.

Driving, piloting or hazardous work:
No problems expected.

Discontinuing:
May be unnecessary to finish medicine. Follow doctor's instructions.

Others:
- Report any rectal bleeding to your doctor.
- Keep cool, but don't freeze.

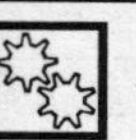

POSSIBLE INTERACTION WITH OTHER DRUGS

GENERIC NAME OR DRUG CLASS	COMBINED EFFECT
Sulfa drugs*	Decreased anti-infective effect of sulfa drugs.

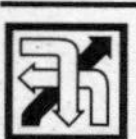

POSSIBLE INTERACTION WITH OTHER SUBSTANCE

INTERACTS WITH	COMBINED EFFECT
Alcohol:	None expected.
Beverages:	None expected.
Cocaine:	Possible nervous system toxicity. Avoid.
Foods:	None expected.
Marijuana:	None expected.
Tobacco:	None expected.

*See Glossary

ANESTHETICS (Topical)

BRAND NAMES

See complete list of brand names in the *Brand Name Directory*, page 893.

BASIC INFORMATION

Habit forming? No
Prescription needed?
High strength: Yes
Low strength: No
Available as generic? Yes
Drug class: Anesthetic (topical)

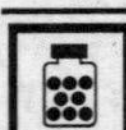

USES

Relieves pain and itch of sunburn, insect bites, scratches and other minor skin irritations.

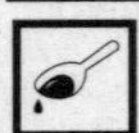

DOSAGE & USAGE INFORMATION

How to use:
All forms—Use only enough to cover irritated area. Follow instructions on label.

When to use:
When needed for discomfort, no more often than every hour.

If you forget an application:
Use as needed.

What drug does:
Blocks pain impulses from skin to brain.

Time lapse before drug works:
3 to 15 minutes.

Don't take with:
Any other medicine without consulting your doctor or pharmacist.

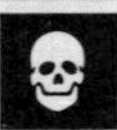

OVERDOSE

SYMPTOMS:
If swallowed or inhaled—Dizziness, nervousness, trembling, seizures.
WHAT TO DO:
- **Dial 911 (emergency) or 0 (operator) for an ambulance or medical help. Then give first aid immediately.**
- **See emergency information on inside covers.**

POSSIBLE ADVERSE REACTIONS OR SIDE EFFECTS

SYMPTOMS	WHAT TO DO
Life-threatening: None expected.	
Common: None expected.	
Infrequent:	
• Nervousness; trembling; hives, rash, itch; inflammation or tenderness not present before application; slow heartbeat.	Discontinue. Call doctor right away.
• Dizziness, blurred vision, swollen feet.	Continue. Call doctor when convenient.
Rare:	
• Blood in urine.	Discontinue. Call doctor right away.
• Increased or painful urination.	Continue. Call doctor when convenient.

WARNINGS & PRECAUTIONS

Don't use if:
You are allergic to any topical anesthetic.

Before you start, consult your doctor:
- If you have skin infection at site of treatment.
- If you have had severe or extensive skin disorders such as eczema or psoriasis.
- If you have bleeding hemorrhoids.

Over age 60:
Adverse reactions and side effects may be more frequent and severe than in younger persons.

Pregnancy:
Risk factors vary for drugs in this group. See category list on page xxii and consult doctor.

Breast-feeding:
No problems expected. Consult doctor.

Infants & children:
Use caution. More likely to be absorbed through skin and cause adverse reactions.

Prolonged use:
Possible excess absorption. Don't use longer than 3 days for any one problem.

Skin & sunlight:
No problems expected.

Driving, piloting or hazardous work:
No problems expected.

Discontinuing:
May be unnecessary to finish medicine. Follow doctor's instructions.

Others:
No problems expected.

POSSIBLE INTERACTION WITH OTHER DRUGS

GENERIC NAME OR DRUG CLASS	COMBINED EFFECT
Sulfa drugs*	Decreased effect of sulfa drugs for infection.

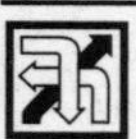

POSSIBLE INTERACTION WITH OTHER SUBSTANCE

INTERACTS WITH	COMBINED EFFECT
Alcohol:	None expected.
Beverages:	None expected.
Cocaine:	Possible nervous system toxicity. Avoid.
Foods:	None expected.
Marijuana:	None expected.
Tobacco:	None expected.

***See Glossary**

ANESTHETICS, MUCOSAL-LOCAL

BRAND AND GENERIC NAMES

Americaine
Anbesol Maximum Strength
Anestacon
Baby Anbesol
Baby Orajel
Baby Oragel Nighttime Formula
BENZOCAINE
Benzodent
BUTACAINE
Butyn
Children's Chloraseptic
Children's Sucrets
Chloraseptic Cool Mint Flavor
Dentocaine
Dyclone
DYCLONINE
Ethyl aminobenzoate
Hurricaine
LIDOCAINE
Maximum Strength Orajel
Orabase with Benzocaine
Orabase-O
Orajel
Pontocaine
Rid-A-Pain
Sabex Teething Syrup
Spec T
Sucrets Wild Cherry Regular Strength
Sucrets Maximum Strength
Supracaine
T-Caine
TETRACAINE
Triamcinolone in Orabase
Tyrobenz
Xylocaine
Xylocaine Viscous

BASIC INFORMATION

Habit forming? No
Prescription needed? Yes, for some.
Available as generic? Yes for lidocaine, no for others
Drug class: Anesthetic (topical)

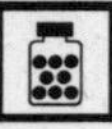

USES

Relieves pain or irritation in mouth caused by toothache, teething, mouth sores, dentures, braces, dental appliances. Also relieves pain of sore throat for short periods of time.

OVERDOSE

SYMPTOMS:
Overabsorption by body—Dizziness, blurred vision, seizures, drowsiness.
WHAT TO DO:
- **Dial 911 (emergency) or 0 (operator) for an ambulance or medical help. Then give first aid immediately.**
- **Not for internal use. If child accidentally swallows, call poison control center.**
- **See emergency information on inside covers.**

DOSAGE & USAGE INFORMATION

How to use:
- For mouth problems—Apply to sore places with cotton-tipped applicator. Don't swallow.
- For throat—Gargle, but don't swallow.
- For aerosol spray—Don't inhale.

When to use:
As directed by physician or label on package.

If you forget a dose:
Use as soon as you remember.

What drug does:
Blocks pain impulses to the brain.

Time lapse before drug works:
Immediately.

Don't use with:
Any other medicine without consulting your doctor or pharmacist.

POSSIBLE ADVERSE REACTIONS OR SIDE EFFECTS

SYMPTOMS	WHAT TO DO
Life-threatening:	
Unusual anxiety, excitement, nervousness, irregular or slow heartbeat.	Discontinue. Seek emergency treatment.
Common:	
None expected.	
Infrequent:	
Redness, irritation, sores not present before treatment, rash, itchy skin, hives.	Discontinue. Call doctor right away.
Rare:	
None expected.	

WARNINGS & PRECAUTIONS

Don't use if:
You are allergic to any of the products listed.

Before you start, consult your doctor:
- If you are allergic to anything.
- If you have infection, canker sores or other sores in your mouth.
- If you take medicine for myasthenia gravis, eye drops for glaucoma or any sulfa medicine.

Over age 60:
Adverse reactions and side effects may be more frequent and severe than in younger persons. Ask doctor about smaller doses.

Pregnancy:
Risk factors vary for drugs in this group. See category list on page xxii and consult doctor.

Breast-feeding:
No problems expected, but check with doctor.

Infants & children:
No problems expected, but check with doctor.

Prolonged use:
Not intended for prolonged use.

Skin & sunlight:
No problems expected.

Driving, piloting or hazardous work:
Wait to see if causes dizziness, sweating, drowsiness or blurred vision. If not, no problems expected.

Discontinuing:
No problems expected.

Others:
- Keep cool, but don't freeze.
- Don't puncture, break or burn aerosol containers.
- Don't eat, drink or chew gum for 1 hour after use.
- Heat and moisture in bathroom medicine cabinet can cause breakdown of medicine. Store someplace else.
- Before anesthesia, tell dentist about any medicines you take or use.

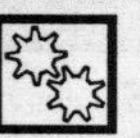

POSSIBLE INTERACTION WITH OTHER DRUGS

GENERIC NAME OR DRUG CLASS	COMBINED EFFECT
So remote, they are not considered clinically significant.	

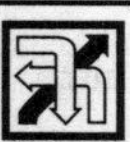

POSSIBLE INTERACTION WITH OTHER SUBSTANCE

INTERACTS WITH	COMBINED EFFECT
Alcohol:	Adverse reactions more common.
Beverages:	None expected.
Cocaine:	May cause too much nervousness and trembling. Avoid.
Foods:	None expected.
Marijuana:	None expected.
Tobacco:	Avoid. Tobacco makes mouth problems worse.

*See Glossary

ANGIOTENSIN-CONVERTING ENZYME (ACE) INHIBITORS

BRAND AND GENERIC NAMES

See complete list of brand and generic names in the *Brand Name Directory*, page 893.

BASIC INFORMATION

Habit forming? No
Prescription needed? Yes
Available as generic? No
Drug class: Antihypertensive, ACE inhibitor

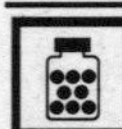

USES

- Treatment for high blood pressure and congestive heart failure.
- Treatment for kidney disease in diabetic patients (captopril).

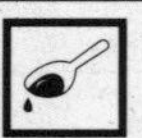

DOSAGE & USAGE INFORMATION

How to take:
Tablet—Swallow with liquid. Instructions to take on empty stomach mean 1 hour before or 2 hours after eating.

When to take:
At the same times each day, usually 2-3 times daily. Take first dose at bedtime and lie down immediately.

If you forget a dose:
Take as soon as you remember up to 2 hours late. If more than 2 hours, wait for next scheduled dose (don't double this dose).

What drug does:
- Reduces resistance in arteries.
- Strengthens heartbeat.

Time lapse before drug works:
60 to 90 minutes.

Don't take with:
Any other medicine without consulting your doctor or pharmacist.

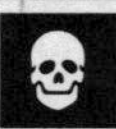

OVERDOSE

SYMPTOMS:
Low blood pressure, fever, chills, sore throat, fainting, convulsions, coma.
WHAT TO DO:
- **Dial 911 (emergency) or 0 (operator) for an ambulance or medical help. Then give first aid immediately.**
- **See emergency information on inside covers.**

POSSIBLE ADVERSE REACTIONS OR SIDE EFFECTS

SYMPTOMS	WHAT TO DO
Life-threatening:	
Hives, rash, intense itching, faintness soon after a dose (anaphylaxis); difficulty breathing.	Seek emergency treatment immediately.
Common:	
Rash, loss of taste.	Discontinue. Call doctor right away.
Infrequent:	
• Swelling of mouth, face, hands or feet.	Discontinue. Seek emergency treatment.
• Dizziness, fainting, chest pain, fast or irregular heartbeat, coughing, confusion, nervousness, numbness and tingling in hands or feet.	Discontinue. Call doctor right away.
• Diarrhea, headache, tiredness.	Continue. Call doctor when convenient.
Rare:	
• Sore throat, cloudy urine, fever, chills.	Discontinue. Call doctor right away.
• Nausea, vomiting, indigestion, abdominal pain.	Continue. Call doctor when convenient.

WARNINGS & PRECAUTIONS

Don't take if:
- You are allergic to any ACE inhibitor*.
- You are receiving blood from a blood bank.
- You will have surgery within 2 months, including dental surgery, requiring general or spinal anesthesia.

Before you start, consult your doctor:
- If you have had a stroke.
- If you have angina or heart or blood vessel disease.
- If you have any autoimmune disease, including AIDS or lupus.
- If you have high level of potassium in blood.
- If you have kidney or liver disease.
- If you are on severe salt-restricted diet.
- If you have a bone marrow disorder.

Over age 60:
Adverse reactions and side effects may be more frequent and severe than in younger persons.

ANGIOTENSIN-CONVERTING ENZYME (ACE) INHIBITORS

Pregnancy:
Risk factors vary for drugs in this group. See category list on page xxii and consult doctor.

Breast-feeding:
Drug passes into milk. Avoid drug or discontinue nursing until you finish medicine. Consult doctor for advice on maintaining milk supply.

Infants & children:
Under close medical supervision only.

Prolonged use:
- May decrease white cells in blood or cause protein loss in urine.
- Request periodic laboratory blood counts and urine tests.

Skin & sunlight:
No problems expected.

Driving, piloting or hazardous work:
Avoid if you become dizzy or faint. Otherwise, no problems expected.

Discontinuing:
Don't discontinue without consulting doctor. Dose may require gradual reduction if you have taken drug for a long time. Doses of other drugs may also require adjustment.

Others:
- Stop taking diuretics or increase salt intake 1 week before starting any ACE inhibitor.
- Avoid exercising in hot weather.
- May affect results in some medical tests.
- Advise any doctor or dentist whom you consult that you take this medicine.

POSSIBLE INTERACTION WITH OTHER DRUGS

GENERIC NAME OR DRUG CLASS	COMBINED EFFECT
Amiloride	Possible excessive potassium in blood.
Antihypertensives, other*	Increased anti-hypertensive effect. Dosage of each may require adjustment.
Beta-adrenergic blocking agents*	Increased anti-hypertensive effect. Dosage of each may require adjustment.
Carteolol	Increased anti-hypertensive effects of both drugs. Dosages may require adjustment.
Chloramphenicol	Possible blood disorders.
Diuretics*	Possible severe blood pressure drop with first dose.
Diclofenac	May decrease ACE inhibitor effect.
Guanfacine	Increased effect of both drugs.
Nicardipine	Possible excessive potassium in blood. Dosages may require adjustment.
Nimodipine	Possible excessive potassium in blood. Dangerous blood pressure drop.
Nitrates*	Possible excessive blood pressure drop.
Nonsteroidal anti-inflammatory drugs (NSAIDs)*	Decreased ACE inhibitor effect.
Pentamidine	May increase bone marrow depression or make kidney damage more likely.
Pentoxifylline	Increased anti-hypertensive effect.
Potassium supplements*	Possible increased potassium in blood.
Potassium iodide	May raise potassium levels in blood to toxic levels.

Continued on page 922

POSSIBLE INTERACTION WITH OTHER SUBSTANCES

INTERACTS WITH	COMBINED EFFECT
Alcohol:	Possible excessive blood pressure drop.
Beverages: Low-salt milk.	Possible excessive potassium in blood.
Cocaine	Increased risk of heart block and high blood pressure.
Foods: Salt substitutes.	Possible excessive potassium.
Marijuana:	Increased dizziness.
Tobacco:	May decrease ACE inhibitor effect.

*See Glossary

ANGIOTENSIN-CONVERTING ENZYME (ACE) INHIBITORS & HYDROCHLOROTHIAZIDE

BRAND AND GENERIC NAMES

See complete list of brand and generic names in the *Brand Names Directory*, page 893.

BASIC INFORMATION

Habit forming? No
Prescription needed? Yes
Available as generic? No
Drug class: Antihypertensive, diuretic (thiazide), ACE inhibitor

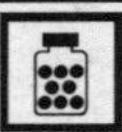

USES

- Treatment for high blood pressure and congestive heart failure.
- Reduces fluid retention.

DOSAGE & USAGE INFORMATION

How to take:
Tablet—Swallow with liquid. Instructions to take on empty stomach mean 1 hour before or 2 hours after eating.

When to take:
At the same times each day, usually 2 to 3 times daily. Take first dose at bedtime and lie down immediately.

If you forget a dose:
Take as soon as you remember up to 2 hours late. If more than 2 hours, wait for next scheduled dose (don't double this dose).

What drug does:
- Forces sodium and water excretion, reducing body fluid.
- Relaxes muscle cells of small arteries.
- Reduced body fluid and relaxed arteries lower blood pressure.
- Reduces resistance in arteries.
- Strengthens heartbeat.

Continued next column

OVERDOSE

SYMPTOMS:
Cramps, weakness, drowsiness, weak pulse, low blood pressure.
WHAT TO DO:
- **Dial 911 (emergency) or 0 (operator) for an ambulance or medical help. Then give first aid immediately.**
- **See emergency information on inside covers.**

Time lapse before drug works:
4 to 6 hours. May require several weeks to lower blood pressure.

Don't take with:
- Nonprescription drugs without consulting doctor.
- See Interaction column and consult doctor.

POSSIBLE ADVERSE REACTIONS OR SIDE EFFECTS

SYMPTOMS	WHAT TO DO
Life-threatening:	
Irregular heartbeat (fast or uneven); hives, rash, intense itching, faintness soon after a dose (anaphylaxis).	Discontinue. Seek emergency treatment.
Common:	
• Dry mouth, thirst, tiredness, weakness, muscle cramps, vomiting, chest pain, skin rash, coughing, weak pulse.	Discontinue. Call doctor right away.
• Taste loss, dizziness.	Continue. Call doctor when convenient.
Infrequent:	
• Face, mouth, hands swell.	Discontinue. Call doctor right away.
• Nausea, diarrhea.	Continue. Call doctor when convenient.
Rare:	
Jaundice (yellow eyes and skin), bruising, back pain.	Discontinue. Call doctor right away.

WARNINGS & PRECAUTIONS

Don't take if:
- You are allergic to any ACE inhibitor or any thiazide diuretic drug.
- You are receiving blood from a blood bank.
- If you will have surgery within 2 months, including dental surgery, requiring general or spinal anesthesia.

Before you start, consult your doctor:
- If you have had a stroke.
- If you have angina, heart or blood vessel disease, a high level of potassium in blood, lupus, gout, liver, pancreas or kidney disorder.
- If you have any autoimmune disease, including AIDS or lupus.
- If you are on severe salt-restricted diet.

ANGIOTENSIN-CONVERTING ENZYME (ACE) INHIBITORS & HYDROCHLOROTHIAZIDE

- If you are allergic to any sulfa drug.
- If you have a bone marrow disorder.

Over age 60:
Adverse reactions and side effects may be more frequent and severe than in younger persons, especially dizziness and excessive potassium loss.

Pregnancy:
Risk factors vary for drugs in this group. See category list on page xxii and consult doctor.

Breast-feeding:
Drug passes into milk. Avoid drug or discontinue nursing until you finish medicine. Consult doctor for advice on maintaining milk supply.

Infants & children:
Not recommended.

Prolonged use:
Talk to your doctor about the need for follow-up medical examinations or laboratory studies to check blood pressure, ECG*, liver function, kidney function.

Skin & sunlight:
May cause rash or intensify sunburn in areas exposed to sun or sunlamp.

Driving, piloting or hazardous work:
Don't drive or pilot aircraft until you learn how medicine affects you. Don't work around dangerous machinery. Don't climb ladders or work in high places. Danger increases if you drink alcohol or take medicine affecting alertness and reflexes, such as antihistamines, tranquilizers, sedatives, pain medicine, narcotics and mind-altering drugs.

Discontinuing:
Don't discontinue without consulting doctor. Dose may require gradual reduction if you have taken drug for a long time. Doses of other drugs may also require adjustment.

Others:
- Hot weather and fever may cause dehydration and drop in blood pressure. Dose may require temporary adjustment. Weigh daily and report any unexpected weight decreases to your doctor.
- May cause rise in uric acid, leading to gout.
- May cause blood-sugar rise in diabetics.

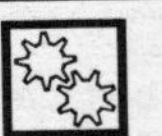

POSSIBLE INTERACTION WITH OTHER DRUGS

GENERIC NAME OR DRUG CLASS	COMBINED EFFECT
Allopurinol	Decreased allopurinol effect.
Amiloride	Possible excessive potassium in blood.
Antidepressants, tricyclic*	Dangerous drop in blood pressure. Avoid combination unless under medical supervision.
Antihypertensives, other*	Increased anti-hypertensive effect. Dosage of each may require adjustment.
Anti-inflammatory drugs nonsteroidal (NSAIDs)*	Decreased captopril effect.
Barbiturates*	Increased hydro-chlorothiazide effect.
Beta-adrenergic blocking agents*	Increased anti-hypertensive effect. Dosage of each may require adjustments.
Carteolol	Increased antihyper-tensive effects of both drugs. Dosages may require adjustment.
Chloramphenicol	Possible blood disorders.
Cholestyramine	Decreased hydro-chlorothiazide effect.
Cortisone drugs*	Excessive potassium loss that causes dan-gerous heart rhythms.

Continued on page 922

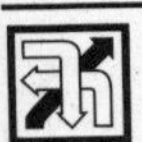

POSSIBLE INTERACTION WITH OTHER SUBSTANCES

INTERACTS WITH	COMBINED EFFECT
Alcohol:	Dangerous blood pressure drop. Avoid.
Beverages: Low-salt milk.	Possible excessive potassium in blood.
Cocaine	Increased risk of heart block and high blood pressure.
Foods: Salt substitutes.	Possible excessive potassium.
Marijuana:	Increased dizziness; may increase blood-pressure.
Tobacco:	May decrease blood pressure lowering effect.

***See Glossary**

ANTACIDS

BRAND AND GENERIC NAMES

See complete list of brand names in the *Brand Names Directory*, page 893.

BASIC INFORMATION

Habit forming? No
Prescription needed? No
Available as generic? Yes, for some.
Drug class: Antacid

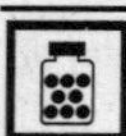

USES

Treatment for hyperacidity in upper gastrointestinal tract, including stomach and esophagus. Symptoms may be heartburn or acid indigestion. Diseases include peptic ulcer, gastritis, esophagitis, hiatal hernia.

DOSAGE & USAGE INFORMATION

How to take:
Follow package instructions.

When to take:
1 to 3 hours after meals unless directed otherwise by your doctor.

If you forget a dose:
Take as soon as you remember, but not simultaneously with any other medicine.

What drug does:
- Neutralizes some of the hydrochloric acid in the stomach.
- Reduces action of pepsin, a digestive enzyme.

Time lapse before drug works:
15 minutes for antacid effect.

Continued next column

OVERDOSE

SYMPTOMS:
Dry mouth, shallow breathing, diarrhea, weakness, fatigue, stupor, bone pain.
WHAT TO DO:
- **Overdose unlikely to threaten life. Depending on severity of symptoms and amount taken, call doctor, poison control center or hospital emergency room for instructions.**
- **Dial 911 (emergency) or 0 (operator) for an ambulance or medical help. Then give first aid immediately.**
- **See emergency information on inside covers.**

Don't take with:
Other medicines at the same time. Decreases absorption of other drugs. Wait 2 hours between doses.

POSSIBLE ADVERSE REACTIONS OR SIDE EFFECTS

SYMPTOMS	WHAT TO DO
Life-threatening:	
Heartbeat irregularity in patient with heart disease.	Discontinue. Seek emergency treatment.
Common:	
• Constipation, headache, appetite loss, distended stomach.	Discontinue. Call doctor right away.
• Unpleasant taste in mouth, abdominal pain, laxative effect, belching, chalky taste.	Continue. Call doctor when convenient.
Infrequent:	
• Bone pain, frequent urination, dizziness, urgent urination, muscle weakness or pain, nausea, weight gain.	Discontinue. Call doctor right away.
• Tiredness or weakness	Continue. Call doctor when convenient.
Rare:	
Mood changes, vomiting, nervousness, swollen feet and ankles.	Discontinue. Call doctor right away.

Note: Side effects are rare unless you take too much medicine for a long time.

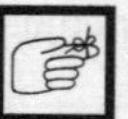

WARNINGS & PRECAUTIONS

Don't take if:
- You are allergic to any antacid.
- You have a high blood-calcium level.

Before you start, consult your doctor:
If you have kidney disease, chronic constipation, colitis, diarrhea, symptoms of appendicitis, stomach or intestinal bleeding, irregular heartbeat.

Over age 60:
Adverse reactions and side effects may be more frequent and severe than in younger persons. Diarrhea or constipation particularly likely.

Pregnancy:
Risk factors vary for drugs in this group. See category list on page xxii and consult doctor.

Breast-feeding:
Drug passes into milk. Consult doctor.

Infants & children:
Use only under medical supervision.

Prolonged use:
- High blood level of calcium (if your antacid contains calcium) which disturbs electrolyte balance.
- Kidney stones, impaired kidney function.
- Talk to your doctor about the need for follow-up medical examinations or laboratory studies to check kidney function, serum calcium, serum potassium.

Skin & sunlight:
No problems expected.

Driving, piloting or hazardous work:
No problems expected.

Discontinuing:
May be unnecessary to finish medicine. Follow doctor's instructions.

Others:
- Don't take longer than 2 weeks unless under medical supervision.
- May affect results in some medical tests.

POSSIBLE INTERACTION WITH OTHER DRUGS

GENERIC NAME OR DRUG CLASS	COMBINED EFFECT
Chlorpromazine	Decreased chlorpromazine effect.
Ciprofloxacin	May cause kidney dysfunction.
Digitalis preparations*	Decreased digitalis effect.
Iron supplements*	Decreased iron effect.
Isoniazid	Decreased isoniazid effect.
Ketoconazole	Reduced ketoconazole effect.
Levodopa	Increased levodopa effect.
Mecamylamine	Increased mecamylamine effect.
Meperidine	Increased meperidine effect.
Methenamine	Reduced methenamine effect.
Nalidixic acid	Decreased nalidixic acid effect.
Nicardipine	Possible decreased nicardipine effect.
Nizatidine	Decreased nizatidine absorption.
Ofloxacin	Decreased ofloxacin effect.
Oxyphenbutazone	Decreased oxyphenbutazone effect.
Para-aminosalicylic acid (PAS)	Decreased PAS effect.
Penicillins*	Decreased penicillin effect.
Pseudoephedrine	Increased pseudoephedrine effect.
Salicylates*	Increased salicylate effect.
Tetracyclines	Decreased tetracycline effect.
Ticlopidine	Decreased ticlopidine effect.

POSSIBLE INTERACTION WITH OTHER SUBSTANCES

INTERACTS WITH	COMBINED EFFECT
Alcohol:	Decreased antacid effect.
Beverages: Milk.	May cause bone discomfort.
Cocaine:	No proven problems.
Foods:	Decreased antacid effect. Wait 1 hour after eating.
Marijuana:	Decreased antacid effect.
Tobacco:	Decreased antacid effect.

*See Glossary

ANTHELMINTICS

BRAND AND GENERIC NAMES

Antiminth
Aut
Cobantril
Combantrin
Foldan
Helmex
Lombriareu
Mebendacin
MEBENDAZOLE
Mebutar
Mintezol
Mintezol (Topical)
Minzolum
Nemasole
Niclocide
NICLOSAMIDE
PYRANTEL
PYRVINIUM
Reese's Pinworm Medicine
THIABENDAZOLE
Triasox
Trilombrin
Vanquin
Vermox
Viprynium

BASIC INFORMATION

Habit forming? No
Prescription needed? Yes
Available as generic? No
Drug class: Anthelmintics

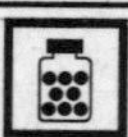

USES

Treatment of roundworms, pinworms, whipworms, hookworms and other intestinal parasites.

DOSAGE & USAGE INFORMATION

How to take or apply:

- Tablet—Swallow with liquid or food to lessen stomach irritation.
- Topical suspension—Apply to end of each tunnel or burrow made by worm.
- Chewable tablets—Chew thoroughly before swallowing.
- Oral suspension—Follow package instructions.

When to take:
Morning and evening with food to increase uptake.

Continued next column

OVERDOSE

SYMPTOMS:
Increased severity of adverse reactions and side effects.
WHAT TO DO:
Overdose unlikely to threaten life. If person takes much larger amount than prescribed, call doctor, poison control center or hospital emergency room for instructions.

If you forget a dose:
Skip dose and begin treatment again. Often only one or two doses are needed to complete treatment.

What drug does:
Kills or paralyzes the parasites. They then pass out of the body in the feces. Usually the type of worm parasite must be identified so the appropriate drug can be prescribed.

Time lapse before drug works:
Some take only hours, others, 1-3 days.

Don't take with:
Any other medicine without consulting your doctor or pharmacist.

POSSIBLE ADVERSE REACTIONS OR SIDE EFFECTS

SYMPTOMS	WHAT TO DO
Life-threatening: None expected.	
Common: None expected.	
Infrequent:	
• Abdominal pain, diarrhea, dizziness, fever, nausea, rectal itching.	Continue. Call doctor when convenient.
• Red stools, asparagus-like urine smell.	No action necessary.
Rare:	
Skin rash, itching, sore throat and fever, weakness (severe), hair loss, headache, blurred vision, seizures.	Discontinue. Call doctor right away.

WARNINGS & PRECAUTIONS

Don't take if:
You are allergic to any anthelmintics.

Before you start, consult your doctor:
- If you have liver disease.
- If you have Crohn's disease.
- If you have ulcerative colitis.

Over age 60:
Adverse reactions and side effects may be more frequent and severe than in younger persons. You may need smaller doses for shorter periods of time.

Pregnancy:
Risk factors vary for drugs in this group. See category list on page xxii and consult doctor.

Breast-feeding:
Unknown effect. Consult your doctor.

Infants & children:
No problems expected. Don't give to a child under age 2 without doctor's approval.

Prolonged use:
- Not intended for long-term use.
- Talk to your doctor about the need for follow-up medical examinations or laboratory studies to check stools, cellophane tape swabs pressed against rectal area to check for parasite eggs, complete blood counts (white blood cell count, platelet count, red blood cell count, hemoglobin, hematocrit).

Skin & sunlight:
No problems expected.

Driving, piloting or hazardous work:
Use caution if the medicine causes you to feel dizzy or weak. Otherwise, no problems expected.

Discontinuing:
No problems expected.

Others:
- Take full course of treatment. Repeat course may be necessary if follow-up examinations reveal persistent infection.
- Wash all bedding after treatment to prevent re-infection.

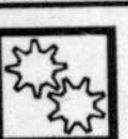

POSSIBLE INTERACTION WITH OTHER DRUGS

GENERIC NAME OR DRUG CLASS	COMBINED EFFECT
Carbamazepine	Decreased effect of mebendazole.
Theophylline	Increased effect of theophylline (with thiabendazole use.)

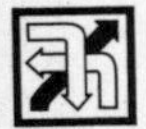

POSSIBLE INTERACTION WITH OTHER SUBSTANCES

INTERACTS WITH	COMBINED EFFECT
Alcohol:	Decreased mebendazole effect. Avoid.
Beverages:	None expected.
Cocaine:	None expected.
Foods:	None expected.
Marijuana:	None expected.
Tobacco:	None expected.

ANTHRALIN (Topical)

BRAND NAMES

Anthra-Derm
Anthraforte
Anthranol
Anthrascalp
Dithranol
Drithocreme
Drithocreme HP
Dritho-Scalp
Lasan
Lasan HP
Lasan Pomade
Lasan Unguent

BASIC INFORMATION

Habit forming? No
Prescription needed? Yes
Available as generic? No
Drug class: Antipsoriasis, hair growth stimulant

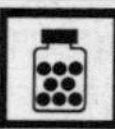

USES

- Treats quiescent or chronic psoriasis.
- Stimulates hair growth in some people (not an approved use by the FDA).

DOSAGE & USAGE INFORMATION

How to use:
- Wear plastic gloves for all applications.
- If directed, apply at night.
- Cream, lotion, ointment—Bathe and dry area before use. Apply small amount and rub gently.
- If for short contact, same as above for cream.
- Leave on 20 to 30 minutes. Then remove medicine by bathing or shampooing.
- If for scalp overnight—Shampoo before use to remove scales or medicine. Dry hair. Part hair several times and apply to scalp. Wear plastic cap on head. Clean off next morning with petroleum jelly, then shampoo.

When to use:
As directed.

If you forget a dose:
Use as soon as you remember.

What drug does:
Reduces growth activity within abnormal cells by inhibiting enzymes.

Continued next column

OVERDOSE

SYMPTOMS:
None expected.
WHAT TO DO:
Not for internal use. If child accidentally swallows, call poison control center.

Time lapse before drug works:
May require several weeks or more.

Don't use with:
Any other medicine without consulting your doctor or pharmacist.

POSSIBLE ADVERSE REACTIONS OR SIDE EFFECTS

SYMPTOMS	WHAT TO DO
Life-threatening: None expected.	
Common: None expected.	
Infrequent: Redness or irritation of skin not present before application, rash.	Discontinue. Call doctor right away.
Rare: None expected.	

WARNINGS & PRECAUTIONS

Don't use if:

- You are allergic to anthralin.
- You have infected skin.

Before you start, consult your doctor:

- If you have chronic kidney disease.
- If you are allergic to anything.

Over age 60:
No problems expected, but check with doctor.

Pregnancy:
Studies in animals and humans have not been done. Consult doctor. Risk category C (see page xxii).

Breast-feeding:
No problems expected, but check with doctor.

Infants & children:
No problems expected, but check with doctor.

Prolonged use:
No problems expected, but check with doctor.

Skin & sunlight:
May cause rash or intensify sunburn in areas exposed to sun or sunlamp. Avoid undue exposure.

Driving, piloting or hazardous work:
No problems expected.

Discontinuing:
No problems expected.

Others:

- Keep cool, but don't freeze.
- Apply petroleum jelly to normal skin or scalp to protect areas not being treated.
- Will stain hair, clothing, shower, bathtub or sheets. Wash as soon as possible.
- Heat and moisture in bathroom medicine cabinet can cause breakdown of medicine. Store someplace else.

POSSIBLE INTERACTION WITH OTHER DRUGS

GENERIC NAME OR DRUG CLASS	COMBINED EFFECT
Antidiabetic agents*	Increased sensitivity to sun exposure.
Coal tar preparations*	Increased sensitivity to sun exposure.
Diuretics, thiazide*	Increased sensitivity to sun exposure.
Griseofulvin	Increased sensitivity to sun exposure.
Methosalen	Increased sensitivity to sun exposure.
Nalidixic acid	Increased sensitivity to sun exposure.
Phenothiazines*	Increased sensitivity to sun exposure.
Sulfa drugs*	Increased sensitivity to sun exposure.
Tetracyclines*	Increased sensitivity to sun exposure.
Trioxsalen	Increased sensitivity to sun exposure.

POSSIBLE INTERACTION WITH OTHER SUBSTANCES

INTERACTS WITH	COMBINED EFFECT
Alcohol:	None expected.
Beverages:	None expected.
Cocaine:	None expected.
Foods:	None expected.
Marijuana:	None expected.
Tobacco:	None expected.

*See Glossary

ANTIACNE, CLEANSING (Topical)

BRAND AND GENERIC NAMES

ALCOHOL AND ACETONE
ALCOHOL AND SULFUR
Liquimat
Postacne
Seba-Nil
SULFURATED LIME
Transact
Trans-Plantar
Tyrosum Liquid
Vlem-Dome
Vlemasque
Vlemickx's solution
Xerac

BASIC INFORMATION

Habit forming? No
Prescription needed? No
Available as generic? Yes
Drug class: Anti-acne agent, cleansing agent

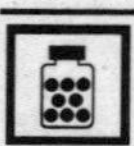

USES

Treats acne or oily skin.

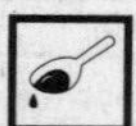

DOSAGE & USAGE INFORMATION

How to use:

- Lotion, gel or pledget—Start with small amount and wipe over face to remove dirt and surface oil. Don't apply to wounds or burns. Don't rinse with water and avoid contact with eyes. Skin may be more sensitive in dry or cold climates.
- Plaster—Follow package instructions.

When to use:
As directed. May increase frequency up to 3 or more times daily as tolerated. Warm, humid weather may allow more frequent use.

If you forget a dose:
Use as soon as you remember and then go back to regular schedule.

Continued next column

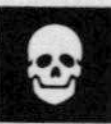

OVERDOSE

SYMPTOMS:
None expected.
WHAT TO DO:

- **Not for internal use. If child accidentally swallows, call poison control center.**
- **Dial 911 (emergency) or 0 (operator) for an ambulance or medical help. Then give first aid immediately.**
- **See emergency information on inside covers.**

What drug does:
Helps remove oil from skin's surface.

Time lapse before drug works:
Works immediately.

Don't use with:

- Other topical acne treatments unless directed by doctor.
- See Interaction column and consult doctor.

POSSIBLE ADVERSE REACTIONS OR SIDE EFFECTS

SYMPTOMS	WHAT TO DO
Life-threatening: None expected.	
Common: None expected.	
Infrequent: Skin infection, pustules or rash; unusual pain, swelling or redness of treated skin; burning or stinging of skin.	Discontinue. Call doctor right away.
Rare: None expected.	

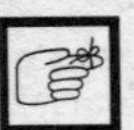

WARNINGS & PRECAUTIONS

Don't use if:
You have to apply over a wounded or burned area.

Before you start, consult your doctor:
If you use benzoyl peroxide, resorcinol, salicylic acid, sulfur or tretinoin (vitamin A acid).

Over age 60:
No problems expected.

Pregnancy:
Risk category not assigned to this drug group. Consult doctor about use.

Breast-feeding:
No problems expected, but check with doctor.

Infants & children:
No problems expected, but check with doctor. Use only under close medical supervision.

Prolonged use:
Excessive drying of skin.

Skin & sunlight:
No problems expected, but check with doctor.

Driving, piloting or hazardous work:
No problems expected, but check with doctor.

Discontinuing:
No problems expected, but check with doctor.

Others:
Some anti-acne agents are flammable. Don't use near fire or while smoking.

POSSIBLE INTERACTION WITH OTHER DRUGS

GENERIC NAME OR DRUG CLASS	COMBINED EFFECT
Abrasive or medicated soaps	Irritation or too much drying.
After-shave lotions	Irritation or too much drying.
Antiacne topical preparations (other)	Irritation or too much drying.
"Cover-up" cosmetics	Irritation or too much drying.
Drying cosmetic soaps	Irritation or too much drying.
Isotretinoin	Irritation or too much drying.
Mercury compounds	May stain skin black and smell bad.
Perfumed toilet water	Irritation or too much drying.
Preparations containing skin-peeling agents such as benzoyl peroxide, resorcinol, salicylic acid, sulfur, tretinoin	Irritation or too much drying.

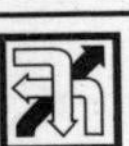

POSSIBLE INTERACTION WITH OTHER SUBSTANCES

INTERACTS WITH	COMBINED EFFECT
Alcohol:	None expected.
Beverages:	None expected.
Cocaine:	None expected.
Foods:	None expected.
Marijuana:	None expected.
Tobacco:	None expected.

*See Glossary

ANTIALLERGIC AGENTS, OPHTHALMIC

BRAND AND GENERIC NAMES

Alomide	Livostin
LEVOCABASTINE	LODOXAMIDE

BASIC INFORMATION

Habit forming? No
Prescription needed? Yes
Available as generic? No
Drug class: Ophthalmic antiallergic agents

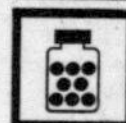

USES

Prevention and treatment of seasonal allergic (hay fever) eye disorders. May be referred to as seasonal conjunctivitis, vernal conjunctivitis, vernal keratitis and vernal keratoconjunctivitis.

DOSAGE & USAGE INFORMATION

How to use:

Eye solution

- Wash hands.
- Apply pressure to inside corner of eye with middle finger.
- Continue pressure for 1 minute after placing medicine in eye.
- Tilt head backward. Pull lower lid away from eye with index finger of the same hand.
- Drop eye drops into pouch and close eye. Don't blink.
- Keep eyes closed for 1 to 2 minutes.

When to use:
1 to 2 drops 4 times a day or as directed by doctor.

If you forget a dose:
Use as soon as you remember, then return to regular schedule.

Time lapse before drug works:
Levocabastine—7 days, with confirmed improvement.
Lodoxamide—3 days.

Continued next column

OVERDOSE

SYMPTOMS:
None expected.
WHAT TO DO:
Not intended for internal use. If child accidentally swallows, call poison control center.

What drug does:

- Lodoxamide acts as a mast cell* stabilizer to prevent a hypersensitivity reaction to certain allergens such as pollen.
- Levocabastine is a histamine H_1 receptor antagonist that blocks hypersensitivity responses to allergens.

Time lapse before drug works:
Relief of symptoms may begin immediately, but full benefit might take a few days.

Don't use with:
Any other medications without first consulting doctor or pharmacist.

POSSIBLE ADVERSE REACTIONS OR SIDE EFFECTS

SYMPTOMS	WHAT TO DO
Life-threatening: None expected.	
Common: Brief and mild burning or stinging when drops are administered.	No action necessary.
Infrequent: Blurred vision, feeling that something is in the eye, redness of eye, eye irritation not present before, eye tearing or discharge.	Discontinue. Call doctor right away.
Rare: • Aching in eye, crusting in corner of eye or eyelid, dryness of eyes or nose, drowsiness or sleepiness, feeling of heat in eye or body, nausea, stomach discomfort, sneezing, sticky or tired feeling of eye.	Continue. Call doctor when convenient.
• Redness or irritation of eyelid, swelling of eye, pain in eye, sensitivity to light, headache, dizziness, skin rash.	Discontinue. Call doctor right away.

WARNINGS & PRECAUTIONS

Don't use if:
You are allergic to levocabastine or lodoxamide.

Before you start, consult your doctor:
- If you wear soft contact lenses.
- You are allergic to any other medications, foods or other substances.

Over age 60:
No special problems expected.

Pregnancy:
Risk category C for levocabastine and B for lodoxamide (see page xxii). Consult doctor.

Breast-feeding:
lodoxamide passes into breast milk after administration into the eye. It is unknown if levocabastine passes into breast milk. Consult doctor.

Infants & children:
No information available on safety or effectiveness for children under age 2 for lodoxamide and under age 12 for levocabastine. Consult doctor.

Prolonged use:
No special problems expected.

Skin & sunlight:
Normally no problems expected, but adverse reaction may cause light sensitivity.

Driving, piloting or hazardous work:
Avoid if you feel dizzy or side effects cause vision problems.

Discontinuing:
No special problems expected.

Others:
- Don't use leftover medicine for other eye problems without your doctor's approval.
- If symptoms don't improve after a few days of use, call your doctor.

POSSIBLE INTERACTION WITH OTHER DRUGS

GENERIC NAME OR DRUG CLASS	COMBINED EFFECT
None significant.	

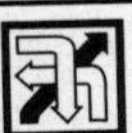

POSSIBLE INTERACTION WITH OTHER SUBSTANCES

INTERACTS WITH	COMBINED EFFECT
Alcohol:	None expected.
Beverages:	None expected.
Cocaine	None expected.
Foods:	None expected.
Marijuana:	None expected.
Tobacco:	None expected.

ANTIBACTERIALS (Ophthalmic)

BRAND AND GENERIC NAMES

See complete list of brand and generic names in the *Brand Name Directory*, page 894.

BASIC INFORMATION

Habit forming? No
Prescription needed? Yes
Available as generic? Yes, for some
Drug class: Antibacterial (ophthalmic)

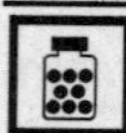

USES

Helps body overcome eye infections on surface tissues of the eye.

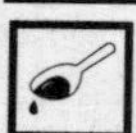

DOSAGE & USAGE INFORMATION

How to use:

Eye drops

- Wash hands.
- Apply pressure to inside corner of eye with middle finger.
- Continue pressure for 1 minute after placing medicine in eye.
- Tilt head backward. Pull lower lid away from eye with index finger of the same hand.
- Drop eye drops into pouch and close eye. Don't blink.
- Keep eyes closed for 1 to 2 minutes.

Eye ointment

- Wash hands.
- Pull lower lid down from eye to form a pouch.
- Squeeze tube to apply thin strip of ointment into pouch.
- Close eye for 1 to 2 minutes.
- Don't touch applicator tip to any surface (including the eye). If you accidentally touch tip, clean with warm soap and water.
- Keep container tightly closed.
- Keep cool, but don't freeze.
- Wash hands immediately after using.

When to use:
As directed. Don't miss doses.

Continued next column

OVERDOSE

SYMPTOMS:
None expected.
WHAT TO DO:
Not intended for internal use. If child accidentally swallows, call poison control center.

If you forget a dose:
Use as soon as you remember.

What drug does:
Penetrates bacterial cell membrane and prevents cells from multiplying.

Time lapse before drug works:
Begins in 1 hour. May require 7 to 10 days to control infection.

Don't use with:
Any other eye drops or ointment without checking with your ophthalmologist.

POSSIBLE ADVERSE REACTIONS OR SIDE EFFECTS

SYMPTOMS	WHAT TO DO
Life-threatening: None expected.	
Common: Ointments cause blurred vision for a few minutes.	Continue. Tell doctor at next visit.
Infrequent: Signs of irritation not present before drug use.	Discontinue. Call doctor right away.
Rare (with chloramphenicol): Sore throat, pale skin, fever, unusual bleeding or bruising.	Discontinue. Call doctor right away.

WARNINGS & PRECAUTIONS

Don't use if:
You are allergic to any antibiotic used on skin, ears, vagina or rectum.

Before you start, consult your doctor:
If you have had an allergic reaction to any medicine, food or other substances.

Over age 60:
No problems expected.

Pregnancy:
Risk factors vary for drugs in this group. See category list on page xxii and consult doctor.

Breast-feeding:
No problems expected, but check with doctor.

Infants & children:
No problems expected. Use only under medical supervision.

Prolonged use:
Sensitivity reaction may develop.

Skin & sunlight:
No problems expected.

Driving, piloting or hazardous work:
No problems expected.

Discontinuing:
Possible rare adverse reaction of bone marrow depression that leads to aplastic anemia may occur after discontinuing chloramphenicol.

Others:
- Notify doctor if symptoms fail to improve in 2 to 4 days.
- Keep cool, but don't freeze.

POSSIBLE INTERACTION WITH OTHER DRUGS

GENERIC NAME OR DRUG CLASS	COMBINED EFFECT
Clinically significant interactions with oral or injected medicines unlikely.	

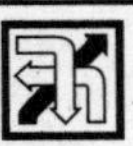

POSSIBLE INTERACTION WITH OTHER SUBSTANCES

INTERACTS WITH	COMBINED EFFECT
Alcohol:	None expected.
Beverages:	None expected.
Cocaine:	None expected.
Foods:	None expected.
Marijuana:	None expected.
Tobacco:	None expected.

ANTIBACTERIALS (Otic)

BRAND AND GENERIC NAMES

CHLORAMPHENICOL
Chloromycetin
COLISTIN, NEOMYCIN & HYDROCORTISONE
Coly-Mycin S
Cortisporin
DESONIDE AND ACETIC ACID
Garamycin Otic Solution
GENTAMICIN (otic)
HYDROCORTISONE AND ACETIC ACID
LazerSporin
NEOMYCIN, POLYMIXIN B AND HYDRO-CORTISONE
Ortega Otic-M
Oticair
Otic Tridesilon Solution
Otobione
Otocort
Otoreid-HC
Pediotic
Sopamycetin
VoSol HC

BASIC INFORMATION

Habit forming? No
Prescription needed? Yes
Available as generic? Yes
Drug class: Antibacterial (otic)

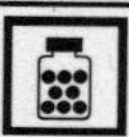

USES

Ear infections in external ear canal (not middle ear) caused by susceptible germs (bacteria, virus, fungus).

DOSAGE & USAGE INFORMATION

How to use:
Ear drops
- Warm ear drops under running water around the unopened bottle.
- Lie down with affected ear up.
- Adults—Pull ear lobe back and up.
- Children—Pull ear lobe down and back.
- Drop medicine into ear canal until canal is full.
- Stay lying down for 2 minutes.
- Gently insert cotton plug into ear to prevent leaking.

Continued next column

Ear ointment
- Apply small amount to skin just inside the ear canal.
- Use finger or piece of sterile gauze.
- Don't use cotton-tipped applicators.

When to use:
As directed on label.

If you forget a dose:
Use as soon as you remember.

What drug does:
Kills germs that infect the skin of the external ear canal.

Time lapse before drug works:
15 minutes.

Don't use with:
Other ear medications unless directed by your doctor.

OVERDOSE

SYMPTOMS:
None expected.
WHAT TO DO:
Not intended for internal use. If child accidentally swallows, call poison control center.

POSSIBLE ADVERSE REACTIONS OR SIDE EFFECTS

SYMPTOMS	WHAT TO DO
Life-threatening: None expected.	
Common: None expected.	
Infrequent: Itching, burning, redness, swelling.	Discontinue. Call doctor right away.
Rare (with chloramphenicol): Pale skin, sore throat, fever, unusual bleeding or bruising, unusual tiredness or weakness.	Discontinue. Call doctor right away.

WARNINGS & PRECAUTIONS

Don't use if:
You are allergic to any of the medicines listed.

Before you start, consult your doctor:
If eardrum is punctured.

Over age 60:
No problems expected.

Pregnancy:
Risk factors vary for drugs in this group. See category list on page xxii and consult doctor.

Breast-feeding:
No problems expected. Consult doctor.

Infants & children:
No problems expected.

Prolonged use:
Not intended for prolonged use.

Skin & sunlight:
Skin sensitivity more likely.

Driving, piloting or hazardous work:
No problems expected.

Discontinuing:
Possible rare adverse reaction of bone marrow depression that leads to aplastic anemia after discontinuing chloramphenicol.

Others:
Keep cool, but don't freeze.

POSSIBLE INTERACTION WITH OTHER DRUGS

GENERIC NAME OR DRUG CLASS	COMBINED EFFECT
None expected.	

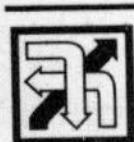

POSSIBLE INTERACTION WITH OTHER SUBSTANCES

INTERACTS WITH	COMBINED EFFECT
Alcohol:	None expected.
Beverages:	None expected.
Cocaine:	None expected.
Foods:	None expected.
Marijuana:	None expected.
Tobacco:	None expected.

*See Glossary

ANTIBACTERIALS (Topical)

BRAND AND GENERIC NAMES

Bactine First Aid Antibiotic
Bactroban
CHLORAMPHENICOL (Topical)
Chloromycetin
Foille
G-Myticin
Garamycin
Gentamar
GENTAMICIN
MUPIROCIN
Mycitracin
NEOMYCIN & POLYMYXIN B
NEOMYCIN, POLYMYXIN B & BACITRACIN
Neo-Polycin
Neosporin
Neosporin Maximum Strength Ointment
Neosporin Ointment
Topisporan

BASIC INFORMATION

Habit forming? No
Prescription needed? Yes
Available as generic? Yes
Drug class: Antibacterial (topical)

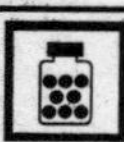

USES

Treats skin infections that may accompany burns, superficial boils, insect bites or stings, skin ulcers, minor surgical wounds.

DOSAGE & USAGE INFORMATION

How to use:
- Cream, lotion, ointment—Bathe and dry area before use. Apply small amount and rub gently.
- May cover with gauze or bandage if desired.

When to use:
3 or 4 times daily, or as directed by doctor.

If you forget a dose:
Use as soon as you remember.

Continued next column

OVERDOSE

SYMPTOMS:
None expected.
WHAT TO DO:
Not for internal use. If child accidentally swallows, call poison control center.
- **Dial 911 (emergency) or 0 (operator) for an ambulance or medical help. Then give first aid immediately.**
- **See emergency information on inside covers.**

What drug does:
Kills susceptible bacteria by interfering with bacterial DNA and RNA.

Time lapse before drug works:
Begins first day. May require treatment for a week or longer to cure infection.

Don't use with:
Any other medicine without consulting your doctor or pharmacist.

POSSIBLE ADVERSE REACTIONS OR SIDE EFFECTS

SYMPTOMS	WHAT TO DO
Life-threatening: None expected.	
Common: None expected.	
Infrequent: Itching, swollen, red skin.	Discontinue. Call doctor right away.
Rare: None expected.	

WARNINGS & PRECAUTIONS

Don't use if:
You are allergic to gentamicin or any topical medication.

Before you start, consult your doctor:
If any of the lesions on the skin are open sores.

Over age 60:
No problems expected.

Pregnancy:
Risk factors vary for drugs in this group. See category list on page xxii and consult doctor.

Breast-feeding:
No problems expected, but check with doctor.

Infants & children:
No problems expected, but check with doctor.

Prolonged use:
No problems expected, but check with doctor.

Skin & sunlight:
No problems expected, but check with doctor.

Driving, piloting or hazardous work:
No problems expected, but check with doctor.

Discontinuing:
No problems expected, but check with doctor.

Others:
- Heat and moisture in bathroom medicine cabinet can cause breakdown of medicine. Store someplace else.
- Keep cool, but don't freeze.

POSSIBLE INTERACTION WITH OTHER DRUGS

GENERIC NAME OR DRUG CLASS	COMBINED EFFECT
Any other topical medication	Hypersensitivity reactions more likely to occur.

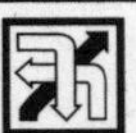

POSSIBLE INTERACTION WITH OTHER SUBSTANCES

INTERACTS WITH	COMBINED EFFECT
Alcohol:	None expected.
Beverages:	None expected.
Cocaine:	None expected.
Foods:	None expected.
Marijuana:	None expected.
Tobacco:	None expected.

ANTIBACTERIALS, ANTIFUNGALS (Topical)

BRAND AND GENERIC NAMES

CLIOQUINOL
CLIOQUINOL & HYDROCORTISONE
Flamazine
Flint SSD
IODOCHLORHYDROXYQUIN
IODOCHLORHYDROXYQUIN & HYDROCORTISONE
Sildimac
Silvadene
SILVER SULFADIAZINE
SSD
SSD AF
Thermazene
Vioform-Hydrocortisone Creme
Vioform-Hydrocortisone Lotion
Vioform-Hydrocortisone Mild Cream
Vioform-Hydrocortisone Mild Ointment
Vioform-Hydrocortisone Ointment

BASIC INFORMATION

Habit forming? No
Prescription needed? Yes
Available as generic? Yes, some are
Drug class: Antibacterial (topical), antifungal (topical)

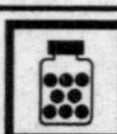

USES

Treats eczema, other inflammatory skin conditions, athlete's foot, skin infections.

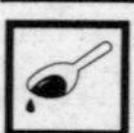

DOSAGE & USAGE INFORMATION

How to use:
- Cream, lotion, ointment—Bathe and dry area before use. Apply small amount and rub gently.
- Keep away from eyes.

When to use:
2 to 4 times a day.

Continued next column

OVERDOSE

SYMPTOMS:
Severe nausea, vomiting, diarrhea.
WHAT TO DO:
- **Not for internal use. If child accidentally swallows, call poison control center.**
- **Dial 911 (emergency) or 0 (operator) for an ambulance or medical help. Then give first aid immediately.**
- **See emergency information on inside covers.**

If you forget a dose:
Use as soon as you remember.

What drug does:
Kills some types of fungus and bacteria on contact.

Time lapse before drug works:
2 to 4 weeks, sometimes longer.

Don't use with:
Other ointments, creams or lotions without consulting doctor.

POSSIBLE ADVERSE REACTIONS OR SIDE EFFECTS

SYMPTOMS	WHAT TO DO
Life-threatening:	
None expected.	
Common:	
May stain skin around nails.	Continue. Tell doctor at next visit.
Infrequent:	
Stomach cramps; hives; itching, burning, peeling, red, stinging, swelling skin.	Discontinue. Call doctor right away.
Rare:	
None expected.	

WARNINGS & PRECAUTIONS

Don't use if:
You are allergic to clioquinol, iodine or any iodine-containing preparation.

Before you start, consult your doctor:
If you are allergic to anything that touches your skin.

Over age 60:
No problems expected.

Pregnancy:
Risk factors vary for drugs in this group. See category list on page xxii and consult doctor.

Breast-feeding:
No problems expected, but check with doctor.

Infants & children:
No problems expected, but check with doctor.

Prolonged use:
No problems expected, but check with doctor.

Skin & sunlight:
No problems expected, but check with doctor.

Driving, piloting or hazardous work:
No problems expected, but check with doctor.

Discontinuing:
No problems expected, but check with doctor.

Others:
- If not improved in 2 weeks, check with doctor.
- May stain clothing or bed linens.
- May stain hair, skin and nails yellow.
- If accidentally gets into eyes, flush with clear water immediately.
- Tests of thyroid function may yield inaccurate results if you use clioquinol within 1 month before testing.

POSSIBLE INTERACTION WITH OTHER DRUGS

GENERIC NAME OR DRUG CLASS	COMBINED EFFECT
None expected.	

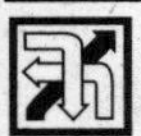

POSSIBLE INTERACTION WITH OTHER SUBSTANCES

INTERACTS WITH	COMBINED EFFECT
Alcohol:	None expected.
Beverages:	None expected.
Cocaine:	None expected.
Foods:	None expected.
Marijuana:	None expected.
Tobacco:	None expected.

ANTIBACTERIALS FOR ACNE (Topical)

BRAND AND GENERIC NAMES

Achromycin
Akne-mycin
A/T/S
Aureomycin
Benzamycin
CHLORTETRACYCLINE (topical)
Cleocin T Gel
Cleocin T Lotion
Cleocin T Topical Solution
Clinda-Derm
CLINDAMYCIN (topical)
Dalacin T Topical Solution
Erycette
EryDerm
Erygel
Erymax
Ery-Sol
ERYTHROMYCIN (topical)
ETS
Meclan
MECLOCYCLINE (topical)
Sans-Acne
Staticin
T-Stat
TETRACYCLINE (topical)
Topicycline

BASIC INFORMATION

Habit forming? No
Prescription needed? Yes
Available as generic? Yes
Drug class: Antibacterial (topical)

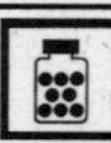

USES

Treats acne by killing skin bacteria that may be part of the cause of acne.

DOSAGE & USAGE INFORMATION

How to use:

- Pledgets and solutions are flammable. Use away from flame or heat.
- Apply medication to entire area, not just to pimples.
- If you use other acne medicines on skin, wait an hour after using erythromycin before applying other medicine.
- Cream, lotion, ointment—Bathe and dry area before use. Apply small amount and rub gently.

Continued next column

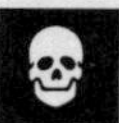

OVERDOSE

SYMPTOMS:
None expected.
WHAT TO DO:
Not for internal use. If child accidentally swallows, call poison control center.

When to use:
2 times a day, morning and evening, or as directed by your doctor.

If you forget a dose:
Use as soon as you remember.

What drug does:
Kills bacteria on skin, skin glands or in hair follicles.

Time lapse before drug works:
3 to 4 weeks to begin improvement.

Don't use with:

- Other skin medicine without telling your doctor.
- See Interaction column and consult doctor.

POSSIBLE ADVERSE REACTIONS OR SIDE EFFECTS

SYMPTOMS	WHAT TO DO
Life-threatening: None expected.	
Common: Stinging or burning of skin for a few minutes after application.	Continue. Tell doctor at next visit.
Infrequent: Red, peeling, itching, irritated skin.	Continue. Call doctor when convenient.
Rare (extremely): Symptoms of excess medicine absorbed by body—Abdominal pain, diarrhea, fever, nausea, vomiting, thirst, weakness, weight loss.	Discontinue. Call doctor right away.

ANTIBACTERIALS FOR ACNE (Topical)

WARNINGS & PRECAUTIONS

Don't use if:
You are allergic to erythromycin.

Before you start, consult your doctor:
- If you are allergic to any substance that touches your skin.
- If you use benzoyl peroxide, resorcinol, salicylic acid, sulfur or tretinoin (vitamin A acid).

Over age 60:
No problems expected.

Pregnancy:
Risk factors vary for drugs in this group. See category list on page xxii and consult doctor.

Breast-feeding:
No problems expected, but check with doctor.

Infants & children:
No problems expected, but check with doctor.

Prolonged use:
Excess irritation to skin.

Skin & sunlight:
No problems expected, but check with doctor.

Driving, piloting or hazardous work:
No problems expected, but check with doctor.

Discontinuing:
No problems expected, but check with doctor.

Others:
- Use water-base cosmetics.
- Keep medicine away from mouth or eyes.
- If accidentally gets into eyes, flush immediately with clear water.
- Keep away from heat or flame.
- Keep cool, but don't freeze.

POSSIBLE INTERACTION WITH OTHER DRUGS

GENERIC NAME OR DRUG CLASS	COMBINED EFFECT
Abrasive or medicated soaps	Irritation or too much drying.
After-shave lotions	Irritation or too much drying.
Anti-acne topical preparations (other)	Irritation or too much drying.
"Cover-up" cosmetics	Irritation or too much drying.
Drying cosmetic soaps	Irritation or too much drying.
Isotretinoin	Irritation or too much drying.
Mercury compounds	May stain skin black and smell bad.
Perfumed toilet water	Irritation or too much drying.
Preparations containing skin peeling agents such as benzoyl peroxide, resorcinol, salicylic acid, sulfur, tretinoin	Irritation or too much drying.

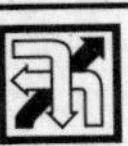

POSSIBLE INTERACTION WITH OTHER SUBSTANCES

INTERACTS WITH	COMBINED EFFECT
Alcohol:	None expected.
Beverages:	None expected.
Cocaine:	None expected.
Foods:	None expected.
Marijuana:	None expected.
Tobacco:	None expected.

ANTICHOLINERGICS

BRAND AND GENERIC NAME

See complete list of brand and generic names in the *Brand Names Directory*, page 894.

BASIC INFORMATION

Habit forming? No
Prescription needed?
Low strength: No
High strength: Yes
Available as generic? Yes
Drug class: Antispasmodic, anticholinergic

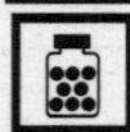

USES

- Reduces spasms of digestive system, bladder and urethra.
- Treatment of bronchial spasms.
- Used as a component in some cough and cold preparations.
- Treatment of peptic ulcers.

DOSAGE & USAGE INFORMATION

How to take:
- Tablet—Swallow with liquid or food to lessen stomach irritation.
- Aerosol—Dilute in saline and inhale as nebulizer.

When to take:
30 minutes before meals (unless directed otherwise by doctor).

If you forget a dose:
Take as soon as you remember up to 2 hours late. If more than 2 hours, wait for next scheduled dose (don't double this dose).

What drug does:
Blocks nerve impulses at parasympathetic nerve endings, preventing muscle contractions and gland secretions of organs involved.

Continued next column

OVERDOSE

SYMPTOMS:
Dilated pupils, rapid pulse and breathing, dizziness, fever, hallucinations, confusion, slurred speech, agitation, flushed face, convulsions, coma.
WHAT TO DO:
- **Dial 911 (emergency) or 0 (operator) for an ambulance or medical help. Then give first aid immediately.**
- **See emergency information on inside covers.**

Time lapse before drug works:
15 to 30 minutes.

Don't take with:
- Antacids* or antidiarrheals*.
- Any other medicine without consulting your doctor or pharmacist.

POSSIBLE ADVERSE REACTIONS OR SIDE EFFECTS

SYMPTOMS	WHAT TO DO
Life-threatening: In case of overdose, see previous column.	
Common:	
• Confusion, delirium, rapid heartbeat.	Discontinue. Call doctor right away.
• Nausea, vomiting, decreased sweating.	Continue. Call doctor when convenient.
• Constipation.	Continue. Tell doctor at next visit.
• Dryness in ears, nose, throat, mouth.	No action necessary.
Infrequent:	
• Headache, difficult or painful urination, nasal congestion, altered taste.	Continue. Call doctor when convenient.
• Lightheadedness.	Discontinue. Call doctor right away.
Rare:	
Rash or hives, eye pain, blurred vision, fever.	Discontinue. Call doctor right away.

WARNINGS & PRECAUTIONS

Don't take if:
- You are allergic to any anticholinergic.
- You have trouble with stomach bloating.
- You have difficulty emptying your bladder completely.
- You have narrow-angle glaucoma.
- You have severe ulcerative colitis.

Before you start, consult your doctor:
- If you have open-angle glaucoma.
- If you have angina or any heart disease or heart rhythm problem.
- If you have chronic bronchitis or asthma.
- If you have liver, kidney or thyroid disease.
- If you have hiatal hernia or esophagitis.
- If you have enlarged prostate or urinary retention.
- If you have myasthenia gravis.
- If you have peptic ulcer.
- If you will have surgery within 2 months, including dental surgery, requiring general or spinal anesthesia.

Over age 60:
Adverse reactions and side effects may be more frequent and severe than in younger persons.

Pregnancy:
Risk factors vary for drugs in this group. See category list on page xxii and consult doctor.

Breast-feeding:
Drug may pass into milk and could affect milk flow. Avoid drug or discontinue nursing until you finish medicine. Consult doctor for advice on maintaining milk supply.

Infants & children:
Use only under medical supervision.

Prolonged use:
Chronic constipation, possible fecal impaction. Consult doctor immediately.

Skin & sunlight:
May increase sensitivity to light.

Driving, piloting or hazardous work:
Use disqualifies you for piloting aircraft. Otherwise, no problems expected.

Discontinuing:
May be unnecessary to finish medicine. Follow doctor's instructions.

Others:
Advise any doctor or dentist whom you consult that you take this medicine.

POSSIBLE INTERACTION WITH OTHER DRUGS

GENERIC NAME OR DRUG CLASS	COMBINED EFFECT
Amantadine	Increased anti-cholinergic effect.
Antacids*	Space doses of the drugs 2 to 3 hours apart.
Anticholinergics, other*	Increased anti-cholinergic effect.
Antidepressants, tricyclic*	Increased anti-cholinergic effect. Increased sedation.
Antihistamines*	Increased anti-cholinergic effect.
Attapulgite	Decreased anti-cholinergic effect.
Cortisone drugs*	Increased internal eye pressure.
Haloperidol	Increased internal eye pressure.
Ketoconazole	Decreased ketoconazole effect.
Methylphenidate	Increased anti-cholinergic effect.
Molindone	Increased anti-cholinergic effect.
Monoamine oxidase (MAO) inhibitors*	Increased anti-cholinergic effect.
Narcotics*	Increased risk of severe constipation.
Orphenadrine	Increased anti-cholinergic effect.
Phenothiazines*	Increased anti-cholinergic effect.
Potassium supplements*	Possible intestinal ulcers with oral potassium tablets.
Quinidine	Increased anti-cholinergic effect.

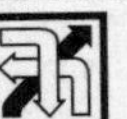

POSSIBLE INTERACTION WITH OTHER SUBSTANCES

INTERACTS WITH	COMBINED EFFECT
Alcohol:	None expected.
Beverages:	None expected.
Cocaine:	Excessively rapid heartbeat. Avoid.
Foods:	None expected.
Marijuana:	Drowsiness and dry mouth.
Tobacco:	None expected.

***See Glossary**

ANTICOAGULANTS (Oral)

BRAND AND GENERIC NAMES

ANISINDIONE
Anthrombin-K
Carfin
Coumadin
DICUMAROL
Miradon
Panwarfin
Sofarin
WARFARIN SODIUM
Warfilone

BASIC INFORMATION

Habit forming? No
Prescription needed? Yes
Available as generic? Yes
Drug class: Anticoagulant

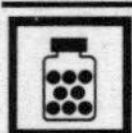

USES

Reduces blood clots. Used for abnormal clotting inside blood vessels.

DOSAGE & USAGE INFORMATION

How to take:
Tablet—Swallow with liquid. If you can't swallow whole, crumble tablet and take with liquid or food.

When to take:
At the same time each day.

If you forget a dose:
Take as soon as you remember up to 12 hours late. If more than 12 hours, wait for next scheduled dose (don't double this dose). Inform your doctor of any missed doses.

What drug does:
Blocks action of vitamin K necessary for blood clotting.

Time lapse before drug works:
36 to 48 hours.

Don't take with:
Any other medicine without consulting your doctor or pharmacist.

OVERDOSE

SYMPTOMS:
Bloody vomit, coughing blood, bloody or black stools, red urine.
WHAT TO DO:

- **Dial 911 (emergency) or 0 (operator) for an ambulance or medical help. Then give first aid immediately.**
- **See emergency information on inside covers.**

POSSIBLE ADVERSE REACTIONS OR SIDE EFFECTS

SYMPTOMS	WHAT TO DO
Life-threatening:	
In case of overdose, see previous column.	
Common:	
Bloating, gas.	Continue. Tell doctor at next visit.
Infrequent:	
• Black stools or bloody vomit, coughing up blood.	Discontinue. Seek emergency treatment.
• Rash, hives, itch, blurred vision, sore throat, easy bruising, bleeding, cloudy or red urine, back pain, jaundice, fever, chills, fatigue, weakness, painful urination, decreased amount of urine, heavy menstruation, bleeding gums.	Discontinue. Call doctor right away.
• Diarrhea, cramps, nausea, vomiting, swollen feet or legs, hair loss.	Continue. Call doctor when convenient.
Rare:	
• Bleeding into and under skin.	Discontinue. Seek emergency treatment.
• Dizziness, headache, mouth sores.	Discontinue. Call doctor right away.

WARNINGS & PRECAUTIONS

Don't take if:

- You have been allergic to any oral anticoagulant.
- You have a bleeding disorder.
- You have an active peptic ulcer.
- You have ulcerative colitis.

Before you start, consult your doctor:

- If you take any other drugs, including nonprescription drugs.
- If you have high blood pressure.
- If you have heavy or prolonged menstrual periods.
- If you have diabetes.
- If you have a bladder catheter.
- If you have serious liver or kidney disease.
- If you will have surgery within 2 months, including dental surgery, requiring general or spinal anesthesia.

Over age 60:
Adverse reactions and side effects may be more frequent and severe than in younger persons.

Pregnancy:
Risk factors vary for drugs in this group. See category list on page xxii and consult doctor.

Breast-feeding:
Drug filters into milk. May harm child. Avoid.

Infants & children:
Use only under doctor's supervision.

Prolonged use:
Talk to your doctor about the need for follow-up medical examinations or laboratory studies to check prothorombin time, stool and urine for blood.

Skin & sunlight:
No problems expected.

Driving, piloting or hazardous work:
- Avoid hazardous activities that could cause injury.
- Don't drive if you feel dizzy or have blurred vision.

Discontinuing:
Don't discontinue without consulting doctor. Dose may require gradual reduction if you have taken drug for a long time. Doses of other drugs may also require adjustment.

Others:
- Carry identification to state that you take anticoagulants.
- Advise any doctor or dentist whom you consult that you take this medicine.

POSSIBLE INTERACTION WITH OTHER DRUGS

GENERIC NAME OR DRUG CLASS	COMBINED EFFECT
Acetaminophen	Increased effect of anticoagulant.
Allopurinol	Increased effect of anticoagulant.
Aminoglutethmide	Decreased effect of anticoagulant.
Amiodarone	Increased effect of anticoagulant.
Androgens*	Increased effect of anticoagulant.
Antacids* (large doses)	Decreased effect of anticoagulant.
Antibiotics*	Increased effect of anticoagulant.
Antidiabetic agents*	Increased effect of anticoagulant.
Antihistamines*	Unpredictable increased or decreased effect of anticoagulant.
Anti-inflammatory drugs, nonsteroidal (NSAIDs)*	Increased risk of bleeding.
Anti-inflammatory drugs, nonsteroidal (ophthalmic)*	May increase bleeding tendency.
Aspirin	Possible spontaneous bleeding.
Barbiturates*	Decreased effect of anticoagulant.
Benzodiazepines*	Unpredictable increased or decreased effect of anticoagulant.
Bismuth subsalicylate	Increased risk of bleeding.
Calcium supplements*	Decreased effect of anticoagulant.
Carbamazepine	Decreased effect of anticoagulant.
Cefixime	Increased effect of anticoagulant.
Chloramphenicol	Increased effect of anticoagulant.
Cholestyramine	Decreased effect of anticoagulant.

Continued on page 923

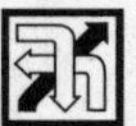

POSSIBLE INTERACTION WITH OTHER SUBSTANCES

INTERACTS WITH	COMBINED EFFECT
Alcohol:	Can increase or decrease effect of anticoagulant. Use with caution.
Beverages:	None expected.
Cocaine:	None expected.
Foods: High in vitamin K such as fish, liver, spinach, cabbage, cauliflower, Brussels sprouts.	May decrease anticoagulant effect.
Marijuana:	None expected.
Tobacco:	Decreased effect of anticoagulant.

***See Glossary**

ANTICONVULSANTS, DIONE

BRAND AND GENERIC NAMES

PARAMETHADIONE	Tridione
Paradione	Tridione-Dulcets
TRIMETHADIONE	

BASIC INFORMATION

Habit forming? No
Prescription needed? Yes
Available as generic? No
Drug class: Anticonvulsant (dione)

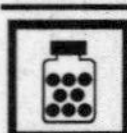

USES

Controls but does not cure petit mal seizures (absence seizures).

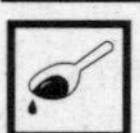

DOSAGE & USAGE INFORMATION

How to take:
Tablets, capsules or liquid: Take with food or milk to lessen stomach irritation.

When to take:
At the same time each day.

If you forget a dose:
Take as soon as you remember up to 2 hours late. If more than 2 hours, wait for next scheduled dose (don't double this dose).

What drug does:
Raises threshold of seizures in cerebral cortex. Does not alter seizure pattern.

Time lapse before drug works:
1 to 3 hours.

Don't take with:
Any other medicine without consulting your doctor or pharmacist.

OVERDOSE

SYMPTOMS:
Bleeding, nausea, drowsiness, ataxia, coma.
WHAT TO DO:

- **Dial 911 (emergency) or 0 (operator) for an ambulance or medical help. Then give first aid immediately.**
- **If patient is unconscious and not breathing, give mouth-to-mouth breathing. If there is no heartbeat, use cardiac massage and mouth-to-mouth breathing (CPR). Don't try to make patient vomit. If you can't get help quickly, take patient to nearest emergency facility.**
- **See emergency information on inside covers.**

POSSIBLE ADVERSE REACTIONS OR SIDE EFFECTS

SYMPTOMS	WHAT TO DO
Life-threatening:	
In case of overdose, see previous column.	
Common:	
Dizziness, drowsiness, headache, rash.	Continue. Call doctor when convenient.
Infrequent:	
Itching, nausea, vomiting, confusion, insomnia, hair loss.	Continue. Call doctor when convenient.
Rare:	
• Changes in vision; sore throat with fever and mouth sores; bleeding gums; easy bleeding or bruising; smoky or bloody urine; jaundice; puffed hands, face, feet or legs; swollen lymph glands; unusual weakness and fatigue.	Continue. Call doctor right away.
• Sensitivity to light.	Continue. Call doctor when convenient.

WARNINGS & PRECAUTIONS

Don't take if:
You are allergic to this drug or any anticonvulsant.

Before you start, consult your doctor:

- If you are pregnant or plan pregnancy.
- If you have blood disease.
- If you have liver or kidney disease.
- If you have disease of optic nerve or eye.
- If you will have surgery within 2 months, including dental surgery, requiring general or spinal anesthesia.

Over age 60:
Adverse reactions and side effects may be more frequent and severe than in younger persons.

Pregnancy:
Risk to unborn child outweighs drug benefits. Don't use. Risk category D (see page xxii).

Breast-feeding:
No problems proven. Avoid if possible. Consult doctor.

Infants & children:
Use only under close medical supervision of doctor experienced in convulsive disorders.

Prolonged use:

- Have regular checkups, especially during early months of treatment.
- Talk to your doctor about the need for follow-up medical examinations or laboratory studies to check complete blood counts (white blood cell count, platelet count, red blood cell count, hemoglobin, hematocrit), liver function, kidney function, eyes, urine.

Skin & sunlight:
Increased sensitivity to sunlight or sun lamp. Avoid overexposure.

Driving, piloting or hazardous work:
Don't drive or pilot aircraft until you learn how medicine affects you. Don't work around dangerous machinery. Don't climb ladders or work in high places. Danger increases if you drink alcohol or take medicine affecting alertness and reflexes, such as antihistamines, tranquilizers, sedatives, pain medicine, narcotics and mind-altering drugs. Be especially careful driving at night because medicine can affect vision.

Discontinuing:
Don't discontinue without consulting doctor. Dose may require gradual reduction if you have taken drug for a long time. Doses of other drugs may also require adjustment.

Others:
Arrange for eye exams every 6 months as well as blood counts and kidney function studies.

POSSIBLE INTERACTION WITH OTHER DRUGS

GENERIC NAME OR DRUG CLASS	COMBINED EFFECT
Any other medicine	Unpredictable effect on seizure prevention.
Amiodarone	Increased or toxic effect of anti-convulsants.
Anticoagulants*	Increased anti-convulsant effect.
Antidepressants, tricyclic*	Greater likelihood of seizures.
Antipsychotic medicines*	Greater likelihood of seizures.
Anticonvulsants* (other)	Increased chance of blood toxicity.
Clozapine	Toxic effect on the central nervous system.
Ethinamate	Dangerous increased effects of ethinamate. Avoid combining.
Fluoxetine	Increased depressant effects of both drugs.
Guanfacine	May increase depressant effects of either drug.
Leucovorin	High alcohol content of leucovorin may cause adverse effects.
Methyprylon	Increased sedative effect, perhaps to dangerous level. Avoid.
Sedatives*, sleeping pills, alcohol, pain medicine, antihistamines*, tranquilizers, narcotics*, mind-altering drugs*.	Extreme drowsiness. Avoid.
Sulfadoxine and pyrimethamine	Increased risk of toxicity.

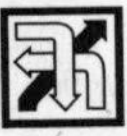

POSSIBLE INTERACTION WITH OTHER SUBSTANCES

INTERACTS WITH	COMBINED EFFECT
Alcohol:	Increased chance of seizures and liver damage. Avoid.
Beverages: Caffeine drinks.	May decrease anti-convulsant effect.
Cocaine:	Increased chance of seizures. Avoid.
Foods:	No problems expected.
Marijuana:	Increased chance of seizures. Avoid.
Tobacco:	Decreased absorption of medicine leading to uneven control of disease.

*See Glossary

ANTICONVULSANTS, HYDANTOIN

BRAND AND GENERIC NAMES

Dilantin	Diphenylhydantoin
Dilantin-30	ETHOTOIN
Dilantin-125	MEPHENYTOIN
Dilantin Infatabs	Mesantoin
Dilantin Kapseals	Peganone
Dilantin-30-Pediatric	Phenytex
Diphenylan	PHENYTOIN

BASIC INFORMATION

Habit forming? No
Prescription needed? Yes
Available as generic? Yes
Drug class: Anticonvulsant (hydantoin)

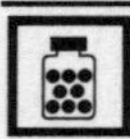

USES

- Prevents some forms of epileptic seizures.
- Stabilizes irregular heartbeat.

DOSAGE & USAGE INFORMATION

How to take:
- Tablet—Swallow with liquid.
- Chewable tablets—Chew well before swallowing.
- Suspension—Shake well before taking with liquid.

When to take:
At the same time each day.

If you forget a dose:
- If drug taken 1 time per day—Take as soon as you remember up to 12 hours late. If more than 12 hours, wait for next scheduled dose (don't double this dose).
- If taken several times per day—Take as soon as possible, then return to regular schedule.

Continued next column

OVERDOSE

SYMPTOMS:
Jerky eye movements; stagger; slurred speech; imbalance; drowsiness; blood pressure drop; slow, shallow breathing; coma.

WHAT TO DO:
- **Dial 911 (emergency) or 0 (operator) for an ambulance or medical help. Then give first aid immediately.**
- **See emergency information on inside covers.**

What drug does:
Promotes sodium loss from nerve fibers. This lessens excitability and inhibits spread of nerve impulses.

Time lapse before drug works:
7 to 10 days continual use.

Don't take with:
Any other medicine without consulting your doctor or pharmacist.

POSSIBLE ADVERSE REACTIONS OR SIDE EFFECTS

SYMPTOMS	WHAT TO DO
Life-threatening:	
Severe allergic reaction (rash, fever, swollen glands, kidney failure).	Seek emergency help.
Common:	
Mild dizziness; drowsiness; nausea; vomiting; constipation; bleeding, swollen or tender gums.	Continue. Call doctor when convenient.
Infrequent:	
• Hallucinations, confusion, slurred speech, stagger, rash, change in vision, agitation.	Continue. Call doctor right away.
• Headache, diarrhea, muscle twitching.	Continue. Call doctor when convenient.
• Increased body and facial hair, breast swelling, insomnia.	Continue. Tell doctor at next visit.
Rare:	
Sore throat, fever, unusual bleeding or bruising, abdominal pain, jaundice.	Continue. Call doctor right away.

WARNINGS & PRECAUTIONS

Don't take if:
You are allergic to any hydantoin anticonvulsant.

Before you start, consult your doctor:
- If you have had impaired liver function or disease.
- If you will have surgery within 2 months, including dental surgery, requiring general or spinal anesthesia.
- If you have diabetes.
- If you have a blood disorder.

Over age 60:
Adverse reactions and side effects may be more frequent and severe than in younger persons.

Pregnancy:
Decide with your doctor if drug benefits justify risk to unborn child. Risk category C (see page xxii).

Breast-feeding:
Drug passes into milk. Avoid drug or discontinue nursing until you finish medicine. Consult doctor for advice on maintaining milk supply.

Infants & children:
Use only under medical supervision.

Prolonged use:
- Weakened bones.
- Lymph gland enlargement.
- Possible liver damage.
- Numbness and tingling of hands and feet.
- Continual back-and-forth eye movements.
- Talk to your doctor about the need for follow-up medical examinations or laboratory studies to check complete blood counts (white blood cell count, platelet count, red blood cell count, hemoglobin, hematocrit), liver function, EEG*.

Skin & sunlight:
May cause rash or intensify sunburn in areas exposed to sun or sunlamp.

Driving, piloting or hazardous work:
Don't drive or pilot aircraft until you learn how medicine affects you. Don't work around dangerous machinery. Don't climb ladders or work in high places. Danger increases if you drink alcohol or take medicine affecting alertness and reflexes.

Discontinuing:
Don't discontinue without consulting doctor. Dose may require gradual reduction if you have taken drug for a long time. Doses of other drugs may also require adjustment.

Others:
May cause learning disability.

POSSIBLE INTERACTION WITH OTHER DRUGS

GENERIC NAME OR DRUG CLASS	COMBINED EFFECT
Amiodarone	Increased anti-convulsant effect.
Antacids*	Decreased anti-convulsant effect.
Anticoagulants*	Increased effect of both drugs.
Antidepressants, tricyclic*	May need to adjust anticonvulsant dose.
Barbiturates*	Changed seizure pattern.
Calcium	Decreased effects of both drugs.
Carbamazepine	Possible increased anticonvulsant metabolism.
Carbonic anhydrase inhibitors*	Increased chance of bone disease.
Central nervous system (CNS) depressants*	Oversedation.
Chloramphenicol	Increased anti-convulsant effect.
Cimetidine	Increased anti-convulsant toxicity.
Contraceptives, oral*	Increased seizures.
Cortisone drugs*	Decreased cortisone effect.
Cyclosporine	May decrease cyclosporine effect.
Digitalis preparations*	Decreased digitalis effect.
Disopyramide	Decreased disopyramide effect.
Disulfiram	Increased anti-convulsant effect.
Estrogens*	Increased estrogen effect.
Felbamate	Increased side effects and adverse reactions.
Fluconazole	Increased anti-convulsant effect.

Continued on page 924

POSSIBLE INTERACTION WITH OTHER SUBSTANCES

INTERACTS WITH	COMBINED EFFECT
Alcohol:	Possible decreased anticonvulsant effect. Use with caution.
Beverages:	None expected.
Cocaine:	Possible seizures.
Foods:	None expected.
Marijuana:	Drowsiness, unsteadiness, decreased anticonvulsant effect.
Tobacco:	None expected.

*See Glossary

ANTICONVULSANTS, SUCCINIMIDE

BRAND AND GENERIC NAMES

Celontin	Milontin
ETHOSUXIMIDE	PHENSUXIMIDE
METHSUXIMIDE	Zarontin

BASIC INFORMATION

Habit forming? No
Prescription needed? Yes
Available as generic? Yes, for some
Drug class: Anticonvulsant (succinimide)

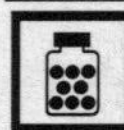

USES

Controls seizures in treatment of some forms of epilepsy.

DOSAGE & USAGE INFORMATION

How to take:
Capsule or syrup—Swallow with liquid or food to lessen stomach irritation.

When to take:
Every day in regularly spaced doses, according to prescription.

If you forget a dose:
Take as soon as you remember up to 2 hours late. If more than 2 hours, wait for next scheduled dose (don't double this dose).

What drug does:
Depresses nerve transmissions in part of brain that controls muscles.

Continued next column

OVERDOSE

SYMPTOMS:
Severe drowsiness, slow or irregular breathing, coma.
WHAT TO DO:
- **Dial 911 (emergency) or 0 (operator) for an ambulance or medical help. Then give first aid immediately.**
- **If patient is unconscious and not breathing, give mouth-to-mouth breathing. If there is no heartbeat, use cardiac massage and mouth-to-mouth breathing (CPR). Don't try to make patient vomit. If you can't get help quickly, take patient to nearest emergency facility.**
- **See emergency information on inside covers.**

Time lapse before drug works:
3 hours.

Don't take with:
Any other medicine without consulting your doctor or pharmacist.

POSSIBLE ADVERSE REACTIONS OR SIDE EFFECTS

SYMPTOMS	WHAT TO DO
Life-threatening:	
In case of overdose, see previous column.	
Common:	
• Nausea, vomiting, appetite loss, dizziness, drowsiness, hiccups, abdominal pain.	Continue. Call doctor when convenient.
• Change in urine color (pink, red, red-brown).	No action necessary.
Infrequent:	
Headache, irritability, mood change, tiredness, increased sex drive.	Continue. Call doctor when convenient.
Rare:	
Sore throat, fever, rash, unusual bleeding or bruising, eye or gum swelling, vaginal bleeding, depression, confusion, swollen lymph glands.	Continue. Call doctor right away.

WARNINGS & PRECAUTIONS

Don't take if:
You are allergic to any succinimide anticonvulsant.

Before you start, consult your doctor:
- If you plan to become pregnant within medication period.
- If you take other anticonvulsants.
- If you have blood disease.
- If you have kidney or liver disease.

Over age 60:
Adverse reactions and side effects may be more frequent and severe than in younger persons.

Pregnancy:
Risk factors vary for drugs in this group. See category list on page xxii and consult doctor.

Breast-feeding:
Drug passes into milk. Avoid drug or discontinue nursing. Consult your doctor about maintaining milk supply.

Infants & children:
Use only under medical supervision.

Prolonged use:
Talk to your doctor about the need for follow-up medical examinations or laboratory studies to check complete blood counts (white blood cell count, platelet count, red blood cell count, hemoglobin, hematocrit), liver function, kidney function, urine.

Skin & sunlight:
No problems expected.

Driving, piloting or hazardous work:
Don't drive or pilot aircraft until you learn how medicine affects you. Don't work around dangerous machinery. Don't climb ladders or work in high places. Danger increases if you drink alcohol or take medicine affecting alertness and reflexes, such as antihistamines, tranquilizers, sedatives, pain medicine, narcotics and mind-altering drugs.

Discontinuing:
Don't discontinue without doctor's advice until you complete prescribed dose, even though symptoms diminish or disappear.

Others:
- Your response to medicine should be checked regularly by your doctor. Dose and schedule may have to be altered frequently to fit individual needs.
- Periodic blood cell counts, kidney and liver function studies recommended.
- May discolor urine pink to red-brown. No action necessary.

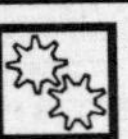

POSSIBLE INTERACTION WITH OTHER DRUGS

GENERIC NAME OR DRUG CLASS	COMBINED EFFECT
Anticonvulsants, other*	Increased effect of both drugs.
Antidepressants, tricyclic*	May provoke seizures.
Antipsychotics*	May provoke seizures.
Central nervous system (CNS) depressants*	Decreased anti-convulsant effect.
Haloperidol	Decreased haloperidol effect; changed seizure pattern.
Phenytoin	Increased phenytoin effect.

POSSIBLE INTERACTION WITH OTHER SUBSTANCES

INTERACTS WITH	COMBINED EFFECT
Alcohol:	May provoke seizures.
Beverages:	None expected.
Cocaine:	May provoke seizures.
Foods:	None expected.
Marijuana:	May provoke seizures.
Tobacco:	None expected.

*See Glossary

ANTIDEPRESSANTS, TRICYCLIC

BRAND AND GENERIC NAMES

See complete list of brand and generic names in the *Brand Name Directory*, page 895.

BASIC INFORMATION

Habit forming? No
Prescription needed? Yes
Available as generic? Yes
Drug class: Antidepressant (tricyclic)

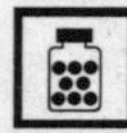

USES

- Gradually relieves, but doesn't cure, symptoms of depression.
- Used to decrease bedwetting.
- Pain relief (sometimes).
- Clomipramine is used to treat obsessive-compulsive disorder.
- Protriptyline may be used to treat attention-deficit disorder.
- Treatment for narcolepsy, ulcers, bulimia, panic attacks, cocaine withdrawal, attention deficit disorder.

DOSAGE & USAGE INFORMATION

How to take:
Tablet, capsule or syrup—Swallow with liquid.

When to take:
At the same time each day, usually at bedtime.

Continued next column

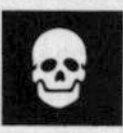

OVERDOSE

SYMPTOMS:
Hallucinations, drowsiness, enlarged pupils, respiratory failure, fever, cardiac arrhythmias, convulsions, coma.
WHAT TO DO:

- **Dial 911 (emergency) or 0 (operator) for an ambulance or medical help. Then give first aid immediately.**
- **If patient is unconscious and not breathing, give mouth-to-mouth breathing. If there is no heartbeat, use cardiac massage and mouth-to-mouth breathing (CPR). Don't try to make patient vomit. If you can't get help quickly, take patient to nearest emergency facility.**
- **See emergency information on inside covers.**

If you forget a dose:
Bedtime dose—If you forget your once-a-day bedtime dose, don't take it more than 3 hours late. If more than 3 hours, wait for next scheduled dose. Don't double this dose.

What drug does:
Probably affects part of brain that controls messages between nerve cells.

Time lapse before drug works:
Begins in 1 to 2 weeks. May require 4 to 6 weeks for maximum benefit.

Don't take with:
Any prescription or nonprescription drugs without consulting your doctor.

POSSIBLE ADVERSE REACTIONS OR SIDE EFFECTS

SYMPTOMS	WHAT TO DO
Life-threatening: In case of overdose, see previous column.	
Common:	
• Tremor.	Discontinue. Call doctor right away.
• Headache, dry mouth or unpleasant taste, constipation or diarrhea, nausea, indigestion, fatigue, weakness, drowsiness, nervousness, anxiety, excessive sweating.	Continue. Call doctor when convenient.
• Insomnia, "sweet tooth."	Continue. Tell doctor at next visit.
Infrequent:	
• Convulsions.	Discontinue. Seek emergency treatment.
• Hallucinations, shakiness, dizziness, fainting, blurred vision, eye pain, vomiting, irregular heartbeat or slow pulse, inflamed tongue, abdominal pain, jaundice, hair loss, rash, fever, chills, joint pain, palpitations, hiccups, visual changes.	Discontinue. Call doctor right away.
• Difficult or frequent urination; decreased sex drive; muscle aches; abnormal dreams; nasal congestion; weakness and faintness when arising from bed or chair; back pain.	Continue. Call doctor when convenient.

Rare:

Itchy skin; sore throat; involuntary movements of jaw, lips and tongue; nightmares; confusion; swollen breasts; swollen testicles.	Discontinue. Call doctor right away.

WARNINGS & PRECAUTIONS

Don't take if:
- You are allergic to any tricyclic antidepressant.
- You drink alcohol.
- You have had a heart attack within 6 weeks.
- You have glaucoma.
- You have taken MAO inhibitors within 2 weeks.
- Patient is younger than 12.

Before you start, consult your doctor:
- If you will have surgery within 2 months, including dental surgery, requiring general or spinal anesthesia.
- If you have an enlarged prostate.
- If you have heart disease or high blood pressure.
- If you have stomach or intestinal problems.
- If you have an overactive thyroid.
- If you have asthma.
- If you have liver disease.

Over age 60:
More likely to develop urination difficulty and side effects such as seizures, hallucinations, shaking, dizziness, fainting, headache, insomnia.

Pregnancy:
Risk factors vary for drugs in this group. See category list on page xxii and consult doctor.

Breast-feeding:
Drug may pass into milk. Avoid drug or discontinue nursing until you finish medicine. Consult doctor about maintaining milk supply.

Infants & children:
Don't give to children younger than 12 except under medical supervision.

Prolonged use:
Talk to your doctor about the need for follow-up medical examinations or laboratory studies to check complete blood counts (white blood cell count, platelet count, red blood cell count, hemoglobin, hematocrit), blood pressure, eyes, teeth.

Skin & sunlight:
May cause rash or intensify sunburn in areas exposed to sun or sunlamp.

Driving, piloting or hazardous work:
Don't drive or pilot aircraft until you learn how medicine affects you. Don't work around dangerous machinery. Don't climb ladders or work in high places. Danger increases if you drink alcohol or take medicine affecting alertness and reflexes.

Discontinuing:
- Don't discontinue without consulting doctor. Dose may require gradual reduction if you have taken drug for a long time. Doses of other drugs may also require adjustment.
- Withdrawal symptoms such as convulsions, muscle cramps, nightmares, insomnia, abdominal pain. Call your physician right away if any of these occur.

Others:
May affect results in some medical tests.

POSSIBLE INTERACTION WITH OTHER DRUGS

GENERIC NAME OR DRUG CLASS	COMBINED EFFECT
Anticoagulants*, oral	Possible increased anticoagulant effect.
Anticholinergics*	Increased anti-cholinergic effect.

Continued on page 925

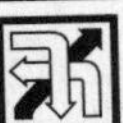

POSSIBLE INTERACTION WITH OTHER SUBSTANCES

INTERACTS WITH	COMBINED EFFECT
Alcohol: Beverages or medicines with alcohol.	Excessive intoxication. Avoid.
Beverages:	None expected.
Cocaine:	Increased risk of heartbeat irregularity.
Foods: Breads, crackers, cookies, cheeses, peanut butter, corn, lentils, cranberries, plums, prunes, peanuts, Brazil nuts, walnuts, pastas, bacon, meat, fowl, eggs, fish (if taken with).	Decreased effectiveness of the antidepressant.
Marijuana:	Excessive drowsiness. Avoid.
Tobacco:	Possible decreased tricyclic anti-depressant effect.

*See Glossary

ANTIDIABETIC AGENTS

BRAND AND GENERIC NAMES

See complete list of brand and generic names in the *Brand Names Directory*, page 895.

BASIC INFORMATION

Habit forming? No
Prescription needed? Yes
Available as generic? Yes, for some.
Drug class: Antidiabetic (oral), sulfonurea

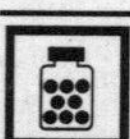

USES

- Treatment for diabetes in adults who can't control blood sugar by diet, weight loss and exercise.
- Treatment for diabetes insipidus.

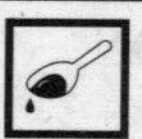

DOSAGE & USAGE INFORMATION

How to take:
- Tablet—Swallow with liquid or food to lessen stomach irritation. If you can't swallow whole, crumble tablet and take with liquid or food.
- Extended-release tablet—Swallow whole with liquid. Do not crush or chew tablet.

When to take:
At the same times each day.

If you forget a dose:
Take as soon as you remember up to 2 hours late. If more than 2 hours, wait for next scheduled dose (don't double this dose).

What drug does:
Stimulates pancreas to produce more insulin. Insulin in blood forces cells to use sugar in blood.

Time lapse before drug works:
3 to 4 hours. May require 2 weeks for maximum benefit.

Don't take with:
Any other medicine without consulting your doctor or pharmacist.

OVERDOSE

SYMPTOMS:
Excessive hunger, nausea, anxiety, cool skin, cold sweats, drowsiness, rapid heartbeat, weakness, unconsciousness, coma.
WHAT TO DO:
- **Dial 911 (emergency) or 0 (operator) for an ambulance or medical help. Then give first aid immediately.**
- **See emergency information on inside covers.**

POSSIBLE ADVERSE REACTIONS OR SIDE EFFECTS

SYMPTOMS	WHAT TO DO
Life-threatening: In case of overdose, see previous column.	
Common:	
• Dizziness.	Discontinue. Call doctor right away.
• Diarrhea, appetite loss, nausea, stomach pain, heartburn, constipation.	Continue. Call doctor when convenient.
Infrequent:	
• Low blood sugar (hunger, anxiety, cold sweats, rapid pulse), shortness of breath.	Discontinue. Seek emergency treatment.
• Headache.	Discontinue. Call doctor right away.
Rare:	
Fatigue, itchy skin or rash, sore throat, fever, ringing in ears, unusual bleeding or bruising, jaundice, edema, weakness, confusion.	Discontinue. Call doctor right away.

WARNINGS & PRECAUTIONS

Don't take if:
- You are allergic to any sulfonurea.
- You have impaired kidney or liver function.

Before you start, consult your doctor:
- If you have a severe infection.
- If you have thyroid disease.
- If you take insulin.
- If you have heart disease.

Over age 60:
Dose usually smaller than for younger adults. Avoid episodes of low blood sugar because repeated ones can damage brain permanently.

Pregnancy:
Discuss any use of these drugs with your doctor. Risk factors vary for drugs in this group. See category list on page xxii and consult doctor.

Breast-feeding:
Drug filters into milk. May lower baby's blood sugar. Avoid.

Infants & children:
Don't give to infants or children.

Prolonged use:
- Adverse effects more likely.

- Talk to your doctor about the need for follow-up medical examinations or laboratory studies to check blood sugar, complete blood counts (white blood cell count, platelet count, redblood cell count, hemoglobin, hematocrit), eyes.

Skin and sunlight:
Increased sensitivity to sunlight.

Driving, piloting or hazardous work:
No problems expected unless you develop hypoglycemia (low blood sugar). If so, avoid driving or hazardous activity.

Discontinuing:
Don't discontinue without consulting doctor. Dose may require gradual reduction if you have taken drug for a long time. Doses of other drugs may also require adjustment.

Others:
- Don't exceed recommended dose. Hypoglycemia (low blood sugar) may occur, even with proper dose schedule. You must balance medicine, diet and exercise.
- May affect results in some medical tests.
- Advise any doctor or dentist whom you consult that you take this medicine.
- Warning: A large study has shown that there is an increase in death rate from heart disease among those who take oral diabetic agents.

POSSIBLE INTERACTION WITH OTHER DRUGS

GENERIC NAME OR DRUG CLASS	COMBINED EFFECT
Androgens*	Increased blood sugar lowering.
Anticoagulants*	Unpredictable prothrombin times.
Anticonvulsants, hydantoin*	Decreased blood sugar lowering.
Anti-inflammatory nonsteriodal drugs (NSAIDs)*	Increased blood-sugar lowering.
Aspirin	Increased blood sugar lowering.
Beta-adrenergic blocking agents*	Increased blood sugar lowering. Possible increased difficulty in regulating blood sugar levels.
Bismuth subsalicylate	Increased insulin effect. May require dosage adjustment.
Chloramphenicol	Increased blood sugar lowering.
Cimetidine	Increased blood sugar lowering.
Clofibrate	Increased blood sugar lowering.
Contraceptives, oral*	Decreased blood sugar lowering.
Cortisone drugs*	Decreased blood sugar lowering.
Dapsone	Increased risk of adverse effect on blood cells.
Desmopressin	May increase desmopressin effect.
Dextrothyroxine	Antidiabetic may require adjustment.
Digoxin	Possible decreased digoxin effect.
Diuretics* (loop, thiazide)	Decreased blood sugar lowering.
Epinephrine	Increased blood sugar lowering.
Estrogens*	Increased blood sugar lowering.
Fluconazole	Greater than expected drop in blood sugar. If any oral antidiabetic drug is taken with fluconazole, blood sugars must be monitored carefully.
Guanethidine	Unpredictable blood sugar lowering effect.
Hemolytics*	Increased risk of adverse effect on blood cells.

Continued on page 926

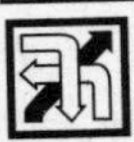

POSSIBLE INTERACTION WITH OTHER SUBSTANCES

INTERACTS WITH	COMBINED EFFECT
Alcohol:	Disulfiram reaction.* Avoid.
Beverages:	None expected.
Cocaine:	No proven problems.
Foods:	None expected.
Marijuana:	Decreased blood sugar lowering. Avoid.
Tobacco:	None expected.

*See Glossary

ANTIDYSKINETICS

BRAND AND GENERIC NAMES

See complete list of brand and generic names in the *Brand Names Directory*, page 895.

BASIC INFORMATION

Habit forming? No
Prescription needed? Yes
Available as generic? Yes
Drug class: Antidyskinetic, antiparkinsonism

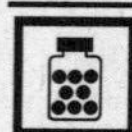

USES

- Treatment of Parkinson's disease.
- Treatment of adverse effects of certain central nervous system drugs.
- Treatment for Tourette's syndrome

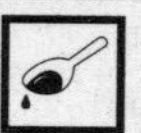

DOSAGE & USAGE INFORMATION

How to take:
- Tablets—Swallow with liquid. If you can't swallow whole, crumble tablet and take with liquid or food to lessen stomach irritation.
- Extended-release capsule or elixir—Take with food to lessen stomach irritation.

When to take:
At the same times each day.

If you forget a dose:
Take as soon as you remember up to 2 hours late. If more than 2 hours, wait for next scheduled dose (don't double this dose).

Continued next column

OVERDOSE

SYMPTOMS:
Agitation, dilated pupils, hallucinations, dry mouth, rapid heartbeat, sleepiness.
WHAT TO DO:
- **Dial 911 (emergency) or 0 (operator) for an ambulance or medical help. Then give first aid immediately.**
- **If patient is unconscious and not breathing, give mouth-to-mouth breathing. If there is no heartbeat, use cardiac massage and mouth-to-mouth breathing (CPR). Don't try to make patient vomit. If you can't get help quickly, take patient to nearest emergency facility.**
- **See emergency information on inside covers.**

What drug does:
- Balances chemical reactions necessary to send nerve impulses within base of brain.
- Improves muscle control and reduces stiffness.

Time lapse before drug works:
1 to 2 hours. Full effect may take 2 to 3 days.

Don't take with:
- Nonprescription drugs for colds, cough or allergy.
- See Interaction column and consult doctor.

POSSIBLE ADVERSE REACTIONS OR SIDE EFFECTS

SYMPTOMS	WHAT TO DO
Life-threatening:	
In case of overdose, see previous column.	
Common:	
• Blurred vision, light sensitivity, constipation, nausea, vomiting.	Continue. Call doctor when convenient.
• Painful or difficult urination, dry mouth.	Continue. Tell doctor at next visit.
Infrequent:	
Headache, memory loss, abdominal pain, nervousness, impotence.	Continue. Call doctor when convenient.
Rare:	
• Rash, eye pain, delusions, hallucinations, amnesia, paranoia, fever, swollen neck glands, weakness and faintness when arising from bed or chair.	Continue. Call hives, doctor right away.
• Confusion, dizziness, sore mouth or tongue, muscle cramps, numbness or tingling in hands or feet.	Continue. Call doctor when convenient.

Note: Most symptoms representing side effects either disappear or decrease when dose is reduced.

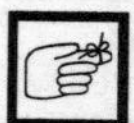

WARNINGS & PRECAUTIONS

Don't take if:
You are allergic to any antidyskinetic.

Before you start, consult your doctor:
- If you have had glaucoma.
- If you have had high blood pressure or heart disease.
- If you have had impaired liver function.
- If you have had kidney disease or urination difficulty.
- If you have had myasthenia gravis.

Over age 60:
More sensitive to drug. Aggravates symptoms of enlarged prostate. Causes impaired thinking, hallucinations, nightmares. Consult doctor about any of these.

Pregnancy:
Decide with your doctor whether drug benefits justify risk to unborn child. Risk category C (see page xxii).

Breast-feeding:
Effects unknown. May inhibit lactation. Consult doctor.

Infants & children:
Not recommended for children 3 and younger. Use for older children only under doctor's supervision.

Prolonged use:
- Possible glaucoma.
- Talk to your doctor about the need for follow-up medical examinations or laboratory studies to check eye pressure.

Skin & sunlight:
May increase sensitivity to sunlight.

Driving, piloting or hazardous work:
Don't drive or pilot aircraft until you learn how medicine affects you. Don't work around dangerous machinery. Don't climb ladders or work in high places. Danger increases if you drink alcohol or take medicine affecting alertness and reflexes, such as antihistamines, tranquilizers, sedatives, pain medicine, narcotics and mind-altering drugs.

Discontinuing:
Don't discontinue without consulting doctor. Dose may require gradual reduction if you have taken drug for a long time. Doses of other drugs may also require adjustment.

Others:
- Internal eye pressure should be measured regularly.
- Avoid becoming overheated.
- Advise any doctor or dentist whom you consult that you take this medicine.

POSSIBLE INTERACTION WITH OTHER DRUGS

GENERIC NAME OR DRUG CLASS	COMBINED EFFECT
Amantadine	Increased amantadine effect.
Antacids*	Possible decreased absorption.
Anticholinergics, others*	Increased anti-cholinergic effect.
Antidepressants, tricyclic*	Increased anti-dyskinetic effect. May cause glaucoma.
Antihistamines*	Increased antidyskinetic effect.
Clozapine	Toxic effect on the central nervous system (except amantadine).
Digoxin	Possible increased toxicity of digoxin.
Disopyramide	Increased anticholinergic effect.
Haloperidol	Possible behavior changes.
Levodopa	Possible increased levodopa effect.
Meperidine	Increased antidyskinetic effect.
Monoamine oxidase (MAO) inhibitors*	Increased antidyskinetic effect.
Nabilone	Greater depression of central nervous system.
Phenothiazines*	Behavior changes.
Primidone	Excessive sedation.
Quinidine	Increased antidyskinetic effect.
Sertraline	Increased depressive effects of both drugs.
Slow-K (extended-release potassium)	Increased risk of gastric irritation.
Tranquilizers*	Excessive sedation.

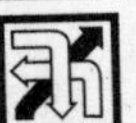

POSSIBLE INTERACTION WITH OTHER SUBSTANCES

INTERACTS WITH	COMBINED EFFECT
Alcohol:	Oversedation. Don't use.
Beverages:	None expected.
Cocaine:	Decreased anti-dyskinetic effect. Avoid.
Foods:	None expected.
Marijuana:	None expected.
Tobacco:	None expected.

*See Glossary

ANTIFIBRINOLYTIC AGENTS

BRAND AND GENERIC NAMES

Amicar
AMINOCAPROIC ACID
Cyclokapron
TRANEXAMIC ACID

BASIC INFORMATION

Habit forming? No
Prescription needed? Yes
Available as generic? Yes
Drug class: Antifibrinolytic, antihemorrhagic

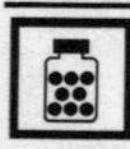

USES

- Treats serious bleeding, especially occurring after surgery, dental or otherwise.
- Sometimes used before surgery in hopes of preventing excessive bleeding in patients with disorders that increase the chance of serious bleeding.

DOSAGE & USAGE INFORMATION

How to take:
- Tablet—Swallow with liquid or food to lessen stomach irritation. If you can't swallow whole, crumble tablet and take with liquid or food.
- Syrup—Take as directed on label.

When to take:
As directed by your doctor.

If you forget a dose:
Take as soon as you remember. Don't double this dose.

What drug does:
Inhibits activation of plasminogen to cause blood clots to disintegrate.

Time lapse before drug works:
Within 2 hours.

Don't take with:
- Thrombolytic chemicals such as streptokinase, urokinase.
- Any other medicine without consulting your doctor or pharmacist.

OVERDOSE

SYMPTOMS:
None expected for oral forms. Injectable forms may cause drop in blood pressure or slow heartbeat.
WHAT TO DO:
Follow doctor's instructions.

POSSIBLE ADVERSE REACTIONS OR SIDE EFFECTS

SYMPTOMS	WHAT TO DO
Life-threatening: Shortness of breath, slurred speech, leg or arm numbness.	Seek emergency treatment.
Common: Diarrhea, nausea, vomiting, severe menstrual cramps.	Continue. Call doctor when convenient.
Infrequent: Dizziness; headache; muscular pain and weakness; red eyes; ringing in ears; skin rash; abdominal pain; stuffy nose; decreased urine; swelling of feet, face, legs; rapid weight gain.	Continue. Call doctor when convenient.
Rare:	
• Unusual tiredness, blurred vision, clotting of menstrual flow.	Continue. Call doctor when convenient.
• Signs of thrombosis (sudden, severe headache; pains in chest, groin or legs; loss of coordination; shortness of breath; slurred speech; vision changes; weakness or numbness in arms or leg).	Seek emergency treatment.

WARNINGS & PRECAUTIONS

Don't take if:
- You are allergic to aminocaproic acid or tranexamic acid.
- You have a diagnosis of disseminated intravascular coagulation (DIC).

Before you start, consult your doctor:
- If you have heart disease.
- If you have bleeding from the kidney.
- If you have had impaired liver function.
- If you have had kidney disease or urination difficulty.
- If you have blood clots in parts of the body.

Over age 60:
No changes from other age groups expected.

Pregnancy:
Risk factors vary for drugs in this group. See category list on page xxii and consult doctor.

Breast-feeding:
No problems documented. Consult doctor.

Infants & children:
Use for children only under doctor's supervision.

Prolonged use:
Talk to your doctor about the need for follow-up medical examinations or laboratory studies to check eyes.

Skin & sunlight:
No problems expected.

Driving, piloting or hazardous work:
Don't drive or pilot aircraft until you learn how medicine affects you. Don't work around dangerous machinery. Don't climb ladders or work in high places. Danger increases if you drink alcohol or take medicine affecting alertness and reflexes, such as antihistamines, tranquilizers, sedatives, pain medicine, narcotics and mind-altering drugs.

Discontinuing:
Don't discontinue without consulting doctor. Dose may require gradual reduction if you have taken drug for a long time. Doses of other drugs may also require adjustment.

Others:
- Should not be used in patients with disseminated intravascular coagulation.
- Have eyes checked frequently.

POSSIBLE INTERACTION WITH OTHER DRUGS

GENERIC NAME OR DRUG CLASS	COMBINED EFFECT
Contraceptives, oral*	Increased possibility of blood clotting.
Estrogens*	Increased possibility of blood clotting.
Thrombolytic agents* (alteplase, streptokinase, urokinase)	Decreased effects of both drugs.

POSSIBLE INTERACTION WITH OTHER SUBSTANCES

INTERACTS WITH	COMBINED EFFECT
Alcohol:	Decreases effectiveness. Avoid.
Beverages:	No problems expected.
Cocaine:	Combined effect unknown. Avoid.
Foods:	No problems expected.
Marijuana:	Combined effect unknown. Avoid.
Tobacco:	Combined effect unknown. Avoid.

*See Glossary

ANTIFUNGALS (Topical)

BRAND AND GENERIC NAMES

See complete list of brand and generic names in the *Brand Name Directory*, page 895.

BASIC INFORMATION

Habit forming? No
Prescription needed? Yes, for some
Available as generic? Yes, for some
Drug class: Antifungal (topical)

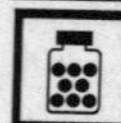

USES

Fights fungus infections such as ringworm of the scalp, athlete's foot, jockey itch, "sun fungus," nail fungus and others.

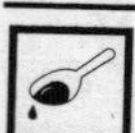

DOSAGE & USAGE INFORMATION

How to use:

- Cream, lotion, ointment, gel—Bathe and dry area before use. Apply small amount and rub gently.
- Powder—Apply lightly to skin.
- Shampoo—Follow package instructions.
- Don't bandage or cover treated areas with plastic wrap.
- Follow other instructions from manufacturer listed on label.

When to use:
Twice a day, morning and evening, unless otherwise directed by your doctor.

If you forget a dose:
Use as soon as you remember.

What drug does:
Kills fungi by damaging the fungal cell wall.

Time lapse before drug works:
May require 6 to 8 weeks for cure.

Don't use with:
Other skin medicines without telling your doctor.

OVERDOSE

SYMPTOMS:
None expected.
WHAT TO DO:

- **Not for internal use. If child accidentally swallows, call poison control center.**
- **Dial 911 (emergency) or 0 (operator) for an ambulance or medical help. Then give first aid immediately.**
- **See emergency information on inside covers.**

POSSIBLE ADVERSE REACTIONS OR SIDE EFFECTS

SYMPTOMS	WHAT TO DO
Life-threatening: None expected.	
Common: None expected.	
Infrequent: Itching, redness, swelling of treated skin not present before treatment.	Discontinue. Call doctor right away.
Rare: None expected.	

WARNINGS & PRECAUTIONS

Don't use if:
You are allergic to any topical antifungal medicine listed.

Before you start, consult your doctor:
If you are allergic to anything that touches your skin.

Over age 60:
No problems expected.

Pregnancy:
Risk factors vary for drugs in this group. See category list on page xxii and consult doctor.

Breast-feeding:
No problems expected, but check with doctor.

Infants & children:
No problems expected, but check with doctor.

Prolonged use:
No problems expected, but check with doctor.

Skin & sunlight:
No problems expected, but check with doctor.

Driving, piloting or hazardous work:
No problems expected, but check with doctor.

Discontinuing:
No problems expected, but check with doctor.

Others:
- Avoid contact with eyes.
- Heat and moisture in bathroom medicine cabinet can cause breakdown of medicine. Store someplace else.
- Keep cool, but don't freeze.
- Store away from heat or sunlight.
- Don't use on other members of the family without consulting your doctor.
- If using for jock itch, avoid wearing tight underwear.
- If using for athlete's foot, dry feet carefully after bathing, wear clean cotton socks with sandals or well-ventilated shoes.

POSSIBLE INTERACTION WITH OTHER DRUGS

GENERIC NAME OR DRUG CLASS	COMBINED EFFECT
None expected.	

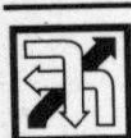

POSSIBLE INTERACTION WITH OTHER SUBSTANCES

INTERACTS WITH	COMBINED EFFECT
Alcohol:	None expected.
Beverages:	None expected.
Cocaine:	None expected.
Foods:	None expected.
Marijuana:	None expected.
Tobacco:	None expected.

ANTIFUNGALS (Vaginal)

BRAND AND GENERIC NAMES

See complete list of brand and generic names in the *Brand Name Directory*, page 896.

BASIC INFORMATION

Habit forming? No
Prescription needed? Yes, for some
Available as generic? Yes, some
Drug class: Antifungal (vaginal)

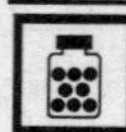

USES

Treats fungus infections of the vagina.

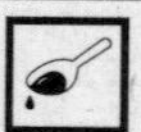

DOSAGE & USAGE INFORMATION

How to use:

- Vaginal creams—Insert into vagina with applicator as illustrated in patient instructions that comes with prescription.
- Vaginal tablets—Insert with applicator as illustrated in instructions.
- Vaginal suppositories—Insert as illustrated in instructions.

When to use:
According to instructions. Usually once or twice daily.

If you forget a dose:
Use as soon as you remember.

What drug does:
Destroys fungus cells membrane causing loss of essential elements to sustain fungus cell life.

Time lapse before drug works:
Begins immediately. May require 2 weeks of treatment to cure vaginal fungus infections. Recurrence common.

Don't use with:
Other vaginal preparations or douches unless otherwise instructed by your doctor.

OVERDOSE

SYMPTOMS:
None expected.
WHAT TO DO:
Overdose unlikely to threaten life.

POSSIBLE ADVERSE REACTIONS OR SIDE EFFECTS

SYMPTOMS	WHAT TO DO
Life-threatening: None expected.	
Common: None expected.	
Infrequent: Vaginal burning, itching, irriation, swelling of labia, redness, increased discharge (not present before starting medicine).	Discontinue. Call doctor right away.
Rare: Skin rash, hives, irritation of sex partner's penis.	Discontinue. Call doctor right away.

WARNINGS & PRECAUTIONS

Don't use if:
- You are allergic to any of the products listed.
- You have pre-existing liver disease.

Before you start, consult your doctor:
If you are pregnant.

Over age 60:
No problems expected.

Pregnancy:
Risk factors vary for drugs in this group. See category list on page xxii and consult doctor.

Breast-feeding:
No problems expected. Consult doctor.

Infants & children:
Use only under close medical supervision.

Prolonged use:
No problems expected.

Skin & sunlight:
No problems expected.

Driving, piloting or hazardous work:
No problems expected.

Discontinuing:
Recurrence likely if you stop before time suggested.

Others:
- Gentian Violet and some of the other products can stain clothing. Sanitary napkins may protect against staining.
- Keep the genital area clean. Use plain unscented soap.
- Take showers rather than tub baths.
- Wear cotton underpants or pantyhose with a cotton crotch. Avoid underpants made from non-ventilating materials. Wear freshly laundered underpants.
- Don't sit around in wet clothing—especially a wet bathing suit.
- If you will take antibiotics in the future, ask your doctor about eating yogurt, sour cream, buttermilk or taking acidophilus tablets.
- After urination or bowel movements, cleanse by wiping or washing from front to back (vagina to anus).
- Don't douche unless your doctor recommends it.
- If urinating causes burning, urinate through a tubular device, such as a toilet-paper roll or plastic cup with the end cut out.

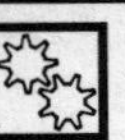

POSSIBLE INTERACTION WITH OTHER DRUGS

GENERIC NAME OR DRUG CLASS	COMBINED EFFECT

Clinically significant interactions with oral or injected medicines unlikely.

POSSIBLE INTERACTION WITH OTHER SUBSTANCES

INTERACTS WITH	COMBINED EFFECT
Alcohol:	None expected.
Beverages:	None expected.
Cocaine:	None expected.
Foods:	None expected.
Marijuana:	None expected.
Tobacco:	None expected.

ANTIGLAUCOMA, LONG-ACTING (Ophthalmic)

BRAND AND GENERIC NAMES

DEMECARIUM	Humorsol
ECHOTHIOPHATE	ISOFLUROPHATE
Floropryl	Phospholine Iodide

BASIC INFORMATION

Habit forming? No
Prescription needed? Yes
Available as generic? No
Drug class: Antiglaucoma (ophthalmic)

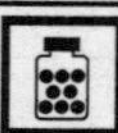

USES

- Treats glaucoma (open-angle type).
- Treats glaucoma after some forms of eye surgery and a few other eye disorders.

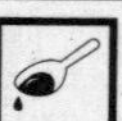

DOSAGE & USAGE INFORMATION

How to use:
Eye drops
- Wash hands.
- Apply pressure to inside corner of eye with middle finger.
- Continue pressure for 1 minute after placing medicine in eye.
- Tilt head backward. Pull lower lid away from eye with index finger of the same hand.
- Drop eye drops into pouch and close eye. Don't blink.
- Keep eyes closed for 1 to 2 minutes.
- Press finger to tear duct in corner of eye for 2 minutes to prevent possible absorption by body.

Eye ointment
- Wash hands.
- Pull lower lid down from eye to form a pouch.
- Squeeze tube to apply thin strip of ointment into pouch.
- Close eye for 1 to 2 minutes.
- Don't touch applicator tip to any surface (including the eye). If you accidentally touch tip, clean with warm soap and water.
- Keep container tightly closed.

Continued next column

OVERDOSE

SYMPTOMS:
None expected.
WHAT TO DO:
Not intended for internal use. If child accidentally swallows, call poison control center.

- Keep cool, but don't freeze.
- Wash hands immediately after using.
- Press finger to tear duct in corner of eye for 2 minutes to prevent possible absorption by body.

When to use:
As directed on label.

If you forget a dose:
Use as soon as you remember.

What drug does:
Inactivates an enzyme to reduce pressure inside the eye.

Time lapse before drug works:
5 to 60 minutes.

Don't use with:
Any other eye medicine without consulting your doctor.

POSSIBLE ADVERSE REACTIONS OR SIDE EFFECTS

SYMPTOMS	WHAT TO DO
Life-threatening:	
None expected.	
Common:	
Pupils become small.	No action necessary.
Infrequent:	
Blurred vision, change in vision, eye pain, eyelids twitch, headache, watery eyes.	Discontinue. Call doctor right away.
Rare:	
Decreased vision with veil or curtain appearing, loss of bladder control, slow heartbeat, increased sweating, weakness, difficult breathing, vomiting, nausea, diarrhea.	Discontinue. Call doctor right away.

ANTIGLAUCOMA, LONG-ACTING (Ophthalmic)

WARNINGS & PRECAUTIONS

Don't use if:
You are allergic to demecarium, echothiophate, isoflurophate.

Before you start, consult your doctor:
- If you have a history of retinal detachment.
- If you plan surgery under general or local anesthesia.
- If you have asthma, epilepsy, Down syndrome, eye infection or other eye disease, heart disease, Parkinson's disease, ulcer in stomach or duodenum.

Over age 60:
No problems expected.

Pregnancy:
Risk factors vary for drugs in this group. See category list on page xxii and consult doctor.

Breast-feeding:
Unknown effect. Consult doctor.

Infants & children:
Use under medical supervision only.

Prolonged use:
No problems expected.

Skin & sunlight:
No problems expected.

Driving, piloting or hazardous work:
Don't drive or pilot aircraft until you learn how medicine affects you. Don't work around dangerous machinery. Don't climb ladders or work in high places. Danger increases if you drink alcohol or take medicine affecting alertness and reflexes, such as antihistamines, tranquilizers, sedatives, pain medicine, narcotics and mind-altering drugs.

Discontinuing:
- Discontinue 2 to 3 weeks prior to eye surgery.
- Otherwise, don't discontinue without consulting your doctor. Dose may require gradual reduction if you have used drug for a long time. Doses of other drugs may also require adjustment.

Others:
- Keep appointments for regular eye examinations to measure pressure in the eye.
- Keep cool, but don't freeze.
- Eyeglass prescription may need changing.

POSSIBLE INTERACTION WITH OTHER DRUGS

GENERIC NAME OR DRUG CLASS	COMBINED EFFECT
Anticholinergics*	Increased risk of toxicity.
Atropine (ophthalmic)	May not be safe. Check with doctor.
Cholinesterase inhibitors*	Increased risk of toxicity.
Cyclopentolate (ophthalmic)	Reduces effect of antiglaucoma eye medicines.
Fibuprofen (ophthalmic)	May decrease antiglaucoma effect.
Insecticides or pesticides with organic phosphates	Increased toxic absorption of pesticides.
Medicines to treat myasthenia gravis	Additive toxicity.
Physostigmine (ophthalmic)	Shortens action of antiglaucoma medicines.
Topical anesthetics	Increased risk of toxic effects of antiglaucoma eye medicines.

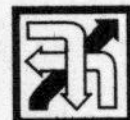

POSSIBLE INTERACTION WITH OTHER SUBSTANCES

INTERACTS WITH	COMBINED EFFECT
Alcohol:	None expected.
Beverages:	None expected.
Cocaine:	None expected.
Foods:	None expected.
Marijuana:	None expected.
Tobacco:	None expected.

*See Glossary

ANTIGLAUCOMA, SHORT-ACTING (Ophthalmic)

BRAND AND GENERIC NAMES

Ayerst Epitrate
CARBACHOL
DIPIVEFRIN
Epifrin
Epinal
EPINEPHRINE
Eppy/N
Eserine
Glaucon
Isopto Carbachol
Isopto Eserine
L-Epinephrine
Miostat
Mytrate
Ophtho-Dipivefrin
PHYSOSTIGMINE
Propine
Propine C Cap B.I.D.
Propine C Cap Q.I.D.

BASIC INFORMATION

Habit forming? No
Prescription needed? Yes
Available as generic? Yes, some are
Drug class: Antiglaucoma (ophthalmic)

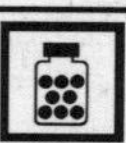

USES

Treats glaucoma (open-angle, secondary, angle-closure during or after eye surgery).

DOSAGE & USAGE INFORMATION

How to use:
Eye drops
- Wash hands.
- Apply pressure to inside corner of eye with middle finger.
- Continue pressure for 1 minute after placing medicine in eye.
- Tilt head backward. Pull lower lid away from eye with index finger of the same hand.
- Drop eye drops into pouch and close eye. Don't blink.
- Keep eyes closed for 1 to 2 minutes.

Eye ointment
- Wash hands.
- Pull lower lid down from eye to form a pouch.
- Squeeze tube to apply thin strip of ointment into pouch.
- Close eye for 1 to 2 minutes.

Continued next column

OVERDOSE

SYMPTOMS:
None expected.
WHAT TO DO:
Not intended for internal use. If child accidentally swallows, call poison control center.

- Don't touch applicator tip to any surface (including the eye). If you accidentally touch tip, clean with warm soap and water.
- Keep container tightly closed.
- Keep cool, but don't freeze.
- Wash hands immediately after using.

When to use:
As directed on label.

If you forget a dose:
Use as soon as you remember.

What drug does:
Inactivates enzyme and facilitates movement of fluid (aqueous humor) into and out of the eye.

Time lapse before drug works:
10-30 minutes.

Don't use with:
Any other medicine without consulting your doctor.

POSSIBLE ADVERSE REACTIONS OR SIDE EFFECTS

SYMPTOMS	WHAT TO DO
Life-threatening: None expected.	
Common: Headache; stinging, burning, watery eyes.	Continue. Call doctor when convenient.
Infrequent: Eye pain, changes in vision, blurred vision.	Discontinue. Call doctor right away.
Rare: Faintness, increased sweating, irregular or fast heartbeat, paleness.	Discontinue. Call doctor right away.

ANTIGLAUCOMA, SHORT-ACTING (Ophthalmic)

WARNINGS & PRECAUTIONS

Don't use if:
You are allergic to any eye medicine for glaucoma.

Before you start, consult your doctor:
- If you plan to have eye or dental surgery.
- If you have any eye disease.
- If you have heart problems or high blood pressure.
- If you have diabetes.

Over age 60:
Adverse reactions and side effects may be more frequent and severe than in younger persons. Ask doctor about smaller doses.

Pregnancy:
Risk factors vary for drugs in this group. See category list on page xxii and consult doctor.

Breast-feeding:
Safety unestablished. Avoid if possible. Consult doctor.

Infants & children:
Use only under close medical supervision.

Prolonged use:
May be necessary.

Skin & sunlight:
No problems expected.

Driving, piloting or hazardous work:
Don't drive or pilot aircraft until you learn how medicine affects you. Don't work around dangerous machinery. Don't climb ladders or work in high places. Danger increases if you drink alcohol or take medicine affecting alertness and reflexes, such as antihistamines, tranquilizers, sedatives, pain medicine, narcotics and mind-altering drugs.

Discontinuing:
Don't discontinue without consulting your doctor. Dose may require gradual reduction if you have used drug for a long time. Doses of other drugs may also require adjustment.

Others:
- Most normal physical activities, including swimming or other exercise, are okay while you use this medicine.
- Keep cool, but don't freeze.
- Keep appointments for regular eye examinations to measure pressure in the eye.

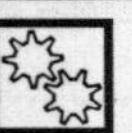

POSSIBLE INTERACTION WITH OTHER DRUGS

GENERIC NAME OR DRUG CLASS	COMBINED EFFECT
Other eye drugs	May decrease antiglaucoma effect.

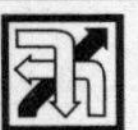

POSSIBLE INTERACTION WITH OTHER SUBSTANCES

INTERACTS WITH	COMBINED EFFECT
Alcohol:	None expected.
Beverages:	None expected.
Cocaine:	None expected.
Foods:	None expected.
Marijuana:	None expected.
Tobacco:	None expected.

ANTIHISTAMINES

BRAND AND GENERIC NAMES

See complete list of brand and generic names in the *Brand Name Directory*, page 896.

BASIC INFORMATION

Habit forming? No
Prescription needed?
High strength: Yes
Low strength: No
Available as generic? Yes
Drug class: Antihistamine

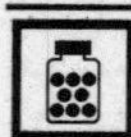

USES

- Reduces allergic symptoms such as hay fever, hives, rash or itching.
- Prevents motion sickness, nausea, vomiting.
- Induces sleep.
- Reduces stiffness and tremors of Parkinson's disease.

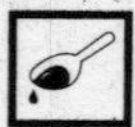

DOSAGE & USAGE INFORMATION

How to take:
Follow label directions.

When to take:
Varies with form. Follow label directions.

If you forget a dose:
Take as soon as you remember up to 2 hours late. If more than 2 hours, wait for next scheduled dose (don't double this dose).

What drug does:
Blocks action of histamine after an allergic response triggers histamine release in sensitive cells.

Time lapse before drug works:
30 minutes.

Don't take with:
Any other medicine without consulting your doctor or pharmacist.

OVERDOSE

SYMPTOMS:
Convulsions, red face, hallucinations, coma.
WHAT TO DO:

- **Dial 911 (emergency) or 0 (operator)for an ambulance or medical help. Then give first aid immediately.**
- **See emergency information on inside covers.**

POSSIBLE ADVERSE REACTIONS OR SIDE EFFECTS

SYMPTOMS	WHAT TO DO
Life-threatening: In case of overdose, see previous column.	
Common: Drowsiness (less likely with loratadine or astemizole); dizziness; dryness of mouth, nose or throat.	Continue. Tell doctor at next visit.
Infrequent:	
• Change in vision, clumsiness, rash.	Discontinue. Call doctor right away.
• Less tolerance for contact lenses, painful or difficult urination.	Continue. Call doctor when convenient.
• Appetite loss.	Continue. Tell doctor at next visit.
Rare: Nightmares, agitation, irritability, sore throat, fever, rapid heartbeat, unusual bleeding or bruising, fatigue, weakness, confusion.	Discontinue. Call doctor right away.

WARNINGS & PRECAUTIONS

Don't take if:
You are allergic to any antihistamine.

Before you start, consult your doctor:

- If you have glaucoma.
- If you have enlarged prostate.
- If you have asthma.
- If you have kidney disease.
- If you have peptic ulcer.
- If you will have surgery within 2 months, including dental surgery, requiring general or spinal anesthesia.

Over age 60:
Don't exceed recommended dose. Adverse reactions and side effects may be more frequent and severe than in younger persons, especially urination difficulty, diminished alertness and other brain and nervous-system symptoms.

Pregnancy:
Risk factors vary for drugs in this group. See category list on page xxii and consult doctor.

Breast-feeding:
Drug passes into milk. Avoid drug or discontinue nursing until you finish medicine. Consult doctor for advice on maintaining milk supply.

Infants & children:
Not recommended for premature or newborn infants. Otherwise, no problems expected.

Prolonged use:
Avoid. May damage bone marrow and nerve cells.

Skin & sunlight:
May cause rash or intensify sunburn in areas exposed to sun or sunlamp.

Driving, piloting or hazardous work:
Don't drive or pilot aircraft until you learn how medicine affects you. Don't work around dangerous machinery. Don't climb ladders or work in high places. Danger increases if you drink alcohol or take medicine affecting alertness and reflexes, such as antihistamines, tranquilizers, sedatives, pain medicine, narcotics and mind-altering drugs.

Discontinuing:
No problems expected.

Others:
- May mask symptoms of hearing damage from aspirin, other salicylates, cisplatin, paromomycin, vancomycin or anticonvulsants. Consult doctor if you use these.
- Advise any doctor or dentist whom you consult that you take this medicine.

POSSIBLE INTERACTION WITH OTHER DRUGS

GENERIC NAME OR DRUG CLASS	COMBINED EFFECT
Anticholinergics*	Increased anti-cholinergic effect.
Anticoagulants, oral*	Decreased anti-histamine effect.
Antidepressants*	Excess sedation. Avoid.
Antihistamines, other*	Excess sedation. Avoid.
Carteolol	Decreased anti-histamine effect.
Central nervous system (CNS) depressants*	May increase sedation.
Clozapine	Toxic effect on the central nervous system.
Dronabinol	Increased effects of both drugs. Avoid.
Erythromycin	Increased risk of cardiac toxicity with astemizole.
Hypnotics*	Excess sedation. Avoid.
Itraconazole	Increased risk of cardiac toxicity and death with astemizole.
Ketocanazole	Increased risk of cardiac toxicity and death with astemizole.
Mind-altering drugs*	Excess sedation. Avoid.
Molindone	Increased sedative and antihistamine effect.
Monoamine oxidase (MAO) inhibitors*	Increased antihistamine effect.
Nabilone	Greater depression of central nervous system.
Narcotics*	Excess sedation. Avoid.
Procarbazine	May increase sedation.
Sedatives*	Excess sedation. Avoid.
Sertraline	Increased depressive effects of both drugs.
Sleep inducers*	Excess sedation. Avoid.
Sotalol	Increased antihistamine effect.
Tranquilizers*	Excess sedation. Avoid.

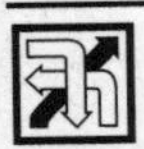

POSSIBLE INTERACTION WITH OTHER SUBSTANCES

INTERACTS WITH	COMBINED EFFECT
Alcohol:	Excess sedation. Avoid.
Beverages: Caffeine drinks.	Less antihistamine sedation.
Cocaine:	Decreased antihistamine effect. Avoid.
Foods:	None expected.
Marijuana:	Excess sedation. Avoid.
Tobacco:	None expected.

*See Glossary

ANTIHISTAMINES, PHENOTHIAZINE-DERIVATIVE

BRAND AND GENERIC NAMES

See complete list of brand and generic names in the *Brand Name Directory*, page 899.

BASIC INFORMATION

Habit forming? No
Prescription needed? Yes
Available as generic? Yes
Drug class: Tranquilizer (phenothiazine), antihistamine

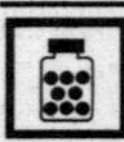

USES

- Relieves itching of hives, skin allergies, chickenpox.
- Treatment for hay fever, motion sickness, vertigo.

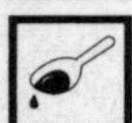

DOSAGE & USAGE INFORMATION

How to take:
- Tablet or syrup—Swallow with liquid or food to lessen stomach irritation.
- Extended-release capsules—Swallow each dose whole. If you take regular tablets, you may chew or crush them.

When to take:
At the same times each day.

If you forget a dose:
Take as soon as you remember up to 2 hours late. If more than 2 hours, wait for next scheduled dose (don't double this dose).

What drug does:
Blocks histamine action in skin.

Time lapse before drug works:
1 to 2 hours.

Continued next column

OVERDOSE

SYMPTOMS:
Fast heartbeat, flushed face, shortness of breath, clumsiness, drowsiness, muscle spasms, jerking movements of head and face.
WHAT TO DO:
- **Dial 911 (emergency) or 0 (operator) for an ambulance or medical help. Then give first aid immediately.**
- **See emergency information on inside covers.**

Don't take with:
- Antacid or medicine for diarrhea.
- Nonprescription drug for cough, cold or allergy.
- Any other medicine without consulting your doctor or pharmacist.

POSSIBLE ADVERSE REACTIONS OR SIDE EFFECTS

SYMPTOMS	WHAT TO DO
Life-threatening:	
In case of overdose, see previous column.	
Common:	
• Restlessness, tremor, drowsiness, tiredness, weakness.	Discontinue. Call doctor right away.
• Decreased sweating, dry mouth, nasal congestion, constipation.	Continue. Call doctor when convenient.
Infrequent:	
• Fainting.	Discontinue. Seek emergency treatment.
• Rash, muscle spasms of face and neck, unsteady gait.	Discontinue. Call doctor right away.
• Difficult urination, less interest in sex, swollen breasts, menstrual irregularities, dizziness, nausea, vomiting.	Continue. Call doctor when convenient.
Rare:	
Change in vision, sore throat, fever, jaundice, confusion, nightmares, unusual excitement.	Discontinue. Call doctor right away.

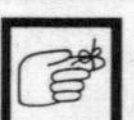

WARNINGS & PRECAUTIONS

Don't take if:
- You are allergic to any phenothiazine.
- You have a blood or bone marrow disease.

Before you start, consult your doctor:
- If you will have surgery within 2 months, including dental surgery, requiring general or spinal anesthesia.
- If you have asthma, emphysema or other lung disorder.
- If you take nonprescription ulcer medicine, asthma medicine or amphetamines.

Over age 60:
Adverse reactions and side effects may be more frequent and severe than in younger persons. More likely to develop tardive dyskinesia (involuntary movement of jaws, lips, tongue, chewing). Report this to your doctor immediately. Early treatment can help.

Pregnancy:
Decide with your doctor if drug benefits justify risk to unborn child. Risk category C (see page xxii).

Breast-feeding:
Drug passes into milk. Avoid drug or discontinue nursing until you finish medicine. Consult doctor for advice on maintaining milk supply.

Infants & children:
Don't give to children younger than 2.

Prolonged use:
- May lead to tardive dyskinesia (involuntary movement of jaws, lips, tongue; chewing).
- Talk to your doctor about the need for follow-up medical examinations or laboratory studies to check complete blood counts (white blood cell count, platelet count, red blood cell count, hemoglobin, hematocrit), liver function, eyes.

Skin & sunlight:
May cause rash or intensify sunburn in areas exposed to sun or sunlamp. Skin may remain sensitive for 3 months after discontinuing.

Driving, piloting or hazardous work:
Don't drive or pilot aircraft until you learn how medicine affects you. Don't work around dangerous machinery. Don't climb ladders or work in high places. Danger increases if you drink alcohol or take medicine affecting alertness and reflexes.

Discontinuing:
May be unnecessary to finish medicine. Follow doctor's instructions.

Others:
May affect results in some medical tests.

POSSIBLE INTERACTION WITH OTHER DRUGS

GENERIC NAME OR DRUG CLASS	COMBINED EFFECT
Antacids*	Decreased anti-histamine effect.
Anticholinergics*	Increased anti-cholinergic effect.
Anticonvulsants, hydantoin*	Increased anti-convulsant effect.
Antidepressants, tricyclic*	Increased anti-histamine effect.
Antihistamines*, other	Increased anti-histamine effect.
Antithyroid drugs*	Increased risk of bone marrow depression.
Appetite suppressants*	Decreased appetite suppressant effect.
Barbiturates*	Oversedation.
Carteolol	Decreased anti-histamine effect.
Central nervous system (CNS) depressants*	Dangerous degree of sedation.
Cisapride	Decreased anti-histamine effect.
Clozapine	Toxic effect on the central nervous system.
Dronabinol	Increased effects of both drugs. Avoid.
Epinephrine	Decreased epinephrine effect.
Ethinamate	Dangerous increased effects of ethina-mate. Avoid combin-ing.
Extrapyramidal reaction*-causing medicines	Increased frequency and severity of extra-pyramidal reactions.
Fluoxetine	Increased depressant effects of both drugs.
Guanethidine	Decreased guanethidine effect.

Continued on page 926

POSSIBLE INTERACTION WITH OTHER SUBSTANCES

INTERACTS WITH	COMBINED EFFECT
Alcohol:	Dangerous oversedation.
Beverages:	None expected.
Cocaine:	Decreased trimeprazine effect. Avoid.
Foods:	None expected.
Marijuana:	Drowsiness.
Tobacco:	None expected.

*See Glossary

ANTI-INFLAMMATORY DRUGS, NONSTEROIDAL (NSAIDs)

BRAND AND GENERIC NAMES

See complete list of brand and generic names in the *Brand Names Directory*, page 899.

BASIC INFORMATION

Habit forming? No
Prescription needed? Yes, for some.
Available as generic? Yes, for some.
Drug class: Anti-inflammatory (nonsteroidal)

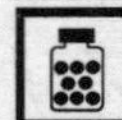

USES

- Treatment for joint pain, stiffness, inflammation and swelling of arthritis and gout.
- Treatment for pain, fever and inflammation.
- Treatment for dysmenorrhea (painful or difficult menstruation).
- Treats juvenile rheumatoid arthritis.

DOSAGE & USAGE INFORMATION

How to take:

- Tablet or capsule—Swallow with liquid or food to lessen stomach irritation. If you can't swallow whole, crumble tablet and take with liquid or food. Don't crumble delayed release tablet.
- Liquid—Take as directed on bottle. Don't freeze.
- Rectal Suppositories—Remove wrapper and moisten suppository with water. Gently insert into rectum, large end first. If suppository is too soft, chill in refrigerator or cool water before removing wrapper.

When to take:
At the same times each day.

If you forget a dose:
Take as soon as you remember up to 2 hours late. If more than 2 hours, wait for next scheduled dose (don't double this dose).

Continued next column

OVERDOSE

SYMPTOMS:
Confusion, agitation, severe headache, incoherence, convulsions, possible hemorrhage from stomach or intestine, coma.
WHAT TO DO:

- **Dial 911 (emergency) or 0 (operator)for an ambulance or medical help. Then give first aid immediately.**
- **See emergency information on inside covers.**

What drug does:
Reduces tissue concentration of prostaglandins (hormones which produce inflammation and pain).

Time lapse before drug works:
Begins in 4 to 24 hours. May require 3 weeks regular use for maximum benefit.

Don't take with:
Any other medicine without consulting your doctor or pharmacist.

POSSIBLE ADVERSE REACTIONS OR SIDE EFFECTS

SYMPTOMS	WHAT TO DO
Life-threatening:	
Hives, rash, intense itching, faintness soon after a dose (anaphylaxis in aspirin-sensitive persons).	Seek emergency treatment immediately.
Common:	
• Dizziness, nausea, pain.	Continue. Call doctor when convenient.
• Headache.	Continue. Tell doctor at next visit.
Infrequent:	
• Depression; drowsiness; ringing in ears; swollen feet, face or legs; constipation or diarrhea; vomiting; gaseousness; dry mouth; tremors; insomnia.	Continue. Call doctor when convenient.
• Muscle cramps, numbness or tingling in hands or feet, mouth ulcers, rapid weight gain.	Discontinue. Call doctor right away.
Rare:	
• Convulsions; confusion; rash, hives or itch; blurred vision; black, bloody, tarry stool; difficult breathing; tightness in chest; rapid heartbeat; unusual bleeding or bruising; blood in urine; jaundice; psychosis; frequent, painful urination; fainting; sore throat; fever; chills; diminished hearing; eye pain; nose bleeds; severe abdominal pain.	Discontinue. Call doctor right away.
• Fatigue, weakness, menstrual irregularities.	Continue. Call doctor when convenient.

ANTI-INFLAMMATORY DRUGS, NONSTEROIDAL (NSAIDs)

WARNINGS & PRECAUTIONS

Don't take if:
- You are allergic to aspirin or any nonsteroidal, anti-inflammatory drug.
- You have gastritis, peptic ulcer, enteritis, ileitis, ulcerative colitis, asthma, heart failure, high blood pressure or bleeding problems.
- Patient is younger than 15.

Before you start, consult your doctor:
- If you have epilepsy.
- If you have Parkinson's disease.
- If you have been mentally ill.
- If you have impaired kidney or liver function.

Over age 60:
Adverse reactions and side effects may be more frequent and severe than in younger persons.

Pregnancy:
Risk factors vary for drugs in this group. See category list on page xxii and consult doctor.

Breast-feeding:
May harm child. Avoid.

Infants & children:
Not recommended for anyone younger than 15. Use only under medical supervision.

Prolonged use:
- Eye damage.
- Reduced hearing.
- Sore throat, fever.
- Weight gain.
- Talk to your doctor about the need for follow-up medical examinations or laboratory studies to check complete blood counts (white blood cell count, platelet count, red blood cell count, hemoglobin, hematocrit), liver function, stools for blood, eyes.

Skin & sunlight:
Possible increased sensitivity to sunlight.

Driving, piloting or hazardous work:
Don't drive or pilot aircraft until you learn how medicine affects you. Don't work around dangerous machinery. Don't climb ladders or work in high places. Danger increases if you drink alcohol or take medicine affecting alertness and reflexes, such as antihistamines, tranquilizers, sedatives, pain medicine, narcotics and mind-altering drugs.

Discontinuing:
Don't discontinue without consulting doctor. Dose may require gradual reduction if you have taken drug for a long time. Doses of other drugs may also require adjustment.

Others:
Advise any doctor or dentist whom you consult that you take this medicine

POSSIBLE INTERACTION WITH OTHER DRUGS

GENERIC NAME OR DRUG CLASS	COMBINED EFFECT
Angiotensin-converting enzyme (ACE) inhibitors*	May decrease ACE inhibitor effect.
Antacids*	Decreased pain relief.
Anticoagulants, oral*	Increased risk of bleeding.
Anticonvulsants, hydantoin*	Increased anti-convulsant effect.
Anti-inflammatory pain relievers (any combination of)	Danger of increased side effects such as stomach bleeding.
Aspirin	Increased risk of stomach ulcer.
Beta-adrenergic blocking agents*	Decreased anti-hypertensive effect.
Carteolol	Decreased anti-hypertensive effect of carteolol.
Cephalosporins*	Increased risk of bleeding.
Cortisone drugs*	Increased risk of stomach ulcer.
Didanosine	Increased risk of pancreatitis (sulindac only).

Continued on page 926

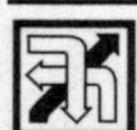

POSSIBLE INTERACTION WITH OTHER SUBSTANCES

INTERACTS WITH	COMBINED EFFECT
Alcohol:	Possible stomach ulcer or bleeding.
Beverages:	None expected.
Cocaine:	None expected.
Foods:	None expected.
Marijuana:	Increased pain relief from NSAIDs.
Tobacco:	None expected.

*See Glossary

ANTI-INFLAMMATORY DRUGS, NONSTEROIDAL (NSAIDs) (Ophthalmic)

BRAND AND GENERIC NAMES

Acular	Ocufen
DICLOFENAC	Profenal
FLURBIPROFEN	SUPROFEN
Indocid	Voltaren Ophtha
INDOMETHACIN	Voltaren Ophthalmic
KETOROLAC	

BASIC INFORMATION

Habit forming? No
Prescription needed? Yes
Available as generic? No
Drug class: Ophthalmic anti-inflammatory agents, nonsteroidal

USES

- Used to prevent problems during and following eye surgery, such as cataract removal.
- Treatment for eye itching caused by seasonal allergic conjunctivitis.

DOSAGE & USAGE INFORMATION

How to use:
Eye solution
- Wash hands.
- Apply pressure to inside corner of eye with middle finger.
- Continue pressure for 1 minute after placing medicine in eye.
- Tilt head backward. Pull lower lid away from eye with index finger of the same hand.
- Drop eye drops into pouch and close eye. Don't blink.
- Keep eyes closed for 1 to 2 minutes.

When to use:
As directed by your doctor or on the label. Your doctor or nurse may instill the drug before an eye operation.

If you forget a dose:
Use as soon as you remember.

Continued next column

OVERDOSE

SYMPTOMS:
None expected.
WHAT TO DO:
Not intended for internal use. If child accidentally swallows, call poison control center.

What drug does:
Blocks prostaglandin production. Prostaglandins cause inflammatory responses and constriction of the pupil.

Time lapse before drug works:
Immediately.

Don't use with:
Any other medications without first consulting doctor or pharmacist.

POSSIBLE ADVERSE REACTIONS OR SIDE EFFECTS

SYMPTOMS	WHAT TO DO
Life-threatening:	
None expected.	
Common:	
Brief and mild burning or stinging when drops are administered.	No action necessary.
Infrequent:	
None expected.	
Rare:	
Allergic reaction (itching, tearing); redness, swelling or bleeding in eye not present before; eye pain; sensitivity to light.	Discontinue. Call doctor right away.

ANTI-INFLAMMATORY DRUGS, NONSTEROIDAL (NSAIDs) (Ophthalmic)

WARNINGS & PRECAUTIONS

Don't use if:
- You are allergic to any eye medication.
- You are allergic to any nonsteroidal anti-inflammatory drugs taken orally, e.g., aspirin.

Before you start, consult your doctor:
- If you have any bleeding disorder such as hemophilia.
- If you have or have had herpes simplex keratitis (an inflammation of the cornea).
- If you have allergies to any medications, foods or other substances.

Over age 60:
No special problems expected.

Pregnancy:
Risk category C (see page xxii). Decide with your doctor whether drug benefit justifies risk to unborn child.

Breast-feeding:
Unknown if drug passes into breast milk after administration into the eye. Consult doctor.

Infants & children:
No information available on safety or effectiveness. Consult doctor.

Prolonged use:
Not intended for long-term use.

Skin & sunlight:
Normally no problems expected, but adverse reaction may cause light sensitivity.

Driving, piloting or hazardous work:
No special problems expected.

Discontinuing:
No special problems expected.

Others:
Don't use leftover medicine for other eye problems without your doctor's approval. Some eye infections could be made worse.

POSSIBLE INTERACTION WITH OTHER DRUGS

GENERIC NAME OR DRUG CLASS	COMBINED EFFECT
Anticoagulants*, oral	May increase bleeding tendency.
Antiglaucoma drugs*	May decrease antiglaucoma effect (with flubiprofen).
Carbachol	Decreased carbachol effect.

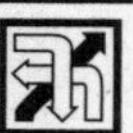

POSSIBLE INTERACTION WITH OTHER SUBSTANCES

INTERACTS WITH	COMBINED EFFECT
Alcohol:	None expected.
Beverages:	None expected.
Cocaine	None expected.
Foods:	None expected.
Marijuana:	None expected.
Tobacco:	None expected.

***See Glossary**

ANTI-INFLAMMATORY DRUGS, STEROIDAL (Ophthalmic)

BRAND AND GENERIC NAMES

See complete list of brand and generic names in the *Brand Name Directory*, page 900.

BASIC INFORMATION

Habit forming? No
Prescription needed? Yes
Available as generic? Yes
Drug class: Adrenocorticoid (ophthalmic); anti-inflammatory, steroidal (ophthalmic)

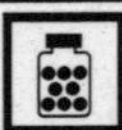

USES

- Relieves redness and irritation due to allergies or other irritants.
- Prevents damage to eye.

DOSAGE & USAGE INFORMATION

How to use:
Eye drops
- Wash hands.
- Apply pressure to inside corner of eye with middle finger.
- Continue pressure for 1 minute after placing medicine in eye.
- Tilt head backward. Pull lower lid away from eye with index finger of the same hand.
- Drop eye drops into pouch and close eye. Don't blink.
- Keep eyes closed for 1 to 2 minutes.

Eye ointment
- Wash hands.
- Pull lower lid down from eye to form a pouch.
- Squeeze tube to apply thin strip of ointment into pouch.
- Close eye for 1 to 2 minutes.
- Don't touch applicator tip to any surface (including the eye). If you accidentally touch tip, clean with warm soap and water.
- Keep container tightly closed.
- Keep cool, but don't freeze.
- Wash hands immediately after using.

Continued next column

When to use:
As directed.

If you forget a dose:
Use as soon as you remember.

What drug does:
Affects cell membranes and decreases response to irritating substances.

Time lapse before drug works:
Immediately.

Don't use with:
Medicines for abdominal cramps or glaucoma without first consulting doctor.

OVERDOSE

SYMPTOMS:
None expected.
WHAT TO DO:
Not intended for internal use. If child accidentally swallows, call poison control center.

POSSIBLE ADVERSE REACTIONS OR SIDE EFFECTS

SYMPTOMS	WHAT TO DO
Life-threatening: None expected.	
Common: None expected.	
Infrequent: Watery, stinging, burning eyes.	Continue. Call doctor when convenient.
Rare (extremely): Eye pain, blurred vision, drooping eyelid, halos around lights, enlarged pupils, flashes of light.	Discontinue. Call doctor right away.

ANTI-INFLAMMATORY DRUGS, STEROIDAL (Ophthalmic)

WARNINGS & PRECAUTIONS

Don't use if:
You are allergic to any cortisone medicine.

Before you start, consult your doctor:
If you have or ever have had any eye infection, glaucoma, virus (herpes) infection of the eye, tuberculosis of the eye.

Over age 60:
No problems expected.

Pregnancy:
Risk factors vary for drugs in this group. See category list on page xxii and consult doctor.

Breast-feeding:
Safety unestablished. Avoid if possible. Consult doctor.

Infants & children:
Use for short periods of time only.

Prolonged use:
Recheck with eye doctor at regular intervals.

Skin & sunlight:
No problems expected.

Driving, piloting or hazardous work:
No problems expected.

Discontinuing:
No problems expected.

Others:

- Cortisone eye medicines should not be used for bacterial, viral, fungal or tubercular infections.
- Keep cool, but don't freeze.
- Notify doctor if condition doesn't improve within 3 days.
- Contact lens wearers have increased risk of infection.

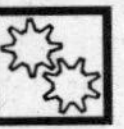

POSSIBLE INTERACTION WITH OTHER DRUGS

GENERIC NAME OR DRUG CLASS	COMBINED EFFECT
Antiglaucoma drugs*, long- and short-acting	Decreased antiglaucoma effect.

POSSIBLE INTERACTION WITH OTHER SUBSTANCES

INTERACTS WITH	COMBINED EFFECT
Alcohol:	None expected.
Beverages:	None expected.
Cocaine:	None expected.
Foods:	None expected.
Marijuana:	None expected.
Tobacco:	None expected.

***See Glossary**

ANTI-INFLAMMATORY DRUGS, STEROIDAL (Otic)

BRAND AND GENERIC NAMES

Ak-Dex	Decadron
BETAMETHASONE (Otic)	DEXAMETHASONE (Otic)
Betnesol	HYDROCORTISONE (Otic)
Cortamed	I-Methasone
Cortisol	

BASIC INFORMATION

Habit forming? No
Prescription needed? Yes
Available as generic? No
Drug class: Anti-inflammatory, steroidal (otic); adrenocorticoid (otic)

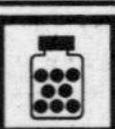

USES

- Treats allergic conditions involving external ear.
- Used together with antibiotics to treat ear infections.
- Treats seborrheic and eczematoid dermatitis involving the ear.

DOSAGE & USAGE INFORMATION

How to use:
Ear drops
- Warm ear drops under running water around the unopened bottle.
- Lie down with affected ear up.
- Adults—Pull ear lobe back and up.
- Children—Pull ear lobe down and back.
- Drop medicine into ear canal until canal is full.
- Stay lying down for 2 minutes.
- Gently insert cotton plug into ear to prevent leaking.

Continued next column

Ear ointment
- Apply small amount to skin just inside the ear canal.
- Use finger or piece of sterile gauze.
- Don't use cotton-tipped applicators.

When to use:
As directed by your doctor.

If you forget a dose:
Use as soon as you remember.

What drug does:
Decreases tissue inflammation, decreases scarring.

Time lapse before drug works:
15 minutes.

Don't use with:
Other ear medications unless directed by your doctor.

OVERDOSE

SYMPTOMS:
None expected.
WHAT TO DO:
Not intended for internal use. If child accidentally swallows, call poison control center.

POSSIBLE ADVERSE REACTIONS OR SIDE EFFECTS

SYMPTOMS	WHAT TO DO
Life-threatening: None expected.	
Common: None expected.	
Infrequent: Itching, burning, redness, swelling.	Discontinue. Call doctor right away.
Rare: None expected.	

ANTI-INFLAMMATORY DRUGS, STEROIDAL (Otic)

WARNINGS & PRECAUTIONS

Don't use if:
You are allergic to any of the medications listed under Brand and Generic Names.

Before you start, consult your doctor:
- If eardrum is punctured.
- If you have a viral infection.
- If you have a fungal ear infection.

Over age 60:
No problems expected.

Pregnancy:
Risk factors vary for drugs in this group. See category list on page xxii and consult doctor.

Breast-feeding:
No problems expected. Consult doctor.

Infants & children:
Use small amounts only.

Prolonged use:
Not intended for prolonged use.

Skin & sunlight:
No problems expected.

Driving, piloting or hazardous work:
No problems expected.

Discontinuing:
No problems expected.

Others:
Keep cool, but don't freeze.

POSSIBLE INTERACTION WITH OTHER DRUGS

GENERIC NAME OR DRUG CLASS	COMBINED EFFECT
None expected.	

POSSIBLE INTERACTION WITH OTHER SUBSTANCES

INTERACTS WITH	COMBINED EFFECT
Alcohol:	None expected.
Beverages:	None expected.
Cocaine:	None expected.
Foods:	None expected.
Marijuana:	None expected.
Tobacco:	None expected.

*See Glossary

ANTISEBORRHEICS (Topical)

BRAND AND GENERIC NAMES

See complete list of brand and generic names in the *Brand Name Directory* page 900.

BASIC INFORMATION

Habit forming? No
Prescription needed? Yes
Available as generic? Yes
Drug class: Antiseborrheic

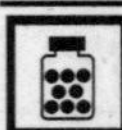

USES

Treats dandruff or seborrheic dermatitis of scalp.

DOSAGE & USAGE INFORMATION

How to use:
- Wet hair and scalp.
- Apply enough medicine to form lather.
- Rub in well. Keep away from eyes.
- Allow to remain on scalp 3 to 5 minutes then rinse.
- Repeat above steps once.

Continued next column

OVERDOSE

SYMPTOMS:
None expected.
WHAT TO DO:
- **Not for internal use. If child accidentally swallows, call poison control center.**
- **Dial 911 (emergency) or 0 (operator) for an ambulance or medical help. Then give first aid immediately.**
- **See emergency information on inside covers.**

When to use:
As directed by doctor. Twice a week for shampoo is average.

If you forget a dose:
Use as soon as you remember.

What drug does:
Slows cell growth in scales on scalp.

Time lapse before drug works:
Varies a great deal. If no improvement in 2 weeks, notify doctor.

Don't use with:
- Other scalp preparations without notifying doctor.
- Any other medicine without consulting your doctor or pharmacist.

POSSIBLE ADVERSE REACTIONS OR SIDE EFFECTS

SYMPTOMS	WHAT TO DO
Life-threatening:	
None expected.	
Common:	
None expected.	
Infrequent:	
• Irritation not present before using, rash.	Discontinue. Call doctor when convenient.
• Dryness or itching scalp.	Continue. Call doctor when convenient.
Rare:	
None expected.	

ANTISEBORRHEICS (Topical)

WARNINGS & PRECAUTIONS

Don't use if:
- You have had an allergic reaction to chloroxine, clioquinol (iodochlorhydroxyquin), iodoquinol (diiodohydroxyquin) or edate sodium.
- Scalp is blistered or infected with oozing or raw areas.

Before you start, consult your doctor:
If you are allergic to anything.

Over age 60:
No problems expected.

Pregnancy:
Risk factors vary for drugs in this group. See category list on page xxii and consult doctor.

Breast-feeding:
No problems expected, but check with doctor.

Infants & children:
No problems expected, but check with doctor.

Prolonged use:
No problems expected, but check with doctor.

Skin & sunlight:
No problems expected, but check with doctor.

Driving, piloting or hazardous work:
No problems expected, but check with doctor.

Discontinuing:
No problems expected, but check with doctor.

Others:
- If medicine accidentally gets into eyes, flush them immediately with cool water.
- Heat and moisture in bathroom medicine cabinet can cause breakdown of medicine. Store someplace else.
- Keep cool, but don't freeze.

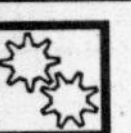

POSSIBLE INTERACTION WITH OTHER DRUGS

GENERIC NAME OR DRUG CLASS	COMBINED EFFECT
Other medical shampoos	May accentuate adverse reactions of each medicine.

POSSIBLE INTERACTION WITH OTHER SUBSTANCES

INTERACTS WITH	COMBINED EFFECT
Alcohol:	None expected.
Beverages:	None expected.
Cocaine:	None expected.
Foods:	None expected.
Marijuana:	None expected.
Tobacco:	None expected.

*See Glossary

ANTITHYROID DRUGS

BRAND AND GENERIC NAMES

METHIMAZOLE	Tapazole
PROPYLTHIOURACIL	Thiamazole
Propyl-Thyracil	

BASIC INFORMATION

Habit forming? No
Prescription needed? Yes
Available as generic? Yes
Drug class: Antihyperthyroid

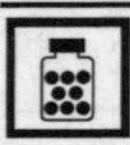

USES

- Treatment of overactive thyroid (hyperthyroidism).
- Treatment of angina in patients who have overactive thyroid.

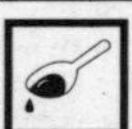

DOSAGE & USAGE INFORMATION

How to take:
Tablet—Swallow with liquid or food to lessen stomach irritation. If you can't swallow whole, crumble tablet and take with liquid or food.

When to take:
At the same times each day.

If you forget a dose:
Take as soon as you remember up to 2 hours late. If more than 2 hours, wait for next scheduled dose (don't double this dose).

What drug does:
Prevents thyroid gland from producing excess thyroid hormone.

Time lapse before drug works:
10 to 20 days.

Don't take with:
- Anticoagulants
- Any other medicine without consulting your doctor or pharmacist.

OVERDOSE

SYMPTOMS:
Bleeding, spots on skin, jaundice (yellow eyes and skin), loss of consciousness.
WHAT TO DO:
Overdose unlikely to threaten life. If person takes much larger amount than prescribed, call doctor, poison control center or hospital emergency room for instructions.

POSSIBLE ADVERSE REACTIONS OR SIDE EFFECTS

SYMPTOMS	WHAT TO DO
Life-threatening: In case of overdose, see previous column.	
Common:	
Skin rash, itching, dryness.	Continue. Call doctor right away.
Infrequent:	
Dizziness, taste loss, sore throat with chills and fever, abdominal pain, constipation, diarrhea.	Continue. Call doctor right away.
Rare:	
Headache; enlarged lymph glands; irregular or rapid heartbeat; unusual bruising or bleeding; backache; numbness or tingling in toes, fingers or face; joint pain; muscle aches; menstrual irregularities; jaundice; tired, weak, sleepy, listless; swollen eyes or feet; black stools; excessive cold feeling; puffy skin; irritability.	Continue. Call doctor right away.

WARNINGS & PRECAUTIONS

Don't take if:
You are allergic to antithyroid medicines.

Before you start, consult your doctor:
- If you have liver disease.
- If you have blood disease.
- If you have an infection.
- If you take anticoagulants.

Over age 60:
Adverse reactions and side effects may be more frequent and severe than in younger persons.

Pregnancy:
Consult doctor. Risk category D (see page xxii).

Breast-feeding:
Drug filters into milk. Consult doctor.

Infants & children:
Use only under special medical supervision by experienced clinician.

Prolonged use:
- Adverse reactions and side effects more common.
- Talk to your doctor about the need for follow-up medical examinations or laboratory studies to check thyroid function, complete blood counts (white blood cell count, platelet count, red blood cell count, hemoglobin, hematocrit).

Skin & sunlight:
No problems expected.

Driving, piloting or hazardous work:
Don't drive or pilot aircraft until you learn how medicine affects you. Don't work around dangerous machinery. Don't climb ladders or work in high places. Danger increases if you drink alcohol or take medicine affecting alertness and reflexes, such as antihistamines, tranquilizers, sedatives, pain medicine, narcotics and mind-altering drugs.

Discontinuing:
Don't discontinue without consulting doctor. Dose may require gradual reduction if you have taken drug for a long time. Doses of other drugs may also require adjustment.

Others:
- Advise any doctor or dentist whom you consult that you take this medicine.
- Ask your doctor about the symptoms of overactive or underactive thyroid and what to do if they occur.

POSSIBLE INTERACTION WITH OTHER DRUGS

GENERIC NAME OR DRUG CLASS	COMBINED EFFECT
Amiodarone	Decreased anti-thyroid effect.
Anticoagulants*	Increased effect of anticoagulants.
Antineoplastic drugs*	Increased chance to suppress bone marrow.
Chloramphenicol	Increased chance to suppress bone marrow.
Clozapine	Toxic effect on bone marrow.
Digitalis preparations*	Increased digitalis effect.
Iodinated glycerol	Decreased anti-thyroid effect.
Iodine	Decreased anti-thyroid effect.
Levamisole	Increased risk of bone marrow depression.
Lithium	Decreased thyroid activity.
Potassium iodide	Decreased anti-thyroid effect.
Tiopronin	Increased risk of toxicity to bone marrow.

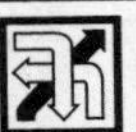

POSSIBLE INTERACTION WITH OTHER SUBSTANCES

INTERACTS WITH	COMBINED EFFECT
Alcohol:	Increased possibility of liver toxicity. Avoid.
Beverages:	No problems expected.
Cocaine:	Increased toxicity potential of medicines. Avoid.
Foods:	No problems expected.
Marijuana:	Increased rapid or irregular heartbeat. Avoid.
Tobacco:	Increased chance of rapid heartbeat. Avoid.

*See Glossary

ANTIVIRALS

BRAND AND GENERIC NAMES

AMANTADINE
Flumadine
RIMANTADINE
Symadine
Symmetrel

BASIC INFORMATION

Habit forming? No
Prescription needed? Yes
Available as generic? Yes
Drug class: Antiviral, antiparkinsonism

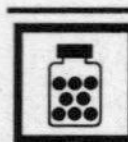

USES

- Prevention and treatment for Type-A flu infections.
- Relief for symptoms of Parkinson's disease.

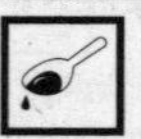

DOSAGE & USAGE INFORMATION

How to take:
- Capsule—Swallow with liquid or food to lessen stomach irritation.
- Syrup—Dilute dose in beverage before swallowing.

When to take:
At the same times each day. For Type-A flu it is especially important to take regular doses as prescribed.

If you forget a dose:
Take as soon as you remember. Wait 4 hours for next dose. Return to schedule.

What drug does:
- Type-A flu—May block penetration of tissue cells by infectious material from virus cells.
- Parkinson's disease and drug-induced extrapyramidal* reactions—Improves muscular condition and coordination.

Continued next column

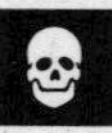

OVERDOSE

SYMPTOMS:
Heart rhythm disturbances, blood pressure drop, convulsions, hallucinations, violent behavior, confusion, slurred speech, rolling eyes.
WHAT TO DO:
- **Dial 911 (emergency) or 0 (operator) for an ambulance or medical help. Then give first aid immediately.**
- **See emergency information on inside covers.**

Time lapse before drug works:
- Type-A flu—48 hours.
- Parkinson's disease—2 days to 2 weeks.

Don't take with:
- Alcohol
- Any other medicine without consulting your doctor or pharmacist.

POSSIBLE ADVERSE REACTIONS OR SIDE EFFECTS

SYMPTOMS	WHAT TO DO
Life-threatening: In case of overdose, see previous column.	
Common: Headache, difficulty in concentrating, dizziness or lightheadedness, insomnia, irritability, nervousness, nightmares (these side effects infrequent with rimantadine).	Continue. Call doctor when convenient.
Infrequent:	
• With amantadine—Blurred or changed vision, confusion, difficult urination, hallucinations, fainting.	Discontinue. Call doctor right away.
• Constipation; dry mouth, nose or throat; vomiting, appetite loss, nausea.	Continue. Call doctor when convenient.
Rare:	
• With amantadine—Swelling or irritated eyes; depression; swelling of hands, legs or feet; skin rash.	Discontinue. Call doctor right away.
• Seizures (may occur in persons with a history of seizures).	Discontinue. Seek emergency help.

WARNINGS & PRECAUTIONS

Don't take if:
You are allergic to amantadine or rimantadine.

Before you start, consult your doctor:
- If you have had epilepsy or other seizures.
- If you have had heart disease or heart failure.
- If you have had liver or kidney disease.
- If you have had peptic ulcers.
- If you have had eczema or skin rashes.
- If you have had emotional or mental disorders or taken drugs for them.

Over age 60:
Adverse reactions and side effects may be more frequent and severe than in younger persons.

Pregnancy:
Decide with your doctor whether benefits justify risk to unborn child. Risk category C (see page xxii).

Breast-feeding:
Drug may pass into milk. Avoid drug or discontinue nursing until you finish medicine. Consult doctor for advice on maintaining milk supply.

Infants & children:
Use only under medical supervision.

Prolonged use:
Skin splotches, feet swelling, rapid weight gain, shortness of breath. Consult doctor.

Skin & sunlight:
No problems expected.

Driving, piloting or hazardous work:
Don't drive or pilot aircraft until you learn how medicine affects you. Don't work around dangerous machinery. Don't climb ladders or work in high places. Danger increases if you drink alcohol or take medicine affecting alertness and reflexes.

Discontinuing:
- Parkinson's disease—Don't discontinue without doctor's advice until you complete prescribed dose, even though symptoms diminish or disappear.
- Type-A flu—Discontinue 48 hours after symptoms disappear.

Others:
- Parkinson's disease—May lose effectiveness in 3 to 6 months. Consult doctor.
- These drugs are not effective for influenza-B virus.
- Drug-resistant strains of the virus may occur within the same household.

POSSIBLE INTERACTION WITH OTHER DRUGS

GENERIC NAME OR DRUG CLASS	COMBINED EFFECT
Acetaminophen	With rimantadine—Decreased antiviral effect.
Anticholinergics*	With amantadine—Increased benefit, but excessive anticholinergic dose produces mental confusion, hallucinations, delirium.
Antidepressants, tricyclic*	With amantadine—Increased risk of confusion, hallucinations, nightmares.
Antidyskinetics*	With amantadine—Increased risk of confusion, hallucinations, nightmares.
Antihistamines*	With amantadine—Increased risk of confusion, hallucinations, nightmares.
Aspirin	With rimantadine—Decreased antiviral effect.
Central nervous system (CNS) stimulants*	With amantadine—Increased risk of adverse reactions.
Levodopa	With amantadine—Increased benefit of levodopa. Can cause agitation.

POSSIBLE INTERACTION WITH OTHER SUBSTANCES

INTERACTS WITH	COMBINED EFFECT
Alcohol:	Increased alcohol effect. Possible fainting.
Beverages:	None expected.
Cocaine:	Dangerous overstimulation.
Foods:	None expected.
Marijuana:	None expected.
Tobacco:	None expected.

*See Glossary

ANTIVIRALS (Ophthalmic)

BRAND AND GENERIC NAMES

Herplex Eye Drops
IDOXURIDINE DROPS & OINTMENT
Liquifilm
Stoxil Eye Ointment
TRIFLURIDINE
Trifluorothymidine
Viroptic

BASIC INFORMATION

Habit forming? No
Prescription needed? Yes
Available as generic? No
Drug class: Antiviral (ophthalmic)

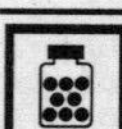

USES

Treats virus infections of the eye (usually herpes simplex virus).

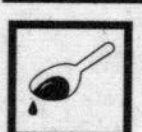

DOSAGE & USAGE INFORMATION

How to use:

Eye drops

- Wash hands.
- Apply pressure to inside corner of eye with middle finger.
- Continue pressure for 1 minute after placing medicine in eye.
- Tilt head backward. Pull lower lid away from eye with index finger of the same hand.
- Drop eye drops into pouch and close eye. Don't blink.
- Keep eyes closed for 1 to 2 minutes.

Eye ointment

- Wash hands.
- Pull lower lid down from eye to form a pouch.
- Squeeze tube to apply thin strip of ointment into pouch.
- Close eye for 1 to 2 minutes.
- Don't touch applicator tip to any surface (including the eye). If you accidentally touch tip, clean with warm soap and water.
- Keep container tightly closed.
- Keep cool, but don't freeze.
- Wash hands immediately after using.

Continued next column

OVERDOSE

SYMPTOMS:
None expected.
WHAT TO DO:
Not intended for internal use. If child accidentally swallows, call poison control center.

When to use:
As directed. Usually 1 drop every 2 hours up to maximum of 9 drops daily.

If you forget a dose:
Use as soon as you remember.

What drug does:
Destroys reproductive capacity of virus.

Time lapse before drug works:
Begins work immediately. Usual course of treatment is 7 days.

Don't use with:
Other eye drops, boric acid or ointment without consulting doctor.

POSSIBLE ADVERSE REACTIONS OR SIDE EFFECTS

SYMPTOMS	WHAT TO DO
Life-threatening	
None expected.	
Common	
Stinging or burning eyes.	Continue. Tell doctor at next visit.
Infrequent	
Blurred vision for a few minutes (with ointment).	No action necessary.
Rare	
Itchy, red eyes; swollen eyelid or eye; excess flow of tears; dimming or haziness of vision.	Discontinue. Call doctor right away.

WARNINGS & PRECAUTIONS

Don't use if:
You are allergic to trifluridine or idoxuridine.

Before you start, consult your doctor:
- If you have had any other eye problems.
- If you use eye drops for glaucoma.

Over age 60:
No problems expected.

Pregnancy:
Risk factors vary for drugs in this group. See category list on page xxii and consult doctor.

Breast-feeding:
No problems expected, but safety not established. Consult doctor.

Infants & children:
Use only under close medical supervision.

Prolonged use:
Avoid unless directed by your eye doctor.

Skin & sunlight:
No problems expected.

Driving, piloting or hazardous work:
No problems expected.

Discontinuing:
Don't discontinue without consulting doctor.

Others:
- Don't use more often or longer than prescribed.
- Keep cool, but don't freeze.
- If problem doesn't improve within a week, notify your doctor.

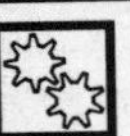

POSSIBLE INTERACTION WITH OTHER DRUGS

GENERIC NAME OR DRUG CLASS	COMBINED EFFECT
Eye products containing boric acid	Increased risk of toxicity to eye.

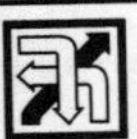

POSSIBLE INTERACTION WITH OTHER SUBSTANCES

INTERACTS WITH	COMBINED EFFECT
Alcohol:	None expected.
Beverages:	None expected.
Cocaine:	None expected.
Foods:	None expected.
Marijuana:	None expected.
Tobacco:	None expected.

*See Glossary

APPETITE SUPPRESSANTS

BRAND AND GENERIC NAMES

See complete list of brand and generic names in the *Brand Name Directory*, page 900.

BASIC INFORMATION

Habit forming? Yes
Prescription needed? Yes
Available as generic? Yes
Drug class: Appetite suppressant

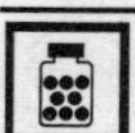

USES

Suppresses appetite. Treatment for obesity.

DOSAGE & USAGE INFORMATION

How to take:

- Tablet or capsule—Swallow with liquid. You may chew or crush tablet.
- Extended-release tablets or capsules—Swallow each dose whole with liquid; do not crush.
- Elixir—Swallow with liquid.

When to take:

- Long-acting forms—10 to 14 hours before bedtime.
- Short-acting forms—1 hour before meals. Last dose no later than 4 to 6 hours before bedtime.

If you forget a dose:

- Long-acting form—Take as soon as you remember up to 2 hours late. If more than 2 hours, wait for next scheduled dose (don't double this dose).
- Short-acting form—Wait for next scheduled dose. Don't double this dose.

What drug does:

Apparently stimulates brain's appetite control center.

Continued next column

OVERDOSE

SYMPTOMS:
Irritability, overactivity, trembling, insomnia, mood changes, fever, rapid heartbeat, confusion, disorientation, hallucinations, convulsions, coma.
WHAT TO DO:

- **Dial 911 (emergency) or 0 (operator) for an ambulance or medical help. Then give first aid immediately.**
- **See emergency information on inside covers.**

Time lapse before drug works:

Begins in 1 hour. Short-acting form lasts 4 hours. Long-acting form lasts 14 hours.

Don't take with:

- Nonprescription drugs without consulting doctor.
- See Interaction column and consult doctor.

POSSIBLE ADVERSE REACTIONS OR SIDE EFFECTS

SYMPTOMS	WHAT TO DO
Life-threatening:	
In case of overdose, see previous column.	
Common:	
Irritability, nervousness, insomnia, false sense of well-being.	Continue. Call doctor when convenient.
Infrequent:	
• Irregular or pounding heartbeat, urgent or difficult urination.	Discontinue. Call doctor right away.
• Blurred vision, unpleasant taste or dry mouth, constipation or diarrhea, nausea, vomiting, cramps, changes in sex drive, increased sweating, headache, nightmares, weakness.	Continue. Call doctor when convenient.
Rare:	
• Rash or hives, breathing difficulty.	Discontinue. Call doctor right away.
• Hair loss.	Continue. Call doctor when convenient.

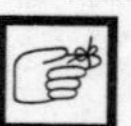

WARNINGS & PRECAUTIONS

Don't take if:

- You are allergic to any sympathomimetic or phenylpropanolamine.
- You have glaucoma.
- You have taken MAO inhibitors within 2 weeks.
- You plan to become pregnant within medication period.
- You have a history of drug or alcohol abuse.
- You have irregular or rapid heartbeat.

APPETITE SUPPRESSANTS

Before you start, consult your doctor:
- If you have high blood pressure or heart disease.
- If you have an overactive thyroid, nervous tension or anxiety.
- If you have epilepsy.
- If you will have surgery within 2 months, including dental surgery, requiring general or spinal anesthesia.
- If you take any other over-the-counter medicine.

Over age 60:
Adverse reactions and side effects may be more frequent and severe than in younger persons.

Pregnancy:
Risk factors vary for drugs in this group. See category list on page xxii and consult doctor.

Breast-feeding:
Safety not established. Consult doctor.

Infants & children:
Don't give to children younger than 12.

Prolonged use:
- Loses effectiveness. Avoid.
- Talk to your doctor about the need for follow-up medical examinations or laboratory studies.

Skin & sunlight:
No problems expected.

Driving, piloting or hazardous work:
Don't drive or pilot aircraft until you learn how medicine affects you. Don't work around dangerous machinery. Don't climb ladders or work in high places. Danger increases if you drink alcohol or take medicine affecting alertness and reflexes, such as antihistamines, tranquilizers, sedatives, pain medicine, narcotics and mind-altering drugs.

Discontinuing:
Don't discontinue without consulting doctor. Dose may require gradual reduction if you have taken drug for a long time. Doses of other drugs may also require adjustment.

Others:
- Don't increase dose.
- Advise any doctor or dentist whom you consult that you take this medicine.

POSSIBLE INTERACTION WITH OTHER DRUGS

GENERIC NAME OR DRUG CLASS	COMBINED EFFECT
Antidiabetic agents*, oral or insulin	May require dosage adjustment of antidiabetic agent.
Antihypertensives*	Decreased antihypertensive effect.
Appetite suppressants, other*	Dangerous overstimulation.
Caffeine	Increased stimulant effect.
Central nervous system (CNS) depressants*	Increased depressive effects of both drugs.
Central nervous system (CNS) stimulants*	Increased stimulant effects of both drugs.
Furazolidine	Sudden severe increase in blood pressure.
Guanethidine	Decreased guanethidine effect.
Hydralazine	Decreased hydralazine effect.
Methyldopa	Decreased methyldopa effect.
Molindone	Decreased suppressant effect.
Monoamine oxidase (MAO) inhibitors*	Dangerous blood pressure rise.
Phenothiazines*	Decreased appetite suppressant effect.
Rauwolfia alkaloids*	Decreased effect of rauwolfia alkaloids.
Sodium bicarbonate	Increased action of appetite suppressants.

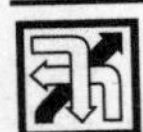

POSSIBLE INTERACTION WITH OTHER SUBSTANCES

INTERACTS WITH	COMBINED EFFECT
Alcohol: Beer, Chianti wines, vermouth.	Increased sedation.
Beverages:	
• Caffeine drinks.	Excessive stimulation.
• Drinks containing tyramine.*	Blood-pressure rise.
Cocaine:	Convulsions or excessive nervousness.
Foods: Foods containing tyramine.*	Blood pressure rise.
Marijuana:	Frequent use—Irregular heartbeat.
Tobacco:	None expected.

*See Glossary

ASPIRIN

BRAND NAMES

See complete list of brand names in the *Brand Name Directory*, page 901.

BASIC INFORMATION

Habit forming? No
Prescription needed? No
Available as generic? Yes
Drug class: Analgesic, anti-inflammatory (nonsteroidal)

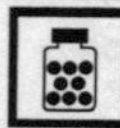

USES

- Reduces pain, fever, inflammation.
- Relieves swelling, stiffness, joint pain of arthritis or rheumatism.
- Antiplatelet effect to reduce chances of heart attack and/or stroke.

DOSAGE & USAGE INFORMATION

How to take:
- Tablet or capsule—Swallow with liquid or food to lessen stomach irritation.
- Extended-release tablets or capsules—Swallow each dose whole.
- Effervescent tablets—Dissolve in water.
- Chewing gum tablets—Chew completely. Don't swallow whole.
- Suppositories—Remove wrapper and moisten suppository with water. Gently insert into rectum, large end first.

When to take:
Pain, fever, inflammation—As needed, no more often than every 4 hours.

If you forget a dose:
- Pain, fever—Take as soon as you remember. Wait 4 hours for next dose.
- Arthritis—Take as soon as you remember up to 2 hours late. Return to regular schedule.

Continued next column

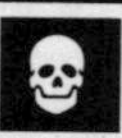

OVERDOSE

SYMPTOMS:
Ringing in ears; nausea; vomiting; dizziness; fever; deep, rapid breathing; hallucinations; convulsions; coma.
WHAT TO DO:
- **Dial 911 (emergency) or 0 (operator) for an ambulance or medical help. Then give first aid immediately.**
- **See emergency information on inside covers.**

What drug does:
- Affects hypothalamus, the part of the brain which regulates temperature by dilating small blood vessels in skin.
- Prevents clumping of platelets (small blood cells) so blood vessels remain open.
- Decreases prostaglandin effect.
- Suppresses body's pain messages.

Time lapse before drug works:
30 minutes for pain, fever, arthritis.

Don't take with:
- Tetracyclines. Space doses 1 hour apart.
- Any other medicine without consulting your doctor or pharmacist.

POSSIBLE ADVERSE REACTIONS OR SIDE EFFECTS

SYMPTOMS	WHAT TO DO
Life-threatening:	
Black or bloody vomit; blood in urine; difficulty breathing; hives, rash, intense itching, faintness soon after a dose (anaphylaxis).	Seek emergency treatment immediately.
Common:	
Heartburn, indigestion, mild nausea or vomiting.	Continue. Call doctor when convenient.
Infrequent:	
Trouble sleeping; rectal irritation (with suppository).	Continue. Call doctor when convenient.
Rare:	
Severe headache, convulsions, extreme drowsiness, flushing or other change in skin color, any loss of hearing, severe vomiting, swelling of face, vision problems, bloody or black stools, ringing in ears, severe stomach cramps or pain (all symptoms more likely with repeated doses for long periods since aspirin can build up in the body).	Discontinue. Call doctor right away or seek emergency treatment

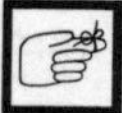

WARNINGS & PRECAUTIONS

Don't take if:
- You need to restrict sodium in your diet. Buffered effervescent tablets and sodium salicylate are high in sodium.
- You are sensitive to aspirin or aspirin has a strong vinegar-like odor, which means it has decomposed.
- You have a peptic ulcer of stomach or duodenum or a bleeding disorder.

Before you start, consult your doctor:
- If you have had stomach or duodenal ulcers.
- If you have had gout.
- If you have asthma or nasal polyps.
- If you have kidney or liver disease.

Over age 60:
More likely to cause hidden bleeding in stomach or intestines. Watch for dark stools.

Pregnancy:
Risk category C; D in third trimester (see page xxii). Consult doctor.

Breast-feeding:
Drug passes into milk. Avoid drug or discontinue nursing until you finish medicine. Consult doctor for advice on maintaining milk supply.

Infants & children:
- Overdose frequent and severe. Keep bottles out of children's reach.
- Consult doctor before giving to persons under age 18 who have fever and discomfort of viral illness, especially chicken pox and influenza. Probably increases risk of Reye's syndrome.

Prolonged use:
Talk to your doctor about the need for follow-up medical examinations or laboratory studies to check liver function, complete blood counts (white blood cell count, platelet count, red blood cell count, hemoglobin, hematocrit).

Skin & sunlight:
Aspirin combined with sunscreen may decrease sunburn.

Driving, piloting or hazardous work:
No restrictions unless you feel drowsy.

Discontinuing:
For chronic illness—Don't discontinue without doctor's advice until you complete prescribed dose, even though symptoms diminish or disappear.

Others:
- Aspirin can complicate surgery, pregnancy, labor and delivery, and illness.
- For arthritis—Don't change dose without consulting doctor.
- Urine tests for blood sugar may be inaccurate.
- Don't take if pills have vinegar-like odor.

POSSIBLE INTERACTION WITH OTHER DRUGS

GENERIC NAME OR DRUG CLASS	COMBINED EFFECT
Acebutolol	Decreased anti-hypertensive effect of acebutolol.
Allopurinol	Decreased allopurinol effect.
Angiotensin-converting enzyme (ACE) inhibitors*	Decreased ACE inhibitor effect.
Antacids*	Decreased aspirin effect.
Anticoagulants*	Increased anti-coagulant effect. Abnormal bleeding.
Antidiabetic agents, oral*	Low blood sugar.
Anti-inflammatory drugs nonsteroidal (NSAIDs)*	Risk of stomach bleeding and ulcers.
Bumetanide	Possible aspirin toxicity.
Carteolol	Decreased anti-hypertensive effect of carteolol.
Cortisone drugs*	Increased cortisone effect. Risk of ulcers and stomach bleeding.
Dextrothyroxine (large doses, continuous use)	Increased dextrothyroxine effect.
Diclofenac	Increased risk of stomach ulcer.
Ethacrynic acid	Possible aspirin toxicity.
Furosemide	Possible aspirin toxicity. May decrease furosemide effect.
Gold compounds*	Increased likelihood of kidney damage.

Continued on page 927

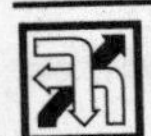

POSSIBLE INTERACTION WITH OTHER SUBSTANCES

INTERACTS WITH	COMBINED EFFECT
Alcohol:	Possible stomach irritation and bleeding. Avoid.
Beverages:	None expected.
Cocaine:	None expected.
Foods:	None expected.
Marijuana:	Possible increased pain relief, but marijuana may slow body's recovery. Avoid.
Tobacco:	None expected.

***See Glossary**

ATOVAQUONE

BRAND NAMES

Mepron

BASIC INFORMATION

Habit forming? No
Prescription needed? Yes
Available as generic? No
Drug class: Antiprotozoal

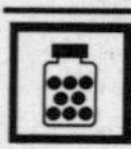

USES

- Treats mild to moderate pneumocystis carinii pneumonia.
- May be effective for other parasitic infections such as toxoplasmosis and malaria.

DOSAGE & USAGE INFORMATION

How to take:
Tablet–Swallow with liquid. If you cannot swallow whole, crumble tablet and take with liquid or food.

When to take:
At the same times each day. Take with meals that are high in fat (eggs, cheese, butter, milk, meat, pizza, nuts) to increase absorption.

If you forget a dose:
Take as soon as you remember up to 2 hours late. If more than 2 hours, wait for next scheduled dose (don't double this dose).

What drug does:
Stops harmful growth of susceptible organisms.

Time lapse before drug works:
3 weeks.

Don't take with:
Any other prescription or nonprescription drug without consulting your doctor or pharmacist.

OVERDOSE

SYMPTOMS:
None expected.
WHAT TO DO:
Overdose unlikely to threaten life. If person takes much larger amount than prescribed, call doctor, poison control center or hospital emergency room for instructions.

POSSIBLE ADVERSE REACTIONS OR SIDE EFFECTS

SYMPTOMS	WHAT TO DO
Life-threatening: None expected.	
Common:	
• Fever, skin rash.	Discontinue. Call doctor right away.
• Nausea or vomiting, diarrhea, headache, cough, trouble sleeping.	Continue. Call doctor when convenient.
Infrequent: None expected.	
Rare: None expected	

WARNINGS & PRECAUTIONS

Don't take if:
You are allergic to atovaquone.

Before you start, consult your doctor:
If you have any gastrointestinal disorder.

Over age 60:
No problems expected.

Pregnancy:
Discuss with your doctor whether drug benefits justify risk to unborn child. Risk category C (see page xxii).

Breast-feeding:
Not known if drug passes into breast milk. Avoid drug or discontinue nursing until you finish medicine. Consult doctor for advice on maintaining milk supply.

Infants & children:
Give only under close medical supervision.

Prolonged use:
Not intended for long-term use.

Skin & sunlight:
No problems expected.

Driving, piloting or hazardous work:
No problems expected.

Discontinuing:
No problems expected.

Others:
- Advise any doctor or dentist whom you consult that you take this medicine.
- May affect the results in some medical tests.
- Talk to your doctor about the need for follow-up medical examinations or laboratory studies to check blood counts and liver function.

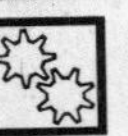

POSSIBLE INTERACTION WITH OTHER DRUGS

GENERIC NAME OR DRUG CLASS	COMBINED EFFECT
None significant.	

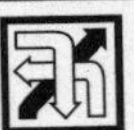

POSSIBLE INTERACTION WITH OTHER SUBSTANCES

INTERACTS WITH	COMBINED EFFECT
Alcohol:	None expected.
Beverages:	None expected.
Cocaine:	None expected.
Foods:	None expected.
Marijuana:	None expected.
Tobacco:	None expected.

ATROPINE, HYOSCYAMINE, METHENAMINE, METHYLENE BLUE, PHENYLSALICYLATE & BENZOIC ACID

BRAND NAMES

Atrosept
Dolsed
Hexalol
Prosed/DS
Trac Tabs 2X
U-Tract
UAA
Uridon Modified
Urimed
Urinary Antiseptic No. 2
Urised
Uriseptic
Uritab
Uritin
Uro-Ves

BASIC INFORMATION

Habit forming? No
Prescription needed? Yes
Available as generic? No
Drug class: Analgesic (urinary), anti-spasmodic, anti-infective (urinary)

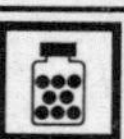

USES

A combination medicine to control infection, spasms and pain caused by urinary tract infections.

DOSAGE & USAGE INFORMATION

How to take:
Tablet—Swallow with liquid or food to lessen stomach irritation.

When to take:
30 minutes before meals (unless directed otherwise by doctor).

If you forget a dose:
Take as soon as you remember up to 2 hours late. If more than 2 hours, wait for next scheduled dose (don't double this dose).

Continued next column

OVERDOSE

SYMPTOMS:
Dilated pupils, rapid pulse and breathing, dizziness, fever, hallucinations, confusion, slurred speech, agitation, flushed face, convulsions, coma.
WHAT TO DO:
- **Dial 911 (emergency) or 0 (operator) for an ambulance or medical help. Then give first aid immediately.**
- **See emergency information on inside covers.**

What drug does:
Makes urine acid. Blocks nerve impulses at parasympathetic nerve endings, preventing muscle contractions and gland secretions of organs involved. Methenamine destroys some germs.

Time lapse before drug works:
15 to 30 minutes.

Don't take with:
- Antacids* or antidiarrheals*.
- Any other medicine without consulting your doctor or pharmacist.

POSSIBLE ADVERSE REACTIONS OR SIDE EFFECTS

SYMPTOMS	WHAT TO DO
Life-threatening:	
Heartbeat irregularity, shortness of breath or difficulty breathing.	Seek emergency treatment immediately.
Common:	
Dry mouth, throat, ears, nose.	Continue. Call doctor when convenient.
Infrequent:	
• Flushed, red face; drowsiness; difficult urination; nausea and vomiting; abdominal pain; ringing or buzzing in ears; severe drowsiness; back pain; lightheadedness.	Discontinue. Call doctor right away.
• Headache, nasal congestion, altered taste.	Continue. Call doctor when convenient.
Rare:	
Blurred vision; pain in eyes; skin rash, hives.	Discontinue. Seek emergency treatment.

WARNINGS & PRECAUTIONS

Don't take if:
- You are allergic to any of the ingredients or aspirin.
- Brain damage in child.
- You have glaucoma.

Before you start, consult your doctor:
- If you are on any special diet such as low-sodium.
- If you have had a hiatal hernia, bronchitis, asthma, liver disease, stomach or duodenal ulcers.
- If you have asthma, nasal polyps, bleeding disorder, glaucoma or enlarged prostate.
- If you will have any surgery within 2 months.
- If you have heart disease.

ATROPINE, HYOSCYAMINE, METHENAMINE, METHYLENE BLUE, PHENYLSALICYLATE & BENZOIC ACID

Over age 60:
- Adverse reactions and side effects may be more frequent and severe than in younger persons.
- More likely to cause hidden bleeding in stomach or intestines. Watch for dark stools.

Pregnancy:
Risk factors vary for drugs in this group. See category list on page xxii and consult doctor.

Breast-feeding:
Drug passes into milk. Avoid or discontinue nursing until you finish medicine.

Infants & children:
Side effects more likely. Not recommended in children under 12.

Prolonged use:
May lead to constipation or kidney damage. Request lab studies to monitor effects of prolonged use.

Skin & sunlight:
No problems expected.

Driving, piloting or hazardous work:
May disqualify for piloting aircraft during time you take medicine.

Discontinuing:
May be unnecessary to finish medicine. Follow your symptoms and doctor's advice.

Others:
- Salicylates can complicate surgery, pregnancy, labor and delivery, and illness.
- Urine tests for blood sugar may be inaccurate.
- Drink cranberry juice or eat prunes or plums to help make urine more acid.

POSSIBLE INTERACTION WITH OTHER DRUGS

GENERIC NAME OR DRUG CLASS	COMBINED EFFECT
Allopurinol	Decreased allopurinol effect.
Amantadine	Increased atropine and belladonna effect.
Antacids*	Decreased salicylate and methenamine effect.
Anticoagulants*	Increased anti-coagulant effect. Abnormal bleeding.
Anticholinergics, other*	Increased atropine and belladonna effect.
Antidepressants, other*	Increased sedation.
Antidiabetics, oral*	Low blood sugar.
Antihistamines*	Increased atropine and hyoscyamine effect.
Anti-inflammatory drugs, nonsteroidal (NSAIDs)*	Risk of stomach bleeding and ulcers.
Aspirin	Likely salicylate toxicity.
Beta-adrenergic blocking agents*	Decreased anti-hypertensive effect.
Carbonic anhydrase inhibitors*	Decreased methenamine effect.
Cortisone drugs*	Increased internal eye pressure, increased cortisone effect. Risk of ulcers and stomach bleeding.
Diuretics, thiazide*	Decreased urine acidity.
Furosemide	Possible salicylate toxicity.
Gold compounds*	Increased likelihood of kidney damage.
Haloperidol	Increased internal eye pressure.

*See Glossary

Continued on page 927

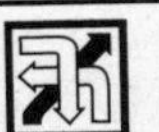

POSSIBLE INTERACTION WITH OTHER SUBSTANCES

INTERACTS WITH	COMBINED EFFECT
Alcohol:	Excessive sedation. Possible stomach irritation and bleeding. Avoid.
Beverages:	None expected.
Cocaine:	Excessively rapid heartbeat. Avoid.
Foods:	None expected.
Marijuana:	Drowsiness and dry mouth. May slow body's recovery.
Tobacco:	Dry mouth.

ATTAPULGITE

BRAND NAMES

Diar-Aid
Diasorb
Fowlers Diarrhea Tablets
Kaopectate
Kaopectate Advanced Formula
Kaopectate Maximum Strength
Rheaban
St. Joseph Antidiarrheal

BASIC INFORMATION

Habit forming? No
Prescription needed? No
Available as generic? Yes
Drug class: Antidiarrheal

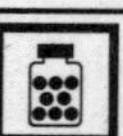

USES

Treats diarrhea. Used in conjunction with fluids, appropriate diet and rest. Treats symptoms only. Does not cure any disorder that causes diarrhea.

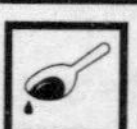

DOSAGE & USAGE INFORMATION

How to take:

- Tablets—Swallow with liquid. If you can't swallow whole, crumble tablet and take with liquid or food. Instructions to take on empty stomach mean 1 hour before or 2 hours after eating.
- Chewable tablets—Chew well before swallowing.

When to take:
2 hours before or 3 hours after taking any other oral medications. Outside of this restriction, take a dose after each loose bowel movement until diarrhea is controlled.

If you forget a dose:
Take as soon as you remember, then resume regular schedule.

What drug does:
Absorbs bacteria and toxins and reduces water loss. Attapulgite does not get absorbed into the body.

Continued next column

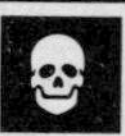

OVERDOSE

SYMPTOMS:
None expected.
WHAT TO DO:
Overdose unlikely to threaten life. If person takes much larger amount than prescribed, call doctor, poison control center or hospital emergency room for instructions.

Time lapse before drug works:
5 to 8 hours.

Don't take with:
See Interaction column and consult doctor.

POSSIBLE ADVERSE REACTIONS OR SIDE EFFECTS

SYMPTOMS	WHAT TO DO
Life-threatening: None expected.	
Common: None expected.	
Infrequent: Constipation (usually mild and of short duration).	Continue. Call doctor when convenient.
Rare: None expected.	

WARNINGS & PRECAUTIONS

Don't take if:
- You are allergic to attapulgite.
- You or your doctor suspects intestinal obstruction.

Before you start, consult your doctor:
If you are dehydrated (signs are a dry mouth, loose skin, sunken eyes and parched lips).

Over age 60:
- Dehydration is more likely in this age group.
- Side effects of constipation are more likely.

Pregnancy:
Risk category not designated. See list on page xxii and consult doctor.

Breast-feeding:
No problems expected, but consult doctor.

Infants & children:
Use only under close medical supervision for children up to 3 years of age. This age group is quite susceptible to fluid and electrolyte loss.

Prolonged use:
Not intended for prolonged use.

Skin & sunlight:
No special problems expected.

Driving, piloting or hazardous work:
No special problems expected.

Discontinuing:
May be unnecessary to finish medicine. Follow doctor's instructions.

Others:
No special problems expected.

POSSIBLE INTERACTION WITH OTHER DRUGS

GENERIC NAME OR DRUG CLASS	COMBINED EFFECT
Digitalis	May decrease effectiveness of digitalis.
Lincomycin*	May decrease effectiveness of lincomycins.
Any other medicine taken by mouth	When taken at the same time, neither drug may be as effective. Take other medicines 2 hours before or 3 hours after attapulgite.

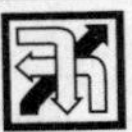

POSSIBLE INTERACTION WITH OTHER SUBSTANCES

INTERACTS WITH	COMBINED EFFECT
Alcohol:	No proven problems.
Beverages:	No proven problems.
Cocaine:	No proven problems.
Foods: Prunes, prune juice and other fruits or foods that may cause diarrhea.	Decreased effect of attapulgite.
Marijuana:	No proven problems.
Tobacco:	No proven problems.

*See Glossary

AZATHIOPRINE

BRAND NAMES

Imuran

BASIC INFORMATION

Habit forming? No
Prescription needed? Yes
Available as generic? Yes
Drug class: Immunosuppressant, antirheumatic

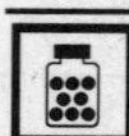

USES

- Protects against rejection of transplanted organs (e.g., kidney, heart).
- Treats severe active rheumatoid arthritis and other immunologic diseases if simpler treatment plans have been ineffective.

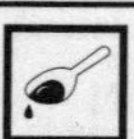

DOSAGE & USAGE INFORMATION

How to take:
Tablets—Swallow with liquid. If you can't swallow whole, crumble tablet and take with liquid or food. Instructions to take on empty stomach mean 1 hour before or 2 hours after eating.

When to take:
Follow your doctor's instructions. Usually once a day.

If you forget a dose:
Take as soon as you remember up to 2 hours late. If more than 2 hours, wait for next scheduled dose (don't double this dose).

What drug does:
Unknown; probably inhibits synthesis of DNA and RNA.

Time lapse before drug works:
6 to 8 weeks.

Don't take with:
Any other medicines (including over-the-counter drugs such as cough and cold medicines, laxatives, antacids, diet pills, caffeine, nose drops or vitamins) without consulting your doctor.

OVERDOSE

SYMPTOMS:
None expected.
WHAT TO DO:
Overdose unlikely to threaten life. If person takes much larger amount than prescribed, call doctor, poison control center or hospital emergency room for instructions.

POSSIBLE ADVERSE REACTIONS OR SIDE EFFECTS

SYMPTOMS	WHAT TO DO
Life-threatening:	
Rapid heart rate, sudden fever, muscle or joint pain, cough, shortness of breath.	Seek emergency treatment immediately.
Common:	
• Infection or low blood count causing fever and chills, back pain cough, painful urination; anemia (tiredness or weakness); nausea; vomiting.	Discontinue. Call doctor right away.
• Appetite loss.	Continue. Call doctor when convenient.
Infrequent:	
Jaundice (yellow eyes, skin), skin rash.	Discontinue. Call doctor right away.
Rare:	
Low platelet count causing bleeding or bruising, tarry or black stools, bloody urine, red spots under skin; severe abdominal pain; mouth sores.	Discontinue. Call doctor right away.

WARNINGS & PRECAUTIONS

Don't take if:
- You are allergic to azathioprine
- You have chicken pox.
- You have shingles (herpes zoster).

Before you start, consult your doctor:
- If you have gout.
- If you have liver or kidney disease.
- If you have an infection.

Over age 60:
Adverse reactions and side effects may be more frequent and severe than in younger persons. You may need smaller doses for shorter periods of time.

Pregnancy:
Risk to unborn child outweighs drug benefits. Don't use. Risk category D (see page xxii).

Breast-feeding:
Drug passes into milk. Avoid drug or discontinue nursing until you finish medicine. Consult doctor for advice on maintaining milk supply.

Infants & children:
No special problems expected.

Prolonged use:
- May increase likelihood of problems upon discontinuing.
- Talk to your doctor about the need for follow-up medical examinations or laboratory studies to check thyroid function, liver function, electrolytes (sodium potassium, chloride), blood pressure and complete blood counts (white blood count, platelet count, red blood cell count, hemoglobin, hematocrit) every week during first two months, then once a month.

Skin & sunlight:
No special problems expected.

Driving, piloting or hazardous work:
Avoid if you feel confused, drowsy or dizzy.

Discontinuing:
May still experience symptoms of bone marrow depression, such as: blood in stools, fever or chills, blood spots under the skin, back pain, hoarseness, bloody urine. If any of these occur, call your doctor right away.

Others:
- Advise any doctor or dentist whom you consult that you take this medicine.
- May affect results in some medical tests.

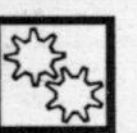

POSSIBLE INTERACTION WITH OTHER DRUGS

GENERIC NAME OR DRUG CLASS	COMBINED EFFECT
Allopurinol	Greatly increased azathioprine activity.
Clozapine	Toxic effect on bone marrow.
Didanosine	Increased risk of pancreatitis.
Tiopronin	Increased risk of toxicity to bone marrow.
Immunosuppressants, other*	Higher risk of developing infection or malignancies.
Levamisole	Increased risk of bone marrow depression.
Vaccines	May decrease effectiveness or cause disease itself.

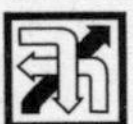

POSSIBLE INTERACTION WITH OTHER SUBSTANCES

INTERACTS WITH	COMBINED EFFECT
Alcohol:	No special problems expected.
Beverages:	No special problems expected.
Cocaine:	Increased likelihood of adverse reactions. Avoid.
Foods:	No special problems expected.
Marijuana:	Increased likelihood of adverse reactions. Avoid.
Tobacco:	No special problems expected.

*See Glossary

AZITHROMYCIN

BRAND NAMES

Zithromax

BASIC INFORMATION

Habit forming? No
Prescription needed? Yes
Available as generic? No
Drug class: Antibiotic (erythromycin)

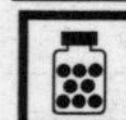

USES

Treatment for mild to moderate bacterial infections responsive to azithromycin.

DOSAGE & USAGE INFORMATION

How to take:
Capsule–Swallow with liquid. Take 1 hour before or 2 hours after meals.

When to take:
At the same time each day.

If you forget a dose:
Take as soon as you remember up to 12 hours late. If more than 12 hours, wait for next scheduled dose (don't double this dose).

What drug does:
Prevents growth and reproduction of susceptible bacteria.

Time lapse before drug works:
2-5 days.

Don't take with:
Any other prescription or nonprescription drug without consulting your doctor or pharmacist.

OVERDOSE

SYMPTOMS:
None reported.
WHAT TO DO:
Overdose unlikely to threaten life. If person takes much larger amount than prescribed, call doctor, poison control center or hospital emergency room for instructions.

POSSIBLE ADVERSE REACTIONS OR SIDE EFFECTS

SYMPTOMS	WHAT TO DO
Life-threatening:	
Rare allergic reaction (breathing difficulty; swelling of hands, feet, face, mouth, neck; skin rash).	Discontinue. Seek emergency treatment.
Common:	
None expected.	
Infrequent:	
Nausea, vomiting, abdominal pain, diarrhea.	Continue. Call doctor when convenient.
Rare:	
Headache, dizziness.	Continue. Call doctor when convenient.

WARNINGS & PRECAUTIONS

Don't take if:
You are allergic to erythromycins or other macrolides*.

Before you start, consult your doctor:
- If you have impaired liver function.
- If you have hypersensitivity*.

Over age 60:
Adverse reactions and side effects may be more frequent and severe than in younger persons.

Pregnancy:
No problems expected. Consult doctor. Risk category B (see page xxii).

Breast-feeding:
Unknown effect. Consult doctor.

Infants & children:
Give only under close medical supervision to those under age 16.

Prolonged use:
Not recommended.

Skin & sunlight:
No problems expected.

Driving, piloting or hazardous work:
Avoid if you feel dizzy. Otherwise, no problems expected.

Discontinuing:
No problems expected.

Others:
No problems expected.

POSSIBLE INTERACTION WITH OTHER DRUGS

GENERIC NAME OR DRUG CLASS	COMBINED EFFECT
Antacids*, aluminum- or magnesium-containing	Decreased azithromycin effect.

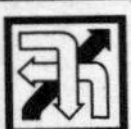

POSSIBLE INTERACTION WITH OTHER SUBSTANCES

INTERACTS WITH	COMBINED EFFECT
Alcohol:	None expected.
Beverages:	None expected.
Cocaine:	None expected.
Foods:	None expected.
Marijuana:	None expected.
Tobacco:	None expected.

***See Glossary**

BACLOFEN

BRAND NAMES

Lioresal

BASIC INFORMATION

Habit forming? No
Prescription needed? Yes
Available as generic? Yes
Drug class: Muscle relaxant for multiple sclerosis

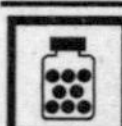

USES

- Relieves spasms, cramps and spasticity of muscles caused by medical problems, including multiple sclerosis and spine injuries.
- Reduces number and severity of trigeminal neuralgia attacks.

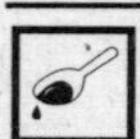

DOSAGE & USAGE INFORMATION

How to take:
Tablet—Swallow with liquid or food to lessen stomach irritation.

When to take:
3 or 4 times daily as directed.

If you forget a dose:
Take as soon as you remember up to 2 hours late. If more than 2 hours, wait for next scheduled dose (don't double this dose).

What drug does:
Blocks body's pain and reflex messages to brain.

Time lapse before drug works:
Variable. Few hours to weeks.

Continued next column

OVERDOSE

SYMPTOMS:
Blurred vision, blindness, difficult breathing, vomiting, drowsiness, muscle weakness, convulsive seizures.
WHAT TO DO:
- **Dial 911 (emergency) or 0 (operator) for an ambulance or medical help. Then give first aid immediately.**
- **If patient is unconscious and not breathing, give mouth-to-mouth breathing. If there is no heartbeat, use cardiac massage and mouth-to-mouth breathing (CPR). Don't try to make patient vomit. If you can't get help quickly, take patient to nearest emergency facility.**
- **See emergency information on inside covers.**

Don't take with:
Any other medicine without consulting your doctor or pharmacist.

POSSIBLE ADVERSE REACTIONS OR SIDE EFFECTS

SYMPTOMS	WHAT TO DO
Life-threatening: In case of overdose, see previous column.	
Common: Dizziness, lightheadedness, confusion, insomnia, drowsiness, nausea.	Continue. Call doctor when convenient.
Infrequent:	
• Rash with itching, numbness or tingling in hands or feet.	Discontinue. Call doctor right away.
• Headache, abdominal pain, diarrhea or constipation, appetite loss, muscle weakness, difficult or painful urination, male sex problems, nasal congestion, clumsiness, slurred speech, insomnia.	Continue. Call doctor when convenient.
Rare:	
• Fainting, weakness, hallucinations, depression, chest pain, muscle pain, pounding heatbeat.	Discontinue. Call doctor right away.
• Ringing in ears, lowered blood pressure, dry mouth, taste disturbance, euphoria, weight gain.	Continue. Call doctor when convenient.

WARNINGS & PRECAUTIONS

Don't take if:
- You are allergic to any muscle relaxant.
- Muscle spasm due to strain or sprain.

Before you start, consult your doctor:
- If you have Parkinson's disease.
- If you have cerebral palsy.
- If you have had a recent stroke.
- If you have had a recent head injury.
- If you have arthritis.
- If you have diabetes.
- If you have epilepsy.
- If you have psychosis.
- If you have kidney disease.
- If you will have surgery within 2 months, including dental surgery, requiring general or spinal anesthesia.

Over age 60:
Adverse reactions and side effects may be more frequent and severe than in younger persons.

Pregnancy:
Decide with your doctor if drug benefits justify risk to unborn child. Risk category C (see page xxii).

Breast-feeding:
Avoid nursing or discontinue until you finish medicine. Consult doctor about maintaining milk supply.

Infants & children:
Not recommended.

Prolonged use:
Epileptic patients should be monitored with EEGs. Diabetics should more closely monitor blood sugar levels. Obtain periodic liver function tests.

Skin & sunlight:
No problems expected.

Driving, piloting or hazardous work:
Don't drive or pilot aircraft until you learn how medicine affects you. Don't work around dangerous machinery. Don't climb ladders or work in high places. Danger increases if you drink alcohol or take medicine affecting alertness and reflexes, such as antihistamines, tranquilizers, sedatives, pain medicine, narcotics and mind-altering drugs.

Discontinuing:
Don't discontinue without consulting doctor. Dose may require gradual reduction if you have taken drug for a long time. Doses of other drugs may also require adjustment.

Others:
No problems expected.

POSSIBLE INTERACTION WITH OTHER DRUGS

GENERIC NAME OR DRUG CLASS	COMBINED EFFECT
Anesthetics, general*	Increased sedation. Low blood pressure. Avoid.
Antidiabetic drugs*, insulin or oral	Need to adjust diabetes medicine dosage.
Central nervous system (CNS) depressants* (antidepressants,* antihistamines,* narcotics,* other muscle relaxants,* sedatives,* sleeping pills,* tranquilizers*)	Increased sedation Low blood pressure. Avoid.
Clozapine	Toxic effect on the central nervous system.
Ethinamate	Dangerous increased effects of ethinamate. Avoid combining.
Fluoxetine	Increased depressant effects of both drugs.
Guanfacine	May increase depressant effects of either drug.
Leucovorin	High alcohol content of leucovorin may cause adverse effects.
Methyprylon	Increased sedative effect, perhaps to dangerous level. Avoid.
Nabilone	Greater depression of the central nervous system.
Sertraline	Increased depressive effects of both drugs.

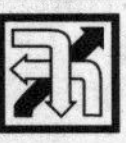

POSSIBLE INTERACTION WITH OTHER SUBSTANCES

INTERACTS WITH	COMBINED EFFECT
Alcohol:	Increased sedation. Low blood pressure. Avoid.
Beverages:	No problems expected.
Cocaine:	Increased spasticity. Avoid.
Foods:	No problems expected.
Marijuana:	Increased spasticity. Avoid.
Tobacco:	May interfere with absorption of medicine.

*See Glossary

BARBITURATES

BRAND AND GENERIC NAMES

See complete list of brand and generic names in the *Brand Names Directory*, page 901.

BASIC INFORMATION

Habit forming? Yes
Prescription needed? Yes
Available as generic? Yes, for some
Drug class: Sedative, hypnotic (barbiturate)

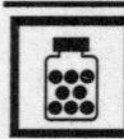

USES

- Reduces anxiety or nervous tension (low dose).
- Reduces likelihood of seizures in epilepsy.
- Aids sleep at night.

DOSAGE & USAGE INFORMATION

How to take:
- Capsule—Swallow with liquid. If you can't swallow whole, open capsule and take with liquid or food. Instructions to take on empty stomach mean 1 hour before or 2 hours after eating.
- Elixir—Swallow with liquid.
- Rectal suppositories—Remove wrapper and moisten suppository with water. Gently insert into rectum, large end first. If suppository is too soft, chill in refrigerator or cool water before removing wrapper.
- Tablet—Swallow with liquid or food to lessen stomach irritation. If you can't swallow whole, crumble tablet and take with liquid or food.

When to take:
At the same times each day.

Continued next column

OVERDOSE

SYMPTOMS:
Deep sleep, trouble breathing, weak pulse, coma.
WHAT TO DO:
- **Dial 911 (emergency) or 0 (operator) for an ambulance or medical help. Then give first aid immediately.**
- **If patient is unconscious and not breathing, give mouth-to-mouth breathing. If there is no heartbeat use cardiac massage and mouth-to-mouth breathing (CPR). Don't try to make patient vomit. If you can't get help quickly, take patient to nearest emergency facility.**
- **See emergency information on inside covers.**

If you forget a dose:
Take as soon as you remember up to 2 hours late. If more than 2 hours, wait for next scheduled dose (don't double this dose).

What drug does:
May partially block nerve impulses at nerve-cell connections.

Time lapse before drug works:
60 minutes.

Don't take with:
- Nonprescription drugs without consulting doctor.
- See Interaction column and consult doctor.

POSSIBLE ADVERSE REACTIONS OR SIDE EFFECTS

SYMPTOMS	WHAT TO DO
Life-threatening:	
In case of overdose, see previous column.	
Common:	
Dizziness, drowsiness, "hangover" effect.	Continue. Call doctor when convenient.
Infrequent:	
• Rash or hives; face, lip or eyelid swelling; sore throat; fever.	Discontinue. Call doctor right away.
• Depression, confusion, diarrhea, nausea, vomiting, joint or muscle pain, slurred speech, hallucinations, headache, decreased sex drive.	Continue. Call doctor when convenient.
Rare:	
• Agitation, slow heartbeat, difficult breathing, jaundice, chest pain.	Discontinue. Call doctor right away.
• Unexplained bleeding or bruising.	Continue. Call doctor when convenient.

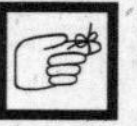

WARNINGS & PRECAUTIONS

Don't take if:
- You are allergic to any barbiturate.
- You have porphyria.

Before you start, consult your doctor:
- If you have epilepsy.
- If you have kidney or liver damage.
- If you have asthma.
- If you have anemia.
- If you have chronic pain.
- If you will have surgery within 2 months, including dental surgery, requiring general or spinal anesthesia.

Over age 60:
Adverse reactions and side effects may be more frequent and severe than in younger persons. Use small doses.

Pregnancy:
Risk to unborn child outweighs drug benefits. Don't use. Risk category D (see page xxii).

Breast-feeding:
Drug passes into milk. Avoid drug or discontinue nursing until you finish medicine. Consult doctor for advice on maintaining milk supply.

Infants & children:
Use only under doctor's supervision.

Prolonged use:
- May cause addiction, anemia, chronic intoxication.
- May lower body temperature, making exposure to cold temperatures hazardous.
- Talk to your doctor about the need for follow-up medical examinations or laboratory studies to check blood sugar, kidney function.

Skin & sunlight:
May cause rash or intensify sunburn in areas exposed to sun or sunlamp.

Driving, piloting or hazardous work:
Don't drive or pilot aircraft until you learn how medicine affects you. Don't work around dangerous machinery. Don't climb ladders or work in high places. Danger increases if you drink alcohol or take medicine affecting alertness and reflexes.

Discontinuing:
If you become addicted, don't stop taking barbiturates suddenly. Seek medical help for safe withdrawal.

Others:
- May affect results in some medical tests.
- Barbiturate addiction is common. Withdrawal effects may be fatal.
- Advise any doctor or dentist whom you consult that you take this medicine.

POSSIBLE INTERACTION WITH OTHER DRUGS

GENERIC NAME OR DRUG CLASS	COMBINED EFFECT
Anticoagulants, oral*	Decreased effect of anticoagulant.
Anticonvulsants*	Changed seizure patterns.
Antidepressants, tricyclic*	Decreased anti-depressant effect. Possible dangerous oversedation.
Antidiabetics, oral*	Increased effect of barbiturate.
Antihistamines*	Dangerous sedation. Avoid.
Aspirin	Decreased aspirin effect.
Beta-adrenergic blocking agents*	Decreased effect of beta-adrenergic blocker.
Carbamazepine	Decreased carba-mazepine effect.
Carteolol	Increased barbiturate effect. Dangerous sedation.
Clozapine	Toxic effect on the central nervous system.
Contraceptives, oral*	Decreased contraceptive effect.
Cortisone drugs*	Decreased cortisone effect.
Dextrothyroxine	Decreased barbiturate effect.
Divalproex	Dangerous sedation. Avoid.
Doxycycline	Decreased doxycycline effect.
Griseofulvin	Decreased griseofulvin effect.
Mind-altering drugs*	Dangerous sedation. Avoid.
Monoamine oxidase (MAO) inhibitors*	Increased barbiturate effect.
Nabilone	Greater depression of central nervous system.

Continued on page 928

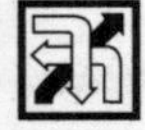

POSSIBLE INTERACTION WITH OTHER SUBSTANCES

INTERACTS WITH	COMBINED EFFECT
Alcohol:	Possible fatal oversedation. Avoid.
Beverages:	None expected.
Cocaine:	Decreased barbiturate effect.
Foods:	None expected.
Marijuana:	Excessive sedation. Avoid.
Tobacco:	None expected.

*See Glossary

BARBITURATES & ASPIRIN (Also contains caffeine)

BRAND AND GENERIC NAMES

See complete list of brand and generic names in the *Brand Names Directory*, page 901.

BASIC INFORMATION

Habit forming? Yes
Prescription needed? Yes
Available as generic? Yes
Drug class: Analgesic, anti-inflammatory (non-steroidal), sedative

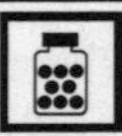

USES

- Reduces anxiety or nervous tension (low dose).
- Reduces pain, fever, inflammation.

DOSAGE & USAGE INFORMATION

How to take:
Tablet or capsule—Swallow with liquid or food to lessen stomach irritation. If you can't swallow whole, crumble tablet or open capsule and take with liquid or food.

When to take:
At the same times each day. No more often than every 4 hours.

If you forget a dose:
Take as soon as you remember up to 2 hours late. If more than 2 hours, wait for next scheduled dose (don't double this dose).

What drug does:
- May partially block nerve impulses at nerve cell connections.
- Affects hypothalamus, the part of the brain which regulates temperature by dilating small blood vessels in skin.
- Prevents clumping of platelets (small blood cells) so blood vessels remain open.
- Decreases prostaglandin effect.
- Suppresses body's pain messages.

Time lapse before drug works:
30 minutes.

Don't take with:
- Nonprescription drugs without consulting doctor.
- See Interaction column and consult doctor.

OVERDOSE

SYMPTOMS:
Deep sleep, weak pulse, ringing in ears, nausea, vomiting, dizziness, fever, deep and rapid breathing, hallucinations, convulsions, coma.
WHAT TO DO:
- **Dial 911 (emergency) or 0 (operator) for an ambulance or medical help. Then give first aid immediately.**
- **See emergency information on inside covers.**

POSSIBLE ADVERSE REACTIONS OR SIDE EFFECTS

SYMPTOMS	WHAT TO DO
Life-threatening:	
Hives, rash, intense itching, faintness soon after a dose (anaphylaxis); wheezing; tightness in chest; black or bloody vomit; black stools; shortness of breath.	Seek emergency treatment immediately.
Common:	
Dizziness, drowsiness, heartburn.	Continue. Call doctor when convenient.
Infrequent:	
Jaundice; vomiting blood; easy bruising; skin rash, hives; confusion; depression; sore throat, fever, mouth sores; hearing loss; slurred speech; decreased vision.	Discontinue. Call doctor right away.
Rare:	
• Diminished vision, blood in urine, unexplained fever.	Discontinue. Call doctor right away.
• Insomnia, nightmares, constipation, headache, jaundice, nervousness.	Continue. Call doctor when convenient.

WARNINGS & PRECAUTIONS

Don't take if:
- You are allergic to any barbiturate or aspirin.
- You have a peptic ulcer of stomach or duodenum, bleeding disorder, porphyria.

Continued next column

BARBITURATES & ASPIRIN (Also contains caffeine)

Before you start, consult your doctor:
- If you have had stomach or duodenal ulcers.
- If you have asthma, nasal polyps, epilepsy, kidney or liver damage, anemia, chronic pain.
- If you will have surgery within 2 months, including dental surgery, requiring general or spinal anesthesia.

Over age 60:
- Adverse reactions and side effects may be more frequent and severe than in younger persons.
- More likely to cause hidden bleeding in stomach or intestines. Watch for dark stools.

Pregnancy:
Risk to unborn child outweighs drug benefits. Don't use. Risk category D (see page xxii).

Breast-feeding:
Drug passes into milk. Avoid drug or discontinue nursing until you finish medicine. Consult doctor for advice on maintaining milk supply.

Infants & children:
- Overdose frequent and severe. Keep bottles out of children's reach.
- Use only under doctor's supervision.
- Consult doctor before giving to persons under age 18 who have fever and discomfort of viral illness, especially chicken pox and influenza. Probably increases risk of Reye's syndrome.

Prolonged use:
- Kidney damage. Periodic kidney function test recommended.
- May cause addiction, anemia, chronic intoxication.
- May lower body temperature, making exposure to cold temperatures hazardous.

Skin & sunlight:
May cause rash or intensify sunburn in areas exposed to sun or sunlamp.

Driving, piloting or hazardous work:
Don't drive or pilot aircraft until you learn how medicine affects you. Don't work around dangerous machinery. Don't climb ladders or work in high places. Danger increases if you drink alcohol or take medicine affecting alertness and reflexes, such as antihistamines, tranquilizers, sedatives, pain medicine, narcotics and mind-altering drugs.

Discontinuing:
May be unnecessary to finish medicine. Follow doctor's instructions. If you develop withdrawal symptoms of hallucinations, agitation or sleeplessness after discontinuing, call doctor right away.

Others:
- Aspirin can complicate surgery; illness; pregnancy, labor and delivery.
- For arthritis—Don't change dose without consulting doctor.
- Urine tests for blood sugar may be inaccurate.
- Great potential for abuse

POSSIBLE INTERACTION WITH OTHER DRUGS

GENERIC NAME OR DRUG CLASS	COMBINED EFFECT
Allopurinol	Decreased allopurinol effect.
Antacids*	Decreased aspirin effect.
Anticoagulants, oral*	Increased anticoagulant effect. Abnormal bleeding.
Anticonvulsants*	Changed seizure patterns.
Antidepressants*	Decreased antidepressant effect. Possible dangerous oversedation.
Antidiabetics, oral*	Increased butalbital effect. Low blood sugar.
Antihistamines*	Dangerous sedation. Avoid.

Continued on page 928

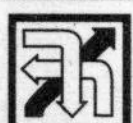

POSSIBLE INTERACTION WITH OTHER SUBSTANCES

INTERACTS WITH	COMBINED EFFECT
Alcohol:	Possible stomach irritation and bleeding, possible fatal oversedation. Avoid.
Beverages:	None expected.
Cocaine:	Decreased butalbital effect.
Foods:	None expected.
Marijuana:	Possible increased pain relief, but marijuana may slow body's recovery. Avoid.
Tobacco:	None expected.

***See Glossary**

BARBITURATES, ASPIRIN & CODEINE (Also contains caffeine)

BRAND AND GENERIC NAMES

See complete list of brand and generic names in the *Brand Name Directory*, page 901.

BASIC INFORMATION

Habit forming? Yes
Prescription needed? Yes
Available as generic? Yes
Drug class: Narcotic, analgesic

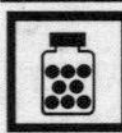

USES

- Reduces anxiety or nervous tension (low dose).
- Reduces pain, fever, inflammation.

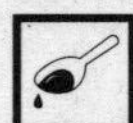

DOSAGE & USAGE INFORMATION

How to take:
- Tablet or capsule—Swallow with liquid or food to lessen stomach irritation. If you can't swallow whole, crumble tablet or open capsule and take with liquid or food.
- Extended-release tablets or capsules—Swallow each dose whole.

When to take:
When needed. No more often than every 4 hours.

If you forget a dose:
Take as soon as you remember. Wait 4 hours for next dose.

Continued next column

OVERDOSE

SYMPTOMS:
Deep sleep, slow and weak pulse, ringing in ears, nausea, vomiting, dizziness, fever, deep and rapid breathing, hallucinations, convulsions, coma.
WHAT TO DO:
- **Dial 911 (emergency) or 0 (operator) for an ambulance or medical help. Then give first aid immediately.**
- **If patient is unconscious and not breathing, give mouth-to-mouth breathing. If there is no heartbeat, use cardiac massage and mouth-to-mouth breathing (CPR). Don't try to make patient vomit. If you can't get help quickly, take patient to nearest emergency facility.**
- **See emergency information on inside covers.**

What drug does:
- May partially block nerve impulses at nerve-cell connections.
- Affects hypothalamus, the part of the brain which regulates temperature by dilating small blood vessels in skin.
- Prevents clumping of platelets (small blood cells) so blood vessels remain open.
- Decreases prostaglandin effect.
- Blocks pain messages to brain and spinal cord.
- Reduces sensitivity of brain's cough-control center.

Time lapse before drug works:
30 minutes.

Don't take with:
- Nonprescription drugs without consulting doctor.
- See Interaction column and consult doctor.

POSSIBLE ADVERSE REACTIONS OR SIDE EFFECTS

SYMPTOMS	WHAT TO DO
Life-threatening: Wheezing, tightness in chest, pinpoint pupils.	Seek emergency treatment immediately.
Common: Dizziness, drowsiness, heartburn, flushed face, depression, false sense of well-being, increased urination.	Continue. Call doctor when convenient.
Infrequent: Jaundice; vomiting blood; easy bruising; skin rash, hives; confusion; depression; sore throat, fever, mouth sores; difficult urination; hearing loss; slurred speech; blood in urine; decreased vision.	Discontinue. Call doctor right away.
Rare: Insomnia, nightmares, constipation, headache, nervousness, flushed face, increased sweating, unusual tiredness.	Continue. Call doctor when convenient.

BARBITURATES, ASPIRIN & CODEINE (Also contains caffeine)

WARNINGS & PRECAUTIONS

Don't take if:
- You are allergic to any barbiturate or narcotic.
- You have a peptic ulcer of stomach or duodenum, bleeding disorder, porphyria.

Before you start, consult your doctor:
- If you have had stomach or duodenal ulcers.
- If you have asthma, epilepsy, kidney or liver damage, anemia, chronic pain, gout.
- If you will have surgery within 2 months, including dental surgery, requiring general or spinal anesthesia.

Over age 60:
- Adverse reactions and side effects may be more frequent and severe than in younger persons.
- More likely to cause hidden bleeding in stomach or intestines. Watch for dark stools.
- More likely to be drowsy, dizzy, unsteady or constipated. Use only if absolutely necessary.

Pregnancy:
Risk factors vary for drugs in this group. See category list on page xxii and consult doctor.

Breast-feeding:
Drug passes into milk. Avoid drug or discontinue nursing until you finish medicine. Consult doctor for advice on maintaining milk supply.

Infants & children:
- Overdose frequent and severe. Keep bottles out of children's reach.
- Use only under doctor's supervision.
- Consult doctor before giving to persons under age 18 who have fever and discomfort of viral illness, especially chicken pox and influenza. Probably increases risk of Reye's syndrome*.

Prolonged use:
- Kidney damage. Periodic kidney function test recommended.
- May cause addiction, anemia, chronic intoxication.
- May lower body temperature, making exposure to cold temperatures hazardous.

Skin & sunlight:
May cause rash or intensify sunburn in areas exposed to sun or sunlamp.

Driving, piloting or hazardous work:
Don't drive or pilot aircraft until you learn how medicine effects you. Don't work around dangerous machinery. Don't climb ladders or work in high places. Danger increases if you drink alcohol or take medicine affecting alertness and reflexes, such as antihistamines, tranquilizers, sedatives, pain medicine, narcotics and mind-altering drugs.

Discontinuing:
May be unnecessary to finish medicine. Follow doctor's instructions. If you develop withdrawal symptoms of hallucinations, agitation or sleeplessness after discontinuing, call doctor right away.

Others:
- Aspirin can complicate surgery; illness; pregnancy, labor and delivery.
- For arthritis—Don't change dose without consulting doctor.
- Urine tests for blood sugar may be inaccurate.
- Great potential for abuse.

POSSIBLE INTERACTION WITH OTHER DRUGS

GENERIC NAME OR DRUG CLASS	COMBINED EFFECT
Allopurinol	Decreased allopurinol effect.
Analgesics, other*	Increased analgesic effect.
Antacids*	Decreased aspirin effect.
Anticoagulants, oral*	Increased anticoagulant effect. Abnormal bleeding.
Anticonvulsants*	Changed seizure patterns.

Continued on page 929

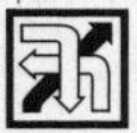

POSSIBLE INTERACTION WITH OTHER SUBSTANCES

INTERACTS WITH	COMBINED EFFECT
Alcohol:	Possible stomach irritation and bleeding, possible fatal oversedation. Avoid.
Beverages:	None expected.
Cocaine:	Increased cocaine toxic effects. Avoid.
Foods:	None expected.
Marijuana:	Possible increased pain relief, but marijuana may slow body's recovery. Impairs physical and mental performance. Avoid.
Tobacco:	None expected.

*See Glossary

BELLADONNA

GENERIC NAME

BELLADONNA

BASIC INFORMATION

Habit forming? No
Prescription needed?
Low strength: No
High strength: Yes
Available as generic? Yes
Drug class: Antispasmodic, anticholinergic

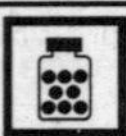

USES

Reduces spasms of digestive system, bladder and urethra.

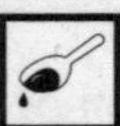

DOSAGE & USAGE INFORMATION

How to take:
- Tablet, elixir or capsule—Swallow with liquid or food to lessen stomach irritation.
- Drops—Dilute dose in beverage before swallowing.

When to take:
30 minutes before meals (unless directed otherwise by doctor).

If you forget a dose:
Take as soon as you remember up to 2 hours late. If more than 2 hours, wait for next scheduled dose (don't double this dose).

What drug does:
Blocks nerve impulses at parasympathetic nerve endings, preventing muscle contractions and gland secretions of organs involved.

Time lapse before drug works:
15 to 30 minutes.

Don't take with:
- Antacids* or antidiarrheals*.
- Any other medicine without consulting your doctor or pharmacist.

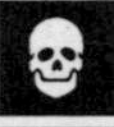

OVERDOSE

SYMPTOMS:
Dilated pupils, rapid pulse and breathing, dizziness, fever, hallucinations, confusion, slurred speech, agitation, flushed face, convulsions, coma.
WHAT TO DO:
- **Dial 911 (emergency) or 0 (operator)for an ambulance or medical help. Then give first aid immediately.**
- **See emergency information on inside covers.**

POSSIBLE ADVERSE REACTIONS OR SIDE EFFECTS

SYMPTOMS	WHAT TO DO
Life-threatening:	
In case of overdose, see previous column.	
Common:	
• Confusion, delirium, rapid heartbeat.	Discontinue. Call doctor right away.
• Nausea, vomiting, decreased sweating,	Continue. Call doctor when convenient.
• Constipation.	Continue. Tell doctor at next visit.
• Dryness in ears, nose, throat, mouth.	No action necessary.
Infrequent:	
• Headache, difficult urination, nasal congestion, altered taste.	Continue. Call doctor when convenient.
• Lightheadedness.	Discontinue. Call doctor right away.
Rare:	
Rash or hives, eye pain, blurred vision.	Discontinue. Call doctor right away.

WARNINGS & PRECAUTIONS

Don't take if:
- You are allergic to any anticholinergic.
- You have trouble with stomach bloating.
- You have difficulty emptying your bladder completely.
- You have narrow-angle glaucoma.
- You have severe ulcerative colitis.

Before you start, consult your doctor:
- If you have open-angle glaucoma.
- If you have angina or fast heartbeat.
- If you have chronic bronchitis or asthma.
- If you have hiatal hernia; liver, kidney orthyroid disease; enlarged prostate ormyasthenia gravis.
- If you will have surgery within 2 months, including dental surgery, requiring general or spinal anesthesia.

Over age 60:
Adverse reactions and side effects may be more frequent and severe than in younger persons.

Pregnancy:
Decide with your doctor whether drug benefits justify risk to unborn child. May cause bleeding in neonate. Risk category C (see page xxii).

Breast-feeding:
Drug passes into milk and decreases milk flow. Avoid drug or discontinue nursing until you finish medicine. Consult doctor for advice on maintaining milk supply.

Infants & children:
Use only under medical supervision. Do not use if under 6 months of age.

Prolonged use:
Chronic constipation, possible fecal impaction. Consult doctor immediately.

Skin & sunlight:
No problems expected.

Driving, piloting or hazardous work:
Use disqualifies you for piloting aircraft. Otherwise, no problems expected.

Discontinuing:
May be unnecessary to finish medicine. Follow doctor's instructions.

Others:
Advise any doctor or dentist whom you consult that you take this medicine.

POSSIBLE INTERACTION WITH OTHER DRUGS

GENERIC NAME OR DRUG CLASS	COMBINED EFFECT
Amantadine	Increased belladonna effect.
Antacids*	Decreased belladonna effect.
Anticholinergics, other*	Increased belladonna effect.
Antidepressants, tricyclic*	Increased belladonna effect. Increased sedation.
Antihistamines*	Increased belladonna effect.
Attapulgite	Decreased belladonna effect.
Cortisone drugs*	Increased internal eye pressure.
Guanethidine	Decreased belladonna effect.
Haloperidol	Increased internal eye pressure.
Ketoconazole	Decreased ketoconazole effect.
Meperidine	Increased belladonna effect.
Methylphenidate	Increased belladonna effect.
Metoclopramide	May decrease metoclopramide effect.
Molindone	Increased anticholinergic effect
Monoamine oxidase (MAO) inhibitors*	Increased belladonna effect..
Nitrates*	Increased internal eye pressure.
Nizatidine	Increased nizatidine effect.
Orphenadrine	Increased belladonna effect.
Phenothiazines*	Increased belladonna effect.
Pilocarpine	Loss of pilocarpine effect in glaucoma treatment.
Potassium supplements*	Possible intestinal ulcers with oral potassium tablets.
Quinidine	Increased belladonna effect.
Reserpine	Decreased belladonna effect.
Sedatives* or central nervous system (CNS) depressants*	Increased sedative effect of both drugs.
Vitamin C	Decreased belladonna effect. Avoid large doses of vitamin C.

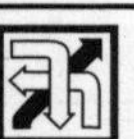

POSSIBLE INTERACTION WITH OTHER SUBSTANCES

INTERACTS WITH	COMBINED EFFECT
Alcohol:	None expected.
Beverages:	None expected.
Cocaine:	Excessively rapid heartbeat. Avoid.
Foods:	None expected.
Marijuana:	Drowsiness and drymouth.
Tobacco:	None expected.

*See Glossary

BELLADONNA ALKALOIDS & BARBITURATES

BRAND AND GENERIC NAMES

See complete list of brand and generic names in the *Brand Name Directory*, page 902.

BASIC INFORMATION

Habit forming? Yes
Prescription needed? Yes
Available as generic? Some yes, some no
Drug class: Antispasmodic, anticholinergic, sedative

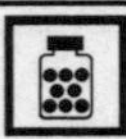

USES

- Reduces spasms of digestive system, bladder and urethra.
- Reduces anxiety or nervous tension (low dose).
- Relieves insomnia (higher bedtime dose).

DOSAGE & USAGE INFORMATION

How to take:
- Tablet, liquid or capsule—Swallow with liquid or food to lessen stomach irritation. If you can't swallow whole, crumble tablet or open capsule and take with liquid or food.
- Extended-release tablets or capsules—Swallow each dose whole.
- Chewable tablets—Chew well before swallowing.
- Drops—Dilute dose in beverage before swallowing.

When to take:
At the same times each day.

If you forget a dose:
Take as soon as you remember up to 2 hours late. If more than 2 hours, wait for next scheduled dose (don't double this dose).

Continued next column

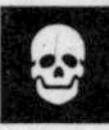

OVERDOSE

SYMPTOMS:
Blurred vision, confusion, convulsions, irregular heartbeat, hallucinations, coma.
WHAT TO DO:
- **Dial 911 (emergency) or 0 (operator) for an ambulance or medical help. Then give first aid immediately.**
- **See emergency information on inside covers.**

What drug does:
- May partially block nerve impulses at nerve cell connections.
- Blocks nerve impulses at parasympathetic nerve endings, preventing muscle contractions and gland secretions of organs involved.

Time lapse before drug works:
15 to 30 minutes.

Don't take with:
- Antacids* or antidiarrheals*.
- Any other medicine without consulting your doctor or pharmacist.

POSSIBLE ADVERSE REACTIONS OR SIDE EFFECTS

SYMPTOMS	WHAT TO DO
Life-threatening:	
Unusual excitement, restlessness, fast heartbeat, breathing difficulty.	Seek emergency treatment immediately.
Common:	
• Dry mouth, throat, nose; drowsiness; constipation; dizziness; nausea; vomiting; "hangover" effect; depression; confusion.	Discontinue. Call doctor right away.
• Reduced sweating, slurred speech, agitation, nasal congestion, altered taste.	Continue. Call doctor when convenient.
Infrequent:	
Difficult urination; difficult swallowing; rash or hives; face, lip or eyelid swelling; joint or muscle pain; lightheadedness.	Discontinue. Call doctor right away.
Rare:	
Jaundice; unusual bruising or bleeding; hives, skin rash; pain in eyes; blurred vision; sore throat, fever, mouth sores; unexplained bleeding or bruising.	Discontinue. Call doctor right away.

BELLADONNA ALKALOIDS & BARBITURATES

WARNINGS & PRECAUTIONS

Don't take if:
- You are allergic to any barbiturate or any anticholinergic.
- You have prophyria, trouble with stomach bloating, difficulty emptying your bladder completely, narrow-angle glaucoma, severe ulcerative colitis.

Before you start, consult your doctor:
- If you have open-angle glaucoma, angina, chronic bronchitis or asthma, hiatal hernia, liver disease, enlarged prostate, myasthenia gravis, peptic ulcer, epilepsy, kidney or liver damage, anemia, chronic pain, thyroid disease.
- If you will have surgery within 2 months, including dental surgery, requiring general or spinal anesthesia.

Over age 60:
Adverse reactions and side effects may be more frequent and severe than in younger persons. Ask your doctor about small doses.

Pregnancy:
Risk factors vary for drugs in this group. See category list on page xxii and consult doctor.

Breast-feeding:
Drug passes into milk. Avoid drug or discontinue nursing until you finish medicine.

Infants & children:
Use only under doctor's supervision.

Prolonged use:
- May cause addiction, anemia, chronic intoxication.
- May lower body temperature, making exposure to cold temperatures hazardous.

Skin & sunlight:
May cause rash or intensify sunburn in areas exposed to sun or sunlamp.

Driving, piloting or hazardous work:
Don't drive or pilot aircraft until you learn how medicine affects you. Don't work around dangerous machinery. Don't climb ladders or work in high places. Danger increases if you drink alcohol or take medicine affecting alertness and reflexes.

Discontinuing:
May be unnecessary to finish medicine. Follow doctor's instructions. If you develop withdrawal symptoms of hallucinations, agitation or sleeplessness after discontinuing, call doctor right away.

Others:
- Great potential for abuse.
- Advise any doctor or dentist whom you consult that you take this medicine.

POSSIBLE INTERACTION WITH OTHER DRUGS

GENERIC NAME OR DRUG CLASS	COMBINED EFFECT
Acetaminophen	Possible decreased barbiturate effect.
Amantadine	Increased belladonna effect.
Antacids*	Decreased belladonna effect.
Anticoagulants, oral*	Decreased anti-coagulant effect.
Anticholinergics, other*	Increased belladonna effect.
Anticonvulsants*	Changed seizure patterns.
Antidepressants, tricyclic*	Possible dangerous oversedation. Avoid.
Antidiabetics, oral*	Increased barbiturate effect.
Antihistamines*	Dangerous sedation. Avoid.
Anti-inflammatory drugs nonsteroidal (NSAIDs)*	Decreased anti-inflammatory effect.
Aspirin	Decreased aspirin effect.

Continued on page 930

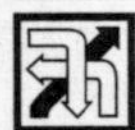

POSSIBLE INTERACTION WITH OTHER SUBSTANCES

INTERACTS WITH	COMBINED EFFECT
Alcohol:	Possible fatal oversedation. Avoid.
Beverages:	None expected.
Cocaine:	Excessively rapid heartbeat. Avoid.
Foods:	None expected.
Marijuana:	Drowsiness and dry mouth. Avoid.
Tobacco:	Decreased effectiveness of acid reduction in stomach.

*See Glossary

BENZODIAZEPINES

BRAND AND GENERIC NAMES

See complete list of brand and generic names in the *Brand Names Directory*, page 902.

BASIC INFORMATION

Habit forming? Yes
Prescription needed? Yes
Available as generic? Yes, for most
Drug class: Tranquilizer (benzodiazepine)

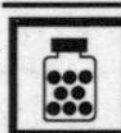

USE

- Treatment for nervousness or tension.
- Treatment for muscle spasm.
- Treatment for convulsive disorders.
- Treatment for insomnia.

DOSAGE & USAGE INFORMATION

How to take:
- Tablet, capsule, extended-release capsule or liquid—Swallow with liquid.
- Sublingual tablet—Do not chew or swallow. Place under tongue until dissolved.

When to take:
At the same time each day, according to instructions on prescription label.

If you forget a dose:
Take as soon as you remember up to 2 hours late. If more than 2 hours, wait for next scheduled dose (don't double this dose).

What drug does:
Affects limbic system of brain, the part that controls emotions.

Continued next column

OVERDOSE

SYMPTOMS:
Drowsiness, weakness, tremor, stupor, coma.
WHAT TO DO:
- **Dial 911 (emergency) or 0 (operator) for an ambulance or medical help. Then give first aid immediately.**
- **If patient is unconscious and not breathing, give mouth-to-mouth breathing. If there is no heartbeat, use cardiac massage and mouth-to-mouth breathing (CPR). Don't try to make patient vomit. If you can't get help quickly, take patient to nearest emergency facility.**
- **See emergency information on inside covers.**

Time lapse before drug works:
2 hours. May take 6 weeks for full benefit.

Don't take with:
Any other medicine without consulting your doctor or pharmacist.

POSSIBLE ADVERSE REACTIONS OR SIDE EFFECTS

SYMPTOMS	WHAT TO DO
Life-threatening:	
In case of overdose, see previous column.	
Common:	
Clumsiness, drowsiness, dizziness.	Continue. Call doctor when convenient.
Infrequent:	
• Hallucinations, confusion, depression, irritability, rash, itch, vision changes, sore throat, fever, chills.	Discontinue. Call doctor right away.
• Constipation or diarrhea, nausea, vomiting, difficult urination, vivid dreams, behavior changes, abdominal pain, headache, dry mouth.	Continue. Call doctor when convenient.
Rare:	
• Slow heartbeat, breathing difficulty.	Discontinue. Seek emergency treatment.
• Mouth, throat ulcers; jaundice.	Discontinue. Call doctor right away.
• Decreased sex drive.	Continue. Call doctor when convenient.

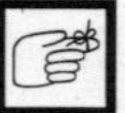

WARNINGS & PRECAUTIONS

Don't take if:
- You are allergic to any benzodiazepine.
- You have myasthenia gravis.
- You are an active or recovering alcoholic.
- Patient is younger than 6 months.

Before you start, consult your doctor:
- If you have liver, kidney or lung disease.
- If you have diabetes, epilepsy or porphyria.
- If you have glaucoma.

Over age 60:
Adverse reactions and side effects may be more frequent and severe than in younger persons. You may need smaller doses for shorter periods of time. You may develop agitation, rage or "hangover" effect.

Pregnancy:
Risk factors vary for drugs in this group. See category list on page xxii and consult doctor.

Breast-feeding:
Drug passes into milk. Avoid drug or discontinue nursing until you finish medicine. Consult doctor for advice on maintaining milk supply.

Infants & children:
Use only under medical supervision for children older than 6 months.

Prolonged use:
May impair liver function.

Skin & sunlight:
No problems expected.

Driving, piloting or hazardous work:
Don't drive or pilot aircraft until you learn how medicine affects you. Don't work around dangerous machinery. Don't climb ladders or work in high places. Danger increases if you drink alcohol or take medicine affecting alertness and reflexes.

Discontinuing:
Don't discontinue without consulting doctor. Dose may require gradual reduction if you have taken drug for a long time. Doses of other drugs may also require adjustment.

Others:
- Hot weather, heavy exercise and profuse sweat may reduce excretion and cause overdose.
- Blood sugar may rise in diabetics, requiring insulin adjustment.
- Don't use for insomnia more than 4-7 days.
- Advise any doctor or dentist whom you consult that you take this medicine.

POSSIBLE INTERACTION WITH OTHER DRUGS

GENERIC NAME OR DRUG CLASS	COMBINED EFFECT
Anticonvulsants*	Change in seizure frequency or severity.
Antidepressants*	Increased sedative effect of both drugs.
Antihistamines*	Increased sedative effect of both drugs.
Antihypertensives*	Excessively low blood pressure.
Clozapine	Toxic effect on the central nervous system.
Contraceptives, oral*	Increased benzodiazepine effect.
Disulfiram	Increased benzodiazepine effect.
Dronabinol	Increased effects of both drugs. Avoid.
Erythromycins*	Increased benzodiazepine effect.
Ketoconazole	Increased benzodiazepine effect.
Levodopa	Possible decreased levodopa effect.
Molindone	Increased tranquilizer effect.
Monoamine oxidase (MAO) inhibitors*	Convulsions, deep sedation, rage.
Nabilone	Greater depression of central nervous system.
Narcotics*	Increased sedative effect of both drugs.
Nicotine	Increased benzodiazepine effect.
Nizatidine	Increased effect and toxicity of benzodiazepine.
Omeprazole	Delayed excretion of benzodiazepine causing increased amount of benzodiazepine in blood.
Probenecid	Increased benzodiazepine effect.
Sedatives*	Increased sedative effect of both drugs.
Sertraline	Increased depressive effects of both drugs.
Sleep inducers*	Increased sedative effect of both drugs.

Continued on page 931

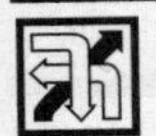

POSSIBLE INTERACTION WITH OTHER SUBSTANCES

INTERACTS WITH	COMBINED EFFECT
Alcohol:	Heavy sedation. Avoid.
Beverages:	None expected.
Cocaine:	Decreased benzodiazepine effect.
Foods:	None expected.
Marijuana:	Heavy sedation. Avoid.
Tobacco:	Decreased benzodiazepine effect.

*See Glossary

BENZOYL PEROXIDE

BRAND NAMES

See complete list of brand names in the *Brand Name Directory*, page 902.

BASIC INFORMATION

Habit forming? No
Prescription needed? No
Available as generic? Yes
Drug class: Anti-acne (topical)

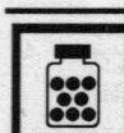

USES

- Treatment for acne.
- Treats pressure sores.

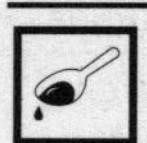

DOSAGE & USAGE INFORMATION

How to use:
Cream, gel, pads, sticks, lotion, cleansing bar or facial mask—Wash affected area with plain soap and water. Dry gently with towel. Rub medicine into affected areas. Keep away from eyes, nose, mouth.

When to use:
Apply 1 or more times daily. If you have a fair complexion, start with single application at bedtime.

If you forget an application:
Use as soon as you remember.

What drug does:
Slowly releases oxygen from skin, which controls some skin bacteria. Also causes peeling and drying, helping control blackheads and whiteheads.

Time lapse before drug works:
1 to 2 weeks.

Don't use with:
Any other medicine without consulting your doctor or pharmacist.

OVERDOSE

SYMPTOMS:
None expected.
WHAT TO DO:
- **If person swallows drug, call doctor, poison control center or hospital emergency room for instructions.**
- **See emergency information on inside covers.**

POSSIBLE ADVERSE REACTIONS OR SIDE EFFECTS

SYMPTOMS	WHAT TO DO
Life-threatening: None expected.	
Common: None expected.	
Infrequent:	
• Rash, excessive dryness, peeling skin.	Discontinue. Call doctor right away.
• Painful skin irritation.	Continue. Call doctor when convenient.
Rare: None expected.	

WARNINGS & PRECAUTIONS

Don't take if:
You are allergic to benzoyl peroxide.

Before you start, consult your doctor:
- If you plan to become pregnant within medication period.
- If you take oral contraceptives.
- If you are using any other prescription or nonprescription medicine for acne.
- If you are using abrasive skin cleansers or medicated cosmetics.

Over age 60:
No problems expected.

Pregnancy:
Consult doctor. Risk category C (see page xxii).

Breast-feeding:
No proven problems. Consult doctor.

Infants & children:
Not recommended.

Prolonged use:
Permanent rash or scarring.

Skin & sunlight:
No problems expected.

Driving, piloting or hazardous work:
No problems expected.

Discontinuing:
- May be unnecessary to finish medicine. Discontinue when acne improves.
- If acne doesn't improve in 2 weeks, call doctor.

Others:
- Keep away from hair and clothing. May bleach.
- Store away from heat in cool, dry place.
- Avoid contact with eyes, lips, nose and sensitive areas of the neck.

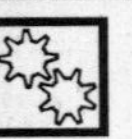

POSSIBLE INTERACTION WITH OTHER DRUGS

GENERIC NAME OR DRUG CLASS	COMBINED EFFECT
Antiacne topical preparations, other	Excessive skin irritation.
Skin-peeling agents (salicylic acid, sulfur, resorcinol, tretinoin)	Excessive skin irritation.

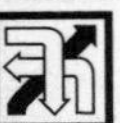

POSSIBLE INTERACTION WITH OTHER SUBSTANCES

INTERACTS WITH	COMBINED EFFECT
Alcohol:	None expected.
Beverages:	None expected.
Cocaine:	None expected.
Foods: Cinnamon, foods with benzoic acid.	Skin rash.
Marijuana:	None expected.
Tobacco:	None expected.

*See Glossary

BETA CAROTENE

BRAND NAMES

Solatene
Numerous multiple vitamin and mineral supplements. Check labels.

BASIC INFORMATION

Habit forming? No
Prescription needed? No
Available as generic? Yes
Drug class: Nutritional supplement

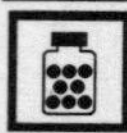

USES

- Used as a nutritional supplement.
- Prevents night blindness.
- Used as an adjunct to the treatment of steatorrhea, chronic fever, obstructive jaundice, pancreatic insufficiency, protein deficiency, total parenteral nutrition and photosensitivity in photo porphyria.

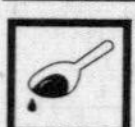

DOSAGE & USAGE INFORMATION

How to take:
Tablet or capsule—Swallow with liquid. If you can't swallow whole, crumble tablet or open capsule and take with liquid or food.

When to take:
At the same time each day, according to directions on package or prescription label.

If you forget a dose:
Take as soon as you remember (don't double this dose).

What drug does:
Enables the body to manufacture vitamin A, which is essential for the normal functioning of the retina, normal growth and development and normal testicular and ovarian function.

Time lapse before drug works:
Total effect may take several weeks.

Don't take with:
No restrictions.

OVERDOSE

SYMPTOMS:
Yellow skin
WHAT TO DO:
Overdose unlikely to threaten life. If person takes much larger amount than prescribed, call doctor, poison control center or hospital emergency room for instructions.

POSSIBLE ADVERSE REACTIONS OR SIDE EFFECTS

SYMPTOMS	WHAT TO DO
Life-threatening:	
None expected.	
Common:	
Yellow palms, hands, soles of feet.	Continue. Call doctor when convenient.
Infrequent:	
None expected.	
Rare:	
• Joint pain, unusual bleeding or bruising.	Discontinue. Call doctor right away.
• Diarrhea, dizziness.	Continue. Call doctor when convenient.

WARNINGS & PRECAUTIONS

Don't take if:
You are hypersensitive to beta carotene

Before you start, consult your doctor:
- If you have liver or kidney disease.
- If you have hypervitaminosis*.

Over age 60:
No problems expected.

Pregnancy:
Consult doctor. Risk category C (see page xxii).

Breast-feeding:
No problems expected.

Infants & children:
No problems expected.

Prolonged use:
No problems expected.

Skin & sunlight:
Beta carotene is not a sunscreen.

Driving, piloting or hazardous work:
No special problems expected.

Discontinuing:
No special problems expected.

Others:
- Some researchers claim that beta carotene may reduce the occurrence of some cancers. There is insufficient data to substantiate this claim.
- May affect results of some medical tests.

POSSIBLE INTERACTION WITH OTHER DRUGS

GENERIC NAME OR DRUG CLASS	COMBINED EFFECT
Cholestyramine	Decreased absorption of beta carotene.
Colestipol	Decreased absorption of beta carotene.
Mineral oil	Decreased absorption of beta carotene.
Neomycin	Decreased absorption of beta carotene.

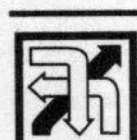

POSSIBLE INTERACTION WITH OTHER SUBSTANCES

INTERACTS WITH	COMBINED EFFECT
Alcohol:	None expected.
Beverages:	None expected.
Cocaine:	None expected.
Foods:	None expected.
Marijuana:	None expected.
Tobacco:	None expected.

*See Glossary

BETA-ADRENERGIC BLOCKING AGENTS

BRAND AND GENERIC NAMES

See complete list of brand and generic names in the *Brand Names Directory*, page 903.

BASIC INFORMATION

Habit forming? No
Prescription needed? Yes
Available as generic? Yes, for some.
Drug class: Beta-adrenergic blocker

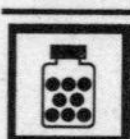

USES

- Reduces angina attacks.
- Stabilizes irregular heartbeat.
- Lowers blood pressure.
- Reduces frequency of vascular headaches. (Does not relieve headache pain.)
- Other uses prescribed by your doctor.

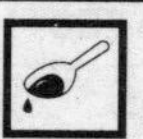

DOSAGE & USAGE INFORMATION

How to take:
Tablet, liquid or extended-release capsule—Swallow with liquid. If you can't swallow whole, crumble tablet or open capsule and take with liquid or food. Don't crush capsule or extended-release tablet.

When to take:
With meals or immediately after.

If you forget a dose:
Take as soon as you remember. Return to regular schedule, but allow 3 hours between doses.

What drug does:
- Blocks certain actions of sympathetic nervous system.
- Lowers heart's oxygen requirements.
- Slows nerve impulses through heart.
- Reduces blood vessel contraction in heart, scalp and other body parts.

Continued next column

OVERDOSE

SYMPTOMS:
Weakness, slow or weak pulse, blood pressure drop, fainting, difficulty breathing, convulsions, cold and sweaty skin.
WHAT TO DO:
- **Dial 911 (emergency) or 0 (operator) for an ambulance or medical help. Then give first aid immediately.**
- **See emergency information on inside covers.**

Time lapse before drug works:
1 to 4 hours.

Don't take with:
Nonprescription drugs or drugs in Interaction column without consulting doctor.

POSSIBLE ADVERSE REACTIONS OR SIDE EFFECTS

SYMPTOMS	WHAT TO DO
Life-threatening:	
Congestive heart failure (severe shortness of breath, rapid heartbeat).	Discontinue. Seek emergency treatment.
Common:	
• Pulse slower than 50 beats per minute.	Discontinue. Call doctor right away.
• Drowsiness, fatigue, numbness or tingling of fingers or toes, dizziness, diarrhea, nausea, weakness.	Continue. Call doctor when convenient.
• Cold hands or feet; dry mouth, eyes and skin.	Continue. Tell doctor at next visit.
Infrequent:	
• Hallucinations, nightmares, insomnia, headache, difficult breathing, joint pain, anxiety, chest pain.	Discontinue. Call doctor right away.
• Confusion, reduced alertness, depression, impotence, abdominal pain.	Continue. Call doctor when convenient.
• Constipation.	Continue. Tell doctor at next visit.
Rare:	
• Rash, sore throat, fever.	Discontinue. Call doctor right away.
• Unusual bleeding and bruising; dry, burning eyes.	Continue. Call doctor when convenient.

BETA-ADRENERGIC BLOCKING AGENTS

WARNINGS & PRECAUTIONS

Don't take if:
- You are allergic to any beta-adrenergic blocker*.
- You have asthma.
- You have hay fever symptoms.
- You have taken a monoamine oxidase (MAO) inhibitor* in the past 2 weeks.

Before you start, consult your doctor:
- If you have heart disease or poor circulation to the extremities.
- If you have hay fever, asthma, chronic bronchitis, emphysema.
- If you have overactive thyroid function.
- If you have impaired liver or kidney function.
- If you will have surgery within 2 months, including dental surgery, requiring general or spinal anesthesia.
- If you have diabetes or hypoglycemia.

Over age 60:
Adverse reactions and side effects may be more frequent and severe than in younger persons.

Pregnancy:
Risk factors vary for drugs in this group. See category list on page xxii and consult doctor.

Breast-feeding:
Drug passes into milk. Avoid drug or discontinue nursing until you finish medicine. Consult doctor for advice on maintaining milk supply.

Infants & children:
Not recommended.

Prolonged use:
- Weakens heart muscle contractions.
- Talk to your doctor about the need for follow-up medical examinations or laboratory studies to check blood pressure, ECG*, kidney function, blood sugar.

Skin & sunlight:
No problems expected.

Driving, piloting or hazardous work:
Don't drive or pilot aircraft until you learn how medicine affects you. Don't work around dangerous machinery. Don't climb ladders or work in high places. Danger increases if you drink alcohol or take medicine affecting alertness and reflexes.

Discontinuing
Don't discontinue without consulting doctor. Dose may require gradual reduction if you have taken drug for a long time. Doses of other drugs may also require adjustment.

Others:
- May mask hypoglycemia.
- May affect results in some medical tests.
- Advise any doctor or dentist whom you consult that you take this medicine.

*See Glossary

POSSIBLE INTERACTION WITH OTHER DRUGS

GENERIC NAME OR DRUG CLASS	COMBINED EFFECT
Angiotensin-converting (ACE) inhibitors*	Increased anti-hypertensive effects of both drugs. Dosages may require adjustment.
Antidiabetics*	Increased anti-diabetic effect.
Antihistamines*	Decreased antihistamine effect.
Antihypertensives*	Increased anti-hypertensive effect.
Anti-inflammatory drugs nonsteroidal (NSAIDs)*	Decreased anti-hypertensive effect of beta blocker.
Barbiturates*	Increased barbiturate effect. Dangerous sedation.
Beta-agonists*	Decreased beta-agonist effect.
Betaxolol eyedrops	Possible increased beta blocker effect.
Calcium channel blockers*	Additional blood pressure drop.
Clonidine	Additional blood pressure drop.

Continued on page 931

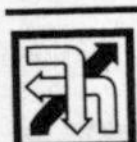

POSSIBLE INTERACTION WITH OTHER SUBSTANCES

INTERACTS WITH	COMBINED EFFECT
Alcohol:	Excessive blood pressure drop. Avoid.
Beverages:	None expected.
Cocaine:	Irregular heartbeat; decreased beta-adrenergic effect. Avoid.
Foods:	None expected.
Marijuana:	Daily use—Impaired circulation to hands and feet.
Tobacco:	Possible irregular heartbeat.

BETA-ADRENERGIC BLOCKING AGENTS (Ophthalmic)

BRAND AND GENERIC NAMES

AKBeta
Apo-Timop
Betagan C Cap B.I.D.
Betagan C Cap Q.D.
Betagan Standard Cap
Beta-Tim
BETAXOLOL (Ophthalmic)
Betoptic
Betoptic S
CARTEOLOL (Ophthalmic)
Gen-Timolol
LEVOBUNOLOL (Ophthalmic)
Med Timolol
METIPRANOLOL (Ophthalmic)
Novo-Timol
Nu-Timolol
Ocupress
OptiPranolol
Timodal
TIMOLOL (Ophthalmic)
Timoptic
Timoptic in Ocudose
Timoptic-XE

BASIC INFORMATION

Habit forming? No
Prescription needed? Yes
Available as generic? Yes, for some
Drug class: Antiglaucoma

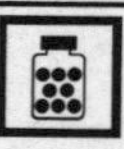

USES

Treatment for glaucoma and ocular hypertension.

DOSAGE & USAGE INFORMATION

How to take:
Eye drops—Follow directions on prescription.

Continued next column

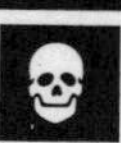

OVERDOSE

SYMPTOMS:
Slow heartbeat, low blood pressure, bronchospasm, heart failure (these symptoms are what might be expected if similar drugs were taken orally).
WHAT TO DO:
- **For overdose in the eye, flush with warm tap water and call doctor immediately.**
- **For accidentally ingested overdose or signs of system toxicity, dial 911 (emergency) or 0 (operator) for an ambulance or medical help. Then give first aid immediately.**
- **See emergency information on inside covers.**

When to take:
At the same time each day according to doctor's instructions.

If you forget a dose:
- Once-a-day dose—Apply as soon as you remember. If almost time for next dose, wait and apply at regular time (don't double this dose).
- More than once-a-day dose—Apply as soon as you remember. If close to time for next dose, wait and apply at regular time (don't double this dose).

What drug does:
Appears to reduce production of aqueous humor (fluid inside eye), thereby reducing pressure inside eye.

Time lapse before drug works:
1 to 6 hours.

Don't take with:
Any other prescription or nonprescription drug without consulting your doctor.

POSSIBLE ADVERSE REACTIONS OR SIDE EFFECTS

SYMPTOMS	WHAT TO DO
Life-threatening:	
In case of overdose, see previous column.	
Common:	
Redness of eye or inside of eyelid, decreased night vision, stinging or irritation of eye when medicine applied.	Continue. Call doctor when convenient.
Infrequent:	
None expected.	
Rare:	
• Changes in vision; blurred vision; sensation of foreign body in eye; dryness, inflammation, discharge or pain in eye; crusty eyelids.	Continue. Call doctor when convenient.
• Symptoms of system absorption may occur.	See information for Possible Adverse Reactions or Side Effects under Beta-Adrenergic Blocking Agents.

BETA-ADRENERGIC BLOCKING AGENTS (Ophthalmic)

WARNINGS & PRECAUTIONS

Don't take if:
You are allergic to any beta-adrenergic blocking agent taken orally or used in the eye.

Before you start, consult your doctor:
- If you have asthma, a bronchial disorder or pulmonary disease.
- If you have any heart disease or heart problem.
- If you have diabetes, low blood pressure, over-active thyroid or myasthenia gravis.

Over age 60:
Adverse reactions and side effects may be more frequent and severe than in younger persons.

Pregnancy:
Decide with your doctor whether drug benefits justify risk to unborn child. Risk category C (see page xxii).

Breast-feeding:
Drug passes into milk. Avoid drug or discontinue nursing until you finish medicine. Consult doctor for advice on maintaining milk supply.

Infants & children:
Give only under close medical supervision. Children may be more sensitive to drug and side effects.

Prolonged use:
Talk to your doctor about the need for follow-up medical examinations to check pressure inside eye.

Skin & sunlight:
May cause increased sensitivity to light.

Driving, piloting or hazardous work:
Don't drive or pilot aircraft until you learn how medicine affects you. Don't work around dangerous machinery. Don't climb ladders or work in high places.

Discontinuing:
- Don't discontinue without doctor's approval.
- May need to discontinue drug temporarily before major surgery. Your doctor will provide instructions.

Others:
Advise any doctor or dentist whom you consult that you take this medicine.

POSSIBLE INTERACTION WITH OTHER DRUGS

GENERIC NAME OR DRUG CLASS	COMBINED EFFECT

Drug interactions are unlikely unless a significant amount of the eye medication is absorbed into the system. Potential interactions that may occur are similar to those listed in Possible Drug Interactions With Other Drugs under Beta-Adrenergic Blocking Agents.

POSSIBLE INTERACTION WITH OTHER SUBSTANCES

INTERACTS WITH	COMBINED EFFECT
Alcohol:	None expected.
Beverages:	None expected.
Cocaine:	None expected.
Foods:	None expected.
Marijuana:	None expected.
Tobacco:	None expected.

BETA-ADRENERGIC BLOCKING AGENTS & THIAZIDE DIURETICS

BRAND AND GENERIC NAMES

See complete list of brand and generic names in the *Brand Names Directory*, page 903.

BASIC INFORMATION

Habit forming? No
Prescription needed? Yes
Available as generic? Yes
Drug class: Beta-adrenergic blocker, diuretic (thiazide)

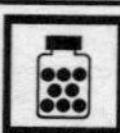

USES

- Controls, but doesn't cure, high blood pressure.
- Reduces fluid retention (edema).
- Reduces angina attacks.
- Stabilizes irregular heartbeat.
- Lowers blood pressure.
- Reduces frequency of migraine headaches. (Does not relieve headache pain.)
- Other uses prescribed by your doctor.

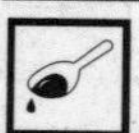

DOSAGE & USAGE INFORMATION

How to take:
Extended-release capsules—Swallow with liquid. If you can't swallow whole, open capsule and take with liquid or food.

When to take:
At the same time each day.

If you forget a dose:
Take as soon as you remember up to 4 hours late. If more than 4 hours, wait for next scheduled dose (don't double this dose).

What drug does:
- Forces sodium and water excretion, reducing body fluid.
- Relaxes muscle cells of small arteries.

Continued next column

- Reduced body fluid and relaxed arteries lower blood pressure.
- Blocks some of the actions of sympathetic nervous system.
- Lowers heart's oxygen requirements.
- Slows nerve impulses through heart.
- Reduces blood vessel contraction in heart, scalp and other body parts.

Time lapse before drug works:
- 1 to 4 hours for beta-blocker effect.
- May require several weeks to lower blood pressure.

Don't take with:
Any other medicines, even over-the-counter drugs such as cough/cold medicines, diet pills, nose drops, caffeine, without consulting your doctor.

OVERDOSE

SYMPTOMS:
Irregular heartbeat (usually too slow), seizures, confusion, fainting, convulsions, coma.
WHAT TO DO:
- **Dial 911 (emergency) or 0 (operator) for an ambulance or medical help. Then give first aid immediately.**
- **See emergency information on inside covers.**

POSSIBLE ADVERSE REACTIONS OR SIDE EFFECTS

SYMPTOMS	WHAT TO DO
Life-threatening:	
Wheezing, chest pain, seizures, irregular heartbeat.	Seek emergency treatment immediately.
Common:	
• Dry mouth, weak pulse, vomiting, muscle cramps, increased thirst, mood changes, nausea.	Discontinue. Call doctor right away.
• Weakness, tiredness, dizziness, mental depression, diminished sex drive, constipation, nightmares, insomnia.	Continue. Call doctor when convenient.
Infrequent:	
• Cold feet and hands, chest pain, breathing difficulty, anxiety, nervousness, headache, appetite loss, abdominal pain, numbness and tingling in fingers and toes, slow heartbeat.	Discontinue. Call doctor right away.
• Confusion, diarrhea.	Continue. Call doctor when convenient.
Rare:	
• Hives, skin rash; joint pain; jaundice; fever, sore throat, mouth ulcers.	Discontinue. Call doctor right away.
• Impotence, back pain.	Continue. Call doctor when convenient.

BETA-ADRENERGIC BLOCKING AGENTS & THIAZIDE DIURETICS

WARNINGS & PRECAUTIONS

Don't take if:
- You are allergic to any beta-adrenergic blocker or any thiazide diuretic drug.
- You have asthma or hay fever symptoms.
- You have taken MAO inhibitors in past two weeks.

Before you start, consult your doctor:
- If you have heart disease or poor circulation to the extremities.
- If you have hay fever, asthma, chronic bronchitis, emphysema, overactive thyroid function, impaired liver or kidney function, gout, diabetes, hypoglycemia, pancreas disorder, systemic lupus erythematosus.
- If you are allergic to any sulfa drug or tartrazine dye.
- If you will have surgery within 2 months, including dental surgery, requiring general or spinal anesthesia.

Over age 60:
Adverse reactions and side effects may be more frequent and severe than in younger persons, especially dizziness and excessive potassium loss.

Pregnancy:
Risk factors vary for drugs in this group. See category list on page xxii and consult doctor.

Breast-feeding:
Drug passes into milk. Avoid drug or discontinue nursing until you finish medicine. Consult doctor for advice on maintaining milk supply.

Infants & children:
Not recommended.

Prolonged use:
- Weakens heart muscle contractions.
- You may need medicine to treat high blood pressure for the rest of your life.
- Talk to your doctor about the need for follow-up medical examinations or laboratory studies.

Skin & sunlight:
May cause rash or intensify sunburn in areas exposed to sun or sunlamp.

Driving, piloting or hazardous work:
Don't drive or pilot aircraft until you learn how medicine affects you. Don't work around dangerous machinery. Don't climb ladders or work in high places. Danger increases if you drink alcohol or take medicine affecting alertness and reflexes, such as antihistamines, tranquilizers, sedatives, pain medicine, narcotics and mind-altering drugs.

Discontinuing:
Don't discontinue without consulting doctor. Dose may require gradual reduction if you have taken drug for a long time. Doses of other drugs may also require adjustment.

Others:
- May mask hypoglycemia symptoms.
- Hot weather and fever may cause dehydration and drop in blood pressure. Dose may require temporary adjustment. Weigh daily and report any unexpected weight decreases to your doctor.
- May cause rise in uric acid, leading to gout.
- May cause blood sugar rise in diabetics.

POSSIBLE INTERACTION WITH OTHER DRUGS

GENERIC NAME OR DRUG CLASS	COMBINED EFFECT
Allopurinol	Decreased allopurinol effect.
Aminophylline	Decreased effectiveness of both.
Antidepressants, tricyclic*	Dangerous drop in blood pressure. Avoid combination unless under medical supervision.

Continued on page 932

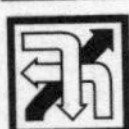

POSSIBLE INTERACTION WITH OTHER SUBSTANCES

INTERACTS WITH	COMBINED EFFECT
Alcohol:	Dangerous blood pressure drop. Avoid.
Beverages:	None expected.
Cocaine:	Irregular heartbeat, decreased beta blocker effect. Avoid.
Foods: Licorice.	Excessive potassium loss that causes dangerous heart rhythms.
Marijuana:	May increase blood pressure.
Tobacco:	May increase blood pressure and make heart work harder. Avoid.

*See Glossary

BETAMETHASONE

BRAND NAMES

See complete list of brand names in the *Brand Name Directory*, page 903.

BASIC INFORMATION

Habit forming? No
Prescription needed? Yes
Available as generic? Yes
Drug class: Cortisone drug (adrenal corticosteroid)

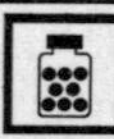

USES

- Reduces inflammation caused by many different medical problems.
- Treatment for some allergic diseases, blood disorders, kidney diseases, asthma and emphysema.
- Replaces corticosteroid deficiencies.

DOSAGE & USAGE INFORMATION

How to take:
- Tablet, extended-release tablet, syrup or liquid—Swallow with liquid or food to lessen stomach irritation. If you can't swallow whole, crumble tablet and take with liquid or food.
- Inhaler—Follow label instructions.

When to take:
At the same times each day. Take once-a-day or once-every-other-day doses in mornings.

If you forget a dose:
- Several-doses-per-day prescription—Take as soon as you remember up to 2 hours late. If more than 2 hours, wait for next scheduled dose (don't double this dose).
- Once-a-day dose or less—Wait for next dose. Double this dose.

What drug does:
Decreases inflammatory responses.

Time lapse before drug works:
2 to 4 days.

Continued next column

OVERDOSE

SYMPTOMS:
Headache, convulsions, heart failure.
WHAT TO DO:
- **Dial 911 (emergency) or 0 (operator) for an ambulance or medical help. Then give first aid immediately.**
- **See emergency information on inside covers.**

Don't take with:
Any other medicine without consulting your doctor or pharmacist.

POSSIBLE ADVERSE REACTIONS OR SIDE EFFECTS

SYMPTOMS	WHAT TO DO
Life-threatening: In case of overdose, see previous column.	
Common:	
Acne, poor wound healing, thirst, indigestion, nausea, vomiting, constipation, gaseousness, unpleasant taste, diarrhea, headache, cough, dizziness, hoarseness, appetite loss.	Continue. Call doctor when convenient.
Infrequent:	
• Bloody or black, tarry stool; various infections; swallowing difficulty; hives.	Discontinue. Seek emergency treatment.
• Blurred vision, halos around lights, sore throat, fever, abdominal pain.	Discontinue. Call doctor right away.
• Mood changes, insomnia, fatigue, restlessness, frequent urination, weight gain, round face, weakness, menstrual irregularities, dry mouth, euphoria, nosebleed.	Continue. Call doctor when convenient.
Rare:	
• Irregular heartbeat.	Discontinue. Seek emergency treatment.
• Rash, TB recurrence.	Discontinue. Call doctor right away.

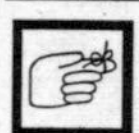

WARNINGS & PRECAUTIONS

Don't take if:
- You are allergic to any cortisone drug.
- You have tuberculosis or fungus infection.
- You have herpes infection of eyes, lips or genitals.
- You have bone disease, thyroid disease, colitis, stomach ulcer, diabetes, myasthenia gravis, liver or kidney disease, diverticulitis, glaucoma, heart disease.

Before you start, consult your doctor:
- If you are taking any other prescription or nonprescription medicine.
- If you have had tuberculosis.

- If you have an infection, congestive heart failure, diabetes, peptic ulcer, glaucoma, underactive thyroid, high blood pressure, myasthenia gravis, blood clots in legs or lungs.

Over age 60:
Adverse reactions and side effects may be more frequent and severe than in younger persons. Likely to aggravate edema, diabetes or ulcers. Likely to cause cataracts and osteoporosis (softening of the bones).

Pregnancy:
Decide with your doctor if drug benefits justify risk to unborn child. Risk category C (see page xxii).

Breast-feeding:
Drug passes into milk. Avoid drug or discontinue nursing until you finish medicine. Consult doctor for advice on maintaining milk supply.

Infants & children:
Use only under medical supervision.

Prolonged use:
- Retards growth in children.
- Possible glaucoma, cataracts, diabetes, fragile bones and thin skin.
- Functional dependence.
- Talk to your doctor about the need for follow-up medical examinations or laboratory studies to check blood pressure, stools for blood, serum electrolytes.

Skin & sunlight:
No problems expected.

Driving, piloting or hazardous work:
No problems expected.

Discontinuing:
- Don't discontinue without doctor's advice until you complete prescribed dose, even though symptoms diminish or disappear.
- Drug affects your response to surgery, illness, injury or stress for up to 2 years after discontinuing. Inform doctor.

Others:
- Avoid immunizations if possible.
- Your resistance to infection is less while taking this medicine.
- Advise any doctor or dentist whom you consult that you take this medicine.

POSSIBLE INTERACTION WITH OTHER DRUGS

GENERIC NAME OR DRUG CLASS	COMBINED EFFECT
Amphotericin B	Potassium depletion.
Anticholinergics*	Possible glaucoma.
Anticoagulants, oral*	Decreased anti-coagulant effect.
Anticonvulsants, hydantoin*	Decreased beta-methasone effect.
Antidiabetics, oral*	Decreased anti-diabetic effect.
Antihistamines*	Decreased beta-methasone effect.
Aspirin	Increased beta-methasone effect.
Barbiturates*	Decreased beta-methasone effect. Oversedation.
Beta-adrenergic blocking agents*	Decreased beta-methasone effect.
Butmetanide	Potassium depletion.
Chloral hydrate	Decreased beta-methasone effect.
Chlorthalidone	Potassium depletion.
Cholestyramine	Decreased beta-methasone effect.
Cholinergics*	Decreased cholinergic effect.
Colestipol	Decreased beta-methasone effect.
Contraceptives, oral*	Increased beta-methasone effect.
Cyclosporine	May increase cyclosporine effect.
Digitalis preparations*	Dangerous potassium depletion. Possible digitalis toxicity.
Diuretics, thiazide*	Potassium depletion.

Continued on page 933

POSSIBLE INTERACTION WITH OTHER SUBSTANCES

INTERACTS WITH	COMBINED EFFECT
Alcohol:	Risk of stomach ulcers.
Beverages:	No proven problems.
Cocaine:	Overstimulation. Avoid.
Foods:	No proven problems.
Marijuana:	Decreased immunity.
Tobacco:	Increased beta-methasone effect. Possible toxicity.

***See Glossary**

BETHANECHOL

BRAND NAMES

Duvoid
Urabeth
Urecholine

BASIC INFORMATION

Habit forming? No
Prescription needed? Yes
Available as generic? Yes
Drug class: Cholinergic

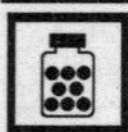

USES

- Helps initiate urination following surgery, or for persons with urinary infections or enlarged prostate.
- Treats reflux esophagitis.

DOSAGE & USAGE INFORMATION

How to take:
Tablet—Swallow with liquid, 1 hour before or 2 hours after eating.

When to take:
At the same times each day.

If you forget a dose:
Take as soon as you remember up to 2 hours late. If more than 2 hours, wait for next scheduled dose (don't double this dose).

What drug does:
Affects chemical reactions in the body that strengthen bladder muscles.

Continued next column

OVERDOSE

SYMPTOMS:
Shortness of breath, wheezing or chest tightness, unconsciousness, coma.
WHAT TO DO:
- **Dial 911 (emergency) or 0 (operator) for an ambulance or medical help. Then give first aid immediately.**
- **If patient is unconscious and not breathing, give mouth-to-mouth breathing. If there is no heartbeat, use cardiac massage and mouth-to-mouth breathing (CPR). Don't try to make patient vomit. If you can't get help quickly, take patient to nearest emergency facility.**
- **See emergency information on inside covers.**

Time lapse before drug works:
30 to 90 minutes.

Don't take with:
Any other medicine without consulting your doctor or pharmacist.

POSSIBLE ADVERSE REACTIONS OR SIDE EFFECTS

SYMPTOMS	WHAT TO DO
Life-threatening: In case of overdose, see previous column.	
Common: None expected.	
Infrequent: Dizziness, headache, faintness, blurred or changed vision, diarrhea, nausea, vomiting, stomach discomfort, belching, excessive urge to urinate.	Continue. Call doctor when convenient.
Rare: Shortness of breath, wheezing, tightness in chest.	Discontinue. Call doctor right away.

WARNINGS & PRECAUTIONS

Don't take if:
You are allergic to any cholinergic.

Before you start, consult your doctor:
- If you plan to become pregnant within medication period.
- If you have asthma.
- If you have epilepsy.
- If you have heart or blood vessel disease.
- If you have high or low blood pressure.
- If you have overactive thyroid.
- If you have intestinal blockage.
- If you have Parkinson's disease.
- If you have stomach problems (including ulcer).
- If you have had bladder or intestinal surgery within 1 month.

Over age 60:
Adverse reactions and side effects may be more frequent and severe than in younger persons.

Pregnancy:
Decide with your doctor if drug benefits justify risk to unborn child. Risk category C (see page xxii).

Breast-feeding:
Unknown effect. Consult doctor.

Infants & children:
Use only under medical supervision.

Prolonged use:
No problems expected.

Skin & sunlight:
No problems expected.

Driving, piloting or hazardous work:
Don't drive or pilot aircraft until you learn how medicine effects you. Don't work around dangerous machinery. Don't climb ladders or work in high places. Danger increases if you drink alcohol or take medicine affecting alertness and reflexes, such as antihistamines, tranquilizers, sedatives, pain medicine, narcotics and mind-altering drugs.

Discontinuing:
May be unnecessary to finish medicine. Follow doctor's instructions.

Others:
- Be cautious about standing up suddenly.
- Interferes with laboratory studies of liver and pancreas function.
- Side effects more likely with injections.

POSSIBLE INTERACTION WITH OTHER DRUGS

GENERIC NAME OR DRUG CLASS	COMBINED EFFECT
Cholinergics, other*	Increased effect of both drugs. Possible toxicity.
Ganglionic blockers*	Decreased blood pressure.
Nitrates*	Decreased bethanechol effect.
Procainamide	Decreased bethanechol effect.
Quinidine	Decreased bethanechol effect.

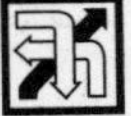

POSSIBLE INTERACTION WITH OTHER SUBSTANCES

INTERACTS WITH	COMBINED EFFECT
Alcohol:	None expected.
Beverages:	None expected.
Cocaine:	None expected.
Foods:	None expected.
Marijuana:	None expected.
Tobacco:	None expected.

*See Glossary

BISACODYL

BRAND NAMES

Bisac-Evac
Bisacolax
Bisco-Lax
Carter's Little Pills
Clysodrast
Dacodyl
Deficol
Dulcodos
Dulcolax
Fleet Bisacodyl
Fleet Bisacodyl Prep
Fleet Laxative
Laxit
Theralax

BASIC INFORMATION

Habit forming? No
Prescription needed? No
Available as generic? Yes
Drug class: Laxative (stimulant)

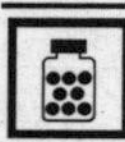

USES

Constipation relief.

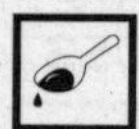

DOSAGE & USAGE INFORMATION

How to take:
- Follow package instructions.
- Tablet—Swallow with liquid, do not crush.
- Suppository—Remove wrapper and moisten suppository with water. Gently insert larger end into rectum. Push well into rectum with finger. Retain in rectum 20-30 minutes.

When to take:
Usually at bedtime with a snack, unless directed otherwise.

If you forget a dose:
Take as soon as you remember.

What drug does:
Acts on smooth muscles of intestine wall to cause vigorous bowel movement.

Time lapse before drug works:
6 to 10 hours.

Don't take with:
- Any other medicine without consulting your doctor or pharmacist.
- Don't take within 2 hours of taking another medicine. Laxative interferes with medicine absorption.

OVERDOSE

SYMPTOMS:
Vomiting, electrolyte depletion.
WHAT TO DO:
Overdose unlikely to threaten life. If person takes much larger amount than prescribed, call doctor, poison control center or hospital emergency room for instructions.

POSSIBLE ADVERSE REACTIONS OR SIDE EFFECTS

SYMPTOMS	WHAT TO DO
Life-threatening:	
None expected.	
Common:	
Rectal irritation.	Continue. Call doctor when convenient.
Infrequent:	
• Dangerous potassium loss (thirst, weakness, heartbeat irregularity, paralysis, nausea and diarrhea).	Discontinue. Call doctor right away.
• Belching, cramps, nausea.	Continue. Call doctor when convenient.
Rare:	
• Irritability, headache, confusion, rash, breathing difficulty, irregular heartbeat, muscle cramps, unusual tiredness or weakness.	Discontinue. Call doctor right away.
• Burning on urination.	Continue. Call doctor when convenient.

WARNINGS & PRECAUTIONS

Don't take if:
- You have symptoms of appendicitis, inflamed bowel or intestinal blockage.
- You are allergic to a stimulant laxative.
- You have missed a bowel movement for only 1 or 2 days.

Before you start, consult your doctor:
- If you have a colostomy or ileostomy.
- If you have congestive heart disease.
- If you have diabetes.
- If you have high blood pressure.
- If you have a laxative habit.
- If you have rectal bleeding.
- If you take other laxatives.

Over age 60:
Adverse reactions and side effects may be more frequent and severe than in younger persons.

Pregnancy:
Decide with your doctor if drug benefits justify risk to unborn child. Risk category C (see page xxii).

Breast-feeding:
Drug passes into milk. Avoid drug or discontinue nursing until you finish medicine. Consult doctor for advice on maintaining milk supply.

Infants & children:
Use only under medical supervision.

Prolonged use:
Don't take for more than 1 week unless under doctor's supervision. May cause laxative dependence.

Skin & sunlight:
No problems expected.

Driving, piloting or hazardous work:
No problems expected.

Discontinuing:
May be unnecessary to finish medicine. Follow doctor's instructions.

Others:
Don't take to "flush out" your system or as a "tonic."

POSSIBLE INTERACTION WITH OTHER DRUGS

GENERIC NAME OR DRUG CLASS	COMBINED EFFECT
Antacids*	Tablet coating may dissolve too rapidly, irritating stomach or bowel.
Antihypertensives*	May cause dangerous low potassium level.
Cimetidine	Stomach or bowel irritation.
Diuretics*	May cause dangerous low potassium level.
Famotidine	Stomach or bowel irritation.
Ranitidine	Stomach or bowel irritation.

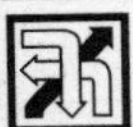

POSSIBLE INTERACTION WITH OTHER SUBSTANCES

INTERACTS WITH	COMBINED EFFECT
Alcohol:	None expected.
Beverages:	None expected.
Cocaine:	None expected.
Foods:	None expected.
Marijuana:	None expected.
Tobacco:	None expected.

*See Glossary

BISMUTH SUBSALICYLATE

BRAND NAMES

Pepto-Bismol

BASIC INFORMATION

Habit forming? No
Prescription needed? No
Available as generic? Yes
Drug class: Antidiarrheal, antacid

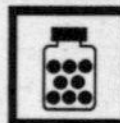

USES

- Treats symptoms of diarrhea, heartburn, nausea, acid indigestion.
- Helps prevent traveler's diarrhea.
- Treats duodenal ulcers.

DOSAGE & USAGE INFORMATION

How to take:
- Chewable tablets—Chew well before swallowing.
- Liquid—Take as directed on label.

When to take:
As directed on label or by your doctor.

If you forget a dose:
Take as soon as you remember. Don't double this dose.

What drug does:
- Binds toxin of some bacteria.
- Stimulates absorption of fluid and electrolytes across the intestinal wall.
- Decreases inflammation and increased motility of the intestinal muscles and lining.

Time lapse before drug works:
30 minutes to 1 hour.

Don't take with:
Any other medicine without consulting your doctor or pharmacist.

OVERDOSE

SYMPTOMS:
Anxiety, confusion, speech difficulty, severe headache, muscle spasms, depression, trembling.
WHAT TO DO:
- **Dial 911 (emergency) or 0 (operator) for an ambulance or medical help. Then give first aid immediately.**
- **See emergency information on inside covers.**

POSSIBLE ADVERSE REACTIONS OR SIDE EFFECTS

SYMPTOMS	WHAT TO DO
Life-threatening: In case of overdose, see previous column.	
Common: Black stools, dark tongue. (These symptoms are normal and medically insignificant.)	No action necessary.
Infrequent: • Hearing loss, confusion, dizziness, fast breathing, headache, increased thirst, ringing or buzzing in ears, vision problems.	Discontinue. Call doctor right away.
• Constipation.	Continue. Call doctor when convenient.
Rare: Flapping movements of hands, abdominal pain, increased sweating, muscle weakness, drowsiness, anxiety, trembling.	Discontinue. Call doctor right away.

WARNINGS & PRECAUTIONS

Don't take if:
- You are allergic to aspirin, salicylates or other nonsteroidal anti-inflammatory drugs.
- You have stomach ulcers that have ever bled.
- The patient is a child with fever.

Before you start, consult your doctor:
- If you are on a low-sodium, low-sugar or other special diet.
- If you have had diarrhea for more than 24 hours. This is especially applicable to infants, children and those over 60.
- If you have had kidney disease.

Over age 60:
- Consult doctor before using.
- May cause severe constipation.

Pregnancy:
Decide with your doctor if drug benefits justify risk to unborn child. Risk category C; D in third trimester (see page xxii).

Breast-feeding:
- Drug passes into milk. Avoid or discontinue nursing until you finish medicine.
- May harm baby if mother takes large amounts.

Infants & children:
Not recommended for children 3 and younger. May cause constipation.

Prolonged use:
May cause constipation.

Skin & sunlight:
No problems expected.

Driving, piloting or hazardous work:
Don't drive or pilot aircraft if you take high or prolonged dose until you learn how medicine affects you. Don't work around dangerous machinery. Don't climb ladders or work in high places. Danger increases if you drink alcohol or take medicine affecting alertness and reflexes, such as antihistamines, tranquilizers, sedatives, pain medicine, narcotics and mind-altering drugs.

Discontinuing:
No problems expected.

Others:
- Pepto-Bismol contains salicylates. When given to children with flu or chicken pox, salicylates may cause a serious illness called Reye's syndrome*. An overdose in children can cause the same problems as aspirin poisoning.
- May cause false urine sugar tests.

POSSIBLE INTERACTION WITH OTHER DRUGS

GENERIC NAME OR DRUG CLASS	COMBINED EFFECT
Anticoagulants*	Increased risk of bleeding.
Insulin or oral antidiabetic drugs*	Increased insulin effect. May require dosage adjustment.
Probenecid	Decreased effect of probenecid.
Salicylates, other*	Increased risk of salicylate toxicity.
Sulfinpyrazone	Decreased effect of sulfinpyrazone.
Tetracylines*	Decreased absorption of tetracycline.
Thrombolytic agents*	Increased risk of bleeding.

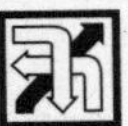

POSSIBLE INTERACTION WITH OTHER SUBSTANCES

INTERACTS WITH	COMBINED EFFECT
Alcohol:	None expected.
Beverages:	None expected.
Cocaine:	Decreased Pepto-Bismol effect. Avoid.
Foods:	None expected.
Marijuana:	None expected.
Tobacco:	None expected.

***See Glossary**

BROMOCRIPTINE

BRAND NAMES

Parlodel

BASIC INFORMATION

Habit forming? No
Prescription needed? Yes
Available as generic? No
Drug class: Antiparkinsonism

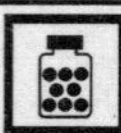

USES

- Controls Parkinson's disease symptoms such as rigidity, tremors and unsteady gait.
- Treats male and female infertility.
- Treats acromegaly.
- Treats some pituitary tumors.

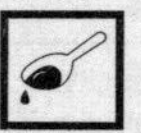

DOSAGE & USAGE INFORMATION

How to take:
Tablet or capsule—Swallow with liquid or food to lessen stomach irritation. If you can't swallow whole, crumble tablet or open capsule and take with liquid or food.

When to take:
At the same times each day.

If you forget a dose:
Take as soon as you remember up to 2 hours late. If more than 2 hours, wait for next scheduled dose (don't double this dose).

Continued next column

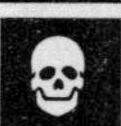

OVERDOSE

SYMPTOMS:
Muscle twitch, spastic eyelid closure, nausea, vomiting, diarrhea, irregular and rapid pulse, weakness, fainting, confusion, agitation, hallucination, coma.
WHAT TO DO:

- **Dial 911 (emergency) or 0 (operator) for an ambulance or medical help. Then give first aid immediately.**
- **If patient is unconscious and not breathing, give mouth-to-mouth breathing. If there is no heartbeat, use cardiac massage and mouth-to-mouth breathing (CPR). Don't try to make patient vomit. If you can't get help quickly, take patient to nearest emergency facility.**
- **See emergency information on inside covers.**

What drug does:
Restores chemical balance necessary for normal nerve impulses.

Time lapse before drug works:
2 to 3 weeks to improve; 6 weeks or longer for maximum benefit.

Don't take with:
Any other medicine without consulting your doctor or pharmacist.

POSSIBLE ADVERSE REACTIONS OR SIDE EFFECTS

SYMPTOMS	WHAT TO DO
Life-threatening:	
In case of overdose, see previous column.	
Common:	
• Mood changes, uncontrollable body movements, diarrhea, nausea.	Continue. Call doctor when convenient.
• Dry mouth, body odor.	No action necessary.
Infrequent:	
• Fainting, severe dizziness, headache, insomnia, nightmares, rash, itch, vomiting, irregular heartbeat.	Discontinue. Call doctor right away.
• Flushed face, blurred vision, muscle twitching, discolored or dark urine, difficult urination, muscle cramps, appetite loss, abdominal discomfort, nasal congestion, tingling and numbness of hands and feet.	Continue. Call doctor when convenient.
• Constipation, tiredness.	Continue. Tell doctor at next visit.
Rare:	
• High blood pressure, hallucinations, psychosis.	Discontinue. Call doctor right away.
• Anemia, impotence.	Continue. Call doctor when convenient.
• Hair loss.	Continue. Tell doctor at next visit.

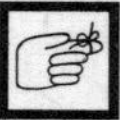

WARNINGS & PRECAUTIONS

Don't take if:

- You are allergic to bromocriptine or ergotamine.
- You have taken a monoamine oxidase (MAO) inhibitor* in the past 2 weeks.
- You have glaucoma (narrow-angle type).

Before you start, consult your doctor:
- If you have diabetes or epilepsy.
- If you have had high blood pressure, heart or lung disease.
- If you have had liver or kidney disease.
- If you have a peptic ulcer.
- If you will have surgery within 2 months, including dental surgery, requiring general or spinal anesthesia.

Over age 60:
Adverse reactions and side effects may be more frequent and severe than in younger persons.

Pregnancy:
Decide with your doctor if drug benefits justify risk to unborn child. Risk category C (see page xxii).

Breast-feeding:
Drug inhibits milk production. Avoid.

Infants & children:
Not recommended if under 15 years old.

Prolonged use:
- May lead to uncontrolled movements of head, face, mouth, tongue, arms or legs.
- Talk to your doctor about the need for follow-up medical examinations or laboratory studies to check blood pressure, x-rays, growth hormone levels.

Skin & sunlight:
No problems expected.

Driving, piloting or hazardous work:
Don't drive or pilot aircraft until you learn how medicine effects you. Don't work around dangerous machinery. Don't climb ladders or work in high places. Danger increases if you drink alcohol or take medicine affecting alertness and reflexes, such as antihistamines, tranquilizers, sedatives, pain medicine, narcotics and mind-altering drugs.

Discontinuing:
Don't discontinue without doctor's advice until you complete prescribed dose, even though symptoms diminish or disappear.

Others:
Expect to start with small doses and increase gradually to lessen frequency and severity of adverse reactions.

POSSIBLE INTERACTION WITH OTHER DRUGS

GENERIC NAME OR DRUG CLASS	COMBINED EFFECT
Antihypertensives*	May decrease blood pressure.
Antiparkinsonism drugs, other*	Increased bromocriptine effect.
Contraceptives, oral*	Decreased bromocriptine effect.
Ergot alkaloids, other	Increased risk of high blood pressure.
Estrogens*	Decreased bromocriptine effect.
Guanfacine	Increased effect of both drugs.
Haloperidol	Decreased bromocriptine effect.
Levodopa	Decreased antiparkinson effect.
Methyldopa	Decreased bromocriptine effect.
Monoamine oxidase (MAO) inhibitors*	Dangerous rise in blood pressure.
Papaverine	Decreased bromocriptine effect.
Phenothiazines*	Decreased bromocriptine effect.
Progestins	Decreased bromocriptine effect.
Pyridoxine (Vitamin B-6)	Decreased bromocriptine effect.
Rauwolfia alkaloids*	Decreased bromocriptine effect.

POSSIBLE INTERACTION WITH OTHER SUBSTANCES

INTERACTS WITH	COMBINED EFFECT
Alcohol:	Decreased alcohol tolerance.
Beverages:	None expected.
Cocaine:	Decreased bromocriptine effect. Avoid.
Foods:	None expected.
Marijuana:	Increased fatigue, lethargy, fainting. Avoid.
Tobacco:	Interferes with absorption. Avoid.

***See Glossary**

BRONCHODILATORS, ADRENERGIC

BRAND AND GENERIC NAMES

See complete list of brand and generic names in the *Brand Name Directory*, page 903.

BASIC INFORMATION

Habit forming? No
Prescription needed? Yes, for most
Available as generic? Yes, for some
Drug class: Sympathomimetic

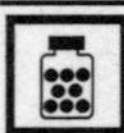

USES

- Relieves bronchial asthma.
- Decreases congestion of breathing passages.
- Suppresses allergic reactions.

DOSAGE & USAGE INFORMATION

How to take:
- Tablet or capsule—Swallow with liquid. You may chew or crush tablet.
- Extended-release tablets—Swallow each dose whole.
- Syrup—Take as directed on bottle.
- Drops—Dilute dose in beverage.
- Aerosal inhalor—Follow directions in package.

When to take:
As needed, no more often than every 4 hours.

If you forget a dose:
Take up to 2 hours late. If more than 2 hours, wait for next dose (don't double this dose).

What drug does:
- Prevents cells from releasing allergy-causing chemicals (histamines).
- Relaxes muscles of bronchial tubes.
- Decreases blood-vessel size and blood flow, thus causing decongestion.

Time lapse before drug works:
30 to 60 minutes.

Continued next column

OVERDOSE

SYMPTOMS:
Severe anxiety, confusion, delirium, muscle tremors, rapid and irregular pulse, severe weakness.
WHAT TO DO:
- **Dial 911 (emergency) or 0 (operator) for an ambulance or medical help. Then give first aid immediately.**
- **See emergency information on inside covers.**

Don't take with:
- Nonprescription drugs with ephedrine, pseudoephedrine or epinephrine.
- Nonprescription drugs for cough, cold, allergy or asthma without consulting doctor.
- Any other medicine without consulting your doctor or pharmacist.

POSSIBLE ADVERSE REACTIONS OR SIDE EFFECTS

SYMPTOMS	WHAT TO DO
Life-threatening: In case of overdose, see previous column.	
Common:	
• Nervousness, anxiety, headache, large pupils, paleness, increased blood pressure, trembling, dry mouth.	Continue. Call doctor when convenient.
• Insomnia.	Continue. Tell doctor at next visit.
Infrequent:	
• Irregular heartbeat, chest pain, hallucinations.	Discontinue. Call doctor right away.
• Dizziness, dry mouth, appetite loss, nausea, vomiting, painful or difficult urination, coughing.	Continue. Call doctor when convenient.
Rare:	
• Muscle cramps, difficulty in breathing, rash, hives, swelling of face or eyelids, wheezing.	Discontinue. Call doctor right away.
• Smell or taste changes.	No action necessary.

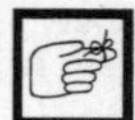

WARNINGS & PRECAUTIONS

Don't take if:
You are allergic to ephedrine or any bronchodilator* drug.

Before you start, consult your doctor:
- If you have high blood pressure.
- If you have diabetes.
- If you have cardiovascular disease.
- If you have overactive thyroid gland.
- If you have difficulty urinating.
- If you have taken any monoamine oxidase(MAO) inhibitor* in past 2 weeks.
- If you have taken digitalis preparations* in the last 7 days.
- If you will have surgery within 2 months, including dental surgery, requiring general or spinal anesthesia.
- If you have pheochromocytoma.

Over age 60:
More likely to develop high blood pressure, heart rhythm disturbances, angina and to feel drug's stimulant effects.

Pregnancy:
Risk factors vary for drugs in this group. See category list on page xxii and consult doctor.

Breast-feeding:
Drug passes into milk. Avoid drug or discontinue nursing until you finish medicine. Consult doctor for advice on maintaining milk supply.

Infants & children:
No problems expected for most. Use only under close medical supervision.

Prolonged use:
- Excessive doses—Rare toxic psychosis.
- Men with enlarged prostate gland may have more urination difficulty.
- Talk to your doctor about the need for follow-up medical examinations or laboratory studies to check ECG*, blood pressure.

Skin & sunlight:
No problems expected.

Driving, piloting or hazardous work:
Avoid if you feel dizzy. Otherwise, no problems expected.

Discontinuing:
May be unnecessary to finish medicine. Follow doctor's instructions.

Others:
May affect results in some medical tests.

POSSIBLE INTERACTION WITH OTHER DRUGS

GENERIC NAME OR DRUG CLASS	COMBINED EFFECT
Antidepressants, tricyclic*	Increased effect of bronchodilator. Excessive stimulation of heart and blood pressure.
Antihypertensives*	Decreased antihypertensive effect.
Beta-adrenergic blocking agents*	Decreased effects of both drugs.
Digitalis preparations*	Serious heart rhythm disturbances.
Epinephrine	Increased bronchodilator effect.
Ergot preparations*	Serious blood-pressure rise.
Finasteride	Decreased finasteride effect.
Furazolidine	Sudden severe increase in blood pressure.
Guanadrel	Decreased effect of both drugs.
Guanethidine	Decreased effect of both drugs.
Maprotiline	Increased heart stimulation.
Methyldopa	Possible increased blood pressure.
Monoamine oxidase (MAO) inhibitors*	Increased bronchodilator effect. Dangerous blood pressure rise.
Nitrates*	Possible decreased effects of both drugs.
Phenothiazines*	Possible increased bronchodilator toxicity. Possible decreased bronchodilator effect.
Pseudoephedrine	Increased bronchodilator effect.
Rauwolfia	Decreased rauwolfia effect.
Sympathomimetics*, other	Increased brochodilator effect.
Terazosin	Decreased effectiveness of terazosin.
Theophylline	Increased gastrointestinal intolerance.
Thyroid drugs	Increased bronchodilator effect.

POSSIBLE INTERACTION WITH OTHER SUBSTANCES

INTERACTS WITH	COMBINED EFFECT
Alcohol:	None expected.
Beverages: Caffeine drinks.	Nervousness or insomnia.
Cocaine:	High risk of heartbeat irregularities and high blood pressure.
Foods:	None expected.
Marijuana:	Rapid heartbeat, possible heart rhythm disturbance.
Tobacco:	None expected.

*See Glossary

BRONCHODILATORS, XANTHINE

BRAND AND GENERIC NAMES

See complete list of brand and generic names in the *Brand Name Directory*, page 903.

BASIC INFORMATION

Habit forming? No
Prescription needed?
U.S.: High strength—Yes
Low strength—No
Canada: No
Available as generic? Yes
Drug class: Bronchodilator (xanthine)

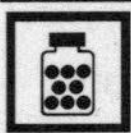

USES

Treatment for bronchial asthma symptoms.

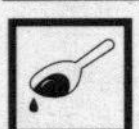

DOSAGE & USAGE INFORMATION

How to take:

- Tablet or capsule—Swallow with liquid.
- Extended-release tablets or capsules—Swallow each dose whole. If you take regular tablets, you may chew or crush them.
- Suppositories—Remove wrapper and moisten suppository with water. Gently insert larger end into rectum. Push well into rectum with finger.
- Syrup—Take as directed on bottle.
- Enema—Use as directed on label.

When to take:
Most effective taken on empty stomach 1 hour before or 2 hours after eating. However, may take with food to lessen stomach upset.

If you forget a dose:
Take as soon as you remember up to 2 hours late. If more than 2 hours, wait for next scheduled dose (don't double this dose).

Continued next column

OVERDOSE

SYMPTOMS:
Restlessness, irritability, confusion, black or tarry stool, breathing difficulty, pounding and irregular heartbeat, vomiting blood, delirium, convulsions, rapid pulse, coma.
WHAT TO DO:

- **Dial 911 (emergency) or 0 (operator) for an ambulance or medical help. Then give first aid immediately.**
- **See emergency information on inside covers.**

What drug does:
Relaxes and expands bronchial tubes.

Time lapse before drug works:
15 to 30 minutes.

Don't take with:
Any other medicine without consulting your doctor or pharmacist.

POSSIBLE ADVERSE REACTIONS OR SIDE EFFECTS

SYMPTOMS	WHAT TO DO
Life-threatening:	
In case of overdose, see previous column.	
Common:	
Headache, irritability, nervousness, nausea, restlessness, insomnia, vomiting, stomach pain.	Continue. Call doctor when convenient.
Infrequent:	
• Rash or hives, flushed face, diarrhea, appetite loss, rapid breathing, irregular heartbeat.	Discontinue. Call doctor right away.
• Dizziness or lightheadedness.	Continue. Call doctor when convenient.
Rare:	
Frequent urination.	Continue. Call doctor when convenient.

WARNINGS & PRECAUTIONS

Don't take if:

- You are allergic to any bronchodilator.
- You have an active peptic ulcer.

Before you start, consult your doctor:

- If you have had impaired kidney or liver function.
- If you have gastritis.
- If you have a peptic ulcer.
- If you have high blood pressure or heart disease.
- If you take medication for gout.

Over age 60:
Adverse reactions and side effects may be more frequent and severe than in younger persons.

Pregnancy:
Decide with your doctor if drug benefits justify risk to unborn child. Risk category C (see page xxii).

Breast-feeding:
Drug passes into milk. Avoid drug or discontinue nursing until you finish medicine. Consult doctor for advice on maintaining milk supply.

Infants & children:
Use only under medical supervision.

Prolonged use:
Stomach irritation may occur.

Skin & sunlight:
No problems expected.

Driving, piloting or hazardous work:
Avoid if lightheaded or dizzy. Otherwise, no problems expected.

Discontinuing:
May be unnecessary to finish medicine. Follow doctor's instructions.

Others:
No problems expected.

POSSIBLE INTERACTION WITH OTHER DRUGS

GENERIC NAME OR DRUG CLASS	COMBINED EFFECT
Allopurinol	Increased theophylline effect.
Aminoglutethimide	Possible decreased bronchodilator effect.
Beta-agonists*	Increased effect of both drugs.
Beta-adrenergic blocking agents*	Decreased bronchodilator effect.
Cimetidine	Increased bronchodilator effect.
Ciprofloxin	Increased xanthine bronchodilator in blood. Dosage adjustments necessary.
Clarithromycin	Increased concentration of theophylline.
Clindamycin	May increase bronchodilator effect.
Corticosteroids*	Possible increased bronchodilator effect.
Erythromicin	Increased bronchodilator effect.
Finasteride	Decreased finasteride effect.
Furosemide	Increased furosemide effect.
Lincomycins*	May increase bronchodilator effect.
Lithium	Decreased lithium effect.
Moricizine	Decreased bronchodilator effect.
Nicotine chewing gum	Possible increased bronchodilator effect.
Norfloxacin	Increased xanthine bronchodilator in blood. Dosage adjustments necessary.
Phenobarbital	Decreased bronchodilator effect.
Phenytoin	Decreased effect of both drugs.
Probenecid	Increased effect of dyphylline.
Ranitidine	Possible increased bronchodilator effect and toxicity.
Rauwolfia alkaloids*	Rapid heartbeat.
Rifampin	Decreased bronchodilator effect.
Sulfinpyrazone	Increased effect of dyphylline.
Sympathomimetics*	Possible increased bronchodilator effect.
Tacrine	Increased bronchodilator effect.
Ticlopidine	Increased theophylline effect.
Troleandomycin	Increased bronchodilator effect.

POSSIBLE INTERACTION WITH OTHER SUBSTANCES

INTERACTS WITH	COMBINED EFFECT
Alcohol:	None expected.
Beverages: Caffeine drinks.	Nervousness and insomnia.
Cocaine:	Excess stimulation. Avoid.
Foods:	None expected.
Marijuana:	Slightly increased antiasthmatic effect of bronchodilator. Decreased effect with chronic use.
Tobacco:	Decreased bronchodilator effect.

***See Glossary**

BUCLIZINE

BRAND NAMES

Bucladin-S

BASIC INFORMATION

Habit forming? No
Prescription needed?
U.S.: No
Canada: Yes
Available as generic? No
Drug class: Antihistamine, antiemetic, anti-motion sickness

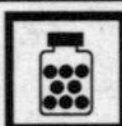

USES

Prevents motion sickness.

DOSAGE & USAGE INFORMATION

How to take:
Tablet—Swallow with liquid or food to lessen stomach irritation. If you can't swallow whole, crumble tablet and chew or take with liquid or food.

When to take:
30 minutes to 1 hour before traveling.

If you forget a dose:
Take as soon as you remember. Wait 4 hours for next dose.

What drug does:
Reduces sensitivity of nerve endings in inner ear, blocking messages to brain's vomiting center.

Time lapse before drug works:
30 to 60 minutes.

Don't take with:
Any other medicine without consulting your doctor or pharmacist.

OVERDOSE

SYMPTOMS:
Drowsiness, confusion, incoordination, stupor, coma, weak pulse, shallow breathing, hallucinations.
WHAT TO DO:

- **Dial 911 (emergency) or 0 (operator) for an ambulance or medical help. Then give first aid immediately.**
- **See emergency information on inside covers.**

POSSIBLE ADVERSE REACTIONS OR SIDE EFFECTS

SYMPTOMS	WHAT TO DO
Life-threatening: In case of overdose, see previous column.	
Common: Drowsiness.	Continue. Tell doctor at next visit.
Infrequent:	
• Headache, diarrhea or constipation, fast heartbeat.	Continue. Call doctor when convenient.
• Dry mouth, nose, throat.	Continue. Tell doctor at next visit.
Rare:	
• Rash or hives.	Discontinue. Call doctor right away.
• Restlessness, excitement, insomnia, blurred vision, frequent urination, difficult urination, hallucinations.	Continue. Call doctor when convenient.
• Appetite loss, nausea.	Continue. Tell doctor at next visit.

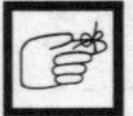

WARNINGS & PRECAUTIONS

Don't take if:

- You are allergic to meclizine, buclizine or cyclizine.
- You have taken a monoamine oxidase (MAO) inhibitor* in the past 2 weeks.

Before you start, consult your doctor:

- If you have glaucoma.
- If you have prostate enlargement.
- If you have reacted badly to any antihistamine.

Over age 60:
Adverse reactions and side effects may be more frequent and severe than in younger persons, especially impaired urination from enlarged prostate gland.

Pregnancy:
Risk category X (see page xxii).

Breast-feeding:
Drug passes into milk. Avoid drug or discontinue nursing until you finish medicine. Consult doctor for advice on maintaining milk supply.

Infants & children:
Safety not established. Avoid if less than 12 years old.

Prolonged use:
No problems expected.

Skin & sunlight:
No problems expected.

Driving, piloting or hazardous work:
Don't fly aircraft. Don't drive until you learn how medicine affects you. Don't work around dangerous machinery. Don't climb ladders or work in high places. Danger increases if you drink alcohol or take medicine affecting alertness and reflexes, such as antihistamines, tranquilizers, sedatives, pain medicine, narcotics and mind-altering drugs.

Discontinuing:
No problems expected.

Others:
Buclizine contains tartrazine dye. Avoid if allergic (especially aspirin hypersensitivity).

POSSIBLE INTERACTION WITH OTHER DRUGS

GENERIC NAME OR DRUG CLASS	COMBINED EFFECT
Amphetamines*	May decrease drowsiness caused by buclizine.
Anticholinergics*	Increased effect of both drugs.
Antidepressants, tricyclic*	Increased effect of both drugs.
Carteolol	Decreased anti-histamine effect.
Cisapride	Decreased buclizine effect.
Clozapine	Toxic effect on the central nervous system.
Dronabinol	Increases effect of buclizine.
Ethinamate	Dangerous increased effects of ethinamate. Avoid combining.
Fluoxetine	Increased depres-sant effects of both drugs.
Guanfacine	May increase depressant effects of either drug.
Methyprylon	Increased sedative effect, perhaps to dangerous level. Avoid.
Monoamine oxidase (MAO) inhibitors*	Increased buclizine effect.
Nabilone	Greater depression of central nervous system.
Narcotics*	Increased effect of both drugs.
Pain relievers*	Increased effect of both drugs.
Sedatives*	Increased effect of both drugs.
Sertraline	Increased depressive effects of both drugs.
Sleep inducers*	Increased effect of both drugs.
Sotalol	Increased antihista-mine effect.
Tranquilizers*	Increased effect of both drugs.

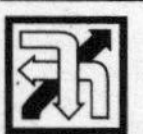

POSSIBLE INTERACTION WITH OTHER SUBSTANCES

INTERACTS WITH	COMBINED EFFECT
Alcohol:	Increased sedation. Avoid.
Beverages: Caffeine drinks.	May decrease drowsiness.
Cocaine:	None expected.
Foods:	None expected.
Marijuana:	Increased drowsi-ness, dry mouth.
Tobacco:	None expected.

*See Glossary

BUPROPION

BRAND AND GENERIC NAMES

AMFEBUTAMONE **Wellbutrin**

BASIC INFORMATION

Habit forming? No
Prescription needed? Yes
Available as generic? No
Drug class: Antidepressant

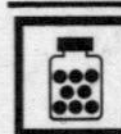

USES

Relieves severe mental depression.

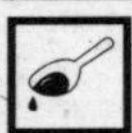

DOSAGE & USAGE INFORMATION

How to take:
Tablets—Swallow with liquid. If you can't swallow whole, crumble tablet and take with liquid or food. May take with food to lessen stomach irritation.

When to take:
At the same time each day, according to instructions on prescription label.

If you forget a dose:
Take as soon as you remember up to 2 hours late. If more than 2 hours, wait for next scheduled dose (don't double this dose).

What drug does:
Blocks certain chemicals that are necessary for nerve transmission in the brain.

Time lapse before drug works:
1 to 3 weeks.

Don't take with:
Any other medicine without consulting your doctor or pharmacist.

OVERDOSE

SYMPTOMS:
Confusion, agitation, seizures, coma.
WHAT TO DO:

- **Dial 911 (emergency) or 0 (operator) for an ambulance or medical help. Then give first aid immediately.**
- **See emergency information on inside covers.**

POSSIBLE ADVERSE REACTIONS OR SIDE EFFECTS

SYMPTOMS	WHAT TO DO
Life-threatening:	
Seizures.	Seek emergency treatment immediately.
Common:	
Excitement, anxiety, insomnia, restlessness, confusion, heartbeat irregularity, headaches.	Continue. Call doctor when convenient.
Infrequent:	
Rash, blurred vision, drowsiness, chills, fever, hallucinations, fatigue, nightmares.	Discontinue. Call doctor right away
Rare:	
Fainting, hostility.	Discontinue. Call doctor right away.

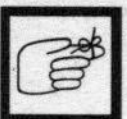

WARNINGS & PRECAUTIONS

Don't take if:
- You have anorexia nervosa or bulimia.
- You have had recent head injury.
- You have convulsions (seizures).
- You have a brain or spinal cord tumor.

Before you start, consult your doctor:
- If you have manic phases to your illness.
- If you abuse drugs.
- If you have liver, kidney or heart disease.

Over age 60:
See Interaction column and consult doctor.

Pregnancy:
No proven harm to unborn child, but avoid if possible. Risk category B (see page xxii).

Breast-feeding:
Drug passes into milk. May cause adverse reactions. Avoid drug or discontinue breast-feeding. Consult doctor about maintaining milk supply.

Infants & children:
Effect not documented. Consult your doctor.

Prolonged use:
Talk to your doctor about the need for follow-up medical examinations or laboratory studies to check kidney function, liver function and serum bupropion levels in blood.

Skin & sunlight:
No problems expected.

Driving, piloting or hazardous work:
Don't drive or pilot aircraft until you learn how medicine affects you. Don't work around dangerous machinery. Don't climb ladders or work in high places. Danger increases if you drink alcohol or take medicine affecting alertness and reflexes.

Discontinuing:
Don't discontinue without doctor's approval. Dose may require gradual reduction to avoid adverse effects.

Others:
- May affect results in some medical tests.
- Advise any doctor or dentist whom you consult that you take this medicine.

POSSIBLE INTERACTION WITH OTHER DRUGS

GENERIC NAME OR DRUG CLASS	COMBINED EFFECT
Antidepressants, tricyclic*	Increased risk of major seizures.
Cimetidine	Increased bupropion effect.
Clozapine	Increased risk of major seizures.
Fluoxetine	Increased risk of major seizures.
Haloperidol	Increased risk of major seizures.
Lithium	Increased risk of major seizures.
Loxapine	Increased risk of major seizures.
Molindone	Increased risk of major seizures.
Monoamine oxidase (MAO) inhibitors*	Increased risk of bupropion toxicity.
Phenothiazines*	Increased risk of major seizures.
Thioxanthenes*	Increased risk of major seizures.
Trazodone	Increased risk of major seizures.

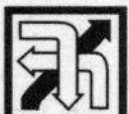

POSSIBLE INTERACTION WITH OTHER SUBSTANCES

INTERACTS WITH	COMBINED EFFECT
Alcohol:	Increased risk of seizures. Avoid.
Beverages: Coffee, tea, cocoa.	Increased side effects such as restlessness, insomnia.
Cocaine:	Increased risk of seizures. Avoid.
Foods:	No special problems expected.
Marijuana:	Increased risk of seizures. Avoid.
Tobacco:	No special problems expected.

***See Glossary**

BUSPIRONE

BRAND NAMES

BuSpar

BASIC INFORMATION

Habit forming? Unknown
Prescription needed? Yes
Available as generic? No
Drug class: Tranquilizer

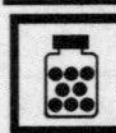

USES

Treats anxiety disorders with nervousness or tension. Not intended for treatment of ordinary stress of daily living. Causes less sedation than some anti-anxiety drugs.

DOSAGE & USAGE INFORMATION

How to take:
Tablets—Take with a glass of liquid.

When to take:
As directed. Usually 3 times daily. Food does not interfere with absorption.

If you forget a dose:
Take as soon as you remember, but skip this dose and don't double the next dose if it is almost time for the next dose.

What drug does:
Chemical family azaspirodecanedione; *not* a benzodiazepine. Probably has an effect on neurotransmitter systems.

Time lapse before drug works:
1 or 2 weeks before beneficial effects may beobserved.

Don't take with:
Alcohol, other tranquilizers, antihistamines, muscle relaxants, sedatives or narcotics.

OVERDOSE

SYMPTOMS:
Severe drowsiness or nausea, vomiting, small pupils, unconsciousness.
WHAT TO DO:

- **Dial 911 (emergency) or 0 (operator) for an ambulance or medical help. Then give first aid immediately.**
- **See emergency information on inside covers.**

POSSIBLE ADVERSE REACTIONS OR SIDE EFFECTS

SYMPTOMS	WHAT TO DO
Life-threatening: Chest pain; pounding, fast heartbeat (rare).	Discontinue. Seek emergency treatment.
Common: Lightheadedness, headache, nausea, restlessness, dizziness.	Discontinue. Call doctor right away.
Infrequent: Drowsiness, dry mouth, ringing in ears, nightmares or vivid dreams, unusual fatigue.	Continue. Call doctor when convenient.
Rare: Numbness or tingling in feet or hands; sore throat; fever; depression or confusion; uncontrollable movements of tongue, lips, arms and legs; slurred speech; psychosis; blurred vision.	Discontinue. Call doctor right away.

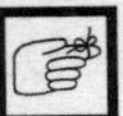

WARNINGS & PRECAUTIONS

Don't take if:
You are allergic to buspirone.

Before you start, consult your doctor:
- If you have ever been addicted to any substance.
- If you have chronic kidney or liver disease.
- If you are already taking *any* medicine.

Over age 60:
Adverse reactions and side effects may be more frequent and severe than in younger persons.

Pregnancy:
No problems expected, but better to avoid if possible. Consult doctor. Risk category B (see page xxii).

Breast-feeding:
Buspirone passes into milk of lactating experimental animals. Avoid if possible.

Infants & children:
Safety and efficacy not established for under 18 years old.

Prolonged use:
- Not recommended for prolonged use. Adverse side effects more likely.
- Request follow-up studies to check kidney function, blood counts, and platelet counts.

Skin & sunlight:
No problems expected.

Driving, piloting or hazardous work:
Don't drive or pilot aircraft until you learn how medicine affects you. Don't work around dangerous machinery. Don't climb ladders or work in high places. Danger increases if you drink alcohol or take medicine affecting alertness and reflexes, such as antihistamines, tranquilizers, sedatives, pain medicine, narcotics and mind-altering drugs.

Discontinuing:
No problems expected.

Others:
Before elective surgery requiring local orgeneral anesthesia, tell your dentist, surgeon or anesthesiologist that you take buspirone.

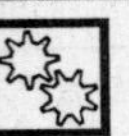

POSSIBLE INTERACTION WITH OTHER DRUGS

GENERIC NAME OR DRUG CLASS	COMBINED EFFECT
Antihistamines*	Excessive sedation. Sedative effect of both drugs may be increased.
Barbiturates*	Excessive sedation. Sedative effect of both drugs may be increased.
Monoamine oxidase MAO inhibitors*	May increase blood pressure.
Muscle relaxants*	Excessive sedation. Sedative effect of both drugs may be increased.
Narcotics*	Excessive sedation. Sedative effect of both drugs may be increased.
Sedatives*	Excessive sedation. Sedative effect of both drugs may be increased.
Tranquilizers, other*	Excessive sedation. Sedative effect of both drugs may be increased.

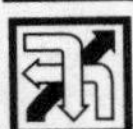

POSSIBLE INTERACTION WITH OTHER SUBSTANCES

INTERACTS WITH	COMBINED EFFECT
Alcohol:	Excess sedation. Avoid.
Beverages: Caffeine-containing drinks.	Avoid. Decreased anti-anxiety effect of busiprone.
Cocaine:	Avoid. Decreased anti-anxiety effect of busiprone.
Foods:	None expected.
Marijuana:	Avoid. Decreased anti-anxiety effect of busiprone.
Tobacco:	Avoid. Decreased anti-anxiety effect of busiprone.

*See Glossary

BUSULFAN

BRAND NAMES

Myleran

BASIC INFORMATION

Habit forming? No
Prescription needed? Yes
Available as generic? No
Drug class: Antineoplastic, immunosuppressant

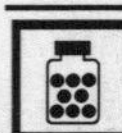

USES

- Treatment for some kinds of cancer.
- Suppresses immune response after transplant and in immune disorders.

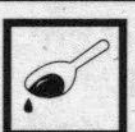

DOSAGE & USAGE INFORMATION

How to take:
Tablet—Swallow with liquid after light meal. Don't drink fluids with meals. Drink extra fluids between meals. Avoid sweet or fatty foods.

When to take:
At the same time each day.

If you forget a dose:
Take as soon as you remember. Don't ever double dose.

What drug does:
Inhibits abnormal cell reproduction. May suppress immune system.

Time lapse before drug works:
Up to 6 weeks for full effect.

Don't take with:
Any other medicine without consulting your doctor or pharmacist.

OVERDOSE

SYMPTOMS:
Bleeding, chills, fever, collapse, stupor, seizure.
WHAT TO DO:

- **Dial 911 (emergency) or 0 (operator) for an ambulance or medical help. Then give first aid immediately.**
- **If patient is unconscious and not breathing, give mouth-to-mouth breathing. If there is no heartbeat, use cardiac massage and mouth-to-mouth breathing (CPR). Don't try to make patient vomit. If you can't get help quickly, take patient to nearest emergency facility.**
- **See emergency information on inside covers.**

POSSIBLE ADVERSE REACTIONS OR SIDE EFFECTS

SYMPTOMS	WHAT TO DO
Life-threatening: In case of overdose, see previous column.	
Common:	
• Unusual bleeding or bruising, mouth sores with sore throat, chills and fever, black stools, lip sores, menstrual irregularities.	Discontinue. Call doctor right away.
• Hair loss.	Continue. Call doctor when convenient.
• Nausea, vomiting, diarrhea (almost always occurs), tiredness, weakness.	Continue. Tell doctor at next visit.
Infrequent:	
• Mental confusion, shortness of breath.	Continue. Call doctor when convenient.
• Cough, joint pain, dizziness, appetite loss.	Continue. Tell doctor at next visit.
Rare:	
• Jaundice, cataracts, symptoms of myasthenia gravis.*	Discontinue. Call doctor right away.
• Swollen breasts.	Continue. Call doctor when convenient.

WARNINGS & PRECAUTIONS

Don't take if:

- You have had hypersensitivity to alkylating antineoplastic drugs.
- Your physician has not explained the serious nature of your medical problem and risks of taking this medicine.

Before you start, consult your doctor:

- If you have gout.
- If you have had kidney stones.
- If you have active infection.
- If you have impaired kidney or liver function.
- If you have taken other antineoplastic drugs or had radiation treatment in last 3 weeks.

Over age 60:
Adverse reactions and side effects may be more frequent and severe than in younger persons.

Pregnancy:
Consult doctor. Risk to child is significant. Risk category D (see page xxii).

Breast-feeding:
Drug passes into milk. Don't nurse.

Infants & children:
Use only under care of medical supervisors who are experienced in anticancer drugs.

Prolonged use:

- Adverse reactions more likely the longer drug is required.
- Talk to your doctor about the need for follow-up medical examinations or laboratory studies to check complete blood counts (white blood cell count, platelet count, red blood cell count, hemoglobin, hematocrit), serum uricacid.

Skin & sunlight:
No problems expected.

Driving, piloting or hazardous work:
No problems expected.

Discontinuing:
Don't discontinue without doctor's advice until you complete prescribed dose, even though symptoms diminish or disappear. Some side effects may follow discontinuing. Report to doctor blurred vision, convulsions, confusion, persistent headache.

Others:

- May cause sterility.
- May increase chance of developing leukemia.

POSSIBLE INTERACTION WITH OTHER DRUGS

GENERIC NAME OR DRUG CLASS	COMBINED EFFECT
Antigout drugs*	Decreased antigout effect.
Antineoplastic drugs, other*	Increased effect of all drugs (may be beneficial).
Chloramphenicol	Increased likelihood of toxic effects of both drugs.
Clozapine	Toxic effect on bone marrow.
Lovastatin	Increased heart and kidney damage.
Tiopronin	Increased risk of toxicity to bone marrow.
Vaccines, live or killed	Increased risk of toxicity or reduced effectiveness of vaccine.

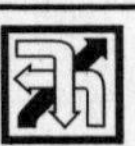

POSSIBLE INTERACTION WITH OTHER SUBSTANCES

INTERACTS WITH	COMBINED EFFECT
Alcohol:	May increase chance of intestinal bleeding.
Beverages:	No problems expected.
Cocaine:	Increases chance of toxicity.
Foods:	Reduces irritation in stomach.
Marijuana:	No problems expected.
Tobacco:	Increases lung toxicity.

*See Glossary

BUTORPHANOL

BRAND NAMES

Stadol NS

BASIC INFORMATION

Habit forming? Yes
Prescription needed? Yes
Available as generic? No
Drug class: Narcotic analgesic

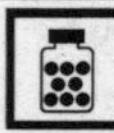

USES

- Treatment for migraine headache pain and postoperative pain.
- Treatment for other types of pain for which a narcotic analgesic is appropriate.

DOSAGE & USAGE INFORMATION

How to take:
Nasal spray—Spray in one nostril using the metered-dose pump.

When to take:
For pain as directed by your doctor. Usual treatment consists of one dose in one nostril followed by a second dose in 60 to 90 minutes if pain persists. Your doctor may direct that the initial 2-dose sequence may be repeated in 3 to 4 hours as needed.

If you forget a dose:
Unlikely to be a problem since the drug is taken for pain and not routinely.

What drug does:
Blocks the pain impulses at specific sites in the brain and spinal cord.

Time lapse before drug works:
Within 15 minutes of the first dose.

Don't take with:
Any other medicine without consulting your doctor or pharmacist.

OVERDOSE

SYMPTOMS:
Heartbeat irregularities, breathing difficulty, coma.
WHAT TO DO:
- **Dial 911 (emergency) or 0 (operator) for an ambulance or medical help. Then give first aid immediately.**
- **See emergency information on inside covers.**

POSSIBLE ADVERSE REACTIONS OR SIDE EFFECTS

SYMPTOMS	WHAT TO DO
Life-threatening:	
In case of overdose, see previous column.	
Common:	
Drowsiness, dizziness, nausea or vomiting, nasal congestion or irritation.	Discontinue. Call doctor when convenient.
Infrequent:	
Constipation (with continued use), faintness, high or low blood pressure.	Discontinue. Call doctor when convenient.
Rare:	
• Taste changes, ear ringing, dry mouth.	No action necessary.
• Difficult breathing, heart palpitations.	Discontinue. Call doctor right away.

WARNINGS & PRECAUTIONS

Don't take if:
You are allergic to butorphanol or the preservative benzethonium chloride*, which is used in the manufacture of the drug.

Before you start, consult your doctor:
- If you have a respiratory disorder or a central nervous system disease.
- If you have had adverse reactions to other narcotics*.
- If you have a history of emotional problems.
- If you have heart, kidney or liver disease.

Over age 60:
Adverse reactions and side effects (particularly dizziness) may be more frequent and severe than in younger persons.

Pregnancy:
Risk category C (see page xxii). Decide with your doctor if drug benefits justify any possible risk to unborn child.

Breast-feeding:
Drug may pass into milk. Decide with your doctor if you should continue breast-feeding while taking this drug.

Infants & children:
Not recommended for children under age 18. Safety and effectiveness have not been established.

Prolonged use:
Long-term use effects are unknown. Probably habit forming. Consult with your doctor on a regular basis while using this drug.

Skin & sunlight:
No special problems expected.

Driving, piloting or hazardous work:
Don't drive or pilot aircraft until you learn how medicine affects you. Don't work around dangerous machinery. Don't climb ladders or work in high places. Danger increases if you drink alcohol or take medicine affecting alertness and reflexes.

Discontinuing:
Don't discontinue this drug after prolonged use without consulting doctor. Dosage may require a gradual reduction before stopping to avoid any withdrawal symptoms.

Others:
- When first using this drug, get up slowly from a sitting or lying position to avoid any dizziness, faintness or lightheadedness.
- Advise any doctor or dentist whom you consult that you take this medicine.
- Take medicine only as directed. Do not increase or reduce dosage without doctor's approval.

POSSIBLE INTERACTION WITH OTHER DRUGS

GENERIC NAME OR DRUG CLASS	COMBINED EFFECT
Central nervous system (CNS) depressants*, other	Increased sedative effect.
Oxymetazoline	Delays start of butorphanol effect.

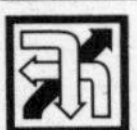

POSSIBLE INTERACTION WITH OTHER SUBSTANCES

INTERACTS WITH	COMBINED EFFECT
Alcohol:	Increased sedative affect. Avoid.
Beverages:	None expected.
Cocaine:	Effect not known. Best to avoid.
Foods:	None expected.
Marijuana:	Effect not known. Best to avoid.
Tobacco:	None expected.

*See Glossary

CAFFEINE

BRAND NAMES

See complete list of brand names in the *Brand Name Directory*, page 904.

BASIC INFORMATION

Habit forming? Yes
Prescription needed? No
Available as generic? Yes
Drug class: Stimulant (xanthine), vasoconstrictor

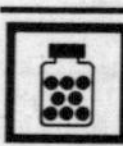

USES

- Treatment for drowsiness and fatigue.
- Treatment for migraine and other vascular headaches in combination with ergot.

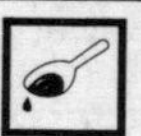

DOSAGE & USAGE INFORMATION

How to take:
- Tablet or liquid—Swallow with liquid or food to lessen stomach irritation. If you can't swallow whole, crumble tablet and take with liquid or food.
- Extended-release capsules—Swallow whole with liquid.

When to take:
At the same times each day.

If you forget a dose:
Take as soon as you remember up to 2 hours late. If more than 2 hours, wait for next scheduled dose (don't double this dose).

What drug does:
- Constricts blood vessel walls.
- Stimulates central nervous system.

Time lapse before drug works:
30 minutes.

Continued next column

OVERDOSE

SYMPTOMS:
Excitement, insomnia, rapid heartbeat (infants can have slow heartbeat), confusion, fever, hallucinations, convulsions, coma.
WHAT TO DO:
- **Dial 911 (emergency) or 0 (operator) for an ambulance or medical help. Then give first aid immediately.**
- **See emergency information on inside covers.**

Don't take with:
- Nonprescription drugs without consulting doctor.
- See Interaction column and consult doctor.

POSSIBLE ADVERSE REACTIONS OR SIDE EFFECTS

SYMPTOMS	WHAT TO DO
Life-threatening: In case of overdose, see previous column.	
Common:	
• Rapid heartbeat, low blood sugar (hunger, anxiety, cold sweats, rapid pulse) with tremor, irritability (mild).	Discontinue. Call doctor right away.
• Nervousness, insomnia.	Continue. Tell doctor at next visit.
• Increased urination.	No action necessary.
Infrequent:	
• Confusion, irritability (severe).	Discontinue. Call doctor right away.
• Nausea, indigestion, burning feeling in stomach.	Continue. Call doctor when convenient.
Rare: None expected.	

WARNINGS & PRECAUTIONS

Don't take if:

- You are allergic to any stimulant.
- You have heart disease.
- You have active peptic ulcer of stomach or duodenum.

Before you start, consult your doctor:

- If you have irregular heartbeat.
- If you have hypoglycemia (low blood sugar).
- If you have epilepsy.
- If you have high blood pressure.
- If you have insomnia.

Over age 60:
Adverse reactions and side effects may be more frequent and severe than in younger persons.

Pregnancy:
Decide with your doctor if drug benefits justify risk to unborn child. Risk category C (see page xxii).

Breast-feeding:
Drug passes into milk. Avoid drug or discontinue nursing until you finish medicine. Consult doctor for advice on maintaining milk supply.

Infants & children:
Not recommended.

Prolonged use:
Stomach ulcers.

Skin & sunlight:
No problems expected.

Driving, piloting or hazardous work:
No problems expected.

Discontinuing:
Will cause withdrawal symptoms of headache, irritability, drowsiness. Discontinue gradually if you use caffeine for a month or more.

Others:
May produce or aggravate fibrocystic disease of the breast in women.

POSSIBLE INTERACTION WITH OTHER DRUGS

GENERIC NAME OR DRUG CLASS	COMBINED EFFECT
Caffeine-containing drugs, other	Increased risk of overstimulation.
Central nervous system (CNS) stimulants*	Increased risk of overstimulation.
Cimetidine	Increased caffeine effect.
Contraceptives, oral*	Increased caffeine effect.
Isoniazid	Increased caffeine effect.
Monoamine oxidase (MAO) inhibitors*	Dangerous blood pressure rise.
Sedatives*	Decreased sedative effect.
Sleep inducers*	Decreased sedative effect.
Sympathomimetics*	Overstimulation.
Thyroid hormones*	Increased thyroid effect.
Tranquilizers*	Decreased tranquilizer effect.

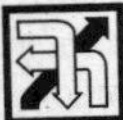

POSSIBLE INTERACTION WITH OTHER SUBSTANCES

INTERACTS WITH	COMBINED EFFECT
Alcohol:	Decreased alcohol effect.
Beverages: Caffeine drinks (coffee, tea, or soft drinks).	Increased caffeine effect.
Cocaine	Convulsions or excessive nervousness.
Foods:	No proven problems.
Marijuana:	Increased effect of both drugs. May lead to dangerous, rapid heartbeat. Avoid.
Tobacco:	Increased heartbeat. Avoid. Decreased caffeine effect.

*See Glossary

CALCIPOTRIENE

BRAND NAMES

Dovonex

BASIC INFORMATION

Habit forming? No
Prescription needed? Yes
Available as generic? No
Drug class: Antipsoriasis

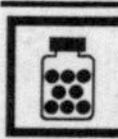

USES

Treats discoid or "plaque" psoriasis, the most common form of the disorder.

DOSAGE & USAGE INFORMATION

How to use:
Ointment—Apply a thin layer to the affected skin. Rub in gently and completely. It should not be used on the face.

When to use:
Twice a day.

If you forget a dose:
Apply ointment as soon as you remember, then return to regular schedule.

What drug does:
Calcipotriene is a vitamin D product that helps regulate skin cell production and development.

Time lapse before drug works:
2 weeks. May take up to 8 weeks for maximum benefits that can include marked improvement in symptoms for most patients or complete clearing for others.

Don't use with:
Other topical or systemic drugs without consulting with your doctor or pharmacist.

OVERDOSE

SYMPTOMS:
May be absorbed into the system through excessive topical application and increase the levels of calcium, which could cause muscle weakness, excess fatigue, depression, loss of appetite and nausea.
WHAT TO DO:
Overdose unlikely to threaten life. If symptoms occur, call doctor for instructions. If child accidentally swallows, call poison control center.

POSSIBLE ADVERSE REACTIONS OR SIDE EFFECTS

SYMPTOMS	WHAT TO DO
Life-threatening: None expected.	
Common: Irritation, burning, itching of the skin.	Discontinue. Call doctor when convenient.
Infrequent: Redness, dryness, peeling or skin rash, worsening of psoriasis.	Discontinue. Call doctor when convenient.
Rare: None expected.	

WARNINGS & PRECAUTIONS

Don't use if:

- You are allergic to calcipotriene or any of its components.
- You have hypercalcemia (excess of calcium in the system).

Before you start, consult your doctor:
If you have had allergic reactions to other topical drugs.

Over age 60:
Adverse reactions and side effects may be more frequent and severe than in younger persons.

Pregnancy:
Decide with your doctor if drug benefits justify any possible risk to unborn child. Risk category C (see page xxii).

Breast-feeding:
Unknown if drug passes into milk. Avoid nursing until you finish medicine. Consult doctor for advice on maintaining milk supply.

Infants & children:
Safety in children has not been established. Use only under close medical supervision. Adverse reactions and side effects may be more frequent and severe.

Prolonged use:
Not intended for long-term use. Usual length of treatment is 8 weeks. If your doctor recommends continued treatment with calcipotriene, discuss the need for follow-up laboratory studies to check calcium levels.

Skin & sunlight:
No special problems expected.

Driving, piloting or hazardous work:
No special problems expected.

Discontinuing:
No special problems expected.

Others:
Wash hands after applying the drug.

POSSIBLE INTERACTION WITH OTHER DRUGS

GENERIC NAME OR DRUG CLASS	COMBINED EFFECT
None expected.	

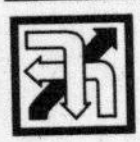

POSSIBLE INTERACTION WITH OTHER SUBSTANCES

INTERACTS WITH	COMBINED EFFECT
Alcohol:	None expected.
Beverages:	None expected.
Cocaine:	None expected.
Foods:	None expected.
Marijuana:	None expected.
Tobacco:	None expected.

CALCIUM CHANNEL BLOCKERS

BRAND AND GENERIC NAMES

See complete list of brand and generic names in *Brand Name Directory*, page 904.

BASIC INFORMATION

Habit forming? No
Prescription needed? Yes
Available as generic? Yes
Drug class: Calcium channel blocker, antiarrhythmic, antianginal

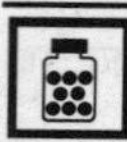

USES

- Prevents angina attacks.
- Stabilizes irregular heartbeat.
- Treats high blood pressure.

DOSAGE & USAGE INFORMATION

How to take:
- Tablet or capsule—Swallow with liquid. You may chew or crush tablet.
- Extended-release tablets or capsules—Swallow each dose whole with liquid; do not crush.

When to take:
At the same times each day. Take verapamil with food.

If you forget a dose:
Take as soon as you remember up to 2 hours late. If more than 2 hours, wait for next scheduled dose (don't double this dose).

Continued next column

OVERDOSE

SYMPTOMS:
Unusually fast or unusually slow heartbeat, loss of consciousness, cardiac arrest.
WHAT TO DO:
- **Dial 911 (emergency) or 0 (operator) for an ambulance or medical help. Then give first aid immediately.**
- **If patient is unconscious and not breathing, give mouth-to-mouth breathing. If there is no heartbeat, use cardiac massage and mouth-to-mouth breathing (CPR). Don't try to make patient vomit. If you can't get help quickly, take patient to nearest emergency facility.**
- **See emergency information on inside covers.**

What drug does:
- Reduces work that heart must perform.
- Reduces normal artery pressure.
- Increases oxygen to heart muscle.

Time lapse before drug works:
1 to 2 hours.

Don't take with:
Any other medicine without consulting your doctor or pharmacist.

POSSIBLE ADVERSE REACTIONS OR SIDE EFFECTS

SYMPTOMS	WHAT TO DO
Life-threatening:	
In case of overdose, see previous column.	
Common:	
Tiredness.	Continue. Tell doctor at next visit.
Infrequent:	
• Unusually fast or unusually slow heartbeat, wheezing, cough, shortness of breath.	Discontinue. Call doctor right away.
• Dizziness; numbness or tingling in hands and feet; swollen feet, ankles or legs; difficult urination.	Continue. Call doctor when convenient.
• Nausea, constipation.	Continue. Tell doctor at next visit.
Rare:	
• Fainting, depression, psychosis, rash, jaundice.	Discontinue. Call doctor right away.
• Headache, insomnia, vivid dreams, hair loss.	Continue. Tell doctor at next visit.

WARNINGS & PRECAUTIONS

Don't take if:
- You are allergic to calcium channel blockers.
- You have very low blood pressure.

Before you start, consult your doctor:
- If you have kidney or liver disease.
- If you have high blood pressure.
- If you have heart disease other than coronary artery disease.

Over age 60:
Adverse reactions and side effects may be more frequent and severe than in younger persons.

Pregnancy:
Decide with your doctor if drug benefits justify risk to unborn child. Risk category C (see page xxii).

Breast-feeding:
Safety not established. Avoid if possible. Consult doctor.

Infants & children:
Not recommended.

Prolonged use:
Talk to your doctor about the need for follow-up medical examinations or laboratory studies to check blood pressure, liver function, kidney function, ECG*.

Skin & sunlight:
No problems expected.

Driving, piloting or hazardous work:
Avoid if you feel dizzy. Otherwise, no problems expected.

Discontinuing:
Don't discontinue without doctor's advice until you complete prescribed dose, even though symptoms diminish or disappear.

Others:
Learn to check your own pulse rate. If it drops to 50 beats per minute or lower, don't take drug until your consult your doctor.

POSSIBLE INTERACTION WITH OTHER DRUGS

GENERIC NAME OR DRUG CLASS	COMBINED EFFECT
Angiotensin-converting (ACE) inhibitors*	Possible excessive potassium in blood. Dosages may require adjustment.
Antiarrhythmics*	Possible increased effect and toxicity of each drug.
Anticoagulants, oral*	Possible increased anticoagulant effect.
Anticonvulsants, hydantoin*	Increased anti-convulsant effect.
Antihypertensives*	Blood pressure drop. Dosages may require adjustment.
Beta-adrenergic blocking agents*	Possible irregular heartbeat and congestive heart failure.
Calcium (large doses)	Possible decreased effect of calcium channel blocker.
Carbamazepine	May increase carbamazepine effect and toxicity.
Cimetidine	Possible increased effect of calcium channel blocker.
Cyclosporine	Increased cyclosporine toxicity.
Digitalis preparations*	Increased digitalis effect. May need to reduce dose.
Disopyramide	May cause dangerously slow, fast or irregular heartbeat.
Diuretics*	Dangerous blood pressure drop. Dosages may require adjustment.
Encainide	Increased effect of toxicity on heart muscle.
Hypokalemia-causing medications*	Increased anti-hypertensive effect.
Lithium	Possible decreased lithium effect.
Nicardipine	Possible increased effect and toxicity of each drug.
Nimodipine	Dangerous blood pressure drop.
Nitrates*	Reduced angina attacks.
Phenytoin	Possible decreased calcium channel blocker effect.
Propafenone	Increased effect of both drugs and increased risk of toxicity.
Quinidine	Increased quinidine effect.

Continued on page 933

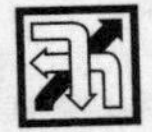

POSSIBLE INTERACTION WITH OTHER SUBSTANCES

INTERACTS WITH	COMBINED EFFECT
Alcohol:	Dangerously low blood pressure. Avoid.
Beverages:	None expected.
Cocaine:	Possible irregular heartbeat. Avoid.
Foods:	None expected.
Marijuana:	Possible irregular heartbeat. Avoid.
Tobacco:	Possible rapid heart-beat. Avoid.

*See Glossary

CALCIUM SUPPLEMENTS

BRAND AND GENERIC NAMES

See complete list of brand and generic names in the *Brand Name Directory*, page 904.

BASIC INFORMATION

Habit forming? No
Prescription needed? For some
Available as generic? Yes
Drug class: Antihypocalcemic, dietary replacement

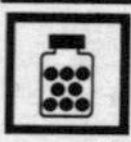

USES

- Treats or prevents osteoporosis (thin, porous, easily fractured bones). Frequently prescribed with estrogen beginning at menopause.
- Helps heart, muscle and nervous system to work properly.
- Dietary supplement when calcium ingestion is insufficient or there is a deficiency such as osteomalacia or rickets.

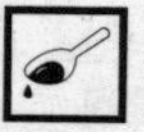

DOSAGE & USAGE INFORMATION

How to take:
- Take in addition to foods high in calcium (milk, yogurt, sardines, cheese, canned salmon, turnip greens, broccoli, shrimp, tofu).
- Tablet—Swallow with liquid or food to lessen stomach irritation. If you can't swallow whole, crumble tablet and take with food or liquid.
- Syrup—Take before meals.
- Suspension—Swallow with liquid or food to lessen stomach irritation.

When to take:
As directed. Don't take within 2 hours of any other medicine you take by mouth.

If you forget a dose:
Use as soon as you remember.

Continued next column

OVERDOSE

SYMPTOMS:
Confusion, irregular heartbeat, depression, bone pain, coma.
WHAT TO DO:
- **Dial 911 (emergency) or 0 (operator) for an ambulance or medical help. Then give first aid immediately.**
- **See emergency information on inside covers.**

What drug does:
- Participates in metabolism of all activities essential for normal life and function of cells.
- Provides calcium necessary for bone, nerve function.

Time lapse before drug works:
15 to 30 minutes.

Don't take with:
- Any other medicine until 2 hours have passed since taking calcium.
- Any other medicine without consulting your doctor or pharmacist.

POSSIBLE ADVERSE REACTIONS OR SIDE EFFECTS

SYMPTOMS	WHAT TO DO
Life-threatening:	
Irregular or very slow heart rate.	Discontinue. Seek emergency treatment.
Common:	
None expected.	
Infrequent:	
Constipation, diarrhea, drowsiness, headache, appetite loss, dry mouth, weakness.	Discontinue. Call doctor right away.
Rare:	
Frequent, painful or difficult urination; increased thirst; nausea, vomiting; rash; urine frequency increased and volume larger; confusion; high blood pressure; eyes sensitive to light.	Discontinue. Call doctor right away.

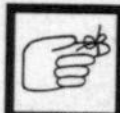

WARNINGS & PRECAUTIONS

Don't take if:
- You are allergic to calcium.
- You have a high blood calcium level.

Before you start, consult your doctor:
If you have diarrhea, heart disease, kidney stones, kidney disease, sarcoidosis, malabsorption.

Over age 60:
No problems expected.

Pregnancy:
Consult doctor. Risk category C (see page xxii).

Breast-feeding:
No problems expected. Consult doctor.

Infants & children:
Use only under close medical supervision.

Prolonged use:
- Side effects more likely.
- Talk to your doctor about the need for follow-up medical examinations or laboratory studies to check serum calcium determinations, blood pressure, urine.

Skin & sunlight:
No problems expected.

Driving, piloting or hazardous work:
No problems expected.

Discontinuing:
No problems expected.

Others:
- Exercise, along with vitamin D from sunshine and calcium, helps prevent osteoporosis.
- Don't use bone meal or dolomite as a source for calcium supplement (they may contain lead).

POSSIBLE INTERACTION WITH OTHER DRUGS

GENERIC NAME OR DRUG CLASS	COMBINED EFFECT
Anticoagulants, oral*	Decreased anti-coagulant effect.
Calcitonin	Decreased calcitonin effect.
Calcium-containing medicines, other	Increased calcium effect.
Chlorpromazine	Decreased chlor-promazine effect.
Contraceptives, oral*	May increase absorption of calcium—frequently a desirable combined effect.
Corticosteroids*	Decreased calcium absorption and effect.
Digitalis preparations*	Decreased digitalis effect.
Diuretics, thiazide*	Increased calcium in blood.
Estrogens*	May increase absorption of calcium—frequently a desirable combined effect.
Etidronate	Decreased etidronate absorption. Take drugs 2 hours apart.
Iron supplements*	Decreased iron effect.
Meperidine	Increased meperidine effect.
Mexiletine	May slow elimination of mexiletine and cause need to adjust dosage.
Nalidixic acid	Decreased effect of nalidixic acid.
Nicardipine	Possible decreased nicardipine effect.
Nimodipine	Possible decreased nimodipine effect.
Oxyphenbutazone	Decreased oxyphen-butazone effect.
Para-aminosalicylic acid (PAS)	Decreased PAS effect.
Penicillins*	Decreased penicillin effect.
Pentobarbital	Decreased pento-barbital effect.
Phenylbutazone	Decreased phenyl-butazone effect.
Phenytoin	Decreased phenytoin absorption.
Pseudoephedrine	Increased pseudo-ephedrine effect.
Quinidine	Increased quinidine effect.
Salicylates*	Increased salicylate effect.
Sulfa drugs*	Decreased sulfa effect.
Tetracyclines*	Decreased tetracy-cline effect.

Continued on page 933

POSSIBLE INTERACTION WITH OTHER SUBSTANCES

INTERACTS WITH	COMBINED EFFECT
Alcohol:	Decreased absorption of calcium.
Beverages:	No problems expected.
Cocaine:	No proven problems.
Foods: Don't take within 1 or 2 hours of eating.	Decreased absorption of calcium.
Marijuana:	Decreased absorption of calcium.
Tobacco:	Decreased absorption of calcium.

***See Glossary**

CAPSAICIN

BRAND NAMES

Axsain
Zotrix
Zotrix-HP

BASIC INFORMATION

Habit forming? No
Prescription needed? No
Available as generic? Yes
Drug class: Analgesic (topical)

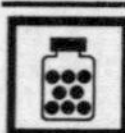

USES

- Treats neuralgias, such as pain that occurs following shingles (herpes zoster) or neuropathy of the feet, ankles and fingers (common in diabetes).
- Treats discomfort caused by arthritis.

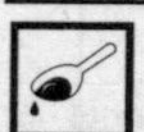

DOSAGE & USAGE INFORMATION

How to use:
Cream—Apply a small amount and rub carefully on the affected areas. Use every day. Wash hands after applying. Don't apply to irritated skin. Don't bandage over treated areas.

When to use:
Apply 3 or 4 times a day.

If you forget a dose:
Use as soon as you remember.

What drug does:
Blocks transmission of pain impulses.

Time lapse before drug works:
Begins to work immediately. Frequently takes 2 to 3 weeks for full benefit, but may take up to 6 or 8 weeks.

Don't use with:
No problems expected.

OVERDOSE

SYMPTOMS:
None expected.
WHAT TO DO:
Not intended for internal use. If child accidentally swallows, call poison control center.

POSSIBLE ADVERSE REACTIONS OR SIDE EFFECTS

SYMPTOMS	WHAT TO DO
Life-threatening: None expected.	
Common: Stinging or burning sensation at application site.	Nothing. It usually improves in 2 to 3 days or becomes less severe the longer you use the drug.
Infrequent: None expected.	
Rare: None expected.	

WARNINGS & PRECAUTIONS

Don't use if:
You are allergic to capsaicin or to the fruit of capsaicin plants (for example, hot peppers).

Before you start, consult your doctor:
If you have any allergies.

Over age 60:
No problems expected.

Pregnancy:
Consult doctor. Risk category C (see page xxii).

Breast-feeding:
No problems expected. Consult doctor.

Infants & children:
Not recommended for children under age 2.

Prolonged use:
No problems expected.

Skin & sunlight:
No problems expected.

Driving, piloting or hazardous work:
No problems expected.

Discontinuing:
Discontinue if there are no signs of improvement within a month.

Others:
- Capsaicin is not a local anesthetic*.
- Although capsaicin may help relieve the pain of neuropathy, it does not cure any disorder.
- If you accidently get some capsaicin in your eye, flush with water.

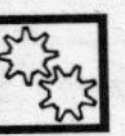

POSSIBLE INTERACTION WITH OTHER DRUGS

GENERIC NAME OR DRUG CLASS	COMBINED EFFECT
None expected	

POSSIBLE INTERACTION WITH OTHER SUBSTANCES

INTERACTS WITH	COMBINED EFFECT
Alcohol:	No proven problems.
Beverages:	No proven problems.
Cocaine:	No proven problems.
Foods:	No proven problems.
Marijuana:	No proven problems.
Tobacco:	No proven problems.

*See Glossary

CARBAMAZEPINE

BRAND NAMES

Apo-Carbamazepine
Epitol
Mazepine
Novocarbamaz
PMS Carbamazepine
Tegretol
Tegretol Chewtabs
Tegretol CR

BASIC INFORMATION

Habit forming? No
Prescription needed? Yes
Available as generic? Yes
Drug class: Analgesic, anticonvulsant

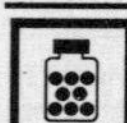

USES

- Decreased frequency, severity and duration of attacks of tic douloureux*.
- Prevents seizures.
- Used for pain relief, alcohol withdrawal, bipolar disorder, diabetes insipidus.

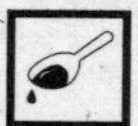

DOSAGE & USAGE INFORMATION

How to take:
Regular or chewable tablet—Swallow with liquid or food to lessen stomach irritation.

When to take:
At the same times each day.

If you forget a dose:
Take as soon as you remember up to 2 hours late. If more than 2 hours, wait for next scheduled dose (don't double this dose).

Continued next column

OVERDOSE

SYMPTOMS:
Involuntary movements, irregular bleeding, decreased urination, decreased blood pressure, dilated pupils, flushed skin, stupor, coma.

WHAT TO DO:
- **Dial 911 (emergency) or 0 (operator) for an ambulance or medical help. Then give first aid immediately.**
- **If patient is unconscious and not breathing, give mouth-to-mouth breathing. If there is no heartbeat, use cardiac massage and mouth-to-mouth breathing (CPR). Don't try to make patient vomit. If you can't get help quickly, take patient to nearest emergency facility.**
- **See emergency information on inside covers.**

What drug does:
- Reduces transmission of pain messages at certain nerve terminals.
- Reduces excitability of nerve fibers in brain, thus inhibiting repetitive spread of nerve impulses.

Time lapse before drug works:
- Tic douloureux—24 to 72 hours.
- Seizures—1 to 2 weeks.

Don't take with:
Any other medicine without consulting your doctor or pharmacist.

POSSIBLE ADVERSE REACTIONS OR SIDE EFFECTS

SYMPTOMS	WHAT TO DO
Life-threatening:	
In case of overdose, see previous column.	
Common:	
• Blurred vision.	Continue. Call doctor when convenient.
• Back-and-forth eye movements.	Discontinue. Call doctor right away.
Infrequent:	
• Confusion, slurred speech, fainting, depression, headache, hallucinations, hives, rash, mouth sores, sore throat, fever, unusual bleeding or bruising, unusual fatigue, jaundice.	Discontinue. Call doctor right away.
• Diarrhea, nausea, vomiting, constipation, dry mouth, impotence.	Continue. Call doctor when convenient.
Rare:	
• Breathing difficulty; irregular, pounding or slow heartbeat; chest pain; uncontrollable body jerks; numbness, weakness or tingling in hands and feet; tender, bluish legs or feet; less urine; swollen lymph glands.	Discontinue. Call doctor right away.
• Frequent urination, muscle pains, joint aches.	Continue. Call doctor when convenient.

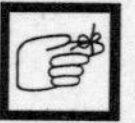

WARNINGS & PRECAUTIONS

Don't take if:
- You are allergic to carbamazepine or any tricyclic antidepressant*.
- You have had liver or bone marrow disease.

- You have taken a monoamine oxidase (MAO) inhibitor* in the past 2 weeks.

Before you start, consult your doctor:
- If you have high blood pressure, thrombophlebitis or heart disease.
- If you have glaucoma.
- If you have emotional or mental problems.
- If you have liver or kidney disease.
- If you drink more than 2 alcoholic drinks per day.

Over age 60:
Adverse reactions and side effects may be more frequent and severe than in younger persons.

Pregnancy:
Decide with your doctor whether drug benefits justify risk to unborn child. Risk category C (see page xxii).

Breast-feeding:
Drug passes into milk. Avoid drug or discontinue nursing until you finish medicine. Consult doctor for advice on maintaining milk supply.

Infants & children:
Not recommended.

Prolonged use:
- Jaundice and liver damage.
- Hair loss.
- Ringing in ears.
- Lower sex drive.
- Talk to your doctor about the need for follow-up medical examinations or laboratory studies to check complete blood counts (white blood cell count, platelet count, red blood cell count, hemoglobin, hematocrit), serum iron.

Skin & sunlight:
May cause rash or intensify sunburn in areas exposed to sun or sunlamp.

Driving, piloting or hazardous work:
Don't drive or pilot aircraft until you learn how medicine effects you. Don't work around dangerous machinery. Don't climb ladders or work in high places. Danger increases if you drink alcohol or take medicine affecting alertness and reflexes.

Discontinuing:
Don't discontinue without doctor's advice until you complete prescribed dose, even though symptoms diminish or disappear.

Others:
- Use only if less hazardous drugs are not effective. Stay under medical supervision.
- Periodic blood tests are needed.

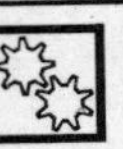

POSSIBLE INTERACTION WITH OTHER DRUGS

GENERIC NAME OR DRUG CLASS	COMBINED EFFECT
Anticoagulants, oral*	Decreased anticoagulant effect.
Anticonvulsants, hydantoin* or succinimide	Decreased effect of both drugs.
Antidepressants, tricyclic*	Confusion. Possible psychosis.
Barbiturates	Possible increased barbiturate metabolism.
Cimetidine	Increased carbamazepine effect.
Cisapride	Decreased carbamazepine effect.
Clozapine	Toxic effect on bone marrow and central nervous system.
Contraceptives, oral*	Reduced contraceptive protection. Use another birth control method.
Cortisone*	Decreased cortisone effect.
Desmopressin	May increase desmopressin effect.
Digitalis preparations*	Excess slowing of heart.

Continued on page 934

POSSIBLE INTERACTION WITH OTHER SUBSTANCES

INTERACTS WITH	COMBINED EFFECT
Alcohol:	Increased sedative effect of alcohol. Avoid.
Beverages:	None expected.
Cocaine:	Increased adverse effects of carbamazepine. Avoid.
Foods:	None expected.
Marijuana:	Increased adverse effects of carbamazepine. Avoid.
Tobacco:	None expected.

*See Glossary

CARBIDOPA & LEVODOPA

BRAND NAMES

Sinemet
Sinemet CR

BASIC INFORMATION

Habit forming? No
Prescription needed? Yes
Available as generic? Yes
Drug class: Antiparkinsonism

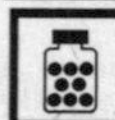

USES

Controls Parkinson's disease symptoms such as rigidity, tremor and unsteady gait.

DOSAGE & USAGE INFORMATION

How to take:
- Tablet—Swallow with liquid or food to lessen stomach irritation. If you can't swallow whole, crumble tablet and take with liquid or food.
- Extended-release tablet—Swallow each dose whole; do not crumble.

When to take:
At the same times each day.

If you forget a dose:
Take as soon as you remember up to 2 hours late. If more than 2 hours, wait for next scheduled dose (don't double this dose).

What drug does:
Restores chemical balance necessary for normal nerve impulses.

Continued next column

OVERDOSE

SYMPTOMS:
Muscle twitch, spastic eyelid closure, nausea, vomiting, diarrhea, irregular and rapid pulse, weakness, fainting, confusion, agitation, hallucination, coma.
WHAT TO DO:
- **Dial 911 (emergency) or 0 (operator) for an ambulance or medical help. Then give first aid immediately.**
- **If patient is unconscious and not breathing, give mouth-to-mouth breathing. If there is no heartbeat, use cardiac massage and mouth-to-mouth breathing (CPR). Don't try to make patient vomit. If you can't get help quickly, take patient to nearest emergency facility.**
- **See emergency information on inside covers.**

Time lapse before drug works:
2 to 3 weeks to improve; 6 weeks or longer for maximum benefit.

Don't take with:
Any other medicine without consulting your doctor or pharmacist.

POSSIBLE ADVERSE REACTIONS OR SIDE EFFECTS

SYMPTOMS	WHAT TO DO
Life-threatening:	
In case of overdose, see previous column.	
Common:	
• Mood changes, uncontrollable body movements, diarrhea.	Continue. Call doctor when convenient.
• Dry mouth, body odor.	No action necessary.
Infrequent:	
• Fainting, severe dizziness, headache, insomnia, nightmares, rash, itch, nausea, vomiting, irregular heartbeat.	Discontinue. Call doctor right away.
• Flushed face, blurred vision, muscle twitching, discolored or dark urine, difficult urination.	Continue. Call doctor when convenient.
• Constipation, tiredness.	Continue. Tell doctor at next visit.
Rare:	
• High blood pressure.	Discontinue. Call doctor right away.
• Upper abdominal pain, anemia.	Continue. Call doctor when convenient.

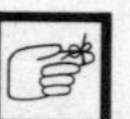

WARNINGS & PRECAUTIONS

Don't take if:
- You are allergic to levodopa or carbidopa.
- You have taken MAO inhibitors in past 2 weeks.
- You have glaucoma (narrow-angle type).

Before you start, consult your doctor:
- You have diabetes or epilepsy.
- If you have had high blood pressure, heart or lung disease.
- If you have had liver or kidney disease.
- If you have a peptic ulcer.
- If you have malignant melanoma.
- If you will have surgery within 2 months, including dental surgery, requiring general or spinal anesthesia.

CARBIDOPA & LEVODOPA

Over age 60:
Adverse reactions and side effects may be more frequent and severe than in younger persons.

Pregnancy:
Decide with your doctor whether drug benefits justify risk to unborn child. Risk category C (see page xxii).

Breast-feeding:
Drug filters into milk. May harm child. Avoid.

Infants & children:
Not recommended.

Prolonged use:
- May lead to uncontrolled movements of head, face, mouth, tongue, arms or legs.
- Talk to your doctor about the need for follow-up medical examinations or laboratory studies to check complete blood counts (white blood cell count, platelet count, red blood cell count, hemoglobin, hematocrit), liver function, eyes, kidney function.

Skin & sunlight:
No problems expected.

Driving, piloting or hazardous work:
Don't drive or pilot aircraft until you learn how medicine affects you. Don't work around dangerous machinery. Don't climb ladders or work in high places. Danger increases if you drink alcohol or take medicine affecting alertness and reflexes, such as antihistamines, tranquilizers, sedatives, pain medicine, narcotics and mind-altering drugs.

Discontinuing:
Don't discontinue without doctor's advice until you complete prescribed dose, even though symptoms diminish or disappear.

Others:
Expect to start with small dose and increase gradually to lessen frequency and severity of adverse reactions.

POSSIBLE INTERACTION WITH OTHER DRUGS

GENERIC NAME OR DRUG CLASS	COMBINED EFFECT
Anticonvulsants*, hydantoin	Decreased effect of carbidopa and levodopa.
Antidepressants*	Weakness or faintness when arising from bed or chair.
Antihypertensives*	Decreased blood pressure and effect of carbidopa and levodopa.
Antiparkinsonism drugs, other*	Increased effect of carbidopa and levodopa.
Haloperidol	Decreased effect of carbidopa and levodopa.
Methyldopa	Decreased effect of carbidopa and levodopa.
Monoamine oxidase (MAO) inhibitors*	Dangerous rise in blood pressure.
Papaverine	Decreased effect of carbidopa and levodopa.
Phenothiazines*	Decreased effect of carbidopa and levodopa.
Phenytoin	Decreased effect of carbidopa and levodopa.
Pyridoxine (Vitamin B-6)	Decreased effect of carbidopa and levodopa.
Rauwolfia alkaloids*	Decreased effect of carbidopa and levodopa.
Selegiline	May require adjustment in dosage of carbidopa and levodopa.

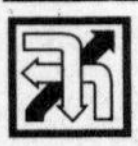

POSSIBLE INTERACTION WITH OTHER SUBSTANCES

INTERACTS WITH	COMBINED EFFECT
Alcohol:	None expected.
Beverages:	None expected.
Cocaine:	Decreased cabidopa and levodopa effect. High rise of hearbeat irregularities. Avoid.
Foods:	None expected.
Marijuana:	Increased fatigue, lethargy, fainting.
Tobacco:	None expected.

***See Glossary**

CARBOHYDRATES & ELECTROLYTES

BRAND NAMES

Gastrolyte
Lytren RHS
Oral rehydration salts
ORS-bicarbonate
ORS-citrate
Pedialyte
Rapolyte
Rehydralyte
Resol
Ricelyte

BASIC INFORMATION

Habit forming? No
Prescription needed? Not for all
Available as generic? Yes
Drug class: Electrolyte replenisher

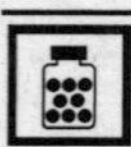

USES

Replenishes fluids and electrolytes (salts) in dehydrated children and adults.

DOSAGE & USAGE INFORMATION

How to take:
Follow package instructions.

When to take:
According to doctor's instructions. Frequency of need varies greatly.

If you forget a dose:
Take as soon as you remember up to 2 hours late. If more than 2 hours, wait for next scheduled dose (don't double this dose).

What drug does:
Prevents and treats electrolyte imbalance due to severe diarrhea.

Time lapse before drug works:
8 to 12 hours.

Don't take with:
Any other medicines (including over-the-counter drugs such as cough and cold medicines, laxatives, antacids, diet pills, caffeine, nose drops or vitamins) without consulting your doctor.

OVERDOSE

SYMPTOMS:
Seizures.
WHAT TO DO:
- **Dial 911 (emergency) or 0 (operator) for an ambulance or medical help. Then give first aid immediately.**
- **See emergency information on inside covers.**

POSSIBLE ADVERSE REACTIONS OR SIDE EFFECTS

SYMPTOMS	WHAT TO DO
Life-threatening:	
In case of overdose, see previous column.	
Common:	
Vomiting.	Continue treatment.
Infrequent:	
Failure to improve.	Continue.
Rare:	
• Too-high blood sodium level, causing convulsions.	Discontinue. Seek emergency treatment.
• Overhydration (puffy eyes).	Discontinue. Call doctor right away.

WARNINGS & PRECAUTIONS

Don't take if:
- Kidneys are not functioning.
- Patient is unable to drink.
- There is severe and sustained vomiting.

Before you start, consult your doctor:
If patient is younger than 6 months.

Over age 60:
No problems expected; well tolerated by older patients.

Pregnancy:
Risk category not designated. See page xxii and consult doctor.

Breast-feeding:
No problems expected. Consult doctor.

Infants & children:
Safe and effective in young; not yet evaluated in premature infants.

Prolonged use:
Talk to your doctor about the need for follow-up medical examinations or laboratory studies to check body weight, blood pressure, serum electrolytes and serum pH.

Skin & sunlight:
No problems expected.

Driving, piloting or hazardous work:
No problems expected.

Discontinuing:
No special problems expected.

Others:
- Advise any doctor or dentist whom you consult that you take this medicine.
- May affect results in some medical tests.

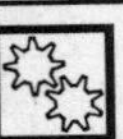

POSSIBLE INTERACTION WITH OTHER DRUGS

GENERIC NAME OR DRUG CLASS	COMBINED EFFECT
None expected.	

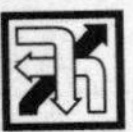

POSSIBLE INTERACTION WITH OTHER SUBSTANCES

INTERACTS WITH	COMBINED EFFECT
Alcohol:	Dangerous. Avoid.
Beverages:	Continuing milk all right. Others as tolerated.
Cocaine:	Dangerous. Avoid.
Foods: Rice, cereal, bananas, cooked potatoes or other carbohydrate-rich foods as tolerated.	Helps maintain nutrition.
Marijuana:	Dangerous. Avoid.
Tobacco:	May increase diarrhea. Avoid.

*See Glossary

CARBOL-FUCHSIN (Topical)

BRAND NAMES

Castellani Paint **Castel Plus**

BASIC INFORMATION

Habit forming? No
Prescription needed? No
Available as generic? Yes
Drug class: Antifungal (topical), drying agent (topical)

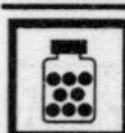

USES

Treats fungus infections of skin and nails.

DOSAGE & USAGE INFORMATION

How to use:
Topical solution—Wash and dry affected areas. Use an applicator or swab to apply to affected areas only. Don't bandage. You may need to apply for several months to cure.

When to use:
As directed, usually 1 to 3 times a day.

If you forget a dose:
Apply as soon as remember.

What drug does:
- Kills spores of fungus and some bacteria.
- Stimulates growth of new skin.

Time lapse before drug works:
2 to 3 weeks or more.

Don't use with:
Any other topical medicine without telling your doctor.

OVERDOSE

SYMPTOMS:
None expected unless accidentally swallowed.
WHAT TO DO:
If accidentally swallowed, call nearest poison control center or your doctor.

POSSIBLE ADVERSE REACTIONS OR SIDE EFFECTS

SYMPTOMS	WHAT TO DO
Life-threatening: None expected.	
Common: Skin irritation.	Discontinue. Call doctor right away.
Infrequent: Mild stinging where applied.	No action necessary.
Rare: None expected.	

WARNINGS & PRECAUTIONS

Don't use if:
No special problems expected.

Before you start, consult your doctor:
If you are taking any other prescription or nonprescription medicine.

Over age 60:
No special problems expected.

Pregnancy:
Consult doctor. Risk category C (see page xxii).

Breast-feeding:
No special problems expected. Consult doctor.

Infants & children:
Don't use more than once daily.

Prolonged use:
No special problems expected.

Skin & sunlight:
No special problems expected.

Driving, piloting or hazardous work:
No special problems expected.

Discontinuing:
No special problems expected.

Others:
Advise any doctor or dentist whom you consult that you take this medicine.

POSSIBLE INTERACTION WITH OTHER DRUGS

GENERIC NAME OR DRUG CLASS	COMBINED EFFECT
None expected.	

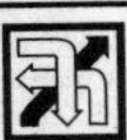

POSSIBLE INTERACTION WITH OTHER SUBSTANCES

INTERACTS WITH	COMBINED EFFECT
Alcohol:	None expected.
Beverages:	None expected.
Cocaine:	None expected.
Foods:	None expected.
Marijuana:	None expected.
Tobacco:	None expected.

*See Glossary

CARBONIC ANHYDRASE INHIBITORS

BRAND AND GENERIC NAMES

Acetazolam
ACETAZOLAMIDE
Ak-Zol
Apo-Acetazolamide
Daranide
Dazamide
Diamox
DICHLORPHENAMIDE
METHAZOLAMIDE
Neptazane

BASIC INFORMATION

Habit forming? No
Prescription needed? Yes
Available as generic? Yes
Drug class: Carbonic anhydrase inhibitor

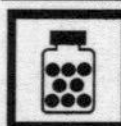

USES

- Treatment of glaucoma.
- Treatment of epileptic seizures.
- Treatment of body fluid retention.
- Treatment for shortness of breath, insomnia and fatigue at high altitudes.
- Treatment for prevention of altitude illness.

DOSAGE & USAGE INFORMATION

How to take:
- Sustained-release tablets—Swallow whole with liquid or food to lessen stomach irritation.
- Extended-release capsules—Swallow whole with liquid.

When to take:
- 1 dose per day—At the same time each morning.
- More than 1 dose per day—Take last dose several hours before bedtime.

If you forget a dose:
Take as soon as you remember. Continue regular schedule.

Continued next column

OVERDOSE

SYMPTOMS:
Drowsiness, confusion, excitement, nausea, vomiting, numbness in hands and feet, coma.
WHAT TO DO:
- **Call your doctor or poison control center for advice if you suspect overdose, even if not sure. Symptoms may not appear until damage has occurred.**
- **See emergency information on inside covers.**

What drug does:
- Inhibits action of carbonic anhydrase, an enzyme. This lowers the internal eye pressure by decreasing fluid formation in the eye.
- Forces sodium and water excretion, reducing body fluid.

Time lapse before drug works:
2 hours.

Don't take with:
- Nonprescription drugs without consulting doctor.
- See Interaction column and consult doctor.

POSSIBLE ADVERSE REACTIONS OR SIDE EFFECTS

SYMPTOMS	WHAT TO DO
Life-threatening:	
Convulsions.	Seek emergency treatment immediately.
Common:	
None expected.	
Infrequent:	
Back pain, sedation, fatigue, weakness, tingling or burning in feet or hands.	Continue. Call doctor when convenient.
Rare:	
• Headache; mood changes; nervousness; clumsiness; trembling; confusion; hives, itch, rash; sores; ringing in ears; hoarseness; dry mouth; thirst; sore throat; fever; appetite change; nausea; vomiting; black, tarry stool; breathing difficulty; irregular or weak heartbeat; easy bleeding or bruising; muscle cramps; painful or frequent urination; blood in urine.	Continue. Call doctor right away.
• Depression, loss of libido.	Continue. Call doctor when convenient.

CARBONIC ANHYDRASE INHIBITORS

WARNINGS & PRECAUTIONS

Don't take if:
- You are allergic to any carbonic anhydrase inhibitor.
- You have liver or kidney disease.
- You have Addison's disease (adrenal gland failure).
- You have diabetes.

Before you start, consult your doctor:
- If you have gout or lupus.
- If you are allergic to any sulfa drug.
- If you will have surgery within 2 months, including dental surgery, requiring general or spinal anesthesia.

Over age 60:
- Don't exceed recommended dose.
- If you take a digitalis preparation, eat foods high in potassium content or take a potassium supplement.

Pregnancy:
Avoid if possible, especially first 3 months. Consult doctor. Risk category C (see page xxii).

Breast-feeding:
Avoid drug or don't nurse your infant. Consult doctor about maintaining milk supply.

Infants & children:
Not recommended for children younger than 12.

Prolonged use:
May cause kidney stones, vision change, loss of taste and smell, jaundice or weight loss.

Skin & sunlight:
No problems expected.

Driving, piloting or hazardous work:
Avoid if you feel drowsy or dizzy. Otherwise, no problems expected.

Discontinuing:
Don't discontinue without medical advice.

Others:
Medicine may increase sugar levels in blood and urine. Diabetics may need insulin adjustment.

POSSIBLE INTERACTION WITH OTHER DRUGS

GENERIC NAME OR DRUG CLASS	COMBINED EFFECT
Amphetamines*	Increased amphetamine effect.
Anticonvulsants*	Increased loss of bone minerals.
Antidepressants, tricyclic*	Increased antidepressant effect.
Antidiabetics, oral*	Increased potassium loss.
Aspirin	Decreased aspirin effect.
Ciprofloxacin	May cause kidney dysfunction.
Cortisone drugs*	Increased potassium loss.
Digitalis preparations*	Possible digitalis toxicity.
Diuretics*	Increased potassium loss.
Lithium	Decreased lithium effect.
Mecamylamine	Increased mecamylamine effect.
Methenamine	Decreased methenamine effect.
Mexiletene	May slow elimination of mexilitene and cause need to adjust dosage.
Quinidine	Increased quinidine effect.
Salicylates*	Salicylate toxicity.
Sympathomimetics*	Increased sympathomimetic effect.

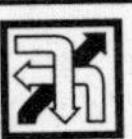

POSSIBLE INTERACTION WITH OTHER SUBSTANCES

INTERACTS WITH	COMBINED EFFECT
Alcohol:	None expected.
Beverages:	None expected.
Cocaine:	Avoid. Decreased carbonic anhydrase inhibitor effect.
Foods: Potassium-rich foods.*	Eat these to decrease potassium loss.
Marijuana:	Avoid. Increased carbonic anhydrase inhibitor effect.
Tobacco:	May decrease absorption of carbonic anhydrase inhibitors.

***See Glossary**

CASCARA

BRAND NAMES

Aromatic Cascara Fluidextract
Cascara Sagrada
Caroid Laxative
Nature's Remedy

BASIC INFORMATION

Habit forming? No
Prescription needed? No
Available as generic? Yes
Drug class: Laxative (stimulant)

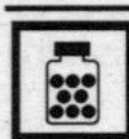

USES

Constipation relief.

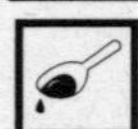

DOSAGE & USAGE INFORMATION

How to take:

- Follow package instructions.
- Tablet—Swallow with liquid. If you can't swallow whole, chew or crumble tablet and take with liquid or food.
- Liquid—Drink 6 to 8 glasses of water each day, in addition to one taken with each dose.

When to take:
Usually at bedtime with a snack, unless directed otherwise.

If you forget a dose:
Take as soon as you remember.

What drug does:
Acts on smooth muscles of intestine wall to cause vigorous bowel movement.

Time lapse before drug works:
6 to 10 hours.

Don't take with:

- Any other medicine without consulting your doctor or pharmacist.
- Don't take within 2 hours of taking another medicine. Laxative interferes with medicine absorption.

OVERDOSE

SYMPTOMS:
Vomiting, electrolyte depletion.
WHAT TO DO:
Overdose unlikely to threaten life. If person takes much larger amount than prescribed, call doctor, poison control center or hospital emergency room for instructions.

POSSIBLE ADVERSE REACTIONS OR SIDE EFFECTS

SYMPTOMS	WHAT TO DO
Life-threatening: None expected.	
Common: Rectal irritation.	Continue. Call doctor when convenient.
Infrequent:	
• Dangerous potassium loss (thirst, weakness, heartbeat irregularity, paralysis, nausea and diarrhea).	Discontinue. Call doctor right away.
• Belching, cramps, nausea.	Continue. Call doctor when convenient.
Rare:	
• Irritability, confusion, headache, rash, breathing difficulty, irregular heartbeat, muscle cramps, unusual tiredness or weakness.	Discontinue. Call doctor right away.
• Burning on urination.	Continue. Call doctor when convenient.
• Discoloration of urine.	No action necessary.

WARNINGS & PRECAUTIONS

Don't take if:
- You have symptoms of appendicitis, inflamed bowel or intestinal blockage.
- You are allergic to a stimulant laxative.
- You have missed a bowel movement for only 1 or 2 days.

Before you start, consult your doctor:
- If you have a colostomy or ileostomy.
- If you have congestive heart disease.
- If you have diabetes.
- If you have high blood pressure.
- If you have a laxative habit.
- If you have rectal bleeding.
- If you take other laxatives.

Over age 60:
Adverse reactions and side effects may be more frequent and severe than in younger persons.

Pregnancy:
Decide with your doctor if drug benefits justify risk to unborn child. Risk category C (see page xxii).

Breast-feeding:
Drug passes into milk. Avoid drug or discontinue nursing until you finish medicine. Consult doctor for advice on maintaining milk supply.

Infants & children:
Use only under medical supervision.

Prolonged use:
Don't take for more than 1 week unless under a doctor's supervision. May cause laxative dependence.

Skin & sunlight:
No problems expected.

Driving, piloting or hazardous work:
No problems expected.

Discontinuing:
May be unnecessary to finish medicine. Follow doctor's instructions.

Others:
Don't take to "flush out" your system or as a "tonic."

POSSIBLE INTERACTION WITH OTHER DRUGS

GENERIC NAME OR DRUG CLASS	COMBINED EFFECT
Antacids*	Irritation of stomach or small intestine.
Digoxin	Increased toxicity due to decreased potassium level.
Diuretics*	May cause dangerous low potassium level.
Ranitidine	Irritation of stomach or small intestine.

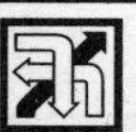

POSSIBLE INTERACTION WITH OTHER SUBSTANCES

INTERACTS WITH	COMBINED EFFECT
Alcohol:	None expected.
Beverages:	None expected.
Cocaine:	None expected.
Foods:	None expected.
Marijuana:	None expected.
Tobacco:	None expected.

***See Glossary**

CASTOR OIL

BRAND NAMES

Alphamul
Emulsoil
Fleet Flavored Castor Oil
Kellogg's Castor Oil
Neoloid
Purge

BASIC INFORMATION

Habit forming? No
Prescription needed? No
Available as generic? Yes
Drug class: Laxative (stimulant)

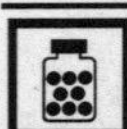

USES

Constipation relief.

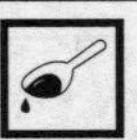

DOSAGE & USAGE INFORMATION

How to take:
- Follow package instructions.
- Liquid or capsules—Drink 6 to 8 glasses of water each day, in addition to one taken with each dose.

When to take:
Usually at bedtime with a snack, unless directed otherwise.

If you forget a dose:
Take as soon as you remember.

What drug does:
Acts on smooth muscles of intestine wall to cause vigorous bowel movement.

Time lapse before drug works:
2 to 6 hours.

Don't take with:
- Any other medicine without consulting your doctor or pharmacist.
- Don't take within 2 hours of taking another medicine. Laxative interferes with medicine absorption.

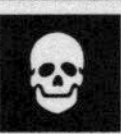

OVERDOSE

SYMPTOMS:
Vomiting, electrolyte depletion.
WHAT TO DO:
Overdose unlikely to threaten life. If person takes much larger amount than prescribed, call doctor, poison control center or hospital emergency room for instructions.

POSSIBLE ADVERSE REACTIONS OR SIDE EFFECTS

SYMPTOMS	WHAT TO DO
Life-threatening:	
None expected.	
Common:	
Rectal irritation.	Continue. Call doctor when convenient.
Infrequent:	
• Dangerous potassium loss (thirst, weakness, heartbeat irregularities, paralysis, nausea and diarrhea).	Discontinue. Call doctor right away.
• Belching, cramps, nausea.	Continue. Call doctor when convenient.
Rare:	
• Irritability, headache, confusion, rash, breathing difficulty, irregular heartbeat, muscle cramps, unusual tiredness or weakness.	Discontinue. Call doctor right away.
• Burning on urination.	Continue. Call doctor when convenient.

WARNINGS & PRECAUTIONS

Don't take if:
- You have symptoms of appendicitis, inflamed bowel or intestinal blockage.
- You are allergic to a stimulant laxative.
- You have missed a bowel movement for only 1 or 2 days.

Before you start, consult your doctor:
- If you have a colostomy or ileostomy.
- If you have congestive heart disease.
- If you have diabetes.
- If you have high blood pressure.
- If you have a laxative habit.
- If you have rectal bleeding.
- If you take other laxatives.

Over age 60:
Adverse reactions and side effects may be more frequent and severe than in younger persons.

Pregnancy:
Risk to mother and unborn child outweighs drug benefits. Don't use. Risk category X (see page xxii).

Breast-feeding:
Drug passes into milk. Avoid drug or discontinue nursing until you finish medicine. Consult doctor for advice on maintaining milk supply.

Infants & children:
Use only under medical supervision.

Prolonged use:
Don't take for more than 1 week unless under doctor's supervision. May cause laxative dependence.

Skin & sunlight:
No problems expected.

Driving, piloting or hazardous work:
No problems expected.

Discontinuing:
May be unnecessary to finish medicine. Follow doctor's instructions.

Others:
Don't take to "flush out" your system or as a "tonic."

POSSIBLE INTERACTION WITH OTHER DRUGS

GENERIC NAME OR DRUG CLASS	COMBINED EFFECT
Antihypertensives*	May cause dangerous low potassium level.
Diuretics*	May caused dangerous low potassium level.

POSSIBLE INTERACTION WITH OTHER SUBSTANCES

INTERACTS WITH	COMBINED EFFECT
Alcohol:	None expected.
Beverages:	None expected.
Cocaine:	None expected.
Foods:	None expected.
Marijuana:	None expected.
Tobacco:	None expected.

CELLULOSE SODIUM PHOSPHATE

BRAND NAMES

Calcibind

BASIC INFORMATION

Habit forming? No
Prescription needed? Yes
Available as generic? No
Drug class: Antiurolithic

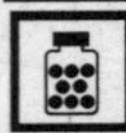

USES

Prevents formation of calcium kidney stones.

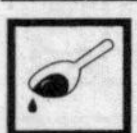

DOSAGE & USAGE INFORMATION

How to take:
Oral suspension—Dissolve in full glass of liquid and swallow. Note: Drink 8 ounces of water or other liquid every hour while you are awake.

When to take:

- According to instructions on prescription label. Usually 3 times a day with meals.
- Don't take within 1-1/2 hours of taking any laxative or antacid containing magnesium.

If you forget a dose:
Take as soon as you remember up to 2 hours late. If more than 2 hours, wait for next scheduled dose (don't double this dose).

What drug does:
Combines with calcium in food to prevent absorption into the bloodstream.

Time lapse before drug works:
None. Works right away.

Don't take with:
Any other medicines (including over-the-counter drugs such as cough and cold medicines, laxatives, antacids, diet pills, caffeine, nose drops or vitamins) without consulting your doctor.

OVERDOSE

SYMPTOMS:
Drowsiness, mental changes, muscle spasms, seizures.
WHAT TO DO:

- **Dial 911 (emergency) or 0 (operator) for an ambulance or medical help. Then give first aid immediately.**
- **See emergency information on inside covers.**

POSSIBLE ADVERSE REACTIONS OR SIDE EFFECTS

SYMPTOMS	WHAT TO DO
Life-threatening: In case of overdose, see previous column.	
Common:	
Loose bowel movements.	Continue. Call doctor when convenient.
Infrequent:	
Abdominal pain.	Discontinue. Call doctor right away.
Rare:	
None expected.	

CELLULOSE SODIUM PHOSPHATE

WARNINGS & PRECAUTIONS

Don't take if:
- You have bone disease.
- You have hyperparathyroidism.
- You have too little calcium in your blood.

Before you start, consult your doctor:
- If you have heart disease.
- If you have kidney disease.

Over age 60:
No special problems expected.

Pregnancy:
Decide with your doctor if drug benefits justify risk to unborn child. Risk category C (see page xxii).

Breast-feeding:
No special problems expected. Consult doctor.

Infants & children:
Not recommended up to age 16.

Prolonged use:
Talk to your doctor about the need for follow-up medical examinations or laboratory studies to check serum calcium and magnesium concentrations (every 6 months), serum parathyroid hormone, urinary calcium and urinary oxalate levels (occasionally).

Skin & sunlight:
No problems expected.

Driving, piloting or hazardous work:
Avoid if you feel confused, drowsy or dizzy.

Discontinuing:
No special problems expected.

Others:
Advise any doctor or dentist whom you consult that you take this medicine.

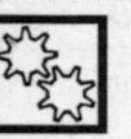

POSSIBLE INTERACTION WITH OTHER DRUGS

GENERIC NAME OR DRUG CLASS	COMBINED EFFECT
Calcium-containing medications	Decreased effect of cellulose sodium phosphate.
Magnesium-containing medicines (includes many laxatives* and antacids*)	Decreased magnesium effect.
Vitamin C (ascorbic acid)	Decreased vitamin C effect.

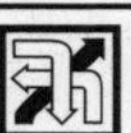

POSSIBLE INTERACTION WITH OTHER SUBSTANCES

INTERACTS WITH	COMBINED EFFECT
Alcohol:	No special problems expected.
Beverages: Milk or other dairy products or tea.	Decreases effectiveness of cellulose sodium phosphate.
Cocaine:	No special problems expected.
Foods: Spinach, broccoli, rhubarb.	Decreases effectiveness of cellulose sodium phosphate.
Marijuana:	No special problems expected.
Tobacco:	No special problems expected.

*See Glossary

CEPHALOSPORINS

BRAND AND GENERIC NAMES

Anspor
Apo-Cephalex
Ceclor
CEFACLOR
CEFADROXIL
Cefanex
CEFIXIME
Cefotan
CEFOTETAN
CEFPODOXIME
CEFPROZIL
Ceftin
CEFUROXIME
Cefzil
CEPHALEXIN
CEPHRADINE
C-Lexin
Ceporex
Duricef
Entacef
Keflet
Keflex
Keftab
Novolexin
Nu-Cephalex
Ro-ceph
Suprax
Ultracef
Vantin
Velosef

BASIC INFORMATION

Habit forming? No
Prescription needed? Yes
Available as generic? Yes
Drug class: Antibiotic (cephalosporin)

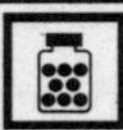

USES

Treatment of bacterial infections. Will not cure viral infections such as cold and flu.

DOSAGE & USAGE INFORMATION

How to take:

- Tablet or capsule—Swallow with liquid. If you can't swallow whole, crumble tablet or open capsule and take with liquid or food.
- Liquid—Use measuring spoon. Mix according to package instructions.

When to take:

- At same times each day, 1 hour before or 2 hours after eating.
- Take until gone or as directed.

Continued next column

OVERDOSE

SYMPTOMS:
Abdominal cramps, nausea, vomiting, severe diarrhea with mucus or blood in stool, convulsions.
WHAT TO DO:
Overdose unlikely to threaten life. If person takes much larger amount than prescribed, call doctor, poison control center or hospital emergency room for instructions.

If you forget a dose:
Take as soon as you remember or double next dose. Return to regular schedule.

What drug does:
Kills susceptible bacteria.

Time lapse before drug works:
May require several days to affect infection.

Don't take with:
Any other medicine without consulting your doctor or pharmacist.

POSSIBLE ADVERSE REACTIONS OR SIDE EFFECTS

SYMPTOMS	WHAT TO DO
Life-threatening:	
Hives, rash, intense itching, faintness soon after a dose (anaphylaxis); difficulty breathing.	Seek emergency treatment immediately.
Common:	
• Rash, redness, itching.	Discontinue. Call doctor right away.
• Diarrhea (mild).	Continue. Call doctor when convenient.
Infrequent:	
Rectal itching, oral or vaginal white spots.	Continue. Call doctor when convenient.
Rare:	
Mild nausea, vomiting, cramps, severe diarrhea with mucus or blood in stool, unusual weakness, tiredness, weight loss, fever, bleeding or bruising, abdominal cramping pain, increased thirst, joint pain, appetite loss.	Discontinue. Call doctor right away.

WARNINGS & PRECAUTIONS

Don't take if:
You are allergic to any cephalosporin antibiotic.

Before you start, consult your doctor:
- If you are allergic to any penicillin antibiotic.
- If you have a kidney disorder.
- If you have colitis or enteritis.

Over age 60:
Adverse reactions and side effects may be more frequent and severe than in younger persons. More likely to itch around rectum and genitals.

Pregnancy:
No proven harm to unborn child. Avoid if possible. Consult doctor. Risk category B (see page xxii).

Breast-feeding:
Drug passes into milk. Avoid drug or discontinue nursing until you finish medicine. Consult doctor for advice on maintaining milk supply.

Infants & children:
No special warnings.

Prolonged use:
- Kills beneficial bacteria that protect body against other germs. Unchecked germs may cause secondary infections.
- Talk to your doctor about the need for follow-up medical examinations or laboratory studies to check prothrombin time.

Skin & sunlight:
No problems expected.

Driving, piloting or hazardous work:
No problems expected.

Discontinuing:
Don't discontinue without doctor's advice until you complete prescribed dose, even though symptoms diminish or disappear.

Others:
No problems expected.

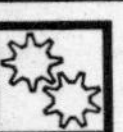

POSSIBLE INTERACTION WITH OTHER DRUGS

GENERIC NAME OR DRUG CLASS	COMBINED EFFECT
Anticoagulants*	Increased anticoagulant effect.
Anti-inflammatory drugs, nonsteroidal (NSAIDs)*	Increased risk of peptic ulcer.
Erythromycins*	Decreased antibiotic effect of cephalosporin.
Chloramphenicol	Decreased antibiotic effect of cephalosporin.
Clindamycin	Decreased antibiotic effect of cephalosporin.
Probenecid	Increased cephalosporin effect.
Tetracyclines*	Decreased antibiotic effect of cephalosporin.

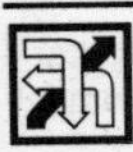

POSSIBLE INTERACTION WITH OTHER SUBSTANCES

INTERACTS WITH	COMBINED EFFECT
Alcohol:	Increased kidney toxicity, likelihood of disulfiram-like* effect.
Beverages:	None expected.
Cocaine:	None expected, but cocaine may slow body's recovery. Avoid.
Foods:	Slow absorption. Take with liquid 1 hour before or 2 hours after eating.
Marijuana:	None expected, but marijuana may slow body's recovery. Avoid.
Tobacco:	None expected.

*See Glossary

CHARCOAL, ACTIVATED

BRAND NAMES

Acta-Char
Acta-Char Liquid
Actidose-Aqua
Actidose with Sorbitol
Aqueous Charcodote
Charac-50
Charac-tol 50
Charcoaid
Charcocaps
Charcodote
Charcodote TFS
Insta-Char
Liqui-Char
Pediatric Aqueous Charcodote
Pediatric Charcodote
SuperChar

BASIC INFORMATION

Habit forming? No
Prescription needed? No
Available as generic? Yes
Drug class: Antidote (adsorbent)

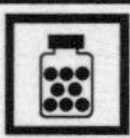

USES

- Treatment of poisonings from medication.
- Treatment (infrequent) for diarrhea or excessive gaseousness.

DOSAGE & USAGE INFORMATION

How to take:
- Tablet or capsule—Swallow with liquid. If you can't swallow whole, crumble tablet or open capsule and take with liquid or food.
- Liquid—Take as directed on label. Don't mix with chocolate syrup, ice cream or sherbet.

When to take:
- For poisoning—Take immediately after poisoning. If your doctor or emergency poison control center has also recommended syrup of ipecac, don't take charcoal for 30 minutes or until vomiting from ipecac stops.
- For diarrhea or gas—Take at same times each day.
- Take 2 or more hours after taking other medicines.

Continued next column

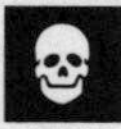

OVERDOSE

SYMPTOMS:
None expected.
WHAT TO DO:
Overdose unlikely to threaten life. If person takes much larger amount than prescribed, call doctor, poison control center or hospital emergency room for instructions.

If you forget a dose:
- For poisonings—Not applicable.
- For diarrhea or gas—Take as soon as you remember up to 2 hours late. If more than 2 hours, wait for next scheduled dose (don't double this dose).

What drug does:
- Helps prevent poison from being absorbed from stomach and intestines.
- Helps absorb gas in intestinal tract.

Time lapse before drug works:
Begins immediately.

Don't take with:
Ice cream or sherbet.

POSSIBLE ADVERSE REACTIONS OR SIDE EFFECTS

SYMPTOMS	WHAT TO DO
Life-threatening: None expected.	
Always: Black bowel movements.	No action necessary.
Infrequent: None expected.	
Rare: Unless taken with cathartic, can cause constipation when taken for overdose of other medicine.	Take a laxative after crisis is over.

WARNINGS & PRECAUTIONS

Don't take if:
The poison was lye or other strong alkali, strong acids (such as sulfuric acid), cyanide, iron, ethyl alcohol or methyl alcohol. Charcoal will not prevent these poisons from causing ill effects.

Before you start, consult your doctor:
If you are taking it as an antidote for poison.

Over age 60:
No problems expected.

Pregnancy:
Consult doctor. Risk category C (see page xxii).

Breast-feeding:
No problems expected. Consult doctor.

Infants & children:
Don't give to children for more than 3 or 4 days for diarrhea. Continuing for longer periods can interfere with normal nutrition.

Prolonged use:
No problems expected.

Skin & sunlight:
No problems expected.

Driving, piloting or hazardous work:
No problems expected.

Discontinuing:
No problems expected.

Others:
No problems expected.

POSSIBLE INTERACTION WITH OTHER DRUGS

GENERIC NAME OR DRUG CLASS	COMBINED EFFECT
Any medicine taken at the same time	May decrease absorption of medicine. Take drugs 2 hours apart.

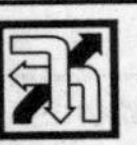

POSSIBLE INTERACTION WITH OTHER SUBSTANCES

INTERACTS WITH	COMBINED EFFECT
Alcohol:	None expected.
Beverages:	None expected.
Cocaine:	None expected.
Foods: Chocolate syrup, ice cream or sherbet.	Decreased charcoal effect.
Marijuana:	None expected.
Tobacco:	None expected.

CHENODIOL

BRAND NAMES

Chenix

BASIC INFORMATION

Habit forming? No
Prescription needed? Yes
Available as generic? No
Drug class: Anticholelithic

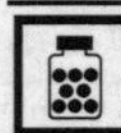

USES

Treats cholesterol gallstone disease in patients who, for any reason, can't have surgery.

DOSAGE & USAGE INFORMATION

How to take:
Tablets—Swallow with liquid. If you can't swallow whole, crumble tablet and take with liquid or food. Instructions to take on empty stomach mean 1 hour before or 2 hours after eating.

When to take:
Usually twice a day (morning and night) with food or milk.

If you forget a dose:
Take as soon as you remember up to 2 hours late. If more than 2 hours, wait for next scheduled dose (don't double this dose).

What drug does:
Reduces cholesterol saturation in blood and dissolves gallstones.

Time lapse before drug works:
1 to 2 hours.

Don't take with:
Any other medicines (including over-the-counter drugs such as cough and cold medicines, laxatives, antacids, diet pills, caffeine, nose drops or vitamins) without consulting your doctor or pharmacist.

OVERDOSE

SYMPTOMS:
None expected.
WHAT TO DO:
Overdose unlikely to threaten life. If person takes much larger amount than prescribed, call doctor, poison control center or hospital emergency room for instructions.

POSSIBLE ADVERSE REACTIONS OR SIDE EFFECTS

SYMPTOMS	WHAT TO DO
Life-threatening: None expected.	
Common: Mild diarrhea.	Continue. Call doctor when convenient.
Infrequent: Constipation, indigestion, appetite loss, abdominal pain, gaseousness.	Continue. Call doctor when convenient.
Rare: Severe diarrhea.	Discontinue. Call doctor right away.

WARNINGS & PRECAUTIONS

Don't take if:
- You have hardening of the arteries (atherosclerosis).
- You are jaundiced.

Before you start, consult your doctor:
- If you have pancreatitis.
- If you have bile duct disease.
- If you have liver disease.
- If you have spastic colitis.

Over age 60:
No special problems expected.

Pregnancy:
Risk category X (see page xxii).

Breast-feeding:
No problems expected. Consult doctor.

Infants & children:
Effect not documented. Consult your pediatrician.

Prolonged use:
Talk to your doctor about the need for follow-up medical examinations or laboratory studies to check continued presence of gallstones (sonograms or cholecystograms), liver function and serum cholesterol levels (every 6 months).

Skin & sunlight:
No problems expected.

Driving, piloting or hazardous work:
No problems expected.

Discontinuing:
No special problems expected.

Others:
- Advise any doctor or dentist whom you consult that you take this medicine.
- May affect results in some medical tests.

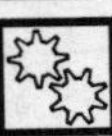

POSSIBLE INTERACTION WITH OTHER DRUGS

GENERIC NAME OR DRUG CLASS	COMBINED EFFECT
Antacids with magnesium*	Severe diarrhea.
Laxatives*	Decreased chenodiol effect.

POSSIBLE INTERACTION WITH OTHER SUBSTANCES

INTERACTS WITH	COMBINED EFFECT
Alcohol:	Decreased chenodiol effect.
Beverages:	No special problems expected.
Cocaine:	No special problems expected.
Foods:	No special problems expected.
Marijuana:	No special problems expected.
Tobacco:	No special problems expected.

***See Glossary**

CHLOPHEDIANOL

BRAND NAMES

Ulone

BASIC INFORMATION

Habit forming? No
Prescription needed? Yes
Available as generic? No
Drug class: Cough suppressant

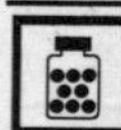

USES

Reduces nonproductive cough due to bronchial irritation.

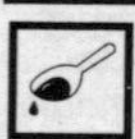

DOSAGE & USAGE INFORMATION

How to take:
Take syrup without diluting. Don't drink fluids immediately after medicine.

When to take:
3 or 4 times a day when needed. No more often than every 3 hours.

If you forget a dose:
Take as soon as you remember up to 2 hours late. If more than 2 hours, wait for next scheduled dose (don't double this dose).

What drug does:
Reduces cough reflex by direct effect on cough center in brain, and by local anesthetic action.

Time lapse before drug works:
30 minutes to 1 hour.

Don't take with:
- Alcohol or brain depressant or stimulant drugs.
- Any other medicine without consulting your doctor or pharmacist.

OVERDOSE

SYMPTOMS:
Blurred vision, hallucinations, coma.
WHAT TO DO:
- **Dial 911 (emergency) or 0 (operator) for an ambulance or medical help. Then give first aid immediately.**
- **If patient is unconscious and not breathing, give mouth-to-mouth breathing. If there is no heartbeat, use cardiac massage and mouth-to-mouth breathing (CPR). Don't try to make patient vomit. If you can't get help quickly, take patient to nearest emergency facility.**
- **See emergency information on inside covers.**

POSSIBLE ADVERSE REACTIONS OR SIDE EFFECTS

SYMPTOMS	WHAT TO DO
Life-threatening: In case of overdose, see previous column.	
Common:	
Difficult urination in older men with enlarged prostate.	Continue. Call doctor when convenient.
Infrequent: None expected.	
Rare:	
• Hallucinations, drowsiness, rash or hives, nausea, vomiting, irregular heartbeat.	Discontinue. Call doctor right away.
• Nightmares, excitement or irritability, blurred vision, dry mouth.	Continue. Call doctor when convenient.

WARNINGS & PRECAUTIONS

Don't take if:
You are allergic to chlophedianol.

Before you start, consult your doctor:
- If medicine is for hyperactive child who takes medicine for treatment.
- If your cough brings up sputum (phlegm).
- If you have heart disease.
- If you will have surgery within 2 months, including dental surgery, requiring general or spinal anesthesia.

Over age 60:
Adverse reactions and side effects may be more frequent and severe than in younger persons.

Pregnancy:
Pregnancy risk not designated. See category list on page xxii and consult doctor.

Breast-feeding:
Unknown whether medicine filters into milk. Consult doctor.

Infants & children:
Not recommended for children under age 2.

Prolonged use:
Not recommended. If cough persists despite medicine, consult doctor.

Skin & sunlight:
No problems expected.

Driving, piloting or hazardous work:
Don't drive or pilot aircraft until you learn how medicine affects you. Don't work around dangerous machinery. Don't climb ladders or work in high places. Danger increases if you drink alcohol or take medicine affecting alertness and reflexes, such as antihistamines, tranquilizers, sedatives, pain medicine, narcotics and mind-altering drugs.

Discontinuing:
May be unnecessary to finish medicine. Follow doctor's instructions.

Others:
Consult doctor if cough persists despite medication for 7 days or if fever, skin rash or headache accompany cough.

POSSIBLE INTERACTION WITH OTHER DRUGS

GENERIC NAME OR DRUG CLASS	COMBINED EFFECT
Anticonvulsants*	Interferes with actions of both.
Antidepressants, tricyclic*	Excess sedation.
Appetite suppressants*	Excess stimulation.
Central nervous system (CNS) depressants*	Excess sedation.
Monoamine oxidase (MAO) inhibitors*	Excess sedation.
Sympathomimetics*	Excess stimulation.

POSSIBLE INTERACTION WITH OTHER SUBSTANCES

INTERACTS WITH	COMBINED EFFECT
Alcohol:	Excess sedation. Avoid.
Beverages: Coffee, tea, cocoa, cola.	Excess stimulation. Avoid.
Cocaine:	Increased chance of toxic stimulation. Avoid.
Foods:	None expected.
Marijuana:	Increased chance of toxic stimulation. Avoid.
Tobacco:	Decreased effect of chlophedianol.

*See Glossary

CHLORAL HYDRATE

BRAND NAMES

Aquachloral
Noctec
Novochlorhydrate

BASIC INFORMATION

Habit forming? Yes
Prescription needed? Yes
Available as generic? Yes
Drug class: Hypnotic

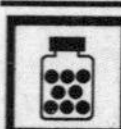

USES

- Reduces anxiety.
- Relieves insomnia.

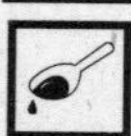

DOSAGE & USAGE INFORMATION

How to take:

- Syrup or capsule—Swallow with liquid or food to lessen stomach irritation.
- Suppositories—Remove wrapper and moisten suppository with water. Gently insert larger end into rectum. Push well into rectum with finger.

When to take:
At the same time each day.

If you forget a dose:
Take as soon as you remember up to 2 hours late. If more than 2 hours, wait for next scheduled dose (don't double this dose).

Continued next column

OVERDOSE

SYMPTOMS:
Confusion, weakness, breathing difficulty, throat irritation, jaundice, stagger, slow or irregular heartbeat, unconsciousness, convulsions, coma.

WHAT TO DO:

- **Dial 911 (emergency) or 0 (operator) for an ambulance or medical help. Then give first aid immediately.**
- **If patient is unconscious and not breathing, give mouth-to-mouth breathing. If there is no heartbeat, use cardiac massage and mouth-to-mouth breathing (CPR). Don't try to make patient vomit. If you can't get help quickly, take patient to nearest emergency facility.**
- **See emergency information on inside covers.**

What drug does:
Affects brain centers that control wakefulness and alertness.

Time lapse before drug works:
30 to 60 minutes.

Don't take with:
Any other medicine without consulting your doctor or pharmacist.

POSSIBLE ADVERSE REACTIONS OR SIDE EFFECTS

SYMPTOMS	WHAT TO DO
Life-threatening: In case of overdose, see previous column.	
Common:	
Nausea, stomach pain, vomiting.	Discontinue. Call doctor right away.
Infrequent:	
"Hangover" effect, clumsiness or unsteadiness, drowsiness, dizziness, lightheadedness, diarrhea.	Continue. Call doctor when convenient.
Rare:	
• Hallucinations, agitation, confusion. leukopenia (white blood cells causing sore throat and fever).	Discontinue. Call doctor right away.
• Hives, rash.	Continue. Call doctor when convenient.

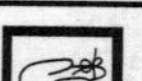

WARNINGS & PRECAUTIONS

Don't take if:
You are allergic to chloral hydrate.

Before you start, consult your doctor:

- If you have had liver, kidney or heart trouble.
- If you are prone to stomach upsets (if medicine is in oral form).
- If you are allergic to tartrazine dye.
- If you have colitis or a rectal inflammation (if medicine is in suppository form).

Over age 60:
Adverse reactions and side effects may be more frequent and severe than in younger persons. More likely to have "hangover" effect.

Pregnancy:
Decide with your doctor if drug benefits justify risk to unborn child. Risk category C (see page xxii).

Breast-feeding:
Drug filters into milk. May harm child. Avoid.

Infants & children:
Use only under medical supervision.

Prolonged use:
Addiction and possible kidney damage.

Skin & sunlight:
No problems expected.

Driving, piloting or hazardous work:
Don't drive or pilot aircraft until you learn how medicine affects you. Don't work around dangerous machinery. Don't climb ladders or work in high places. Danger increases if you drink alcohol or take medicine affecting alertness and reflexes, such as antihistamines, tranquilizers, sedatives, pain medicine, narcotics and mind-altering drugs.

Discontinuing:
Don't discontinue without consulting doctor. Dose may require gradual reduction if you have taken drug for a long time. Doses of other drugs may also require adjustment.

Others:
Frequent kidney-function tests recommended when drug is used for long time.

POSSIBLE INTERACTION WITH OTHER DRUGS

GENERIC NAME OR DRUG CLASS	COMBINED EFFECT
Anticoagulants, oral*	Possible hemorrhaging.
Antidepressants*	Increased chloral hydrate effect.
Antihistamines*	Increased chloral hydrate effect.
Clozapine	Toxic effect on the central nervous system.
Ethinamate	Dangerous increased effects of ethinamate. Avoid combining.
Fluoxetine	Increased depressant effects of both drugs.
Guanfacine	May increase depressant effects of either drug.
Leucovorin	High alcohol content of leucovorin may cause adverse effects.
Methyprylon	Increased sedative effect, perhaps to dangerous level. Avoid.
Mind-altering drugs*	Increased chloral hydrate effect.
Molindone	Increased tranquilizer effect.
Monoamine oxidase (MAO) inhibitors*	Increased chloral hydrate effect.
Nabilone	Greater depression of central nervous system.
Narcotics*	Increased chloral hydrate effect.
Pain relievers*	Increased chloral hydrate effect.
Phenothiazines*	Increased chloral hydrate effect.
Sedatives*	Increased chloral hydrate effect.
Sertraline	Increased depressive effects of both drugs.
Sleep inducers*	Increased chloral hydrate effect.
Tranquilizers*	Increased chloral hydrate effect.

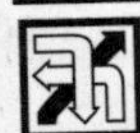

POSSIBLE INTERACTION WITH OTHER SUBSTANCES

INTERACTS WITH	COMBINED EFFECT
Alcohol:	Increased sedative effect of both. Avoid.
Beverages:	None expected.
Cocaine:	Decreased chloral hydrate effect. Avoid.
Foods:	None expected.
Marijuana:	May severely impair mental and physical functioning. Avoid.
Tobacco:	None expected.

*See Glossary

CHLORAMBUCIL

BRAND NAMES

Leukeran

BASIC INFORMATION

Habit forming? No
Prescription needed? Yes
Available as generic? No
Drug class: Antineoplastic, immunosuppressant

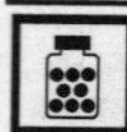

USES

- Treatment for some kinds of cancer.
- Suppresses immune response after transplant and in immune disorders.

DOSAGE & USAGE INFORMATION

How to take:
Tablet—Swallow with liquid after light meal. Don't drink fluids with meals. Drink extra fluids between meals. Avoid sweet or fatty foods.

When to take:
At the same time each day.

If you forget a dose:
Take as soon as you remember. Don't ever double dose.

What drug does:
Inhibits abnormal cell reproduction. May suppress immune system.

Time lapse before drug works:
Up to 6 weeks for full effect.

Don't take with:
Any other medicine without consulting your doctor or pharmacist.

OVERDOSE

SYMPTOMS:
Bleeding, chills, fever, vomiting, abdominal pain, ataxia, collapse, stupor, seizure.
WHAT TO DO:

- **Dial 911 (emergency) or 0 (operator) for an ambulance or medical help. Then give first aid immediately.**
- **If patient is unconscious and not breathing, give mouth-to-mouth breathing. If there is no heartbeat, use cardiac massage and mouth-to-mouth breathing (CPR). Don't try to make patient vomit. If you can't get help quickly, take patient to nearest emergency facility.**
- **See emergency information on inside covers.**

POSSIBLE ADVERSE REACTIONS OR SIDE EFFECTS

SYMPTOMS	WHAT TO DO
Life-threatening: In case of overdose, see previous column.	
Common:	
• Unusual bleeding or bruising, mouth sores with sore throat, chills and fever, black stools, mouth and lip sores, menstrual irregularities, back pain.	Discontinue. Call doctor right away.
• Hair loss, joint pain.	Continue. Call doctor when convenient.
• Nausea, vomiting, diarrhea, tiredness, weakness.	Continue. Tell doctor at next visit.
Infrequent:	
• Mental confusion, shortness of breath.	Continue. Call doctor when convenient.
• Cough, rash, foot swelling.	Continue. Tell doctor at next visit.
Rare:	
Jaundice, convulsions, hallucinations, muscle twitching.	Discontinue. Call doctor right away.

WARNINGS & PRECAUTIONS

Don't take if:
- You have had hypersensitivity to alkylating antineoplastic drugs.
- Your physician has not explained serious nature of your medical problem and risks of taking this medicine.

Before you start, consult your doctor:
- If you have gout.
- If you have had kidney stones.
- If you have active infection.
- If you have impaired kidney or liver function.
- If you have taken other antineoplastic drugs or had radiation treatment in last 3 weeks.

Over age 60:
Adverse reactions and side effects may be more frequent and severe than in younger persons.

Pregnancy:
Consult doctor. Risk to unborn child is significant. Risk category D (see page xxii).

Breast-feeding:
Safety not established. Consult doctor.

Infants & children:
Use only under care of medical supervisors who are experienced in anticancer drugs.

Prolonged use:
- Adverse reactions more likely the longer drug is required.
- Talk to your doctor about the need for follow-up medical examinations or laboratory studies to check complete blood counts (white blood cell count, platelet count, red blood cell count, hemoglobin, hematocrit).

Skin & sunlight:
No problems expected.

Driving, piloting or hazardous work:
No problems expected.

Discontinuing:
Don't discontinue without doctor's advice until you complete prescribed dose, even though symptoms diminish or disappear. Some side effects may follow discontinuing. Report to doctor blurred vision, convulsions, confusion, persistent headache.

Others:
- May cause sterility.
- May increase chance of developing leukemia.
- Consult your doctor before you or a household member gets any immunization.

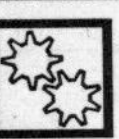

POSSIBLE INTERACTION WITH OTHER DRUGS

GENERIC NAME OR DRUG CLASS	COMBINED EFFECT
Antigout drugs*	Decreased antigout effect.
Antineoplastic drugs, other*	Increased effect of all drugs (may be beneficial).
Chloramphenicol	Increased likelihood of toxic effects of both drugs.
Clozapine	Toxic effect on bone marrow.
Cyclosporine	May increase risk of infection.
Immuno-suppressants*	Increased chance of infection.
Lovastatin	Increased heart and kidney damage.
Tiopronin	Increased risk of toxicity to bone marrow.

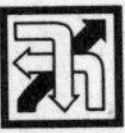

POSSIBLE INTERACTION WITH OTHER SUBSTANCES

INTERACTS WITH	COMBINED EFFECT
Alcohol:	May increase chance of intestinal bleeding.
Beverages:	No problems expected.
Cocaine:	Increases chance of toxicity.
Foods:	Reduces irritation in stomach.
Marijuana:	No problems expected.
Tobacco:	Increases lung toxicity.

*See Glossary

CHLORAMPHENICOL

BRAND NAMES

Chloromycetin Novochlorocap

BASIC INFORMATION

Habit forming? No
Prescription needed? Yes
Available as generic? Yes
Drug class: Antibiotic (antibacterial)

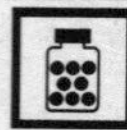

USES

Treatment of infections susceptible to chloramphenicol.

DOSAGE & USAGE INFORMATION

How to take:
Suspension or capsule—Take with a full glass of water.

When to take:
Capsule or suspension—1 hour before or 2 hours after eating.

If you forget a dose:
Take as soon as you remember up to 2 hours late. If more than 2 hours, wait for next scheduled dose (don't double this dose).

What drug does:
Prevents bacteria from growing and reproducing. Will not kill viruses.

Time lapse before drug works:
2 to 5 days, depending on type and severity of infection.

Don't take with:
Any other medicine without consulting your doctor or pharmacist.

OVERDOSE

SYMPTOMS:
Nausea, vomiting, diarrhea.
WHAT TO DO:
Overdose unlikely to threaten life. If person takes much larger amount than prescribed, call doctor, poison control center or hospital emergency room for instructions.

POSSIBLE ADVERSE REACTIONS OR SIDE EFFECTS

SYMPTOMS	WHAT TO DO
Life-threatening:	
Hives, rash, intense itching, faintness soon after a dose (anaphylaxis).	Seek emergency treatment immediately.
Common:	
None expected.	
Infrequent:	
• Swollen face or extremities; diarrhea; nausea; vomiting; numbness, tingling, burning pain or weakness in hands and feet; pale skin; unusual bleeding or bruising.	Discontinue. Call doctor right away.
• Headache, confusion.	Continue. Call doctor when convenient.
Rare:	
• Pain, blurred vision, possible vision loss, delirium, rash, sore throat, fever, jaundice, anemia.	Discontinue. Call doctor right away.
• In babies: Bloated stomach, uneven breathing, drowsiness, low temperature, gray skin.	Discontinue. Call doctor right away.

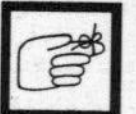

WARNINGS & PRECAUTIONS

Don't take if:
- You are allergic to chloramphenicol.
- It is prescribed for a minor disorder such as flu, cold or mild sore throat.

Before you start, consult your doctor:
- If you have had a blood disorder or bone-marrow disease.
- If you have had kidney or liver disease.
- If you have diabetes.

Over age 60:
Adverse reactions and side effects may be more frequent and severe than in younger persons, particularly skin irritation around rectum.

Pregnancy:
Decide with your doctor if drug benefits justify risk to unborn child. Risk category C (see page xxii).

Breast-feeding:
Drug passes into milk. Avoid drug or discontinue nursing until you finish medicine. Consult doctor for advice on maintaining milk supply.

Infants & children:
Use only under close medical supervision, especially in infants younger than 2.

Prolonged use:
- You may become more susceptible to infections caused by germs not responsive to chloramphenicol.
- Talk to your doctor about the need for follow-up medical examinations or laboratory studies to check complete blood counts (white blood cell count, platelet count, red blood cell count, hemoglobin, hematocrit), chloramphenicol serum levels.

Skin & sunlight:
No problems expected.

Driving, piloting or hazardous work:
Don't drive or pilot aircraft until you learn how medicine affects you. Don't work around dangerous machinery. Don't climb ladders or work in high places. Danger increases if you drink alcohol or take medicine affecting alertness and reflexes.

Discontinuing:
Don't discontinue without doctor's advice until you complete prescribed dose, even though symptoms diminish or disappear.

Others:
- Chloramphenicol can cause serious anemia. Frequent laboratory blood studies, liver and kidney tests recommended.
- Second medical opinion recommended before starting.

POSSIBLE INTERACTION WITH OTHER DRUGS

GENERIC NAME OR DRUG CLASS	COMBINED EFFECT
Anticoagulants*	Increased anti-coagulant effect.
Antidiabetics, oral*	Increased antidiabetic effect.
Anticonvulsants*	Increased chance of toxicity to bone marrow.
Cefiximine	Decreased antibiotic effect of cefiximine.
Cephalosporins*	Decreased chloramphenicol effect.
Clindamycin	Decreased clindamycin effect.
Clozapine	Toxic effect on bone marrow.
Cyclophosphamide	Increased cyclophosphamide effect.
Didanosine	Increased risk of peripheral neuropathy.
Erythromycins	Decreased erythromycin effect.
Flecainide	Possible decreased blood cell production in bone marrow.
Levamisole	Increased risk of bone marrow depression.
Lincomycin	Decreased lincomycin effect.
Lisinopril	Possible blood disorders.
Penicillins*	Decreased penicillin effect.
Phenobarbital	Increased phenobarbital effect.
Phenytoin	Increased phenytoin effect.
Rifampin	Decreased chloramphenicol effect.
Thioguanine	More likelihood of toxicity of both drugs.
Tiopronin	Increased risk of toxicity to bone marrow.
Tocainide	Possible decreased blood cell production in bone marrow.

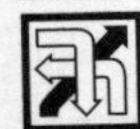

POSSIBLE INTERACTION WITH OTHER SUBSTANCES

INTERACTS WITH	COMBINED EFFECT
Alcohol:	Possible liver problems. May cause disulfiram reaction.*
Beverages:	None expected.
Cocaine:	No proven problems.
Foods:	None expected.
Marijuana:	None expected.
Tobacco:	None expected.

*See Glossary

CHLORHEXIDINE

BRAND NAMES

Peridex
Periogard

BASIC INFORMATION

Habit forming? No
Prescription needed? Yes
Available as generic? No
Drug class: Antibacterial (dental)

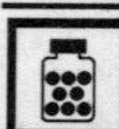

USES

Treatment for gingivitis (inflammation of the gums) and other infections of the mouth.

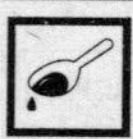

DOSAGE & USAGE INFORMATION

How to use:
Oral rinse—Swish in mouth for 30 seconds, then spit out. Do not swallow the solution, and do not rinse mouth with water after using. Use product at full strength; do not dilute.

When to use:
Twice a day after brushing and flossing teeth.

If you forget a dose:
Use as soon as you remember, then return to regular schedule.

What drug does:
Kills or prevents growth of susceptible bacteria.

Time lapse before drug works:
Antibacterial action begins within an hour, but full benefit may take several weeks.

Don't use with:
Other mouthwashes without consulting your dentist or pharmacist.

OVERDOSE

SYMPTOMS:
None expected. If a child swallows several ounces of the solution, may have slurred speech, staggering or stumbling walk, sleepiness.
WHAT TO DO:
If symptoms occur, call doctor for instructions. If child weighing under 22 pounds accidentally swallows more than 4 ounces, seek emergency help. Dial 911 (emergency) or 0 (operator) for an ambulance or medical help. Then give first aid immediately.

POSSIBLE ADVERSE REACTIONS OR SIDE EFFECTS

SYMPTOMS	WHAT TO DO
Life-threatening: None expected.	
Common: Staining of teeth and other oral surfaces, increased tartar, taste changes, minor mouth irritation.	Continue. Call dentist when convenient.
Infrequent: None expected.	
Rare: Allergic reaction (stuffy nose, shortness of breath, skin rash, hives, itching, face swelling); swollen glands on side of face or neck.	Discontinue. Call doctor right away.

WARNINGS & PRECAUTIONS

Don't take if:
You are allergic to chlorhexidine or skin cleaners that contain chlorhexidine.

Before you start, consult your dentist:
- If you have front tooth fillings (may become discolored).
- If you have periodontitis.

Over age 60:
No special problems expected.

Pregnancy:
Consult doctor. Risk category B (see page xxii).

Breast-feeding:
It is unknown if drug passes into milk. Consult doctor.

Infants & children:
Safety in children under age 18 has not been established.

Prolonged use:
See your dentist every 6 months.

Skin & sunlight:
No special problems expected.

Driving, piloting or hazardous work:
No special problems expected.

Discontinuing:
No special problems expected.

Others:
Brush teeth with a tartar-control toothpaste, and floss daily to help reduce tartar buildup.

POSSIBLE INTERACTION WITH OTHER DRUGS

GENERIC NAME OR DRUG CLASS	COMBINED EFFECT
None expected.	

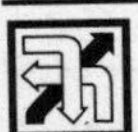

POSSIBLE INTERACTION WITH OTHER SUBSTANCES

INTERACTS WITH	COMBINED EFFECT
Alcohol:	None expected.
Beverages:	Avoid drinking any fluids for several hours after using mouthwash.
Cocaine:	None expected.
Foods:	Avoid eating any foods for several hours after using mouthwash.
Marijuana:	None expected.
Tobacco:	None expected.

*See Glossary

CHLOROQUINE

BRAND NAMES

Aralen

BASIC INFORMATION

Habit forming? No
Prescription needed? Yes
Available as generic? Yes
Drug class: Antiprotozoal, antirheumatic

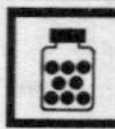

USES

- Treatment for protozoal infections, such as malaria and amebiasis.
- Treatment for some forms of arthritis and lupus.

DOSAGE & USAGE INFORMATION

How to take:
Tablet—Swallow with food or milk to lessen stomach irritation.

When to take:
- Depends on condition. Is adjusted during treatment.
- Malaria prevention—Begin taking medicine 2 weeks before traveling to areas where malaria is present.

If you forget a dose:
- 1 or more doses a day—Take as soon as you remember up to 2 hours late. If more than 2 hours, wait for next scheduled dose (don't double this dose).
- 1 dose weekly—Take as soon as possible, then return to regular dosing schedule.

What drug does:
- Inhibits parasite multiplication.
- Decreases inflammatory response in diseased joint.

Continued next column

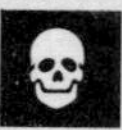

OVERDOSE

SYMPTOMS:
Severe breathing difficulty, drowsiness, faintness, headache, seizures.
WHAT TO DO:
- **Dial 911 (emergency) or 0 (operator) for an ambulance or medical help. Then give first aid immediately.**
- **See emergency information on inside covers.**

Time lapse before drug works:
1 to 2 hours. For treatment of arthritis symptoms, may take up to 6 months for maximum effectiveness.

Don't take with:
Any other medicine without consulting your doctor or pharmacist.

POSSIBLE ADVERSE REACTIONS OR SIDE EFFECTS

SYMPTOMS	WHAT TO DO
Life-threatening:	
In case of overdose, see previous column.	
Common:	
Headache, appetite loss, abdominal pain.	Continue. Tell doctor at next visit.
Infrequent:	
• Blurred or changed vision.	Discontinue. Call doctor right away.
• Rash or itch, diarrhea, nausea, vomiting, decreased blood pressure, hair loss, blue-black skin or mouth, dizziness, nervousness.	Continue. Call doctor when convenient.
Rare:	
• Mood or mental changes, seizures, sore throat, fever, unusual bleeding or bruising, muscle weakness, convulsions.	Discontinue. Call doctor right away.
• Ringing or buzzing in ears, hearing loss.	Continue. Call doctor when convenient.

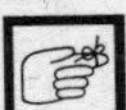

WARNINGS & PRECAUTIONS

Don't take if:
You are allergic to chloroquine or hydroxychloroquine.

Before you start, consult your doctor:
- If you plan to become pregnant within the medication period.
- If you have blood disease.
- If you have eye or vision problems.
- If you have a G6PD deficiency.
- If you have liver disease.
- If you have nerve or brain disease (including seizure disorders).
- If you have porphyria.
- If you have psoriasis.
- If you have stomach or intestinal disease.
- If you drink more than 3 oz. of alcohol daily.

Over age 60:
Adverse reactions and side effects may be more frequent and severe than in younger persons.

Pregnancy:
Decide with your doctor if drug benefits justify risk to unborn child. Risk category C (see page xxii).

Breast-feeding:
Drug passes into milk. Avoid drug or discontinue nursing. Consult doctor about maintaining milk supply.

Infants & children:
Not recommended. Dangerous.

Prolonged use:
- Permanent damage to the retina (back part of the eye) or nerve deafness.
- Talk to your doctor about the need for follow-up medical examinations or laboratory studies to check complete blood counts (white blood cell count, platelet count, red blood cell count, hemoglobin, hematocrit), eyes.

Skin & sunlight:
May cause rash or intensify sunburn in areas exposed to sun or sunlamp.

Driving, piloting or hazardous work:
Don't drive or pilot aircraft until you learn how medicine affects you. Don't work around dangerous machinery. Don't climb ladders or work in high places. Danger increases if you drink alcohol or take medicine affecting alertness and reflexes.

Discontinuing:
Don't discontinue without doctor's advice until you complete prescribed dose, even though symptoms diminish or disappear.

Others:
- Periodic physical and blood examinations recommended.
- If you are in a malaria area for a long time, you may need to change to another preventive drug every 2 years.

POSSIBLE INTERACTION WITH OTHER DRUGS

GENERIC NAME OR DRUG CLASS	COMBINED EFFECT
Penicillamine	Possible blood or kidney toxicity.

POSSIBLE INTERACTION WITH OTHER SUBSTANCES

INTERACTS WITH	COMBINED EFFECT
Alcohol:	Possible liver toxicity. Avoid.
Beverages:	None expected.
Cocaine:	None expected.
Foods:	None expected.
Marijuana:	None expected.
Tobacco:	None expected.

*See Glossary

CHLORPROTHIXENE

BRAND NAMES

Taractan
Tarasan

BASIC INFORMATION

Habit forming? No
Prescription needed? Yes
Available as generic? No
Drug class: Tranquilizer (thioxanthene), antiemetic

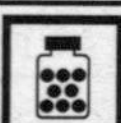

USES

- Reduces anxiety, agitation, psychosis.
- Stops vomiting, hiccups.

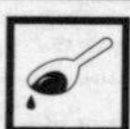

DOSAGE & USAGE INFORMATION

How to take:
- Tablet—Swallow with liquid. If you can't swallow whole, crumble tablet and take with liquid or food.
- Oral suspension—Dilute dose in beverage before swallowing.

When to take:
At the same time each day.

If you forget a dose:
Take as soon as you remember up to 2 hours late. If more than 2 hours, wait for next scheduled dose (don't double this dose).

What drug does:
Corrects imbalance of nerve impulses.

Continued next column

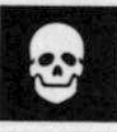

OVERDOSE

SYMPTOMS:
Drowsiness, dizziness, weakness, muscle rigidity, twitching, tremors, confusion, dry mouth, blurred vision, rapid pulse, shallow breathing, low blood pressure, convulsions, coma.

WHAT TO DO:
- **Dial 911 (emergency) or 0 (operator) for an ambulance or medical help. Then give first aid immediately.**
- **If patient is unconscious and not breathing, give mouth-to-mouth breathing. If there is no heartbeat, use cardiac massage and mouth-to-mouth breathing (CPR). Don't try to make patient vomit. If you can't get help quickly, take patient to nearest emergency facility.**
- **See emergency information on inside covers.**

Time lapse before drug works:
3 weeks.

Don't take with:
Any other medicine without consulting your doctor or pharmacist.

POSSIBLE ADVERSE REACTIONS OR SIDE EFFECTS

SYMPTOMS	WHAT TO DO
Life-threatening:	
Uncontrollable movements of head, neck, arms, legs (rarely).	Discontinue. Seek emergency treatment.
Common:	
• Fainting; jerky, involuntary movements; restlessness; blurred vision; rapid heartbeat.	Discontinue. Call doctor right away.
• Dizziness, drowsiness, constipation, muscle spasms, shuffling walk, decreased sweating, increased appetite, weight gain, sensitivity to light.	Continue. Call doctor when convenient.
• Dry mouth, stuffy nose.	Continue. Tell doctor at next visit.
Infrequent:	
• Rash.	Discontinue. Call doctor right away.
• Less sexual ability, difficult urination.	Continue. Call doctor when convenient.
• Menstrual irregularities, swollen breasts, breast milk secretion.	Continue. Tell doctor at next visit.
Rare:	
Sore throat, fever, jaundice, abdominal pain, lip smacking, cheek puffing, chewing movements of mouth, heatstroke, unusual bleeding or bruising.	Discontinue. Call doctor right away.

WARNINGS & PRECAUTIONS

Don't take if:
- You are allergic to any thioxanthine or phenothiazine tranquilizer.
- You have serious blood disorder.
- You have Parkinson's disease.
- Patient is younger than 12.

Before you start, consult your doctor:
- If you have had liver or kidney disease.
- If you have epilepsy, glaucoma or prostate trouble.
- If you have high blood pressure or heart disease (especially angina).

- If you use alcohol daily.
- If you will have surgery within 2 months, including dental surgery, requiring general or spinal anesthesia.

Over age 60:
Adverse reactions and side effects may be more frequent and severe than in younger persons.

Pregnancy:
Safety not established. Avoid if possible. Consult doctor. Risk category C (see page xxii).

Breast-feeding:
Studies inconclusive. Consult your doctor.

Infants & children:
Not recommended.

Prolonged use:
- Pigment deposits in lens and retina of eye.
- Involuntary movements of jaws, lips, tongue (tardive dyskinesia).
- Talk to your doctor about the need for follow-up medical examinations or laboratory studies to check complete blood counts (white blood cell count, platelet count, red blood cell count, hemoglobin, hematocrit), liver function, eyes.

Skin & sunlight:
May cause rash or intensify sunburn in areas exposed to sun or sunlamp.

Driving, piloting or hazardous work:
Don't drive or pilot aircraft until you learn how medicine affects you. Don't work around dangerous machinery. Don't climb ladders or work in high places. Danger increases if you drink alcohol or take medicine affecting alertness and reflexes.

Discontinuing:
Don't discontinue without consulting doctor. Dose may require gradual reduction if you have taken drug for a long time. Doses of other drugs may also require adjustment.

Others:
Hot temperatures increase chance of heat stroke.

POSSIBLE INTERACTION WITH OTHER DRUGS

GENERIC NAME OR DRUG CLASS	COMBINED EFFECT
Anticholinergics*	Increased anti-cholinergic effect.
Anticonvulsants*	Change in seizure pattern.
Antidepressants, tricyclic*	Increased chlor-prothixene effect. Excessive sedation.
Antihistamines*	Increased chlor-prothixene effect. Excessive sedation.
Antihypertensives*	Excessively low blood pressure.
Barbiturates*	Increased chlor-prothixene effect Excessive sedation.
Bethanechol	Decreased bethanechol effect.
Bupropion	Increased risk of major seizures.
Dronabinol	Increased effects of both drugs. Avoid.
Epinephrine	Low blood pressure and rapid heartbeat.
Guanethidine	Decreased guanethidine effect.
Levodopa	Decreased levodopa effect.
Mind-altering drugs*	Increased chlor-prothixene effect. Excessive sedation.
Monoamine oxidase (MAO) inhibitors*	Excessive sedation.
Narcotics*	Increased chlor-prothixene effect. Excessive sedation.
Pergolide	Decreased pergolide effect.
Procarbazine	Increased sedation.
Sedatives*	Increased chlor-prothixene effect. Excessive sedation.

Continued on page 934

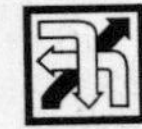

POSSIBLE INTERACTION WITH OTHER SUBSTANCES

INTERACTS WITH	COMBINED EFFECT
Alcohol:	Excessive brain depression. Avoid.
Beverages:	None expected.
Cocaine:	Decreased chlor-prothixene effect. Avoid.
Foods:	None expected.
Marijuana:	Daily use—Fainting likely, possible psychosis.
Tobacco:	None expected.

*See Glossary

CHLORZOXAZONE & ACETAMINOPHEN

BRAND NAMES

Parafon Forte

BASIC INFORMATION

Habit forming? Possibly
Prescription needed? Yes
Available as generic? Yes
Drug class: Muscle relaxant, analgesic, fever-reducer

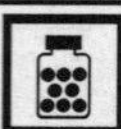

USES

- Adjunctive treatment to rest, analgesics and physical therapy for muscle spasms.
- Treatment of mild to moderate pain and fever.

DOSAGE & USAGE INFORMATION

How to take:
Tablet—Swallow with liquid.

When to take:
As needed, no more often than every 3 hours.

If you forget a dose:
Take as soon as you remember. Wait 3 hours for next dose.

What drug does:
- Blocks body's pain messages to brain. Also causes sedation.
- May affect hypothalamus, the part of the brain that helps regulate body heat and receives body's pain messages.

Time lapse before drug works:
15 to 30 minutes. May last 4 hours.

Continued next column

OVERDOSE

SYMPTOMS:
Nausea, vomiting, diarrhea, anorexia, headache, severe weakness, unusual increase in sweating, fainting, breathing difficulty, irritability, convulsions, sensation of paralysis, coma.
WHAT TO DO:
- **Overdose unlikely to threaten life. Depending on severity of symptoms and amount taken, call doctor, poison control center or hospital emergency room for instructions.**
- **Dial 911 (emergency) or 0 (operator) for an ambulance or medical help. Then give first aid immediately.**
- **See emergency information on inside covers.**

Don't take with:
- Other drugs with acetaminophen. Too much acetaminophen can damage liver and kidneys.
- Any other medicine without consulting your doctor or pharmacist.

POSSIBLE ADVERSE REACTIONS OR SIDE EFFECTS

SYMPTOMS	WHAT TO DO
Life-threatening:	
Hives, rash, intense itching, faintness soon after a dose (anaphylaxis); extreme weakness, transient paralysis, temporary loss of vision.	Seek emergency treatment immediately.
Common:	
Dizziness, lightheadedness, drowsiness.	Discontinue. Call doctor right away.
Infrequent:	
• Difficult or frequent urination, severe back pain, cloudy urine.	Discontinue. Call doctor right away.
• Nervousness, restlessness, irritability, headache, indigestion, depression, agitation, constipation, tiredness, weakness.	Continue. Call doctor when convenient.
Rare:	
• Sudden decrease in urine output; swelling of lips, face or tongue.	Discontinue. Seek emergency treatment.
• Bloody or black stools, jaundice, unusual bleeding or bruising, sore mouth or throat, fever, hiccups, skin rash, hives.	Discontinue. Call doctor right away.

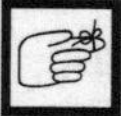

WARNINGS & PRECAUTIONS

Don't take if:
- You are allergic to any skeletal muscle relaxant or acetaminophen.
- Your symptoms don't improve after 2 days use. Call your doctor.

Before you start, consult your doctor:
- If you have had liver disease.
- If you have kidney disease or liver damage.
- If you plan pregnancy within medication period.
- If you are allergic to tartrazine dye*.

CHLORZOXAZONE & ACETAMINOPHEN

Over age 60:
- Adverse reactions and side effects may be more frequent and severe than in younger persons.
- Don't exceed recommended dose. You can't eliminate drug as efficiently as younger persons.

Pregnancy:
Safety not proven. Avoid if possible. Consult doctor. Risk category C (see page xxii)

Breast-feeding:
Drug passes into milk. Avoid drug or discontinue nursing until you finish medicine. Consult doctor for advice on maintaining milk supply.

Infants & children:
Not recommended.

Prolonged use:
- May affect blood system and cause anemia. Limit use to 5 days for children 12 and under, and 10 days for adults.
- Talk to your doctor about the need for follow-up medical examinations or laboratory studies to check complete blood counts (white blood cell count, platelet count, red blood cell count, hemoglobin, hematocrit), liver function.

Skin & sunlight:
No problems expected.

Driving, piloting or hazardous work:
Don't drive or pilot aircraft until you learn how medicine affects you. Don't work around dangerous machinery. Don't climb ladders or work in high places. Danger increases if you drink alcohol or take medicine affecting alertness and reflexes, such as antihistamines, tranquilizers, sedatives, pain medicine, narcotics and mind-altering drugs.

Discontinuing:
Don't discontinue without consulting your doctor. Dose may require gradual reduction if you have taken drug for a long time. Doses of other drugs may also require adjustment.

Others:
Periodic liver-function tests recommended if you use this drug for a long time.

POSSIBLE INTERACTION WITH OTHER DRUGS

GENERIC NAME OR DRUG CLASS	COMBINED EFFECT
Anticoagulants, oral*	May increase anticoagulant effect. If combined frequently, prothrombin time should be monitored.
Antidepressants*	Increased sedation.
Antihistamines*	Increased sedation.
Clozapine	Toxic effect on the central nervous system.
Dronabinol	Increased effect of dronabinol on central nervous system. Avoid combination.
Mind-altering drugs*	Increased sedation.
Monoamine oxidase (MAO) inhibitors*	Increased effect of both drugs (but safety not established).
Muscle relaxants, others*	Increased sedation.
Narcotics*	Increased sedation.
Phenobarbital	Quicker elimination and decreased effects of acetaminophen.
Sedatives*	Increased sedation.
Sertraline	Increased depressive effects of both drugs.
Sleep inducers*	Increased sedation.
Tetracyclines* (effervescent granules or tablets)	May slow tetracycline absorption. Space doses 2 hours apart.

Continued on page 934

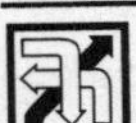

POSSIBLE INTERACTION WITH OTHER SUBSTANCES

INTERACTS WITH	COMBINED EFFECT
Alcohol:	Drowsiness, increased sedation. Long-term use may cause toxic effect in liver.
Beverages:	No problems expected.
Cocaine:	Lack of coordination. May slow body's recovery. Avoid.
Foods:	No problems expected.
Marijuana:	Increased pain relief, lack of coordination, drowsiness, fainting. May slow body's recovery. Avoid.
Tobacco:	No problems expected.

*See Glossary

CHOLESTYRAMINE

BRAND NAMES

Cholybar
Questran
Questran Light

BASIC INFORMATION

Habit forming? No
Prescription needed? Yes
Available as generic? Yes
Drug class: Antihyperlipidemic, antipruritic

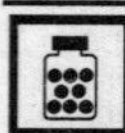

USES

- Removes excess bile acids that occur with some liver problems. Reduces persistent itch caused by bile acids.
- Lowers cholesterol level.
- Treatment of one form of colitis (rare).

DOSAGE & USAGE INFORMATION

How to take:
Powder, granules—Sprinkle into 8 oz. liquid. Let stand for 2 minutes, then mix with liquid before swallowing. Or mix with cereal, soup or pulpy fruit. Don't swallow dry.

When to take:
- 3 or 4 times a day on an empty stomach, 1 hour before or 2 hours after eating.
- If taking other medicines, take 1 hour before or 4 to 6 hours after taking cholestyramine.

If you forget a dose:
Take as soon as you remember up to 2 hours late. If more than 2 hours, wait for next scheduled dose (don't double this dose).

What drug does:
Binds with bile acids to prevent their absorption.

Time lapse before drug works:
- Cholesterol reduction—1 day.
- Bile-acid reduction—3 to 4 weeks.

Continued next column

OVERDOSE

SYMPTOMS:
Increased side effects and adverse reactions.
WHAT TO DO:
Overdose unlikely to threaten life. Depending on severity of symptoms and amount taken, call doctor, poison control center or hospital emergency room for instructions.

Don't take with:
- Any drug or vitamin simultaneously. Space doses 2 hours apart.
- Any other medicine without consulting your doctor or pharmacist.

POSSIBLE ADVERSE REACTIONS OR SIDE EFFECTS

SYMPTOMS	WHAT TO DO
Life-threatening: In case of overdose, see previous column.	
Common: Constipation.	Continue. Call doctor when convenient.
Infrequent:	
• Belching, bloating, diarrhea, mild nausea, vomiting, stomach pain, rapid weight gain.	Discontinue. Call doctor right away.
• Heartburn (mild).	Continue. Call doctor when convenient.
Rare:	
• Severe stomach pain; black, tarry stool.	Discontinue. Seek emergency treatment.
• Rash, hives, hiccups.	Discontinue. Call doctor right away.
• Sore tongue.	Continue. Call doctor when convenient.

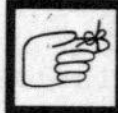

WARNINGS & PRECAUTIONS

Don't take if:
You are allergic to cholestyramine.

Before you start, consult your doctor:
- If you plan to become pregnant within medication period.
- If you have angina, heart or blood-vessel disease.
- If you have stomach problems (including ulcer).
- If you have tartrazine sensitivity.
- If you have constipation or hemorrhoids.
- If you have kidney disease.

Over age 60:
Adverse reactions and side effects may be more frequent and severe than in younger persons.

Pregnancy:
Decide with your doctor whether drug benefits justify risk to unborn child. Risk category C (see page xxii).

Breast-feeding:
No problems expected, but consult doctor.

Infants & children:
Not recommended.

Prolonged use:
- May decrease absorption of folic acid.
- Talk to your doctor about the need for follow-up medical examinations or laboratory studies to check serum cholesterol and triglycerides.

Skin & sunlight:
No problems expected.

Driving, piloting or hazardous work:
No problems expected.

Discontinuing:
Don't discontinue without doctor's advice until you complete prescribed dose, even though symptoms diminish or disappear.

Others:
No problems expected.

POSSIBLE INTERACTION WITH OTHER DRUGS

GENERIC NAME OR DRUG CLASS	COMBINED EFFECT
Anticoagulants, oral*	Increased anticoagulant effect.
Beta carotene	Decreased absorption of beta carotene.
Dextrothyroxine	Decreased dextrothyroxine effect.
Digitalis preparations*	Decreased digitalis effect.
Indapamide	Decreased indapamide effect.
Penicillins*	May decrease penicillin effect.
Thiazides*	Decreased absorption of cholestyramine.
Thyroid hormones*	Decreased thyroid effect.
Trimethoprim	Decreased absorption of cholestyramine.
Ursodiol	Decreased absorption of ursodiol.
Vancomycin	Increased chance of hearing loss or kidney damage. Decreased therapeutic effect of vancomycin.
Vitamins	Decreased absorption of fat-soluble vitamins (A,D,E,K).
All other medicines	Decreased absorption, so dosages or dosage intervals may require adjustment.

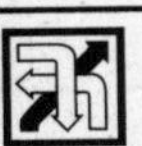

POSSIBLE INTERACTION WITH OTHER SUBSTANCES

INTERACTS WITH	COMBINED EFFECT
Alcohol:	None expected.
Beverages:	None expected.
Cocaine:	None expected.
Foods:	Absorption of vitamins in foods decreased. Take vitamin supplements, particularly A, D, E & K.
Marijuana:	None expected.
Tobacco:	None expected.

***See Glossary**

CINOXACIN

BRAND NAMES

Cinobac

BASIC INFORMATION

Habit forming? No
Prescription needed? Yes
Available as generic? No
Drug class: Anti-infective (urinary)

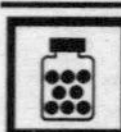

USES

Treatment for urinary tract infections.

DOSAGE & USAGE INFORMATION

How to take:
Capsules—Swallow with food or milk to lessen stomach irritation. If you can't swallow whole, open capsule and take with liquid or food.

When to take:
At the same times each day.

If you forget a dose:
Take as soon as you remember up to 2 hours late. If more than 2 hours, wait for next scheduled dose (don't double this dose).

What drug does:
Destroys bacteria susceptible to cinoxacin.

Time lapse before drug works:
1 to 2 weeks.

Don't take with:
Any other medicine without consulting your doctor or pharmacist.

OVERDOSE

SYMPTOMS:
Lethargy, stomach upset, behavioral changes, convulsions and stupor.
WHAT TO DO:

- **Dial 911 (emergency) or 0 (operator) for an ambulance or medical help. Then give first aid immediately.**
- **If patient is unconscious and not breathing, give mouth-to-mouth breathing. If there is no heartbeat, use cardiac massage and mouth-to-mouth breathing (CPR). Don't try to make patient vomit. If you can't get help quickly, take patient to nearest emergency facility.**
- **See emergency information on inside covers.**

POSSIBLE ADVERSE REACTIONS OR SIDE EFFECTS

SYMPTOMS	WHAT TO DO
Life-threatening:	
Hives, rash, intense itching, faintness soon after a dose (anaphylaxis).	Seek emergency treatment immediately.
Common:	
Rash, itch; decreased, blurred or double vision; halos around lights or excess brightness; changes in color vision; nausea, vomiting, diarrhea.	Discontinue. Call doctor right away.
Infrequent:	
Dizziness, drowsiness, headache, ringing in ears, insomnia, appetite loss.	Continue. Call doctor when convenient.
Rare:	
Severe stomach pain, seizures, psychosis, joint pain, numbness or tingling in hands or feet (infants and children).	Discontinue. Call doctor right away.

WARNINGS & PRECAUTIONS

Don't take if:
- You are allergic to cinoxacin or nalidixic acid.
- You have a seizure disorder (epilepsy, convulsions).

Before you start, consult your doctor:
- If you plan to become pregnant during medication period.
- If you have or have had kidney or liver disease.
- If you have impaired circulation to the brain (hardened arteries).

Over age 60:
Adverse reactions and side effects may be more frequent and severe than in younger persons.

Pregnancy:
Decide with your doctor if drug benefits justify risk to unborn child. Risk category C (see page xxii).

Breast-feeding:
Unknown effect. Avoid drug or discontinue nursing until you finish medicine. Consult doctor for advice on maintaining milk supply.

Infants & children:
Give only under close medical supervision.

Prolonged use:
Talk to your doctor about the need for follow-up medical examinations or laboratory studies to check kidney function, liver function.

Skin & sunlight:
- May cause sunlight to hurt eyes.
- May cause rash or intensify sunburn in areas exposed to sun or sunlamp.

Driving, piloting or hazardous work:
Avoid if you feel drowsy, dizzy or have vision problems. Otherwise, no problems expected.

Discontinuing:
Don't discontinue without consulting doctor. Dose may require gradual reduction if you have taken drug for a long time. Doses of other drugs may also require adjustment.

Others:
May interfere with the accuracy of some medical tests.

POSSIBLE INTERACTION WITH OTHER DRUGS

GENERIC NAME OR DRUG CLASS	COMBINED EFFECT
Probenecid	Decreased cinoxacin effect.

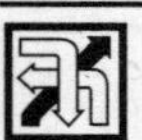

POSSIBLE INTERACTION WITH OTHER SUBSTANCES

INTERACTS WITH	COMBINED EFFECT
Alcohol:	Impaired alertness, judgment and coordination.
Beverages:	None expected.
Cocaine:	Impaired judgment and coordination.
Foods:	None expected.
Marijuana:	Impaired alertness, judgment and coordination.
Tobacco:	None expected.

***See Glossary**

CISAPRIDE

BRAND NAMES

Propulsid

BASIC INFORMATION

Habit forming? No
Prescription needed? Yes
Available as generic? No
Drug class: Cholinergic

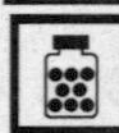

USES

- Treatment and prevention of gastro-esophageal reflux or heartburn.
- Treatment for gastroparesis (a stomach disorder).

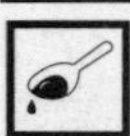

DOSAGE & USAGE INFORMATION

How to take:
- Tablet–Swallow with liquid.
- Oral suspension–Take as directed on label.

When to take:
At the same times each day. Take 15 minutes before meals and at bedtime.

If you forget a dose:
Take as soon as you remember up to 2 hours late. If more than 2 hours, wait for next scheduled dose (don't double this dose).

What drug does:
Restores the normal anti-reflux mechanism of the esophagus, helping prevent reflux of gastric contents into the esophagus.

Time lapse before drug works:
30 to 60 minutes.

Don't take with:
- Any other prescription or nonprescription drug without consulting your doctor.
- See Interaction column and consult doctor.

OVERDOSE

SYMPTOMS:
None expected.
WHAT TO DO:
Overdose unlikely to threaten life. If person takes much larger amount than prescribed, call doctor, poison control center or hospital emergency room for instructions.

POSSIBLE ADVERSE REACTIONS OR SIDE EFFECTS

SYMPTOMS	WHAT TO DO
Life-threatening: None expected.	
Common: None expected.	
Infrequent: Stomach cramps, diarrhea, constipation, unusual tiredness or weakness, headache, nausea, drowsiness.	Continue. Call doctor when convenient.
Rare: Seizures (in patients with a history of seizures).	Discontinue. Call doctor right away.

WARNINGS & PRECAUTIONS

Don't take if:
You are allergic to cisapride.

Before you start, consult your doctor:
- If you have bleeding from the stomach or abdomen.
- If you have epilepsy or a history of seizures.
- If you have kidney or liver disease.

Over age 60:
Adverse reactions and side effects may be more frequent and severe than in younger persons.

Pregnancy:
Discuss with your doctor whether drug benefits justify risk to unborn child. Risk category C (see page xxii).

Breast-feeding:
Drug passes into milk. Avoid drug or discontinue nursing until you finish medicine. Consult doctor for advice on maintaining milk supply.

Infants & children:
No problems expected. Use only under close medical supervision.

Prolonged use:
Your body may develop a tolerance* to the drug, which can decrease its effectiveness.

Skin & sunlight:
No problems expected.

Driving, piloting or hazardous work:
Don't drive or pilot aircraft until you learn how medicine affects you. Don't work around dangerous machinery. Don't climb ladders or work in high places. Danger increases if you drink alcohol or take other medicines affecting alertness and reflexes.

Discontinuing:
No problems expected.

Others:
Advise any doctor or dentist whom you consult that you take this medicine.

POSSIBLE INTERACTION WITH OTHER DRUGS

GENERIC NAME OR DRUG CLASS	COMBINED EFFECT
Amantadine	Decreased amantadine effect.
Anticholinergics*	Decreased anti-cholinergic effect.
Antidepressants*	Decreased anti-depressant effect.
Antidyskinetics*	Decreased anti-dyskinetic effect.
Antihistamines*	Decreased anti-histamine effect.
Antipsychotics*	Decreased anti-psychotic effect.
Buclizine	Decreased buclizine effect.
Carbamazepine	Decreased carba-mazepine effect.
Cimetidine	Increased cimetidine effect.
Cyclobenzaprine	Decreased cycloben-zaprine effect.
Disopyramide	Decreased disopyra-mide effect.
Flavoxate	Decreased flavoxate effect.
Meclizine	Decreased meclizine effect.
Methylphenidate	Decreased methyl-phenidate effect.
Orphenadrine	Decreased orphenadrine effect.
Procainamide	Decreased pro-cainamide effect.
Quinidine	Decreased quinidine effect.
Ranitidine	Increased ranitidine effect.
Trimeprazine	Decreased trimeprazine effect.

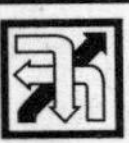

POSSIBLE INTERACTION WITH OTHER SUBSTANCES

INTERACTS WITH	COMBINED EFFECT
Alcohol:	Increased absorption of alcohol. Avoid.
Beverages:	None expected.
Cocaine:	None expected.
Foods:	None expected.
Marijuana:	None expected.
Tobacco:	None expected.

***See Glossary**

CITRATES

BRAND AND GENERIC NAMES

Albright's Solution
Bicitra
Citra Forte
Citrolith
Efricon Expectorant Liquid
Lanatuss Expectorant
Modified Shohl's Solution
Oracit
Phanadex
Phanatuss
Polycitra
Polycitra-K
Polycitra-LC-Sugar-free
POTASSIUM CITRATE
POTASSIUM CITRATE & CITRIC ACID
POTASSIUM CITRATE & SODIUM CITRATE
SODIUM CITRATE & CITRIC ACID
TRICITRATES
Tricodene NN Cough & Cold Medication
Tussirex with Codeine liquid
Urocit-K

BASIC INFORMATION

Habit forming? No
Prescription needed? Yes
Available as generic? No
Drug class: Urinary alkalizer, antiurolithic

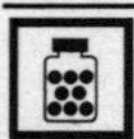

USES

- To make urine more alkaline (less acid).
- To treat or prevent recurrence of some types of kidney stones.

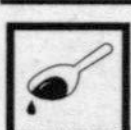

DOSAGE & USAGE INFORMATION

How to take:
Tablets or liquid—Take right after a meal or with a bedtime snack.

When to take:
On full stomach, usually after meals or with food.

If you forget a dose:
Take as soon as you remember up to 2 hours late. If more than 2 hours, wait for next scheduled dose (don't double this dose).

Continued next column

OVERDOSE

SYMPTOMS:
Convulsions, coma.
WHAT TO DO:
- **Dial 911 (emergency) or 0 (operator) for an ambulance or medical help. Then give first aid immediately.**
- **See emergency information on inside covers.**

What drug does:
Increases urinary alkalinity by excretion of bicarbonate ions.

Time lapse before drug works:
1 hour.

Don't take with:
- Any medicine that will decrease mental alertness or reflexes, such as alcohol, other mind-altering drugs, cough/cold medicines, antihistamines, allergy medicine, sedatives, tranquilizers (sleeping pills or "downers"), barbiturates, seizure medicine, narcotics, other prescription medicine for pain, muscle relaxants, anesthetics.
- See Interaction column and consult doctor.

POSSIBLE ADVERSE REACTIONS OR SIDE EFFECTS

SYMPTOMS	WHAT TO DO
Life-threatening:	
Black, tarry stools; vomiting blood; severe abdominal cramps; irregular heartbeat; shortness of breath.	Discontinue. Seek emergency treatment.
Common:	
Nausea or vomiting.	Continue. Call doctor when convenient.
Infrequent:	
Confusion, dizziness, swollen feet and ankles, irritability, depression, muscle pain, nervousness, numbness or tingling in hands or feet, unpleasant taste, weakness.	Discontinue. Call doctor right away.
Rare:	
Slow breathing, tiredness.	Discontinue. Call doctor right away.

WARNINGS & PRECAUTIONS

Don't take if:
You are allergic to any citrate.

Before you start, consult your doctor:
- If you have any disease involving the adrenal glands, diabetes, chronic diarrhea, heart problems, hypertension, kidney disease, stomach ulcer or gastritis, urinary tract infection, toxemia of pregnancy.
- If you plan strenuous exercise.

Over age 60:
Adverse reactions and side effects may be more frequent and severe than in younger persons. Ask doctor about smaller doses.

Pregnancy:
Avoid if possible. Consult doctor. Risk category C (see page xxii).

Breast-feeding:
Safety during lactation not established. Consult doctor.

Infants & children:
Use only under close medical supervision.

Prolonged use:
- Adverse reactions more likely.
- Talk to your doctor about the need for follow-up medical examinations or laboratory studies to check complete blood counts (white blood cell count, platelet count, red blood cell count, hemoglobin, hematocrit), serum electrolytes, urine.

Skin & sunlight:
No problems expected.

Driving, piloting or hazardous work:
Don't drive or pilot aircraft until you learn how medicine affects you. Don't work around dangerous machinery. Don't climb ladders or work in high places. Danger increases if you drink alcohol or take medicine affecting alertness and reflexes, such as antihistamines, tranquilizers, sedatives, pain medicine, narcotics and mind-altering drugs.

Discontinuing:
Don't discontinue without consulting doctor. Dose may require gradual reduction if you have taken drug for a long time. Doses of other drugs may also require adjustment.

Others:
- Drink at least 8 ounces of water or other liquid (except milk) every hour while awake.
- Liquid may be chilled (don't freeze) to improve taste.
- Monitor potassium in blood with frequent laboratory studies.

POSSIBLE INTERACTION WITH OTHER DRUGS

GENERIC NAME OR DRUG CLASS	COMBINED EFFECT
Amphetamines*	Increased amphetamine effect.
Antacids*	Toxic effect of citrates (alkalosis).
Calcium supplements*	Increased risk of kidney stones.
Digitalis preparations*	Increased risk of too much potassium in blood.
Methenamine	Decreased effects of methenamine.
Mexiletine	May slow elimination of mexiletine and cause need to adjust dosage.
Quinidine	Prolonged quinidine effect.

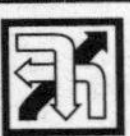

POSSIBLE INTERACTION WITH OTHER SUBSTANCES

INTERACTS WITH	COMBINED EFFECT
Alcohol:	Decreased mental alertness.
Beverages: Salt-free milk.	May cause potassium toxicity.
Cocaine:	No proven problems.
Foods: Milk, cheese, ice cream, yogurt, buttermilk, salty foods, salt, salt substitutes.	May increase likelihood of kidney stones.
Marijuana:	No proven problems.
Tobacco:	Increased likelihood of stomach irritation.

***See Glossary**

CLARITHROMYCIN

BRAND NAMES

Biaxin

BASIC INFORMATION

Habit forming? No
Prescription needed? Yes
Available as generic? No
Drug class: Antibacterial (erythromycin)

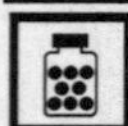

USES

Treats infections including bronchitis, pharyngitis, pneumonia, sinusitis, skin infections and Legionnaire's disease.

DOSAGE & USAGE INFORMATION

How to take:
Tablets—Swallow with liquid. If you can't swallow whole, crumble tablet and take with liquid or food.

When to take:
At the same time each day.

If you forget a dose:
- If you take 3 or more doses daily—Take as soon as you remember, then resume regular schedule.
- If you take 2 doses daily—Take as soon as you remember. Wait 5 to 6 hours for next dose. Return to regular schedule.

What drug does:
Prevents growth and reproduction of susceptible bacteria.

Time lapse before drug works:
Usually within 2 hours. Will take 2 to 5 days for noticeable effect.

Don't take with:
Any other medicine without consulting your doctor.

OVERDOSE

SYMPTOMS:
Nausea, vomiting, abdominal discomfort, diarrhea.
WHAT TO DO:
Overdose unlikely to threaten life. If person takes much larger amount than prescribed, call doctor, poison control center or hospital emergency room for instructions.

POSSIBLE ADVERSE REACTIONS OR SIDE EFFECTS

SYMPTOMS	WHAT TO DO
Life-threatening: None expected.	
Common: None expected.	
Infrequent: Abdominal discomfort, diarrhea, nausea, headache, change in taste.	Continue. Call doctor when convenient.
Rare: None expected.	

WARNINGS & PRECAUTIONS

Don't take if:
You are allergic to clarithromycin or erythromycins*.

Before you start, consult your doctor:
If you have significant kidney disease.

Over age 60:
Adverse reactions and side effects may be more frequent and severe than in younger persons.

Pregnancy:
Decide with your doctor if drug benefits justify risk to unborn child. Risk category C (see page xxii).

Breast-feeding:
Drug passes into milk. Avoid drug or discontinue nursing until you finish medicine. Consult doctor for advice on maintaining milk supply.

Infants & children:
Use only under medical supervision.

Prolonged use:
- You may become more susceptible to infections caused by germs that are not responsive to clarithromycin.
- Talk to your doctor about the need for follow-up medical examinations or laboratory studies to check liver function.

Skin & sunlight:
No special problems expected.

Driving, piloting or hazardous work:
No special problems expected.

Discontinuing:
Take drug for the full amount of time prescribed by doctor.

Others:
No problems expected.

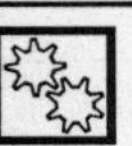

POSSIBLE INTERACTION WITH OTHER DRUGS

GENERIC NAME OR DRUG CLASS	COMBINED EFFECT
Theophylline	Increased concentration of theophylline.
Zidovudine	Decreased effect of zidovudine.

POSSIBLE INTERACTION WITH OTHER SUBSTANCES

INTERACTS WITH	COMBINED EFFECT
Alcohol:	Possible liver damage.
Beverages: Caffeine drinks.	Increased caffeine toxicity. Avoid.
Cocaine:	No proven problems.
Foods:	No proven problems.
Marijuana:	No proven problems.
Tobacco:	No proven problems.

*See Glossary

CLIDINIUM

BRAND NAMES

Apo-Chlorax
Clindex
Clinoxide
Corium
Librax
Lidox
Lodoxide
Quarzan
Zebrax

BASIC INFORMATION

Habit forming? No
Prescription needed?
Low strength: No
High strength: Yes
Available as generic? No
Drug class: Antispasmodic, anticholinergic

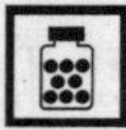

USES

Reduces spasms of digestive system, bladder and urethra.

DOSAGE & USAGE INFORMATION

How to take:
Capsule—Swallow with liquid or food to lessen stomach irritation.

When to take:
30 minutes before meals (unless directed otherwise by doctor).

If you forget a dose:
Take as soon as you remember up to 2 hours late. If more than 2 hours, wait for next scheduled dose (don't double this dose).

What drug does:
Blocks nerve impulses at parasympathetic nerve endings, preventing muscle contractions and gland secretions of organs involved.

Time lapse before drug works:
15 to 30 minutes.

Continued next column

OVERDOSE

SYMPTOMS:
Dilated pupils, rapid pulse and breathing, dizziness, fever, hallucinations, confusion, slurred speech, agitation, flushed face, convulsions, coma.
WHAT TO DO:
- **Dial 911 (emergency) or 0 (operator) for an ambulance or medical help. Then give first aid immediately.**
- **See emergency information on inside covers.**

Don't take with:
Any other medicine without consulting your doctor or pharmacist.

POSSIBLE ADVERSE REACTIONS OR SIDE EFFECTS

SYMPTOMS	WHAT TO DO
Life-threatening:	
In case of overdose, see previous column.	
Common:	
• Confusion, delirium, rapid heartbeat.	Discontinue. Call doctor right away.
• Nausea, vomiting, decreased sweating.	Continue. Call doctor when convenient.
• Constipation.	Continue. Tell doctor at next visit.
• Dryness in ears, nose, throat, mouth.	No action necessary.
Infrequent:	
• Nasal congestion, altered taste, difficult urination, headache, impotence.	Continue. Call doctor when convenient.
• Lightheadedness.	Discontinue. Call doctor right away.
Rare:	
Rash or hives, eye pain, blurred vision.	Discontinue. Call doctor right away.

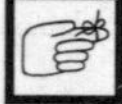

WARNINGS & PRECAUTIONS

Don't take if:
- You are allergic to any anticholinergic.
- You have trouble with stomach bloating.
- You have difficulty emptying your bladder completely (enlarged prostate).
- You have narrow-angle glaucoma.
- You have severe ulcerative colitis.

Before you start, consult your doctor:
- If you have open-angle glaucoma.
- If you have angina, chronic bronchitis or asthma, kidney or thyroid disease, hiatal hernia, liver disease, enlarged prostate, myasthenia gravis, peptic ulcer.
- If you will have surgery within 2 months, including dental surgery, requiring general or spinal anesthesia.

Over age 60:
Adverse reactions and side effects may be more frequent and severe than in younger persons.

Pregnancy:
Decide with your doctor whether drug benefits justify risk to unborn child. Risk category C (see page xxii).

Breast-feeding:
Drug passes into milk and decreases milk flow. Avoid drug or discontinue nursing until you finish medicine. Consult doctor for advice on maintaining milk supply.

Infants & children:
Use only under medical supervision.

Prolonged use:
Chronic constipation, possible fecal impaction. Consult doctor immediately.

Skin & sunlight:
No problems expected.

Driving, piloting or hazardous work:
Don't drive or pilot aircraft until you learn how medicine affects you. Don't work around dangerous machinery. Don't climb ladders or work in high places. Danger increases if you drink alcohol or take medicine affecting alertness and reflexes, such as antihistamines, tranquilizers, sedatives, pain medicine, narcotics, or mind-altering drugs.

Discontinuing:
May be unnecessary to finish medicine. Follow doctor's instructions.

Others:
Advise any doctor or dentist whom you consult that you take this medicine.

POSSIBLE INTERACTION WITH OTHER DRUGS

GENERIC NAME OR DRUG CLASS	COMBINED EFFECT
Amantadine	Increased clidinium effect.
Antacids*	Decreased clidinium effect.
Anticholinergics, other*	Increased clidinium effect.
Antidepressants, tricyclic*	Increased clidinium effect. Increased sedation.
Antidiarrheals*	Increased clidinium effect.
Antihistamines*	Increased clidinium effect.
Attapulgite	Decreased clidinium effect.
Haloperidol	Increased internal eye pressure.
Ketoconazole	Decreased ketoconazole effect.
Meperidine	Increased clidinium effect.
Methylphenidate	Increased clidinium effect.
Molindone	Increased anti-cholinergic effect.
Monoamine oxidase (MAO) inhibitors*	Increased clidinium effect.
Nitrates*	Increased internal eye pressure.
Nizatidine	Increased nizatidine effect.
Orphenadrine	Increased clidinium effect.
Pilocarpine	Loss of pilocarpine effect in glaucoma treatment.
Potassium supplements*	Possible intestinal ulcers with oral potassium tablets.
Tranquilizers*	Increased clidinium effect.
Vitamin C	Decreased clidinium effect. Avoid large doses of vitamin C.

POSSIBLE INTERACTION WITH OTHER SUBSTANCES

INTERACTS WITH	COMBINED EFFECT
Alcohol:	None expected.
Beverages:	None expected.
Cocaine:	Excessively rapid heartbeat. Avoid.
Foods:	None expected.
Marijuana:	Drowsiness and dry mouth.
Tobacco:	None expected.

*See Glossary

CLINDAMYCIN

BRAND NAMES

Cleocin
Cleocin Pediatric
Dalacin C
Dalacin C Palmitate
Dalacin C Phosphate

BASIC INFORMATION

Habit forming? No
Prescription needed? Yes
Available as generic? Yes
Drug class: Antibiotic (lincomycin)

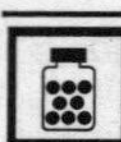

USES

Treatment of bacterial infections that are susceptible to clindamycin.

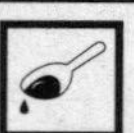

DOSAGE & USAGE INFORMATION

How to take:
Capsule or liquid—Swallow with liquid. Take with a full glass of water or a meal to avoid gastric irritation.

When to take:
At the same times each day.

If you forget a dose:
Take as soon as you remember up to 2 hours late. If more than 2 hours, wait for next scheduled dose (don't double this dose).

What drug does:
Destroys susceptible bacteria. Does not kill viruses.

Time lapse before drug works:
3 to 5 days.

Don't take with:
Any other medicine without consulting your doctor or pharmacist.

OVERDOSE

SYMPTOMS:
Severe nausea, vomiting, diarrhea.
WHAT TO DO:
Overdose unlikely to threaten life. If person takes much larger amount than prescribed, call doctor, poison control center or hospital emergency room for instructions.

POSSIBLE ADVERSE REACTIONS OR SIDE EFFECTS

SYMPTOMS	WHAT TO DO
Life-threatening:	
Hives, wheezing, faintness, itching, coma.	Seek emergency treatment immediately.
Common:	
Bloating.	Discontinue. Call doctor right away.
Infrequent:	
• Unusual thirst; vomiting; stomach cramps; severe and watery diarrhea with blood or mucus; painful, swollen joints; fever; jaundice; tiredness; weakness.	Discontinue. Call doctor right away.
• White patches in mouth; rash, itch around groin, rectum or armpits; vaginal discharge, itching.	Continue. Call doctor when convenient.
Rare:	
None expected.	

WARNINGS & PRECAUTIONS

Don't take if:
- You are allergic to lincomycins.
- You have had ulcerative colitis.

Before you start, consult your doctor:
- If you have had yeast infections of mouth, skin or vagina.
- If you will have surgery within 2 months, including dental surgery, requiring general or spinal anesthesia.
- If you have kidney or liver disease.
- If you have allergies of any kind.

Over age 60:
Adverse reactions and side effects may be more frequent and severe than in younger persons.

Pregnancy:
Decide with your doctor if drug benefits justify risk to unborn child. Risk category C (see page xxii).

Breast-feeding:
Drug passes into milk. Avoid drug or discontinue nursing until you finish medicine. Consult doctor for advice on maintaining milk supply.

Infants & children:
Don't give to infants younger than 1 month. Use for children only under medical supervision.

Prolonged use:
- Severe colitis with diarrhea and bleeding.
- You may become more susceptible to infections caused by germs not responsive to clindamycin.
- Talk to your doctor about the need for follow-up medical examinations or laboratory studies to check stool exams and perform proctosigmoidoscopy.

Skin & sunlight:
No problems expected.

Driving, piloting or hazardous work:
No problems expected.

Discontinuing:
Don't discontinue without doctor's advice until you complete prescribed dose, even though symptoms diminish or disappear.

Others:
May interfere with the accuracy of some medical tests.

POSSIBLE INTERACTION WITH OTHER DRUGS

GENERIC NAME OR DRUG CLASS	COMBINED EFFECT
Antidiarrheal preparations*	Decreased clindamycin effect.
Cefixime	Decreased antibiotic effect of cefixime.
Chloramphenicol	Decreased clindamycin effect.
Diphenoxylate	May delay removal of toxins from colon in cases of diarrhea caused by side effects of clindamycin.
Erythromycins*	Decreased clindamycin effect.
Loperamide	May delay removal of toxins from colon in cases of diarrhea caused by side effects of clindamycin.
Muscle blockers*	Increased actions of muscle blockers to unsafe degree. Avoid.

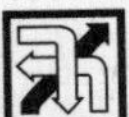

POSSIBLE INTERACTION WITH OTHER SUBSTANCES

INTERACTS WITH	COMBINED EFFECT
Alcohol:	None expected.
Beverages:	None expected.
Cocaine:	None expected.
Foods:	None expected.
Marijuana:	None expected.
Tobacco:	None expected.

*See Glossary

CLOFIBRATE

BRAND NAMES

Abitrate
Atromid-S
Claripex
Novofibrate

BASIC INFORMATION

Habit forming? No
Prescription needed? Yes
Available as generic? Yes
Drug class: Antihyperlipidemic

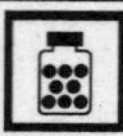

USES

Reduces fatty substances in the blood (triglycerides).

DOSAGE & USAGE INFORMATION

How to take:
Capsule—Swallow with liquid or food to lessen stomach irritation.

When to take:
At the same times each day.

If you forget a dose:
Take as soon as you remember up to 2 hours late. If more than 2 hours, wait for next scheduled dose (don't double this dose).

What drug does:
Inhibits formation of fatty substances.

Time lapse before drug works:
3 months or more.

Don't take with:
Any other medicine without consulting your doctor or pharmacist.

OVERDOSE

SYMPTOMS:
Diarrhea, headache, muscle pain.
WHAT TO DO:
Overdose unlikely to threaten life. If person takes much larger amount than prescribed, call doctor, poison control center or hospital emergency room for instructions.

POSSIBLE ADVERSE REACTIONS OR SIDE EFFECTS

SYMPTOMS	WHAT TO DO
Life-threatening: None expected.	
Common: None expected.	
Infrequent:	
• Chest pain, shortness of breath, irregular heartbeat, nausea, flu-like illness, vomiting.	Discontinue. Call doctor right away.
• Diarrhea, abdominal pain.	Continue. Call doctor when convenient.
Rare:	
• Cardiac arrhythmias, angina.	Discontinue. Seek emergency treatment.
• Rash, itch; mouth or lip sores; sore throat; swollen feet, legs; blood in urine; painful urination; fever; chills, anemia.	Discontinue. Call doctor right away.
• Dizziness, weakness, drowsiness, muscle cramps, headache, diminished sex drive, hair loss, dry mouth.	Continue. Call doctor when convenient.

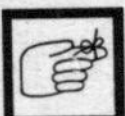

WARNINGS & PRECAUTIONS

Don't take if:
- You are allergic to any clofibrate.
- You have had serious liver disease.

Before you start, consult your doctor:
- If you have had liver or kidney disease.
- If you have had peptic ulcer disease.
- If you have diabetes.

Over age 60:
Adverse reactions and side effects may be more frequent and severe than in younger persons. May develop flu-like symptoms.

Pregnancy:
Decide with your doctor if drug benefits justify risk to unborn child. Risk category C (see page xxii).

Breast-feeding:
May harm child. Avoid. Consult doctor.

Infants & children:
Not recommended.

Prolonged use:
- May cause gall bladder infection.
- Possible cause of stomach cancer.
- Talk to your doctor about the need for follow-up medical examinations or laboratory studies to check complete blood counts (white blood cell count, platelet count, red blood cell count, hemoglobin, hematocrit), serum low-density lipoprotein.

Skin & sunlight:
No problems expected.

Driving, piloting or hazardous work:
Avoid if you feel drowsy or dizzy. Otherwise, no problems expected.

Discontinuing:
Don't discontinue without doctor's advice until you complete prescribed dose, even though symptoms diminish or disappear.

Others:
- Periodic blood-cell counts and liver-function studies recommended if you take clofibrate for a long time.
- Some studies question effectiveness. Many studies warn against toxicity.

POSSIBLE INTERACTION WITH OTHER DRUGS

GENERIC NAME OR DRUG CLASS	COMBINED EFFECT
Anticoagulants, oral*	Increased anti-coagulant effect. Dose reduction of anticoagulant necessary.
Antidiabetics, oral*	Increased antidiabetic effect.
Contraceptives, oral*	Decreased clofibrate effect.
Desmopressin	May decrease desmopressin effect.
Estrogens*	Decreased clofibrate effect.
Furosemide	Possible toxicity of both drugs.
Insulin	Increased insulin effect.
Probenecid	Increased effect and toxicity of clofibrate.
Thyroid hormones*	Increased clofibrate effect.
Ursodiol	Decreased effect of ursodiol.

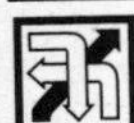

POSSIBLE INTERACTION WITH OTHER SUBSTANCES

INTERACTS WITH	COMBINED EFFECT
Alcohol:	None expected.
Beverages:	None expected.
Cocaine:	None expected.
Foods: Fatty foods.	Decreased clofibrate effect.
Marijuana:	None expected.
Tobacco:	None expected.

*See Glossary

CLOMIPHENE

BRAND NAMES

Clomid
Milophene
Serophene

BASIC INFORMATION

Habit forming? No
Prescription needed? Yes
Available as generic? Yes
Drug class: Gonad stimulant

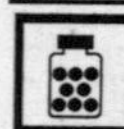

USES

- Treatment for men with low sperm counts.
- Treatment for ovulatory failure in women who wish to become pregnant.

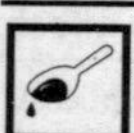

DOSAGE & USAGE INFORMATION

How to take:
Tablet—Swallow with liquid.

When to take:
- Men—Take at the same time each day.
- Women—Follow physician's instructions carefully.

If you forget a dose:
Take as soon as you remember. If you forget a day, double next dose. If you miss 2 or more doses, consult doctor.

What drug does:
Antiestrogen effect stimulates ovulation and sperm production.

Time lapse before drug works:
Usually 3 to 6 months. Ovulation may occur 6 to 10 days after last day of treatment in any cycle.

Don't take with:
No restrictions.

OVERDOSE

SYMPTOMS:
Increased severity of adverse reactions and side effects.
WHAT TO DO:
Overdose unlikely to threaten life. If person takes much larger amount than prescribed, call doctor, poison control center or hospital emergency room for instructions.

POSSIBLE ADVERSE REACTIONS OR SIDE EFFECTS

SYMPTOMS	WHAT TO DO
Life-threatening:	
Sudden shortness of breath.	Seek emergency treatment.
Common:	
• Bloating, abdominal pain, pelvic pain.	Discontinue. Call doctor right away.
• Hot flashes.	Continue. Tell doctor at next visit.
Infrequent:	
• Rash, itch, vomiting, jaundice.	Discontinue. Call doctor right away.
• Constipation, diarrhea, increased appetite, heavy menstrual flow, frequent urination, breast discomfort, weight change, hair loss, nausea.	Continue. Call doctor when convenient.
Rare:	
• Vision changes.	Discontinue. Call doctor right away.
• Dizziness, headache, tiredness, depression, nervousness.	Continue. Call doctor when convenient.

WARNINGS & PRECAUTIONS

Don't take if:
You are allergic to clomiphene.

Before you start, consult your doctor:
- If you have an ovarian cyst, fibroid uterine tumors or unusual vaginal bleeding.
- If you have inflamed veins caused by blood clots.
- If you have liver disease.
- If you are depressed.

Over age 60:
Not recommended.

Pregnancy:
Stop taking at first sign of pregnancy. Consult doctor. Risk category C (see page xxii).

Breast-feeding:
Not used.

Infants & children:
Not used.

Prolonged use:
- Not recommended.
- Talk to your doctor about the need for follow-up medical examinations or laboratory studies to check basal body temperature, endometrial biopsy, kidney function, eyes.

Skin & sunlight:
Eyes more sensitive to light.

Driving, piloting or hazardous work:
- Avoid if you feel dizzy.
- May cause blurred vision.

Discontinuing:
May be unnecessary to finish medicine. Follow doctor's instructions.

Others:
- Have a complete pelvic examination before treatment.
- If you become pregnant, twins or triplets are possible.

POSSIBLE INTERACTION WITH OTHER DRUGS

GENERIC NAME OR DRUG CLASS	COMBINED EFFECT
Thyroglobulin	May increase serum thyroglobulin.
Thyroxine (T-4)	May increase serum thyroxine.

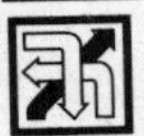

POSSIBLE INTERACTION WITH OTHER SUBSTANCES

INTERACTS WITH	COMBINED EFFECT
Alcohol:	None expected.
Beverages:	None expected.
Cocaine:	None expected.
Foods:	None expected.
Marijuana:	None expected.
Tobacco:	None expected.

CLONIDINE

BRAND NAMES

Catapres
Catapres-TTS
Dixarit

BASIC INFORMATION

Habit forming? No
Prescription needed? Yes
Available as generic? Yes
Drug class: Antihypertensive

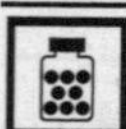

USES

- Treatment of high blood pressure and congestive heart failure.
- Treatment of dysmenorrhea and menopausal "hot flashes."
- Treatment of narcotic withdrawal syndrome.
- Prevention of vascular headaches.

DOSAGE & USAGE INFORMATION

How to take:

- Tablet—Swallow with liquid.
- Patches that attach to skin—Apply to clean, dry, hairless skin on arm or trunk.

When to take:
Daily dose at bedtime.

If you forget a dose:
Bedtime dose—If you forget your once-a-day dose, take it as soon as you remember. *Don't* double dose.

Continued next column

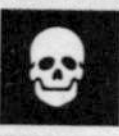

OVERDOSE

SYMPTOMS:
Vomiting, fainting, slow heartbeat, coma, diminished reflexes, shortness of breath, dizziness, extreme tiredness.
WHAT TO DO:

- **Dial 911 (emergency) or 0 (operator) for an ambulance or medical help. Then give first aid immediately.**
- **If patient is unconscious and not breathing, give mouth-to-mouth breathing. If there is no heartbeat, use cardiac massage and mouth-to-mouth breathing (CPR). Don't try to make patient vomit. If you can't get help quickly, take patient to nearest emergency facility.**
- **See emergency information on inside covers.**

What drug does:
Relaxes and allows expansion of blood vessel walls.

Time lapse before drug works:
1 to 3 hours.

Don't take with:

- Nonprescription medicines containing alcohol.
- Any other medicine without consulting your doctor or pharmacist.

POSSIBLE ADVERSE REACTIONS OR SIDE EFFECTS

SYMPTOMS	WHAT TO DO
Life-threatening:	
In case of overdose, see previous column.	
Common:	
• Dizziness, weight gain, drowsiness, lightheadedness upon rising from sitting or lying, swollen breasts.	Continue. Call doctor when convenient.
• Dry mouth, tiredness.	Continue. Tell doctor at next visit.
Infrequent:	
• Abnormal heart rhythm.	Discontinue. Call doctor right away.
• Headache; painful glands in neck; nightmares; nausea; vomiting; cold fingers and toes; dry, burning eyes; depression.	Continue. Call doctor when convenient.
• Insomnia, constipation, appetite loss, diminished sex drive, nervousness.	Continue. Tell doctor at next visit.
Rare:	
Rash, itch.	Discontinue. Call doctor right away.

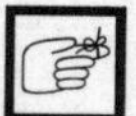

WARNINGS & PRECAUTIONS

Don't take if:

- You are allergic to any alpha-adrenergic blocker.
- You are under age 12.

Before you start, consult your doctor:

- If you will have surgery within 2 months, including dental surgery, requiring general or spinal anesthesia.
- If you have heart disease or chronic kidney disease.
- If you have a peripheral circulation disorder (intermittent claudication, Buerger's disease).
- If you have history of depression.

Over age 60:
Adverse reactions and side effects may be more frequent and severe than in younger persons.

Pregnancy:
Decide with your doctor whether drug benefits justify risk to unborn child. Risk category C (see page xxii).

Breast-feeding:
Unknown whether safe or not. Consult doctor.

Infants & children:
Use only under careful medical supervision after age 12. Avoid before age 12.

Prolonged use:
- Don't discontinue without consulting doctor. Dose may require gradual reduction if you have taken drug for a long time. Doses of other drugs may also require adjustment.
- Continued use may cause fluid retention, requiring addition of diuretic to treatment program.
- Request yearly eye examinations.
- Talk to your doctor about the need for follow-up medical examinations or laboratory studies.

Skin & sunlight:
No problems expected.

Driving, piloting or hazardous work:
Don't drive or pilot aircraft until you learn how medicine affects you. Don't work around dangerous machinery. Don't climb ladders or work in high places. Danger increases if you drink alcohol or take medicine affecting alertness and reflexes.

Discontinuing:
Don't discontinue abruptly. May cause rebound high blood pressure, anxiety, chest pain, insomnia, headache, nausea, irregular heartbeat, flushed face, sweating.

Others:
No problems expected.

POSSIBLE INTERACTION WITH OTHER DRUGS

GENERIC NAME OR DRUG CLASS	COMBINED EFFECT
Angiotensin-converting enzyme (ACE) inhibitors*	Possible excessive potassium in blood.
Antidepressants, tricyclic*	Decreased clonidine effect.
Antihypertensives, other*	Excessive blood pressure drop.
Appetite suppressants*	Decreased clonidine effect.
Beta-adrenergic blocking agents*	Possible precipitous change in blood pressure.
Carteolol	Increased anti-hypertensive effect.
Central nervous system (CNS) depressants*	Increased sedative effect.
Clozapine	Toxic effect on the central nervous system.
Diuretics*	Excessive blood pressure drop.
Ethinamate	Dangerous increased effects of ethinamate. Avoid combining.
Fenfluramine	Possible increased clonidine effect.
Fluoxetine	Increased depressant effects of both drugs.
Guanfacine	Blood pressure control impaired.
Leucovorin	High alcohol content of leucovorin may cause adverse effects.

Continued on page 934

POSSIBLE INTERACTION WITH OTHER SUBSTANCES

INTERACTS WITH	COMBINED EFFECT
Alcohol:	Increased sensitivity to sedative effect of alcohol and very low blood pressure. Avoid.
Beverages: Caffeine-containing drinks.	Decreased clonidine effect.
Cocaine:	Increased risk of heart block and high blood pressure.
Foods:	No problems expected.
Marijuana:	Weakness on standing.
Tobacco:	No problems expected.

*See Glossary

CLONIDINE & CHLORTHALIDONE

BRAND NAMES

Combipres

BASIC INFORMATION

Habit forming? No
Prescription needed? Yes
Available as generic? Yes
Drug class: Antihypertensive

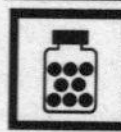

USES

- Treatment of high blood pressure.
- Reduces fluid retention (edema) caused by conditions such as heart disorders and liver disease.

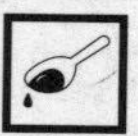

DOSAGE & USAGE INFORMATION

How to take:
Tablet—Swallow with liquid. If you can't swallow whole, crumble tablet and take with liquid or food. Don't exceed dose.

When to take:
At the same time each day.

If you forget a dose:
Take as soon as you remember up to 2 hours late. If more than 2 hours, wait for next scheduled dose (don't double this dose).

What drug does:
- Relaxes and allows expansion of blood vessel walls.

Continued next column

OVERDOSE

SYMPTOMS:
Vomiting; fainting; rapid, irregular, slow heartbeat; diminished reflexes; cramps; shortness of breath; weakness; drowsiness; weak pulse; coma.
WHAT TO DO:
- **Dial 911 (emergency) or 0 (operator) for an ambulance or medical help. Then give first aid immediately.**
- **If patient is unconscious and not breathing, give mouth-to-mouth breathing. If there is no heartbeat, use cardiac massage and mouth-to-mouth breathing (CPR). Don't try to make patient vomit. If you can't get help quickly, take patient to nearest emergency facility.**
- **See emergency information on inside covers.**

- Forces sodium and water excretion, reducing body fluid.
- Reduced body fluid and relaxed arteries lower blood pressure.

Time lapse before drug works:
4 to 6 hours. May require several weeks to lower blood pressure.

Don't take with:
Any medicine that will decrease mental alertness such as alcohol, antihistamines, cold/cough medicines, sedatives, tranquilizers, narcotics, prescription pain medicine, barbiturates, seizure medicine, anesthetics.

POSSIBLE ADVERSE REACTIONS OR SIDE EFFECTS

SYMPTOMS	WHAT TO DO
Life-threatening:	
Irregular heartbeat, weak pulse.	Discontinue. Seek emergency treatment.
Common:	
Dry mouth, increased thirst, muscle cramps, nausea or vomiting, mood changes, drowsiness.	Discontinue. Call doctor right away.
Infrequent:	
Vomiting, diminished sex desire and performance, insomnia, dizziness, diarrhea, constipation, appetite loss.	Continue. Call doctor when convenient.
Rare:	
• Jaundice; easy bruising or bleeding; sore throat, fever, mouth ulcers; rash or hives; joint pain; flank pain; abdominal pain.	Discontinue. Call doctor right away.
• Cold fingers and toes, nightmares.	Continue. Call doctor when convenient.

WARNINGS & PRECAUTIONS

Don't take if:
- You are allergic to any thiazide diuretic drug or alpha-adrenergic blocker.
- You are under age 12.

Before you start, consult your doctor:
- If you are allergic to any sulfa drug.
- If you have gout, liver, pancreas or kidney disorder, a peripheral circulation disorder (intermittent claudication, Buerger's disease), history of depression, heart disease.

- If you will have surgery within 2 months, including dental surgery, requiring general or spinal anesthesia.

Over age 60:
Adverse reactions and side effects may be more frequent and severe than in younger persons, especially dizziness and excessive potassium loss.

Pregnancy:
Decide with your doctor if drug benefits justify risk to unborn child. Risk category C (see page xxii).

Breast-feeding:
Drug passes into milk. Avoid drug or discontinue nursing until you finish medicine. Consult doctor for advice on maintaining milk supply.

Infants & children:
Use only after careful medical supervision after age 12. Avoid before age 12.

Prolonged use:
- Don't discontinue without consulting doctor. Dose may require gradual reduction if you have taken drug for a long time. Doses of other drugs may also require adjustment.
- Continued use may cause fluid retention, requiring addition of diuretic to treatment program.
- Request yearly eye examinations.
- Talk to your doctor about the need for follow-up medical examinations or laboratory studies.

Skin & sunlight:
May cause rash or intensify sunburn in areas exposed to sun or sunlamp.

Driving, piloting or hazardous work:
Don't drive or pilot aircraft until you learn how medicine affects you. Don't work around dangerous machinery. Don't climb ladders or work in high places. Danger increases if you drink alcohol or take medicine affecting alertness and reflexes, such as antihistamines, tranquilizers, sedatives, pain medicine, narcotics and mind-altering drugs.

Discontinuing:
Don't discontinue abruptly. May cause rebound high blood pressure, anxiety, chest pain, insomnia, headache, nausea, irregular heartbeat, flushed face, sweating.

Others:
- Hot weather and fever may cause dehydration and drop in blood pressure. Dose may require temporary adjustment. Weigh daily and report any unexpected weight decreases to your doctor.
- May cause rise in uric acid, leading to gout.
- May cause blood-sugar rise in diabetics.

POSSIBLE INTERACTION WITH OTHER DRUGS

GENERIC NAME OR DRUG CLASS	COMBINED EFFECT
Allopurinol	Decreased allopurinol effect.
Angiotensin-converting enzyme (ACE) inhibitors*	Possible excessive potassium in blood.
Antidepressants, tricyclic*	Dangerous drop in blood pressure. Avoid combination unless under medical supervision.
Antihypertensives, other*	Excessive blood pressure drop.
Appetite suppressants*	Decreased clonidine effect.
Barbiturates*	Increased chlorthalidone effect.
Beta-adrenergic blocking agents*	Possible precipitous change in blood pressure.
Carteolol	Increased anti-hypertensive effect.

Continued on page 935

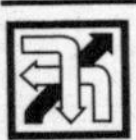

POSSIBLE INTERACTION WITH OTHER SUBSTANCES

INTERACTS WITH	COMBINED EFFECT
Alcohol:	Increased sensitivity to sedative effect of alcohol and very low blood pressure. Avoid.
Beverages: Caffeine-containing drinks.	Decreased clonidine effect.
Cocaine:	Increased risk of heart block and high blood pressure.
Foods: Licorice.	Excessive potassium loss that causes dangerous heart rhythm.
Marijuana:	Weakness on standing. May increase blood pressure.
Tobacco:	None expected.

*See Glossary

CLOTRIMAZOLE (Oral-Local)

BRAND NAMES

Mycelex Troches

BASIC INFORMATION

Habit forming? No
Prescription needed? Yes
Available as generic? No
Drug class: Antifungal

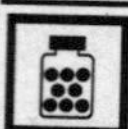

USES

- Treats thrush, white mouth (candidiasis).
- Used primarily in immunosuppressed patients to treat and prevent mouth infection.

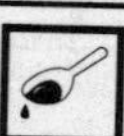

DOSAGE & USAGE INFORMATION

How to take:
Lozenges—Dissolve slowly and completely in the mouth, 5 times a day. Swallow saliva during this time. Don't swallow lozenge whole and don't chew.

When to take:
14 days or longer.

If you forget a dose:
Take as soon as you remember up to 2 hours late. If more than 2 hours, wait for next scheduled dose (don't double this dose).

What drug does:
Kills fungus by interfering with cell wall membrane and its permeability.

Time lapse before drug works:
1 to 3 hours.

Don't take with:
Any other medicine without consulting your doctor or pharmacist.

OVERDOSE

SYMPTOMS:
None expected, but if large dose has been taken, follow instructions below.
WHAT TO DO:

- **Dial 911 (emergency) or 0 (operator) for an ambulance or medical help. Then give first aid immediately.**
- **See emergency information on inside covers.**

POSSIBLE ADVERSE REACTIONS OR SIDE EFFECTS

SYMPTOMS	WHAT TO DO
Life-threatening: None expected.	
Common: None expected.	
Infrequent: Abdominal pain, diarrhea, nausea, vomiting.	Discontinue. Call doctor right away.
Rare: None expected.	

WARNINGS & PRECAUTIONS

Don't take if:
You have severe liver disease.

Before you start, consult your doctor:
If you have had a recent organ transplant.

Over age 60:
Adverse reactions and side effects may be more frequent and severe than in younger persons. You may need smaller doses for shorter periods of time.

Pregnancy:
Decide with your doctor if drug benefits justify risk to unborn child. Risk category C (see page xxii).

Breast-feeding:
Unknown effect. Consult doctor.

Infants & children:
Use only under medical supervision for children younger than 4 or 5 years.

Prolonged use:
No problems expected.

Skin & sunlight:
No problems expected.

Driving, piloting or hazardous work:
Don't drive or pilot aircraft until you learn how medicine affects you. Don't work around dangerous machinery. Don't climb ladders or work in high places. Danger increases if you drink alcohol or take medicine affecting alertness and reflexes.

Discontinuing:
Don't discontinue without consulting doctor. Dose may require gradual reduction if you have taken drug for a long time. Doses of other drugs may also require adjustment.

Others:
- Continue for full term of treatment. May require several months.
- Check with physician if not improved in 1 week.

POSSIBLE INTERACTION WITH OTHER DRUGS

GENERIC NAME OR DRUG CLASS	COMBINED EFFECT
None expected.	

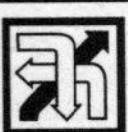

POSSIBLE INTERACTION WITH OTHER SUBSTANCES

INTERACTS WITH	COMBINED EFFECT
Alcohol:	Decreased effects of clotrimazole.
Beverages:	None expected.
Cocaine:	Decreased effects of clotrimazole.
Foods:	None expected.
Marijuana:	Decreased effects of clotrimazole.
Tobacco:	Decreased effects of clotrimazole.

CLOZAPINE

BRAND NAMES

Clozaril
Leponex

BASIC INFORMATION

Habit forming? No
Prescription needed? Yes. Prescribed only through a special program.
Available as generic? No
Drug class: Antipsychotic

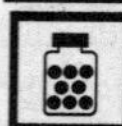

USES

Treats severe schizophrenia in patients not helped by other medicines.

DOSAGE & USAGE INFORMATION

How to take:
Tablet—Swallow with liquid. If you can't swallow whole, crumble tablet and take with liquid or food.

When to take:
Once or twice daily as directed.

If you forget a dose:
Take as soon as you remember up to 2 hours late. If more than 2 hours, wait for next scheduled dose (don't double this dose).

What drug does:
Interferes with binding of dopamine. May produce significant improvement, but may at times also make schizophrenia worse.

Time lapse before drug works:
1 to 6 hours.

Don't take with:
Any other prescription drug, nonprescription drug or alcohol without first checking with your doctor.

OVERDOSE

SYMPTOMS:
Heartbeat fast, slow, irregular; hallucinations; restlessness; excitement; drowsiness; breathing difficulty.
WHAT TO DO:
- **Dial 911 (emergency) or 0 (operator) for an ambulance or medical help. Then give first aid immediately.**
- **See emergency information on inside covers.**

POSSIBLE ADVERSE REACTIONS OR SIDE EFFECTS

SYMPTOMS	WHAT TO DO
Life-threatening:	
Seizures (rare).	Seek emergency treatment immediately.
Common:	
• Fast or irregular heartbeat, dizziness or fainting, fever.	Continue, but call doctor right away.
• Constipation, lightheadedness, increased salivation, heartburn, nausea, weight gain.	Continue. Call doctor when convenient.
Infrequent:	
Abdominal discomfort, increased sweating, anxiety, confusion, mild restlessness, blurred vision, unusual bleeding.	Continue, but call doctor right away.
Rare:	
Chills, fever, sore throat, mouth ulcers; difficult urination; rigid muscles; muscle tremors; mental depression; insomnia; lip-smacking, cheek puffing, uncontrolled tongue movements.	Continue, but call doctor right away.

WARNINGS & PRECAUTIONS

Don't take if:
- You are significantly mentally depressed.
- You have bone marrow depression from other drugs.
- You have glaucoma.

Before you start, consult your doctor:
- If you have an enlarged prostate gland.
- If you have ever had seizures from any cause.
- If you have liver, heart or gastrointestinal disease.

Over age 60:
Possible greater risk of weakness or dizziness upon standing after sitting or lying down. Greater risk of excitement, confusion. Great risk of difficulty in urination.

Pregnancy:
Risk category B (see page xxii).

Breast-feeding:
May cause sedation, restlessness or irritability in the nursing infant. Avoid.

Infants & children:
Safety not established. Consult doctor.

Prolonged use:
Effects unknown.

Skin & sunlight:
No problems expected.

Driving, piloting or hazardous work:
Don't drive or pilot aircraft until you learn how medicine affects you. Don't work around dangerous machinery. Don't climb ladders or work in high places. Danger increases if you drink alcohol or take medicine affecting alertness and reflexes.

Discontinuing:
Don't discontinue without consulting doctor. Dose may require gradual reduction if you have taken drug for a long time. Doses of other drugs may also require adjustment.

Others:
- This medicine is available only through a special management program for monitoring and distributing this drug.
- You will need laboratory studies each week for white blood cell and differential counts.

POSSIBLE INTERACTION WITH OTHER DRUGS

GENERIC NAME OR DRUG CLASS	COMBINED EFFECT
Bone marrow depressants*	Toxic bone marrow depression.
Central nervous system (CNS) depressants*	Toxic effects on the central nervous system.
Lithium	Increased risk of seizures.
Risperidone	Increased risperidone effect.

POSSIBLE INTERACTION WITH OTHER SUBSTANCES

INTERACTS WITH	COMBINED EFFECT
Alcohol:	Avoid. Increases toxic effect on the central nervous system.
Beverages: Caffeine drinks.	Excess (more than 3 cups of coffee or equivalent) increases risk of heartbeat irregularities.
Cocaine:	Increased risk of heartbeat irregularities.
Foods:	No special problems expected.
Marijuana:	Increased risk of heartbeat irregularities.
Tobacco:	Decreased serum concentration of clozapine. Avoid.

***See Glossary**

COAL TAR (Topical)

BRAND AND GENERIC NAMES

See complete list of brand and generic names in the *Brand Name Directory*, page 905.

BASIC INFORMATION

Habit forming? No
Prescription needed? No (for most)
Available as generic? Yes
Drug class: Antiseborrheic, antipsoriatic, keratolytic

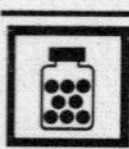

USES

Applied to the skin to treat dandruff, seborrhea, dermatitis, eczema and other skin diseases.

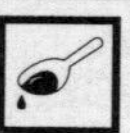

DOSAGE & USAGE INFORMATION

How to use:
- Follow package instructions.
- Don't apply to blistered, oozing, infected or raw skin.
- Keep away from eyes.
- Protect treated area from sunshine for 72 hours.

When to use:
According to package instructions.

If you forget a dose:
Use as soon as you remember.

What drug does:
- Kills bacteria and fungus organisms on contact.
- Suppresses overproduction of skin cells.

Time lapse before drug works:
None. Works immediately. May take several days before maximum effect.

Don't take with:
Any other medicine without consulting your doctor or pharmacist.

OVERDOSE

SYMPTOMS:
None expected.
WHAT TO DO:
Overdose unlikely to threaten life. If person takes much larger amount than prescribed, call doctor, poison control center or hospital emergency room for instructions.

POSSIBLE ADVERSE REACTIONS OR SIDE EFFECTS

SYMPTOMS	WHAT TO DO
Life-threatening: None expected.	
Common: Skin stinging.	Continue. Call doctor when convenient.
Infrequent: Skin more irritated.	Continue. Call doctor when convenient.
Rare: Pus forms in lesions on skin.	Continue. Call doctor when convenient.

WARNINGS & PRECAUTIONS

Don't use if:
You have intolerance to coal tar.

Before you start, consult your doctor:
If you have infected skin or open wounds.

Over age 60:
No special problems expected.

Pregnancy:
Consult doctor. Risk category C (see page xxii).

Breast-feeding:
No special problems expected. Consult doctor.

Infants & children:
Don't use on infants.

Prolonged use:
No special problems expected.

Skin & sunlight:
Protect treated area from direct sunlight for 72 hours.

Driving, piloting or hazardous work:
No problems expected.

Discontinuing:
No special problems expected.

Others:
May affect results in some medical tests.

POSSIBLE INTERACTION WITH OTHER DRUGS

GENERIC NAME OR DRUG CLASS	COMBINED EFFECT
Psoralens (methoxsalen, trioxsalen)	Excess sensitivity to sun.

POSSIBLE INTERACTION WITH OTHER SUBSTANCES

INTERACTS WITH	COMBINED EFFECT
Alcohol:	No special problems expected.
Beverages:	No special problems expected.
Cocaine:	No special problems expected.
Foods:	No special problems expected.
Marijuana:	No special problems expected.
Tobacco:	No special problems expected.

***See Glossary**

COCAINE

GENERIC NAME

COCAINE

BASIC INFORMATION

Habit forming? Yes
Prescription needed? Yes
Available as generic? Yes
Drug class: Anesthetic (local)

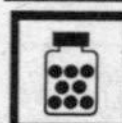

USES

Provides local anesthesia to the nose, mouth or throat to allow some types of surgery or examinations without pain.

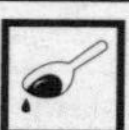

DOSAGE & USAGE INFORMATION

How to use:
Used only under doctor's supervision, it's applied by spray or cotton swab directly to the area being anesthetized.

When to use:
Immediately before special examinations or surgery.

If you forget a dose:
Not applicable.

What drug does:
- Blocks conduction of nerve impulses to brain.
- Reduces swelling, bleeding and congestion at operation site.

Time lapse before drug works:
Immediate.

Don't use with:
Any other medicine without consulting your doctor or pharmacist.

OVERDOSE

SYMPTOMS:
Abdominal pain, chills, confusion, lightheadedness, dizziness, severe nervousness or restlessness, fast or irregular heartbeat, severe headache, sweating, twitching, dilated pupils, bulging eyes.
WHAT TO DO:
- **Tell your doctor immediately if any of the above occurs after cocaine has been applied.**
- **Dial 911 (emergency) or 0 (operator) for an ambulance or medical help. Then give first aid immediately.**
- **See emergency information on inside covers.**

POSSIBLE ADVERSE REACTIONS OR SIDE EFFECTS

SYMPTOMS	WHAT TO DO
Life-threatening: Blue discoloration of skin, lips, nails; irregular, weak heartbeat; chest pain; seizure; loss of bowel and bladder control.	Seek emergency treatment immediately.
Common: Abdominal pain, dizziness, confusion, agitation, irritability, hallucinations, fast or irregular heartbeat, headache, euphoria, psychotic behavior, trembling, large pupils, chills and fever, twitching, stuffy nose.	Discontinue. Seek medical help if symptoms don't quickly subside.
Infrequent: Loss of taste or smell after application to nose or mouth.	Nothing. This is a normal effect.
Rare: Death.	

WARNINGS & PRECAUTIONS

Don't take if:
You are allergic to cocaine.

Before you start, consult your doctor:
- If you are allergic to anything.
- If you are taking any other medicine.
- If you have any acute illness or history of cancer, convulsions, irregular heartbeat, heart disease, blood vessel disease, high blood pressure, liver disease, heart attack history, hyperthyroidism (overactive thyroid gland).
- If you have recently used an insecticide.
- If you have had glaucoma or are using eye drops for glaucoma (such as Betoptic, Betagan, Timoptic).
- If you have a throat infection.

Over age 60:
More sensitive to drug. May cause impaired thinking, hallucinations, nightmares. Consult doctor about any of these.

Pregnancy:
Decide with your doctor if drug benefits justify risk to unborn child. Risk category C (see page xxii).

Breast-feeding:
Risk outweighs any possible drug benefits. Don't use.

Infants & children:
Not recommended for children 6 and younger. Use for older children only under doctor's supervision.

Prolonged use:
Addiction.

Skin & sunlight:
No problems expected.

Driving, piloting or hazardous work:
Don't drive or pilot aircraft for 24 hours after cocaine has been used for local anesthesia. Don't work around dangerous machinery. Don't climb ladders or work in high places. Danger increases if you drink alcohol or take medicine affecting alertness and reflexes, such as antihistamines, tranquilizers, sedatives, pain medicine, narcotics and mind-altering drugs.

Discontinuing:
No problems expected.

Others:
- In some people, even small amounts of cocaine can cause serious adverse reactions.
- Cocaine is used only under the direct supervision of your doctor.
- May interfere with the accuracy of some medical tests, such as blood sugar, blood pressure, heart rate.

POSSIBLE INTERACTION WITH OTHER DRUGS

GENERIC NAME OR DRUG CLASS	COMBINED EFFECT
Anesthetics*	Increased risk of heartbeat irregularity.
Antidepressants, tricyclic*	Increased risk of heartbeat irregularity.
Antihypertensives*	Increased risk of heart block and high blood pressure.
Beta-adrenergic blocking agents*	Decreased beta-blocker effect.
Central nervous system (CNS) stimulants*	Convulsions or excessive nervousness.
Digitalis preparations*	Increased risk of heartbeat irregularity.
Insecticides	Increased risk of toxicity.
Levodopa	Increased risk of heartbeat irregularity.
Methyldopa	Increased risk of heartbeat irregularity.
Monoamine oxidase (MAO) inhibitors*	Increased risk of toxicity.
Nitrates*	Reduced effectiveness of nitrates.
Sympathomimetics*	High risk of heart-beat irregularities and high blood pressure.

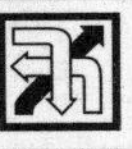

POSSIBLE INTERACTION WITH OTHER SUBSTANCES

INTERACTS WITH	COMBINED EFFECT
Alcohol:	Dangerous inter-action. Don't use.
Beverages: Caffeine drinks.	Dangerous inter-action. Don't use.
Cocaine: Orally.	Increased chance of adverse reactions or death.
Foods:	No proven problems.
Marijuana:	Dangerous inter-action. Don't use.
Tobacco:	Increased likelihood of irregular or rapid heartbeat.

*See Glossary

COLCHICINE

GENERIC NAMES

COLCHICINE

BASIC INFORMATION

Habit forming? No
Prescription needed? Yes
Available as generic? Yes
Drug class: Antigout

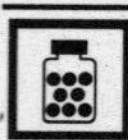

USES

- Relieves joint pain, inflammation, swelling of gout.
- Also used for familial Mediterranean fever, dermatitis herpetiformis, calcium pyrophosphate deposition disease, amyloidosis, Paget's disease of bone, recurrent pericarditis, Behcet's syndrome.

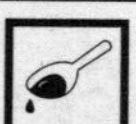

DOSAGE & USAGE INFORMATION

How to take:
Tablet—Swallow with liquid or food to lessen stomach irritation.

When to take:
- As prescribed. Stop taking when pain stops or at first sign of digestive upset. Wait at least 3 days between treatments.
- Don't take more than 8 doses.

If you forget a dose:
Don't double next dose. Consult doctor.

What drug does:
Decreases acidity of joint tissues and prevents deposits of uric-acid crystals.

Time lapse before drug works:
12 to 48 hours.

Don't take with:
Any other medicine without consulting your doctor or pharmacist.

OVERDOSE

SYMPTOMS:
Bloody urine; diarrhea; burning feeling in the throat, skin or stomach; nausea or vomiting; muscle weakness; fever; shortness of breath; stupor; convulsions; coma.
WHAT TO DO:
- **Dial 911 (emergency) or 0 (operator) for an ambulance or medical help. Then give first aid immediately.**
- **See emergency information on inside covers.**

POSSIBLE ADVERSE REACTIONS OR SIDE EFFECTS

SYMPTOMS	WHAT TO DO
Life-threatening: In case of overdose, see previous column.	
Common: Diarrhea, nausea, vomiting, abdominal pain.	Discontinue. Call doctor right away.
Infrequent: Hair loss with long-term use.	Continue. Call doctor when convenient.
Rare: Jaundice, black or tarry stool, blood in urine, breathing difficulty, fever, chills, headache, hives, mouth or lip sores, sore throat, unusual bruising or bleeding, unusual tiredness or weakness.	Discontinue. Call doctor right away.

WARNINGS & PRECAUTIONS

Don't take if:
You are allergic to colchicine.

Before you start, consult your doctor:
- If you have had peptic ulcers or ulcerative colitis.
- If you have heart, liver or kidney disease.
- If you will have surgery within 2 months, including dental surgery, requiring general or spinal anesthesia.
- If you have a gastrointestinal disorder.
- If you drink large amounts of alcohol.

Over age 60:
Adverse reactions and side effects may be more frequent and severe than in younger persons. Colchicine has a narrow margin of safety for people in this age group.

Pregnancy:
Consult doctor. Risk category D (see page xxii).

Breast-feeding:
Drug passes into breast milk. Effect unknown. Consult doctor.

Infants & children:
Not recommended.

Prolonged use:
- Hair loss.
- Numbness or tingling in hands and feet.
- Talk to your doctor about the need for follow-up medical examinations or laboratory studies to check complete blood counts (white blood cell count, platelet count, red blood cell count, hemoglobin, hematocrit).

Skin & sunlight:
No problems expected.

Driving, piloting or hazardous work:
Don't drive or pilot aircraft until you learn how medicine affects you. Don't work around dangerous machinery. Don't climb ladders or work in high places. Danger increases if you drink alcohol or take medicine affecting alertness and reflexes, such as antihistamines, tranquilizers, sedatives, pain medicine, narcotics and mind-altering drugs.

Discontinuing:
- May be unnecessary to finish medicine. Follow doctor's instructions.
- Stop taking if digestive upsets occur before symptoms are relieved.

Others:
- Limit each course of treatment to 8 mg. Don't exceed 3 mg. per 24 hours.
- May cause decreased sperm production in males.
- May interfere with the accuracy of some medical tests.

POSSIBLE INTERACTION WITH OTHER DRUGS

GENERIC NAME OR DRUG CLASS	COMBINED EFFECT
Anticoagulants*	Increased anticoagulant effect.
Anti-inflammatory drugs, nonsteroidal (NSAIDs)*	Increased risk of gastrointestinal problems.
Blood dyscrasia-causing medications*	Increased bone marrow depressant effect.
Bone marrow depressants,* other	Increased bone marrow depressant effect.
Phenylbutazone	Increased chance of ulcers in gastrointestinal tract.
Thioguanine	May need increased dosage of colchicine.
Vitamin B-12	Decreased absorption of vitamin B-12.

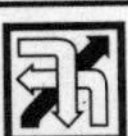

POSSIBLE INTERACTION WITH OTHER SUBSTANCES

INTERACTS WITH	COMBINED EFFECT
Alcohol:	Increased risk of gastrointestinal toxicity.
Beverages: Herbal teas.	Increased colchicine effect. Avoid.
Cocaine:	Overstimulation Avoid.
Foods:	No proven problems.
Marijuana:	Decreased colchicine effect.
Tobacco:	No proven problems.

*See Glossary

COLESTIPOL

BRAND NAMES

Colestid

BASIC INFORMATION

Habit forming? No
Prescription needed? Yes
Available as generic? No
Drug class: Antihyperlipidemic

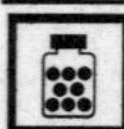

USES

- Reduces cholesterol level in blood in patients with type IIa hyperlipidemia.
- Treats overdose of digitalis.
- Reduces skin itching associated with some forms of liver disease.
- Treats diarrhea after some surgical operations.
- Treatment of one form of colitis (rare).

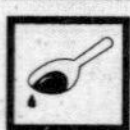

DOSAGE & USAGE INFORMATION

How to take:
Oral suspension—Mix well with 6 ounces or more or water or liquid, or in soups, pulpy fruits, with milk or in cereals. Will not dissolve.

When to take:
- Before meals.
- If taking other medicine, take it 1 hour before or 4 to 6 hours after taking colestipol.

If you forget a dose:
Take as soon as you remember up to 2 hours late. If more than 2 hours, wait for next scheduled dose (don't double this dose).

What drug does:
Binds with bile acids in intestines, preventing reabsorption.

Time lapse before drug works:
3 to 12 months.

Don't take with:
Any other medicine without consulting your doctor or pharmacist.

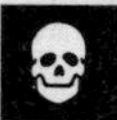

OVERDOSE

SYMPTOMS:
Fecal impaction.
WHAT TO DO:
Overdose unlikely to threaten life. If person takes much larger amount than prescribed, call doctor, poison control center or hospital emergency room for instructions.

POSSIBLE ADVERSE REACTIONS OR SIDE EFFECTS

SYMPTOMS	WHAT TO DO
Life-threatening: None expected.	
Common: None expected.	
Infrequent:	
• Black, tarry stools from gastrointestinal bleeding.	Discontinue. Seek emergency treatment.
• Severe abdominal pain.	Discontinue. Call doctor right away.
• Constipation, belching, diarrhea, nausea, unexpected weight loss.	Continue. Call doctor when convenient.
Rare:	
Hives, skin rash, hiccups.	Discontinue. Call doctor right away.

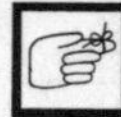

WARNINGS & PRECAUTIONS

Don't take if:
You are allergic to colestipol.

Before you start, consult your doctor:
- If you have liver disease such as cirrhosis.
- If you are jaundiced.
- If you will have surgery within 2 months, including dental surgery, requiring general or spinal anesthesia.
- If you are constipated.
- If you have peptic ulcer.
- If you have coronary artery disease.

Over age 60:
Constipation more likely. Other adverse effects more likely.

Pregnancy:
Safety not established. Consult doctor. Risk category C (see page xxii).

Breast-feeding:
No proven harm to child. Consult doctor.

Infants & children:
Only under expert medical supervision.

Prolonged use:
- Request lab studies to determine serum cholesterol and serum triglycerides.
- May decrease absorption of folic acid.

Skin & sunlight:
No problems expected.

Driving, piloting or hazardous work:
No problems expected.

Discontinuing:
Don't discontinue without consulting doctor. Dose may require gradual reduction if you have taken drug for a long time. Doses of other drugs may also require adjustment, particularly digitalis.

Others:
- This medicine does not cure disorders, but helps to control them.
- May interfere with the accuracy of some medical tests.

POSSIBLE INTERACTION WITH OTHER DRUGS

GENERIC NAME OR DRUG CLASS	COMBINED EFFECT
Anticoagulants, oral*	Decreased anti-coagulant effect.
Beta carotene	Decreased absorption of beta carotene.
Dextrothyroxine	Decreased dextrothyroxine effect.
Digitalis preparations*	Decreased absorption of digitalis preparations.
Diuretics, thiazide*	Decreased absorption of thiazide diuretics.
Penicillins*	Decreased absorption of penicillins.
Tetracyclines*	Decreased absorption of tetracyclines.
Thiazides*	Decreased absorption of colestipol.
Thyroid hormones*	Decreased thyroid effect.
Trimethoprim	Decreased absorption of colestipol.
Ursodiol	Decreased absorption of ursodiol.
Vancomycin	Increased chance of hearing loss or kidney damage. Decreased therapeutic effect of vancomycin.
Vitamins	Decreased absorption of fat-soluble vitamins (A,D,E,K).
Other medicines	May delay or reduce absorption.

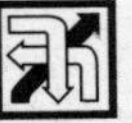

POSSIBLE INTERACTION WITH OTHER SUBSTANCES

INTERACTS WITH	COMBINED EFFECT
Alcohol:	None expected.
Beverages:	None expected.
Cocaine:	None expected.
Foods:	Interferes with absorption of vitamins. Take supplements.
Marijuana:	None expected.
Tobacco:	None expected.

***See Glossary**

CONTRACEPTIVES, ORAL

BRAND AND GENERIC NAMES

See complete list of brand and generic names in the *Brand Name Directory*, page 905.

BASIC INFORMATION

Habit forming? No
Prescription needed? Yes
Available as generic? No
Drug class: Female sex hormone, contraceptive (oral)

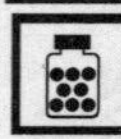

USES

- Prevents pregnancy.
- Regulates menstrual periods.

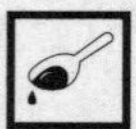

DOSAGE & USAGE INFORMATION

How to take:
Tablet—Swallow with liquid or food to lessen stomach irritation.

When to take:
At same time each day according to prescribed instructions, usually for 21 days of 28-day cycle.

If you forget a dose:
Call doctor's office for advice about additional protection against pregnancy.

What drug does:
- Alters mucus at cervix entrance to prevent sperm entry.
- Alters uterus lining to resist implantation of fertilized egg.
- Creates same chemical atmosphere in blood that exists during pregnancy, suppressing pituitary hormones which stimulate ovulation.

Time lapse before drug works:
10 days or more to provide contraception.

Don't take with:
- Tobacco
- Any other medicine without consulting your doctor or pharmacist.

OVERDOSE

SYMPTOMS:
Drowsiness, nausea, vomiting, vaginal bleeding.
WHAT TO DO:
Overdose unlikely to threaten life. If person takes much larger amount than prescribed, call doctor, poison control center or hospital emergency room for instructions.

POSSIBLE ADVERSE REACTIONS OR SIDE EFFECTS

SYMPTOMS	WHAT TO DO
Life-threatening:	
Stroke, chest pain, coughing blood, sudden severe headache, severe leg pain, shortness of breath.	Seek emergency treatment immediately.
Common:	
Brown blotches on skin; vaginal discharge, itch; fluid retention; break-through bleeding; acne.	Continue. Call doctor when convenient.
Infrequent:	
• Headache; pain, swelling in leg (possible blood clots in leg vein); muscle, joint pain; depression; severe abdominal pain; bulging eyes; fainting; frequent urination; breast lumps.	Discontinue. Call doctor right away.
• Blue tinge to objects, lights; appetite change; nausea; bloating; vomiting; pain; changed sex drive.	Continue. Call doctor when convenient.
Rare:	
• Jaundice, rash, hives, itch, fever, hyper-calcemia in breast cancer, intolerance of contact lenses, excess hair growth, voice change, enlarged clitoris in women.	Discontinue. Call doctor right away.
• Amenorrhea, insom-nia, hair loss.	Continue. Call doctor when convenient.

WARNINGS & PRECAUTIONS

Don't take if:
- You are allergic to any female hormone.
- You have had heart disease, blood clots or stroke.
- You have liver disease.
- You have cancer of breast, uterus or ovaries.
- You have unexplained vaginal bleeding.
- You smoke cigarettes.

Before you start, consult your doctor:
- If you have fibrocystic disease of breast.
- If you have migraine headaches.
- If you have fibroid tumors of uterus.
- If you have epilepsy.

- If you have asthma.
- If you have high blood pressure.
- If you will have surgery within 2 months, including dental surgery, requiring general or spinal anesthesia.
- If you have endometriosis.
- If you have diabetes.
- If you have sickle-cell anemia.
- If you are over age 35.

Over age 60:
Not used.

Pregnancy:
Discontinue at first sign of pregnancy. Risk category X (see page xxii).

Breast-feeding:
Drug passes into milk. Avoid drug or discontinue nursing.

Infants & children:
Not recommended.

Prolonged use:
- Gallstones.
- Gradual blood pressure rise.
- Possible difficulty becoming pregnant after discontinuing.
- Talk to your doctor about the need for follow-up medical examinations or laboratory studies to check blood pressure, liver function, pap smear.

Skin & sunlight:
May cause rash or intensify sunburn in areas exposed to sun or sunlamp.

Driving, piloting or hazardous work:
No problems expected.

Discontinuing:
Don't become pregnant for 6 months after discontinuing.

Others:
- Failure to take oral contraceptives for 1 day may cancel pregnancy protection. If you forget a dose, use other contraceptive measures and call doctor for instructions on re-starting oral contraceptive.
- May interfere with the accuracy of some medical tests.
- May cause some vitamin deficiencies.

POSSIBLE INTERACTION WITH OTHER DRUGS

GENERIC NAME OR DRUG CLASS	COMBINED EFFECT
Ampicillin	Decreased contraceptive effect.
Anticoagulants*	Decreased anticoagulant effect.
Anticonvulsants, hydantoin*	Decreased contraceptive effect.
Antidepressants, tricyclic*	Increased toxicity of antidepressants.
Antidiabetics* oral	Decreased antidiabetic effect.
Antifibronolytic agents*	Increased possibility of blood clotting.
Anti-inflammatory drugs nonsteroidal (NSAIDs)*	Decreased contraceptive effect.
Antihistamines*	Decreased contraceptive effect.
Barbiturates*	Decreased contraceptive effect.
Chloramphenicol	Decreased contraceptive effect.
Clofibrate	Decreased clofibrate effect.
Dextrothyroxine	Decreased dextrothyroxine effect.
Guanethidine	Decreased guanethidine effect.
Hypoglycemics, oral*	Decreased effect of hypoglycemics.
Insulin	Possibly decreased insulin effect.
Meperidine	Increased meperidine effect.

Continued on page 935

POSSIBLE INTERACTION WITH OTHER SUBSTANCES

INTERACTS WITH	COMBINED EFFECT
Alcohol:	No proven problems.
Beverages:	No proven problems.
Cocaine:	No proven problems.
Foods: Salt.	Increased edema (fluid retention).
Marijuana:	Increased bleeding between periods. Avoid.
Tobacco:	Possible heart attack, blood clots and stroke. If you take "the pill," *don't smoke.*

***See Glossary**

CONTRACEPTIVES, VAGINAL (Spermicides)

BRAND AND GENERIC NAMES

See complete list of brand and generic names in the *Brand Name Directory* page 905.

BASIC INFORMATION

Habit forming? No
Prescription needed? Not for most
Available as generic? Most aren't
Drug class: Contraceptive (vaginal)

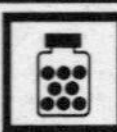

USES

- Provides a degree of protection against pregnancy.
- May help to protect against some sexually transmitted diseases, such as those caused by chlamydia, gardnerella, mycoplasma, neisseria, trichomonas, ureaplasma and possibly herpes virus.

DOSAGE & USAGE INFORMATION

How to take:
- Read package insert carefully. Some cautions to remember:
- Do not douche for 6 to 8 hours after intercourse.
- Do not remove sponge, cervical cap or diaphragm for 6 to 8 hours after intercourse.
- Follow product label instructions for storage.

When to take:
Consistently with every sexual exposure.

If you forget to use:
Contact your doctor to consider using another form of pregnancy protection, such as the "morning-after" pill.

What drug does:
Forms a chemical barrier between sperm in semen and the mucous membranes in the vagina. The chemical acts to inactivate viable sperm and also kills some bacteria, viruses, yeast and fungus.

Time lapse before vaginal contraceptive works:
- Immediate for foam, gels, jellies and sponges.
- 5 to 15 minutes for film and suppositories.

Don't use with:
Not applicable.

OVERDOSE

SYMPTOMS:
None expected.

POSSIBLE ADVERSE REACTIONS OR SIDE EFFECTS

SYMPTOMS	WHAT TO DO
Life-threatening:	
Toxic shock syndrome (chills; fever; skin rash; muscle aches; extreme weakness; confusion; redness of vagina, inside of mouth, nose, throat or eyes). (Very rare.)	Seek emergency treatment immediately.
Common:	
None expected.	
Infrequent:	
None expected.	
Rare:	
Vaginal discharge, irritation or rash; painful urination; cloudy or bloody urine.	Discontinue. Call doctor right away.

CONTRACEPTIVES, VAGINAL (Spermicides)

WARNINGS & PRECAUTIONS

Don't take if:
You are allergic to any form of octoxynol, nonoxynol or benzalkonium chloride.

Before you start, consult your doctor:
If you desire complete protection against pregnancy, a combination of methods gives better protection than vaginal contraceptives alone.

Over age 60:
Adverse reactions and side effects may be more frequent and severe than in younger persons.

Pregnancy:
Risk factor not designated. See categories on page xxii and consult doctor.

Breast-feeding:
Safety not established. Consult doctor.

Infants & children:
Not recommended.

Prolonged use:
Allergic reactions and irritation more likely.

Skin & sunlight:
No problems expected.

Driving, piloting or hazardous work:
No special problems expected.

Discontinuing:
No special problems expected.

Others:
- Failure rate when used alone is relatively high. Therefore a vaginal cream, sponge, suppository, foam, gel, jelly or other product should be used with a mechanical barrier, such as a condom, cervical cap, vaginal diaphragm or other form of pregnancy protection.
- Don't use a cervical cap, sponge or diaphragm during menstruation. Consider using a condom instead if additional protection is desired.
- Vaginal contraceptives usually also have spermicidal effects and may partially protect against sexually transmitted diseases.

POSSIBLE INTERACTION WITH OTHER DRUGS

GENERIC NAME OR DRUG CLASS	COMBINED EFFECT
Topical vaginal medications that include any of the following: sulfa drugs, soaps or disinfectants, nitrates*, permanganates, lanolin, hydrogen peroxide, iodides, cotton dressings, aluminum citrates, salicylates*	Spermicidal activity may be reduced or negated. Avoid combinations.
Vaginal douche products	May prevent spermicidal effect. Avoid until 8 hours following intercourse.

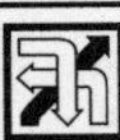

POSSIBLE INTERACTION WITH OTHER SUBSTANCES

INTERACTS WITH	COMBINED EFFECT
Alcohol:	None expected.
Beverages:	None expected.
Cocaine:	None expected.
Foods:	None expected.
Marijuana:	None expected.
Tobacco:	None expected.

***See Glossary**

CORTISONE

BRAND NAMES

Cortone
Cortone Acetate

BASIC INFORMATION

Habit forming? No
Prescription needed? Yes
Available as generic? Yes
Drug class: Cortisone drug (adrenal corticosteroid)

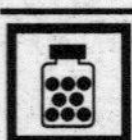

USES

- Reduces inflammation caused by many different medical problems.
- Treatment for some allergic diseases, blood disorders, kidney diseases, asthma and emphysema.
- Replaces corticosteroid deficiencies.

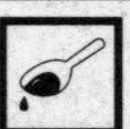

DOSAGE & USAGE INFORMATION

How to take:
Tablet—Swallow with liquid or food to lessen stomach irritation. If you can't swallow whole, crumble tablet and take with liquid or food.

When to take:
At the same times each day. Take once-a-day or once-every-other-day doses in mornings.

If you forget a dose:
- Several-doses-per-day prescription—Take as soon as you remember up to 2 hours late. If more than 2 hours, wait for next scheduled dose (don't double this dose).
- Once-a-day dose or less—Wait for next dose. Double this dose.

What drug does:
- Decreases inflammatory responses.
- Replaces cortisone in patients with adrenal insufficiency.

Time lapse before drug works:
2 to 4 days.

Continued next column

OVERDOSE

SYMPTOMS:
Headache, convulsions, fluid retention, heart failure.
WHAT TO DO:
- **Dial 911 (emergency) or 0 (operator) for an ambulance or medical help. Then give first aid immediately.**
- **See emergency information on inside covers.**

Don't take with:
Any other medicine without consulting your doctor or pharmacist.

POSSIBLE ADVERSE REACTIONS OR SIDE EFFECTS

SYMPTOMS	WHAT TO DO
Life-threatening:	
Hives, rash, intense itching, faintness soon after a dose (anaphylaxis).	Seek emergency treatment immediately.
Common:	
Acne, thirst, nausea, indigestion, vomiting, poor wound healing.	Continue. Call doctor when convenient.
Infrequent:	
• Bloody or black, tarry stool.	Discontinue. Seek emergency treatment.
• Blurred vision; halos around lights; sore throat, fever; muscle cramps; swollen legs, feet.	Discontinue. Call doctor right away.
• Mood changes, insomnia, fatigue, restlessness, frequent urination, weight gain, round face, weakness, irregular menstrual periods.	Continue. Call doctor when convenient.
Rare:	
• Irregular heartbeat.	Discontinue. Seek emergency treatment.
• Rash, hallucinations, thrombophlebitis, pancreatitis, numbness or tingling in hands or feet, convulsions.	Discontinue. Call doctor right away.

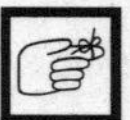

WARNINGS & PRECAUTIONS

Don't take if:
- You are allergic to any cortisone drug.
- You have tuberculosis or fungus infection.
- You have herpes infection of eyes, lips or genitals.

Before you start, consult your doctor:
- If you have had tuberculosis.
- If you have congestive heart failure.
- If you have diabetes, peptic ulcer, glaucoma, underactive thyroid, high blood pressure, myasthenia gravis, blood clots in legs or lungs.

Over age 60:
- Adverse reactions and side effects may be more frequent and severe than in younger persons.
- Likely to aggravate edema, diabetes or ulcers.
- Likely to cause cataracts and osteoporosis (softening of the bones).

Pregnancy:
Decide with your doctor if drug benefits justify risk to unborn child. Risk category C (see page xxii).

Breast-feeding:
Drug passes into milk. Avoid drug or discontinue nursing until you finish medicine. Consult doctor for advice on maintaining milk supply.

Infants & children:
Use only under medical supervision.

Prolonged use:
- Retards growth in children.
- Possible glaucoma, cataracts, diabetes, fragile bones and thin skin.
- Functional dependence.
- Talk to your doctor about the need for follow-up medical examinations or laboratory studies to check blood sugar, eyes, serum electrolytes, stools for blood.

Skin & sunlight:
No problems expected.

Driving, piloting or hazardous work:
No problems expected.

Discontinuing:
- Don't discontinue without doctor's advice until you complete prescribed dose, even though symptoms diminish or disappear.
- Drug affects your response to surgery, illness, injury or stress for 2 years after discontinuing. Tell anyone who takes medical care of you within 2 years about drug.

Others:
- Avoid immunizations if possible.
- Your resistance to infection is less while taking this medicine.
- Advise any doctor or dentist whom you consult that you take this medicine.
- Those who have inactive or "cured" tuberculosis may be subjected to a possible recurrence of active tuberculosis.
- Children who must take cortisone drugs may grow less well.

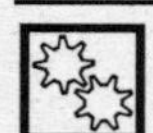

POSSIBLE INTERACTION WITH OTHER DRUGS

GENERIC NAME OR DRUG CLASS	COMBINED EFFECT
Amphotericin B	Potassium depletion.
Anticholinergics*	Possible glaucoma.
Anticoagulants, oral*	Decreased anti-coagulant effect.
Anticonvulsants, hydantoin*	Decreased cortisone effect.
Antidiabetics, oral*	Decreased anti-diabetic effect.
Antihistamines*	Decreased cortisone effect.
Anti-inflammatory drugs nonsteroidal (NSAIDs)*	Increased risk of ulcers, increased cortisone effect.
Aspirin	Increased cortisone effect.
Attenuated virus vaccines*	Possible viral infection.
Barbiturates*	Decreased cortisone effect. Oversedation.
Chloral hydrate	Decreased cortisone effect.
Chlorthalidone	Potassium depletion.
Cholinergics*	Decreased cholinergic effect.
Cholestyramine	Decreased cortisone absorption effect.
Colestipol	Decreased cortisone absorption effect.
Contraceptives, oral*	Increased cortisone effect.
Cyclosporine	Increased risk of infection.
Diclofenac	Increased risk of stomach ulcer.

Continued on page 936

POSSIBLE INTERACTION WITH OTHER SUBSTANCES

INTERACTS WITH	COMBINED EFFECT
Alcohol:	Risk of stomach ulcers.
Beverages:	No proven problems.
Cocaine:	Overstimulation. Avoid.
Foods:	No proven problems.
Marijuana:	Decreased immunity.
Tobacco:	Increased cortisone effect. Possible toxicity.

*See Glossary

CROMOLYN

BRAND NAMES

Fivent
Gastrocrom
Intal
Nalcrom
Nasalcrom
Rynacrom
Sodium Cromoglycate
Vistacrom

BASIC INFORMATION

Habit forming? No
Prescription needed? Yes
Available as generic? Yes, for some
Drug class: Antiasthmatic, anti-inflammatory (nonsteroidal)

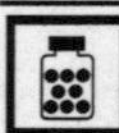

USES

- Powdered form and nebulizer solution prevent asthma attacks. Will not stop an active asthma attack.
- Eye drops treat inflammation of covering to eye and cornea.
- Nasal spray reduces nasal allergic symptoms.
- Capsules may help prevent allergic symptoms.

DOSAGE & USAGE INFORMATION

How to take:
Inhaler
Follow instructions enclosed with inhaler. Don't swallow cartridges for inhaler. Gargle and rinse mouth after inhalations.
Eye drops
- Wash hands.
- Apply pressure to inside corner of eye with middle finger.
- Continue pressure for 1 minute after placing medicine in eye.
- Tilt head backward. Pull lower lid away from eye with index finger of the same hand.
- Drop eye drops into pouch and close eye.
- Don't blink. Keep eyes closed for 1 to 2 minutes.

Continued next column

- Don't touch applicator tip to any surface (including the eye). If you accidentally touch tip, clean with warm soap and water.
- Keep container tightly closed.
- Keep cool, but don't freeze.
- Wash hands immediately after using.

Nasal solution
Follow prescription instructions.
Capsules
Open capsule and dissolve contents in 4 ounces of hot water, then add equal amount of cold water. Drink all the liquid.

When to take:
At the same times each day. If you also use a bronchodilator inhaler, use the bronchodilator before the cromolyn.

If you forget a dose:
Take as soon as you remember up to 2 hours late. If more than 2 hours, wait for next scheduled dose (don't double this dose).

What drug does:
Blocks histamine release from mast cells.

Time lapse before drug works:
- For inhaler forms: 4 weeks for prevention of asthma attacks. However, if taken 10-15 minutes after exercise or exposure to known allergens, may prevent wheezing.
- 1 to 2 weeks for nasal symptoms; only a few days for eye symptoms.

Don't take with:
Any other medicine without consulting your doctor or pharmacist.

OVERDOSE

SYMPTOMS:
Increased side effects and adverse reactions listed.
WHAT TO DO:
Overdose unlikely to threaten life. If person inhales much larger amount than prescribed, call doctor, poison control center or hospital emergency room for instructions.

POSSIBLE ADVERSE REACTIONS OR SIDE EFFECTS

SYMPTOMS	WHAT TO DO
Life-threatening:	
Hives, rash, intense itching, faintness soon after a dose (anaphylaxis).	Seek emergency treatment immediately.
Common:	
Cough, dry mouth.	Continue. Call doctor when convenient.
Infrequent:	
• Rash, hives, swallowing difficulty, nausea, vomiting, increased wheezing, joint pain or swelling, sneezing, nasal burning, weakness, muscle pain, difficult or painful urination.	Discontinue. Call doctor right away.
• Drowsiness, dizziness, headache, watery eyes, stuffy nose, throat irritation, insomnia.	Continue. Call doctor when convenient.

Rare:	
Nosebleed, numbness or tingling in feet or hands, hoarseness.	Continue. Call doctor when convenient.

WARNINGS & PRECAUTIONS

Don't take if:
You use the dry powder form of cromolyn and if you are allergic to cromolyn, lactose, milk or milk products.

Before you start, consult your doctor:
- If you plan to become pregnant within medication period.
- If you have kidney or liver disease.

Over age 60:
Adverse reactions and side effects may be more frequent and severe than in younger persons.

Pregnancy:
No proven harm to unborn child, but avoid if possible. Consult doctor. Risk category B (see page xxii).

Breast-feeding:
Effects unknown. Confer with your doctor.

Infants & children:
Use only under medical supervision.

Prolonged use:
No problems expected.

Skin & sunlight:
No problems expected.

Driving, piloting or hazardous work:
No problems expected.

Discontinuing:
No problems expected.

Others:
- Inhaler must be cleaned and work well for drug to be effective.
- Treatment with inhalation cromolyn does not stop an acute asthma attack. It may aggravate it.

POSSIBLE INTERACTION WITH OTHER DRUGS

GENERIC NAME OR DRUG CLASS	COMBINED EFFECT
None significant.	

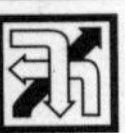

POSSIBLE INTERACTION WITH OTHER SUBSTANCES

INTERACTS WITH	COMBINED EFFECT
Alcohol:	None expected.
Beverages:	None expected.
Cocaine:	None expected.
Foods:	None expected.
Marijuana:	None expected.
Tobacco:	None expected, but tobacco smoke aggravates asthma and eye irritation. Avoid.

CYCLANDELATE

BRAND NAMES

Cyclospasmol　　Cyraso-400

BASIC INFORMATION

Habit forming? No
Prescription needed?
U.S.: Yes
Canada: No
Available as generic? Yes
Drug class: Vasodilator

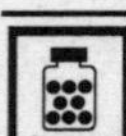

USES

May improve poor blood flow to extremities.

DOSAGE & USAGE INFORMATION

How to take:
Tablet or capsule—Swallow with liquid. If you can't swallow whole, crumble tablet or open capsule and take with liquid or food.

When to take:
At the same time each day.

If you forget a dose:
Take as soon as you remember up to 2 hours late. If more than 2 hours, wait for next scheduled dose (don't double this dose).

What drug does:
Increases blood flow by relaxing and expanding blood-vessel walls.

Time lapse before drug works:
3 weeks.

Don't take with:
Any other medicine without consulting your doctor or pharmacist.

OVERDOSE

SYMPTOMS:
Severe headache, dizziness; nausea, vomiting; flushed, hot face.
WHAT TO DO:
Overdose unlikely to threaten life. If person takes much larger amount than prescribed, call doctor, poison control center or hospital emergency room for instructions.

POSSIBLE ADVERSE REACTIONS OR SIDE EFFECTS

SYMPTOMS	WHAT TO DO
Life-threatening: In case of overdose, see previous column.	
Common: None expected.	
Infrequent:	
• Rapid heartbeat.	Discontinue. Call doctor right away.
• Dizziness; headache; weakness; flushed face; tingling in face, fingers or toes; unusual sweating.	Continue. Call doctor when convenient.
• Belching, heartburn, nausea or stomach pain.	Continue. Tell doctor at next visit.
Rare: None expected.	

WARNINGS & PRECAUTIONS

Don't take if:
You have had allergic reaction to cyclandelate.

Before you start, consult your doctor:
- If you have glaucoma.
- If you have had heart attack or stroke.

Over age 60:
Adverse reactions and side effects may be more frequent and severe than in younger persons.

Pregnancy:
Consult doctor. Risk category C (see page xxii).

Breast-feeding:
No proven problems. Consult doctor.

Infants & children:
Not recommended.

Prolonged use:
No problems expected.

Skin & sunlight:
No problems expected.

Driving, piloting or hazardous work:
Avoid if you feel dizzy or weak. Otherwise, no problems expected.

Discontinuing:
Don't discontinue without doctor's advice until you complete prescribed dose, even though symptoms diminish or disappear.

Others:
Response to drug varies. If your symptoms don't improve after 3 weeks of use, consult doctor.

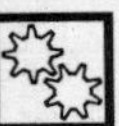

POSSIBLE INTERACTION WITH OTHER DRUGS

GENERIC NAME OR DRUG CLASS	COMBINED EFFECT
None expected.	

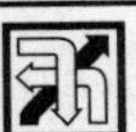

POSSIBLE INTERACTION WITH OTHER SUBSTANCES

INTERACTS WITH	COMBINED EFFECT
Alcohol:	None expected.
Beverages:	None expected.
Cocaine:	Decreased cyclandelate effect. Avoid.
Foods:	None expected.
Marijuana:	None expected.
Tobacco:	May decrease cyclandelate effect.

CYCLIZINE

BRAND NAMES

Marezine
Marzine

BASIC INFORMATION

Habit forming? No
Prescription needed?
U.S.: No
Canada: Yes
Available as generic? No
Drug class: Antiemetic, anti-motion sickness

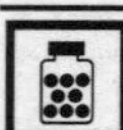

USES

Prevention and treatment for motion sickness.

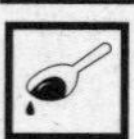

DOSAGE & USAGE INFORMATION

How to take:
Tablet—Swallow with liquid or food to lessen stomach irritation. If you can't swallow whole, crumble tablet and chew or take with liquid or food.

When to take:
30 minutes to 1 hour before traveling.

If you forget a dose:
Take as soon as you remember. Wait 4 hours for next dose.

What drug does:
Reduces sensitivity of nerve endings in inner ear, blocking messages to brain's vomiting center.

Time lapse before drug works:
30 to 60 minutes.

Don't take with:
Any other medicine without consulting your doctor or pharmacist.

OVERDOSE

SYMPTOMS:
Drowsiness, confusion, incoordination, stupor, coma, weak pulse, shallow breathing, hallucinations.
WHAT TO DO:
- **Dial 911 (emergency) or 0 (operator) for an ambulance or medical help. Then give first aid immediately.**
- **See emergency information on inside covers.**

POSSIBLE ADVERSE REACTIONS OR SIDE EFFECTS

SYMPTOMS	WHAT TO DO
Life-threatening:	
In case of overdose, see previous column.	
Common:	
Drowsiness.	Continue. Tell doctor at next visit.
Infrequent:	
• Headache, diarrhea or constipation, nausea, fast heartbeat.	Continue. Call doctor when convenient.
• Dry mouth, nose, throat; dizziness.	Continue. Tell doctor at next visit.
Rare:	
• Rash or hives, jaundice.	Discontinue. Call doctor right away.
• Restlessness, excitement, insomnia, blurred vision, frequent or difficult urination, hallucinations.	Continue. Call doctor when convenient.
• Appetite loss, nausea.	Continue. Tell doctor at next visit.

WARNINGS & PRECAUTIONS

Don't take if:
- You are allergic to meclizine, buclizine or cyclizine.
- You have taken a monoamine oxidase (MAO) inhibitor* in the past 2 weeks.

Before you start, consult your doctor:
- If you have glaucoma.
- If you have prostate enlargement.
- If you have reacted badly to any antihistamine
- If you have asthma.

Over age 60:
Adverse reactions and side effects may be more frequent and severe than in younger persons, especially impaired urination from enlarged prostate gland.

Pregnancy:
Consult doctor. Risk category B (see page xxii).

Breast-feeding:
Drug passes into milk. Avoid drug or discontinue nursing until you finish medicine. Consult doctor for advice on maintaining milk supply.

Infants & children:
Avoid if under age 6.

Prolonged use:
No problems expected.

Skin & sunlight:
No problems expected.

Driving, piloting or hazardous work:
Don't fly aircraft. Don't drive until you learn how medicine affects you. Don't work around dangerous machinery. Don't climb ladders or work in high places. Danger increases if you drink alcohol or take medicine affecting alertness and reflexes, such as antihistamines, tranquilizers, sedatives, pain medicine, narcotics and mind-altering drugs.

Discontinuing:
No problems expected.

Others:
- Some products contain tartrazine dye. Avoid if allergic (especially aspirin hypersensitivity).
- May interfere with the accuracy of some medical tests.

POSSIBLE INTERACTION WITH OTHER DRUGS

GENERIC NAME OR DRUG CLASS	COMBINED EFFECT
Amphetamines*	May decrease drowsiness caused by cyclizine.
Anticholinergics*	Increased effect of both drugs.
Antidepressants, tricyclic*	Increased effect of both drugs.
Carteolol	Decreased antihistamine effect.
Clozapine	Toxic effect on the central nervous system.
Dronabinol	Increased cyclizine effect.
Ethinamate	Dangerous increased effects of ethinamate. Avoid combining.
Fluoxetine	Increased depressant effects of both drugs.
Guanfacine	May increase depressant effects of either drug.
Leucovorin	High alcohol content of leucovorin may cause adverse effects.
Methyprylon	Increased sedative effect, perhaps to dangerous level. Avoid.
Monoamine oxidase (MAO) inhibitors*	Increased cyclizine effect.
Nabilone	Greater depression of central nervous system.
Narcotics*	Increased effect of both drugs.
Pain relievers*	Increased effect of both drugs.
Sedatives*	Increased effect of both drugs.
Sertraline	Increased depressive effect of both drugs.
Sleep inducers*	Increased effect of both drugs.
Sotalol	Increased antihistamine effect.
Tranquilizers*	Increased effect of both drugs.

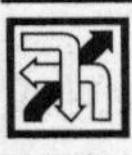

POSSIBLE INTERACTION WITH OTHER SUBSTANCES

INTERACTS WITH	COMBINED EFFECT
Alcohol:	Increased sedation. Avoid.
Beverages: Caffeine drinks.	May decrease drowsiness.
Cocaine:	None expected.
Foods:	None expected.
Marijuana:	Increased drowsiness, dry mouth.
Tobacco:	None expected.

CYCLOBENZAPRINE

BRAND NAMES

Cycoflex
Flexeril

BASIC INFORMATION

Habit forming? No
Prescription needed? Yes
Available as generic? Yes
Drug class: Muscle relaxant

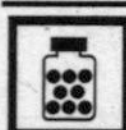

USES

Treatment for pain and limited motion caused by spasms in voluntary muscles.

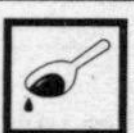

DOSAGE & USAGE INFORMATION

How to take:
Tablet—Swallow with liquid.

When to take:
At the same time each day or according to label instructions.

If you forget a dose:
Take as soon as you remember. Wait 4 hours for next dose.

What drug does:
Blocks body's pain messages to brain. May also sedate.

Time lapse before drug works:
30 to 60 minutes.

Continued next column

OVERDOSE

SYMPTOMS:
Drowsiness, confusion, difficulty concentrating, visual problems, vomiting, blood pressure drop, low body temperature, weak and rapid pulse, convulsions, coma.
WHAT TO DO:
- **Dial 911 (emergency) or 0 (operator) for an ambulance or medical help. Then give first aid immediately.**
- **If patient is unconscious and not breathing, give mouth-to-mouth breathing. If there is no heartbeat, use cardiac massage and mouth-to-mouth breathing (CPR). Don't try to make patient vomit. If you can't get help quickly, take patient to nearest emergency facility.**
- **See emergency information on inside covers.**

Don't take with:
- Nonprescription drugs without consulting doctor.
- See Interaction column and consult doctor.

POSSIBLE ADVERSE REACTIONS OR SIDE EFFECTS

SYMPTOMS	WHAT TO DO
Life-threatening:	
In case of overdose, see previous column.	
Common:	
Drowsiness, dizziness, dry mouth.	Continue. Call doctor when convenient.
Infrequent:	
• Blurred vision, fast heartbeat.	Discontinue. Call doctor right away.
• Insomnia, numbness in extremities, bad taste in mouth, fatigue, nausea, sweating.	Continue. Call doctor when convenient.
Rare:	
• Unsteadiness, confusion, depression, hallucinations, rash, itch, swelling, breathing difficulty.	Discontinue. Call doctor right away.
• Difficult urination, rash.	Continue. Call doctor when convenient.

WARNINGS & PRECAUTIONS

Don't take if:
- You are allergic to any skeletal muscle relaxant*.
- You have taken a monoamine oxidase (MAO) inhibitor* in last 2 weeks.
- You have had a heart attack within 6 weeks, or suffer from congestive heart failure.
- You have an overactive thyroid.

Before you start, consult your doctor:
- If you have a heart problem.
- If you have reacted to tricyclic anti-depressants.
- If you have glaucoma.
- If you have a prostate condition and urination difficulty.
- If you intend to pilot aircraft.

Over age 60:
Adverse reactions and side effects may be more frequent and severe than in younger persons. Avoid extremes of heat and cold.

Pregnancy:
No problems expected. Consult doctor. Risk category B (see page xxii).

Breast-feeding:
Drug may pass into milk. Avoid drug or discontinue nursing until you finish medicine. Consult doctor for advice on maintaining milk supply.

Infants & children:
Don't use for children younger than 15.

Prolonged use:
Do not take for longer than 2 to 3 weeks.

Skin & sunlight:
May cause rash or intensify sunburn in areas exposed to sun or sunlamp.

Driving, piloting or hazardous work:
Don't drive or pilot aircraft until you learn how medicine affects you. Don't work around dangerous machinery. Don't climb ladders or work in high places. Danger increases if you drink alcohol or take medicine affecting alertness and reflexes.

Discontinuing:
May be unnecessary to finish medicine. Follow doctor's instructions.

Others:
No problems expected.

POSSIBLE INTERACTION WITH OTHER DRUGS

GENERIC NAME OR DRUG CLASS	COMBINED EFFECT
Anticholinergics*	Increased anticholinergic effect.
Antidepressants*	Increased sedation.
Antihistamines*	Increased antihistamine effect.
Barbiturates*	Increased sedation.
Central nervous system (CNS) depressants*	Increased sedation.
Cimetidine	Possible increased cyclobenzaprine effect.
Cisapride	Decreased cyclobenzaprine effect.
Clonidine	Decreased clonidine effect.
Dronabinol	Increased effect of dronabinol on central nervous system. Avoid combination.
Guanethidine	Decreased guanethidine effect.
Methyldopa	Decreased methyldopa effect.
Mind-altering drugs*	Increased mind-altering effect.
Monoamine oxidase (MAO) inhibitors*	High fever, convulsions, possible death.
Narcotics*	Increased sedation.
Pain relievers*	Increased pain reliever effect.
Procainamide	Possible increased conduction disturbance.
Quinidine	Possible increased conduction disturbance.
Rauwolfia alkaloids*	Decreased effect of rauwolfia alkaloids.
Sedatives*	Increased sedative effect.
Sleep inducers*	Increased sedation.
Tranquilizers*	Increased tranquilizer effect.

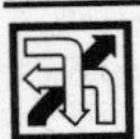

POSSIBLE INTERACTION WITH OTHER SUBSTANCES

INTERACTS WITH	COMBINED EFFECT
Alcohol:	Depressed brain function. Avoid.
Beverages:	None expected.
Cocaine:	Decreased cyclobenzaprine effect.
Foods:	None expected.
Marijuana:	Occasional use—Drowsiness. Frequent use—Severe mental and physical impairment.
Tobacco:	None expected.

*See Glossary

CYCLOPEGIC, MYDRIATIC (Ophthalmic)

BRAND AND GENERIC NAMES

AK Homatropine
Atropair
ATROPINE
Atropine Care Eye Drops & Ointment
Atropine Sulfate S.O.P.
Atropisol
Dispersa
Homatrine
HOMATROPINE
I-Homatropine
Isopto
Isopto Atropine
Isopto Homatropine
Isopto Hyoscine
I-Tropine
Minims Homatropine
Minims Atropine
Ocu-Tropine
S.M.P. Atropine
SCOPOLAMINE
Spectro-Homatropine

BASIC INFORMATION

Habit forming? No
Prescription needed? Yes
Available as generic? Yes, some
Drug class: Cyclopegic, mydriatic

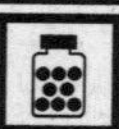

USES

- Dilates pupil of the eye.
- Used before some eye examinations, before and after some eye surgical procedures and, rarely, to treat some eye problems such as glaucoma.

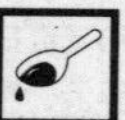

DOSAGE & USAGE INFORMATION

How to use:
Eye drops
- Wash hands.
- Apply pressure to inside corner of eye with middle finger.
- Continue pressure for 1 minute after placing medicine in eye.
- Tilt head backward. Pull lower lid away from eye with index finger of the same hand.
- Drop eye drops into pouch and close eye. Don't blink.
- Keep eyes closed for 1 to 2 minutes.

Continued next column

Eye ointment
- Wash hands.
- Pull lower lid down from eye to form a pouch.
- Squeeze tube to apply thin strip of ointment into pouch.
- Close eye for 1 to 2 minutes.
- Don't touch applicator tip to any surface (including the eye). If you accidentally touch tip, clean with warm soap and water.
- Keep container tightly closed.
- Keep cool, but don't freeze.
- Wash hands immediately after using.

When to use:
As directed on label.

If you forget a dose:
Use as soon as you remember.

What drug does:
Blocks normal response to sphincter muscle of the iris of the eye and the accommodative muscle of the ciliary body.

Time lapse before drug works:
Begins within 1 minute. Residual effects may last up to 14 days.

Don't use with:
Other eye medicines such as carbachol, demecarium, echothiopate, isoflurophate, physostigmine, pilocarpine.

OVERDOSE

SYMPTOMS:
None expected.
WHAT TO DO:
Not intended for internal use. If child accidentally swallows, call poison control center.

POSSIBLE ADVERSE REACTIONS OR SIDE EFFECTS

SYMPTOMS	WHAT TO DO
Life-threatening:	
None expected.	
Common:	
• Increased sensitivity to light.	Continue. Call doctor when convenient.
• Burning eyes.	Continue. Tell doctor at next visit.
Infrequent:	
None expected.	
Rare (extremely):	
Symptoms of excess medicine absorbed by the body—Clumsiness, confusion, fever, flushed face, hallucinations, rash, slurred speech, swollen stomach (children), unusual drowsiness, fast heartbeat.	Discontinue. Call doctor right away.

CYCLOPEGIC, MYDRIATIC (Ophthalmic)

WARNINGS & PRECAUTIONS

Don't use if:
You are allergic to cyclopentolate.

Before you start, consult your doctor:
- If medicine is for a brain-damaged child or child with Down's syndrome.
- If prescribed for a child with spastic paralysis.

Over age 60:
No problems expected.

Pregnancy:
Decide with your doctor if drug benefits justify risk to unborn child. Risk category C (see page xxii).

Breast-feeding:
Safety unestablished. Avoid if possible.

Infants & children:
Use only under close medical supervision.

Prolonged use:
Avoid. May increase absorption into body.

Skin & sunlight:
Wear sunglasses to protect from sunlight and bright light.

Driving, piloting or hazardous work:
Don't drive or pilot aircraft until you learn how medicine affects you. Don't work around dangerous machinery. Don't climb ladders or work in high places. Danger increases if you drink alcohol or take medicine affecting alertness and reflexes, such as antihistamines, tranquilizers, sedatives, pain medicine, narcotics and mind-altering drugs.

Discontinuing:
Effects may last up to 14 days later.

Others:
Keep cool, but don't freeze.

POSSIBLE INTERACTION WITH OTHER DRUGS

GENERIC NAME OR DRUG CLASS	COMBINED EFFECT
Clinically significant interactions with oral or injected medicines unlikely.	

POSSIBLE INTERACTION WITH OTHER SUBSTANCES

INTERACTS WITH	COMBINED EFFECT
Alcohol:	None expected.
Beverages:	None expected.
Cocaine:	None expected.
Foods:	None expected.
Marijuana:	None expected.
Tobacco:	None expected.

*See Glossary

CYCLOPENTOLATE (Ophthalmic)

BRAND NAMES

Ak-Pentolate
Cyclogyl
I-Pentolate
Minims
  Cyclopentolate
Ocu-Pentolate
Pentolair
Spectro-Pentolate

BASIC INFORMATION

Habit forming? No
Prescription needed? Yes
Available as generic? Yes
Drug class: Cyclopegic, mydriatic

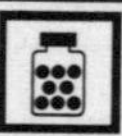

USES

- Enlarges (dilates) pupil.
- Temporarily paralyzes the normal pupil accommodation to light before eye examinations and to treat some eye conditions.

DOSAGE & USAGE INFORMATION

How to use:
Eye drops
- Wash hands.
- Apply pressure to inside corner of eye with middle finger.
- Continue pressure for 1 minute after placing medicine in eye.
- Tilt head backward. Pull lower lid away from eye with index finger of the same hand.
- Drop eye drops into pouch and close eye. Don't blink.
- Keep eyes closed for 1 to 2 minutes.
- Don't touch applicator tip to any surface (including the eye). If you accidentally touch tip, clean with warm soap and water.
- Keep container tightly closed.
- Keep cool, but don't freeze.
- Wash hands immediately after using.

When to use:
As directed on bottle.

Continued next column

OVERDOSE

SYMPTOMS:
None expected.
WHAT TO DO:
Not intended for internal use. If child accidentally swallows, call poison control center.

If you forget a dose:
Use as soon as you remember.

What drug does:
Blocks sphincter muscle of the iris and ciliary body.

Time lapse before drug works:
Within 30 to 60 minutes. Effects usually disappear in 24 hours.

Don't use with:
Other eye medicines such as carbachol, demecarium, echothiopate, isoflurophate, physostigmine, pilocarpine without doctor's approval.

POSSIBLE ADVERSE REACTIONS OR SIDE EFFECTS

SYMPTOMS	WHAT TO DO
Life-threatening:	
None expected.	
Common:	
• Increased sensitivity to light.	Continue. Call doctor when convenient.
• Burning eyes.	Continue. Tell doctor at next visit.
Infrequent:	
None expected.	
Rare (extremely):	
Symptoms of excess medicine absorbed by the body—Clumsiness, confusion, fever, flushed face, hallucinations, rash, slurred speech, swollen stomach (children), drowsiness, fast heartbeat.	Discontinue. Call doctor right away.

CYCLOPENTOLATE (Ophthalmic)

WARNINGS & PRECAUTIONS

Don't use if:
You are allergic to cyclopentolate.

Before you start, consult your doctor:
- If medicine is for a brain-damaged child or child with Down syndrome.
- If prescribed for a child with spastic paralysis.

Over age 60:
No problems expected.

Pregnancy:
Avoid if possible. Consult doctor. Risk category C (see page xxii).

Breast-feeding:
Safety unestablished. Avoid if possible. Consult doctor.

Infants & children:
Use only under close medical supervision.

Prolonged use:
Avoid. May increase absorption into body.

Skin & sunlight:
Wear sunglasses to protect from sunlight and bright light.

Driving, piloting or hazardous work:
Don't drive or pilot aircraft until you learn how medicine affects you. Don't work around dangerous machinery. Don't climb ladders or work in high places. Danger increases if you drink alcohol or take medicine affecting alertness and reflexes, such as antihistamines, tranquilizers, sedatives, pain medicine, narcotics and mind-altering drugs.

Discontinuing:
If effects last longer than 36 hours after last drops, consult doctor.

Others:
Keep cool, but don't freeze.

POSSIBLE INTERACTION WITH OTHER DRUGS

GENERIC NAME OR DRUG CLASS	COMBINED EFFECT

Clinically significant interactions with oral or injected medicines unlikely.

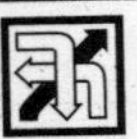

POSSIBLE INTERACTION WITH OTHER SUBSTANCES

INTERACTS WITH	COMBINED EFFECT
Alcohol:	None expected.
Beverages:	None expected.
Cocaine:	None expected.
Foods:	None expected.
Marijuana:	None expected.
Tobacco:	None expected.

*See Glossary

CYCLOPHOSPHAMIDE

BRAND NAMES

Cytoxan
Neosar
Procytox

BASIC INFORMATION

Habit forming? No
Prescription needed? Yes
Available as generic? No
Drug class: Immunosuppressant, antineoplastic

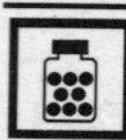

USES

- Treatment for cancer.
- Treatment for severe rheumatoid arthritis.
- Treatment for blood-vessel disease.
- Treatment for skin disease.

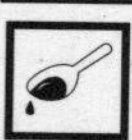

DOSAGE & USAGE INFORMATION

How to take:
Tablet or liquid—Swallow with liquid. If you can't swallow whole, crumble tablet and take with liquid or food.

When to take:
Works best if taken first thing in morning. Should be taken on an empty stomach. However, may take with food to lessen stomach irritation. Don't take at bedtime.

If you forget a dose:
Take as soon as you remember up to 12 hours late. If more than 12 hours, wait for next scheduled dose (don't double this dose).

What drug does:
- Kills cancer cells.
- Suppresses spread of cancer cells.
- Suppresses immune system.

Time lapse before drug works:
7 to 10 days continual use.

Don't take with:
Any other medicine without consulting your doctor or pharmacist.

OVERDOSE

SYMPTOMS:
Bloody urine, water retention, weight gain, severe infection.
WHAT TO DO:
Overdose unlikely to threaten life. If person takes much larger amount than prescribed, call doctor, poison control center or hospital emergency room for instructions.

POSSIBLE ADVERSE REACTIONS OR SIDE EFFECTS

SYMPTOMS	WHAT TO DO
Life-threatening:	
Hives, rash, intense itching, faintness soon after a dose (anaphylaxis).	Seek emergency treatment immediately.
Common:	
• Sore throat, fever.	Continue, but call doctor right away.
• Dark skin, nails; nausea; appetite loss; vomiting; missed menstrual period.	Continue. Call doctor when convenient.
Infrequent:	
• Rash, hives, itch; shortness of breath; rapid heartbeat; cough; blood in urine, painful urination; pain in side; bleeding, bruising; increased sweating; hoarseness; foot or ankle swelling.	Continue, but call doctor right away.
• Confusion, agitation, headache, dizziness, flushed face, stomach pain, joint pain, fatigue, weakness, diarrhea.	Continue. Call doctor when convenient.
Rare:	
• Mouth, lip sores; black stool; unusual thirst; jaundice.	Continue, but call doctor right away.
• Blurred vision, increased urination, hair loss.	Continue. Call doctor when convenient.

WARNINGS & PRECAUTIONS

Don't take if:
- You are allergic to any alkylating agent.
- You have an infection.
- You have bloody urine.
- You will have surgery within 2 months, including dental surgery, requiring general or spinal anesthesia.

Before you start, consult your doctor:
- If you have impaired liver or kidney function.
- If you have impaired bone marrow or blood cell production.
- If you have had chemotherapy or x-ray therapy.
- If you have taken cortisone drugs in the past year.
- If you plan to become pregnant.

Over age 60:
Adverse reactions and side effects may be more frequent and severe than in younger persons. To reduce risk of chemical bladder inflammation, drink 8 to 10 glasses of water daily.

Pregnancy:
Risk to unborn child outweighs drug benefits. Don't use. Risk category D (see page xxii).

Breast-feeding:
Drug passes into milk. Avoid drug or discontinue nursing until you finish medicine. Consult doctor for advice on maintaining milk supply.

Infants & children:
Use only under medical supervision.

Prolonged use:
- Development of fibrous lung tissue.
- Possible jaundice.
- Swelling of feet, lower legs.
- Cancer.
- Infertility in men.
- Talk to your doctor about the need for follow-up medical examinations or laboratory studies to check complete blood counts (white blood cell count, platelet count, red blood cell count, hemoglobin, hematocrit), urine, liver function.

Skin & sunlight:
No problems expected.

Driving, piloting or hazardous work:
Avoid if you feel dizzy or have blurred vision. Otherwise, no problems expected.

Discontinuing:
Don't discontinue without consulting doctor. Dose may require gradual reduction if you have taken drug for a long time. Doses of other drugs may also require adjustment.

Others:
- Frequently causes hair loss. After treatment ends, hair should grow back.
- Avoid vaccinations.

POSSIBLE INTERACTION WITH OTHER DRUGS

GENERIC NAME OR DRUG CLASS	COMBINED EFFECT
Allopurinol or other medicines to treat gout	Possible anemia; decreased anti-gout effect.
Antidiabetics, oral*	Increased antidiabetic effect.
Bone marrow depressants,* other	Increased bone marrow depressant effect.
Clozapine	Toxic effect on bone marrow.
Cyclosporine	May increase risk of infection.
Digoxin	Possible decreased digoxin absorption.
Immuno-suppressants,* other	Increased risk of infection.
Insulin	Increased insulin effect.
Levamisole	Increased risk of bone marrow depression.
Lovastatin	Increased heart and kidney damage.
Phenobarbital	Increased cyclophosphamide effect.
Probenecid	Increased blood uric acid.
Sulfinpyrazone	Increased blood uric acid.
Tiopronin	Increased risk of toxicity to bone marrow.

POSSIBLE INTERACTION WITH OTHER SUBSTANCES

INTERACTS WITH	COMBINED EFFECT
Alcohol:	No problems expected.
Beverages:	No problems expected. Drink at least 2 quarts fluid every day.
Cocaine:	Increased danger of brain damage.
Foods:	None expected.
Marijuana:	Increased impairment of immunity.
Tobacco:	None expected.

*See Glossary

CYCLOSERINE

BRAND NAMES

Seromycin

BASIC INFORMATION

Habit forming? No
Prescription needed? Yes
Available as generic? No
Drug class: Antibacterial (antibiotic)

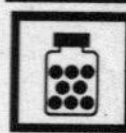

USES

- Treats urinary tract infections.
- Treats tuberculosis.

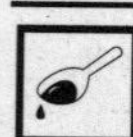

DOSAGE & USAGE INFORMATION

How to take:
Capsules—Swallow with liquid or food to lessen stomach irritation. If you can't swallow whole, open capsule and take with liquid or food.

When to take:
- Once or twice daily.
- At the same time each day after meals to prevent stomach irritation.

If you forget a dose:
Take as soon as you remember up to 2 hours late. If more than 2 hours, wait for next scheduled dose (don't double this dose).

What drug does:
Interferes with bacterial wall synthesis and keeps germs from multiplying.

Time lapse before drug works:
3 to 4 hours.

Don't take with:
Any other medicine without consulting your doctor or pharmacist.

OVERDOSE

SYMPTOMS:
Seizures.
WHAT TO DO:
- **Dial 911 (emergency) or 0 (operator) for an ambulance or medical help. Then give first aid immediately.**
- **See emergency information on inside covers.**

POSSIBLE ADVERSE REACTIONS OR SIDE EFFECTS

SYMPTOMS	WHAT TO DO
Life-threatening: Seizures, muscle twitching or trembling.	Seek emergency treatment immediately.
Common: Gum inflammation, pale skin, depression, confusion, dizziness, restlessness, anxiety, nightmares, severe headache, drowsiness.	Continue, but call doctor right away.
Infrequent: Visual changes; sun sensitivity; skin rash; numbness, tingling or burning in hands and feet; jaundice; eye pain.	Continue. Call doctor when convenient.
Rare: Seizures, thoughts of suicide.	Discontinue. Seek emergency treatment.

WARNINGS & PRECAUTIONS

Don't take if:
- You are a frequent user of alcohol.
- You have a convulsive disorder.

Before you start, consult your doctor:
- If you are depressed.
- If you have kidney disease.
- If you have severe anxiety.

Over age 60:
Adverse reactions and side effects may be more frequent and severe than in younger persons. You may need smaller doses for shorter periods of time.

Pregnancy:
Decide with your doctor if drug benefits justify risk to unborn child. Risk category C (see page xxii).

Breast-feeding:
Drug passes into milk. Avoid drug or discontinue nursing until you finish medicine. Consult doctor for advice on maintaining milk supply.

Infants & children:
No information available.

Prolonged use:
- May cause liver or kidney damage.
- May cause anemia.

Skin & sunlight:
May cause hypersensitivity to sun exposure.

Driving, piloting or hazardous work:
Don't drive or pilot aircraft until you learn how medicine affects you. Don't work around dangerous machinery. Don't climb ladders or work in high places. Danger increases if you drink alcohol or take medicine affecting alertness and reflexes.

Discontinuing:
Don't discontinue without consulting doctor. Dose may require gradual reduction if you have taken drug for a long time. Doses of other drugs may also require adjustment.

Others:
- May have to take anticonvulsants, sedatives and/or pyridoxine to prevent or minimize toxic effects on the brain.
- If you must take more than 500 mg per day, toxicity is much more likely to occur.
- Talk to your doctor about taking pyridoxine as a supplement.

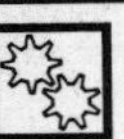

POSSIBLE INTERACTION WITH OTHER DRUGS

GENERIC NAME OR DRUG CLASS	COMBINED EFFECT
Ethionamide	Increased risk of seizures.
Isoniazid	Increased risk of central nervous system effects.
Pyridoxine	Reduces effects of pyridoxine. Since pyridoxine is a vital vitamin, patients on cycloserine require pyridoxine supplements to prevent anemia or peripheral neuritis.

POSSIBLE INTERACTION WITH OTHER SUBSTANCES

INTERACTS WITH	COMBINED EFFECT
Alcohol:	Toxic. May increase risk of seizures. Avoid.
Beverages:	None expected. All beverages except those with alcohol.
Cocaine:	Toxic. Avoid.
Foods:	None expected.
Marijuana:	May increase risk of seizures.
Tobacco:	May decrease effect of cycloserine.

*See Glossary

CYCLOSPORINE

BRAND NAMES

Sandimmune

BASIC INFORMATION

Habit forming? No
Prescription needed? Yes
Available as generic? No
Drug class: Immunosuppressant

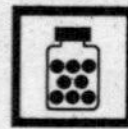

USES

- Suppresses the immune response in patients who have transplants of the heart, lung, kidney, liver, pancreas. Cyclosporine treats rejection as well as helps prevent it.
- Treatment for severe psoriasis when regular treatment is ineffective or not appropriate.

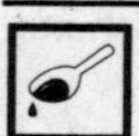

DOSAGE & USAGE INFORMATION

How to take:
- Oral solution—Take after meals with liquid to decrease stomach irritation. May mix with milk, chocolate milk or orange juice. Don't mix in styrofoam cups. Use special dropper for exact dosage.
- Capsules—Take with water or other fluid. Don't break capsule open.

When to take:
At the same time each day, according to instructions on prescription label.

If you forget a dose:
Take as soon as you remember up to 2 hours late. If more than 2 hours, wait for next scheduled dose (don't double this dose).

What drug does:
Exact mechanism is unknown, but believed to inhibit interluken II to affect T-lymphocytes.

Time lapse before drug works:
3 to 3-1/2 hours.

Don't take with:
Any other medicine without consulting your doctor or pharmacist.

OVERDOSE

SYMPTOMS:
Irregular heartbeat, seizures, coma.
WHAT TO DO:
- **Dial 911 (emergency) or 0 (operator) for an ambulance or medical help. Then give first aid immediately.**
- **See emergency information on inside covers.**

POSSIBLE ADVERSE REACTIONS OR SIDE EFFECTS

SYMPTOMS	WHAT TO DO
Life-threatening:	
Seizures, wheezing with shortness of breath, convulsions.	Discontinue. Seek emergency treatment.
Common:	
• Gum inflammation, blood in urine, jaundice, tremors.	Continue. Call doctor when convenient.
• Increased hair growth.	Continue. Tell doctor at next visit.
Infrequent:	
• Fever, chills, sore throat, shortness of breath.	Call doctor right away.
• Frequent urination, headache, leg cramps.	Continue. Call doctor when convenient.
Rare:	
• Confusion, irregular heartbeat, numbness of hands and feet, nervousness, face flushing, severe abdominal pain, weakness.	Call doctor right away.
• Acne, headache.	Continue. Call doctor when convenient.

WARNINGS & PRECAUTIONS

Don't take if:
- You have chicken pox.
- You have shingles (herpes zoster).

Before you start, consult your doctor:
- If you have liver problems.
- If you have an infection.
- If you have kidney disease.

Over age 60:
No special problems expected.

Pregnancy:
Decide with your doctor if drug benefits justify risk to unborn child. Risk category C (see page xxii).

Breast-feeding:
Drug passes into milk. Avoid drug or discontinue nursing until you finish medicine. Consult doctor for advice on maintaining milk supply.

Infants & children:
No problems expected.

Prolonged use:
- Can cause reduced function of kidney.
- Talk to your doctor about the need for follow-up medical examinations or laboratory studies to check blood pressure, kidney function, liver function.

Skin & sunlight:
No problems expected.

Driving, piloting or hazardous work:
Don't drive or pilot aircraft until you learn how medicine affects you. Don't work around dangerous machinery. Don't climb ladders or work in high places. Danger increases if you drink alcohol or take medicine affecting alertness and reflexes.

Discontinuing:
Don't discontinue without consulting doctor. You probably will require this medicine for the remainder of your life.

Others:
- Request regular laboratory studies to measure levels of potassium and cyclosporine in blood and to evaluate liver and kidney function.
- Check blood pressure. Cyclosporine sometimes causes hypertension.
- Don't store solution in the refrigerator.
- Avoid any immunizations except those specifically recommended by your doctor.
- Maintain good dental hygiene. Cyclosporine can cause gum problems.
- Kidney toxicity occurs commonly after 12 months of taking cyclosporine.
- Don't mix in styrofoam cups.

POSSIBLE INTERACTION WITH OTHER DRUGS

GENERIC NAME OR DRUG CLASS	COMBINED EFFECT
Androgens	Increased effect of cyclosporine.
Anticonvulsants*	Decreased effect of cyclosporine.
Cimetidine	Increased effect of cyclosporine.
Danazol	Increased effect of cyclosporine.
Diltiazem	Increased effect of cyclosporine.
Diuretics, potassium-sparing	Increased effect of cyclosporine.
Erythromycin	Increased effect of cyclosporine.
Estrogens	Increased effect of cyclosporine.
Fluconazole	Increased effect of cyclosporine. Cyclosporine dosage must be adjusted.
Immuno-suppressants* (adrenocorticoids, azathioprine, chlorambucil, cyclophosphamide, mercaptopurine, muromonab-CD3)	May increase risk of infection.
Itraconazole	Increased cyclosporine toxicity.
Ketoconazole	Increased risk of toxicity to kidney.
Lovastatin	Increased heart and kidney damage.
Medicines that may be toxic to kidneys (gold*, NSAIDs*, sulfonamides*)	Increased risk of toxicity to kidneys.
Nimodipine	Increased cyclosporine toxicity.
Rifampin	Decreased effect of cyclosporine.
Tiopronin	Increased risk of toxicity to kidneys.
Vancomycin	Increased chance of hearing loss or kidney damage.
Virus vaccines	Increased adverse reactions to vaccine.

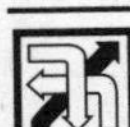

POSSIBLE INTERACTION WITH OTHER SUBSTANCES

INTERACTS WITH	COMBINED EFFECT
Alcohol:	May increase possibility of toxic effects. Avoid.
Beverages:	None expected.
Cocaine:	May increase possibility of toxic effects. Avoid.
Foods:	None expected.
Marijuana:	May increase possibility of toxic effects. Avoid.
Tobacco:	May increase possibility of toxic effects. Avoid.

*See Glossary

DANAZOL

BRAND NAMES

Cyclomen
Danocrine

BASIC INFORMATION

Habit forming? No
Prescription needed? Yes
Available as generic? No
Drug class: Gonadotropin inhibitor

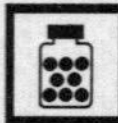

USES

Treatment of endometriosis, fibrocystic breast disease, angioneurotic edema except in pregnant women, gynecomastia, infertility, excessive menstruation, precocious puberty.

DOSAGE & USAGE INFORMATION

How to take:
Capsule—Swallow with liquid or food to lessen stomach irritation. If you can't swallow whole, open capsule and take with liquid or food.

When to take:
At the same times each day.

If you forget a dose:
Take as soon as you remember (don't double dose).

What drug does:
Partially prevents output of pituitary follicle-stimulating hormone and lutenizing hormone reducing estrogen production.

Time lapse before drug works:
- 2 to 3 months to treat endometriosis.
- 1 to 2 months to treat other disorders.

Don't take with:
- Birth control pills.
- Any other medicine without consulting your doctor or pharmacist.

OVERDOSE

SYMPTOMS:
None expected.
WHAT TO DO:
Overdose unlikely to threaten life. If person takes much larger amount than prescribed, call doctor, poison control center or hospital emergency room for instructions.

POSSIBLE ADVERSE REACTIONS OR SIDE EFFECTS

SYMPTOMS	WHAT TO DO
Life-threatening: None expected.	
Common: Menstrual irregularities.	Continue. Call doctor when convenient.
Infrequent:	
• Unnatural hair growth in women, nosebleeds, bleeding gums, sore throat and chills.	Discontinue. Call doctor right away.
• Dizziness; deepened voice; hoarseness; flushed or red skin; muscle cramps; enlarged clitoris; decreased testicle size; vaginal burning, itching; swollen feet; decreased breast size; increased or decreased sex drive.	Continue. Call doctor when convenient.
• Headache, acne, weight gain, vision changes.	Continue. Tell doctor at next visit.
Rare: Jaundice, flushing, sweating, vaginitis, rash, nausea, vomiting, constipation, abdominal pain.	Discontinue. Call doctor right away.

WARNINGS & PRECAUTIONS

Don't take if:
- You become pregnant.
- You have breast cancer.

Before you start, consult your doctor:
- If you take birth control pills.
- If you have diabetes.
- If you have heart disease.
- If you have epilepsy.
- If you have kidney disease.
- If you have liver disease.
- If you have migraine headaches.

Over age 60:
Adverse reactions and side effects may be more frequent and severe than in younger persons.

Pregnancy:
Risk to unborn child outweighs drug benefits. Don't use. Stop if you get pregnant. Risk category X (see page xxii).

Breast-feeding:
Unknown whether medicine filters into milk. Consult doctor.

Infants & children:
Not recommended.

Prolonged use:
- Required for full effect. Don't discontinue without consulting doctor.
- Talk to your doctor about the need for follow-up medical examinations or laboratory studies to check liver function, mammogram.

Skin & sunlight:
No problems expected.

Driving, piloting or hazardous work:
No problems expected.

Discontinuing:
Don't discontinue without consulting doctor. Menstrual periods may be absent for 2 to 3 months after discontinuation.

Others:
- May alter blood sugar levels in diabetic persons.
- May interfere with the accuracy of some medical tests.

POSSIBLE INTERACTION WITH OTHER DRUGS

GENERIC NAME OR DRUG CLASS	COMBINED EFFECT
Anticoagulants, oral*	Increased anti-coagulant effect.
Antidiabetic agents, oral*	Decreased anti-diabetic effect.
Cyclosporine	Increased risk of kidney damage.
Insulin	Decreased insulin effect.

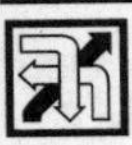

POSSIBLE INTERACTION WITH OTHER SUBSTANCES

INTERACTS WITH	COMBINED EFFECT
Alcohol:	Excessive nervous system depression. Avoid.
Beverages: Caffeine.	Rapid, irregular heartbeat. Avoid.
Cocaine:	May interfere with expected action of danazol. Avoid.
Foods:	No problems expected.
Marijuana:	May interfere with expected action of danazol. Avoid.
Tobacco:	Rapid, irregular heartbeat. Avoid. Increased leg cramps.

***See Glossary**

DANTROLENE

BRAND NAMES

Dantrium

BASIC INFORMATION

Habit forming? No
Prescription needed? Yes
Available as generic? No
Drug class: Muscle relaxant, antispastic

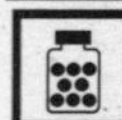

USES

- Relieves muscle spasticity caused by diseases such as multiple sclerosis, cerebral palsy, stroke.
- Relieves muscle spasticity caused by injury to spinal cord.
- Relieves or prevents excess body temperature brought on by some surgical procedures.

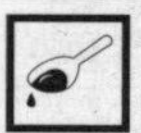

DOSAGE & USAGE INFORMATION

How to take:
Capsules—Swallow with liquid.

When to take:
Once a day for muscle spasticity during first 6 days. Later, every 6 hours. For excess body temperature, follow label instructions.

If you forget a dose:
Take as soon as you remember up to 2 hours late. If more than 2 hours, wait for next scheduled dose (don't double this dose).

Continued next column

OVERDOSE

SYMPTOMS:
Shortness of breath, bloody urine, chest pain, convulsions.
WHAT TO DO:
- **Dial 911 (emergency) or 0 (operator) for an ambulance or medical help. Then give first aid immediately.**
- **If patient is unconscious and not breathing, give mouth-to-mouth breathing. If there is no heartbeat, use cardiac massage and mouth-to-mouth breathing (CPR). Don't try to make patient vomit. If you can't get help quickly, take patient to nearest emergency facility.**
- **See emergency information on inside covers.**

What drug does:
Acts directly on muscles to prevent excess contractions.

Time lapse before drug works:
1 or more weeks.

Don't take with:
Any other medicine without consulting your doctor or pharmacist.

POSSIBLE ADVERSE REACTIONS OR SIDE EFFECTS

SYMPTOMS	WHAT TO DO
Life-threatening:	
Seizure.	Seek emergency treatment immediately.
Common:	
Drowsiness, dizziness, weakness.	Discontinue. Call doctor right away.
Infrequent:	
• Rash, hives; black or bloody stools; chest pain; fast heartbeat; backache; blood in urine; painful, swollen feet; chills; fever; shortness of breath.	Discontinue. Call doctor right away.
• Depression, confusion, headache, slurred speech, insomnia, nervousness, diarrhea, blurred vision, difficult swallowing, appetite loss, difficult urination, decreased sexual function in males.	Continue. Call doctor when convenient.
Rare:	
• Jaundice, abdominal cramps, double vision.	Discontinue. Call doctor right away.
• Constipation.	Continue. Call doctor when convenient.

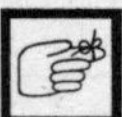

WARNINGS & PRECAUTIONS

Don't take if:
You are allergic to dantrolene or any muscle relaxant or antispastic medication.

Before you start, consult your doctor:
- If you have liver disease.
- If you have heart disease.
- If you have lung disease (especially emphysema).
- If you are over age 35.
- If you will have surgery within 2 months, including dental surgery, requiring general or spinal anesthesia.

Over age 60:
Adverse reactions and side effects may be more frequent and severe than in younger persons.

Pregnancy:
Decide with your doctor if drug benefits justify risk to unborn child. Risk category C (see page xxii).

Breast-feeding:
Avoid nursing or discontinue until you finish drug. Consult doctor.

Infants & children:
Only under close medical supervision.

Prolonged use:
Recommended periodically during prolonged use—Blood counts, G6PD* tests before treatment begins in Negroes and Caucasians of Mediterranean heritage, liver function studies.

Skin & sunlight:
May cause rash or intensify sunburn in areas exposed to sun or sunlamp.

Driving, piloting or hazardous work:
Don't drive or pilot aircraft until you learn how medicine affects you. Don't work around dangerous machinery. Don't climb ladders or work in high places. Danger increases if you drink alcohol or take medicine affecting alertness and reflexes, such as antihistamines, tranquilizers, sedatives, pain medicine, narcotics and mind-altering drugs.

Discontinuing:
Don't discontinue without consulting doctor. Dose may require gradual reduction if you have taken drug for a long time. Doses of other drugs may also require adjustment.

Others:
- No problems expected.
- Advise any doctor or dentist whom you consult that you take this medicine.

POSSIBLE INTERACTION WITH OTHER DRUGS

GENERIC NAME OR DRUG CLASS	COMBINED EFFECT
Central nervous system (CNS) depressants *	Increased sedation, low blood pressure. Avoid.
Dronabinol	Increased effect of dronabinol on central nervous system. Avoid.

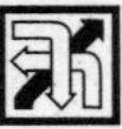

POSSIBLE INTERACTION WITH OTHER SUBSTANCES

INTERACTS WITH	COMBINED EFFECT
Alcohol:	Increased sedation, low blood pressure. Avoid.
Beverages:	No problems expected.
Cocaine:	Increased spasticity. Avoid.
Foods:	No problems expected.
Marijuana:	Increased spasticity. Avoid.
Tobacco:	May interfere with absorption of medicine.

***See Glossary**

DAPSONE

BRAND NAMES

Avlosulfon DDS

BASIC INFORMATION

Habit forming? No
Prescription needed? Yes
Available as generic? Yes
Drug class: Antibacterial (antileprosy), sulfone

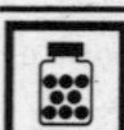

USES

- Treatment of dermatitis herpetiformis.
- Treatment of leprosy.
- Prevention and treatment of pneumocystis carnii pneumonia.
- Other uses include granuloma annulare, pemphigoid, pyoderma gangrenosum, polychondritis, eye ulcerations, systemic lupus erythematosus.

DOSAGE & USAGE INFORMATION

How to take:
Tablet—Swallow with liquid or food to lessen stomach irritation.

When to take:
Once a day at same time.

If you forget a dose:
Take as soon as you remember up to 2 hours late. If more than 2 hours, wait for next scheduled dose (don't double this dose).

Continued next column

OVERDOSE

SYMPTOMS:
Bleeding, vomiting, seizures, cyanosis, coma.
WHAT TO DO:
- **Dial 911 (emergency) or 0 (operator) for an ambulance or medical help. Then give first aid immediately.**
- **If patient is unconscious and not breathing, give mouth-to-mouth breathing. If there is no heartbeat, use cardiac massage and mouth-to-mouth breathing (CPR). Don't try to make patient vomit. If you can't get help quickly, take patient to nearest emergency facility.**
- **See emergency information on inside covers.**

What drug does:
Inhibits enzymes. Kills leprosy germs.

Time lapse before drug works:
- 3 years for leprosy.
- 1 to 2 weeks for dermatitis herpetiformis.

Don't take with:
Any other medicine without consulting your doctor or pharmacist.

POSSIBLE ADVERSE REACTIONS OR SIDE EFFECTS

SYMPTOMS	WHAT TO DO
Life-threatening:	
In case of overdose, see previous column.	
Common:	
• Rash, abdominal pain.	Discontinue. Call doctor right away.
• Appetite loss.	Continue. Call doctor when convenient.
Infrequent:	
Pale.	Discontinue. Call doctor right away.
Rare:	
• Dizziness; mental changes; sore throat; fever; difficult breathing; bleeding; jaundice; numbness, tingling, pain or burning in hands or feet; swelling of feet, hands, eyelids; blurred vision; anemia; peeling skin.	Discontinue. Call doctor right away.
• Headache; itching; nausea; vomiting; blue fingernails, lips.	Continue. Call doctor when convenient.

WARNINGS & PRECAUTIONS

Don't take if:
- You have G6PD* deficiency.
- You are allergic to furosemide, thiazide diuretics, sulfonureas, carbonic anhydrase inhibitors, sulfonamides.

Before you start, consult your doctor:
- If you take any other medicine.
- If you are anemic.
- If you have liver or kidney disease.
- If you are Negro or Caucasian with Mediterranean heritage.
- If you will have surgery within 2 months, including dental surgery, requiring general or spinal anesthesia.

Over age 60:
Adverse reactions and side effects may be more frequent and severe than in younger persons.

Pregnancy:
Decide with your doctor if drug benefits justify risk to unborn child. Risk category C (see page xxii).

Breast-feeding:
Consult doctor. Avoid drug or discontinue nursing.

Infants & children:
Under close medical supervision only.

Prolonged use:
- Request liver function studies.
- Talk to your doctor about the need for follow-up medical examinations or laboratory studies to check complete blood counts (white blood cell count, platelet count, red blood cell count, hemoglobin, hematocrit).

Skin & sunlight:
Exposure may cause illness with swelling, spots on skin, fever.

Driving, piloting or hazardous work:
Don't drive or pilot aircraft until you learn how medicine affects you. Don't work around dangerous machinery. Don't climb ladders or work in high places. Danger increases if you drink alcohol or take medicine affecting alertness and reflexes, such as antihistamines, tranquilizers, sedatives, pain medicine, narcotics and mind-altering drugs.

Discontinuing:
Don't discontinue without consulting doctor. Dose may require gradual reduction if you have taken drug for a long time. Doses of other drugs may also require adjustment.

Others:
- Dapsone may rarely cause liver damage.
- For full effect you may need to take dapsone for many months or years.

POSSIBLE INTERACTION WITH OTHER DRUGS

GENERIC NAME OR DRUG CLASS	COMBINED EFFECT
Aminobenzoic acid (PABA)	Decreased dapsone effect. Avoid.
Didanosine	Increased risk of peripheral neuropathy. Reduced absorption of both drugs.
Dideoxyinosine (ddl)	Decreased dapsone effect.
Hemolytics*	May increase adverse effects on blood cells.
Methotrexate	May increase blood toxicity.
Probenecid	Increased toxicity of dapsone.
Pyrimethamine	May increase blood toxicity.
Rifampin	Decreased effect of dapsone.
Trimethoprim	May increase blood toxicity.

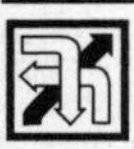

POSSIBLE INTERACTION WITH OTHER SUBSTANCES

INTERACTS WITH	COMBINED EFFECT
Alcohol:	Increased chance of toxicity to liver.
Beverages:	No problems expected.
Cocaine:	Increased chance of toxicity. Avoid.
Foods:	No problems expected.
Marijuana:	Increased chance of toxicity. Avoid.
Tobacco:	May interfere with absorption of medicine.

*See Glossary

DECONGESTANTS (Ophthalmic)

BRAND AND GENERIC NAMES

Ak-Con
Albalon
Albalon Liquifilm
Allerest
Allergy Drops
Clear Eyes
Comfort Eye Drops
Degest 2
Estivin II
I-Naphline
Murine Plus
Muro's Opcon
Nafazair
NAPHAZOLINE
Naphcon
Naphcon Forte
Napholine
OcuClear
Ocu-Zoline
Opcon
OXYMETAZOLINE
TETRAHYDROZILINE
VasoClear
VasoClear A
Vasocon
Vasocon Regular
Visine L.R.

BASIC INFORMATION

Habit forming? No
Prescription needed? Yes, for some
Available as generic? Yes
Drug class: Decongestant (ophthalmic)

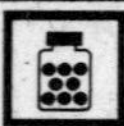

USES

Treats eye redness, itching, burning or other irritation due to dust, colds, allergies, rubbing eyes, wearing contact lenses, swimming or eye strain from close work, watching TV, reading.

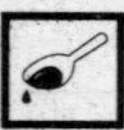

DOSAGE & USAGE INFORMATION

How to use:
Eye drops
- Wash hands.
- Apply pressure to inside corner of eye with middle finger.
- Tilt head backward. Pull lower lid away from eye with index finger of the same hand.
- Drop eye drops into pouch and close eye. Don't blink.
- Keep eyes closed for 1 to 2 minutes.
- Continue pressure for 1 minute after placing medicine in eye.

Continued next column

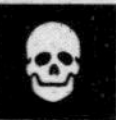

OVERDOSE

SYMPTOMS:
None expected.
WHAT TO DO:
Not intended for internal use. If child accidentally swallows, call poison control center.

- Don't touch applicator tip to any surface (including the eye). If you accidentally touch tip, clean with warm soap and water.
- Keep container tightly closed.
- Keep cool, but don't freeze.
- Wash hands immediately after using.

When to use:
As directed. Usually every 3 or 4 hours.

If you forget a dose:
Use as soon as you remember.

What drug does:
Acts on small blood vessels to make them constrict or become smaller.

Time lapse before drug works:
2 to 10 minutes.

Don't use with:
Other eye drops without consulting your doctor.

POSSIBLE ADVERSE REACTIONS OR SIDE EFFECTS

SYMPTOMS	WHAT TO DO
Life-threatening:	
None expected.	
Common:	
Increased eye irritation.	Discontinue. Call doctor right away.
Infrequent:	
None expected.	
Rare:	
Blurred vision, large pupils, weakness, drowsiness, decreased body temperature, slow heartbeat, dizziness, headache, nervousness, nausea.	Discontinue. Call doctor right away.

WARNINGS & PRECAUTIONS

Don't use if:
You are allergic to any decongestant eye drops.

Before you start, consult your doctor:
- If you take antidepressants or maprolitine.
- If you have glaucoma, eye disease, infection or injury.
- If you have heart disease, high blood pressure, thyroid disease.

Over age 60:
No problems expected.

Pregnancy:
Decide with your doctor if drug benefits justify risk to unborn child. Risk category C (see page xxii).

Breast-feeding:
No problems expected, but check with doctor.

Infants & children:
Don't use.

Prolonged use:
Don't use for more than 3 or 4 days.

Skin & sunlight:
No problems expected.

Driving, piloting or hazardous work:
No problems expected.

Discontinuing:
May not need all the medicine in container. If symptoms disappear, stop using.

Others:
- Keep cool, but don't freeze.
- Check with your doctor if eye irritation continues or becomes worse.

POSSIBLE INTERACTION WITH OTHER DRUGS

GENERIC NAME OR DRUG CLASS	COMBINED EFFECT

Clinically significant interactions with oral or injected medicines unlikely.

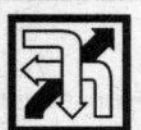

POSSIBLE INTERACTION WITH OTHER SUBSTANCES

INTERACTS WITH	COMBINED EFFECT
Alcohol:	None expected.
Beverages:	None expected.
Cocaine:	None expected.
Foods:	None expected.
Marijuana:	None expected.
Tobacco:	Smoke may increase eye irritation. Avoid.

DEHYDROCHOLIC ACID

BRAND NAMES

Bilax
Cholan-HMB
Decholin
Hepahydrin
Neolax
Trilax

BASIC INFORMATION

Habit forming? No
Prescription needed? No
Available as generic? Yes
Drug class: Laxative (stimulant)

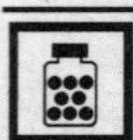

USES

Constipation relief.

DOSAGE & USAGE INFORMATION

How to take:
Tablet or capsule—Swallow with liquid.

When to take:
Usually at bedtime with a snack, unless directed otherwise.

If you forget a dose:
Take as soon as you remember.

What drug does:
Acts on smooth muscles of intestine wall to cause vigorous bowel movement.

Time lapse before drug works:
6 to 10 hours.

Don't take with:
- Any other medicine without consulting your doctor or pharmacist.
- Don't take within 2 hours of taking another medicine. Laxative interferes with medicine absorption.

OVERDOSE

SYMPTOMS:
Vomiting, electrolyte depletion.
WHAT TO DO:
Overdose unlikely to threaten life. If person takes much larger amount than prescribed, call doctor, poison control center or hospital emergency room for instructions.

POSSIBLE ADVERSE REACTIONS OR SIDE EFFECTS

SYMPTOMS	WHAT TO DO
Life-threatening:	
None expected.	
Common:	
Rectal irritation.	Continue. Call doctor when convenient.
Infrequent:	
• Dangerous potassium loss (thirst, weakness, heartbeat irregularity, paralysis and diarrhea).	Discontinue. Call doctor right away.
• Belching, cramps, nausea.	Continue. Call doctor when convenient.
Rare:	
• Irritability, confusion, headache, rash, breathing difficulty, irregular heartbeat, muscle cramps, unusual tiredness or weakness.	Discontinue. Call doctor right away.
• Burning on urination.	Continue. Call doctor when convenient.

WARNINGS & PRECAUTIONS

Don't take if:
- You have symptoms of appendicitis, inflamed bowel or intestinal blockage.
- You are allergic to a stimulant laxative.
- You have missed a bowel movement for only 1 or 2 days.
- You have liver disease.

Before you start, consult your doctor:
- If you have a colostomy or ileostomy.
- If you have congestive heart disease.
- If you have diabetes.
- If you have an enlarged prostate.
- If you have a laxative habit.
- If you have rectal bleeding.
- If you take other laxatives.

Over age 60:
Adverse reactions and side effects may be more frequent and severe than in younger persons.

Pregnancy:
Decide with your doctor if drug benefits justify risk to unborn child. Risk category C (see page xxii).

Breast-feeding:
Drug passes into milk. Avoid drug or discontinue nursing until you finish medicine. Consult doctor for advice on maintaining milk supply.

Infants & children:
Use only under medical supervision.

Prolonged use:
Don't take for more than 1 week unless under a doctor's supervision. May cause laxative dependence.

Skin & sunlight:
No problems expected.

Driving, piloting or hazardous work:
No problems expected.

Discontinuing:
May be unnecessary to finish medicine. Follow doctor's instructions.

Others:
Don't take to "flush out" your system or as a "tonic."

POSSIBLE INTERACTION WITH OTHER DRUGS

GENERIC NAME OR DRUG CLASS	COMBINED EFFECT
Antihypertensives*	May cause dangerous low potassium level.
Diuretics*	May cause dangerous low potassium level.

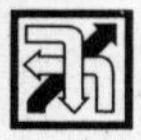

POSSIBLE INTERACTION WITH OTHER SUBSTANCES

INTERACTS WITH	COMBINED EFFECT
Alcohol:	None expected.
Beverages:	None expected.
Cocaine:	None expected.
Foods:	None expected.
Marijuana:	None expected.
Tobacco:	None expected.

***See Glossary**

DESMOPRESSIN

BRAND NAMES

DDAVP
Stimate

BASIC INFORMATION

Habit forming? No
Prescription needed? Yes
Available as generic? No
Drug class: Antidiuretic, antihemorrhagic

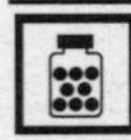

USES

- Prevents and controls symptoms associated with central diabetes insipidus.
- Treats primary nocturnal enuresis (bedwetting during sleep).

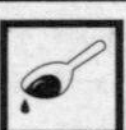

DOSAGE & USAGE INFORMATION

How to take:
Nasal spray—Fill the rhinyle (a flexible, calibrated catheter) with a measured dose of the nasal spray. Blow on the other end of the catheter to deposit the solution deep in the nasal cavity. For infants and children, an air-filled syringe may be used.

When to take:
At the same time each day, according to instructions on prescription label.

If you forget a dose:
Take as soon as you remember up to 2 hours late. If more than 2 hours, wait for next scheduled dose. Don't double this dose.

What drug does:
Increases water reabsorption in the kidney and decreases urine output.

Time lapse before drug works:
Within 1 hour. Effect may last from 6 to 24 hours.

Don't take with:
Any other medicine without consulting your doctor or pharmacist.

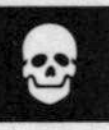

OVERDOSE

SYMPTOMS:
Confusion, coma, seizures.
WHAT TO DO:
Overdose unlikely to threaten life. If person takes much larger amount than prescribed, call doctor, poison control center or hospital emergency room for instructions.

POSSIBLE ADVERSE REACTIONS OR SIDE EFFECTS

SYMPTOMS	WHAT TO DO
Life-threatening: None expected.	
Common: Headache.	Continue. Call doctor when convenient.
Infrequent:	
• Flushed or red skin, nausea.	Discontinue. Call doctor right away.
• Abdominal cramps.	Continue. Call doctor when convenient.
Rare:	
• Water intoxication (confusion, drowsiness, headache, seizures, rapid weight gain).	Discontinue. Seek emergency treatment.
• Increased blood pressure.	Discontinue. Call doctor right away.

WARNINGS & PRECAUTIONS

Don't take if:
You know that you are sensitive to desmopressin.

Before you start, consult your doctor:
- If you have allergic rhinitis.
- If you have nasal congestion.
- If you have a cold or other upper respiratory infection.
- If you have heart disease or high blood pressure.

Over age 60:
Increased risk of water intoxication.

Pregnancy:
No proven harm to unborn child, but avoid if possible. Consult doctor. Risk category B (see page xxii).

Breast-feeding:
Drug passes into milk. Avoid drug or discontinue nursing until you finish medicine. Consult doctor for advice on maintaining milk supply.

Infants & children:
More sensitive to effect. Use only under close medical supervision.

Prolonged use:
May require increasing dosage for same effect.

Skin & sunlight:
No special problems expected.

Driving, piloting or hazardous work:
Don't drive or pilot aircraft until you learn how medicine affects you. Don't work around dangerous machinery. Don't climb ladders or work in high places. Danger increases if you drink alcohol or take medicine affecting alertness and reflexes.

Discontinuing:
No special problems expected.

Others:
- Advise any doctor or dentist whom you consult that you take this medicine.
- Fluid intake may need to be adjusted.

POSSIBLE INTERACTION WITH OTHER DRUGS

GENERIC NAME OR DRUG CLASS	COMBINED EFFECT
Carbamazepine	May increase desmopressin effect.
Chlorpropamide	May increase desmopressin effect.
Clofibrate	May increase desmopressin effect.
Demeclocycline	May decrease desmopressin effect.
Lithium	May decrease desmopressin effect.
Norepinephrine	May decrease desmopressin effect.

POSSIBLE INTERACTION WITH OTHER SUBSTANCES

INTERACTS WITH	COMBINED EFFECT
Alcohol:	May decrease desmopressin effect.
Beverages: Caffeine drinks.	May decrease desmopressin effect.
Cocaine:	May decrease desmopressin effect.
Foods:	None expected.
Marijuana:	May decrease desmopressin effect.
Tobacco:	May decrease desmopressin effect.

*See Glossary

DEXAMETHASONE

BRAND NAMES

See complete list of brand names in the *Brand Name Directory*, page 905.

BASIC INFORMATION

Habit forming? No
Prescription needed? Yes
Available as generic? Yes
Drug class: Cortisone drug (adrenal corticosteroid)

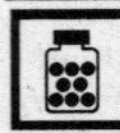

USES

- Reduces inflammation caused by many different medical problems.
- Treatment for some allergic diseases, blood disorders, kidney diseases, asthma and emphysema.
- Replaces corticosteroid deficiencies.

DOSAGE & USAGE INFORMATION

How to take:
- Tablet or liquid—Swallow with liquid or food to lessen stomach irritation. If you can't swallow whole, crumble tablet and take with liquid or food.
- Inhaler—Follow label instructions.

When to take:
At the same times each day. Take once-a-day or once-every-other-day doses in mornings.

If you forget a dose:
- Several-doses-per-day prescription—Take as soon as you remember up to 2 hours late. If more than 2 hours, wait for next scheduled dose (don't double this dose).
- Once-a-day dose or less—Wait for next dose. Double this dose.

What drug does:
Decreases inflammatory responses.

Continued next column

Time lapse before drug works:
2 to 4 days.

Don't take with:
Any other medicine without consulting your doctor or pharmacist.

OVERDOSE

SYMPTOMS:
Headache, convulsions, fluid retention, heart failure.
WHAT TO DO:
- **Dial 911 (emergency) or 0 (operator) for an ambulance or medical help. Then give first aid immediately.**
- **See emergency information on inside covers.**

POSSIBLE ADVERSE REACTIONS OR SIDE EFFECTS

SYMPTOMS	WHAT TO DO
Life-threatening:	
Hives, rash, intense itching, faintness soon after a dose (anaphylaxis).	Seek emergency treatment immediately.
Common:	
Poor wound healing, acne, thirst, nausea, indigestion, vomiting.	Continue. Call doctor when convenient.
Infrequent:	
• Bloody or black, tarry stool.	Discontinue. Seek emergency treatment.
• Blurred vision; halos around lights; sore throat, fever; muscle cramps; swollen legs, feet.	Discontinue. Call doctor right away.
• Mood changes, insomnia, fatigue, restlessness, frequent urination, weight gain, round face, weakness, irregular menstrual periods.	Continue. Call doctor when convenient.
Rare:	
• Irregular heartbeat.	Discontinue. Seek emergency treatment.
• Rash, pancreatitis, numbness or tingling in hands or feet, thrombophlebitis, hallucinations, hiccups, convulsions.	Discontinue. Call doctor right away.

WARNINGS & PRECAUTIONS

Don't take if:
- You are allergic to any cortisone drug.
- You have tuberculosis or fungus infection.
- You have herpes infection of eyes, lips or genitals.

Before you start, consult your doctor:
- If you have had tuberculosis.
- If you have congestive heart failure, diabetes, peptic ulcer, glaucoma, underactive thyroid, high blood pressure, myasthenia gravis.
- If you have blood clots in legs or lungs.

Over age 60:
Adverse reactions and side effects may be more frequent and severe than in younger persons. Likely to aggravate edema, diabetes or ulcers. Likely to cause cataracts and osteoporosis (softening of the bones).

Pregnancy:
Decide with your doctor if drug benefits justify risk to unborn child. Risk category C (see page xxii).

Breast-feeding:
Drug passes into milk. Avoid drug or discontinue nursing until you finish medicine. Consult doctor for advice on maintaining milk supply.

Infants & children:
Use only under medical supervision.

Prolonged use:
- Retards growth in children.
- Possible glaucoma, cataracts, diabetes, fragile bones and thin skin.
- Functional dependence.
- Talk to your doctor about the need for follow-up medical examinations or laboratory studies to check blood sugar, eyes, serum electrolytes, stools for blood.

Skin & sunlight:
No problems expected.

Driving, piloting or hazardous work:
No problems expected.

Discontinuing:
- Don't discontinue without doctor's advice until you complete prescribed dose, even though symptoms diminish or disappear.
- Drug affects your response to surgery, illness, injury or stress for 2 years after discontinuing. Tell anyone who takes medical care of you within 2 years about drug.

Others:
- Avoid immunizations if possible.
- Your resistance to infection is less while taking this medicine.
- Advise any doctor or dentist whom you consult that you take this medicine.
- Those who have inactive or "cured" tuberculosis* may be subjected to a possible recurrence of active tuberculosis.
- Children who must take cortisone drugs may grow less well.

POSSIBLE INTERACTION WITH OTHER DRUGS

GENERIC NAME OR DRUG CLASS	COMBINED EFFECT
Aminoglutethimide	Dexamethasone effect decreased by half.
Amphotericin B	Potassium depletion.
Anticholinergics*	Possible glaucoma.
Anticoagulants, oral*	Decreased anti-coagulant effect.
Anticonvulsants, hydantoin*	Decreased dexa-methasone effect.
Antidiabetics, oral*	Decreased anti-diabetic effect.
Antihistamines*	Decreased dexa-methasone effect.
Anti-inflammatory drugs, nonsteroidal (NSAIDs)*	Increased risk of ulcers and dexa-methasone effect.
Aspirin	Increased dexa-methasone effect.
Attenuated virus vaccines*	Possible viral infection.
Barbiturates*	Decreased dexa-methasone effect. Oversedation.
Chloral hydrate	Decreased dexa-methasone effect.
Chlorthalidone	Potassium depletion.
Cholestyramine	Decreased dexa-methasone effect.
Cholinergics*	Decreased cholinergic effect.
Colestipol	Decreased dexa-methasone absorption.
Contraceptives, oral*	Increased dexa-methasone effect.

Continued on page 936

POSSIBLE INTERACTION WITH OTHER SUBSTANCES

INTERACTS WITH	COMBINED EFFECT
Alcohol:	Risk of stomach ulcers.
Beverages:	No proven problems.
Cocaine:	Overstimulation. Avoid.
Foods:	No proven problems.
Marijuana:	Decreased immunity.
Tobacco:	Increased dexa-methasone effect. Possible toxicity.

***See Glossary**

DEXTROMETHORPHAN

BRAND NAMES

See complete list of brand names in the *Brand Name Directory*, page 906.

BASIC INFORMATION

Habit forming? No
Prescription needed? No
Available as generic? Yes
Drug class: Cough suppressant

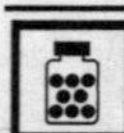

USES

Suppresses cough associated with allergies or infections such as colds, bronchitis, flu and lung disorders.

DOSAGE & USAGE INFORMATION

How to take:

- Chewable tablet—Chew well before swallowing.
- Lozenges or syrups—Take as directed on label.
- Capsules—Swallow with liquid.

When to take:
As needed, no more often than every 3 hours.

If you forget a dose:
Take as soon as you remember. Wait 3 hours for next dose.

What drug does:
Reduces sensitivity of brain's cough control center, suppressing urge to cough.

Time lapse before drug works:
15 to 30 minutes.

Don't take with:
Any other medicine without consulting your doctor or pharmacist.

OVERDOSE

SYMPTOMS:
Euphoria, overactivity, sense of intoxication, visual and auditory hallucinations, lack of coordination, stagger, stupor, shallow breathing.
WHAT TO DO:

- **Dial 911 (emergency) or 0 (operator) for an ambulance or medical help. Then give first aid immediately.**
- **See emergency information on inside covers.**

POSSIBLE ADVERSE REACTIONS OR SIDE EFFECTS

SYMPTOMS	WHAT TO DO
Life-threatening: In case of overdose, see previous column.	
Common: None expected.	
Infrequent: Confusion, excitement or nervousness.	Discontinue. Call doctor right away.
Rare: Dizziness, drowsiness, rash, diarrhea, nausea or vomiting, abdominal pain.	Discontinue. Call doctor right away.

WARNINGS & PRECAUTIONS

Don't take if:
You are allergic to any cough syrup containing dextromethorphan.

Before you start, consult your doctor:
- If you have asthma attacks.
- If you have impaired liver function.

Over age 60:
Adverse reactions and side effects may be more frequent and severe than in younger persons. You may require smaller doses for shorter periods of time.

Pregnancy:
Decide with your doctor if drug benefits justify risk to unborn child. Risk category C (see page xxii).

Breast-feeding:
No proven problems. Consult doctor.

Infants & children:
Use only as label directs.

Prolonged use:
No problems expected.

Skin & sunlight:
No problems expected.

Driving, piloting or hazardous work:
Don't drive or pilot aircraft until you learn how medicine affects you. Don't work around dangerous machinery. Don't climb ladders or work in high places. Danger increases if you drink alcohol or take medicine affecting alertness and reflexes, such as antihistamines, tranquilizers, sedatives, pain medicine, narcotics and mind-altering drugs.

Discontinuing:
May be unnecessary to finish medicine. Follow doctor's instructions.

Others:
- If cough persists or if you cough blood or brown-yellow, thick mucus, call your doctor.
- Excessive use may lead to functional dependence.

POSSIBLE INTERACTION WITH OTHER DRUGS

GENERIC NAME OR DRUG CLASS	COMBINED EFFECT
Monozmine oxidase (MAO) inhibitors*	Disorientation, high fever, drop in blood pressure and loss of consciousness.
Sedatives* and other central nervous system (CNS) depressants*	Increased sedative effect of both drugs.

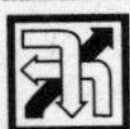

POSSIBLE INTERACTION WITH OTHER SUBSTANCES

INTERACTS WITH	COMBINED EFFECT
Alcohol:	None expected.
Beverages:	None expected.
Cocaine:	Decreased dextromethorphan effect. Avoid.
Foods:	None expected.
Marijuana:	None expected.
Tobacco:	None expected.

*See Glossary

DEXTROTHYROXINE

BRAND NAMES

Choloxin

BASIC INFORMATION

Habit forming? No
Prescription needed? Yes
Available as generic? No
Drug class: Antihyperlipidemic, thyroid hormone

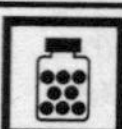

USES

- Lowers blood cholesterol and low-density lipoproteins in patients who don't respond to low-fat diet and weight loss alone.
- Treats hypothyroidism in patients with heart disease.

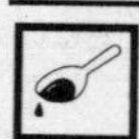

DOSAGE & USAGE INFORMATION

How to take:
Tablets—Swallow with liquid. If you can't swallow whole, crumble tablet and take with liquid or food. Instructions to take on empty stomach mean 1 hour before or 2 hours after eating.

When to take:
According to your doctor's instructions.

If you forget a dose:
Take as soon as you remember up to 2 hours late. If more than 2 hours, wait for next scheduled dose (don't double this dose).

What drug does:
Increases breakdown of LDL (low-density lipoprotein).

Time lapse before drug works:
1 to 2 months.

Don't take with:
Any other medicines (including over-the-counter drugs such as cough and cold medicines, laxatives, antacids, diet pills, caffeine, nose drops or vitamins) without consulting your doctor.

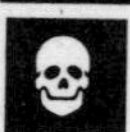

OVERDOSE

SYMPTOMS:
None expected.
WHAT TO DO:
Overdose unlikely to threaten life. If person takes much larger amount than prescribed, call doctor, poison control center or hospital emergency room for instructions.

POSSIBLE ADVERSE REACTIONS OR SIDE EFFECTS

SYMPTOMS	WHAT TO DO
Life-threatening: None expected.	
Common:	
• Tremor, headache, irritability, insomnia.	Discontinue. Call doctor right away.
• Appetite change, diarrhea, leg cramps, menstrual irregularities, fever, heat sensitivity, unusual sweating, weight loss.	Continue. Call doctor when convenient.
Infrequent: Hives, rash, vomiting, chest pain, rapid and irregular heartbeat, shortness of breath.	Discontinue. Call doctor right away.
Rare: None expected.	

WARNINGS & PRECAUTIONS

Don't take if:
- You have had a heart attack within 6 weeks.
- You have no thyroid deficiency, but want to use this to lose weight.

Before you start, consult your doctor:
- If you have heart disease or high blood pressure.
- If you have diabetes.
- If you have Addison's disease, have had adrenal gland deficiency or use epinephrine, ephedrine or isoproterenol for asthma.

Over age 60:
More sensitive to thyroid hormone. May need smaller doses.

Pregnancy:
Consult doctor. Risk category B (see page xxii).

Breast-feeding:
Present in milk. Considered safe if dose is correct.

Infants & children:
Use only under medical supervision.

Prolonged use:
- No problems expected, if dose is correct.
- Talk to your doctor about the need for follow-up medical examinations or laboratory studies to check serum cholesterol and triglycerides.

Skin & sunlight:
No problems expected.

Driving, piloting or hazardous work:
No problems expected.

Discontinuing:
Don't discontinue without consulting doctor. Dose may require gradual reduction if you have taken drug for a long time. Doses of other drugs may also require adjustment.

Others:
- Digestive upsets, tremors, cramps, nervousness, insomnia or diarrhea may indicate need for dose adjustment.
- Advise any doctor or dentist whom you consult that you take this medicine.
- May affect results in some medical tests.
- Stay on a low-fat diet.

POSSIBLE INTERACTION WITH OTHER DRUGS

GENERIC NAME OR DRUG CLASS	COMBINED EFFECT
Amphetamines*	Increased amphetamine effect.
Anticoagulants, oral*	Increased anticoagulant effect.
Antidepressants, tricyclic*	Increased antidepressant effect. Irregular heartbeat.
Antidiabetics*	Antidiabetic may require adjustment.
Aspirin (large doses, continuous use)	Increased dextrothyroxine effect.
Barbiturates*	Decreased barbiturate effect.
Beta-adrenergic blocking agents*	Possible decreased beta blocker effect.
Cholestyramine	Decreased dextrothyroxine effect.
Colestipol	Decreased dextrothyroxine effect.
Contraceptives, oral*	Decreased dextrothyroxine effect.
Cortisone drugs*	Requires dose adjustment to prevent cortisone deficiency.
Digitalis preparations*	Decreased digitalis effect.
Ephedrine	Increased ephedrine effect.
Epinephrine	Increased epinephrine effect.
Estrogens*	Decreased dextrothyroxine effect.
Methylphenidate	Increased methylphenidate effect.
Phenytoin	Possible decreased dextrothyroxine effect.

POSSIBLE INTERACTION WITH OTHER SUBSTANCES

INTERACTS WITH	COMBINED EFFECT
Alcohol:	None expected.
Beverages:	None expected.
Cocaine:	Excess stimulation. Avoid.
Foods: Soybeans.	Heavy consumption interferes with thyroid function.
Marijuana:	None expected.
Tobacco:	None expected.

*See Glossary

DICYCLOMINE

BRAND NAMES

See complete list of brand names in the *Brand Name Directory*, page 907.

BASIC INFORMATION

Habit forming? No
Prescription needed? Yes
Available as generic? Yes
Drug class: Antispasmodic, anticholinergic

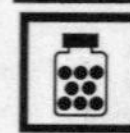

USES

- Reduces spasms of digestive system, bladder and urethra.
- Treats irritable bowel syndrome.

DOSAGE & USAGE INFORMATION

How to take:
Tablet, syrup or capsule—Swallow with liquid or food to lessen stomach irritation.

When to take:
30 minutes before meals (unless directed otherwise by doctor).

If you forget a dose:
Take as soon as you remember up to 2 hours late. If more than 2 hours, wait for next scheduled dose (don't double this dose).

What drug does:
Blocks nerve impulses at parasympathetic nerve endings, preventing muscle contractions and gland secretions of organs involved.

Time lapse before drug works:
15 to 30 minutes.

Don't take with:
Any other medicine without consulting your doctor or pharmacist.

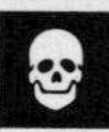

OVERDOSE

SYMPTOMS:
Dilated pupils, blurred vision, rapid pulse and breathing, dizziness, fever, hallucinations, confusion, slurred speech, agitation, flushed face, convulsions, coma.
WHAT TO DO:
- **Dial 911 (emergency) or 0 (operator) for an ambulance or medical help. Then give first aid immediately.**
- **See emergency information on inside covers.**

POSSIBLE ADVERSE REACTIONS OR SIDE EFFECTS

SYMPTOMS	WHAT TO DO
Life-threatening:	
Hives, rash, intense itching, faintness soon after a dose (anaphylaxis).	Seek emergency treatment immediately.
Common:	
• Confusion, delirium, rapid heartbeat.	Discontinue. Call doctor right away.
• Nausea, vomiting, decreased sweating.	Continue. Call doctor when convenient.
• Constipation, loss of taste.	Continue. Tell doctor at next visit.
• Dry ears, nose, throat, mouth.	No action necessary.
Infrequent:	
• Headache, difficult urination, nasal congestion, altered taste.	Continue. Call doctor when convenient.
• Lightheadedness.	Discontinue. Call doctor right away.
Rare:	
Rash or hives, eye pain, blurred vision.	Discontinue. Call doctor right away.

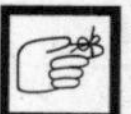

WARNINGS & PRECAUTIONS

Don't take if:
- You are allergic to any anticholinergic.
- You have trouble with stomach bloating.
- You have difficulty emptying your bladder completely.
- You have narrow-angle glaucoma.
- You have severe ulcerative colitis.

Before you start, consult your doctor:
- If you have open-angle glaucoma.
- If you have angina, chronic bronchitis or asthma.
- If you have hiatal hernia, liver disease, kidney or thyroid disease, enlarged prostate, myasthenia gravis, peptic ulcer.
- If you will have surgery within 2 months, including dental surgery, requiring general or spinal anesthesia.

Over age 60:
Adverse reactions and side effects may be more frequent and severe than in younger persons.

Pregnancy:
Decide with your doctor whether drug benefits justify risk to unborn child. Risk category C (see page xxii).

Breast-feeding:
Drug passes into milk and decreases milk flow. Avoid drug or discontinue nursing until you finish medicine. Consult doctor for advice on maintaining milk supply.

Infants & children:
Use only under medical supervision.

Prolonged use:
Chronic constipation, possible fecal impaction. Consult doctor immediately.

Skin & sunlight:
No problems expected.

Driving, piloting or hazardous work:
Use disqualifies you for piloting aircraft. Otherwise, no problems expected.

Discontinuing:
May be unnecessary to finish medicine. Follow doctor's instructions.

Others:
Advise any doctor or dentist whom you consult that you take this medicine.

POSSIBLE INTERACTION WITH OTHER DRUGS

GENERIC NAME OR DRUG CLASS	COMBINED EFFECT
Amantadine	Increased dicyclomine effect.
Antacids*	Decreased dicyclomine effect.
Anticholinergics, other*	Increased dicyclomine effect.
Antidepressants, tricyclic*	Increased dicyclomine effect. Increased sedation.
Antidiarrheals*	Decreased dicyclomine effect.
Antihistamines*	Increased dicyclomine effect.
Attapulgite	Decreased dicyclomine effect.
Buclizine	Increased dicyclomine effect.
Cortisone drugs*	Increased internal eye pressure.
Digitalis	Possible decreased absorption of digitalis.
Haloperidol	Increased internal eye pressure.
Ketoconazole	Decreased ketoconazole effect.
Meperidine	Increased dicyclomine effect.
Methylphenidate	Increased dicyclomine effect.
Monoamine oxidase (MAO) inhibitors*	Increased dicyclomine effect.
Nitrates*	Increased internal eye pressure.
Nizatidine	Increased nizatidine effect.
Orphenadrine	Increased dicyclomine effect.
Phenothiazines*	Increased dicyclomine effect.
Pilocarpine	Loss of pilocarpine effect in glaucoma treatment.
Potassium supplements*	Possible intestinal ulcers with oral potassium tablets.
Quinidine	Increased dicyclomine effect.
Sedatives* or central nervous system (CNS) depressants*	Increased sedative effect of both drugs.
Vitamin C	Decreased dicyclomine effect. Avoid large doses of vitamin C.

POSSIBLE INTERACTION WITH OTHER SUBSTANCES

INTERACTS WITH	COMBINED EFFECT
Alcohol:	None expected.
Beverages:	None expected.
Cocaine:	Excessively rapid heartbeat. Avoid.
Foods:	None expected.
Marijuana:	Drowsiness and dry mouth.
Tobacco:	None expected.

*See Glossary

DIDANOSINE

BRAND NAMES

Videx

BASIC INFORMATION

Habit forming? No
Prescription needed? Yes
Available as generic? No
Drug class: Antiviral

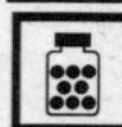

USES

- Treats human immunodeficiency virus (HIV).
- Treats acquired immunodeficiency syndrome (AIDS).

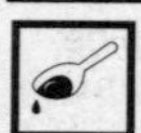

DOSAGE & USAGE INFORMATION

How to take:
- Tablets—Chew or manually crush tablet. If crumble tablet, mix with at least 1 ounce of water and swallow immediately.
- Buffered didanosine for oral solution—Dissolve packet contents in 4 ounces of water.

When to take:
At the same times each day, according to instructions on prescription label.

If you forget a dose:
Take as soon as you remember up to 2 hours late. If more than 2 hours, wait for next scheduled dose (don't double this dose).

What drug does:
Suppresses replication of human immunodeficiency virus.

Time lapse before drug works:
90 minutes.

Don't take with:
See Interaction column and consult doctor.

OVERDOSE

SYMPTOMS:
Seizures.
WHAT TO DO:
- **Dial 911 (emergency) or 0 (operator) for an ambulance or medical help. Then give first aid immediately.**
- **See emergency information on inside covers.**

POSSIBLE ADVERSE REACTIONS OR SIDE EFFECTS

SYMPTOMS	WHAT TO DO
Life-threatening:	
Seizures.	Seek emergency treatment immediately.
Common:	
• Tingling, numbness and burning in the feet and ankles.	Discontinue. Call doctor right away.
• Headache, anxiety, restlessness, digestive disturbances, diarrhea.	Continue. Call doctor when convenient.
Infrequent:	
Unusual tiredness and weakness, fever, chills, sore throat, unusual bleeding or bruising, yellow skin and eyes, skin rash.	Discontinue. Call doctor right away.
Rare:	
None expected.	

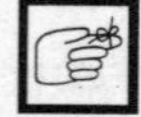

WARNINGS & PRECAUTIONS

Don't take if:
You are allergic to didanosine.

Before you start, consult your doctor:
- If you are an alcoholic.
- If you have hypertriglyceridemia or pancreatitis.
- If you have any condition requiring sodium restriction.
- If you have liver disease, impaired liver function or peripheral neuropathy.
- If you have gout.

Over age 60:
No special problems expected.

Pregnancy:
Consult doctor. Risk category B (see page xxii).

Breast-feeding:
Unknown effect. Consult doctor.

Infants & children:
May cause depigmentation of the retina. Children should have eye exams every 3-6 months to check for vision changes.

Prolonged use:
Talk with your doctor about the need for follow-up medical examination or laboratory studies to check blood serum and uric acid levels.

Skin & sunlight:
No special problems expected.

Driving, piloting or hazardous work:
Don't drive or pilot aircraft until you learn how medicine affects you. Don't work around dangerous machinery. Don't climb ladders or work in high places. Danger increases if you drink alcohol or take medicine affecting alertness and reflexes, such as antihistamines, tranquilizers, sedatives, pain medicines, narcotics and mind-altering drugs.

Discontinuing:
Don't discontinue without consulting doctor. Dose may require gradual reduction if you have taken drug for a long time. Doses of other drugs may require adjustment.

Others:
- Advise any doctor or dentist whom you consult that you take this medicine.
- Avoid sexual intercourse or use condoms to help prevent the transmission of HIV.
- Don't share needles or injectable equipment with other persons.
- The drug zidovudine should be used as the initial treatment for HIV infection since there are no controlled studies as yet on the effectiveness of didanosine in prolonging survival or decreasing the incidence of opportunistic infections.

POSSIBLE INTERACTION WITH OTHER DRUGS

GENERIC NAME OR DRUG CLASS	COMBINED EFFECT
Asparaginase	Increased risk of pancreatitis.
Azathioprine	Increased risk of pancreatitis.
Chloramphenicol	Increased risk of peripheral neuropathy.
Dapsone	Increased risk of peripheral neuropathy. Reduced absorption of both drugs.
Diuretics, thiazide*	Increased risk of pancreatitis.
Estrogens*	Increased risk of pancreatitis.
Ethambutol	Increased risk of peripheral neuropathy.
Ethionamide	Increased risk of peripheral neuropathy.
Fluoroquinolone antibacterials (antibiotics)*	Reduced antibiotic effect.
Furosemide	Increased risk of pancreatitis.
Hydralazine	Increased risk of peripheral neuropathy.
Isoniazid	Increased risk of peripheral neuropathy.
Itraconazole	Decreased absorption of itraconazole.
Ketoconazole	Reduced absorption of both drugs. Increased risk of pancreatitis.
Lithium	Increased risk of peripheral neuropathy.
Methyldopa	Increased risk of pancreatitis.
Metronidazole	Increased risk of peripheral neuropathy.
Nitrofurantoin	Increased risk of pancreatitis and peripheral neuropathy.
Phenytoin	Increased risk of peripheral neuropathy.
Sulfonamides*	Increased risk of pancreatitis.
Sulindac	Increased risk of pancreatitis.

Continued on page 937

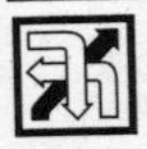

POSSIBLE INTERACTION WITH OTHER SUBSTANCES

INTERACTS WITH	COMBINED EFFECT
Alcohol:	Increased chance of pancreatitis or peripheral neuropathy.
Beverages:	No proven problems.
Cocaine:	No proven problems.
Foods:	No proven problems.
Marijuana:	No proven problems.
Tobacco:	No proven problems.

***See Glossary**

DIFENOXIN & ATROPINE

BRAND NAMES

Motofen

BASIC INFORMATION

Habit forming? Yes
Prescription needed? Yes
Available as generic? No
Drug class: Antidiarrheal

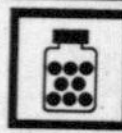

USES

- Reduces spasms of digestive system.
- Treats severe diarrhea.

DOSAGE & USAGE INFORMATION

How to take:
Tablet—Swallow with liquid or food to lessen stomach irritation.

When to take:
After each loose stool or every 3 to 4 hours. No more than 5 tablets in 12 hours.

If you forget a dose:
Take as soon as you remember. Don't double this dose.

What drug does:
- Blocks nerve impulses at parasympathetic nerve endings, preventing muscle contractions and gland secretions of organs involved.
- Acts on brain to decrease spasm of smooth muscle.

Time lapse before drug works:
40 to 60 minutes.

Continued next column

OVERDOSE

SYMPTOMS:
Dilated pupils, rapid pulse and breathing, dizziness, fever, hallucinations, confusion, slurred speech, agitation, flushed face, convulsions, coma.
WHAT TO DO:
- **Dial 911 (emergency) or 0 (operator) for an ambulance or medical help. Then give first aid immediately.**
- **See emergency information on inside covers.**

Don't take with:
- Any medicine that will decrease mental alertness or reflexes, such as alcohol, other mind-altering drugs, cough/cold medicines, antihistamines, allergy medicine, sedatives, tranquilizers (sleeping pills or "downers") barbiturates, seizure medicine, narcotics, other prescription medicines for pain, muscle relaxants, anesthetics.
- See Interaction column and consult doctor.

POSSIBLE ADVERSE REACTIONS OR SIDE EFFECTS

SYMPTOMS	WHAT TO DO
Life-threatening:	
Shortness of breath, agitation, nervousness.	Discontinue. Seek emergency treatment.
Common:	
Dizziness, drowsiness.	Continue. Call doctor when convenient.
Infrequent:	
• Bloating; constipation; appetite loss; abdominal pain; blurred vision; warm, flushed skin; fast heartbeat; dry mouth.	Discontinue. Call doctor right away.
• Frequent urination, lightheadedness, dry skin, headache, insomnia.	Continue. Call doctor when convenient.
Rare:	
Weakness, confusion, fever.	Continue. Call doctor when convenient.

WARNINGS & PRECAUTIONS

Don't take if:
- You are allergic to any anticholinergic.
- You have trouble with stomach bloating, difficulty emptying your bladder completely, narrow-angle glaucoma, severe ulcerative colitis.
- You are dehydrated.

Before you start, consult your doctor:
- If you have open-angle glaucoma, angina, chronic bronchitis, asthma, liver disease, hiatal hernia, enlarged prostate, myasthenia gravis, peptic ulcer.
- If you will have surgery within 2 months, including dental surgery, requiring general or spinal anesthesia.

Over age 60:
Adverse reactions and side effects may be more frequent and severe than in younger persons.

Pregnancy:
Decide with your doctor whether drug benefits justify risk to unborn child. Risk category C (see page xxii).

Breast-feeding:
Drug passes into milk. Avoid drug or discontinue nursing until you finish medicine. Consult doctor for advice on maintaining milk supply.

Infants & children:
Use only under medical supervision.

Prolonged use:
- Chronic constipation, possible fecal impaction. Consult doctor immediately.
- Talk to your doctor about the need for follow-up medical examinations or laboratory studies to check liver function.

Skin & sunlight:
No problems expected.

Driving, piloting or hazardous work:
Use disqualifies you for piloting aircraft. Don't drive until you learn how medicine affects you. Don't work around dangerous machinery. Don't climb ladders or work in high places. Danger increases if you drink alcohol or take medicine affecting alertness and reflexes, such as antihistamines, tranquilizers, sedatives, pain medicine, narcotics and mind-altering drugs.

Discontinuing:
May be unnecessary to finish medicine. Follow doctor's instructions.

Others:
Atropine included at doses below therapeutic level to prevent abuse.

POSSIBLE INTERACTION WITH OTHER DRUGS

GENERIC NAME OR DRUG CLASS	COMBINED EFFECT
Addictive substances (narcotics,* others)	Increased chance of abuse.
Amantadine	Increased atropine effect.
Anticholinergics, other*	Increased atropine effect.
Antidepressants, tricyclic (TCA)*	Increased atropine effect. Increased sedation.
Antihistamines*	Increased atropine effect.
Antihypertensives*	Increased sedation.
Clozapine	Toxic effect on the central nervous system.
Cortisone drugs*	Increased internal eye pressure.
Ethinamate	Dangerous increased effects of ethinamate. Avoid combining.
Fluoxetine	Increased depressant effects of both drugs.
Guanfacine	May increase depressant effects of either drug.
Haloperidol	Increased internal eye pressure.
Leucovorin	High alcohol content of leucovorin may cause adverse effects.
Meperidine	Increased atropine effect.
Methylphenidate	Increased atropine effect.
Methyprylon	Increased sedative effect, perhaps to dangerous level. Avoid.
Monozmine oxidase (MAO) inhibitors*	Increased atropine effect.
Nabilone	Greater depression of central nervous system.
Naltrexone	Triggers withdrawal symptoms.
Narcotics*	Increased sedation. Avoid.

Continued on page 937

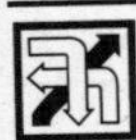

POSSIBLE INTERACTION WITH OTHER SUBSTANCES

INTERACTS WITH	COMBINED EFFECT
Alcohol:	Increased sedation. Avoid.
Beverages:	None expected.
Cocaine:	Excessively rapid heartbeat. Avoid.
Foods:	None expected.
Marijuana:	Drowsiness and dry mouth.
Tobacco:	May increase diarrhea. Avoid.

*See Glossary

DIGITALIS PREPARATIONS (Digitalis Glycosides)

BRAND AND GENERIC NAMES

Cedilanid
Crystodigin
DIGITALIS
DIGITOXIN
DIGOXIN
Lanoxicaps
Lanoxin
Novodigoxin

BASIC INFORMATION

Habit forming? No
Prescription needed? Yes
Available as generic? Yes
Drug class: Digitalis preparation

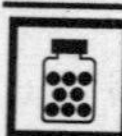

USES

- Strengthens weak heart muscle contractions to prevent congestive heart failure.
- Corrects irregular heartbeat.

DOSAGE & USAGE INFORMATION

How to take:

- Tablet or capsule—Swallow with liquid. If you can't swallow whole, crumble tablet or open capsule and take with liquid or food.
- Liquid—Dilute dose in beverage before swallowing.

When to take:
At the same time each day.

If you forget a dose:
Take as soon as you remember up to 12 hours late. If more than 12 hours, wait for next scheduled dose (don't double this dose).

What drug does:

- Strengthens heart muscle contraction.
- Delays nerve impulses to heart.

Time lapse before drug works:
May require regular use for a week or more.

Continued next column

OVERDOSE

SYMPTOMS:
Nausea, vomiting, diarrhea, vision disturbances, halos around lights, fatigue, irregular heartbeat, confusion, hallucinations, convulsions.

WHAT TO DO:

- **Dial 911 (emergency) or 0 (operator) for an ambulance or medical help. Then give first aid immediately.**
- **See emergency information on inside covers.**

Don't take with:

- Nonprescription drugs without consulting doctor.
- See Interaction column and consult doctor.

POSSIBLE ADVERSE REACTIONS OR SIDE EFFECTS

SYMPTOMS	WHAT TO DO
Life-threatening: In case of overdose, see previous column.	
Common:	
Appetite loss, diarrhea.	Continue. Call doctor when convenient.
Infrequent:	
Extreme drowsiness, lethargy, disorientation, headache, fainting.	Discontinue. Call doctor right away.
Rare:	
• Rash, hives, cardiac arrhythmias, hallucinations, psychosis.	Discontinue. Call doctor right away.
• Double or yellow-green vision; enlarged, sensitive male breasts; tiredness; weakness; depression; decreased sex drive.	Continue. Call doctor when convenient.

WARNINGS & PRECAUTIONS

Don't take if:

- You are allergic to any digitalis preparation.
- Your heartbeat is slower than 50 beats per minute.

Before you start, consult your doctor:

- If you have taken another digitalis preparation in past 2 weeks.
- If you have taken a diuretic within 2 weeks.
- If you have liver or kidney disease.
- If you have a thyroid disorder.
- If you will have surgery within 2 months, including dental surgery, requiring general or spinal anesthesia.

Over age 60:
Adverse reactions and side effects may be more frequent and severe than in younger persons.

Pregnancy:
Decide with you doctor if drug benefits justify risk to unborn child. Risk category C (see page xxii).

Breast-feeding:
Drug filters into milk. May harm child. Avoid.

Infants & children:
Use only under medical supervision.

Prolonged use:
Talk to your doctor about the need for follow-up medical examinations or laboratory studies to check ECG*, liver function, kidney function, serum electrolytes.

Skin & sunlight:
No problems expected.

Driving, piloting or hazardous work:
Possible vision disturbances. Otherwise, no problems expected.

Discontinuing:
Don't stop without doctor's advice.

Others:
Some digitalis products contain tartrazine dye. Avoid, especially if you are allergic to aspirin.

POSSIBLE INTERACTION WITH OTHER DRUGS

GENERIC NAME OR DRUG CLASS	COMBINED EFFECT
Amiodarone	Increased digitalis effect.
Amphotericin B	Decreased potassium. Increased toxicity of amphotericin B.
Antacids*	Decreased digitalis effect.
Anticonvulsants, hydantoin*	Increased digitalis effect at first, then decreased.
Anticholinergics*	Possible increased digitalis effect.
Attapulgite	May decrease effectiveness of digitalis.
Beta-adrenergic blocking agents*	Increased digitalis effect.
Beta-agonists*	Increased risk of heartbeat irregularity.
Calcium supplements*	Decreased digitalis effects.
Carteolol	Can either increase or decrease heart rate. Improves irregular heartbeat.
Cholestyramine	Decreased digitalis effect.
Colestipol	Decreased digitalis effect.
Cortisone drugs*	Digitalis toxicity.
Dextrothyroxine	Decreased digitalis effect.
Disopyramide	Possible decreased digitalis effect.
Diuretics*	Possible digitalis toxicity. Excessive potassium loss that may cause irregular heartbeat.
Ephedrine	Disturbed heart rhythm. Avoid.
Epinephrine	Disturbed heart rhythm. Avoid.
Erythromycins*	May increase digitalis absorption.
Flecainide	May increase digitalis blood level.
Fluoxetine	May cause confusion, agitation, convulsions and high blood pressure. Avoid combining.
Hydroxychloroquine	Possible increased digitalis toxicity.
Itraconazole	Possible toxic levels of digitalis.
Laxatives*	Decreased digitalis effect.
Metoclopramide	Decreased digitalis absorption.

Continued on page 937

POSSIBLE INTERACTION WITH OTHER SUBSTANCES

INTERACTS WITH	COMBINED EFFECT
Alcohol:	None expected.
Beverages: Caffeine drinks.	Irregular heartbeat. Avoid.
Cocaine:	Irregular heartbeat. Avoid.
Foods: Prune juice, bran cereals, foods high in fiber.	Decreased digitalis effect.
Marijuana:	Decreased digitalis effect.
Tobacco:	Irregular heartbeat. Avoid.

*See Glossary

DIMETHYL SULFOXIDE (DMSO)

BRAND NAMES

Rimso-50

BASIC INFORMATION

Habit forming? No
Prescription needed? Yes
Available as generic? Yes
Drug class: Anti-inflammatory (local)

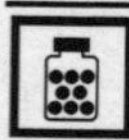

USES

When applied directly to the bladder's membrane lining, DMSO relieves symptoms of bladder inflammation.

DOSAGE & USAGE INFORMATION

How to use:
Under doctor's guidance, directly instill into urinary bladder using a catheter or aseptic syringe. Allow to remain in bladder about 15 minutes, then void. *Note:* Follow doctor's instructions.

When to use:
Follow doctor's instructions.

If you forget a dose:
Take as soon as you remember up to 2 hours late. If more than 2 hours, wait for next scheduled dose (don't double this dose).

What drug does:
Reduces inflammation by unknown mechanism.

Time lapse before drug works:
Works quickly (within minutes).

Don't take with:
Any other medicines (including over-the-counter drugs such as cough and cold medicines, laxatives, antacids, diet pills, caffeine, nose drops or vitamins) without consulting your doctor.

OVERDOSE

SYMPTOMS:
None expected.
WHAT TO DO:
Overdose unlikely to threaten life. If person takes much larger amount than prescribed, call doctor, poison control center or hospital emergency room for instructions.

POSSIBLE ADVERSE REACTIONS OR SIDE EFFECTS

SYMPTOMS	WHAT TO DO
Life-threatening: Breathing difficulty.	Seek emergency treatment immediately.
Common: Garlic-like taste for up to 72 hours.	No action necessary.
Infrequent: Vision problems (not documented in humans, but well documented in animals).	Continue. Call doctor when convenient.
Rare: Nasal congestion, itching, hives, facial swelling.	Discontinue. Seek emergency treatment.

DIMETHYL SULFOXIDE (DMSO)

WARNINGS & PRECAUTIONS

Don't use if:

- You have a bladder malignancy.
- You are allergic to DMSO.

Before you start, consult your doctor:
If you have visual problems.

Over age 60:
No special problems expected.

Pregnancy:
Decide with you doctor if drug benefits justify risk to unborn child. Risk category C (see page xxii).

Breast-feeding:
Effect not documented. Consult your doctor.

Infants & children:
Not recommended.

Prolonged use:
Talk to your doctor about the need for follow-up medical examinations or laboratory studies to check liver and kidney function, complete blood counts (white blood cell count, platelet count, red blood cell count, hemoglobin, hematocrit) and vision.

Skin & sunlight:
No special problems expected.

Driving, piloting or hazardous work:
No special problems expected.

Discontinuing:
No special problems expected.

Others:
Although readily available in impure forms, DMSO has not proven effective or safe for sprains, strains, arthritis, scleroderma, gout, skin infections, burns or other uses. Many studies are underway for safety and efficacy for conditions other than bladder inflammation.

POSSIBLE INTERACTION WITH OTHER DRUGS

GENERIC NAME OR DRUG CLASS	COMBINED EFFECT
Any other drug used inside the bladder	Increased effect of both medicines.

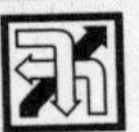

POSSIBLE INTERACTION WITH OTHER SUBSTANCES

INTERACTS WITH	COMBINED EFFECT
Alcohol:	No special problems expected.
Beverages:	No special problems expected.
Cocaine:	No special problems expected.
Foods:	No special problems expected.
Marijuana:	No special problems expected.
Tobacco:	No special problems expected.

*See Glossary

DIPHENIDOL

BRAND NAMES

Vontrol

BASIC INFORMATION

Habit forming? No
Prescription needed? Yes
Available as generic? No
Drug class: Antiemetic, antivertigo

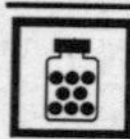

USES

- Prevents motion sickness.
- Controls nausea and vomiting (do not use during pregnancy).

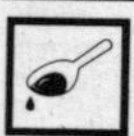

DOSAGE & USAGE INFORMATION

How to take:
Tablet—Swallow with liquid or food to lessen stomach irritation. If you can't swallow whole, crumble tablet and chew or take with liquid or food.

When to take:
30 to 60 minutes before traveling.

If you forget a dose:
Take as soon as you remember. Wait 4 hours for next dose.

What drug does:
Reduces sensitivity of nerve endings in inner ear, blocking messages to brain's vomiting center.

Time lapse before drug works:
30 to 60 minutes.

Don't take with:
Any other medicine without consulting your doctor or pharmacist.

OVERDOSE

SYMPTOMS:
Drowsiness, confusion, incoordination, weak pulse, shallow breathing, stupor, coma.
WHAT TO DO:
- **Dial 911 (emergency) or 0 (operator) for an ambulance or medical help. Then give first aid immediately.**
- **See emergency information on inside covers.**

POSSIBLE ADVERSE REACTIONS OR SIDE EFFECTS

SYMPTOMS	WHAT TO DO
Life-threatening: In case of overdose, see previous column.	
Common: Drowsiness.	Continue. Tell doctor at next visit.
Infrequent:	
• Headache, diarrhea or constipation, heartburn.	Continue. Call doctor when convenient.
• Dry mouth, nose or throat; dizziness.	Continue. Tell doctor at next visit.
Rare:	
• Hallucinations, confusion.	Discontinue. Seek emergency treatment.
• Rash or hives, depression, jaundice.	Discontinue. Call doctor right away.
• Restlessness; excitement; insomnia; blurred vision; urgent, painful or difficult urination.	Continue. Call doctor when convenient.
• Appetite loss, nausea, weakness.	Continue. Tell doctor at next visit.

WARNINGS & PRECAUTIONS

Don't take if:
- You have severe kidney disease.
- You are allergic to diphenidol or meclizine.

Before you start, consult your doctor:
- If you have prostate enlargement.
- If you have glaucoma.
- If you have heart disease.
- If you have intestinal obstruction or ulcers in the gastrointestinal tract.
- If you have kidney disease.
- If you have low blood pressure.
- If you will have surgery within 2 months, including dental surgery, requiring general or spinal anesthesia.

Over age 60:
Adverse reactions and side effects may be more frequent and severe than in younger persons.

Pregnancy:
Decide with your doctor whether drug benefits justify risk to unborn child. Risk category C (see page xxii).

Breast-feeding:
Drug passes into milk. Avoid drug or discontinue nursing until you finish medicine. Consult doctor for advice on maintaining milk supply.

Infants & children:
No problems expected.

Prolonged use:
No problems expected.

Skin & sunlight:
No problems expected.

Driving, piloting or hazardous work:
Don't fly aircraft. Don't drive until you learn how medicine affects you. Don't work around dangerous machinery. Don't climb ladders or work in high places. Danger increases if you drink alcohol or take medicine affecting alertness and reflexes, such as antihistamines, tranquilizers, sedatives, pain medicine, narcotics and mind-altering drugs.

Discontinuing:
No problems expected.

Others:
No problems expected.

POSSIBLE INTERACTION WITH OTHER DRUGS

GENERIC NAME OR DRUG CLASS	COMBINED EFFECT
Anticonvulsants*	Increased effect of both drugs.
Antidepressants, tricyclic*	Increased sedative effect of both drugs.
Antihistamines*	Increased sedative effect of both drugs.
Atropine	Increased chance of toxic effect of atropine and atropine-like medicines.
Narcotics*	Increased sedative effect of both drugs.
Sedatives*	Increased sedative effect of both drugs.
Tranquilizers*	Increased sedative effect of both drugs.

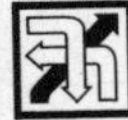

POSSIBLE INTERACTION WITH OTHER SUBSTANCES

INTERACTS WITH	COMBINED EFFECT
Alcohol:	Increased sedation. Avoid.
Beverages: Caffeine.	May decrease drowsiness.
Cocaine:	Increased chance of toxic effects of cocaine. Avoid.
Foods:	None expected.
Marijuana:	Increased drowsiness, dry mouth.
Tobacco:	None expected.

*See Glossary

DIPHENOXYLATE & ATROPINE

BRAND NAMES

Diphenatol
Lofene
Logen
Lomanate
Lomotil
Lonox
Lo-Trol
Nor-Mil

BASIC INFORMATION

Habit forming? Yes
Prescription needed? Yes
Available as generic? Yes
Drug class: Antidiarrheal

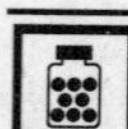

USES

Relieves diarrhea and intestinal cramps.

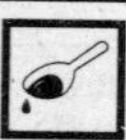

DOSAGE & USAGE INFORMATION

How to take:

- Tablet—Swallow with liquid or food to lessen stomach irritation.
- Drops or liquid—Follow label instructions and use marked dropper.

When to take:
No more often than directed on label.

If you forget a dose:
Take as soon as you remember up to 2 hours late. If more than 2 hours, wait for next scheduled dose (don't double this dose).

What drug does:
Blocks digestive tract's nerve supply, which reduces propelling movements.

Continued next column

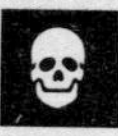

OVERDOSE

SYMPTOMS:
Excitement, constricted pupils, shallow breathing, coma.
WHAT TO DO:

- **Dial 911 (emergency) or 0 (operator) for an ambulance or medical help. Then give first aid immediately.**
- **If patient is unconscious and not breathing, give mouth-to-mouth breathing. If there is no heartbeat, use cardiac massage and mouth-to-mouth breathing (CPR). Don't try to make patient vomit. If you can't get help quickly, take patient to nearest emergency facility.**
- **See emergency information on inside covers.**

Time lapse before drug works:
May require 12 to 24 hours of regular doses to control diarrhea.

Don't take with:
Any other medicine without consulting your doctor or pharmacist.

POSSIBLE ADVERSE REACTIONS OR SIDE EFFECTS

SYMPTOMS	WHAT TO DO
Life-threatening:	
Hives, rash, intense itching, faintness soon after a dose (anaphylaxis).	Seek emergency treatment immediately.
Common:	
None expected.	
Infrequent:	
• Dry mouth, swollen gums, rapid heartbeat.	Discontinue. Call doctor right away.
• Dizziness, depression, drowsiness, rash or itch, blurred vision, decreased urination.	Continue. Call doctor when convenient.
Rare:	
Restlessness, flush, fever, headache, stomach pain, nausea, vomiting, bloating, constipation, numbness of hands or feet.	Discontinue. Call doctor right away.

WARNINGS & PRECAUTIONS

Don't take if:

- You are allergic to diphenoxylate and atropine or any narcotic or anticholinergic.
- You have jaundice.
- You have infectious diarrhea or antibiotic-associated diarrhea.
- Patient is younger than 2.

Before you start, consult your doctor:

- If you have had liver problems.
- If you have ulcerative colitis.
- If you plan to become pregnant within medication period.
- If you have any medical disorder.
- If you take any medication, including nonprescription drugs.

Over age 60:
Adverse reactions and side effects may be more frequent and severe than in younger persons.

Pregnancy:
Decide with your doctor if drug benefits justify risk to unborn child. Risk category C (see page xxii).

Breast-feeding:
Drug passes into milk. Avoid drug or discontinue nursing until you finish medicine. Consult doctor for advice on maintaining milk supply.

Infants & children:
Don't give to infants or toddlers. Use only under doctor's supervision for children older than 2.

Prolonged use:
- Habit forming.
- Talk to your doctor about the need for follow-up medical examinations or laboratory studies to check liver function.

Skin & sunlight:
No problems expected.

Driving, piloting or hazardous work:
Don't drive or pilot aircraft until you learn how medicine affects you. Don't work around dangerous machinery. Don't climb ladders or work in high places. Danger increases if you drink alcohol or take medicine affecting alertness and reflexes.

Discontinuing:
- May be unnecessary to finish medicine. Follow doctor's instructions.
- After discontinuing, consult doctor if you experience muscle cramps, nausea, vomiting, trembling, stomach cramps or unusual sweating.

Others:
If diarrhea lasts longer than 4 days, discontinue and call doctor.

POSSIBLE INTERACTION WITH OTHER DRUGS

GENERIC NAME OR DRUG CLASS	COMBINED EFFECT
Barbiturates*	Increased effect of both drugs.
Clozapine	Toxic effect on the central nervous system.
Ethinamate	Dangerous increased effects of ethinamate. Avoid combining.
Fluoxetine	Increased depressant effects of both drugs.
Guanfacine	May increase depressant effects of either drug.
Leucovorin	High alcohol content of leucovorin may cause adverse effects.
Methyprylon	Increased sedative effect, perhaps to dangerous level. Avoid.
Monozmine oxidase (MAO) inhibitors*	May increase blood pressure excessively.
Naltrexone	Triggers withdrawal symptoms.
Narcotics*	Increased sedation. Avoid.
Sedatives*	Increased effect of both drugs.
Sertraline	Increased depressive effects of both drugs.
Tranquilizers*	Increased effect of both drugs.

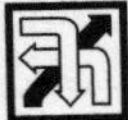

POSSIBLE INTERACTION WITH OTHER SUBSTANCES

INTERACTS WITH	COMBINED EFFECT
Alcohol:	Depressed brain function. Avoid.
Beverages:	None expected.
Cocaine:	Decreased effect of diphenoxylate and atropine.
Foods:	None expected.
Marijuana:	None expected.
Tobacco:	None expected.

*See Glossary

DIPYRIDAMOLE

BRAND NAMES

Apo-Dipyridamole
Dipimol
Dipridacot
Novodipiradol
Persantine
Pyridamole

BASIC INFORMATION

Habit forming? No
Prescription needed?
U.S.: Yes
Canada: No
Available as generic? Yes
Drug class: Platelet aggregation inhibitor

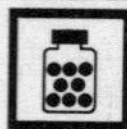

USES

- May reduce frequency and intensity of angina attacks.
- Prevents blood clots after heart surgery.

DOSAGE & USAGE INFORMATION

How to take:
Tablet—Swallow with a full glass of water. If you can't swallow whole, crumble tablet and take with liquid.

When to take:
1 hour before or 2 hours after meals.

If you forget a dose:
Take as soon as you remember up to 2 hours late. If more than 2 hours, wait for next scheduled dose (don't double this dose).

Continued next column

OVERDOSE

SYMPTOMS:
Decreased blood pressure; weak, rapid pulse; cold, clammy skin; collapse.
WHAT TO DO:

- **Dial 911 (emergency) or 0 (operator) for an ambulance or medical help. Then give first aid immediately.**
- **If patient is unconscious and not breathing, give mouth-to-mouth breathing. If there is no heartbeat, use cardiac massage and mouth-to-mouth breathing (CPR). Don't try to make patient vomit. If you can't get help quickly, take patient to nearest emergency facility.**
- **See emergency information on inside covers.**

What drug does:

- Probably dilates blood vessels to increase oxygen to heart.
- Prevents platelet clumping, which causes blood clots.

Time lapse before drug works:
3 months of continual use.

Don't take with:
Any other medicine without consulting your doctor or pharmacist.

POSSIBLE ADVERSE REACTIONS OR SIDE EFFECTS

SYMPTOMS	WHAT TO DO
Life-threatening: In case of overdose, see previous column.	
Common:	
Dizziness.	Continue. Call doctor when convenient.
Infrequent:	
• Fainting, headache.	Discontinue. Call doctor right away.
• Red flush, rash, nausea, vomiting, cramps, weakness.	Continue. Call doctor when convenient.
Rare:	
Chest pain.	Discontinue. Call doctor right away.

WARNINGS & PRECAUTIONS

Don't take if:
- You are allergic to dipyridamole.
- You are recovering from a heart attack.

Before you start, consult your doctor:
- If you have low blood pressure.
- If you have liver disease.

Over age 60:
Begin treatment with small doses.

Pregnancy:
No proven harm to unborn child. Avoid if possible. Consult doctor. Risk category B (see page xxii).

Breast-feeding:
No proven problems. Consult doctor.

Infants & children:
Not recommended.

Prolonged use:
Talk to your doctor about the need for follow-up medical examinations or laboratory studies.

Skin & sunlight:
No problems expected.

Driving, piloting or hazardous work:
Avoid if you feel dizzy. Otherwise, no problems expected.

Discontinuing:
Don't discontinue without doctor's advice until you complete prescribed dose, even though symptoms diminish or disappear.

Others:
- Drug increases your ability to be active without angina pain. Avoid excessive physical exertion that might injure heart.
- Advise any doctor or dentist whom you consult that you take this medicine.

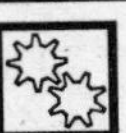

POSSIBLE INTERACTION WITH OTHER DRUGS

GENERIC NAME OR DRUG CLASS	COMBINED EFFECT
Anticoagulants, oral*	Increased anti-coagulant effect. Bleeding tendency.
Aspirin and combination drugs containing aspirin	Increased dipyridamole effect. Dose may need adjustment.

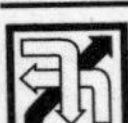

POSSIBLE INTERACTION WITH OTHER SUBSTANCES

INTERACTS WITH	COMBINED EFFECT
Alcohol:	May lower blood pressure excessively.
Beverages:	None expected.
Cocaine:	No proven problems.
Foods:	Decreased dipyridamole absorption unless taken 1 hour before eating.
Marijuana:	Daily use—Decreased dipyridamole effect.
Tobacco: Nicotine.	May decrease dipyridamole effect.

*See Glossary

DISOPYRAMIDE

BRAND NAMES

Norpace
Norpace CR
Rythmodan
Rythmodan-LA

BASIC INFORMATION

Habit forming? No
Prescription needed? Yes
Available as generic? Yes
Drug class: Antiarrhythmic

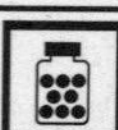

USES

Corrects heart rhythm disorders.

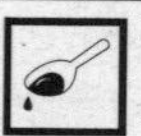

DOSAGE & USAGE INFORMATION

How to take:

- Extended-release tablet or capsule—Swallow with liquid. Do not crush tablet or open capsule.
- Capsule—Swallow with liquid. If you can't swallow whole, ask your pharmacist to prepare a liquid suspension for your use.

When to take:
At the same times each day.

If you forget a dose:
Take as soon as you remember up to 2 hours late. If more than 2 hours, wait for next scheduled dose (don't double this dose).

What drug does:
Delays nerve impulses to heart to regulate heartbeat.

Continued next column

OVERDOSE

SYMPTOMS:
Blood-pressure drop, irregular heartbeat, apnea, loss of consciousness.
WHAT TO DO:

- **Dial 911 (emergency) or 0 (operator) for an ambulance or medical help. Then give first aid immediately.**
- **If patient is unconscious and not breathing, give mouth-to-mouth breathing. If there is no heartbeat, use cardiac massage and mouth-to-mouth breathing (CPR). Don't try to make patient vomit. If you can't get help quickly, take patient to nearest emergency facility.**
- **See emergency information on inside covers.**

Time lapse before drug works:
Begins in 30 to 60 minutes. Must use for 5 to 7 days to determine effectiveness.

Don't take with:
Any other medicine without consulting your doctor or pharmacist.

POSSIBLE ADVERSE REACTIONS OR SIDE EFFECTS

SYMPTOMS	WHAT TO DO
Life-threatening:	
Hives, rash, intense itching, faintness soon after a dose (anaphylaxis).	Seek emergency treatment immediately.
Common:	
• Hypoglycemia (cold sweats, fast heartbeat, extreme hunger, shakiness and nervousness, anxiety, cool and pale skin, drowsiness, headache).	Discontinue. Call doctor right away.
• Dry mouth, constipation, painful or difficult urination, rapid weight gain, blurred vision.	Continue. Call doctor when convenient.
Infrequent:	
• Dizziness, fainting, confusion, chest pain, nervousness, depression, slow or fast heartbeat.	Discontinue. Call doctor right away.
• Swollen feet.	Continue. Call doctor when convenient.
Rare:	
• Shortness of breath, psychosis.	Discontinue. Seek emergency treatment.
• Rash, sore throat, fever, headache, jaundice, muscle weakness.	Discontinue. Call doctor right away.
• Eye pain, diminished sex drive, numbness or tingling of hands and feet, bleeding tendency.	Continue. Call doctor when convenient.

WARNINGS & PRECAUTIONS

Don't take if:

- You are allergic to disopyramide or any antiarrhythmic.
- You have second- or third-degree heart block.
- You have heart failure.

Before you start, consult your doctor:

- If you react unfavorably to other anti-arrhythmic drugs.
- If you have had heart disease.
- If you have low blood pressure.
- If you have liver disease.
- If you have glaucoma.
- If you have enlarged prostate.
- If you have myasthenia gravis.
- If you take digitalis preparations or diuretics.

Over age 60:

- May require reduced dose.
- More likely to have difficulty urinating or be constipated.
- More likely to have blood pressure drop.

Pregnancy:
Decide with your doctor if drug benefits justify risk to unborn child. Risk category C (see page xxii).

Breast-feeding:
Drug passes into milk. Avoid drug or discontinue nursing until you finish medicine. Consult doctor for advice on maintaining milk supply.

Infants & children:
Safety not established. Don't use.

Prolonged use:
Talk to your doctor about the need for follow-up medical examinations or laboratory studies to check liver function, kidney function, ECG*, blood pressure, serum potassium.

Skin & sunlight:
No problems expected.

Driving, piloting or hazardous work:
Don't drive or pilot aircraft until you learn how medicine affects you. Don't work around dangerous machinery. Don't climb ladders or work in high places. Danger increases if you drink alcohol or take medicine affecting alertness and reflexes, such as antihistamines, tranquilizers, sedatives, pain medicine, narcotics, or mind-altering drugs.

Discontinuing:
Don't discontinue without doctor's advice until you complete prescribed dose, even though symptoms diminish or disappear.

Others:
If new illness, injury or surgery occurs, tell doctors of disopyramide use.

POSSIBLE INTERACTION WITH OTHER DRUGS

GENERIC NAME OR DRUG CLASS	COMBINED EFFECT
Antiarrhythmics*	May increase effect and toxicity of each drug.
Anticholinergics*	Increased anticholinergic effect.
Anticoagulants, oral*	Possible increased anticoagulant effect.
Antihypertensives*	Increased anti-hypertensive effect.
Cisapride	Decreased disopyramide effect.
Encainide	Increased effect of toxicity on the heart muscle.
Flecainide	Possible irregular heartbeat.
Nicardipine	May cause dangerously slow, fast or irregular heartbeat.
Nimodipine	May cause dangerous irregular, slow or fast heartbeat.
Phenobarbital	Increased metabolism, decreased disopyramide effect.
Phenytoin	Increased metabolism, decreased disopyramide effect.
Propafenone	Increased effect of both drugs and increased risk of toxicity.
Rifampin	Increased metabolism, decreased disopyramide effect.
Tocainide	Increased likelihood of adverse reactions with either drug.

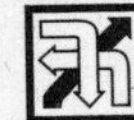

POSSIBLE INTERACTION WITH OTHER SUBSTANCES

INTERACTS WITH	COMBINED EFFECT
Alcohol:	Decreased blood pressure and blood sugar. Use caution.
Beverages:	None expected.
Cocaine:	Irregular heartbeat.
Foods:	None expected.
Marijuana:	Unpredictable. May decrease disopyramide effect.
Tobacco:	May decrease disopyramide effect.

***See Glossary**

DISULFIRAM

BRAND NAMES

Antabuse

BASIC INFORMATION

Habit forming? No
Prescription needed? Yes
Available as generic? Yes
Drug class: None

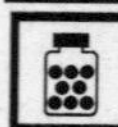

USES

Treatment for alcoholism. Will not cure alcoholism, but is a powerful deterrent to drinking.

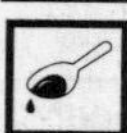

DOSAGE & USAGE INFORMATION

How to take:
Tablet—Swallow with liquid.

When to take:
Morning or bedtime. Avoid if you have used *any* alcohol, tonics, cough syrups, fermented vinegar, after-shave lotion or backrub solutions within 12 hours.

If you forget a dose:
Take as soon as you remember up to 12 hours late. If more than 12 hours, wait for next scheduled dose (don't double this dose).

What drug does:
In combination with alcohol, produces a metabolic change that causes severe, temporary toxicity.

Time lapse before drug works:
3 to 12 hours.

Continued next column

OVERDOSE

SYMPTOMS:
Memory loss, behavior disturbances, lethargy, confusion and headaches; nausea, vomiting, stomach pain and diarrhea; weakness and unsteady walk; temporary paralysis.

WHAT TO DO:
- **Dial 911 (emergency) or 0 (operator) for an ambulance or medical help. Then give first aid immediately.**
- **See emergency information on inside covers.**

Don't take with:
- See Interaction column and consult doctor.
- Nonprescription drugs that contain *any* alcohol.
- Any other central nervous system (CNS) depressant drugs*.

POSSIBLE ADVERSE REACTIONS OR SIDE EFFECTS

SYMPTOMS	WHAT TO DO
Life-threatening:	
In case of overdose, see previous column.	
Common:	
Drowsiness.	Continue. Tell doctor at next visit.
Infrequent:	
• Eye pain, vision changes, abdominal discomfort, throbbing headache, numbness in hands and feet.	Continue. Call doctor when convenient.
• Mood change, decreased sexual ability in men, tiredness.	Continue. Tell doctor at next visit.
• Bad taste in mouth (metal or garlic).	No action necessary.
Rare:	
Rash, jaundice.	Discontinue. Call doctor right away.

WARNINGS & PRECAUTIONS

Don't take if:
- You are allergic to disulfiram (alcohol-disulfiram combination is not an allergic reaction).
- You have used alcohol in any form or amount within 12 hours.
- You have taken paraldehyde within 1 week.
- You have heart disease.

Before you start, consult your doctor:
- If you have allergies.
- If you plan to become pregnant within medication period.
- If no one has explained to you how disulfiram reacts.
- If you think you cannot avoid drinking.
- If you have diabetes, epilepsy, liver or kidney disease.
- If you take other drugs.

Over age 60:
Adverse reactions and side effects may be more frequent and severe than in younger persons.

Pregnancy:
Decide with your doctor if drug benefits justify risk to unborn child. Risk category C (see page xxii).

Breast-feeding:
Studies inconclusive. Consult your doctor.

Infants & children:
Not recommended.

Prolonged use:
Periodic blood cell counts and liver function tests recommended if you take this drug a long time.

Skin & sunlight:
No problems expected.

Driving, piloting or hazardous work:
Avoid if you feel drowsy or have vision side effects. Otherwise, no restrictions.

Discontinuing:
Don't discontinue without consulting doctor. Dose may require gradual reduction if you have taken drug for a long time. Doses of other drugs may also require adjustment. Avoid alcohol at least 14 days following last dose.

Others:
Check all liquids that you take or rub on for presence of alcohol.

POSSIBLE INTERACTION WITH OTHER DRUGS

GENERIC NAME OR DRUG CLASS	COMBINED EFFECT
Anticoagulants*	Possible unexplained bleeding.
Anticonvulsants*	Excessive sedation.
Barbiturates*	Excessive sedation.
Cephalosporins*	Disulfiram reaction.*
Clozapine	Toxic effect on the central nervous system.
Ethinamate	Dangerous increased effects of ethinamate. Avoid combining.
Fluoxetine	Increased depressant effects of both drugs.
Guanfacine	May increase depressant effects of either drug.
Isoniazid	Unsteady walk and disturbed behavior.
Leucovorin	High alcohol content of leucovorin may cause adverse effects.
Methyprylon	Increased sedative effect, perhaps to dangerous level. Avoid.
Metronidazole	Disulfiram reaction.*
Nabilone	Greater depression of central nervous system.
Paraldehyde	Increased paraldehyde effect. Avoid simultaneous use.
Sedatives*	Excessive sedation.
Sertraline	Increased depressive effects of both drugs.

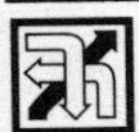

POSSIBLE INTERACTION WITH OTHER SUBSTANCES

INTERACTS WITH	COMBINED EFFECT
Alcohol: *Any* form or amount.	Possible life-threatening toxicity. See disulfiram reaction.*
Beverages: Punch or fruit drink that may contain alcohol.	Disulfiram reaction.*
Cocaine:	Increased disulfiram effect.
Foods: Sauces, fermented vinegar, marinades, desserts or other foods prepared with *any* alcohol.	Disulfiram reaction.*
Marijuana:	None expected.
Tobacco:	None expected.

*See Glossary

DIURETICS, LOOP

BRAND AND GENERIC NAMES

Apo-Furosemide
Bumex
BUMETANIDE
Demadex
Edecrin
ETHACRYNIC ACID
FUROSEMIDE
Furoside
Lasix
Lasix Special
Myrosemide
Novosemide
TORSEMIDE
Uritol

BASIC INFORMATION

Habit forming? No
Prescription needed? Yes
Available as generic? Yes
Drug class: Diuretic (loop), antihypertensive

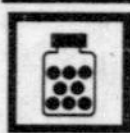

USES

- Lowers high blood pressure.
- Decreases fluid retention.

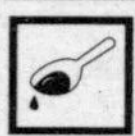

DOSAGE & USAGE INFORMATION

How to take:
Tablet or liquid—Swallow with liquid. If you can't swallow whole, crumble tablet and take with liquid or food.

When to take:
- 1 dose a day—Take after breakfast.
- More than 1 dose a day—Take last dose no later than 6 p.m. unless otherwise directed.

If you forget a dose:
- 1 dose a day—Take as soon as you remember up to 12 hours late. If more than 12 hours, wait for next scheduled dose (don't double this dose).
- More than 1 dose a day—Take as soon as you remember up to 2 hours late. If more than 2 hours, wait for next scheduled dose (don't double this dose).

Continued next column

OVERDOSE

SYMPTOMS:
Weakness, lethargy, dizziness, confusion, nausea, vomiting, leg muscle cramps, thirst, stupor, deep sleep, weak and rapid pulse, cardiac arrest.
WHAT TO DO:
- **Dial 911 (emergency) or 0 (operator) for an ambulance or medical help. Then give first aid immediately.**
- **See emergency information on inside covers.**

What drug does:
Increases elimination of sodium and water from body. Decreased body fluid reduces blood pressure.

Time lapse before drug works:
1 hour to increase water loss. Requires 2 to 3 weeks to lower blood pressure.

Don't take with:
- Nonprescription drugs with aspirin.
- Any other medicine without consulting your doctor.

POSSIBLE ADVERSE REACTIONS OR SIDE EFFECTS

SYMPTOMS	WHAT TO DO
Life-threatening: In case of overdose, see previous column.	
Common: Dizziness.	Continue. Call doctor when convenient.
Infrequent: Mood change, fatigue, appetite loss, diarrhea, irregular heartbeat, muscle cramps, low blood pressure, abdominal pain, weakness.	Discontinue. Call doctor right away.
Rare: Rash or hives, yellow vision, ringing in ears, hearing loss, sore throat, fever, dry mouth, thirst, side or stomach pain, nausea, vomiting, unusual bleeding or bruising, joint pain, jaundice, numbness or tingling in hands or feet.	Discontinue. Call doctor right away.

WARNINGS & PRECAUTIONS

Don't take if:
You are allergic to loop diuretics.

Before you start, consult your doctor:
- If you are taking any other prescription or nonprescription medicine.
- If you are allergic to any sulfa drug.
- If you have liver or kidney disease.
- If you have gout, diabetes or impaired hearing.
- If you will have surgery within 2 months, including dental surgery, requiring general or spinal anesthesia.

Over age 60:
Adverse reactions and side effects may be more frequent and severe than in younger persons.

Pregnancy:
Risk factors vary for drugs in this group. See category list on page xxii and consult doctor.

Breast-feeding:
Drug filters into milk. May harm child. Avoid.

Infants & children:
Use only under medical supervision.

Prolonged use:
- Impaired balance of water, salt and potassium in blood and body tissues.
- Possible diabetes.

Skin & sunlight:
May cause rash or intensify sunburn in areas exposed to sun or sunlamp.

Driving, piloting or hazardous work:
Avoid if you feel dizzy; otherwise no problems expected.

Discontinuing:
Don't discontinue without doctor's advice until you complete prescribed dose, even though symptoms diminish or disappear.

Others:
Frequent laboratory studies to monitor potassium level in blood recommended. Eat foods rich in potassium or take potassium supplements. Consult doctor.

POSSIBLE INTERACTION WITH OTHER DRUGS

GENERIC NAME OR DRUG CLASS	COMBINED EFFECT
Allopurinol	Decreased allopurinol effect.
Amiodarone	Increased risk of heartbeat irregularity due to low potassium.
Angiotensin-converting enzyme (ACE) inhibitors*	Possible excessive potassium in blood.
Anticoagulants*	Abnormal clotting.
Antidepressants, tricyclic*	Excessive blood pressure drop.
Antidiabetics, oral*	Decreased anti-diabetic effect.
Antihypertensives*	Increased anti-hypertensive effect. Dosages may require adjustment.
Anti-inflammatory drugs, nonsteroidal (NSAIDs)*	Decreased diuretic effect.
Barbiturates*	Low blood pressure.
Beta-adrenergic blocking agents*	Increased anti-hypertensive effect. Dosages may require adjustment.
Corticosteroids*	Decreased potassium.
Cortisone drugs*	Excessive potassium loss.
Digitalis preparations*	Excessive potassium loss could lead to serious heart rhythm disorders.
Diuretics, other*	Increased diuretic effect.
Hypokalemia-causing medicines*	Increased risk of excessive potassium loss.
Insulin	Decreased insulin effect.
Lithium	Increased lithium toxicity.
Narcotics*	Dangerous low blood pressure. Avoid.
Nephrotoxics*	Increased risk of toxicity.
Nimodipine	Dangerous blood pressure drop.
Nitrates*	Excessive blood pressure drop.
Phenytoin	Decreased diuretic effect.
Potassium supplements*	Decreased potassium effect.

Continued on page 938

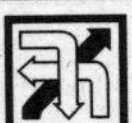

POSSIBLE INTERACTION WITH OTHER SUBSTANCES

INTERACTS WITH	COMBINED EFFECT
Alcohol:	Blood pressure drop. Avoid.
Beverages:	None expected.
Cocaine:	Dangerous blood pressure drop. Avoid.
Foods:	None expected.
Marijuana:	Increased thirst and urinary frequency, fainting.
Tobacco:	Decreased furosemide effect.

***See Glossary**

DIURETICS, THIAZIDE

BRAND AND GENERIC NAMES

See complete list of brand and generic names in the *Brand Names Directory*, page 907.

BASIC INFORMATION

Habit forming? No
Prescription needed? Yes
Available as generic? Yes, for some.
Drug class: Antihypertensive, diuretic (thiazide)

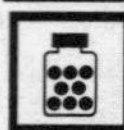

USES

- Controls, but doesn't cure, high blood pressure.
- Reduces fluid retention (edema) caused by conditions such as heart disorders and liver disease.

DOSAGE & USAGE INFORMATION

How to take:
Tablet or liquid—Swallow with liquid. If you can't swallow whole, crumble tablet and take with liquid or food. Don't exceed dose.

When to take:
At the same time each day.

If you forget a dose:
Take as soon as you remember up to 2 hours late. If more than 2 hours, wait for next scheduled dose (don't double this dose).

What drug does:
- Forces sodium and water excretion, reducing body fluid.
- Relaxes muscle cells of small arteries.
- Reduced body fluid and relaxed arteries lower blood pressure.

Time lapse before drug works:
4 to 6 hours. May require several weeks to lower blood pressure.

Continued next column

OVERDOSE

SYMPTOMS:
Cramps, weakness, drowsiness, weak pulse, coma.
WHAT TO DO:
- **Dial 911 (emergency) or 0 (operator) for an ambulance or medical help. Then give first aid immediately.**
- **See emergency information on inside covers.**

Don't take with:
- Nonprescription drugs without consulting doctor.
- See Interaction column and consult doctor.

POSSIBLE ADVERSE REACTIONS OR SIDE EFFECTS

SYMPTOMS	WHAT TO DO
Life-threatening:	
In case of overdose, see previous column.	
Common:	
Muscle cramps.	Discontinue. Call doctor right away.
Infrequent:	
• Blurred vision, severe abdominal pain, nausea, vomiting, irregular heartbeat, weak pulse.	Discontinue. Call doctor right away.
• Dizziness, mood changes, headaches, weakness, tiredness, weight changes, decreased sex drive, diarrhea.	Continue. Call doctor when convenient.
• Dry mouth, thirst.	Continue. Tell doctor at next visit.
Rare:	
• Rash or hives.	Discontinue. Seek emergency treatment.
• Jaundice, joint pain, black stools.	Discontinue. Call doctor right away.
• Sore throat, fever.	Continue. Tell doctor at next visit.

WARNINGS & PRECAUTIONS

Don't take if:
You are allergic to any thiazide diuretic drug.

Before you start, consult your doctor:
- If you are allergic to any sulfa drug or tartrazine dye.
- If you have gout, systemic lupus erythematosis.
- If you have liver, pancreas, diabetes or kidney disorder.

Over age 60:
Adverse reactions and side effects may be more frequent and severe than in younger persons, especially dizziness and excessive potassium loss.

Pregnancy:
Risk factors vary for drugs in this group. See category list on page xxii and consult doctor.

Breast-feeding:
Drug passes into milk. Avoid drug or discontinue nursing.

Infants & children:
No problems expected.

Prolonged use:
- You may need medicine to treat high blood pressure for the rest of your life.
- Talk to your doctor about the need for follow-up medical examinations or laboratory studies to check blood sugar, kidney function, blood pressure, serum electrolytes.

Skin & sunlight:
May cause rash or intensify sunburn in areas exposed to sun or sunlamp.

Driving, piloting or hazardous work:
Don't drive or pilot aircraft until you learn how medicine affects you. Don't work around dangerous machinery. Don't climb ladders or work in high places. Danger increases if you drink alcohol or take medicine affecting alertness and reflexes, such as antihistamines, tranquilizers, sedatives, pain medicine, narcotics and mind-altering drugs.

Discontinuing:
Don't discontinue without medical advice.

Others:
- Hot weather and fever may cause dehydration and drop in blood pressure. Dose may require temporary adjustment. Weigh daily and report any unexpected weight decreases to your doctor.
- May cause rise in uric acid, leading to gout.
- May cause blood-sugar rise in diabetics.
- May affect results in some medical tests.
- Advise any doctor or dentist whom you consult that you take this medicine.

POSSIBLE INTERACTION WITH OTHER DRUGS

GENERIC NAME OR DRUG CLASS	COMBINED EFFECT
Allopurinol	Decreased allopurinol effect.
Amiodarone	Increased risk of heartbeat irregularity due to low potassium.
Amphotericin B	Increased potassium.
Angiotensin-converting enzyme (ACE) inhibitors*	Decreased blood pressure.
Antidepressants, tricyclic*	Dangerous drop in blood pressure. Avoid combination unless under medical supervision.
Antidiabetic agents, oral*	Increased blood sugar.
Antihypertensives*	Increased hypertensive effect.
Barbiturates*	Increased anti-hypertensive effect.
Beta-adrenergic blocking agents*	Increased anti-hypertensive effect. Dosages of both drugs may require adjustments.
Calcium supplements*	Increased calcium in blood.
Carteolol	Increased anti-hypertensive effect.
Cholestyramine	Decreased anti-hypertensive effect.
Colestipol	Decreased anti-hypertensive effect.
Cortisone drugs*	Excessive potassium loss that causes dangerous heart rhythms.
Didanosine	Increased risk of pancreatitis.
Digitalis preparations*	Excessive potassium loss that causes dangerous heart rhythms.
Diuretics, thiazide*, other	Increased effect of other thiazide diuretics.

Continued on page 938

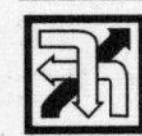

POSSIBLE INTERACTION WITH OTHER SUBSTANCES

INTERACTS WITH	COMBINED EFFECT
Alcohol:	Dangerous blood pressure drop.
Beverages:	None expected.
Cocaine	Increased risk of heart block and high blood pressure.
Foods: Licorice.	Excessive potassium loss that causes dangerous heart rhythms.
Marijuana:	May increase blood pressure.
Tobacco:	None expected.

DIVALPROEX

BRAND NAMES

Depakote
Depakote Sprinkle
Epival

BASIC INFORMATION

Habit forming? No
Prescription needed? Yes
Available as generic? No
Drug class: Anticonvulsant

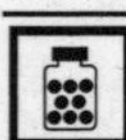

USES

Controls petit mal (absence) seizures in treatment of epilepsy.

DOSAGE & USAGE INFORMATION

How to take:
Delayed-release capsule or delayed-release tablet—Swallow with liquid or food to lessen stomach irritation. Do not crumble capsule or crush tablet.

When to take:
Once or twice a day as directed by your doctor.

If you forget a dose:
Take as soon as you remember. Don't ever double dose.

What drug does:
Increases concentration of gamma aminobutyric acid, which inhibits nerve transmission in parts of brain.

Time lapse before drug works:
1 to 4 hours.

Don't take with:
Any other medicine without consulting your doctor or pharmacist.

OVERDOSE

SYMPTOMS:
Coma.
WHAT TO DO:

- **Dial 911 (emergency) or 0 (operator) for an ambulance or medical help. Then give first aid immediately.**
- **If patient is unconscious and not breathing, give mouth-to-mouth breathing. If there is no heartbeat, use cardiac massage and mouth-to-mouth breathing (CPR). Don't try to make patient vomit. If you can't get help quickly, take patient to nearest emergency facility.**
- **See emergency information on inside covers.**

POSSIBLE ADVERSE REACTIONS OR SIDE EFFECTS

SYMPTOMS	WHAT TO DO
Life-threatening: In case of overdose, see previous column.	
Common:	
Menstrual irregularities, nausea, vomiting, abdominal cramps, diarrhea, tremor, weight gain.	Continue. Call doctor when convenient.
Infrequent:	
• Rash, bloody spots under skin, hair loss, bleeding, easy bruising.	Continue, but call doctor right away.
• Drowsiness, weakness, easily upset emotionally, depression, psychic changes, headache, incoordination, appetite change, constipation.	Continue. Call doctor when convenient.
Rare:	
• Double vision, unusual movements of eyes (nystagmus), jaundice, increased bleeding tendency, edema (swelling of feet and legs).	Continue, but call doctor right away.
• Anemia (paleness, fatigue).	Continue. Call doctor when convenient.

WARNINGS & PRECAUTIONS

Don't take if:
You are allergic to divalproex.

Before you start, consult your doctor:
- If you have blood, kidney or liver disease.
- If you will have surgery within 2 months, including dental surgery, requiring general or spinal anesthesia.

Over age 60:
Adverse reactions and side effects may be more frequent and severe than in younger persons.

Pregnancy:
Risk to unborn child outweighs drug benefits. Don't use. Risk category D (see page xxii).

Breast-feeding:
Unknown effect. Consult doctor.

Infants & children:
Under close medical supervision only.

Prolonged use:
Request periodic blood tests, liver and kidney function tests.

Skin & sunlight:
No problems expected.

Driving, piloting or hazardous work:
Don't drive or pilot aircraft until you learn how medicine affects you. Don't work around dangerous machinery. Don't climb ladders or work in high places. Danger increases if you drink alcohol or take medicine affecting alertness and reflexes, such as antihistamines, tranquilizers, sedatives, pain medicine, narcotics and mind-altering drugs.

Discontinuing:
Don't discontinue without consulting doctor. Dose may require gradual reduction if you have taken drug for a long time. Doses of other drugs may also require adjustment.

Others:
Advise any doctor or dentist whom you consult that you take this medicine.

POSSIBLE INTERACTION WITH OTHER DRUGS

GENERIC NAME OR DRUG CLASS	COMBINED EFFECT
Anticoagulants*	Increases chance of bleeding.
Aspirin	Increases chance of bleeding.
Central nervous system (CNS) depressants* (antidepressants,* antihistamines,* muscle relaxants,* narcotics,* sedatives,* sleeping pills,* tranquilizers*)	Increases sedative effect.
Clonazepam	May cause or prolong seizure.
Dipyridamole	Increases chance of bleeding.
Monoamine oxidase (MAO) inhibitors*	Increases sedative effect.
Nabilone	Greater depression of central nervous system.
Phenobarbital	Increases chance of toxicity.
Phenytoin	Unpredictable. May require increased or decreased dosage.
Primidone	Increases chance of toxicity.
Sertraline	Increased depressive effect of both drugs.
Sulfinpyrazone	Increases chance of bleeding.

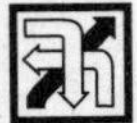

POSSIBLE INTERACTION WITH OTHER SUBSTANCES

INTERACTS WITH	COMBINED EFFECT
Alcohol:	Deep sedation. Avoid.
Beverages:	No problems expected.
Cocaine:	Increased brain sensitivity. Avoid.
Foods:	No problems expected.
Marijuana:	Increased brain sensitivity. Avoid.
Tobacco:	Increased brain sensitivity. Avoid.

*See Glossary

DOCUSATES

BRAND AND GENERIC NAMES

See complete list of brand names in the *Brand Name Directory*, page 907.

BASIC INFORMATION

Habit forming? No
Prescription needed? No
Available as generic? Yes
Drug class: Laxative (stool softener)

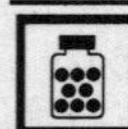

USES

Constipation relief.

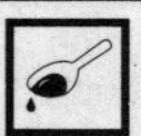

DOSAGE & USAGE INFORMATION

How to take:

- Tablet or capsule—Swallow with liquid. Don't open capsules.
- Syrup—Take as directed on bottle.
- Effervescent granules—Dissolve granules in 4 oz. cool water. Drink all the water.
- Rectal dosage—Follow instructions on package

When to take:
At the same time each day, preferably bedtime. Follow doctor's instructions for a prescribed laxative.

If you forget a dose:
Take as soon as you remember. Wait 12 hours for next dose. Return to regular schedule.

What drug does:
Makes stool hold fluid so it is easier to pass.

Time lapse before drug works:
2 to 3 days of continual use.

Don't take with:

- Other medicines at same time. Wait 2 hours.
- Any other medicine without consulting your doctor or pharmacist.

OVERDOSE

SYMPTOMS:
Appetite loss, nausea, vomiting, diarrhea.
WHAT TO DO:
Overdose unlikely to threaten life. If person takes much larger amount than prescribed, call doctor, poison control center or hospital emergency room for instructions.

POSSIBLE ADVERSE REACTIONS OR SIDE EFFECTS

SYMPTOMS	WHAT TO DO
Life-threatening: None expected.	
Common: None expected.	
Infrequent: Throat irritation (liquid only), intestinal and stomach cramps.	Continue. Call doctor when convenient.
Rare: Rash.	Discontinue. Call doctor right away.

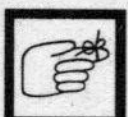

WARNINGS & PRECAUTIONS

Don't take if:
- You are allergic to any emollient laxative.
- You have abdominal pain and fever that might be appendicitis.

Before you start, consult your doctor:
- If you are taking other laxatives.
- To be sure constipation isn't a sign of a serious disorder.

Over age 60:
You must drink 6 to 8 glasses of fluid every 24 hours for drug to work.

Pregnancy:
Consult doctor. Risk category C (see page xxii).

Breast-feeding:
No problems expected. Consult doctor.

Infants & children:
No problems expected. Do not give laxatives to a child under age 6 without doctor's approval.

Prolonged use:
Avoid. Overuse of laxatives may damage intestine lining.

Skin & sunlight:
No problems expected.

Driving, piloting or hazardous work:
No problems expected.

Discontinuing:
May be unnecessary to finish medicine. Follow doctor's instructions.

Others:
No problems expected.

POSSIBLE INTERACTION WITH OTHER DRUGS

GENERIC NAME OR DRUG CLASS	COMBINED EFFECT
Danthron	Possible liver damage.
Digitalis preparations*	Toxic absorption of digitalis.
Mineral oil	Increased mineral oil absorption into bloodstream. Avoid. May cause tumor-like deposits in tissues.
Phenolphthalein	Increased phenolphthalein absorption. Possible toxicity.

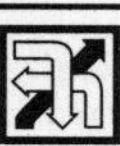

POSSIBLE INTERACTION WITH OTHER SUBSTANCES

INTERACTS WITH	COMBINED EFFECT
Alcohol:	None expected.
Beverages:	None expected.
Cocaine:	None expected.
Foods:	None expected.
Marijuana:	None expected.
Tobacco:	None expected.

*See Glossary

DOXAZOSIN

BRAND NAMES

Cardura

BASIC INFORMATION

Habit forming? No
Prescription needed? Yes
Available as generic? Yes
Drug class: Antihypertensive

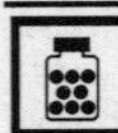

USES

- Treatment for high blood pressure.
- May improve congestive heart failure.
- Treatment for Raynaud's disease.

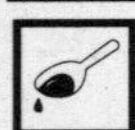

DOSAGE & USAGE INFORMATION

How to take:
Tablet—Swallow with liquid. If you can't swallow whole, crumble tablet and take with liquid or food.

When to take:
At the same times each day.

If you forget a dose:
Take as soon as you remember up to 2 hours late. If more than 2 hours, wait for next scheduled dose (don't double this dose).

What drug does:
Expands and relaxes blood vessel walls to lower blood pressure.

Time lapse before drug works:
30 minutes.

Don't take with:
Any other medicine without consulting your doctor or pharmacist.

OVERDOSE

SYMPTOMS:
Extreme weakness; loss of consciousness; cold, sweaty skin; weak, rapid pulse; coma.
WHAT TO DO:

- **Dial 911 (emergency) or 0 (operator) for an ambulance or medical help. Then give first aid immediately.**
- **If patient is unconscious and not breathing, give mouth-to-mouth breathing. If there is no heartbeat, use cardiac massage and mouth-to-mouth breathing (CPR). Don't try to make patient vomit. If you can't get help quickly, take patient to nearest emergency facility.**
- **See emergency information on inside covers.**

POSSIBLE ADVERSE REACTIONS OR SIDE EFFECTS

SYMPTOMS	WHAT TO DO
Life-threatening: In case of overdose, see previous column.	
Common:	
• Rapid heartbeat.	Discontinue. Call doctor right away.
• Vivid dreams, drowsiness, dizziness.	Continue. Call doctor when convenient.
Infrequent:	
• Rash or itchy skin, blurred vision, shortness of breath, difficult breathing, chest pain.	Discontinue. Call doctor right away.
• Appetite loss, constipation or diarrhea, abdominal pain, nausea, vomiting, fluid retention, joint or muscle aches, weakness and faintness when arising from bed or chair.	Continue. Call doctor when convenient.
• Headache, irritability, depression, dry mouth, stuffy nose, increased urination.	Continue. Tell doctor at next visit.
Rare:	
Decreased sexual function, numbness or tingling in hands or feet.	Continue. Call doctor when convenient.

WARNINGS & PRECAUTIONS

Don't take if:
- You are allergic to prazosin.
- You are depressed.
- You will have surgery within 2 months, including dental surgery, requiring general or spinal anesthesia.

Before you start, consult your doctor:
- If you experience lightheadedness or fainting with other antihypertensive drugs.
- If you are easily depressed.
- If you have impaired brain circulation or have had a stroke.
- If you have coronary heart disease (with or without angina).
- If you have kidney disease or impaired liver function.

Over age 60:
Begin with no more than 1 mg. per day for first 3 days. Increases should be gradual and supervised by your doctor. Don't stand while taking. Sudden changes in position may cause falls. Sit or lie down promptly if you feel dizzy. If you have impaired brain circulation or coronary heart disease, excessive lowering of blood pressure should be avoided. Report problems to your doctor immediately.

Pregnancy:
Consult doctor. Risk category B (see page xxii).

Breast-feeding:
No proven problems. Consult doctor.

Infants & children:
Not recommended.

Prolonged use:
Talk to your doctor about the need for follow-up medical examinations or laboratory studies.

Skin & sunlight:
No problems expected.

Driving, piloting or hazardous work:
Don't drive or pilot aircraft until you learn how medicine affects you. Don't work around dangerous machinery. Don't climb ladders or work in high places.

Discontinuing:
Don't discontinue without doctor's advice until you complete prescribed dose, even though symptoms diminish or disappear.

Others:
First dose likely to cause dizziness or lightheadedness. Take drug at night and get out of bed slowly next morning.

POSSIBLE INTERACTION WITH OTHER DRUGS

GENERIC NAME OR DRUG CLASS	COMBINED EFFECT
Amphetamines*	Decreased doxazosin effect.
Antihypertensives, other*	Increased anti-hypertensive effect. Dosages may require adjustments.
Anti-inflammatory drugs, nonsteroidal (NSAIDs)*	Decreased effect of doxazosin.
Estrogen	Decreased effect of doxazosin.
Sympathomimetics*	Decreased effect of doxazosin.

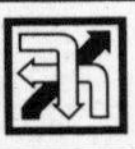

POSSIBLE INTERACTION WITH OTHER SUBSTANCES

INTERACTS WITH	COMBINED EFFECT
Alcohol:	Excessive blood pressure drop.
Beverages:	None expected.
Cocaine:	Increased risk of heart block and high blood pressure.
Foods:	None expected.
Marijuana:	Possible fainting. Avoid.
Tobacco:	Possible spasm of coronary arteries. Avoid.

DRONABINOL (THC, Marijuana)

BRAND NAMES

Marinol

BASIC INFORMATION

Habit forming? Yes
Prescription needed? Yes
Available as generic? No
Drug class: Antiemetic

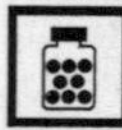

USES

- Prevents nausea and vomiting that may accompany taking anticancer medication (cancer chemotherapy). Should not be used unless other antinausea medicines fail.
- Appetite stimulant.

DOSAGE & USAGE INFORMATION

How to take:
Capsule—Swallow with liquid.

When to take:
Under supervision, a total of no more than 4 to 6 doses per day, every 2 to 4 hours after cancer chemotherapy for prescribed number of days.

If you forget a dose:
Take as soon as you remember up to 2 hours late. If more than 2 hours, wait for next scheduled dose (don't double this dose).

What drug does:
Affects nausea and vomiting center in brain to make it less irritable following cancer chemotherapy. Exact mechanism is unknown.

Time lapse before drug works:
2 to 4 hours.

Don't take with:
- Nonprescription drugs without consulting doctor.
- Drugs in interaction column without consulting doctor.

OVERDOSE

SYMPTOMS:
Pounding, rapid heart rate; high or low blood pressure; confusion; hallucinations; drastic mood changes; nervousness or anxiety.
WHAT TO DO:
Overdose unlikely to threaten life. If person takes much larger amount than prescribed, call doctor, poison control center or hospital emergency room for instructions.

POSSIBLE ADVERSE REACTIONS OR SIDE EFFECTS

SYMPTOMS	WHAT TO DO
Life-threatening:	
In case of overdose, see previous column.	
Common:	
• Rapid, pounding heartbeat.	Discontinue. Call doctor right away.
• Dizziness, irritability, drowsiness, euphoria, decreased coordination.	Continue. Call doctor when convenient.
• Red eyes, dry mouth.	No action necessary.
Infrequent:	
• Depression, anxiety, nervousness, headache, hallucinations, dramatic mood changes.	Discontinue. Call doctor right away.
• Blurred or changed vision.	Continue. Call doctor when convenient.
Rare:	
• Rapid heartbeat, fainting, frequent or difficult urination, convulsions, shortness of breath.	Discontinue. Call doctor right away.
• Paranoia, nausea, loss of appetite, dizziness when standing after sitting or lying down, diarrhea.	Continue. Call doctor when convenient.

WARNINGS & PRECAUTIONS

Don't take if:
- Your nausea and vomiting is caused by anything other than cancer chemotherapy.
- You are sensitive or allergic to any form of marijuana or sesame oil.
- Your cycle of chemotherapy is longer than 7 consecutive days. Harmful side effects may occur.

Before you start, consult your doctor:
- If you have heart disease or high blood pressure.
- If you are an alcoholic or drug addict.
- If you are pregnant or intend to become pregnant.
- If you are nursing an infant.
- If you have schizophrenia or a manic-depressive disorder.

Over age 60:
Adverse reactions and side effects may be more frequent and severe than in younger persons.

Pregnancy:
Decide with your doctor if drug benefits justify risk to unborn child. Risk category C (see page xxii).

Breast-feeding:
Drug passes into milk. Avoid drug or discontinue nursing until you finish medicine. Consult doctor about maintaining milk supply.

Infants & children:
Not recommended.

Prolonged use:
- Avoid. Habit forming.
- Talk to your doctor about the need for follow-up medical examinations or laboratory studies to check heart function.

Skin & sunlight:
No problems expected.

Driving, piloting or hazardous work:
Don't drive or pilot aircraft until you learn how medicine affects you. Don't work around dangerous machinery. Don't climb ladders or work in high places. Danger increases if you drink alcohol or take medicine affecting alertness and reflexes, such as antihistamines, tranquilizers, sedatives, pain medicine, narcotics and mind-altering drugs.

Discontinuing:
Withdrawal effects such as irritability, insomnia, restlessness, sweating, diarrhea, hiccups, loss of appetite and hot flashes may follow abrupt withdrawal within 12 hours. Should they occur, these symptoms will probably subside within 96 hours.

Others:
Store in refrigerator.

POSSIBLE INTERACTION WITH OTHER DRUGS

GENERIC NAME OR DRUG CLASS	COMBINED EFFECT
Anesthetics*	Oversedation.
Anticonvulsants*	Oversedation.
Antidepressants, tricyclic*	Oversedation.
Antihistamines*	Oversedation.
Barbiturates*	Oversedation.
Clozapine	Toxic effect on the central nervous system.
Ethinamate	Dangerous increased effects of ethinamate. Avoid combining.
Fluoxetine	Increased depressant effects of both drugs.
Guanfacine	May increase depressant effects of either drug.
Leucovorin	High alcohol content of leucovorin may cause adverse effects.
Methyprylon	Increased sedative effect, perhaps to dangerous level. Avoid.
Molindone	Increased effects of both drugs. Avoid.
Muscle relaxants*	Oversedation.
Nabilone	Greater depression of central nervous system.
Narcotics*	Oversedation.
Sedatives*	Oversedation.
Sertraline	Increased depressive effects of both drugs.
Tranquilizers*	Oversedation.

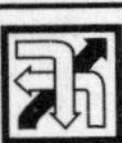

POSSIBLE INTERACTION WITH OTHER SUBSTANCES

INTERACTS WITH	COMBINED EFFECT
Alcohol:	Oversedation.
Beverages:	No problems expected.
Cocaine:	No problems expected.
Foods:	No problems expected.
Marijuana:	Oversedation.
Tobacco:	No problems expected.

*See Glossary

EPHEDRINE

BRAND NAMES

See complete list of brand names in the *Brand Name Directory*, page 907.

BASIC INFORMATION

Habit forming? No
Prescription needed?
Low Strength: No
High Strength: Yes
Available as generic? Yes, for some.
Drug class: Sympathomimetic

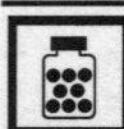

USES

- Relieves bronchial asthma.
- Decreases congestion of breathing passages.
- Suppresses allergic reactions.

DOSAGE & USAGE INFORMATION

How to take:
- Tablet or capsule—Swallow with liquid. You may chew or crush tablet.
- Extended-release tablets or capsules—Swallow each dose whole.
- Syrup—Take as directed on bottle.
- Drops—Dilute dose in beverage.

When to take:
As needed, no more often than every 4 hours. To prevent insomnia, take last dose at least 2 hours before bedtime.

If you forget a dose:
Take up to 2 hours late. If more than 2 hours, wait for next dose (don't double this dose).

What drug does:
- Prevents cells from releasing allergy-causing chemicals (histamines).
- Relaxes muscles of bronchial tubes.
- Decreases blood vessel size and blood flow, thus causing decongestion.

Continued next column

OVERDOSE

SYMPTOMS:
Severe anxiety, confusion, delirium, muscle tremors, rapid and irregular pulse.
WHAT TO DO:
- **Dial 911 (emergency) or 0 (operator) for an ambulance or medical help. Then give first aid immediately.**
- **See emergency information on inside covers.**

Time lapse before drug works:
30 to 60 minutes.

Don't take with:
- Nonprescription drugs with ephedrine, pseudoephedrine or epinephrine.
- Nonprescription drugs for cough, cold, allergy or asthma without consulting doctor.
- See Interaction column and consult doctor.

POSSIBLE ADVERSE REACTIONS OR SIDE EFFECTS

SYMPTOMS	WHAT TO DO
Life-threatening:	
In case of overdose, see previous column.	
Common:	
• Nervousness, headache, paleness, rapid heartbeat.	Continue. Call doctor when convenient.
• Insomnia.	Continue. Tell doctor at next visit.
Infrequent:	
• Irregular heartbeat.	Discontinue. Call doctor right away.
• Dizziness, appetite loss, nausea, vomiting, painful or difficult urination.	Continue. Call doctor when convenient.
Rare:	
None expected.	

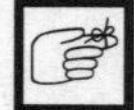

WARNINGS & PRECAUTIONS

Don't take if:
You are allergic to ephedrine or any sympathomimetic* drug.

Before you start, consult your doctor:
- If you have high blood pressure.
- If you have diabetes.
- If you have overactive thyroid gland.
- If you have difficulty urinating.
- If you have taken any MAO inhibitor in past 2 weeks.
- If you have taken digitalis preparations in the last 7 days.
- If you will have surgery within 2 months, including dental surgery, requiring general or spinal anesthesia.

Over age 60:
More likely to develop high blood pressure, heart-rhythm disturbances, angina and to feel drug's stimulant effects.

Pregnancy:
Decide with your doctor if drug benefits justify risk to unborn child. Risk category C (see page xxii).

Breast-feeding:
Drug passes into milk. Avoid drug or discontinue nursing until you finish medicine. Consult doctor for advice on maintaining milk supply.

Infants & children:
No problems expected.

Prolonged use:
- Excessive doses—Rare toxic psychosis.
- Men with enlarged prostate gland may have more urination difficulty.

Skin & sunlight:
No problems expected.

Driving, piloting or hazardous work:
Avoid if you feel dizzy. Otherwise, no problems expected.

Discontinuing:
May be unnecessary to finish medicine. Follow doctor's instructions.

Others:
No problems expected.

POSSIBLE INTERACTION WITH OTHER DRUGS

GENERIC NAME OR DRUG CLASS	COMBINED EFFECT
Antidepressants, tricyclic*	Increased effect of ephedrine. Excessive stimulation of heart and blood pressure.
Antihypertensives*	Decreased anti-hypertensive effect.
Beta-adrenergic blocking agents*	Decreased effects of both drugs.
Dextrothyroxine	Increased ephedrine effect.
Digitalis preparations*	Serious heart rhythm disturbances.
Epinephrine	Increased epinephrine effect.
Ergot preparations*	Serious blood pressure rise.
Furazolidine	Sudden, severe increase in blood pressure.
Guanadrel	Decreased effect of both drugs.
Guanethidine	Decreased effect of both drugs.
Methyldopa	Possible increased blood pressure.
Monoamine oxidase (MAO) inhibitors*	Increased ephedrine effect. Dangerous blood pressure rise.
Nitrates*	Possible decreased effects of both drugs.
Phenothiazines*	Possible increased ephedrine toxicity. Possible decreased ephedrine effect.
Pseudoephedrine	Increased pseudo-ephedrine effect.
Rauwolfia	Decreased rauwolfia effect.
Sympathomimetics*	Increased ephedrine effect.
Terazosin	Decreases effective-ness of terazosin.
Theophylline	Increased gastro-intestinal intolerance.

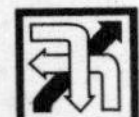

POSSIBLE INTERACTION WITH OTHER SUBSTANCES

INTERACTS WITH	COMBINED EFFECT
Alcohol:	None expected.
Beverages: Caffeine drinks.	Nervousness or insomnia.
Cocaine:	High risk of heart-beat irregularities and high blood pressure.
Foods:	None expected.
Marijuana:	Rapid heartbeat, possible heart rhythm disturbance.
Tobacco:	None expected.

*See Glossary

ERGOLOID MESYLATES

BRAND NAMES

Gerimal
Hydergine
Hydergine LC
Niloric

BASIC INFORMATION

Habit forming? No
Prescription needed? Yes
Available as generic? Yes
Drug class: Ergot preparation

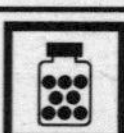

USES

Treatment for reduced alertness, poor memory, confusion, depression or lack of motivation in the elderly.

DOSAGE & USAGE INFORMATION

How to take:

- Tablet or capsule—Swallow with liquid. If you can't swallow whole, crumble tablet or open capsule and take with liquid or food.
- Liquid—Take as directed on label.
- Sublingual tablets—Dissolve tablet under tongue.

When to take:
At the same times each day.

If you forget a dose:
Take as soon as you remember up to 2 hours late. If more than 2 hours, wait for next scheduled dose (don't double this dose).

What drug does:
Stimulates brain-cell metabolism to increase use of oxygen and nutrients.

Time lapse before drug works:
Gradual improvements over 3 to 4 months.

Continued next column

OVERDOSE

SYMPTOMS:
Headache, flushed face, nasal congestion, nausea, vomiting, blood pressure drop, blurred vision, weakness, collapse, coma.
WHAT TO DO:

- **Dial 911 (emergency) or 0 (operator) for an ambulance or medical help. Then give first aid immediately.**
- **See emergency information on inside covers.**

Don't take with:

- Nonprescription drugs containing alcohol without consulting doctor.
- Any other medication without consulting your doctor or pharmacist.

POSSIBLE ADVERSE REACTIONS OR SIDE EFFECTS

SYMPTOMS	WHAT TO DO
Life-threatening:	
In case of overdose, see previous column.	
Common:	
Runny nose, skin flushing, headache.	Continue. Tell doctor at next visit.
Infrequent:	
• Slow heartbeat, tingling fingers.	Discontinue. Call doctor right away.
• Blurred vision.	Continue. Call doctor when convenient.
Rare:	
• Fainting.	Discontinue. Seek emergency treatment.
• Rash, nausea, vomiting, stomach cramps, dizziness when getting up, drowsiness, soreness under tongue, appetite loss.	Continue. Call doctor when convenient.

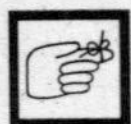

WARNINGS & PRECAUTIONS

Don't use if:
- If you are allergic to any ergot preparation.
- Your heartbeat is less than 60 beats per minute.
- Your systolic blood pressure is consistently below 100.

Before you start, consult your doctor:
- If you have had low blood pressure.
- If you have liver disease.
- If you have severe mental illness.

Over age 60:
Primarily used in persons older than 60. Results unpredictable, but many patients show improved brain function.

Pregnancy:
Decide with your doctor if drug benefits justify risk to unborn child. Risk category C (see page xxii).

Breast-feeding:
Risk to nursing child outweighs drug benefits. Don't use.

Infants & children:
Not recommended.

Prolonged use:
Talk to your doctor about the need for follow-up medical examinations or laboratory studies.

Skin & sunlight:
No problems expected.

Driving, piloting or hazardous work:
Avoid if you feel dizzy, faint or have blurred vision. Otherwise, no problems expected.

Discontinuing:
No problems expected.

Others:
May lessen your body's ability to adjust to cold temperatures.

POSSIBLE INTERACTION WITH OTHER DRUGS

GENERIC NAME OR DRUG CLASS	COMBINED EFFECT
Ergot preparations, other	May cause decreased circulation to arms, legs, feet and hands. Avoid.
Sympathomimetics*	May cause decreased circulation to arms, legs, feet and hands. Avoid.

POSSIBLE INTERACTION WITH OTHER SUBSTANCES

INTERACTS WITH	COMBINED EFFECT
Alcohol:	Use caution. May drop blood pressure excessively.
Beverages:	None expected.
Cocaine:	Overstimulation. Avoid.
Foods:	None expected.
Marijuana:	Decreased effect of ergot alkaloids.
Tobacco:	Decreased ergoloid effect. Don't smoke.

*See Glossary

ERGONOVINE

BRAND NAMES

Ergometrine
Ergotrate
Ergotrate Maleate

BASIC INFORMATION

Habit forming? No
Prescription needed? Yes
Available as generic? Yes
Drug class: Ergot preparation (uterine stimulant)

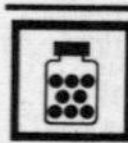

USES

Retards excessive post-delivery bleeding.

DOSAGE & USAGE INFORMATION

How to take:
Tablet—Swallow with liquid or food to lessen stomach irritation.

When to take:
At the same times each day.

If you forget a dose:
Don't take missed dose and don't double next one. Wait for next scheduled dose.

What drug does:
Causes smooth muscle cells of uterine wall to contract and surround bleeding blood vessels of relaxed uterus.

Time lapse before drug works:
Tablets—20 to 30 minutes.

Don't take with:
Any other medicine without consulting your doctor or pharmacist.

OVERDOSE

SYMPTOMS:
Vomiting, diarrhea, weak pulse, low blood pressure, difficult breathing, angina, convulsions.
WHAT TO DO:
- **Dial 911 (emergency) or 0 (operator) for an ambulance or medical help. Then give first aid immediately.**
- **If patient is unconscious and not breathing, give mouth-to-mouth breathing. If there is no heartbeat, use cardiac massage and mouth-to-mouth breathing (CPR). Don't try to make patient vomit. If you can't get help quickly, take patient to nearest emergency facility.**
- **See emergency information on inside covers.**

POSSIBLE ADVERSE REACTIONS OR SIDE EFFECTS

SYMPTOMS	WHAT TO DO
Life-threatening: In case of overdose, see previous column.	
Common: Nausea, vomiting, severe lower abdominal menstrual-like cramps.	Discontinue. Call doctor right away.
Infrequent: • Confusion, ringing in ears, diarrhea, muscle cramps.	Discontinue. Call doctor right away.
• Unusual sweating.	Continue. Call doctor when convenient.
Rare: Sudden, severe headache; shortness of breath; chest pain; numb, cold hands and feet.	Discontinue. Seek emergency treatment.

WARNINGS & PRECAUTIONS

Don't take if:
You are allergic to any ergot preparation.

Before you start, consult your doctor:
- If you have coronary artery or blood vessel disease.
- If you have liver or kidney disease.
- If you have high blood pressure.
- If you have postpartum infection.

Over age 60:
Not recommended.

Pregnancy:
Risk to unborn child outweighs drug benefits. Don't use. Risk category X (see page xxii).

Breast-feeding:
Drug passes into milk. Avoid drug or discontinue nursing until you finish medicine. Consult doctor for advice on maintaining milk supply.

Infants & children:
Not recommended.

Prolonged use:
Talk to your doctor about the need for follow-up medical examinations or laboratory studies to check blood pressure, ECG*.

Skin & sunlight:
No problems expected.

Driving, piloting or hazardous work:
No problems expected.

Discontinuing:
May be unnecessary to finish medicine. Follow doctor's instructions.

Others:
Drug should be used for short time only following childbirth or miscarriage.

POSSIBLE INTERACTION WITH OTHER DRUGS

GENERIC NAME OR DRUG CLASS	COMBINED EFFECT
Beta-adrenergic blocking agents*	Possible vasospasm (peripheral and cardiac).
Ergot preparations, other	May cause decreased circulation to arms, legs, feet and hands. Avoid.
Sympathomimetics*	May cause decreased circulation to arms, legs, feet and hands. Avoid.

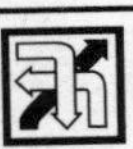

POSSIBLE INTERACTION WITH OTHER SUBSTANCES

INTERACTS WITH	COMBINED EFFECT
Alcohol:	None expected.
Beverages:	None expected.
Cocaine:	None expected.
Foods:	None expected.
Marijuana:	None expected.
Tobacco:	Decreased ergonovine effect. Don't smoke.

*See Glossary

ERGOTAMINE

BRAND NAMES

Ergomar
Ergostat
Gynergen
Medihaler Ergotamine

BASIC INFORMATION

Habit forming? No
Prescription needed? Yes
Available as generic? No
Drug class: Vasoconstrictor, ergot preparation

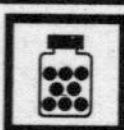

USES

Relieves pain of migraines and other headaches caused by dilated blood vessels. Will not prevent headaches.

DOSAGE & USAGE INFORMATION

How to take:

- Tablet—Swallow with liquid. If you can't swallow whole, crumble tablet and take with liquid or food.
- Sublingual tablet—Don't swallow whole. Let dissolve under tongue. Don't eat or drink while tablet is dissolving.
- Suppositories—Remove wrapper and moisten suppository with water. Gently insert larger end into rectum. Push well into rectum with finger.
- Aerosol inhaler—Use only as directed on prescription label.
- Lie down in quiet, dark room after taking.

When to take:
At first sign of vascular or migraine headache.

If you forget a dose:
Take as soon as you remember. Wait 4 hours for next dose.

Continued next column

OVERDOSE

SYMPTOMS:
Tingling, cold extremities and muscle pain. Progresses to nausea, vomiting, diarrhea, cold skin, rapid and weak pulse, severe numbness of extremities, confusion, convulsions, coma.

WHAT TO DO:

- **Dial 911 (emergency) or 0 (operator) for an ambulance or medical help. Then give first aid immediately.**
- **See emergency information on inside covers.**

What drug does:
Constricts blood vessels in the head.

Time lapse before drug works:
30 to 60 minutes.

Don't take with:
Any other medicine without consulting your doctor or pharmacist.

POSSIBLE ADVERSE REACTIONS OR SIDE EFFECTS

SYMPTOMS	WHAT TO DO
Life-threatening: In case of overdose, see previous column.	
Common:	
• Dizziness, nausea, diarrhea, vomiting, increased frequency or severity of headaches.	Continue. Call doctor when convenient.
• Feet and ankle swelling.	Discontinue. Call doctor right away.
Infrequent: Itchy or swollen skin; cold, pale hands or feet; pain or weakness in arms, legs, back.	Discontinue. Call doctor right away.
Rare: Anxiety or confusion; red or purple blisters, especially on hands, feet; change in vision; extreme thirst; stomach pain or bloating; unusually fast or slow heartbeat; chest pain; numbness or tingling in face, fingers, toes.	Discontinue. Call doctor right away.

WARNINGS & PRECAUTIONS

Don't take if:
You are allergic to any ergot preparation.

Before you start, consult your doctor:
- If you plan to become pregnant within medication period.
- If you have an infection.
- If you have angina, heart problems, high blood pressure, hardening of the arteries or vein problems.
- If you have kidney or liver disease.
- If you are allergic to other spray inhalants.

Over age 60:
Adverse reactions and side effects may be more frequent and severe than in younger persons.

Pregnancy:
Risk to unborn child outweighs drug benefits. Don't use. Risk category X (see page xxii).

Breast-feeding:
Drug filters into milk. May harm child. Avoid.

Infants & children:
Studies inconclusive on harm to children. Consult your doctor.

Prolonged use:
Cold skin, muscle pain, gangrene of hands and feet. This medicine not intended for uninterrupted use.

Skin & sunlight:
No problems expected.

Driving, piloting or hazardous work:
Don't drive or pilot aircraft until you learn how medicine affects you. Don't work around dangerous machinery. Don't climb ladders or work in high places. Danger increases if you drink alcohol or take medicine affecting alertness and reflexes, such as antihistamines, tranquilizers, sedatives, pain medicine, narcotics and mind-altering drugs.

Discontinuing:
May be unnecessary to finish medicine. Follow doctor's instructions.

Others:
- Impaired blood circulation can lead to gangrene in intestines or extremities. Never exceed recommended dose.
- May affect results in some medical tests.

POSSIBLE INTERACTION WITH OTHER DRUGS

GENERIC NAME OR DRUG CLASS	COMBINED EFFECT
Amphetamines*	Dangerous blood pressure rise.
Beta-adrenergic blocking agents*	Narrowed arteries in heart if ergotamine is taken in high doses.
Ephedrine	Dangerous blood pressure rise.
Epinephrine	Dangerous blood pressure rise.
Ergot preparations, other	May cause decreased circulation to arms, legs, feet and hands. Avoid.
Erythromycin	Decreased ergotamine effect.
Nitroglycerin	Decreased nitroglycerin effect.
Pseudoephedrine	Dangerous blood pressure rise.
Sumatriptan	Increased vasoconstriction. Delay 24 hours between drugs.
Sympathomimetics*	May cause decreased circulation to arms, legs, feet and hands. Avoid.
Troleandomycin	Decreased ergotamine effect.

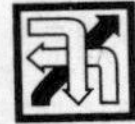

POSSIBLE INTERACTION WITH OTHER SUBSTANCES

INTERACTS WITH	COMBINED EFFECT
Alcohol:	Dilates blood vessels. Makes headache worse.
Beverages: Caffeine drinks.	May help relieve headache.
Cocaine:	Decreased ergotamine effect.
Foods: Any to which you are allergic.	May make headache worse. Avoid.
Marijuana:	Occasional use—Cool extremities. Regular use—Persistent chill.
Tobacco:	Decreased effect of ergotamine. Makes headache worse.

*See Glossary

ERGOTAMINE, BELLADONNA & PHENOBARBITAL

BRAND NAMES

Bellergal
Bellergal-S
Bellergal Spacetabs

BASIC INFORMATION

Habit forming? Yes
Prescription needed? Yes
Available as generic? No
Drug class: Analgesic, antispasmodic, vasoconstrictor

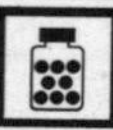

USES

- Reduces anxiety or nervous tension (low dose).
- Prevents vascular headaches.

DOSAGE & USAGE INFORMATION

How to take:
- Tablet or extended-release tablet—Swallow with liquid, or let dissolve under tongue.
- Lie down in quiet, dark room after taking.

When to take:
At first sign of vascular or migraine headache.

If you forget a dose:
Take as soon as you remember. Wait 4 hours for next dose.

What drug does:
- Constricts blood vessels in the head.
- Blocks nerve impulses at parasympathetic nerve endings, preventing muscle contractions and gland secretions of organs involved.

Continued next column

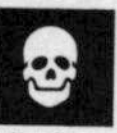

OVERDOSE

SYMPTOMS:
Tingling, cold extremities; muscle pain; nausea; vomiting; diarrhea; cold skin; rapid and weak pulse; severe numbness of extremities; confusion; dilated pupils; rapid pulse and breathing; dizziness; fever; hallucinations; slurred speech; agitation; flushed face; convulsions; coma.
WHAT TO DO:
- **Dial 911 (emergency) or 0 (operator) for an ambulance or medical help. Then give first aid immediately.**
- **See emergency information on inside covers.**

Time lapse before drug works:
15 to 30 minutes.

Don't take with:
Nonprescription drugs without consulting doctor.

POSSIBLE ADVERSE REACTIONS OR SIDE EFFECTS

SYMPTOMS	WHAT TO DO
Life-threatening:	
In case of overdose, see previous column.	
Common:	
• Flushed skin, fever, drowsiness, bloating, depression, frequent urination.	Discontinue. Call doctor right away.
• Constipation, dizziness, drowsiness, "hangover" effect, increased frequency or severity of headaches.	Continue. Call doctor when convenient.
Infrequent:	
• Swollen feet and ankles, numbness or tingling in hands or feet, cold hands and feet, rash.	Discontinue. Call doctor right away.
• Nasal congestion, altered taste.	Continue. Call doctor when convenient.
Rare:	
Jaundice, weak legs, swallowing difficulty, dry mouth, increased sensitivity to sunlight, nausea, vomiting, decreased sweating.	Discontinue. Call doctor right away.

WARNINGS & PRECAUTIONS

Don't take if:
- You are allergic to any barbiturate, tartrazine dye, anticholinergic or ergot preparation.
- You have porphyria, trouble with stomach bloating, difficulty emptying your bladder completely, narrow-angle glaucoma, severe ulcerative colitis, enlarged prostate.

Before you start, consult your doctor:
- If you have epilepsy; kidney, thyroid or liver damage; anemia; chronic pain; open-angle glaucoma; angina; fast heartbeat; heart problems; high blood pressure; hardening of the arteries; vein problems; chronic bronchitis; asthma; hiatal hernia; enlarged prostate; myasthenia gravis; peptic ulcer; an infection.
- If you plan to become pregnant within medication period.

ERGOTAMINE, BELLADONNA & PHENOBARBITAL

- If you will have surgery within 2 months, including dental surgery, requiring general or spinal anesthesia.

Over age 60:
Adverse reactions and side effects may be more frequent and severe than in younger persons.

Pregnancy:
Risk to unborn child outweighs drug benefits. Don't use. Risk category X (see page xxii).

Breast-feeding:
Drug passes into milk. Avoid drug or discontinue nursing until you finish medicine. Consult doctor for advice on maintaining milk supply.

Infants & children:
Not recommended.

Prolonged use:
- May cause addiction, anemia, chronic intoxication.
- May lower body temperature, making exposure to cold temperatures hazardous.
- Chronic constipation, possible fecal impaction.
- Cold skin, muscle pain, gangrene of hands and feet. This medicine not intended for uninterrupted use.

Skin & sunlight:
May cause rash or intensify sunburn in areas exposed to sun or sunlamp.

Driving, piloting or hazardous work:
Don't drive or pilot aircraft until you learn how medicine affects you. Don't work around dangerous machinery. Don't climb ladders or work in high places. Danger increases if you drink alcohol or take medicine affecting alertness and reflexes, such as antihistamines, tranquilizers, sedatives, pain medicine, narcotics and mind-altering drugs.

Discontinuing:
May be unnecessary to finish medicine. Follow doctor's instructions. If you develop withdrawal symptoms of hallucinations, agitation or sleeplessness after discontinuing, call doctor right away.

Others:
- Impaired blood circulation can lead to gangrene in intestines or extremities. Never exceed recommended dose.
- May affect results in some medical tests.

POSSIBLE INTERACTION WITH OTHER DRUGS

GENERIC NAME OR DRUG CLASS	COMBINED EFFECT
Amantadine	Increased belladonna effect.
Amphetamines*	Dangerous blood pressure rise.
Anticholinergics, other*	Increased belladonna effect.
Anticoagulants, oral*	Decreased anticoagulant effect.
Anticonvulsants*	Changed seizure patterns.
Antidepressants, tricyclic*	Decreased anti-depressant effect. Possible dangerous oversedation.
Antidiabetics, oral*	Increased phenobarbital effect.
Antihistamines*	Dangerous sedation. Avoid.
Aspirin	Decreased aspirin effect.
Beta-adrenergic blocking agents*	Narrowed arteries in heart if taken in large doses.
Contraceptives, oral*	Decreased contraceptive effect.
Cortisone drugs*	Decreased cortisone effect. Increased internal eye pressure.
Digitoxin	Decreased digitoxin effect.
Doxycycline	Decreased doxycycline effect.
Dronabinol	Increased effect of drugs.

Continued on page 938

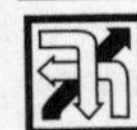

POSSIBLE INTERACTION WITH OTHER SUBSTANCES

INTERACTS WITH	COMBINED EFFECT
Alcohol:	Possible fatal oversedation. Avoid.
Beverages:	None expected.
Cocaine:	Excessively rapid heartbeat. Avoid.
Foods:	None expected.
Marijuana:	Drowsiness and dry mouth, excessive sedation. Avoid.
Tobacco:	None expected.

***See Glossary**

ERGOTAMINE & CAFFEINE

BRAND NAMES

Cafergot
Cafertine
Cafetrate
Ercaf
Ergo-Caff
Gotamine
Migergot
Wigraine

BASIC INFORMATION

Habit forming? No
Prescription needed? Yes
Available as generic? No
Drug class: Analgesic, stimulant (xanthine), vasoconstrictor

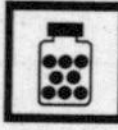

USES

Relieves pain of migraines and other headaches caused by dilated blood vessels. Will not prevent headaches.

DOSAGE & USAGE INFORMATION

How to take:
- Tablet—Swallow with liquid, or let dissolve under tongue. If you can't swallow whole, crumble tablet and take with liquid or food.
- Suppositories—Remove wrapper and moisten suppository with water. Gently insert larger end into rectum. Push well into rectum with finger.
- Lie down in quiet, dark room after taking.

When to take:
At first sign of vascular or migraine headache.

If you forget a dose:
Take as soon as you remember up to 2 hours late. If more than 2 hours, wait for next scheduled dose (don't double this dose).

What drug does:
- Constricts blood vessels in the head.

Continued next column

OVERDOSE

SYMPTOMS:
Tingling, cold extremities; muscle pain; nausea; vomiting; diarrhea; cold skin; severe numbness of extremities; confusion; excitement; rapid heartbeat; insomnia, hallucinations; convulsions; coma.
WHAT TO DO:
- **Dial 911 (emergency) or 0 (operator) for an ambulance or medical help. Then give first aid immediately.**
- **See emergency information on inside covers.**

- Constricts blood vessel walls.
- Stimulates central nervous system.

Time lapse before drug works:
30 to 60 minutes.

Don't take with:
- Nonprescription drugs containing alcohol without consulting doctor.
- Any other medicine without consulting your doctor or pharmacist.

POSSIBLE ADVERSE REACTIONS OR SIDE EFFECTS

SYMPTOMS	WHAT TO DO
Life-threatening:	
In case of overdose, see previous column.	
Common:	
• Fast heartbeat, feet or ankle swelling.	Discontinue. Call doctor right away.
• Dizziness, nausea, diarrhea, vomiting, nervousness, increased frequency or severity of headaches.	Continue. Call doctor when convenient.
Infrequent:	
Itchy skin; abdominal pain; cold hands and feet; weakness in arms, legs, back; confusion; irritability; indigestion; low blood sugar with weakness and trembling.	Discontinue. Call doctor right away.
Rare:	
Anxiety; red or purple blisters, especially on on hands and feet; change in vision; extreme thirst; numbness or tingling in hands or feet.	Discontinue. Call doctor right away.

WARNINGS & PRECAUTIONS

Don't take if:
- You are allergic to any stimulant or any ergot preparation.
- You have heart disease.
- You have active peptic ulcer of stomach or duodenum.

Before you start, consult your doctor:
- If you have irregular heartbeat, angina, heart problems, high blood pressure, hardening of the arteries or vein problems.
- If you have hypoglycemia (low blood sugar), epilepsy, an infection, kidney or liver disease.
- If you are allergic to spray inhalants.
- If you plan to become pregnant within medication period.

Over age 60:
Adverse reactions and side effects may be more frequent and severe than in younger persons, especially dizziness and excessive potassium loss.

Pregnancy:
Risk to unborn child outweighs drug benefits. Don't use. Risk category X (see page xxii).

Breast-feeding:
Drug passes into milk. Avoid drug or discontinue nursing until you finish medicine. Consult doctor for advice on maintaining milk supply.

Infants & children:
Not recommended.

Prolonged use:
Cold skin, muscle pain, stomach ulcers, gangrene of hands and feet. This medicine not intended for uninterrupted use.

Skin & sunlight:
No problems expected.

Driving, piloting or hazardous work:
Don't drive or pilot aircraft until you learn how medicine affects you. Don't work around dangerous machinery. Don't climb ladders or work in high places. Danger increases if you drink alcohol or take medicine affecting alertness and reflexes, such as antihistamines, tranquilizers, sedatives, pain medicine, narcotics and mind-altering drugs.

Discontinuing:
Will cause withdrawal symptoms of headache, irritability, drowsiness. Discontinue gradually if you use caffeine for a month or more.

Others:
- May produce or aggravate fibrocystic breast disease in women.
- Impaired blood circulation can lead to gangrene in intestines or extremities. Never exceed recommended dose.

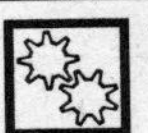

POSSIBLE INTERACTION WITH OTHER DRUGS

GENERIC NAME OR DRUG CLASS	COMBINED EFFECT
Amphetamines*	Dangerous blood pressure rise.
Beta-adrenergic blocking agents*	Narrowed arteries in heart if taken in large doses.
Cimetidine	Increased caffeine effect.
Contraceptives, oral*	Increased caffeine effect.
Ephedrine	Dangerous blood pressure rise.
Epinephrine	Dangerous blood pressure rise.
Erythromycin	Decreased ergotamine effect.
Isoniazid	Increased caffeine effect.
Monoamine oxidase (MAO) inhibitors*	Dangerous blood pressure rise.
Nitroglycerin	Decreased nitro-glycerin effect.
Pseudoephedrine	Dangerous blood pressure rise.
Sedatives*	Decreased sedative effect.
Sleep inducers*	Decreased sedative effect.
Sumatriptan	Increased vasocon-striction. Delay 24 hours between drugs.
Sympathomimetics*	Overstimulation.
Thyroid hormones*	Increased thyroid effect.

Continued on page 939

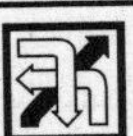

POSSIBLE INTERACTION WITH OTHER SUBSTANCES

INTERACTS WITH	COMBINED EFFECT
Alcohol:	Dilates blood vessels. Makes headache worse.
Beverages: Caffeine drinks.	May help relieve headache.
Cocaine:	Overstimulation. Avoid.
Foods: Any to which you are allergic.	May make headache worse. Avoid.
Marijuana:	Occasional use—Cool extremities. Regular use—Persistent chill. Increased effect of both drugs. May lead to dangerous, rapid heartbeat. Avoid.
Tobacco:	Decreased effect of ergotamine and caffeine. Makes headache worse. Avoid.

*See Glossary

ERGOTAMINE, CAFFEINE, BELLADONNA & PENTOBARBITAL

BRAND NAMES

Cafergot-PB

BASIC INFORMATION

Habit forming? Yes
Prescription needed? Yes
Available as generic? No
Drug class: Vasoconstrictor, stimulant (xanthine), sedative, antispasmodic

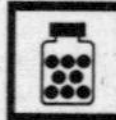

USES

- Relieves pain of migraines and other headaches caused by dilated blood vessels. Will not prevent headaches.
- Reduces anxiety, nervous tension (low dose).

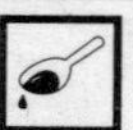

DOSAGE & USAGE INFORMATION

How to take:
- Tablet—Swallow with liquid, or let dissolve under tongue. If you can't swallow whole, crumble tablet and take with liquid or food.
- Suppositories—Remove wrapper; moisten suppository with water. Gently insert larger end into rectum. Push into rectum with finger.
- Lie down in quiet, dark room after taking.

When to take:
At first sign of vascular or migraine headache.

If you forget a dose:
Take as soon as you remember up to 2 hours late. If more than 2 hours, wait for next scheduled dose (don't double this dose).

What drug does:
- Blocks nerve impulses at parasympathetic nerve endings, preventing muscle contractions and gland secretions of organs involved.

Continued next column

OVERDOSE

SYMPTOMS:
Tingling, cold extremities and muscle pain. Progresses to nausea, vomiting, diarrhea, insomnia, cold skin, rapid and weak pulse, severe numbness of extremities, confusion, convulsions, coma.
WHAT TO DO:
- **Dial 911 (emergency) or 0 (operator) for an ambulance or medical help. Then give first aid immediately.**
- **See emergency information on inside covers.**

- May partially block nerve impulses at nerve cell connections.
- Constricts blood vessel walls.
- Stimulates central nervous system.

Time lapse before drug works:
15 to 30 minutes.

Don't take with:
- Nonprescription drugs without consulting doctor.
- Any other medicine without consulting your doctor or pharmacist.

POSSIBLE ADVERSE REACTIONS OR SIDE EFFECTS

SYMPTOMS	WHAT TO DO
Life-threatening:	
In case of overdose, see previous column.	
Common:	
• Moderately fast heartbeat.	Discontinue. Call doctor right away.
• Dizziness, nausea, diarrhea, vomiting, nervousness, "hang-over" effect, increased frequency or severity of headaches.	Continue. Call doctor when convenient.
Infrequent:	
• Itchy skin; rash; abdominal pain; cold hands and feet; weakness in arms, back legs; confusion; irritability; indigestion; low blood sugar with weakness and trembling.	Discontinue. Call doctor right away.
• Nasal congestion, altered taste.	Continue. Call doctor when convenient.
Rare:	
Anxiety; red or purple blisters, especially in hands and feet; change in vision; extreme thirst; numbness or tingling in hands or feet; jaundice.	Discontinue. Call doctor right away.

WARNINGS & PRECAUTIONS

Don't take if:
- You are allergic to any stimulant, ergot preparation, barbiturate or anticholinergic.

- You have heart disease, peptic ulcer of stomach or duodenum, porphyria, trouble with stomach bloating, difficulty emptying your bladder completely, narrow-angle glaucoma, severe ulcerative colitis.

Before you start, consult your doctor:
- If you have hypoglycemia (low blood sugar), an infection, angina, heart problems, high blood pressure, hardening of the arteries, vein problems, kidney or liver disease, epilepsy, asthma, anemia, chronic pain, open-angle glaucoma, chronic bronchitis, hiatal hernia, enlarged prostate, myasthenia gravis, peptic ulcer.
- If you plan to become pregnant within medication period.
- If you will have surgery within 2 months, including dental surgery, requiring general or spinal anesthesia.

Over age 60:
Adverse reactions and side effects may be more frequent and severe than in younger persons, especially dizziness and excessive potassium loss.

Pregnancy:
Risk to unborn child outweighs drug benefits. Don't use. Risk category X (see page xxii).

Breast-feeding:
Drug filters into milk. May harm child. Avoid.

Infants & children:
Not recommended.

Prolonged use:
- Stomach ulcers.
- Cold skin, muscle pain, gangrene of hands and feet. This medicine not intended for uninterrupted use.
- May cause addiction, anemia, chronic intoxication.
- May lower body temperature, making exposure to cold temperatures hazardous.
- Chronic constipation, possible fecal impaction.

Skin & sunlight:
May cause rash or intensify sunburn in areas exposed to sun or sunlamp.

Driving, piloting or hazardous work:
Don't drive or pilot aircraft until you learn how medicine affects you. Don't work around dangerous machinery. Don't climb ladders or work in high places. Danger increases if you drink alcohol or take medicine affecting alertness and reflexes, such as antihistamines, tranquilizers, sedatives, pain medicine, narcotics and mind-altering drugs.

Discontinuing:
May be unnecessary to finish medicine. Follow doctor's instructions. If you develop withdrawal symptoms of hallucinations, headache, agitation or sleeplessness after discontinuing, call doctor right away.

Others:
- Great potential for abuse.
- May produce or aggravate fibrocystic breast disease in women.
- Impaired blood circulation can lead to gangrene in intestines or extremities. Never exceed recommended dose.

POSSIBLE INTERACTION WITH OTHER DRUGS

GENERIC NAME OR DRUG CLASS	COMBINED EFFECT
Amantadine	Increased belladonna effect.
Amphetamines*	Dangerous blood pressure rise.
Anticoagulants, oral*	Decreased anticoagulant effect.

Continued on page 939

POSSIBLE INTERACTION WITH OTHER SUBSTANCES

INTERACTS WITH	COMBINED EFFECT
Alcohol:	Dilates blood vessels. Makes headache worse. Possible fatal oversedation. Avoid.
Beverages: Caffeine drinks.	May help relieve headache.
Cocaine:	Excessively rapid heartbeat. Avoid.
Foods: Any to which you are allergic.	May make headache worse. Avoid.
Marijuana:	Drowsiness and dry mouth, excessive sedation. Avoid. Occasional use—Cool extremities. Regular use—Persistent chill.
Tobacco:	Decreased effect of ergotamine. Makes headache worse.

*See Glossary

ERYTHROMYCINS

BRAND AND GENERIC NAMES

See complete list of brand and generic names in the *Brand Name Directory*, page 907.

BASIC INFORMATION

Habit forming? No
Prescription needed? Yes
Available as generic? Yes
Drug class: Antibiotic (erythromycin)

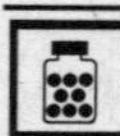

USES

Treatment of infections responsive to erythromycin.

DOSAGE & USAGE INFORMATION

How to take:

- Tablet or capsule—Swallow with liquid. You may chew or crush.
- Extended-release tablets or capsules—Swallow each dose whole.
- Oral suspension—Shake well before using. Use dropper supplied with prescription or use a specially marked measuring spoon to measure dose.

When to take:
At the same times each day, 1 hour before or 2 hours after eating. May be taken with food if stomach upset occurs.

If you forget a dose:

- If you take 3 or more doses daily—Take as soon as you remember. Return to regular schedule.
- If you take 2 doses daily—Take as soon as you remember. Wait 5 to 6 hours for next dose. Return to regular schedule.

What drug does:
Prevents growth and reproduction of susceptible bacteria.

Continued next column

OVERDOSE

SYMPTOMS:
Nausea, vomiting, abdominal discomfort, diarrhea.
WHAT TO DO:
Overdose unlikely to threaten life. If person takes much larger amount than prescribed, call doctor, poison control center or hospital emergency room for instructions.

Time lapse before drug works:
2 to 5 days.

Don't take with:
Any other medicine without consulting your doctor or pharmacist.

POSSIBLE ADVERSE REACTIONS OR SIDE EFFECTS

SYMPTOMS	WHAT TO DO
Life-threatening:	
None expected.	
Common:	
Mild nausea.	Continue. Call doctor when convenient.
Infrequent:	
• Diarrhea, abdominal cramps, discomfort, vomiting, rash.	Discontinue. Call doctor right away.
• Sore mouth or tongue.	Continue. Call doctor
Rare:	
• Jaundice in adults, hearing loss.	Discontinue. Call doctor right away.
• Unusual tiredness or weakness.	Continue. Call doctor when convenient.

WARNINGS & PRECAUTIONS

Don't take if:
- You are allergic to any erythromycin.
- You have had liver disease or impaired liver function.

Before you start, consult your doctor:
If you have taken erythromycin estolate in the past.

Over age 60:
Adverse reactions and side effects may be more frequent and severe than in younger persons, especially skin reactions around genitals and anus.

Pregnancy:
Decide with your doctor if drug benefits justify risk to unborn child. Risk category C (see page xxii).

Breast-feeding:
Drug passes into milk. Avoid drug or discontinue nursing until you finish medicine. Consult doctor for advice on maintaining milk supply.

Infants & children:
Use only under medical supervision.

Prolonged use:
- You may become more susceptible to infections caused by germs not responsive to erythromycin.
- Talk to your doctor about the need for follow-up medical examinations or laboratory studies to check liver function.

Skin & sunlight:
No problems expected.

Driving, piloting or hazardous work:
No problems expected.

Discontinuing:
You must take full dose at least 10 consecutive days for streptococcal or staphylococcal infections.

Others:
No problems expected.

POSSIBLE INTERACTION WITH OTHER DRUGS

GENERIC NAME OR DRUG CLASS	COMBINED EFFECT
Aminophylline	Increased effect of aminophylline in blood.
Astemizole	Increased risk of heart toxicity.
Caffeine	Increased effect of caffeine.
Carbamazepine	Increased risk of carbamazepine toxicity.
Cefixime	Decreased antibiotic effect of cefixime.
Cyclosporins	May increase cyclosporin toxicity.
Hepatotoxics*	Increased risk of liver toxicity.
Ketoconazole	Possible heartbeat irregularity
Lincomycins*	Decreased lincomycin effect.
Oxtriphylline	Increased level of oxtriphylline in blood.
Penicillins*	Decreased penicillin effect.
Terfenadine	Increased risk of heart toxicity.
Theophylline	Increased level of theophylline in blood.
Warfarin	Increased risk of bleeding.

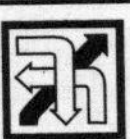

POSSIBLE INTERACTION WITH OTHER SUBSTANCES

INTERACTS WITH	COMBINED EFFECT
Alcohol:	Possible liver damage.
Beverages: Caffeine-containing.	Increased caffeine toxicity. Avoid.
Cocaine:	None expected.
Foods: Wines, syrup, acidic fruits or juices (if taken with).	Decreased antibiotic effect.
Marijuana:	None expected.
Tobacco:	None expected.

*See Glossary

ERYTHROMYCIN & SULFISOXAZOLE

BRAND NAMES

Eryzole
Pediazole
Sulfimycin

BASIC INFORMATION

Habit forming? No
Prescription needed? Yes
Available as generic? Yes
Drug class: Antibiotic (erythromycin), sulfa (sulfonamide)

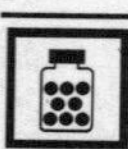

USES

Treatment of infections responsive to erythromycin and sulfa.

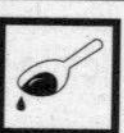

DOSAGE & USAGE INFORMATION

How to take:
Suspension—Swallow with liquid. Instructions to take on empty stomach mean 1 hour before or 2 hours after eating. Shake carefully before measuring.

When to take:
At the same times each day, 1 hour before or 2 hours after eating.

If you forget a dose:
Take as soon as you remember up to 2 hours late. If more than 2 hours, wait for next scheduled dose (don't double this dose).

What drug does:
Prevents growth and reproduction of susceptible bacteria.

Time lapse before drug works:
2 to 5 days to affect infection.

Don't take with:
Any other medicine without consulting your doctor or pharmacist.

OVERDOSE

SYMPTOMS:
Less urine, bloody urine, nausea, skin rash, vomiting, abdominal discomfort, diarrhea, coma.
WHAT TO DO:
- **Dial 911 (emergency) or 0 (operator) for an ambulance or medical help. Then give first aid immediately.**
- **See emergency information on inside covers.**

POSSIBLE ADVERSE REACTIONS OR SIDE EFFECTS

SYMPTOMS	WHAT TO DO
Life-threatening: In case of overdose, see previous column.	
Common:	
• Headache, dizziness, itchy skin, rash, appetite loss, vomiting.	Discontinue. Call doctor right away.
• Mild nausea.	Continue. Call doctor when convenient.
Infrequent:	
• Dryness, irritation, stinging with use of skin solution, mouth or tongue sore.	Continue. Call doctor when convenient.
• Diarrhea, nausea, abdominal cramps, swallowing difficulty.	Discontinue. Call doctor right away.
Rare:	
• Jaundice, painful or difficult urination, muscle or joint pain, unusual tiredness, blood in urine, swelling of neck.	Discontinue. Call doctor right away.
• Weakness.	Continue. Call doctor when convenient.

WARNINGS & PRECAUTIONS

Don't take if:
- You are allergic to any sulfa drug or any erythromycin.
- You have had liver disease or impaired liver function.

Before you start, consult your doctor:
- If you are allergic to carbonic anhydrase inhibitors, oral antidiabetics or thiazide diuretics.
- If you are allergic by nature.
- If you have liver or kidney disease or porphyria, developed anemia from use of any drug, taken erythromycin estolate in the past.

Over age 60:
Adverse reactions and side effects may be more frequent and severe than in younger persons, especially skin reactions around genitals and anus.

Pregnancy:
Decide with your doctor if drug benefits justify risk to unborn child. Risk category C (see page xxii).

ERYTHROMYCIN & SULFISOXAZOLE

Breast-feeding:
Drug passes into milk. Avoid drug or discontinue nursing until you finish medicine. Consult doctor for advice on maintaining milk supply.

Infants & children:
Don't give to infants younger than 1 month.

Prolonged use:
- May enlarge thyroid gland.
- Request frequent blood counts, liver and kidney function studies.
- You may become more susceptible to infections caused by germs not responsive to erythromycin or sulfa.

Skin & sunlight:
May cause rash or intensify sunburn in areas exposed to sun or sunlamp.

Driving, piloting or hazardous work:
Avoid if you feel dizzy. Otherwise, no problems expected.

Discontinuing:
Don't discontinue without doctor's advice until you complete prescribed dose, even though symptoms diminish or disappear.

Others:
- Drink extra liquid each day to prevent adverse reactions, such as kidney damage.
- If you require surgery, tell anesthetist you take sulfa.

POSSIBLE INTERACTION WITH OTHER DRUGS

GENERIC NAME OR DRUG CLASS	COMBINED EFFECT
Aminobenzoate potassium	Possible decreased sulfisoxazole effect.
Aminophylline	Increased effect of aminophylline in blood.
Anticoagulants, oral*	Increased anticoagulant effect.
Anticonvulsants, hydantoin*	Toxic effect on brain.
Aspirin	Increased sulfa effect.
Astemizole	Increased risk of heart toxicity.
Carbamazepine	Increased risk of carbamazepine toxicity.
Flecainide	Possible decreased blood cell production in bone marrow.
Hepatotoxics*	Increased risk of liver toxicity.
Isoniazid	Possible anemia.
Lincomycins*	Decreased lincomycin effect.
Methenamine	Possible kidney blockage.
Methotrexate	Increased possibility of toxic side effects from methotrexate.
Oxtriphylline	Increased level of oxtriphylline in blood.
Oxyphenbutazone	Increased sulfa effect.
Para-aminosalicylic acid (PAS)	Decreased sulfa effect.
Penicillins*	Decreased penicillin effect.
Phenylbutazone	Increased sulfa effect.
Probenecid	Increased sulfa effect.
Sulfinpyrazone	Increased sulfa effect.
Terfenadine	Increased risk of heart toxicity.
Theophylline	Increased level of theophylline in blood.
Tocainide	Possible decreased blood cell production in bone marrow.
Trimethoprim	Increased sulfa effect.

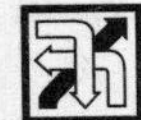

POSSIBLE INTERACTION WITH OTHER SUBSTANCES

INTERACTS WITH	COMBINED EFFECT
Alcohol:	Increased alcohol effect. Possible liver damage.
Beverages:	None expected.
Cocaine:	None expected.
Foods: Wines, syrups, acidic fruits or juices (if taken with).	Decreased antibiotic effect.
Marijuana:	None expected.
Tobacco:	None expected.

***See Glossary**

ESTRAMUSTINE

BRAND NAMES

Emcyt

BASIC INFORMATION

Habit forming? No
Prescription needed? Yes
Available as generic? No
Drug class: Antineoplastic

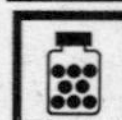

USES

Treats prostate cancer.

DOSAGE & USAGE INFORMATION

How to take:
Capsule—Swallow with liquid. If you can't swallow whole, open capsule and take with liquid or food. Instructions to take on empty stomach mean 1 hour before or 2 hours after eating.

When to take:
According to doctor's instructions. Try to take 1 hour before or 2 hours after eating or drinking any milk products.

If you forget a dose:
Skip dose. Never double dose.

What drug does:
Suppresses growth of cancer cells.

Time lapse before drug works:
Within 20 hours.

Don't take with:
Any other medicines (including over-the-counter drugs such as cough and cold medicines, laxatives, antacids, diet pills, caffeine, nose drops or vitamins) without consulting your doctor.

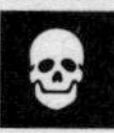

OVERDOSE

SYMPTOMS:
None expected.
WHAT TO DO:
Overdose unlikely to threaten life. If person takes much larger amount than prescribed, call doctor, poison control center or hospital emergency room for instructions.

POSSIBLE ADVERSE REACTIONS OR SIDE EFFECTS

SYMPTOMS	WHAT TO DO
Life-threatening:	
Sudden headaches, chest pain, shortness of breath, leg pain, vision changes, slurred speech.	Seek emergency treatment immediately.
Common:	
• Skin rash, itching.	Discontinue. Call doctor right away.
• Increased sun sensitivity.	Decrease sun exposure. Call doctor when convenient.
• Diarrhea, dizziness, nausea, vomiting, headache, swelling in hands or feet.	Continue. Call doctor when convenient.
Infrequent:	
• Joint or muscle pain, difficulty swallowing, sore throat and fever, peeling skin, jaundice.	Discontinue. Call doctor right away.
• Mouth or tongue irritation, breast tenderness or enlargement, decreased interest in sex.	Continue. Call doctor when convenient.
Rare:	
Bloody urine, hearing loss, back pain, abdominal pain.	Discontinue. Call doctor right away.

WARNINGS & PRECAUTIONS

Don't take if:
You have active thrombophlebitis.

Before you start, consult your doctor:
- If you have jaundice.
- If you have history of thrombophlebitis.
- If you have peptic ulcer.
- If you have mental depression.
- If you have migraine headaches.
- If you have or recently had chicken pox.
- If you have shingles (herpes zoster).
- If you have had a recent heart attack.

Over age 60:
Adverse reactions and side effects may be more frequent and severe than in younger persons. You may need smaller doses for shorter periods of time.

Pregnancy:
Used in men only.

Breast-feeding:
Used in men only.

Infants & children:
Not used.

Prolonged use:
Talk to your doctor about the need for follow-up medical examinations or laboratory studies to check complete blood counts (white blood cell count, platelet count, red blood cell count, hemoglobin, hematocrit), blood pressure, liver function, serum acid, serum calcium and alkaline phosphatase.

Skin & sunlight:
No problems expected.

Driving, piloting or hazardous work:
No special problems expected.

Discontinuing:
No special problems expected.

Others:
- Advise any doctor or dentist whom you consult that you take this medicine.
- May affect results in some medical tests.
- May decrease sperm count in males.

POSSIBLE INTERACTION WITH OTHER DRUGS

GENERIC NAME OR DRUG CLASS	COMBINED EFFECT
Calcium supplements*	Decreased absorption of estramustine.
Hepatotoxic medications*	Increased risk of liver toxicity.

POSSIBLE INTERACTION WITH OTHER SUBSTANCES

INTERACTS WITH	COMBINED EFFECT
Alcohol:	Increased "hangover effect" and other gastrointestinal symptoms.
Beverages: Milk and milk products.	Decreased absorption of estramustine.
Cocaine:	No special problems expected.
Foods: Foods high in calcium.	Decreased absorption of estramustine.
Marijuana:	No special problems expected.
Tobacco:	Increased risk of heart attack and blood clots.

***See Glossary**

ESTROGENS

BRAND AND GENERIC NAMES

See complete list of brand and generic names in *Brand Name Directory*, page 908.

BASIC INFORMATION

Habit forming? No
Prescription needed? Yes
Available as generic? Yes
Drug class: Female sex hormone (estrogen)

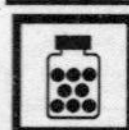

USES

- Treatment for estrogen deficiency.
- Treatment for symptoms of menopause and menstrual cycle irregularity.
- Treatment for estrogen-deficiency osteoporosis (bone softening from calcium loss).
- Treatment for vulvar squamous hyperplasia.
- Treatment for atrophic vaginitis.
- Treatment for prostate cancer.

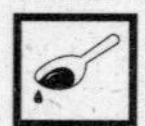

DOSAGE & USAGE INFORMATION

How to take:

- Tablet or capsule—Take with or after food to reduce nausea. Swallow with liquid. If you can't swallow whole, crumble tablet or open capsule and take with liquid or food.
- Vaginal cream or suppositories—Use as directed on label.
- By injection under medical supervision.
- Transdermal patches—Follow package instructions.

When to take:
At the same time each day.

If you forget a dose:
Take as soon as you remember up to 12 hours late. If more than 12 hours, wait for next scheduled dose (don't double this dose).

Continued next column

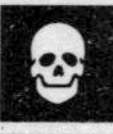

OVERDOSE

SYMPTOMS:
Nausea, vomiting, fluid retention, breast enlargement and discomfort, abnormal vaginal bleeding.
WHAT TO DO:
Overdose unlikely to threaten life. If person takes much larger amount than prescribed, call doctor, poison control center or hospital emergency room for instructions.

What drug does:

- Restores normal estrogen level in tissues.
- Combined with progestins for contraception.

Time lapse before drug works:
10 to 20 days.

Don't take with:
Any other medicine without consulting your doctor or pharmacist.

POSSIBLE ADVERSE REACTIONS OR SIDE EFFECTS

SYMPTOMS	WHAT TO DO
Life-threatening:	
Profuse bleeding.	Seek emergency treatment.
Common:	
• Stomach cramps.	Discontinue. Call doctor right away.
• Appetite loss.	Continue. Call doctor when convenient.
• Nausea; diarrhea; swollen feet and ankles; tender, swollen breasts; acne; intolerance of contact lenses; change in menstruation.	Continue. Tell doctor at next visit.
Infrequent:	
• Rash, stomach or side pain, joint or muscle pain, bloody skin blisters, breast lumps.	Discontinue. Call doctor right away.
• Depression, dizziness, migraine headache, irritability, vomiting.	Continue. Call doctor when convenient.
• Brown blotches, hair loss, vaginal discharge or bleeding, changes in sex drive.	Continue. Tell doctor at next visit.
Rare:	
• Jaundice, hypercalcemia in breast cancer. • Involuntary movements.	Discontinue. Call doctor right away.

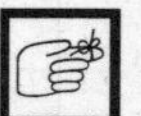

WARNINGS & PRECAUTIONS

Don't take if:

- You are allergic to any estrogen-containing drugs.
- You have impaired liver function.
- You have had blood clots, stroke or heart attack.
- You have unexplained vaginal bleeding.

Before you start, consult your doctor:

- If you have had cancer of the breast or reproductive organs, fibrocystic breast disease, fibroid tumors of the uterus or endometriosis.

- If you have had migraine headaches, epilepsy or porphyria.
- If you have diabetes, high blood pressure, asthma, congestive heart failure, kidney disease or gallstones.
- If you plan to become pregnant within 3 months.

Over age 60:
Controversial. You and your doctor must decide if risks of drug outweigh benefits.

Pregnancy:
Risk to unborn child outweighs benefits of drug. Don't use. Risk category X (see page xxii).

Breast-feeding:
Drug filters into milk. May harm child. Avoid.

Infants & children:
Not recommended.

Prolonged use:
- Increased growth of fibroid tumors of uterus. Possible association with cancer of uterus.
- Talk to your doctor about the need for follow-up medical examinations or laboratory studies to check pap smear, liver function, mammogram.

Skin & sunlight:
May cause rash or intensify sunburn in areas exposed to sun or sunlamp.

Driving, piloting or hazardous work:
No problems expected.

Discontinuing:
You may need to discontinue estrogens periodically. Consult your doctor.

Others:
- In rare instances, may cause blood clot in lung, brain or leg. Symptoms are sudden severe headache, coordination loss, vision change, chest pain, breathing difficulty, slurred speech, pain in legs or groin. Seek emergency treatment immediately.
- Carefully read the paper called "Information for the Patient" that was given to you with your prescription. If you lose it, ask your pharmacist for a copy.

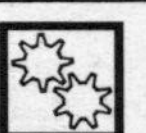

POSSIBLE INTERACTION WITH OTHER DRUGS

GENERIC NAME OR DRUG CLASS	COMBINED EFFECT
Anticoagulants, oral*	Decreased anti-coagulant effect.
Anticonvulsants, hydantoin*	Decreased estrogen effect.
Antidepressants, tricyclic*	Increased toxicity of antidepressants.
Antidiabetics, oral*	Unpredictable increase or decrease in blood sugar.
Antifibrinolytic agents*	Increased possibility of blood clotting.
Carbamazepine	Decreased estrogen effect.
Clofibrate	Decreased clofibrate effect.
Dextrothyroxine	Decreased dextrothyroxine effect.
Didanosine	Increased risk of pancreatitis.
Guanfacine	May decrease antihypertensive effects of guanfacine.
Insulin	Possible decreased insulin effect. May require dosage adjustment.
Meprobamate	Increased estrogen effect.
Phenobarbital	Decreased estrogen effect.
Primidone	Decreased estrogen effect.
Pyridoxine (vitamin B-6)	Decreased pyridoxine effect.
Rifampin	Decreased estrogen effect.
Tamoxifen	Decreased tamoxifen effect.

Continued on page 940

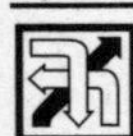

POSSIBLE INTERACTION WITH OTHER SUBSTANCES

INTERACTS WITH	COMBINED EFFECT
Alcohol:	None expected.
Beverages:	None expected.
Cocaine:	No proven problems.
Foods:	None expected.
Marijuana:	Possible menstrual irregularities and bleeding between periods.
Tobacco:	Increased risk of blood clots leading to stroke or heart attack.

***See Glossary**

ETHCHLORVYNOL

BRAND NAMES

Placidyl

BASIC INFORMATION

Habit forming? Yes
Prescription needed? Yes
Available as generic? No
Drug class: Sleep inducer (hypnotic)

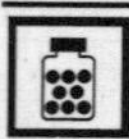

USES

Treatment of insomnia for short periods. Prolonged use is not recommended.

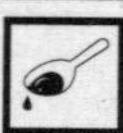

DOSAGE & USAGE INFORMATION

How to take:
Capsules—Take with food or milk to lessen side effects.

When to take:
At or near bedtime.

If you forget a dose:
Bedtime dose—If you forget your once-a-day bedtime dose, don't take it more than 3 hours late.

What drug does:
Affects brain centers that control waking and sleeping.

Time lapse before drug works:
30 to 60 minutes.

Don't take with:
Any other medicine without consulting your doctor or pharmacist.

OVERDOSE

SYMPTOMS:
Excitement, delirium, incoordination, shortness of breath, slow heartbeat, excessive drowsiness, deep coma.
WHAT TO DO:

- **Dial 911 (emergency) or 0 (operator) for an ambulance or medical help. Then give first aid immediately.**
- **If patient is unconscious and not breathing, give mouth-to-mouth breathing. If there is no heartbeat, use cardiac massage and mouth-to-mouth breathing (CPR). Don't try to make patient vomit. If you can't get help quickly, take patient to nearest emergency facility.**
- **See emergency information on inside covers.**

POSSIBLE ADVERSE REACTIONS OR SIDE EFFECTS

SYMPTOMS	WHAT TO DO
Life-threatening: In case of overdose, see previous column.	
Common:	
• Indigestion, nausea, vomiting, stomach pain.	Discontinue. Call doctor right away.
• Blurred vision, dizziness.	Continue. Call doctor when convenient.
• Unpleasant taste in mouth, fatigue, weakness.	Continue. Tell doctor at next visit.
Infrequent:	
Jitters, clumsiness, unsteadiness, drowsiness, confusion, rash, hives, unusual bleeding or bruising, facial numbness.	Discontinue. Call doctor right away.
Rare:	
Slow heartbeat, difficult breathing, fainting, jaundice, slurred speech, trembling, uncontrolled eye movements.	Discontinue. Call doctor right away.

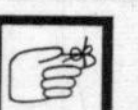

WARNINGS & PRECAUTIONS

Don't take if:

- You are allergic to any hypnotic.
- You have porphyria.
- Patient is younger than 12.

Before you start, consult your doctor:

- If you plan to become pregnant within medication period.
- If you have kidney or liver disease.

Over age 60:
Adverse reactions and side effects, especially a "hangover" effect, may be more frequent and severe than in younger persons.

Pregnancy:
Decide with your doctor if drug benefits justify risk to unborn child. Risk category C (see page xxii).

Breast-feeding:
No problems expected, but observe child and ask doctor for guidance.

Infants & children:
Not recommended.

Prolonged use:
Impaired vision.

Skin & sunlight:
No problems expected.

Driving, piloting or hazardous work:
Don't drive or pilot aircraft until you learn how medicine affects you. Don't work around dangerous machinery. Don't climb ladders or work in high places. Danger increases if you drink alcohol or take medicine affecting alertness and reflexes.

Discontinuing:
- Don't discontinue without consulting doctor. Dose may require gradual reduction if you have taken drug for a long time. Doses of other drugs may also require adjustment.
- Many side effects may occur when you stop taking this drug, including irritability, muscle twitching, hallucinations or seizures. Consult your doctor.

Others:
No problems expected.

POSSIBLE INTERACTION WITH OTHER DRUGS

GENERIC NAME OR DRUG CLASS	COMBINED EFFECT
Anticoagulants, oral*	Decreased anticoagulant effect.
Antidepressants, tricyclic* (especially amitriptyline)	Delirium and deep sedation.
Antihistamines*	Increased antihistamine effect.
Clozapine	Toxic effect on the central nervous system.
Ethinamate	Dangerous increased effects of ethinamate. Avoid combining.
Fluoxetine	Increased depressant effects of both drugs.
Guanfacine	May increase depressant effects of either drug.
Leucovorin	High alcohol content of leucovorin may cause adverse effects.
Methyprylon	Increased sedative effect, perhaps to dangerous level. Avoid.
Molindone	Increased sedative effect.
Monoamine oxidase (MAO) inhibitors*	Increased sedation.
Nabilone	Greater depression of central nervous system.
Narcotics*	Increased narcotic effect.
Pain relievers*	Increased effect of pain reliever.
Sedatives*	Increased sedative effect.
Sertraline	Increased depressive effects of both drugs.
Tranquilizers*	Increased tranquilizer effect.

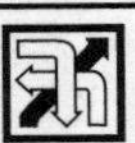

POSSIBLE INTERACTION WITH OTHER SUBSTANCES

INTERACTS WITH	COMBINED EFFECT
Alcohol:	Excessive depressant and sedative effect. Avoid.
Beverages:	None expected.
Cocaine:	Decreased ethchlorvynol effect.
Foods:	None expected.
Marijuana:	Occasional use—Drowsiness, unsteadiness, depressed function. Frequent use—Severe drowsiness, impaired physical and mental function.
Tobacco:	None expected.

***See Glossary**

ETHINAMATE

BRAND NAMES

Valmid

BASIC INFORMATION

Habit forming? Yes
Prescription needed? Yes
Available as generic? No
Drug class: Sedative (hypnotic)

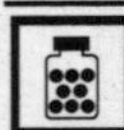

USES

Treats insomnia for short periods. Prolonged use is not recommended.

DOSAGE & USAGE INFORMATION

How to take:
Capsules—Swallow with liquid or food to lessen stomach irritation. If you can't swallow whole, open capsule and take with liquid or food.

When to take:
At bedtime.

If you forget a dose:
Skip dose. Never double dose.

What drug does:
Helps sleeplessness by an unknown mechanism of action.

Time lapse before drug works:
30 to 40 minutes.

Don't take with:
Any other medicine without consulting your doctor or pharmacist.

OVERDOSE

SYMPTOMS:
Oversedation, slow heartbeat, difficult breathing, coma.
WHAT TO DO:

- **Dial 911 (emergency) or 0 (operator) for an ambulance or medical help. Then give first aid immediately.**
- **See emergency information on inside covers.**

POSSIBLE ADVERSE REACTIONS OR SIDE EFFECTS

SYMPTOMS	WHAT TO DO
Life-threatening:	
Coma, shortness of breath, slow heartbeat.	Seek emergency treatment immediately.
Common:	
Confusion, staggering.	Discontinue. Call doctor right away.
Infrequent:	
• Unusual excitement (especially in children).	Discontinue. Seek emergency treatment.
• Skin rash, upper abdominal discomfort, vomiting.	Discontinue. Call doctor right away.
Rare:	
• Excessive bleeding.	Discontinue. Call doctor right away.
• Daytime drowsiness.	Continue. Call doctor when convenient.

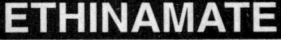

WARNINGS & PRECAUTIONS

Don't take if:
- You are an alcoholic.
- You have a history of drug abuse of any sort.

Before you start, consult your doctor:
- If you have ever had significant depression.
- If you have uncontrolled pain.

Over age 60:
Adverse reactions and side effects may be more frequent and severe than in younger persons. You may need smaller doses for shorter periods of time.

Pregnancy:
Decide with your doctor if drug benefits justify risk to unborn child. Risk category C (see page xxii).

Breast-feeding:
Unknown effects. Avoid.

Infants & children:
Not recommended.

Prolonged use:
May lead to habituation.

Skin & sunlight:
No problems expected.

Driving, piloting or hazardous work:
Don't drive or pilot aircraft until you learn how medicine affects you. Don't work around dangerous machinery. Don't climb ladders or work in high places. Danger increases if you drink alcohol or take medicine affecting alertness and reflexes.

Discontinuing:
Discontinue after maximum of 7 days. Don't resume without your doctor's recommendation.

Others:
Has not been shown to be effective after 1 week. If treatment must be repeated, allow 1 or more weeks between treatment periods.

POSSIBLE INTERACTION WITH OTHER DRUGS

GENERIC NAME OR DRUG CLASS	COMBINED EFFECT
Central nervous system (CNS) depressants*	Will dangerously increase the effects of ethinamate and any of the CNS drugs. Avoid combining.
Clozapine	Toxic effect on the central nervous system.
Fluoxetine	Increased depressant effects of both drugs.
Guanfacine	May increase depressant effects of either drug.
Leucovorin	High alcohol content of leucovorin may cause adverse effects.
Methyprylon	Increased sedative effect, perhaps to dangerous level. Avoid.
Nabilone	Greater depression of central nervous system.
Sertraline	Increased depressive effects of both drugs.

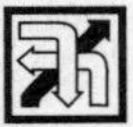

POSSIBLE INTERACTION WITH OTHER SUBSTANCES

INTERACTS WITH	COMBINED EFFECT
Alcohol:	Dangerous oversedation. Avoid.
Beverages: Any containing caffeine, such as coffee, tea or cocoa.	Decreases effects of ethinamate.
Cocaine:	Decreases effects of ethinamate and increases chance of toxicity. Avoid.
Foods:	No special problems expected.
Marijuana:	Decreases effects of ethinamate.
Tobacco:	No special problems expected.

***See Glossary**

ETHIONAMIDE

BRAND NAMES

Trecator-SC

BASIC INFORMATION

Habit forming? No
Prescription needed? Yes
Available as generic? No
Drug class: Antimycobacterial (antituberculosis)

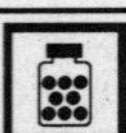

USES

Treats tuberculosis. Used in combination with other antituberculosis drugs such as isoniazid, streptomycin, rifampin, ethambutol.

DOSAGE & USAGE INFORMATION

How to take:
Tablets—Swallow with liquid or food to lessen stomach irritation. If you can't swallow whole, crumble tablet and take with liquid or food.

When to take:
Usually every 8 to 12 hours, with or after meals.

If you forget a dose:
Take as soon as you remember up to 2 hours late. If more than 2 hours, wait for next scheduled dose. Don't double this dose.

What drug does:
Kills germs that cause tuberculosis.

Time lapse before drug works:
Within 3 hours.

Don't take with:
Any other medicine without consulting your doctor or pharmacist.

OVERDOSE

SYMPTOMS:
None expected.
WHAT TO DO:
Overdose unlikely to threaten life. If person takes much larger amount than prescribed, call doctor, poison control center or hospital emergency room for instructions.

POSSIBLE ADVERSE REACTIONS OR SIDE EFFECTS

SYMPTOMS	WHAT TO DO
Life-threatening: None expected.	
Common:	
• Vomiting.	Discontinue. Call doctor right away.
• Dizziness, sore mouth, nausea, metallic taste.	Continue. Call doctor when convenient.
Infrequent: Jaundice (yellow eyes and skin); numbness, tingling, pain in hands or feet; depression; confusion.	Discontinue. Call doctor right away.
Rare:	
• Hunger, shakiness, rapid heartbeat; blurred vision; vision changes; skin rash.	Discontinue. Call doctor right away.
• Gradual swelling in the neck (thyroid gland).	Continue. Call doctor when convenient.
• Enlargement of breasts (male).	No action necessary.

WARNINGS & PRECAUTIONS

Don't take if:
You know you are hypersensitive to ethionamide.

Before you start, consult your doctor:
- If you have diabetes mellitus.
- If you have liver disease.

Over age 60:
No information available.

Pregnancy:
Decide with your doctor if drug benefits justify risk to unborn child. Risk category C (see page xxii).

Breast-feeding:
Effect not documented. Consult your family doctor or pediatrician.

Infants & children:
Effect not documented. Consult your family doctor or pediatrician.

Prolonged use:
No special problems expected.

Skin & sunlight:
No special problems expected.

Driving, piloting or hazardous work:
Don't drive or pilot aircraft until you learn how medicine affects you. Don't work around dangerous machinery. Don't climb ladders or work in high places. Danger increases if you drink alcohol or take medicine affecting alertness and reflexes.

Discontinuing:
Don't discontinue without consulting doctor.

Others:
- Advise any doctor or dentist whom you consult that you take this medicine.
- Request occasional laboratory studies for liver function.
- Request occasional eye examinations.
- Treatment may take months or years.
- You should take pyridoxine (vitamin B-6) supplements while taking ethionamide.

POSSIBLE INTERACTION WITH OTHER DRUGS

GENERIC NAME OR DRUG CLASS	COMBINED EFFECT
Cycloserine	Increased risk of seizures.
Pyridoxine	Increased excretion by kidney. (Should take pyridoxine supplements while on ethionamide to prevent development of neuritis in feet and hands).

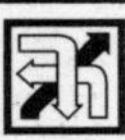

POSSIBLE INTERACTION WITH OTHER SUBSTANCES

INTERACTS WITH	COMBINED EFFECT
Alcohol:	Increased incidence of liver diseases.
Beverages: Any alcoholic beverage.	Increased incidence of liver diseases.
Cocaine:	None expected.
Foods:	None expected.
Marijuana:	No interaction expected, but may slow body's recovery.
Tobacco:	No interaction expected, but may slow body's recovery.

*See Glossary

ETIDRONATE

BRAND NAMES

Didronel
EHDP

BASIC INFORMATION

Habit forming? No
Prescription needed? Yes
Available as generic? No
Drug class: Antihypercalcemic

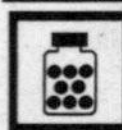

USES

- Treats Paget's disease of the bone.
- Aids healing following hip replacement or spinal cord injury.
- Treats postmenopausal osteoporosis.

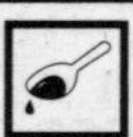

DOSAGE & USAGE INFORMATION

How to take:
Tablet—Swallow with water. Do not take with milk.

When to take:
According to doctor's instructions. Take 1 hour before or 2 hours after eating.

If you forget a dose:
Take as soon as you remember up to 6 hours late. If more than 6 hours, wait for next dose (don't double this dose).

What drug does:
Unknown. Appears to retard bone loss and stimulates bone formation.

Time lapse before drug works:
- Paget's disease—1 month.
- Other uses—1 day to several months.

Don't take with:
Any other medicine without consulting your doctor or pharmacist.

OVERDOSE

SYMPTOMS:
None expected.
WHAT TO DO:
Overdose unlikely to threaten life. If person takes much larger amount than prescribed, call doctor, poison control center or hospital emergency room for instructions.

POSSIBLE ADVERSE REACTIONS OR SIDE EFFECTS

SYMPTOMS	WHAT TO DO
Life-threatening: None expected.	
Common: Tenderness or pain in bones, diarrhea, nausea.	Continue. Call doctor when convenient.
Infrequent: None expected.	
Rare: Rash; hives; swelling of hands, feet, lips, throat.	Discontinue. Call doctor right away.

WARNINGS & PRECAUTIONS

Don't take if:
You are allergic to etidronate.

Before you start, consult your doctor:
If you have kidney disease, heart failure, bone fractures or colitis.

Over age 60:
No special problems expected.

Pregnancy:
Consult doctor. Risk category B (see page xxii).

Breast-feeding:
Safety not established. Consult doctor.

Infants & children:
Use only under supervision of a medical professional.

Prolonged use:
No special problems expected.

Skin & sunlight:
No special problems expected.

Driving, piloting or hazardous work:
No special problems expected.

Discontinuing:
Don't discontinue without doctor's advice, even though symptoms diminish or disappear.

Others:
- Medicine may be prescribed for 2 weeks, stopped for 2 to 3 months, then started again.
- Have regular check-ups with your doctor even if you currently are not undergoing treatment.

POSSIBLE INTERACTION WITH OTHER DRUGS

GENERIC NAME OR DRUG CLASS	COMBINED EFFECT
Antacids*	Decreased effect of etidronate.
Mineral supplements*	Decreased effect of etidronate.

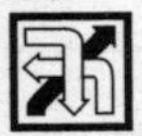

POSSIBLE INTERACTION WITH OTHER SUBSTANCES

INTERACTS WITH	COMBINED EFFECT
Alcohol:	None expected.
Beverages: Milk.	Decreased effect of etidronate.
Cocaine:	None expected.
Foods: Dairy products or foods containing high levels of calcium.	Decreased effect of etidronate.
Marijuana:	None expected.
Tobacco:	None expected.

ETOPOSIDE

BRAND NAMES

VePesid VP-16

BASIC INFORMATION

Habit forming? No
Prescription needed? Yes
Available as generic? No
Drug class: Antineoplastic

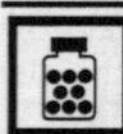

USES

- Treats testicle, lung and bladder cancer.
- Treats Hodgkin's disease and some other forms of cancer.

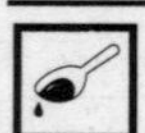

DOSAGE & USAGE INFORMATION

How to take:
- Capsules—Swallow with liquid. If you can't swallow whole, open capsule and take with liquid or food. Instructions to take on empty stomach mean 1 hour before or 2 hours after eating.
- Injection—Given under doctor's supervision.

When to take:
According to your doctor's instructions.

If you forget a dose:
Skip this dose. Never double dose. Resume regular schedule.

What drug does:
Inhibits DNA in cancer cells.

Time lapse before drug works:
Unpredictable.

Don't take with:
Any other medicines (including over-the-counter drugs such as cough and cold medicines, laxatives, antacids, diet pills, caffeine, nose drops or vitamins) without consulting your doctor.

OVERDOSE

SYMPTOMS:
Rapid pulse, shortness of breath, wheezing, fainting, coma.
WHAT TO DO:
- **Dial 911 (emergency) or 0 (operator) for an ambulance or medical help. Then give first aid immediately.**
- **See emergency information on inside covers.**

POSSIBLE ADVERSE REACTIONS OR SIDE EFFECTS

SYMPTOMS	WHAT TO DO
Life-threatening:	
In case of overdose, see previous column.	
Common:	
• Appetite loss, nausea, vomiting.	Continue. Call doctor when convenient.
• Loss of hair	No action necessary.
Infrequent:	
Symptoms of low white blood cell count and low platelet count: black, tarry stools; bloody urine; cough; chills or fever; low back pain; bruising.	Discontinue. Call doctor right away.
Rare:	
Mouth sores.	Continue. Call doctor when convenient.

WARNINGS & PRECAUTIONS

Don't take if:
- You have chicken pox.
- You have shingles (herpes zoster).

Before you start, consult your doctor:
If you have liver or kidney disease.

Over age 60:
No special problems expected.

Pregnancy:
Risk to unborn child outweighs drug benefits. Don't use. Risk category D (see page xxii).

Breast-feeding:
Drug passes into milk. Avoid drug or discontinue nursing until you finish medicine. Consult doctor for advice on maintaining milk supply.

Infants & children:
Effect not documented. Consult your doctor.

Prolonged use:
- Talk to your doctor about the need for follow-up medical examinations or laboratory studies to check complete blood counts (white blood cell count, platelet count, red blood cell count, hemoglobin, hematocrit).
- Check mouth frequently for ulcers.

Skin & sunlight:
No problems expected.

Driving, piloting or hazardous work:
Avoid if you feel confused, drowsy or dizzy.

Discontinuing:
May still experience symptoms of bone marrow depression, such as: blood in stools, fever or chills, blood spots under the skin, back pain, hoarseness, bloody urine. If any of these occur, call your doctor right away.

Others:
- Advise any doctor or dentist whom you consult that you take this medicine.
- May affect results in some medical tests.
- Etoposide may be used in combinations with other antineoplastic treatment plans. The incidence and severity of side effects may be different when used in combinations such as doxorubicin, procarbazine and etoposide (APE); etoposide, cyclophosphamide, doxorubicin and vincristine (CAVE, ECHO, CAPO, EVAC or VOCA); cyclophosphamide, doxorubicin and etoposide (CAE or ACE); cisplatin, bleomycin, doxorubicin and etoposide; cisplatin, bleomycin and etoposide; cisplatin and etoposide. For further information regarding these combinations, consult your doctor.

POSSIBLE INTERACTION WITH OTHER DRUGS

GENERIC NAME OR DRUG CLASS	COMBINED EFFECT
Angiotensin-converting enzyme (ACE) inhibitors*	May increase bone marrow depression or make kidney damage more likely.
Antineoplastic (cancer-treating) drugs*	May increase bone marrow depression or make kidney damage more likely.
Clozapine	Toxic effect on bone marrow.
Tiopronin	Increased risk of toxicity to bone marrow.
Vaccines, live or killed virus	Increased likelihood of toxicity or reduced effectiveness of vaccine. Wait 3 months to 1 year after etoposide treatment before getting vaccine.

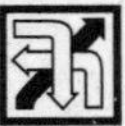

POSSIBLE INTERACTION WITH OTHER SUBSTANCES

INTERACTS WITH	COMBINED EFFECT
Alcohol:	Increased likelihood of adverse reactions. Avoid.
Beverages:	No special problems expected.
Cocaine:	Increased likelihood of adverse reactions. Avoid.
Foods:	No special problems expected.
Marijuana:	Increased likelihood of adverse reactions. Avoid.
Tobacco:	No special problems expected.

*See Glossary

ETRETINATE

BRAND NAMES

Tegison

BASIC INFORMATION

Habit forming? No
Prescription needed? Yes
Available as generic? No
Drug class: Antipsoriatic

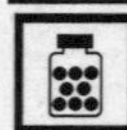

USES

- Treats psoriasis in patients who don't respond well to standard or usual treatment.
- Treats arthritic symptoms sometimes associated with psoriasis.
- Treats ichthyosis.

DOSAGE & USAGE INFORMATION

How to take:
Capsules—Swallow with liquid or food to lessen stomach irritation. If you can't swallow whole, open capsule and take with liquid or food.

When to take:
At the same time each day, according to instructions on prescription label.

If you forget a dose:
Take as soon as you remember up to 2 hours late. If more than 2 hours, wait for next scheduled dose (don't double this dose).

What drug does:
- Mechanism of action on skin is unknown, but positive effects on the disease have been documented. It probably reduces the production of protein in the outer layers of skin. It is chemically related to tretinoin (Retin-A).
- Also functions as an anti-inflammatory agent.

Continued next column

OVERDOSE

SYMPTOMS:
None documented. If overdose is suspected, follow instructions below.
WHAT TO DO:
- **Dial 911 (emergency) or 0 (operator) for an ambulance or medical help. Then give first aid immediately.**
- **See emergency information on inside covers.**

Time lapse before drug works:
- 2 to 6 hours for effects to begin.
- Prolonged treatment, up to 2 to 4 weeks (sometimes with psoralens, ultraviolet light may be necessary to develop maximum benefit).

Don't take with:
Any other medicine without consulting your doctor or pharmacist.

POSSIBLE ADVERSE REACTIONS OR SIDE EFFECTS

SYMPTOMS	WHAT TO DO
Life-threatening:	
None expected.	
Common:	
• Bone and joint pain, eye irritation on exposure to sunlight.	Discontinue. Call doctor right away.
• Dry skin and eyes, nosebleeds, hair loss.	Continue. Call doctor when convenient.
Infrequent:	
Muscle cramps, blurred vision, hearing loss, dark-colored urine, jaundice, unusual bleeding or bruising.	Discontinue. Call doctor right away.
Rare:	
• Itching, peeling skin; inflamed nails; nausea; vomiting; headache.	Discontinue. Call doctor right away.
• Confusion, depression, anxiety, erection difficulties in males.	Continue. Call doctor when convenient.

WARNINGS & PRECAUTIONS

Don't take if:
If you are pregnant or expect to get pregnant in the future. Fetal abnormalies have occurred as long as 2 years after discontinuing drug.

Before you start, consult your doctor:
- If you have heart or blood vessel disease.
- If you have immediate family members with heart or blood vessel disease.
- If you have high plasma triglycerides.
- If you are an alcoholic.
- If you have diabetes mellitus.
- If you have liver disease.

Over age 60:
Adverse reactions and side effects may be more frequent and severe than in younger persons. You may need smaller doses for shorter periods of time.

Pregnancy:
Risk to unborn child outweighs drug benefits. Etretinate has caused major human fetal abnormalities. Don't use. Risk category X (see page xxii).

Breast-feeding:
Drug passes into milk. Avoid drug or discontinue nursing until you finish medicine. Consult doctor for advice on maintaining milk supply.

Infants & children:
Don't use.

Prolonged use:
- No problems expected, if used for no more than 4 months per treatment session.
- Talk to your doctor about the need for follow-up medical examinations or laboratory studies to check blood lipids, liver function.

Skin & sunlight:
May cause increased sensitivity to sunlight. Avoid when possible.

Driving, piloting or hazardous work:
Don't drive or pilot aircraft until you learn how medicine affects you. Don't work around dangerous machinery. Don't climb ladders or work in high places. Danger increases if you drink alcohol or take medicine affecting alertness and reflexes.

Discontinuing:
Don't discontinue without consulting doctor. Dose may require gradual reduction if you have taken drug for a long time. Doses of other drugs may also require adjustment.

Others:
- Courses of treatment are usually limited to 4 months, and repeating, if necessary, after a 4-month rest period.
- Don't donate blood during treatment or for several years thereafter.
- Likelihood of producing cancer is very low.
- During early treatment, psoriasis may appear to worsen.
- May cause changes in cholesterol levels in blood.
- May cause calcium deposits in tendons and ligaments.

POSSIBLE INTERACTION WITH OTHER DRUGS

GENERIC NAME OR DRUG CLASS	COMBINED EFFECT
Abrasive soaps or cleaners	Excessive drying effect on skin.
Acne preparations*	Excessive drying effect on skin.
Any topical preparation containing alcohol such as after-shave lotions	Excessive drying effect on skin.
Isoniazid	Increased risk of liver damage.
Isotretinoin	Increased toxicity.
Medicated cosmetics	Excessive drying effect on skin.
Methotrexate	Increased toxicity to liver.
Tetracyclines*	Increased adverse reactions of etretinate.
Tretinoin	Increased toxicity.
Vitamin A	Increased toxicity.

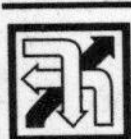

POSSIBLE INTERACTION WITH OTHER SUBSTANCES

INTERACTS WITH	COMBINED EFFECT
Alcohol:	May cause hypertriglyceridemia.
Beverages: Milk.	Aids absorption of etretinate.
Cocaine:	None expected.
Foods: High-fat diet or milk products.	Aids absorption of etretinate.
Marijuana:	None expected.
Tobacco:	None expected.

*See Glossary

FAMCICLOVIR

BRAND NAMES

Famvir

BASIC INFORMATION

Habit forming? No
Prescription needed? Yes
Available as generic? No
Drug class: Antiviral (systemic)

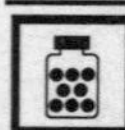

USES

- Treatment for acute herpes zoster (also known as shingles), a viral infection of the skin.
- May be used for treatment and prevention of genital herpes simplex infection.

DOSAGE & USAGE INFORMATION

How to take:
Tablet—Swallow with liquid. May be taken on a full or empty stomach.

When to take:
At the same times each day and night. Drug works best if started within 48 hours of diagnosis (or when symptoms first appear).

If you forget a dose:
Take as soon as you remember up to 2 hours late. If more than 2 hours, wait for next dose (don't double this dose).

What drug does:
Relieves the acute pain of herpes zoster and helps the blisters heal faster.

Time lapse before drug works:
Begins the first day, but may take several days for symptoms (pain, burning and blisters) to improve.

Don't take with:
Any other medicine without consulting your doctor or pharmacist.

OVERDOSE

SYMPTOMS:
None expected.
WHAT TO DO:
Overdose unlikely to threaten life. If person takes much larger amount than prescribed, call doctor, poison control center or hospital emergency room for instructions.

POSSIBLE ADVERSE REACTIONS OR SIDE EFFECTS

SYMPTOMS	WHAT TO DO
Life-threatening:	
None expected.	
Common:	
None expected.	
Infrequent:	
Headache, nausea, diarrhea, vomiting, tiredness, dizziness.	Continue. Call doctor when convenient.
Rare:	
None expected.	

WARNINGS & PRECAUTIONS

Don't take if:
You are allergic to famciclovir.

Before you start, consult your doctor:
If you have kidney disease.

Over age 60:
No special problems expected.

Pregnancy:
Consult doctor about safety of use during pregnancy. Risk category B (see page xxii).

Breast-feeding:
Unknown effects. Avoid nursing until you finish medicine. Consult doctor for advice on maintaining milk supply.

Infants & children:
Safety and dosage have not been established. Use only under medical supervision.

Prolonged use:
Not intended for long-term use.

Skin & sunlight:
No special problems expected.

Driving, piloting or hazardous work:
No special problems expected.

Discontinuing:
Follow doctor's instructions.

Others:
- Keep affected skin area clean and dry.
- Decrease blister irritation by wearing loose-fitting clothing.

POSSIBLE INTERACTION WITH OTHER DRUGS

GENERIC NAME OR DRUG CLASS	COMBINED EFFECT
None significant.	

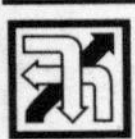

POSSIBLE INTERACTION WITH OTHER SUBSTANCES

INTERACTS WITH	COMBINED EFFECT
Alcohol:	None expected.
Beverages:	None expected.
Cocaine:	None expected.
Foods:	None expected.
Marijuana:	None expected.
Tobacco:	None expected.

*See Glossary

FELBAMATE

BRAND AND GENERIC NAMES

Felbatol FBM

BASIC INFORMATION

Habit forming? No
Prescription needed? Yes
Available as generic? No
Drug class: Anticonvulsant

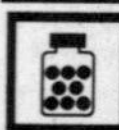

USES

- Treatment for partial epileptic seizures.
- Treatment for Lennox-Gastaut syndrome (a severe form of epilepsy in children).

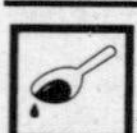

DOSAGE & USAGE INFORMATION

How to take:
- Tablet–Swallow with liquid.
- Oral suspension–Follow instructions on package label.

When to take:
At the same times each day. Your doctor will determine the best schedule. Dosages will gradually be increased over the first 3 weeks.

If you forget a dose:
Take as soon as you remember up to 2 hours late. If more than 2 hours, wait for next scheduled dose (don't double this dose).

What drug does:
- Decreases the frequency of partial seizures that start in a localized part of the brain, including those that progress into more generalized grand mal seizures.
- Decreases seizure activity and improves quality of life in children with Lennox-Gastaut syndrome.

Time lapse before drug works:
May take several weeks for maximum effectiveness.

Don't take with:
- Any other prescription or nonprescription drug without consulting your doctor.
- See Interaction column and consult doctor.

OVERDOSE

SYMPTOMS:
Gastric distress, increased heart rate.
WHAT TO DO:
Overdose unlikely to threaten life. If person takes much larger amount than prescribed, call doctor, poison control center or hospital emergency room for instructions.

POSSIBLE ADVERSE REACTIONS OR SIDE EFFECTS

SYMPTOMS	WHAT TO DO
Life-threatening: None expected.	
Common:	
• Fever, red or purple spots on skin, walking in unusual manner.	Continue, but call doctor right away.
• Abdominal pain, taste changes, constipation, sleeping difficulty, dizziness, headache, nausea or vomiting, indigestion, appetite loss.	Continue. Call doctor when convenient.
Infrequent:	
• Mood or mental changes, clumsiness, skin rash, tremor.	Continue, but call doctor right away.
• Vision changes, diarrhea, drowsiness, coughing or sneezing, ear pain or fullness, runny nose, weight loss.	Continue. Call doctor when convenient.
Rare:	
Black or tarry stools, bloody or dark-colored urine, unusual bruising or bleeding, breathing difficulty, wheezing, pain or tightness in chest, sore throat, mouth or lip sores, swollen face, swollen or painful glands or lymph nodes, yellow skin or eyes, chills, general tired feeling, continuing headache or abdominal pain, hives, itching, muscle cramps, stuffy nose, skin reaction to sunlight.	Continue, but call doctor right away.

WARNINGS & PRECAUTIONS

Don't take if:
You are allergic to felbamate.

Before you start, consult your doctor:
- If you have a sensitivity to other carbamate drugs*, other medications or other substances.
- If you have any blood disorder.
- If you have a history of bone marrow depression.
- If you have or have had any liver disease.

Over age 60:
Adverse reactions and side effects may be more frequent and severe than in younger persons.

Pregnancy:
Decide with your doctor if drug benefits justify risks to unborn child. Risk category B (see page xxii).

Breast-feeding:
Drug passes into milk. Unknown effect. Consult your doctor.

Infants & children:
Give only under close medical supervision.

Prolonged use:
Talk to your doctor about the need for follow-up medical examinations or laboratory studies to check complete blood counts (white blood cell count, platelet count, red blood cell count, hemoglobin, hematocrit), iron concentrations and liver function studies.

Skin & sunlight:
No problems expected.

Driving, piloting or hazardous work:
Don't drive or pilot aircraft until you learn how medicine affects you. Don't work around dangerous machinery. Don't climb ladders or work in high places. Danger increases if you drink alcohol or take other medicines affecting alertness and reflexes such as antihistamines, tranquilizers, sedatives, pain medicine, narcotics and mind-altering drugs.

Discontinuing:
Don't discontinue without doctor's approval due to risk of increased seizure activity.

Others:
- Felbamate may cause serious side effects including blood problems and liver problems (rarely fatal). Decide with your doctor if drug benefits justify risks.
- Advise any doctor or dentist whom you consult that you take this medicine.
- Felbamate may be used alone or combined with other antiepileptic drugs. The dosages of other antiepileptic drugs you currently use will be reduced to minimize side effects and adverse reactions due to interactions.

*See Glossary

POSSIBLE INTERACTION WITH OTHER DRUGS

GENERIC NAME OR DRUG CLASS	COMBINED EFFECT
Carbamazepine	Increased side effects and adverse reactions.
Phenytoin	Increased side effects and adverse reactions.
Valproic acid	Increased side effects and adverse reactions.

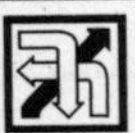

POSSIBLE INTERACTION WITH OTHER SUBSTANCES

INTERACTS WITH	COMBINED EFFECT
Alcohol:	None expected.
Beverages:	None expected.
Cocaine:	None expected.
Foods:	None expected.
Marijuana:	None expected.
Tobacco:	None expected.

FINASTERIDE

BRAND NAMES

Proscar

BASIC INFORMATION

Habit forming? No
Prescription needed? Yes
Available as generic? No
Drug class: Dihydrotestosterone inhibitor

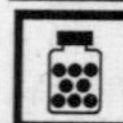

USES

- Treats noncancerous enlargement of the prostate gland in men (benign prostatic hypertrophy or BPH).
- Theoretically, may prevent the development of prostate cancer.

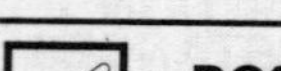

DOSAGE & USAGE INFORMATION

How to take:
Tablets—Swallow with liquid. If you can't swallow whole, crumble tablet and take with liquid or food.

When to take:
Once a day or as directed, with or without meals.

If you forget a dose:
Take as soon as you remember up to 2 hours late. If more than 2 hours, wait for next scheduled dose (don't double this dose).

What drug does:
Inhibits the enzyme needed for the conversion of testosterone to dihydrotestosterone. Dihydrotestosterone is required for the development of benign prostatic hypertrophy.

Time lapse before drug works:
May require up to 6 months for full therapeutic effect.

Don't take with:
Any other medicine without consulting your doctor or pharmacist, especially nonprescription decongestants.

OVERDOSE

SYMPTOMS:
None expected.
WHAT TO DO:
Overdose unlikely to threaten life.

POSSIBLE ADVERSE REACTIONS OR SIDE EFFECTS

SYMPTOMS	WHAT TO DO
Life-threatening: None expected.	
Common: None expected.	
Infrequent: Decreased volume of ejaculation.	Continue. Tell doctor at next visit.
Rare: Impotence, decreased libido.	Continue. Call doctor when convenient.

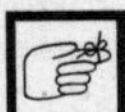

WARNINGS & PRECAUTIONS

Don't take if:
You are allergic to finasteride.

Before you start, consult your doctor:
- If you have not had a blood test to check for prostate cancer.
- If your wife is pregnant or may become pregnant.
- If you have a liver disorder.
- If you have reduced urinary flow.
- If you have large residual urinary volume.

Over age 60:
No special problems expected.

Pregnancy:
- Not recommended for women.
- Pregnant women should not handle the crushed tablets.
- Avoid exposure to mate's semen if he takes finasteride.
- Risk category X (see page xxii).

Breast-feeding:
Not recommended for women.

Infants & children:
Not recommended.

Prolonged use:
Talk to your doctor about the need for follow-up medical examinations or laboratory studies to check the effectiveness of the treatment.

Skin & sunlight:
No special problems expected.

Driving, piloting or hazardous work:
No special problems expected.

Discontinuing:
Don't discontinue without medical advice.

Others:
- Advise any doctor or dentist whom you consult that you take this medicine.
- May affect results of some medical tests.
- For those who respond well, the drug must be continued indefinitely.

POSSIBLE INTERACTION WITH OTHER DRUGS

GENERIC NAME OR DRUG CLASS	COMBINED EFFECT
Anticholinergics*	Decreased finasteride effect.
Bronchodilators, adrenergic	Decreased finasteride effect.
Bronchodilators, xanthine	Decreased finasteride effect.
Ephedrine	Decreased finasteride effect.
Phenylpropanolamine	Decreased finasteride effect.
Pseudoephedrine	Decreased finasteride effect.

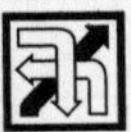

POSSIBLE INTERACTION WITH OTHER SUBSTANCES

INTERACTS WITH	COMBINED EFFECT
Alcohol:	No proven problems.
Beverages:	No proven problems.
Cocaine:	No proven problems.
Foods:	No proven problems.
Marijuana:	No proven problems.
Tobacco:	No proven problems.

***See Glossary**

FLAVOXATE

BRAND NAMES

Urispas

BASIC INFORMATION

Habit forming? No
Prescription needed? Yes
Available as generic? No
Drug class: Antispasmodic (urinary tract)

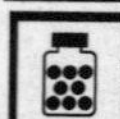

USES

Relieves urinary pain, urgency, nighttime urination, unusual frequency of urination associated with urinary system disorders.

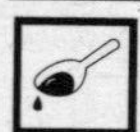

DOSAGE & USAGE INFORMATION

How to take:
Tablet—Swallow with liquid or food to lessen stomach irritation.

When to take:
30 minutes before meals (unless directed otherwise by doctor).

If you forget a dose:
Take as soon as you remember up to 2 hours late. If more than 2 hours, wait for next scheduled dose (don't double this dose).

What drug does:
Blocks nerve impulses at smooth muscle nerve endings, preventing muscle contractions and gland secretions of organs involved.

Time lapse before drug works:
15 to 30 minutes.

Don't take with:
Any other medicine without consulting your doctor or pharmacist.

OVERDOSE

SYMPTOMS:
Dilated pupils, rapid pulse and breathing, dizziness, fever, hallucinations, confusion, slurred speech, agitation, flushed face, convulsions, coma.
WHAT TO DO:
- **Dial 911 (emergency) or 0 (operator) for an ambulance or medical help. Then give first aid immediately.**
- **See emergency information on inside covers.**

POSSIBLE ADVERSE REACTIONS OR SIDE EFFECTS

SYMPTOMS	WHAT TO DO
Life-threatening:	
In case of overdose, see previous column.	
Common:	
• Confusion, delirium, rapid heartbeat.	Discontinue. Call doctor right away.
• Nausea, vomiting, less perspiration, drowsiness.	Continue. Call doctor when convenient.
• Constipation.	Continue. Tell doctor at next visit.
• Dry ears, nose, throat.	No action necessary.
Infrequent:	
• Unusual excitement, irritability, restlessness, clumsiness, hallucinations.	Discontinue. Call doctor right away.
• Headache, increased sensitivity to light, painful or difficult urination.	Continue. Call doctor when convenient.
Rare:	
• Shortness of breath.	Discontinue. Seek emergency treatment.
• Rash or hives; eye pain; blurred vision; sore throat, fever, mouth sores; abdominal pain.	Discontinue. Call doctor right away.
• Dizziness.	Continue. Call doctor when convenient.

WARNINGS & PRECAUTIONS

Don't take if:
- You are allergic to any anticholinergic.
- You have trouble with stomach bloating.
- You have difficulty emptying your bladder completely.
- You have narrow-angle glaucoma.
- You have severe ulcerative colitis.

Before you start, consult your doctor:
- If you have open-angle glaucoma.
- If you have angina.
- If you have chronic bronchitis or asthma.
- If you have liver disease.
- If you have hiatal hernia.
- If you have enlarged prostate.
- If you have myasthenia gravis.
- If you have peptic ulcer.
- If you will have surgery within 2 months, including dental surgery, requiring general or spinal anesthesia.

Over age 60:
Adverse reactions and side effects, particularly mental confusion, may be more frequent and severe than in younger persons.

Pregnancy:
Consult doctor. Risk category B (see page xxii).

Breast-feeding:
Drug passes into milk. Avoid drug or discontinue nursing until you finish medicine. Consult doctor for advice on maintaining milk supply.

Infants & children:
Use only under medical supervision.

Prolonged use:
Chronic constipation, possible fecal impaction. Consult doctor immediately.

Skin & sunlight:
No problems expected.

Driving, piloting or hazardous work:
Use disqualifies you for piloting aircraft. Don't drive until you learn how medicine affects you. Don't work around dangerous machinery. Don't climb ladders or work in high places. Danger increases if you drink alcohol or take medicine affecting alertness and reflexes, such as antihistamines, tranquilizers, sedatives, pain medicine, narcotics and mind-altering drugs.

Discontinuing:
May be unnecessary to finish medicine. Follow doctor's instructions.

Others:
No problems expected.

POSSIBLE INTERACTION WITH OTHER DRUGS

GENERIC NAME OR DRUG CLASS	COMBINED EFFECT
Antimuscarinics*	Increased effect of flavoxate.
Central nervous system (CNS) depressants, other*	Increased effect of both drugs.
Clozapine	Toxic effect on the central nervous system.
Ethinamate	Dangerous increased effects of ethinamate. Avoid combining.
Fluoxetine	Increased depressant effects of both drugs.
Guanfacine	May increase depressant effects of either drug.
Leucovorin	High alcohol content of leucovorin may cause adverse effects.
Methyprylon	Increased sedative effect, perhaps to dangerous level. Avoid.
Nabilone	Greater depression of central nervous system.
Nizatidine	Increased nizatidine effect.
Sertraline	Increased depressive effects of both drugs.

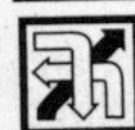

POSSIBLE INTERACTION WITH OTHER SUBSTANCES

INTERACTS WITH	COMBINED EFFECT
Alcohol:	None expected.
Beverages:	None expected.
Cocaine:	Excessively rapid heartbeat. Avoid.
Foods:	None expected.
Marijuana:	Drowsiness, dry mouth.
Tobacco:	None expected.

*See Glossary

FLECAINIDE ACETATE

BRAND NAMES

Tambocor

BASIC INFORMATION

Habit forming? No
Prescription needed? Yes
Available as generic? No
Drug class: Antiarrhythmic

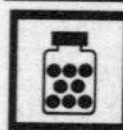

USES

Stabilizes irregular heartbeat.

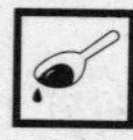

DOSAGE & USAGE INFORMATION

How to take:
Tablet—Swallow with liquid. If you can't swallow whole, crumble tablet and take with liquid or food.

When to take:
At the same time each day, according to instructions on prescription label. Take tablets approximately 12 hours apart.

If you forget a dose:
Take as soon as you remember up to 4 hours late. If more than 4 hours, wait for next scheduled dose (don't double this dose).

What drug does:
Decreases conduction of abnormal electrical activity in the heart muscle or its regulating systems.

Continued next column

OVERDOSE

SYMPTOMS:
Low blood pressure or unconsciousness, irregular or rapid heartbeat, sleepiness, tremor, sweating.
WHAT TO DO:

- **Dial 911 (emergency) or 0 (operator) for an ambulance or medical help. Then give first aid immediately.**
- **If patient is unconscious and not breathing, give mouth-to-mouth breathing. If there is no heartbeat, use cardiac massage and mouth-to-mouth breathing (CPR). Don't try to make patient vomit. If you can't get help quickly, take patient to nearest emergency facility.**
- **See emergency information on inside covers.**

Time lapse before drug works:
1 to 6 hours. May need doses daily for 2 to 3 days for maximum effect.

Don't take with:
Any other medicine without consulting your doctor or pharmacist.

POSSIBLE ADVERSE REACTIONS OR SIDE EFFECTS

SYMPTOMS	WHAT TO DO
Life-threatening:	
In case of overdose, see previous column.	
Common:	
Blurred vision, dizziness.	Continue. Call doctor when convenient.
Infrequent:	
• Chest pain, irregular heartbeat.	Discontinue. Seek emergency treatment.
• Shakiness, rash, nausea, vomiting.	Continue, but call doctor right away.
• Anxiety; depression; weakness; headache; appetite loss; weakness in muscles, bones, joints; swollen feet, ankles or legs; loss of taste; numbness or tingling in hands or feet, abdominal pain.	Continue. Call doctor when convenient.
• Constipation.	Continue. Tell doctor at next visit.
Rare:	
• Shortness of breath.	Discontinue. Seek emergency treatment.
• Sore throat, jaundice, fever.	Continue, but call doctor right away.

WARNINGS & PRECAUTIONS

Don't take if:
You are allergic to flecainide or a local anesthetic such as novocaine, xylocaine or other drug whose generic name ends with "caine."

Before you start, consult your doctor:

- If you have kidney disease.
- If you have liver disease.
- If you have had a heart attack in past 3 weeks.
- If you have a pacemaker.

Over age 60:
Adverse reactions and side effects may be more frequent and severe than in younger persons.

Pregnancy:
Decide with your doctor whether drug benefits justify risk to unborn child. Risk category C (see page xxii).

Breast-feeding:
Drug passes into milk. Avoid drug or discontinue nursing until you finish medicine. Consult doctor for advice on maintaining milk supply.

Infants & children:
Not recommended. Safety and dosage have not been established.

Prolonged use:
Talk to your doctor about the need for follow-up medical examinations or laboratory studies to check complete blood counts (white blood cell count, platelet count, red blood cell count, hemoglobin, hematocrit), ECG*.

Skin & sunlight:
No problems expected.

Driving, piloting or hazardous work:
Don't drive or pilot aircraft until you learn how medicine affects you. Don't work around dangerous machinery. Don't climb ladders or work in high places. Danger increases if you drink alcohol or take medicine affecting alertness and reflexes, such as antihistamines, tranquilizers, sedatives, pain medicine, narcotics and mind-altering drugs.

Discontinuing:
Don't discontinue without consulting doctor. Dose may require gradual reduction if you have taken drug for a long time. Doses of other drugs may also require adjustment.

Others:
Wear identification bracelet or carry an identification card with inscription of medicine you take.

POSSIBLE INTERACTION WITH OTHER DRUGS

GENERIC NAME OR DRUG CLASS	COMBINED EFFECT
Antacids* (high dose)	Possible increased flecainide acetate effect.
Antiarrhythmics, other*	Possible irregular heartbeat.
Beta-adrenergic blocking agents*	Possible decreased efficiency of heart muscle contraction, leading to congestive heart failure.
Bone marrow depressants*	Possible decreased production of blood cells in bone marrow.
Carbonic anhydrase inhibitors*	Possible increased flecainide acetate effect.
Cimetidine	Increased effect of flecainide.
Digitalis preparations*	Possible increased digitalis effect. Possible irregular heartbeat.
Disopyramide	Possible decreased efficiency of heart muscle contraction, leading to congestive heart failure.
Encainide	Increased effect of toxicity on the heart muscle.
Nicardipine	Possible increased effect and toxicity of each drug.
Paroxetine	Increased effect of both drugs.
Propafenone	Increased effect of both drugs and increased risk of toxicity.
Sodium bicarbonate	Possible increased flecainide acetate effect.
Verapamil	Possible decreased efficiency of heart muscle contraction, leading to congestive heart failure.

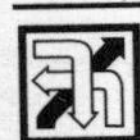

POSSIBLE INTERACTION WITH OTHER SUBSTANCES

INTERACTS WITH	COMBINED EFFECT
Alcohol:	May further depress normal heart function.
Beverages: Caffeine-containing beverages.	Possible decreased flecainide effect.
Cocaine:	Possible decreased flecainide effect.
Foods:	None expected.
Marijuana:	Possible decreased flecainide effect.
Tobacco:	Possible decreased flecainide effect.

*See Glossary

FLUCONAZOLE

BRAND NAMES

Diflucan

BASIC INFORMATION

Habit forming? No
Prescription needed? Yes
Available as generic? No
Drug class: Antifungal

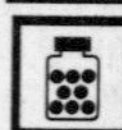

USES

- Treats meningitis.
- Treats candidiasis (thrush) whether in the mouth, esophagus or vagina or widely disseminated throughout the body.

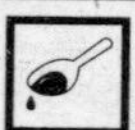

DOSAGE & USAGE INFORMATION

How to take:
Tablets—Swallow with liquid. If you can't swallow whole, crumble tablet and take with liquid or food. Instructions to take on empty stomach mean 1 hour before or 2 hours after eating.

When to take:
Once a day, probably for 10 to 12 weeks, depending on the disease being treated and your kidney function status.

If you forget a dose:
Take as soon as you remember up to 2 hours late. If more than 2 hours, wait for next scheduled dose (don't double this dose).

What drug does:
Changes the cell membranes of susceptible fungus germs.

Time lapse before drug works:
1 to 2 hours. Several weeks of treatment are necessary for full benefit.

Don't take with:
Other antifungal drugs in the azole family (ketoconazole, miconazole or itraconazole).

OVERDOSE

SYMPTOMS:
Overdose not expected to threaten life, but if accidental or purposeful overdose occurs, follow the directions below.
WHAT TO DO:

- **Dial 911 (emergency) or 0 (operator) for an ambulance or medical help. Then give first aid immediately.**
- **See emergency information on inside covers.**

POSSIBLE ADVERSE REACTIONS OR SIDE EFFECTS

SYMPTOMS	WHAT TO DO
Life-threatening: In case of overdose, see previous column.	
Common: None expected.	
Infrequent: Diarrhea, nausea, vomiting.	Continue. Call doctor when convenient.
Rare: Skin rash, blistering, peeling skin, dark urine, yellow skin or eyes, abdominal pain, unusual bleeding or bruising.	Discontinue. Call doctor right away.

WARNINGS & PRECAUTIONS

Don't take if:
You are allergic to similar drugs, such as ketoconazole, miconazole or itraconazole.

Before you start, consult your doctor:
- If you have kidney disease.
- If you have liver disease.

Over age 60:
No studies available, but dosage may need adjustment if there is any age-related kidney impairment

Pregnancy:
Decide with your doctor if drug benefits justify risk to unborn child. Risk category C (see page xxii).

Breast-feeding:
Safety not established. Consult doctor.

Infants & children:
Safety not established. Consult doctor.

Prolonged use:
No special problems expected.

Skin & sunlight:
No special problems expected.

Driving, piloting or hazardous work:
No special problems expected

Discontinuing:
Don't discontinue without consulting doctor. Dose may require gradual reduction if you have taken drug for a long time. Doses of other drugs may also require adjustment.

Others:
- Advise any doctor or dentist whom you consult that you take this medicine.
- May affect results of some medical tests.
- Does not alter male hormone activity. (A similar drug, ketoconazole, does alter male hormone activity.)

POSSIBLE INTERACTION WITH OTHER DRUGS

GENERIC NAME OR DRUG CLASS	COMBINED EFFECT
Antidiabetics, oral*	Greater than expected drop in blood sugar. If any antidiabetic agent is taken with fluconazole, blood sugars must be monitored carefully.
Cyclosporine	Increased cyclosporine effect.
Phenytoin	Increased phenytoin effect.
Rifampin	Decreased fluconazole effect.
Warfarin	Increased warfarin effect.

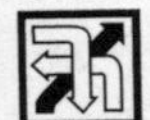

POSSIBLE INTERACTION WITH OTHER SUBSTANCES

INTERACTS WITH	COMBINED EFFECT
Alcohol:	None expected.
Beverages:	None expected.
Cocaine:	None expected.
Foods:	None expected.
Marijuana:	None expected.
Tobacco:	None expected.

*See Glossary

FLUOROQUINOLONES

BRAND AND GENERIC NAMES

Cipro	Maxaquin
CIPROFLOXACIN	NORFLOXACIN
ENOXACIN	Noroxin
Floxin	OFLOXACIN
LOMEFLOXACIN	Penetrex

BASIC INFORMATION

Habit forming? No
Prescription needed? Yes
Available as generic? No
Drug class: Antibacterial (antibiotic), fluoroquinolone

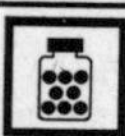

USES

Treats a wide range of bacteria that may cause diarrhea, pneumonia, skin and soft tissue infections, urinary tract infections, bone infections.

DOSAGE & USAGE INFORMATION

How to take:
Tablets—Take with full glass of water on empty stomach (ciprofloxacin or lomefloxacin may be taken with meals).

When to take:
As directed by your doctor.

If you forget a dose:
Take as soon as you remember up to 2 hours late. If more than 2 hours, wait for next scheduled dose (don't double this dose).

Continued next column

OVERDOSE

SYMPTOMS:
Convulsions.
WHAT TO DO:
- **Dial 911 (emergency) or 0 (operator) for an ambulance or medical help. Then give first aid immediately.**
- **If patient is unconscious and not breathing, give mouth-to-mouth breathing. If there is no heartbeat, use cardiac massage and mouth-to-mouth breathing (CPR). Don't try to make patient vomit. If you can't get help quickly, take patient to nearest emergency facility.**
- **See emergency information on inside covers.**

What drug does:
Destroys bacteria in the body, probably by promoting DNA breakage in germs.

Time lapse before drug works:
1 to 2 hours.

Don't take with:
- Antacids.
- Any other medicine without consulting your doctor or pharmacist.

POSSIBLE ADVERSE REACTIONS OR SIDE EFFECTS

SYMPTOMS	WHAT TO DO
Life-threatening:	
Hives, rash, intense itching, faintness soon after a dose (anaphylaxis).	Seek emergency treatment immediately.
Common:	
None expected.	
Infrequent:	
Dizziness, light-headedness, headache, nervousness, drowsiness or insomnia, stomach pain, diarrhea, nausea or vomiting.	Continue. Call doctor when convenient.
Rare:	
Agitation, confusion, hallucinations, tremors, skin rash or redness, shortness of breath, neck or face swelling, bloody or cloudy urine, swelling of feet or legs.	Discontinue. Call doctor right away.

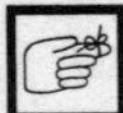

WARNINGS & PRECAUTIONS

Don't take if:
You are allergic to fluoroquinolones or quinolone derivatives.

Before you start, consult your doctor:
- If you have any disorder of the central nervous system such as epilepsy or stroke.
- If you have liver or kidney disease.

Over age 60:
Adverse reactions and side effects may be more frequent and severe than in younger persons. You may need smaller doses for shorter periods of time.

Pregnancy:
Decide with your doctor if drug benefits justify risk to unborn child. Risk category C (see page xxii).

Breast-feeding:
Drug passes into milk. Avoid drug or discontinue nursing until you finish medicine. Consult doctor for advice on maintaining milk supply.

Infants & children:
Not recommended.

Prolonged use:
No documented problems.

Skin & sunlight:
Rare adverse reaction to sunlight or sun lamp. Avoid over-exposure.

Driving, piloting or hazardous work:
Don't drive or pilot aircraft until you learn how medicine affects you. Don't work around dangerous machinery. Don't climb ladders or work in high places. Danger increases if you drink alcohol or take medicine affecting alertness and reflexes, such as antihistamines, tranquilizers, sedatives, pain medicine, narcotics and mind-altering drugs.

Discontinuing:
Don't discontinue without consulting doctor. Dose may require gradual reduction if you have taken drug for a long time. Doses of other drugs may also require adjustment.

Others:
May affect accuracy of laboratory test values for SGOT*, serum bilirubin, serum creatinine and LDH*.

POSSIBLE INTERACTION WITH OTHER DRUGS

GENERIC NAME OR DRUG CLASS	COMBINED EFFECT
Aminophylline	Increased risk of aminophylline toxicity.
Antacids*	Decreased fluoro-quinolone effect.
Caffeine	With enoxacin or norfloxacin—Increased risk of central nervous system side effects.
Carbonic anyhdrase inhibitors*	May cause kidney dysfunction.
Didanosine	Decreased fluoro-quinolone effect.
Oxtriphylline	Increased risk of oxtriphylline toxicity.
Probenecid	May cause kidney dysfunction.
Sucralfate	Decreased fluoro-quinolone effect.
Theophylline	Increased risk of theophylline toxicity.
Warfarin	Increased warfarin effect.

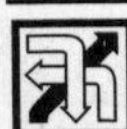

POSSIBLE INTERACTION WITH OTHER SUBSTANCES

INTERACTS WITH	COMBINED EFFECT
Alcohol:	Increased possibility of central nervous system side effects.
Beverages:	None expected.
Cocaine:	Increased possibility of central nervous system side effects.
Foods:	None expected.
Marijuana:	Increased possibility of central nervous system side effects.
Tobacco:	Increased possibility of central nervous system side effects.

FLUOROURACIL (Topical)

BRAND NAMES

5-FU
Efudex
Fluoroplex

BASIC INFORMATION

Habit forming? No
Prescription needed? Yes
Available as generic? No
Drug class: Antineoplastic (topical)

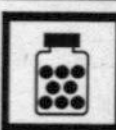

USES

- Treats precancerous actinic keratoses on skin.
- Treats superficial basal cell carcinomas (skin cancers that don't spread to distant organs and, therefore, do not threaten life).

DOSAGE & USAGE INFORMATION

How to use:
- Apply with cotton-tipped applicator.
- Cream, lotion, ointment—Bathe and dry area before use. Apply small amount and rub gently.
- Wash hands (if fingertips are used to apply) after applying medicine to other parts of body.

When to use:
Once or twice a day or as directed by doctor.

If you forget a dose:
Apply as soon as you remember. Resume basic schedule.

What drug does:
Selectively destroys actively proliferating cells.

Time lapse before drug works:
2 to 3 days.

Don't use with:
Other topical medications unless prescribed by your doctor.

OVERDOSE

SYMPTOMS:
None expected.
WHAT TO DO:
Not for internal use. If child accidentally swallows, call poison control center.

POSSIBLE ADVERSE REACTIONS OR SIDE EFFECTS

SYMPTOMS	WHAT TO DO
Life-threatening	
None expected.	
Common	
• Skin redness or swelling.	Discontinue. Call doctor right away.
• After 1 or 2 weeks of use—Skin itching or oozing; rash, tenderness, soreness.	Continue. Call doctor when convenient.
Infrequent	
Skin darkening or scaling.	Continue. Call doctor when convenient.
Rare	
Watery eyes.	Discontinue. Call doctor right away.

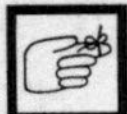

WARNINGS & PRECAUTIONS

Don't use if:
You are allergic to fluorouracil.

Before you start, consult your doctor:
- If you have cloasma or acne rosacea.
- If you have any other skin problems.

Over age 60:
No problems expected.

Pregnancy:
Consult doctor. Risk category X (see page xxii).

Breast-feeding:
Avoid drug or discontinue nursing until you finish medicine. Consult doctor for advice on maintaining milk supply.

Infants & children:
No problems expected, but check with doctor.

Prolonged use:
No problems expected, but check with doctor.

Skin & sunlight:
Increased sensitivity to sunlight during treatment and for 1 to 2 months following. Avoid exposure if possible.

Driving, piloting or hazardous work:
No problems expected, but check with doctor.

Discontinuing:
Pink, smooth area remains after treatment (usually fades in 1 to 2 months).

Others:
- Skin lesions may need biopsy before treatment.
- Keep medicine out of eyes or mouth.
- Heat and moisture in bathroom medicine cabinet can cause breakdown of medicine. Store someplace else.

POSSIBLE INTERACTION WITH OTHER DRUGS

GENERIC NAME OR DRUG CLASS	COMBINED EFFECT
None significant.	

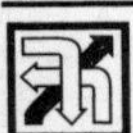

POSSIBLE INTERACTION WITH OTHER SUBSTANCES

INTERACTS WITH	COMBINED EFFECT
Alcohol:	None expected.
Beverages:	None expected.
Cocaine:	None expected.
Foods:	None expected.
Marijuana:	None expected.
Tobacco:	None expected.

FLUOXETINE

BRAND NAMES

Prozac

BASIC INFORMATION

Habit forming? No
Prescription needed? Yes
Available as generic? No
Drug class: Antidepressant

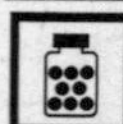

USES

- Treats mental depression, particularly in people who do not tolerate tricyclic antidepressants.
- Treats obsessive-compulsive disorder.
- Treats bulimia.
- May be used to treat obesity.

DOSAGE & USAGE INFORMATION

How to take:
- Capsules—Swallow with liquid or food to lessen stomach irritation. If you can't swallow whole, open capsule and take with liquid or food.
- Oral solution—Follow Instructions on prescription.

When to take:
In the morning at the same time each day.

If you forget a dose:
Take as soon as you remember up to 2 hours late. If more than 2 hours, wait for next scheduled dose (don't double this dose).

What drug does:
- Inhibits serotonin uptake in the central nervous system, preventing depression.
- Causes loss of appetite.

Time lapse before drug works:
1 to 3 weeks.

Don't take with:
- Any medicine that will change your level of consciousness or reflexes.
- Any other medicine without consulting your doctor or pharmacist.

Continued next column

OVERDOSE

SYMPTOMS:
Seizures, agitation, violent vomiting.
WHAT TO DO:
- **Dial 911 (emergency) or 0 (operator) for an ambulance or medical help. Then give first aid immediately.**
- **See emergency information on inside covers.**

POSSIBLE ADVERSE REACTIONS OR SIDE EFFECTS

SYMPTOMS	WHAT TO DO
Life-threatening: Rash, itchy skin, breathing difficulty (allergic reaction), chest pain.	Seek emergency treatment immediately.
Common: Diarrhea, nervousness, drowsiness, headache, increased sweating, insomnia.	Continue. Call doctor when convenient.
Infrequent:	
• Chills, fever, joint or muscle pain, enlarged lymph glands, unusual excitability, blurred vision, chest pain.	Discontinue. Call doctor right away.
• Nightmares, taste changes, vision changes, decreased sex drive, dry mouth, skin flushing, urinating frequently, dysmenorrhea, stuffy nose, tremors.	Continue. Call doctor when convenient.
Rare:	
• Convulsions.	Discontinue. Seek emergency treatment.
• Fast heartbeat, abdominal pain.	Discontinue. Call doctor right away.
• Nausea, vomiting, constipation, cough, increased appetite.	Continue. Call doctor when convenient.

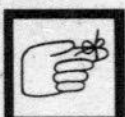

WARNINGS & PRECAUTIONS

Don't take if:
You are allergic to fluoxetine.

Before you start, consult your doctor:
- If you have history of seizure disorders.
- If you have severe liver or kidney disease.

Over age 60:
Adverse reactions and side effects may be more frequent and severe than in younger persons. You may need smaller doses for shorter periods of time.

Pregnancy:
No proven effects. Don't take unless essential. Consult doctor. Risk category B (see page xxii).

Breast-feeding:
Unknown effects. Consult doctor.

Infants & children:
Not recommended.

Prolonged use:
No problems expected.

Skin & sunlight:
No problems expected.

Driving, piloting or hazardous work:
Don't drive or pilot aircraft until you learn how medicine affects you. Don't work around dangerous machinery. Don't climb ladders or work in high places. Danger increases if you drink alcohol or take medicine affecting alertness and reflexes.

Discontinuing:
Don't discontinue without consulting doctor. Dose may require gradual reduction if you have taken drug for a long time. Doses of other drugs may also require adjustment.

Others:
No problems expected.

POSSIBLE INTERACTION WITH OTHER DRUGS

GENERIC NAME OR DRUG CLASS	COMBINED EFFECT
Anticoagulants, oral*	May cause confusion, agitation, convulsions, high blood pressure.
Central nervous system (CNS) depressants*	Increases depressant effect of both drugs.
Digitalis preparations*	May cause confusion, agitation, convulsions, high blood pressure.
Lithium	Increased risk of lithium toxicity.
Monoamine oxidase (MAO) inhibitors*	May cause confusion, agitation, convulsions, high blood pressure.
Tryptophan	Increased chance of agitation, restlessness, stomach upsets.

POSSIBLE INTERACTION WITH OTHER SUBSTANCES

INTERACTS WITH	COMBINED EFFECT
Alcohol:	Possible toxicity of both drugs. Avoid.
Beverages:	Decreases effect of fluoxetine.
Cocaine:	Decreases effect of fluoxetine.
Foods:	None expected.
Marijuana:	Decreases effect of fluoxetine.
Tobacco:	Decreases effect of fluoxetine.

***See Glossary**

FLUTAMIDE

BRAND NAMES

Eulexin
Euflex

BASIC INFORMATION

Habit forming? No
Prescription needed? Yes
Available as generic? No
Drug class: Antineoplastic

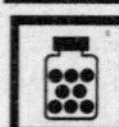

USES

Treats prostate cancer when used with leuteinizing hormone-releasing hormone (LHRH).

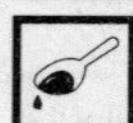

DOSAGE & USAGE INFORMATION

How to take:
Tablet or capsule—Swallow with liquid.

When to take:
According to doctor's instructions.

If you forget a dose:
Take as soon as you remember up to 2 hours late. If more than 2 hours, wait for next scheduled dose (don't double this dose).

What drug does:
Interferes with utilization of androgen (testosterone) by body cells.

Time lapse before drug works:
2 hours.

Don't take with:
Any other medicines (including over-the-counter drugs such as cough and cold medicines, laxatives, antacids, diet pills, caffeine, nose drops or vitamins) without consulting your doctor.

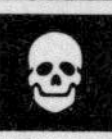

OVERDOSE

SYMPTOMS:
None expected.
WHAT TO DO:
Overdose unlikely to threaten life. If person takes much larger amount than prescribed, call doctor, poison control center or hospital emergency room for instructions.

POSSIBLE ADVERSE REACTIONS OR SIDE EFFECTS

SYMPTOMS	WHAT TO DO
Life-threatening: None expected.	
Common: Decreased sex drive, diarrhea, appetite loss, sweating and hot flashes, nausea, vomiting.	Continue. Call doctor when convenient.
Infrequent: Hands and feet tingling or numb, swollen breasts, swollen feet and legs.	Continue. Call doctor when convenient.
Rare: Jaundice (yellow eyes and skin).	Continue. Call doctor right away.

WARNINGS & PRECAUTIONS

Don't take if:
You can't tolerate flutamide.

Before you start, consult your doctor:
If you have liver disease.

Over age 60:
Adverse reactions and side effects may be more frequent and severe than in younger persons. You may need smaller doses for shorter periods of time.

Pregnancy:
Not intended for use in women. Risk category D (see page xxii).

Breast-feeding:
Not intended for use in women.

Infants & children:
Not intended for use in infants and children.

Prolonged use:
Talk to your doctor about the need for follow-up medical examinations or laboratory studies to check liver function.

Skin & sunlight:
No problems expected.

Driving, piloting or hazardous work:
No problems expected.

Discontinuing:
No special problems expected. Don't discontinue drug without doctor's approval.

Others:
- Advise any doctor or dentist whom you consult that you take this medicine.
- May affect results in some medical tests.
- May decrease sperm count.

POSSIBLE INTERACTION WITH OTHER DRUGS

GENERIC NAME OR DRUG CLASS	COMBINED EFFECT
None significant.	

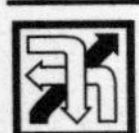

POSSIBLE INTERACTION WITH OTHER SUBSTANCES

INTERACTS WITH	COMBINED EFFECT
Alcohol:	Jaundice more likely.
Beverages:	No special problems expected.
Cocaine:	No special problems expected.
Foods:	No special problems expected.
Marijuana:	No special problems expected.
Tobacco:	No special problems expected.

FOLIC ACID (Vitamin B-9)

BRAND NAMES

Apo-Folic
Folvite
Novo-Folacid

Numerous other multiple vitamin-mineral supplements. Check labels.

BASIC INFORMATION

Habit forming? No
Prescription needed?
High strength: Yes
Vitamin mixtures: No
Available as generic? Yes
Drug class: Vitamin supplement

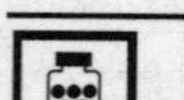

USES

- Dietary supplement to promote normal growth, development and good health.
- Treatment for anemias due to folic acid deficiency occurring from alcoholism, liver disease, hemolytic anemia, sprue, infants on artificial formula, pregnancy, breast feeding and use of oral contraceptives.

DOSAGE & USAGE INFORMATION

How to take:
Tablet—Swallow with liquid or food to lessen stomach irritation. If you can't swallow whole, crumble tablet and take with liquid or food.

When to take:
At the same time each day.

If you forget a dose:
Take when you remember. Don't double next dose. Resume regular schedule.

What drug does:
Essential to normal red blood cell formation.

Time lapse before drug works:
Not determined.

Don't take with:
Any other medicine without consulting your doctor or pharmacist.

OVERDOSE

SYMPTOMS:
None expected.
WHAT TO DO:
Overdose unlikely to threaten life.

POSSIBLE ADVERSE REACTIONS OR SIDE EFFECTS

SYMPTOMS	WHAT TO DO
Life-threatening: None expected.	
Common: Large dose may produce yellow urine.	Continue. Tell doctor at next visit.
Infrequent: None expected.	
Rare: Rash, itching, bronchospasm.	Discontinue. Call doctor right away.

WARNINGS & PRECAUTIONS

Don't take if:
You are allergic to any B vitamin.

Before you start, consult your doctor:
- If you have liver disease.
- If you have pernicious anemia. (Folic acid corrects anemia, but nerve damage of pernicious anemia continues.)

Over age 60:
No problems expected.

Pregnancy:
No problems expected. Consult doctor. Risk category A (see page xxii).

Breast-feeding:
No problems expected. Consult doctor.

Infants & children:
No problems expected.

Prolonged use:
No problems expected.

Skin & sunlight:
No problems expected.

Driving, piloting or hazardous work:
No problems expected.

Discontinuing:
Don't discontinue without doctor's advice until you complete prescribed dose, even though symptoms diminish or disappear.

Others:
- Folic acid removed by kidney dialysis. Dialysis patients should increase intake to 300% of RDA or take as directed.
- A balanced diet should provide all the folic acid a healthy person needs and make supplements unnecessary. Best sources are green, leafy vegetables; fruits; liver and kidney.

POSSIBLE INTERACTION WITH OTHER DRUGS

GENERIC NAME OR DRUG CLASS	COMBINED EFFECT
Analgesics*	Decreased effect of folic acid.
Anticonvulsants, hydantoin*	Decreased effect of folic acid. Possible increased seizure frequency.
Chloramphenicol	Possible decreased folic acid effect.
Contraceptives, oral*	Decreased effect of folic acid.
Cortisone drugs*	Decreased effect of folic acid.
Methotrexate	Decreased effect of folic acid.
Para-aminosalicylic acid (PAS)	Decreased effect of folic acid.
Pyrimethamine	Decreased effect of folic acid.
Sulfasalazine	Decreased dietary absorption of folic acid.
Triamterene	Decreased effect of folic acid.
Trimethoprim	Decreased effect of folic acid.
Zinc supplements	Increased need for zinc.

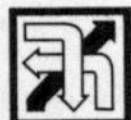

POSSIBLE INTERACTION WITH OTHER SUBSTANCES

INTERACTS WITH	COMBINED EFFECT
Alcohol:	None expected.
Beverages:	None expected.
Cocaine:	None expected.
Foods:	None expected.
Marijuana:	None expected.
Tobacco:	None expected.

*See Glossary

FURAZOLIDONE

BRAND NAMES

Furoxone
Furoxone Liquid

BASIC INFORMATION

Habit forming? No
Prescription needed? Yes
Available as generic? No
Drug class: Antiprotozoal, antibacterial

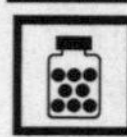

USES

- As an adjunct in treating most germs that infect the gastrointestinal tract such as cholera, salmonellosis, E. coli, proteus infections, and other bacterial causes of diarrhea.
- Treats giardiasis.

DOSAGE & USAGE INFORMATION

How to take:
- Liquid—Use a measuring spoon to ensure correct dose.
- Tablet—Swallow with liquid or food to lessen stomach irritation. If you can't swallow whole, crumble tablet and take with liquid or food.

When to take:
At the same time each day, according to instructions on prescription label.

If you forget a dose:
Take as soon as you remember up to 2 hours late. If more than 2 hours, wait for next scheduled dose. Don't double this dose.

What drug does:
Kills microscopic germs.

Time lapse before drug works:
Immediate.

Don't take with:
Any other medicine without consulting your doctor or pharmacist.

OVERDOSE

SYMPTOMS:
None expected.
WHAT TO DO:
Overdose unlikely to threaten life. If person takes much larger amount than prescribed, call doctor, poison control center or hospital emergency room for instructions.

POSSIBLE ADVERSE REACTIONS OR SIDE EFFECTS

SYMPTOMS	WHAT TO DO
Life-threatening: None expected except when taken with forbidden foods (see Possible Interaction with Other Substances).	
Common:	
• Nausea, vomiting.	Continue. Call doctor when convenient.
• Dark yellow or brown urine.	No action necessary.
Infrequent:	
• Abdominal pain.	Discontinue. Call doctor right away.
• Headache.	Continue. Call doctor when convenient.
Rare:	
Sore throat, fever, skin rash, itching, joint pain.	Discontinue. Call doctor right away.

WARNINGS & PRECAUTIONS

Don't take if:

- You have G6PD* deficiency.
- You have hypersensitivity to furazolidone, nitrofurantoin (Furadantin), or nitrofurazone (Furacin).

Before you start, consult your doctor:
If you are taking any other prescription or nonprescription medicine.

Over age 60:
No special problems expected.

Pregnancy:
Decide with your doctor if drug benefits justify risk to unborn child. Risk category C (see page xxii).

Breast-feeding:
Drug may pass into milk. Avoid drug or discontinue nursing until you finish medicine. Consult doctor for advice on maintaining milk supply.

Infants & children:
Don't use for infants without specific instructions from your doctor.

Prolonged use:
No special problems expected.

Skin & sunlight:
No special problems expected.

Driving, piloting or hazardous work:
No special problems expected.

Discontinuing:
Food restrictions outlined in Possible Interaction with Other Substances must be continued for at least 2 weeks after furazolidone is discontinued.

Others:

- Should not be taken with foods or drinks high in tyramine (see Possible Interaction with Other Substances).
- Advise any doctor or dentist whom you consult that you take this medicine.

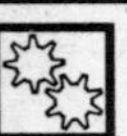

POSSIBLE INTERACTION WITH OTHER DRUGS

GENERIC NAME OR DRUG CLASS	COMBINED EFFECT
Antidepressants, tricyclic*	Sudden, severe increase in blood pressure.
Monoamine oxidase (MAO) inhibitors*	Sudden, severe increase in blood pressure.
Sumatriptan	Adverse effects unknown. Avoid.
Sympathomimetics*	Sudden, severe increase in blood pressure.

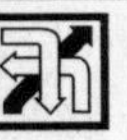

POSSIBLE INTERACTION WITH OTHER SUBSTANCES

INTERACTS WITH	COMBINED EFFECT
Alcohol:	Flushed face, shortness of breath, fever, tightness in chest. Avoid.
Beverages: Any alcoholic beverage.	Flushed face, shortness of breath, fever, tightness in chest. Avoid.
Cocaine:	High blood pressure. Avoid.
Foods: Aged cheese; dark beer; red wine (especially Chianti); sherry; liqueurs; caviar; yeast or protein extracts; fava beans; smoked or pickled meat, poultry, fish; pepperoni, salami, summer sausage; over-ripe fruit.	Sudden, severe high blood pressure that may be life-threatening. Avoid.
Marijuana:	High blood pressure. Avoid.
Tobacco:	No special problems expected.

*See Glossary

GABAPENTIN

BRAND NAMES

Neurontin

BASIC INFORMATION

Habit forming? No
Prescription needed? Yes
Available as generic? No
Drug class: Anticonvulsant, antiepileptic

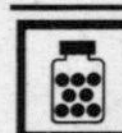

USES

Treatment for partial (focal) epileptic seizures. Used in combination with other antiepileptic drugs.

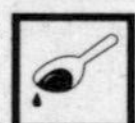

DOSAGE & USAGE INFORMATION

How to take:
Capsule–Swallow with liquid. May be taken with or without food.

When to take:
Your doctor will determine the best schedule. Dosages will be increased rapidly over the first 3 days of use. Further increases may be necessary to achieve maximum benefits.

If you forget a dose:
Take as soon as you remember. If it is almost time for the next dose, skip the missed dose and wait for your next scheduled dose (don't double this dose).

What drug does:
The exact mechanism is unknown. The anticonvulsant action may result from an altered transport of brain amino acids. Amino acids play an important part in chemical reactions within the cells.

Time lapse before drug works:
May take several weeks for effectiveness.

Don't take with:
- Any other prescription or nonprescription drug without consulting your doctor.
- See Interaction column and consult doctor.

OVERDOSE

SYMPTOMS:
Double vision, slurred speech, drowsiness, tiredness, diarrhea.
WHAT TO DO:
Overdose unlikely to threaten life. If person takes much larger amount than prescribed, call doctor, poison control center or hospital emergency room for instructions.

POSSIBLE ADVERSE REACTIONS OR SIDE EFFECTS

SYMPTOMS	WHAT TO DO
Life-threatening: None expected.	
Common: Sleepiness, dizziness, fatigue, clumsiness, lack of coordination.	Continue. Call doctor when convenient.
Infrequent: Rapid eye movement (nystagmus), double or blurred vision.	Continue. Call doctor when convenient.
Rare: Rash; nervousness; depression; twitching or swelling in hands, feet or legs; runny nose; dry or sore throat; nausea; vomiting, coughing; dry mouth; constipation; impotence; increased appetite, weight gain; muscle or back ache; forgetfulness; indigestion.	Continue. Call doctor when convenient.

WARNINGS & PRECAUTIONS

Don't take if:
You are allergic to gabapentin.

Before you start, consult your doctor:
If you have kidney disease.

Over age 60:
No special problems expected.

Pregnancy:
Decide with your doctor if drug benefits justify risks to unborn child. Risk category C (see page xxii).

Breast-feeding:
It is unknown if drug passes into milk. Consult your doctor.

Infants & children:
Not recommended for children under age 12.

Prolonged use:
No special problems expected. Follow-up laboratory blood studies may be recommended by your doctor.

Skin & sunlight:
No problems expected.

Driving, piloting or hazardous work:
Don't drive or pilot aircraft until you learn how medicine affects you. Don't work around dangerous machinery. Don't climb ladders or work in high places. Danger increases if you drink alcohol or take other medicines affecting alertness and reflexes such as antihistamines, tranquilizers, sedatives, pain medicine, narcotics and mind-altering drugs.

Discontinuing:
Don't discontinue without doctor's approval due to risk of increased seizure activity.

Others:
- Advise any doctor or dentist whom you consult that you take this medicine.
- Side effects of gabapentin are usually mild to moderate. Because it is normally used with other anticonvulsant drugs, additional side effects may also occur. If they do, discuss them with your doctor.

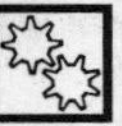

POSSIBLE INTERACTION WITH OTHER DRUGS

GENERIC NAME OR DRUG CLASS	COMBINED EFFECT
Antacids*	Allow at least 2 hours between the 2 drugs.

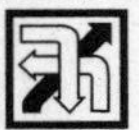

POSSIBLE INTERACTION WITH OTHER SUBSTANCES

INTERACTS WITH	COMBINED EFFECT
Alcohol:	None expected.
Beverages:	None expected.
Cocaine:	None expected.
Foods:	None expected.
Marijuana:	None expected.
Tobacco:	None expected.

*See Glossary

GALLBLADDER X-RAY TEST DRUGS (Cholecystographic Agents)

BRAND AND GENERIC NAMES

Bilivist	**IPODATE**
Bilopaque	**Oragrafin Calcium**
Cholebrine	**Oragrafin Sodium**
IOCETAMIC ACID	**Telepaque**
IOPANOIC ACID	**TYROPANOATE**

BASIC INFORMATION

Habit forming? No
Prescription needed? Yes
Available as generic? No
Drug class: Diagnostic aid, radiopaque

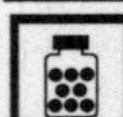

USES

To check for problems with the gallbladder or the bile ducts.

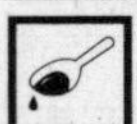

DOSAGE & USAGE INFORMATION

How to take:
- Take tablets or liquid as directed after the evening meal on the evening before special x-rays will be taken.
- Don't eat or drink anything (except water) after taking.

When to take:
As directed.

If you forget a dose:
Take as soon as you remember.

What drug does:
These are organic iodine compounds which get absorbed into the bloodstream, get concentrated in a healthy gallbladder and make the gallbladder and gallstones (if present) visible on special x-rays.

Time lapse before drug works:
10 to 15 hours.

Continued next column

OVERDOSE

SYMPTOMS:
Severe diarrhea, nausea or vomiting; difficult urination.
WHAT TO DO:
Not life-threatening. Discontinue and call doctor right away.

Don't take with:
- Other medicines unless directed by your doctor or x-ray specialist.
- If you take cholestyramine, discontinue it for 48 hours before taking the radiopaque drug.

POSSIBLE ADVERSE REACTIONS OR SIDE EFFECTS

SYMPTOMS	WHAT TO DO
Life-threatening:	
Faintness; swelling of lips, hands, face; difficult breathing.	Discontinue. Seek emergency treatment.
Common:	
Difficult or painful urination, increased urinary frequency.	No action necessary.
Infrequent:	
Abdominal cramps, diarrhea, dizziness, headache, indigestion, vomiting, nausea.	Discontinue. Call doctor right away.
Rare:	
Itching, unusual bleeding or bruising, hives or rash.	Discontinue. Call doctor right away.

GALLBLADDER X-RAY TEST DRUGS (Cholecystographic Agents)

WARNINGS & PRECAUTIONS

Don't take if:
You are allergic to any iodine compound or other radiopaque chemicals.

Before you start, consult your doctor:
If you are allergic to anything, including shellfish, cabbage, kale, turnips, iodized salt.

Over age 60:
Adverse reactions and side effects may be more frequent and severe than in younger persons. Ask doctor about smaller doses.

Pregnancy:
- X-rays should not be taken unless absolutely necessary during pregnancy. Consult doctor.
- Risk factors vary for drugs in this group. See category list on page xxii and consult doctor.

Breast-feeding:
No problems expected, but ask doctor.

Infants & children:
No problems expected, but ask doctor.

Prolonged use:
Not intended for prolonged use.

Skin & sunlight:
No problems expected.

Driving, piloting or hazardous work:
Don't drive or pilot aircraft until you learn how medicine affects you. Don't work around dangerous machinery. Don't climb ladders or work in high places. Danger increases if you drink alcohol or take medicine affecting alertness and reflexes, such as antihistamines, tranquilizers, sedatives, pain medicine, narcotics and mind-altering drugs.

Discontinuing:
No problems expected.

Others:
- Special diets and laxatives or enemas before x-rays may be ordered. Follow instructions.
- Tests on your thyroid gland may be made inaccurate for 8 weeks because of the iodine contained in radiopaque substances. Keep this in mind if your doctor orders thyroid tests.
- Results of other lab studies may be inaccurate.

POSSIBLE INTERACTION WITH OTHER DRUGS

GENERIC NAME OR DRUG CLASS	COMBINED EFFECT
Cholestyramine	Unsuccessful gallbladder test.

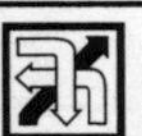

POSSIBLE INTERACTION WITH OTHER SUBSTANCES

INTERACTS WITH	COMBINED EFFECT
Alcohol:	None expected.
Beverages:	None expected.
Cocaine:	None expected.
Foods:	None expected.
Marijuana:	None expected.
Tobacco:	None expected.

GEMFIBROZIL

BRAND NAMES

Lopid

BASIC INFORMATION

Habit forming? No
Prescription needed? Yes
Available as generic? No
Drug class: Antihyperlipidemic

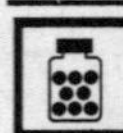

USES

Reduces fatty substances in the blood (triglycerides).

DOSAGE & USAGE INFORMATION

How to take:
Tablet or capsule—Swallow with liquid or food to lessen stomach irritation.

When to take:
At the same times each day.

If you forget a dose:
Take as soon as you remember up to 2 hours late. If more than 2 hours, wait for next scheduled dose (don't double this dose).

What drug does:
Inhibits formation of fatty substances.

Time lapse before drug works:
3 months or more.

Don't take with:
Any other medicine without consulting your doctor or pharmacist.

OVERDOSE

SYMPTOMS:
Diarrhea, headache, muscle pain.
WHAT TO DO:
Overdose unlikely to threaten life. If person takes much larger amount than prescribed, call doctor, poison control center or hospital emergency room for instructions.

POSSIBLE ADVERSE REACTIONS OR SIDE EFFECTS

SYMPTOMS	WHAT TO DO
Life-threatening: None expected.	
Common: Indigestion.	Continue. Call doctor when convenient.
Infrequent: Chest pain, shortness of breath, irregular heartbeat, nausea, vomiting, diarrhea, stomach pain.	Discontinue. Call doctor right away.
Rare:	
• Rash, itch; sores in mouth, on lips; sore throat; swollen feet, legs; blood in urine; painful urination; fever; chills.	Discontinue. Call doctor right away.
• Dizziness, headache, drowsiness, muscle cramps, dry skin, backache, unusual tiredness, decreased sex drive.	Continue. Call doctor when convenient.

WARNINGS & PRECAUTIONS

Don't take if:
You are allergic to any antihyperlipidemic.

Before you start, consult your doctor:
- If you have had liver or kidney disease.
- If you have had peptic-ulcer disease.
- If you have diabetes.

Over age 60:
Adverse reactions and side effects may be more frequent and severe than in younger persons.

Pregnancy:
Decide with your doctor if drug benefits justify risks to unborn child. Risk category C (see page xxii).

Breast-feeding:
May harm child. Avoid. Consult doctor.

Infants & children:
Not recommended.

Prolonged use:
Periodic blood cell counts and liver function studies recommended if you take gemfibrozil for a long time.

Skin & sunlight:
No problems expected.

Driving, piloting or hazardous work:
Avoid if you feel drowsy or dizzy. Otherwise, no problems expected.

Discontinuing:
Don't discontinue without doctor's advice until you complete prescribed dose, even though symptoms diminish or disappear.

Others:
- Some studies question effectiveness. Many studies warn against toxicity.
- May affect results in some medical tests.

POSSIBLE INTERACTION WITH OTHER DRUGS

GENERIC NAME OR DRUG CLASS	COMBINED EFFECT
Anticoagulants, oral*	Increased anti-coagulant effect. Dose reduction of anticoagulant necessary.
Antidiabetics, oral*	Increased antidiabetic effect.
Contraceptives, oral*	Decreased gemfibrozil effect.
Estrogens*	Decreased gemfibrozil effect.
Furosemide	Possible toxicity of both drugs.
HMG-CoA reductase inhibitors	Increased risk of muscle inflammation and kidney failure.
Insulin	Increased insulin effect.
Lovastatin	Increased risk of kidney problems.
Thyroid hormones*	Increased gemfibrozil effect.

POSSIBLE INTERACTION WITH OTHER SUBSTANCES

INTERACTS WITH	COMBINED EFFECT
Alcohol:	None expected.
Beverages:	None expected.
Cocaine:	Decreased effect of gemfibrozil. Avoid.
Foods: Fatty foods.	Decreased gemfibrozil effect.
Marijuana:	None expected.
Tobacco:	Decreased gemfibrozil absorption. Avoid.

*See Glossary

GLUCAGON

BRAND NAMES

Glucagon for Injection

BASIC INFORMATION

Habit forming? No
Prescription needed? Yes
Available as generic? Yes
Drug class: Antihypoglycemic, diagnostic aid

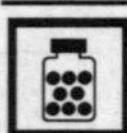

USES

- Treats low blood sugar in diabetics.
- Used as antidote for overdose of beta-adrenergic blockers, quinidine and tricyclic antidepressants.

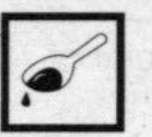

DOSAGE & USAGE INFORMATION

How to take:
Injection—As directed by your doctor.

When to take:
When there are signs of low blood sugar (anxiety; chills; cool, pale skin; hunger; nausea; tremors; sweating; weakness; unconsciousness) in diabetics who don't respond to eating some form of sugar.

If you forget a dose:
Single dose only.

What drug does:
Forces liver to make more sugar and release it into the bloodstream.

Time lapse before drug works:
- For hypoglycemic condition—5 to 20 minutes.
- For muscle relaxant—1 to 10 minutes.

Don't take with:
Any other medicines (including over-the-counter drugs such as cough and cold medicines, laxatives, antacids, diet pills, caffeine, nose drops or vitamins) without consulting your doctor.

OVERDOSE

SYMPTOMS:
Nausea, vomiting, severe weakness, irregular heartbeat, hoarseness, cramps.
WHAT TO DO:
- **Dial 911 (emergency) or 0 (operator) for an ambulance or medical help. Then give first aid immediately.**
- **See emergency information on inside covers.**

POSSIBLE ADVERSE REACTIONS OR SIDE EFFECTS

SYMPTOMS	WHAT TO DO
Life-threatening:	
Unconsciousness.	Seek emergency treatment immediately.
Common:	
Nausea.	Continue. Call doctor when convenient.
Infrequent:	
Lightheadedness, breathing difficulty.	Discontinue. Call doctor right away.
Rare:	
Skin rash.	Discontinue. Call doctor right away.

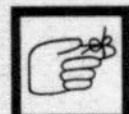

WARNINGS & PRECAUTIONS

Don't take if:
You can't tolerate glucagon.

Before you start, consult your doctor:
- If you are allergic to beef or pork.
- If you have pheochromocytoma.*

Over age 60:
No special problems expected.

Pregnancy:
No proven harm to unborn child, but avoid if possible. Consult doctor. Risk category B (see page xxii).

Breast-feeding:
No special problems expected. Consult doctor.

Infants & children:
No special problems expected.

Prolonged use:
To be used intermittently and not for prolonged periods.

Skin & sunlight:
No problems expected.

Driving, piloting or hazardous work:
Don't drive or pilot aircraft until you learn how medicine affects you. Don't work around dangerous machinery. Don't climb ladders or work in high places. Danger increases if you drink alcohol or take medicine affecting alertness and reflexes.

Discontinuing:
No special problems expected.

Others:
- May affect results in some medical tests.
- Explain to other family members how to inject glucagon.
- Before injecting, try to eat some form of sugar, such as glucose tablets, corn syrup, honey, orange juice, hard candy or sugar cubes.
- Store glucagon in refrigerator, but don't freeze.

POSSIBLE INTERACTION WITH OTHER DRUGS

GENERIC NAME OR DRUG CLASS	COMBINED EFFECT
Anticoagulants*	Increased anticoagulant effect.

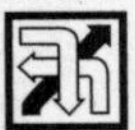

POSSIBLE INTERACTION WITH OTHER SUBSTANCES

INTERACTS WITH	COMBINED EFFECT
Alcohol:	Decreased glucagon effect.
Beverages:	No special problems expected.
Cocaine:	Increased adverse reactions.
Foods: Sugar, fruit juice, candy.	Enhances glucagon effect.
Marijuana:	Increased adverse reactions.
Tobacco:	No special problems expected.

GLYCOPYRROLATE

BRAND NAMES

Robinul
Robinul Forte

BASIC INFORMATION

Habit forming? No
Prescription needed? Yes
Available as generic? Yes
Drug class: Antispasmodic, anticholinergic

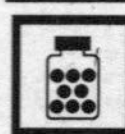

USES

- Reduces spasms of digestive system.
- Reduces production of saliva during dental procedures.
- Treats peptic ulcer by reducing gastric acid secretion.

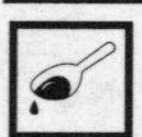

DOSAGE & USAGE INFORMATION

How to take:
Tablet—Swallow with liquid. If you can't swallow whole, crumble tablet and take with small amount of liquid or food.

When to take:
30 minutes before meals (unless directed otherwise by doctor).

If you forget a dose:
Wait for next scheduled dose (don't double this dose).

What drug does:
Blocks nerve impulses at parasympathetic nerve endings, preventing smooth (involuntary) muscle contractions and gland secretions of organs involved.

Time lapse before drug works:
15 to 30 minutes.

Don't take with:
Any other medicine without consulting your doctor or pharmacist.

OVERDOSE

SYMPTOMS:
Dry mouth, blurred vision, low blood pressure, decreased breathing rate, rapid heartbeat, flushed skin, drowsiness.
WHAT TO DO:
- **Dial 911 (emergency) or 0 (operator) for an ambulance or medical help. Then give first aid immediately.**
- **See emergency information on inside covers.**

POSSIBLE ADVERSE REACTIONS OR SIDE EFFECTS

SYMPTOMS	WHAT TO DO
Life-threatening:	
Hives, rash, intense itching, faintness soon after a dose (anaphylaxis).	Seek emergency treatment immediately.
Common:	
Dry mouth, loss of taste, constipation, difficult urination.	Continue. Call doctor when convenient.
Infrequent:	
• Confusion; dizziness; drowsiness; eye pain; headache; rash; sleep disturbance such as nightmares, frequent waking; nausea; vomiting; rapid heartbeat; lightheadedness.	Discontinue. Call doctor right away.
• Insomnia, blurred vision, diminished sex drive, decreased sweating, nasal congestion, altered taste.	Continue. Call doctor when convenient.
Rare:	
Rash, hives.	Discontinue. Call doctor right away.

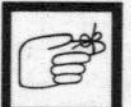

WARNINGS & PRECAUTIONS

Don't take if:
- You are allergic to any anticholinergic.
- You have trouble with stomach bloating.
- You have difficulty emptying your bladder completely.
- You have narrow-angle glaucoma.
- You have severe ulcerative colitis.

Before you start, consult your doctor:
- If you have open-angle glaucoma.
- If you have angina, chronic bronchitis or asthma, liver disease, hiatal hernia, enlarged prostate, myasthenia gravis, peptic ulcer, kidney or thyroid disease.
- If you will have surgery within 2 months, including dental surgery, requiring general or spinal anesthesia.

Over age 60:
Adverse reactions and side effects may be more frequent and severe than in younger persons.

Pregnancy:
Consult doctor. Risk category B (see page xxii).

Breast-feeding:
Drug passes into milk and decreases milk flow. Avoid drug or discontinue nursing until you finish medicine. Consult doctor for advice on maintaining milk supply.

Infants & children:
Use only under medical supervision.

Prolonged use:
Chronic constipation, possible fecal impaction. Consult doctor immediately.

Skin & sunlight:
No problems expected.

Driving, piloting or hazardous work:
Use disqualifies you for piloting aircraft. Otherwise, no problems expected.

Discontinuing:
May be unnecessary to finish medicine. Follow doctor's instructions.

Others:
- Heatstroke more likely if you become overheated during exertion.
- Advise any doctor or dentist whom you consult that you take this medicine.

POSSIBLE INTERACTION WITH OTHER DRUGS

GENERIC NAME OR DRUG CLASS	COMBINED EFFECT
Antacids*	Decreased glycopyrrolate absorption effect.
Amantadine	Increased glycopyrrolate effect.
Anticholinergics, other*	Increased glycopyrrolate effect.
Antidepressants, tricyclic*	Increased glycopyrrolate effect.
Antidiarrheals*	Decreased glycopyrrolate absorption effect.
Attapulgite	Decreased effect of anticholinergic.
Buclizine	Increased glycopyrrolate effect.
Cortisone drugs*	Increased internal eye pressure.
Digitalis	Possible decreased absorption of digitalis.
Haloperidol	Increased internal eye pressure.
Ketoconazole	Decreased ketoconazole effect.
Meperidine	Increased glycopyrrolate effect.
Methylphenidate	Increased anticholinergic effect.
Molindone	Increased nizatidine effect.
Monoamine oxidase (MAO) inhibitors*	Increased glycopyrrolate effect.
Orphenadrine	Increased glycopyrrolate effect
Phenothiazines	Increased glycopyrrolate effect.
Pilocarpine	Increased glycopyrrolate effect. Loss of pilocarpine effect in glaucoma treatment.
Potassium chloride tabs	Increased side effects of potassium tablets.
Quinidine	Increased glycopyrrolate effect.
Retocunazole	Decreased absorption of both.
Sedatives* or central nervous system (CNS) depressants*	Increased sedative effect of both drugs.
Vitamin C	Increased glycopyrrolate effect. Avoid large vitamin C doses.

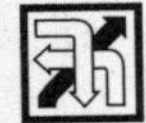

POSSIBLE INTERACTION WITH OTHER SUBSTANCES

INTERACTS WITH	COMBINED EFFECT
Alcohol:	None expected.
Beverages:	None expected.
Cocaine:	Excessively rapid heartbeat.
Foods:	None exected.
Marijuana:	Drowsiness and dry mouth.
Tobacco:	None expected.

*See Glossary

GOLD COMPOUNDS

BRAND AND GENERIC NAMES

AURANOFIN
AUROTHIOGLUCOSE
Gold Sodium Thiomalate
Myochrysine—injection
Myocrisin
Ridaura—oral
SODIUM AUROTHIOMALATE

BASIC INFORMATION

Habit forming? No
Prescription needed? Yes
Available as generic? No
Drug class: Gold compounds

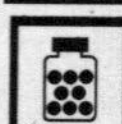

USES

Treatment for rheumatoid arthritis and juvenile arthritis.

DOSAGE & USAGE INFORMATION

How to take:
- Capsules—Swallow with full glass of fluid. Follow prescription directions. Taking too much can cause serious adverse reactions.
- Injections—Under medical supervision.

When to take:
Once or twice daily, morning and night.

If you forget a dose:
Take as soon as you remember up to 6 hours late, then go back to usual schedule.

What drug does:
Modifies disease activity of rheumatoid arthritis by mechanisms not yet understood.

Time lapse before drug works:
3 to 6 months.

Don't take with:
Any other medicine without consulting your doctor or pharmacist.

OVERDOSE

SYMPTOMS:
Confusion, delirium, numbness and tingling in feet and hands.
WHAT TO DO:
- **Induce vomiting with syrup of ipecac if available.**
- **Dial 911 (emergency) or 0 (operator) for an ambulance or medical help. Then give first aid immediately.**
- **See emergency information on inside covers.**

POSSIBLE ADVERSE REACTIONS OR SIDE EFFECTS

SYMPTOMS	WHAT TO DO
Life-threatening:	
Hives, rash, intense itching, faintness soon after a dose (anaphylaxis).	Seek emergency treatment immediately.
Common:	
• Itch; hives; sores or white spots in mouth, throat; appetite loss; diarrhea; vomiting; skin rashes; fever.	Discontinue. Call doctor right away.
• Indigestion, constipation.	Continue. Call doctor when convenient.
Infrequent:	
• Excessive fatigue; sore tongue, mouth or gums; metallic or odd taste; unusual bleeding or bruising; blood in urine; vaginal discharge; flushing; fainting; dizziness; sweating after injection.	Discontinue. Call doctor right away.
• Hair loss; pain in muscles, bones and joints (with injections).	Continue. Call doctor when convenient.
Rare:	
• Blood in stool, difficult breathing, coughing, seizures.	Discontinue. Seek emergency treatment.
• Abdominal pain, jaundice, numbness or tingling in hands or feet, muscle weakness.	Discontinue. Call doctor right away.
• "Pink eye."	Continue. Call doctor when convenient.

WARNINGS & PRECAUTIONS

Don't take if:
- You have history of allergy to gold or other metals.
- You have any blood disorder.
- You have kidney disease.

Before you start, consult your doctor:
- If you are pregnant or may become pregnant.
- If you have lupus erythematosus.
- If you have Sjögren's syndrome.
- If you have chronic skin disease.
- If you are debilitated.
- If you have blood dyscrasias.

Over age 60:
Adverse reactions and side effects may be more frequent and severe than in younger persons.

Pregnancy:
Decide with your doctor if drug benefits justify risks to unborn child. Risk category C (see page xxii).

Breast-feeding:
Drug may filter into milk, causing side effects in infants. Avoid. Consult doctor.

Infants & children:
Not recommended. Safety and dosage have not been established.

Prolonged use:
Request periodic laboratory studies of blood counts, urine and liver function. These should be done before use and at least once a month during treatment.

Skin & sunlight:
- Skin rash may be aggravated by sunlight.
- Blue-gray pigmentation in skin exposed to sunlight.

Driving, piloting or hazardous work:
Avoid if you have serious adverse reactions or side effects. Otherwise, no problems expected.

Discontinuing:
Don't discontinue without doctor's advice until you complete prescribed dose.

Others:
- Side effects and adverse reactions may appear during treatment or for many months after discontinuing.
- Gold has been shown to cause kidney tumors and kidney cancer in animals given excessive doses.
- May interfere with the accuracy of some medical tests.

POSSIBLE INTERACTION WITH OTHER DRUGS

GENERIC NAME OR DRUG CLASS	COMBINED EFFECT
Bone marrow depressants*	Increased risk of toxicity of both drugs.
Hepatotoxics*	Increased risk of toxicity of both drugs.
Nephrotoxics*	Increased risk of toxicity of both drugs.
Penicillamine	Increased likelihood of kidney damage.
Phenytoin	Increased phenytoin blood levels. Phenytoin dosage may require adjustment.

POSSIBLE INTERACTION WITH OTHER SUBSTANCES

INTERACTS WITH	COMBINED EFFECT
Alcohol:	None expected.
Beverages:	None expected.
Cocaine:	None expected.
Foods:	None expected.
Marijuana:	None expected.
Tobacco:	None expected.

*See Glossary

GRISEOFULVIN

BRAND NAMES

Fulvicin P/G
Fulvicin U/F
Grifulvin V
Gris-PEG
Grisactin
Grisactin Ultra
Grisovin-FP

BASIC INFORMATION

Habit forming? No
Prescription needed? Yes
Available as generic? Yes
Drug class: Antibiotic (antifungal)

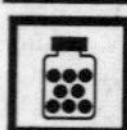

USES

Treatment for fungal infections susceptible to griseofulvin.

DOSAGE & USAGE INFORMATION

How to take:
- Tablet or capsule—Swallow with liquid or food to lessen stomach irritation. If you can't swallow whole, crumble tablet or open capsule and take with liquid or food.
- Liquid—Follow label instructions.

When to take:
With or immediately after meals.

If you forget a dose:
Take as soon as you remember up to 2 hours late. If more than 2 hours, wait for next scheduled dose (don't double this dose).

What drug does:
Prevents fungi from growing and reproducing.

Time lapse before drug works:
2 to 10 days for skin infections. 2 to 4 weeks for infections of fingernails or toenails. Complete cure of either may require several months.

Don't take with:
Any other medicine without consulting your doctor or pharmacist.

OVERDOSE

SYMPTOMS:
Nausea, vomiting, diarrhea. In sensitive individuals, severe diarrhea may occur without overdosing.
WHAT TO DO:
Overdose unlikely to threaten life. If person takes much larger amount than prescribed, call doctor, poison control center or hospital emergency room for instructions.

POSSIBLE ADVERSE REACTIONS OR SIDE EFFECTS

SYMPTOMS	WHAT TO DO
Life-threatening: In case of overdose, see previous column.	
Common: Headache.	Continue. Tell doctor at next visit.
Infrequent: • Confusion; rash, hives, itch; mouth or tongue irritation; soreness; nausea; vomiting; diarrhea; stomach pain.	Discontinue. Call doctor right away.
• Insomnia, tiredness.	Continue. Call doctor when convenient.
Rare: Sore throat, fever, numbness or tingling in hands or feet, cloudy urine, sensitivity to sunlight, jaundice.	Discontinue. Call doctor right away.

WARNINGS & PRECAUTIONS

Don't take if:
- You are allergic to any antifungal medicine.
- You are allergic to penicillin.
- You have liver disease.
- You have porphyria.
- The infection is minor and will respond to less potent drugs.

Before you start, consult your doctor:
- If you plan to become pregnant within medication period.
- If you have liver disease.
- If you have lupus.

Over age 60:
Adverse reactions and side effects may be more frequent and severe than in younger persons.

Pregnancy:
Risk to unborn child outweighs drug benefits. Don't use. Risk category X (see page xxii).

Breast-feeding:
No problems expected, but consult your doctor.

Infants & children:
Not recommended for children younger than 2.

Prolonged use:
- You may become susceptible to infections caused by germs not responsive to griseofulvin.
- Talk to your doctor about the need for follow-up medical examinations or laboratory studies to check complete blood counts (white blood cell count, platelet count, red blood cell count, hemoglobin, hematocrit), liver function, kidney function.

Skin & sunlight:
May cause rash or intensify sunburn in areas exposed to sun or sunlamp.

Driving, piloting or hazardous work:
- Don't drive if you feel dizzy or have vision problems.
- Don't pilot aircraft.

Discontinuing:
Don't discontinue without doctor's advice until you complete prescribed dose, even though symptoms diminish or disappear.

Others:
Periodic laboratory blood studies and liver and kidney function tests recommended.

POSSIBLE INTERACTION WITH OTHER DRUGS

GENERIC NAME OR DRUG CLASS	COMBINED EFFECT
Anticoagulants, oral*	Decreased anti-anticoagulant effect.
Barbiturates*	Decreased griseofulvin effect.
Contraceptives, oral*	Decreased contraceptive effect.
Drugs that increase sensitivity to sunlight	Increased sun hazard.

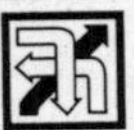

POSSIBLE INTERACTION WITH OTHER SUBSTANCES

INTERACTS WITH	COMBINED EFFECT
Alcohol:	Increased intoxication. Possible disulfiram reaction.*
Beverages:	None expected.
Cocaine:	None expected.
Foods:	None expected, but foods high in fat will improve drug absorption.
Marijuana:	None expected.
Tobacco:	None expected.

*See Glossary

GUAIFENESIN

BRAND NAMES

See complete list of brand names in the *Brand Name Directory*, page 908.

BASIC INFORMATION

Habit forming? No
Prescription needed? No
Available as generic? Yes
Drug class: Cough/cold preparation

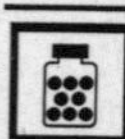

USES

Loosens mucus in respiratory passages from allergies and infections (hay fever, cough, cold).

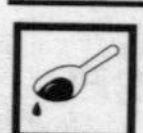

DOSAGE & USAGE INFORMATION

How to take:

- Tablet or capsule—Swallow with liquid. If you can't swallow whole, crumble tablet or open capsule and take with liquid or food.
- Extended-release tablet or extended-release capsule—Swallow with liquid.
- Syrup, oral solution or lozenge—Take as directed on label. Follow with 8 oz. water.

When to take:
As needed, no more often than every 3 hours.

If you forget a dose:
Take as soon as you remember. Wait 3 hours for next dose.

What drug does:
Increases production of watery fluids to thin mucus so it can be coughed out or absorbed.

Time lapse before drug works:
15 to 30 minutes. Regular use for 5 to 7 days necessary for maximum benefit.

Don't take with:
Any other medicine without consulting your doctor or pharmacist.

OVERDOSE

SYMPTOMS:
Drowsiness, mild weakness, nausea, vomiting.
WHAT TO DO:
Overdose unlikely to threaten life. If person takes much larger amount than prescribed, call doctor, poison control center or hospital emergency room for instructions.

POSSIBLE ADVERSE REACTIONS OR SIDE EFFECTS

SYMPTOMS	WHAT TO DO
Life-threatening: None expected.	
Common: None expected.	
Infrequent:	
• Rash, stomach pain, diarrhea, nausea, vomiting.	Discontinue. Call doctor right away.
• Drowsiness.	Continue. Call doctor when convenient.
Rare: None expected.	

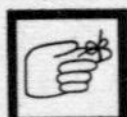

WARNINGS & PRECAUTIONS

Don't take if:
You are allergic to any cough or cold preparation containing guaifenesin.

Before you start, consult your doctor:
If you are allergic to any medicine, food or other substance.

Over age 60:
Adverse reactions and side effects may be more frequent and severe than in younger persons. For drug to work, you must drink 8 to 10 glasses of fluid per day.

Pregnancy:
Decide with your doctor if drug benefits justify risks to unborn child. Risk category C (see page xxii).

Breast-feeding:
No proven problems. Consult your doctor.

Infants & children:
No problems expected.

Prolonged use:
No problems expected.

Skin & sunlight:
No problems expected.

Driving, piloting or hazardous work:
Avoid if you feel drowsy. Otherwise, no problems expected.

Discontinuing:
May be unnecessary to finish medicine. Discontinue when symptoms disappear. If symptoms persist more than 1 week, consult doctor.

Others:
No problems expected.

POSSIBLE INTERACTION WITH OTHER DRUGS

GENERIC NAME OR DRUG CLASS	COMBINED EFFECT
Anticoagulants*	Possible risk of bleeding.

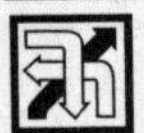

POSSIBLE INTERACTION WITH OTHER SUBSTANCES

INTERACTS WITH	COMBINED EFFECT
Alcohol:	No proven problems.
Beverages:	You must drink 8 to 10 glasses of fluid per day for drug to work.
Cocaine:	No proven problems.
Foods:	None expected.
Marijuana:	No proven problems.
Tobacco:	No proven problems.

*See Glossary

GUANABENZ

BRAND NAMES

Wytensin

BASIC INFORMATION

Habit forming? No
Prescription needed? Yes
Available as generic? No
Drug class: Antihypertensive

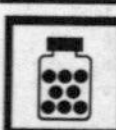

USES

Controls, but doesn't cure, high blood pressure.

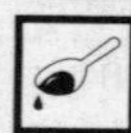

DOSAGE & USAGE INFORMATION

How to take:
Tablet—Swallow with liquid or food to lessen stomach irritation. If you can't swallow whole, crumble tablet and take with liquid or food.

When to take:
At the same times each day.

If you forget a dose:
Take as soon as you remember up to 2 hours late. If more than 2 hours, wait for next scheduled dose (don't double this dose).

What drug does:
- Relaxes muscle cells of small arteries.
- Slows heartbeat.

Time lapse before drug works:
1 hour.

Don't take with:
Any other medicine without consulting your doctor or pharmacist.

OVERDOSE

SYMPTOMS:
Severe dizziness, slow heartbeat, unusual tiredness or weakness, pinpoint pupils, fainting, coma.
WHAT TO DO:
- **Dial 911 (emergency) or 0 (operator) for an ambulance or medical help. Then give first aid immediately.**
- **If patient is unconscious and not breathing, give mouth-to-mouth breathing. If there is no heartbeat, use cardiac massage and mouth-to-mouth breathing (CPR). Don't try to make patient vomit. If you can't get help quickly, take patient to nearest emergency facility.**
- **See emergency information on inside covers.**

POSSIBLE ADVERSE REACTIONS OR SIDE EFFECTS

SYMPTOMS	WHAT TO DO
Life-threatening:	
In case of overdose, see previous column.	
Common:	
• Dry mouth, drowsiness.	Continue. Call doctor when convenient.
• Insomnia, weakness.	Continue. Tell doctor at next visit.
Infrequent:	
• Irregular heartbeat, shakiness in hands.	Discontinue. Call doctor right away.
• Dizziness, appetite loss, nausea, vomiting, painful or difficult urination, headache.	Continue. Call doctor when convenient.
Rare:	
Decreased sex drive.	Continue. Call doctor when convenient.

WARNINGS & PRECAUTIONS

Don't take if:
You are allergic to any sympathomimetic drug.

Before you start, consult your doctor:
- If you have blood disease.
- If you have heart disease.
- If you have liver disease.
- If you have diabetes or overactive thyroid.
- If you will have surgery within 2 months, including dental surgery, requiring general or spinal anesthesia.

Over age 60:
Adverse reactions and side effects may be more frequent and severe than in younger persons. Hot weather may cause need to reduce dosage.

Pregnancy:
Decide with your doctor if drug benefits justify risks to unborn child. Risk category C (see page xxii).

Breast-feeding:
Unknown effect. Consult doctor.

Infants & children:
Not recommended.

Prolonged use:
Side effects tend to diminish. Request uric acid and kidney function studies periodically.

Skin & sunlight:
No problems expected.

Driving, piloting or hazardous work:
Avoid if you feel dizzy; otherwise, no problems expected.

Discontinuing:
Don't discontinue without consulting doctor. Dose may require gradual reduction if you have taken drug for a long time. Doses of other drugs may also require adjustment. Abruptly discontinuing may cause anxiety, chest pain, salivation, headache, abdominal cramps, fast heartbeat, increased sweating, tremors, insomnia.

Others:
- Stay away from high-sodium foods. Lose weight if you are overweight.
- May interfere with the accuracy of some medical tests.

POSSIBLE INTERACTION WITH OTHER DRUGS

GENERIC NAME OR DRUG CLASS	COMBINED EFFECT
Angiotensin-converting enzyme (ACE) inhibitors*	Possible excessive potassium in blood.
Antihypertensives, other*	Decreases blood pressure more than either alone. May be beneficial, but requires dosage adjustment.
Beta-adrenergic blocking agents*	Blood pressure control more difficult.
Central nervous system (CNS) depressants* (sedatives,* sleeping pills,* tranquilizers,* antidepressants,* narcotics*)	Increased brain depression. Avoid.
Clozapine	Toxic effect on the central nervous system.
Diuretics*	Decreases blood pressure more than either alone. May be beneficial, but requires dosage adjustment.
Ethinamate	Dangerous increased effects of ethinamate. Avoid combining.
Fluoxetine	Increased depressant effects of both drugs.
Guanfacine	May increase depressant effects of either drug.
Leucovorin	High alcohol content of leucovorin may cause adverse effects.
Methyprylon	Increased sedative effect, perhaps to dangerous level. Avoid.
Nabilone	Greater depression of central nervous system.
Nicardipine	Blood pressure drop. Dosages may require adjustment.
Nimodipine	Dangerous blood pressure drop.
Sertraline	Increased depressive effects of both drugs.

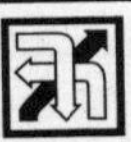

POSSIBLE INTERACTION WITH OTHER SUBSTANCES

INTERACTS WITH	COMBINED EFFECT
Alcohol:	Oversedation. Avoid.
Beverages: Caffeine.	Overstimulation. Avoid.
Cocaine:	Overstimulation. Avoid.
Foods: Salt.	Decrease salt intake to increase beneficial effects of guanabenz.
Marijuana:	Overstimulation. Avoid.
Tobacco:	Decreased guanabenz effect.

*See Glossary

GUANADREL

BRAND NAMES

Hylorel

BASIC INFORMATION

Habit forming? No
Prescription needed? Yes
Available as generic? No
Drug class: Antihypertensive

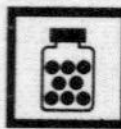

USES

Controls, but doesn't cure, high blood pressure.

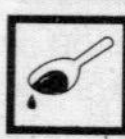

DOSAGE & USAGE INFORMATION

How to take:
Tablet—Swallow with liquid or food to lessen stomach irritation. If you can't swallow whole, crumble tablet and take with liquid or food.

When to take:
At the same time each day.

If you forget a dose:
Take as soon as you remember up to 2 hours late. If more than 2 hours, wait for next scheduled dose (don't double this dose).

What drug does:
Relaxes muscle cells of small arteries.

Time lapse before drug works:
4 to 6 hours. May need to take for lifetime.

Don't take with:
Any other medicine without consulting your doctor or pharmacist.

OVERDOSE

SYMPTOMS:
Severe blood pressure drop; fainting; blurred vision; slow, weak pulse; cold, sweaty skin; loss of consciousness.
WHAT TO DO:
- **Dial 911 (emergency) or 0 (operator) for an ambulance or medical help. Then give first aid immediately.**
- **See emergency information on inside covers.**

POSSIBLE ADVERSE REACTIONS OR SIDE EFFECTS

SYMPTOMS	WHAT TO DO
Life-threatening:	
In case of overdose, see previous column.	
Common:	
• Diarrhea, more bowel movements, fatigue, weakness.	Continue. Call doctor when convenient.
• Dizziness, lower sex drive, feet and ankle swelling, drowsiness.	Continue. Tell doctor at next visit.
• Stuffy nose, dry mouth.	No action necessary.
Infrequent:	
• Rash, blurred vision, drooping eyelids, chest pain or shortness of breath, muscle pain or tremor.	Discontinue. Call doctor right away.
• Nausea or vomiting, headache.	Continue. Call doctor when convenient.
• Impotence, nighttime urination.	Continue. Tell doctor at next visit.
Rare:	
Decreased white blood cells causing sore throat, fever.	Discontinue. Call doctor right away.

WARNINGS & PRECAUTIONS

Don't take if:
- You are allergic to guanadrel.
- You have taken MAO inhibitors within 2 weeks.

Before you start, consult your doctor:
- If you have stroke or heart disease.
- If you have asthma.
- If you have had kidney disease.
- If you have peptic ulcer or chronic acid indigestion.
- If you will have surgery within 2 months, including dental surgery, requiring general or spinal anesthesia.

Over age 60:
Adverse reactions and side effects may be more frequent and severe than in younger persons. Start with small doses and monitor blood pressure frequently.

Pregnancy:
No proven harm to unborn child. Avoid if possible. Consult doctor. Risk category B (see page xxii).

Breast-feeding:
No proven harm to nursing infant. Avoid if possible. Consult doctor.

Infants & children:
Not recommended.

Prolonged use:
- Due to drug's cumulative effect, dose will require adjustment to prevent wide fluctuations in blood pressure.
- Talk to your doctor about the need for follow-up medical examinations or laboratory studies.

Skin & sunlight:
No problems expected.

Driving, piloting or hazardous work:
Don't drive or pilot aircraft until you learn how medicine affects you. Don't work around dangerous machinery. Don't climb ladders or work in high places. Danger increases if you drink alcohol or take medicine affecting alertness and reflexes, such as antihistamines, tranquilizers, sedatives, pain medicine, narcotics and mind-altering drugs.

Discontinuing:
Don't discontinue without consulting doctor. Dose may require gradual reduction if you have taken drug for a long time. Doses of other drugs may also require adjustment.

Others:
- Hot weather further lowers blood pressure, particularly in patients over 60.
- Advise any doctor or dentist whom you consult that you take this medicine.

POSSIBLE INTERACTION WITH OTHER DRUGS

GENERIC NAME OR DRUG CLASS	COMBINED EFFECT
Angiotensin-converting enzyme (ACE) inhibitors*	Possible excessive potassium in blood.
Antidepressants, tricyclic*	Decreased effect of guanadrel.
Antihypertensives, other*	Increased effect of guanadrel.
Beta-adrenergic blocking agents*	Increased likelihood of dizziness and fainting.
Carteolol	Increased anti-hypertensive effect.
Contraceptives, oral*	Increased side effects of oral contraceptives.
Central nervous system (CNS) depressants* (anticonvulsants,* antihistamines,* muscle relaxants,* narcotics,* sedatives,* tranquilizers*)	Decreased effect of guanadrel.
Diuretics*	Increased likelihood of dizziness and fainting.
Haloperidol	Decreased effect of guanadrel.
Insulin	Increased insulin effect.
Loxapine	Decreased effect of guanadrel.
Monoamine oxidase (MAO) inhibitors*	Severe high blood pressure. Avoid.
Nicardipine	Blood pressure drop. Dosages may require adjustment.
Nimodipine	Dangerous blood pressure drop.
Phenothiazines*	Decreased effect of guanadrel.
Rauwolfia alkaloids*	Increased likelihood of dizziness and fainting.
Sotalol	Increased anti-hypertensive effect.
Sympathomimetics*	Decreased effect of guanadrel.
Terazosin	Decreases effectiveness of terazosin.
Thioxanthenes*	Decreased effect of guanadrel.
Trimeprazine	Decreased effect of guanadrel.

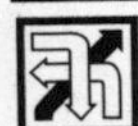

POSSIBLE INTERACTION WITH OTHER SUBSTANCES

INTERACTS WITH	COMBINED EFFECT
Alcohol:	Decreased effect of guanadrel. Avoid.
Beverages: Caffeine.	Decreased effect of guanadrel.
Cocaine:	Increased risk of heart block and high blood pressure.
Foods:	No problems expected.
Marijuana:	Higher blood pressure. Avoid.
Tobacco:	Higher blood pressure. Avoid.

*See Glossary

GUANETHIDINE

BRAND NAMES

Apo-Guanethidine   Ismelin

BASIC INFORMATION

Habit forming? No
Prescription needed? Yes
Available as generic? Yes
Drug class: Antihypertensive

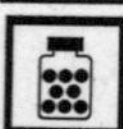

USES

Reduces high blood pressure.

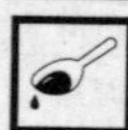

DOSAGE & USAGE INFORMATION

How to take:
Tablet—Swallow with liquid. If you can't swallow tablet whole, crumble and take with liquid or food.

When to take:
At the same time each day.

If you forget a dose:
Take as soon as you remember up to 2 hours late. If more than 2 hours, wait for next scheduled dose (don't double this dose).

What drug does:
Displaces norepinephrine—hormone necessary to maintain small blood vessel tone. Blood vessels relax and high blood pressure drops.

Time lapse before drug works:
Regular use for several weeks may be necessary to determine effectiveness.

Don't take with:
- Nonprescription drugs containing alcohol without consulting doctor.
- Any other medicine without consulting your doctor or pharmacist.

OVERDOSE

SYMPTOMS:
Severe blood pressure drop; fainting; blurred vision; slow, weak pulse; cold, sweaty skin; loss of consciousness.
WHAT TO DO:
- **Dial 911 (emergency) or 0 (operator) for an ambulance or medical help. Then give first aid immediately.**
- **See emergency information on inside covers.**

POSSIBLE ADVERSE REACTIONS OR SIDE EFFECTS

SYMPTOMS	WHAT TO DO
Life-threatening:	
In case of overdose, see previous column.	
Common:	
• Unusually slow heartbeat.	Discontinue. Call doctor right away.
• Diarrhea; more bowel movements; swollen feet, legs; fatigue, weakness.	Continue. Call doctor when convenient.
• Dizziness, lower sex drive.	Continue. Tell doctor at next visit.
• Stuffy nose, dry mouth.	No action necessary.
Infrequent:	
• Rash, blurred vision, drooping eyelids, chest pain or shortness of breath, muscle pain or tremor.	Discontinue. Call doctor right away.
• Nausea or vomiting, headache.	Continue. Call doctor when convenient.
• Impotence, nighttime urination, hair loss.	Continue. Tell doctor at next visit.
Rare:	
Decreased white blood cells causing sore throat, fever.	Discontinue. Call doctor right away.

WARNINGS & PRECAUTIONS

Don't take if:
- You are allergic to guanethidine.
- You have taken MAO inhibitors within 2 weeks.

Before you start, consult your doctor:
- If you have had stroke or heart disease.
- If you have asthma.
- If you have had kidney disease.
- If you have peptic ulcer or chronic acid indigestion.
- If you will have surgery within 2 months, including dental surgery, requiring general or spinal anesthesia.

Over age 60:
Adverse reactions and side effects may be more frequent and severe than in younger persons. Start with small doses and monitor blood pressure frequently.

Pregnancy:
Decide with your doctor if drug benefits justify risk to unborn child. Risk category C (see page xxii).

Breast-feeding:
Unknown effect. Consult doctor.

Infants & children:
Not recommended.

Prolonged use:
- Due to drug's cumulative effect, dose will require adjustment to prevent wide fluctuations in blood pressure.
- Talk to your doctor about the need for follow-up medical examinations or laboratory studies.

Skin & sunlight:
No problems expected.

Driving, piloting or hazardous work:
Don't drive or pilot aircraft until you learn how medicine affects you. Don't work around dangerous machinery. Don't climb ladders or work in high places. Danger increases if you drink alcohol or take medicine affecting alertness and reflexes, such as antihistamines, tranquilizers, sedatives,pain medicine, narcotics and mind-altering drugs.

Discontinuing:
Don't discontinue without consulting doctor. Dose may require gradual reduction if you have taken drug for a long time. Doses of other drugs may also require adjustment.

Others:
Hot weather further lowers blood pressure.

POSSIBLE INTERACTION WITH OTHER DRUGS

GENERIC NAME OR DRUG CLASS	COMBINED EFFECT
Amphetamines*	Decreased guanethidine effect.
Angiotensin-converting enzyme (ACE) inhibitors*	Possible excessive potassium in blood.
Antidepressants, tricyclic*	Decreased guanethidine effect.
Antidiabetics, oral*	Increased guanethidine effect.
Antihistamines*	Decreased guanethidine effect.
Carteolol	Increased anti-hypertensive effect.
Contraceptives, oral*	Decreased guanethidine effect. Increased side effects of oral contraceptives.
Digitalis preparations*	Slower heartbeat.
Diuretics, thiazide*	Increased guanethidine effect.
Haloperidol	Decreased guanethidine effect.
Indapamide	Possible increased effects of both drugs. When monitored carefully, combination may be beneficial in controlling hypertension.
Insulin	Increased insulin effect.
Loxapine	Decreased effect of guanethidine.
Minoxidil	Dosage adjustments may be necessary to keep blood pressure at proper level.
Monoamine oxidase (MAO) inhibitors*	Increased blood pressure.
Nicardipine	Blood pressure drop. Dosages may require adjustment.
Nimodipine	Dangerous blood pressure drop.
Phenothiazines*	Decreased guanethidine effect.

Continued on page 940

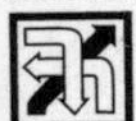

POSSIBLE INTERACTION WITH OTHER SUBSTANCES

INTERACTS WITH	COMBINED EFFECT
Alcohol:	Use caution. Decreases blood pressure.
Beverages: Carbonated drinks.	Use sparingly. Sodium content increases blood pressure.
Cocaine:	Increased risk of heart block and high blood pressure.
Foods: Spicy or acid foods.	Avoid if subject to indigestion or peptic ulcer.
Marijuana:	Excessively low blood pressure. Avoid.
Tobacco:	Possible blood pressure rise. Avoid.

*See Glossary

GUANETHIDINE & HYDROCHLOROTHIAZIDE

BRAND NAMES

Esimil **Ismelin-Esidrix**

BASIC INFORMATION

Habit forming? No
Prescription needed? Yes
Available as generic? No
Drug class: Antihypertensive, diuretic

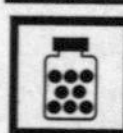

USES

- Controls, but doesn't cure, high blood pressure.
- Reduces fluid retention (edema).

DOSAGE & USAGE INFORMATION

How to take:
Tablet—Swallow with liquid. If you can't swallow whole, crumble tablet and take with liquid or food.

When to take:
At the same time each day.

If you forget a dose:
Take as soon as you remember up to 2 hours late. If more than 2 hours, wait for next scheduled dose (don't double this dose).

What drug does:
- Forces sodium and water secretion, reducing body fluid.
- Displaces norepinephrine—hormone necessary to maintain small blood vessel tone. Blood vessels relax and high blood pressure drops.

Time lapse before drug works:
Regular use for several weeks may be necessary to determine effectiveness.

Continued next column

OVERDOSE

SYMPTOMS:
Cramps, weakness, drowsiness, blurred vision, weak pulse, severe blood pressure drop, fainting, cold and sweaty skin, loss of consciousness, coma.
WHAT TO DO:
- **Dial 911 (emergency) or 0 (operator) for an ambulance or medical help. Then give first aid immediately.**
- **See emergency information on inside covers.**

Don't take with:
- Nonprescription drugs containing alcohol without consulting doctor.
- Any other medicine without consulting your doctor or pharmacist.

POSSIBLE ADVERSE REACTIONS OR SIDE EFFECTS

SYMPTOMS	WHAT TO DO
Life-threatening:	
Chest pain, shortness of breath, irregular heartbeat.	Discontinue. Seek emergency treatment.
Common:	
• Slow heartbeat, swollen feet and ankles, fatigue, weakness.	Discontinue. Call doctor right away.
• Dizziness, stuffy nose, dry mouth, diarrhea, diminished sex drive.	Continue. Call doctor when convenient.
Infrequent:	
• Mood change, rash or hives, blurred vision, drooping eyelids, muscle pain or tremors.	Discontinue. Call doctor right away.
• Increased nighttime urination, abdominal pain, vomiting, nausea, headache, weakness.	Continue. Call doctor when convenient.
• Impotence, nighttime urination, hair loss.	Continue. Tell doctor at next visit.
Rare:	
• Decreased white blood cells causing sore throat, fever; jaundice.	Discontinue. Call doctor right away.
• Weight gain or loss.	Continue. Call doctor when convenient.

WARNINGS & PRECAUTIONS

Don't take if:
- You are allergic to any thiazide diuretic drug or guanethidine.
- You have taken MAO inhibitors within 2 weeks.

Before you start, consult your doctor:
- If you are allergic to any sulfa drug.
- If you have gout, asthma, liver, pancreas or kidney disorder, peptic ulcer or chronic acid indigestion.
- If you have had stroke or heart disease.
- If you will have surgery within 2 months, including dental surgery, requiring general or spinal anesthesia.

GUANETHIDINE & HYDROCHLOROTHIAZIDE

Over age 60:
Adverse reactions and side effects may be more frequent and severe than in younger persons, especially dizziness and excessive potassium loss.

Pregnancy:
Decide with your doctor if drug benefits justify risk to unborn child. Risk category C (see page xxii).

Breast-feeding:
Drug passes into milk. Avoid drug or discontinue nursing until you finish medicine. Consult doctor for advice on maintaining milk supply.

Infants & children:
Not recommended.

Prolonged use:
- Due to drug's cumulative effect, dose will require adjustment to prevent wide fluctuations in blood pressure.
- Talk to your doctor about the need for follow-up medical examinations or laboratory studies.

Skin & sunlight:
May cause rash or intensify sunburn in areas exposed to sun or sunlamp.

Driving, piloting or hazardous work:
Don't drive or pilot aircraft until you learn how medicine affects you. Don't work around dangerous machinery. Don't climb ladders or work in high places. Danger increases if you drink alcohol or take medicine affecting alertness and reflexes, such as antihistamines, tranquilizers, sedatives, pain medicine, narcotics and mind-altering drugs.

Discontinuing:
Don't discontinue without consulting doctor. Dose may require gradual reduction if you have taken drug for a long time. Doses of other drugs may also require adjustment.

Others:
- Hot weather and fever may cause dehydration and drop in blood pressure. Dose may require temporary adjustment. Weigh daily and report any unexpected weight decreases to your doctor.
- May cause rise in uric acid, leading to gout.
- May cause blood sugar rise in diabetics.

POSSIBLE INTERACTION WITH OTHER DRUGS

GENERIC NAME OR DRUG CLASS	COMBINED EFFECT
Allopurinol	Decreased allopurinol effect.
Amphetamines*	Decreased guanethidine effect.
Antidepressants, tricyclic*	Dangerous drop in blood pressure. Avoid combination unless under medical supervision.
Antihistamines*	Decreased guanethidine effect.
Barbiturates*	Increased hydrochlorothiazide effect.
Beta-adrenergic blocking agents*	Increased anti-hypertensive effect. Dosages of both drugs may require adjustments.
Carteolol	Increased anti-hypertensive effect.
Cholestyramine	Decreased hydrochlorothiazide effect.
Contraceptives, oral*	Decreased guanethidine effect.

Continued on page 940

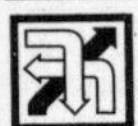

POSSIBLE INTERACTION WITH OTHER SUBSTANCES

INTERACTS WITH	COMBINED EFFECT
Alcohol:	Use caution Decreases blood pressure.
Beverages: Carbonated drinks.	Use sparingly. Sodium content increases blood pressure.
Cocaine:	Raises blood pressure. Avoid.
Foods: Spicy or acid foods.	Avoid if subject to indigestion or peptic ulcer.
Licorice.	Excessive potassium loss that causes dangerous heart rhythms.
Marijuana:	Effect on blood pressure unpredictable.
Tobacco:	Possible blood pressure rise. Avoid.

*See Glossary

GUANFACINE

BRAND NAMES

Tenex

BASIC INFORMATION

Habit forming? No
Prescription needed? Yes
Available as generic? No
Drug class: Antihypertensive

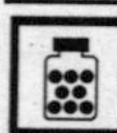

USES

Treats high blood pressure, usually in combination with a diuretic drug.

DOSAGE & USAGE INFORMATION

How to take:
Tablets—Swallow with liquid or food to lessen stomach irritation. If you can't swallow whole, crumble tablet and take with liquid or food.

When to take:
Usually at bedtime to minimize daytime drowsiness.

If you forget a dose:
Take as soon as you remember up to 2 hours late. If more than 2 hours, wait for next scheduled dose (don't double this dose).

What drug does:
- Decreases stimulating effects of the sympathetic nervous system on the heart, kidneys and arteries throughout the body.
- Decreases both systolic and diastolic blood pressure.

Time lapse before drug works:
Within 1 week.

Don't take with:
Any other medicine without consulting your doctor or pharmacist.

OVERDOSE

SYMPTOMS:
Difficulty breathing, loss of consciousness, dizziness, very slow heartbeat.
WHAT TO DO:
- **Dial 911 (emergency) or 0 (operator) for an ambulance or medical help. Then give first aid immediately.**
- **See emergency information on inside covers.**

POSSIBLE ADVERSE REACTIONS OR SIDE EFFECTS

SYMPTOMS	WHAT TO DO
Life-threatening:	
Shortness of breath.	Seek emergency treatment immediately.
Common:	
• Decreased sexual function, drowsiness, constipation.	Continue. Call doctor when convenient.
• Increased dental problems because of dry mouth and less salivation.	Consult your dentist about a prevention program.
Infrequent:	
• Confusion, dizziness or fainting, slow heartbeat.	Continue, but call doctor right away.
• Mental depression, eye irritation, insomnia, tiredness or weakness, headache, nausea and/or vomiting.	Continue. Call doctor when convenient.
Rare:	
May occur if medicine is abruptly discontinued—Anxiety, chest pain, heartbeat irregularities, excess salivation, sleep problems, nervousness, sweating.	Seek emergency treatment.

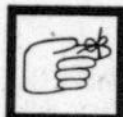

WARNINGS & PRECAUTIONS

Don't take if:
You have had a recent heart attack.

Before you start, consult your doctor:
- If you have heart disease or liver disease.
- If you have coronary insufficiency.
- If you have mental depression.

Over age 60:
None significant.

Pregnancy:
No proven harm to unborn child, but avoid if possible. Consult doctor. Risk category B (see page xxii).

Breast-feeding:
Effect not documented. Consult your doctor.

Infants & children:
Effect not documented. Consult your pediatrician.

Prolonged use:
Talk to your doctor about the need for follow-up medical examinations or laboratory studies to check blood pressure.

Skin & sunlight:
No problems expected.

Driving, piloting or hazardous work:
Don't drive or pilot aircraft until you learn how medicine affects you. Don't work around dangerous machinery. Don't climb ladders or work in high places. Danger increases if you drink alcohol or take medicine affecting alertness and reflexes.

Discontinuing:
- Don't discontinue without consulting doctor. Dose may require gradual reduction if you have taken drug for a long time. Doses of other drugs may also require adjustment.
- May occur if medicine is discontinued abruptly: anxiety, chest pain, heartbeat irregularities, excess salivation, sleep problems, nervousness, sweating.

Others:
- This medication works better if you attempt to reduce your weight to normal, exercise regularly, restrict salt in your diet and reduce stress wherever possible. Continue taking medicine even when you feel good.
- Adverse reactions are usually dose-related and diminish when dosage is reduced.

POSSIBLE INTERACTION WITH OTHER DRUGS

GENERIC NAME OR DRUG CLASS	COMBINED EFFECT
Antihypertensives, other*	May increase effects of guanfacine and other medicines.
Anti-inflammatory drugs, nonsteroidal (NSAIDs)*	May decrease anti-hypertensive effects of guanfacine.
Carteolol	Increased anti-hypertensive effect.
Central nervous system (CNS) depressants*	Increases depressant effect of both drugs.
Clozapine	Toxic effect on the central nervous system.
Estrogens*	May decrease anti-hypertensive effects of guanfacine.
Ethinamate	Dangerous increased effects of ethinamate. Avoid combining.
Fluoxetine	Increased depressant effects of both drugs.
Leucovorin	High alcohol content of leucovorin may cause adverse effects.
Lisinopril	Increased anti-hypertensive effect. Dosage of each may require adjustment.
Methyprylon	Increased sedative effect, perhaps to dangerous level. Avoid.
Nabilone	Greater depression of central nervous system.
Nicardipine	Blood pressure drop. Dosages may require adjustment.
Nimodipine	Dangerous blood pressure drop.
Propafenone	Increased effect of both drugs and increased risk of toxicity.
Sertraline	Increased depressive effects of both drugs.
Sotalol	Increased anti-hypertensive effect.

Continued on page 941

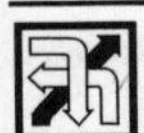

POSSIBLE INTERACTION WITH OTHER SUBSTANCES

INTERACTS WITH	COMBINED EFFECT
Alcohol:	Excess use may lead to dangerous drop in blood pressure.
Beverages: Any containing caffeine, such as coffee, tea or cocoa.	May decrease anti-hypertensive effect of guanfacine.
Cocaine:	Increased risk of heart block and high blood pressure.
Foods:	None expected.
Marijuana:	May decrease anti-hypertensive effect of guanfacine.
Tobacco:	May decrease anti-hypertensive effect of guanfacine

***See Glossary**

HALOPERIDOL

BRAND NAMES

Apo-Haloperidol
Haldol
Haldol Decanoate
Haldol LA
Halperon
Novo-Peridol
Peridol
PMS-Haloperidol

BASIC INFORMATION

Habit forming? No
Prescription needed? Yes
Available as generic? Yes
Drug class: Tranquilizer (antipsychotic)

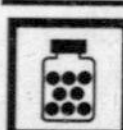

USES

- Reduces severe anxiety, agitation and psychotic behavior.
- Treatment for Tourette's syndrome
- Treatment for infantile autism.
- Treatment for Huntington's chorea.

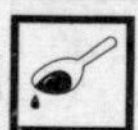

DOSAGE & USAGE INFORMATION

How to take:
- Tablet—Swallow with liquid. If you can't swallow whole, crumble tablet and take with liquid or food.
- Drops—Dilute dose in beverage before swallowing.

When to take:
At the same times each day.

Continued next column

OVERDOSE

SYMPTOMS:
Weak, rapid pulse; shallow, slow breathing; tremor or muscle weakness; very low blood pressure; convulsions; deep sleep ending in coma.
WHAT TO DO:
- **Dial 911 (emergency) or 0 (operator) for an ambulance or medical help. Then give first aid immediately.**
- **If patient is unconscious and not breathing, give mouth-to-mouth breathing. If there is no heartbeat, use cardiac massage and mouth-to-mouth breathing (CPR). Don't try to make patient vomit. If you can't get help quickly, take patient to nearest emergency facility.**
- **See emergency information on inside covers.**

If you forget a dose:
Take as soon as you remember up to 2 hours late. If more than 2 hours, wait for next scheduled dose (don't double this dose).

What drug does:
Corrects an imbalance in nerve impulses from brain.

Time lapse before drug works:
3 weeks to 2 months for maximum benefit.

Don't take with:
- Nonprescription drugs without consulting doctor.
- Any other medicine without consulting your doctor or pharmacist.

POSSIBLE ADVERSE REACTIONS OR SIDE EFFECTS

SYMPTOMS	WHAT TO DO
Life-threatening:	
Uncontrolled muscle movements of tongue, face and other muscles (neuroleptic malignant syndrome, rare).	Discontinue. Seek emergency treatment.
Common:	
• Blurred vision, loss of balance, muscle spasms, severe restlessness.	Discontinue. Call doctor right away.
• Shuffling, stiffness, jerkiness, shakiness, constipation, weight gain.	Continue. Call doctor when convenient.
• Dry mouth.	No action necessary.
Infrequent:	
• Rash, circling motions of tongue, hallucinations, lip smacking.	Discontinue. Call doctor right away.
• Dizziness, faintness, drowsiness, difficult urination, decreased sexual ability, nausea or vomiting.	Continue. Call doctor when convenient.
Rare:	
Sore throat; fever; jaundice; abdominal pain; dry, warm skin.	Discontinue. Call doctor right away.

WARNINGS & PRECAUTIONS

Don't take if:
- You have ever been allergic to haloperidol.
- You are depressed.
- You have Parkinson's disease.
- Patient is younger than 3 years old.

Before you start, consult your doctor:
- If you take sedatives, sleeping pills, tranquilizers, antidepressants, antihistamines, narcotics or mind-altering drugs.
- If you have a history of mental depression.
- If you have had kidney or liver problems.
- If you have diabetes, epilepsy, glaucoma, high blood pressure or heart disease, prostate trouble.
- If you drink alcoholic beverages frequently.

Over age 60:
Adverse reactions and side effects may be more frequent and severe than in younger persons.

Pregnancy:
Decide with your doctor if drug benefits justify risk to unborn child. Risk category C (see page xxii).

Breast-feeding:
Drug passes into milk. Avoid drug or discontinue nursing until you finish medicine. Consult doctor about maintaining milk supply.

Infants & children:
Not recommended.

Prolonged use:
- May develop tardive dyskinesia (involuntary movements of jaws, lips and tongue).
- Talk to your doctor about the need for follow-up medical examinations or laboratory studies to check blood pressure, liver function.

Skin & sunlight:
May cause rash or intensify sunburn in areas exposed to sun or sunlamp.

Driving, piloting or hazardous work:
Don't drive or pilot aircraft until you learn how medicine affects you. Don't work around dangerous machinery. Don't climb ladders or work in high places. Danger increases if you drink alcohol or take medicine affecting alertness and reflexes.

Discontinuing:
Don't discontinue without consulting doctor. Dose may require gradual reduction if you have taken drug for a long time. Doses of other drugs may also require adjustment.

Others:
No problems expected.

POSSIBLE INTERACTION WITH OTHER DRUGS

GENERIC NAME OR DRUG CLASS	COMBINED EFFECT
Anticholinergics*	Increased anti-cholinergic effect. May cause pressure within the eye.
Anticonvulsants*	Changed seizure pattern.
Antidepressants*	Excessive sedation.
Antihistamines*	Excessive sedation.
Antihypertensives*	May cause severe blood pressure drop.
Barbiturates*	Excessive sedation.
Bupropion	Increased risk of major seizures.
Central nervous system (CNS) depressants*	Increased CNS depression; increased blood pressure drop.
Clozapine	Toxic effect on the central nervous system.
Dronabinol	Increased effects of both drugs. Avoid.
Ethinamate	Dangerous increased effects of ethinamate. Avoid combining.
Fluoxetine	Increased depressant effects of both drugs.
Guanethidine	Decreased guanethidine effect.
Guanfacine	May increase depressant effects of either drug.
Leucovorin	High alcohol content of leucovorin may cause adverse effects.

Continued on page 941

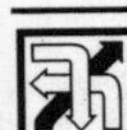

POSSIBLE INTERACTION WITH OTHER SUBSTANCES

INTERACTS WITH	COMBINED EFFECT
Alcohol:	Excessive sedation and depressed brain function. Avoid.
Beverages:	None expected.
Cocaine:	Decreased effect of haloperidol. Avoid.
Foods:	None expected.
Marijuana:	Occasional use—Increased sedation. Frequent use—Possible toxic psychosis.
Tobacco:	None expected.

***See Glossary**

HISTAMINE H_2 RECEPTOR ANTAGONISTS

BRAND AND GENERIC NAMES

Apo-Cimetidine
Apo-Ranitidine
Axid
CIMETIDINE
FAMOTIDINE
NIZATIDINE
Novocimetine
Pepcid
Peptol
RANITIDINE
Tagamet
Zantac
Zantac-C

BASIC INFORMATION

Habit forming? No
Prescription needed? Yes
Available as generic? No
Drug class: Histamine H_2 antagonist

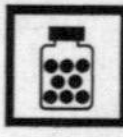

USES

Treatment for duodenal and gastric ulcers and other conditions in which stomach produces excess hydrochloric acid.

DOSAGE & USAGE INFORMATION

How to take:
- Tablet, capsule or liquid—Swallow with liquid.
- Oral suspension—Follow instructions on prescription.

When to take:
- 1 dose per day—Take at bedtime.
- 2 or more doses per day—Take at the same times each day.

If you forget a dose:
Take as soon as you remember up to 2 hours late. If more than 2 hours, wait for next scheduled dose (don't double this dose).

What drug does:
Blocks histamine release so stomach secretes less acid.

Time lapse before drug works:
Begins in 30 minutes. May require several days to relieve pain.

Continued next column

OVERDOSE

SYMPTOMS:
Confusion, slurred speech, breathing difficulty, rapid heartbeat, delirium.
WHAT TO DO:
Overdose unlikely to threaten life. If person takes much larger amount than prescribed, call doctor, poison control center or hospital emergency room for instructions.

Don't take with:
Any other medicine without consulting your doctor or pharmacist.

POSSIBLE ADVERSE REACTIONS OR SIDE EFFECTS

SYMPTOMS	WHAT TO DO
Life-threatening: In case of overdose, see previous column.	
Common: None expected.	
Infrequent:	
• Dizziness or headache, diarrhea.	Continue. Call doctor when convenient.
• Diminished sex drive, unusual milk flow in females, hair loss.	Continue. Tell doctor at next visit.
Rare:	
• Confusion; rash, hives; sore throat, fever; slow, fast or irregular heartbeat; unusual bleeding or bruising; muscle cramps or pain; fatigue; weakness.	Discontinue. Call doctor right away.
• Constipation.	Continue. Call doctor when convenient.

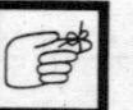

WARNINGS & PRECAUTIONS

Don't take if:
You are allergic to any histamine H_2 antagonist.

Before you start, consult your doctor:
- If you plan to become pregnant while on medication.
- If you take aspirin. Aspirin may irritate stomach.

Over age 60:
Adverse reactions and side effects may be more frequent and severe than in younger persons.

Pregnancy:
Risk factors vary for drugs in this group. See category list on page xxii and consult doctor.

Breast-feeding:
Drug passes into milk. Avoid drug or discontinue nursing until you finish medicine. Consult doctor about maintaining milk supply.

Infants & children:
Not recommended.

Prolonged use:
- Possible liver damage.
- Talk to your doctor about the need for follow-up medical examinations or laboratory studies to check blood levels of vitamin B-12.

Skin & sunlight:
No problems expected.

Driving, piloting or hazardous work:
Don't drive or pilot aircraft until you learn how medicine affects you. Don't work around dangerous machinery. Don't climb ladders or work in high places. Danger increases if you drink alcohol or take medicine affecting alertness and reflexes, such as antihistamines, tranquilizers, sedatives, pain medicine, narcotics and mind-altering drugs.

Discontinuing:
Don't discontinue without consulting a doctor. Dose may require gradual reduction if you have taken drug for a long time. Doses of other drugs may also require adjustment.

Others:
- Patients on kidney dialysis—Take at end of dialysis treatment.
- May interfere with the accuracy of some medical tests.

POSSIBLE INTERACTION WITH OTHER DRUGS

GENERIC NAME OR DRUG CLASS	COMBINED EFFECT
Alprazolam	Increased effect and toxicity of alprazolam.
Antacids*	Decreased absorption of histamine H_2 receptor antagonist.
Anticoagulants, oral*	Increased anticoagulant effect.
Anticholinergics*	Increased histamine H_2 receptor antagonist effect.
Bupropion	Increased bupropion effect.
Carbamazepine	Increased effect and toxicity of carbamazepine.
Carmustine (BCNU)	Severe impairment of red blood cell production; some interference with white blood cell formation.
Chlordiazepoxide	Increased effect and toxicity of chlordiazepoxide.
Cisapride	Decreased histamine H_2 receptor effect.
Diazepam	Increased effect and toxicity of diazepam.
Digitalis preparations*	Increased digitalis effect.
Encainide	Increased effect of histamine H_2 receptor antagonist.
Flurazepam	Increased effect and toxicity of flurazepam.
Glipizide	Increased effect and toxicity of glipizide.
Itraconazole	Decreased absorption of itraconazole.
Ketoconazole	Decreased ketoconazole absorption.
Labetalol	Increased antihypertensive effects.

Continued on page 941

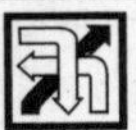

POSSIBLE INTERACTION WITH OTHER SUBSTANCES

INTERACTS WITH	COMBINED EFFECT
Alcohol:	No interactions expected, but alcohol may slow body's recovery. Avoid.
Beverages:	
Milk.	Enhanced effectiveness. Small amounts useful for taking medication.
Caffeine drinks.	May increase acid secretion and delay healing.
Cocaine:	Decreased effect of histamine H_2 receptor antagonist.
Foods:	Enhanced effectiveness. Protein-rich foods should be eaten in moderation to minimize secretion of stomach acid.
Marijuana:	Increased chance of low sperm count. Marijuana may slow body's recovery. Avoid.
Tobacco:	Reversed effect of histamine H_2 receptor antagonist. Tobacco may slow body's recovery. Avoid.

***See Glossary**

HMG-CoA REDUCTASE INHIBITORS

BRAND AND GENERIC NAMES

Epistatin
Eptastatin
FLUVASTATIN
Lescol
LOVASTATIN
Mevacor
Mevinolin
Pravachol
PRAVASTATIN
SIMVASTATIN
Synvinolin
Zocor

BASIC INFORMATION

Habit forming? No
Prescription needed? Yes
Available as generic? No
Drug class: Antihyperlipidemic

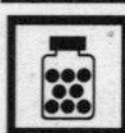

USES

Lowers blood cholesterol levels caused by low-density lipoproteins (LDL) in persons who haven't improved by exercising, dieting or using other measures.

DOSAGE & USAGE INFORMATION

How to take:
Tablet or capsule—Swallow with liquid. If you can't swallow whole, crumble tablet and take with liquid or food.

When to take:
According to directions on prescription.

If you forget a dose:
Take as soon as you remember up to 2 hours late. If more than 2 hours, wait for next scheduled dose (don't double this dose).

What drug does:
Inhibits an enzyme in the liver.

Time lapse before drug works:
Within 2 weeks.

Don't take with:
- A high-fat diet.
- Any other medicine without consulting your doctor or pharmacist.

OVERDOSE

SYMPTOMS:
None expected.
WHAT TO DO:
Overdose not expected to threaten life. If person takes much larger amount than prescribed, call doctor, poison control center or hospital emergency room for instructions.

POSSIBLE ADVERSE REACTIONS OR SIDE EFFECTS

SYMPTOMS	WHAT TO DO
Life-threatening: None expected.	
Common: None expected.	
Infrequent:	
• Aching muscles, fever, blurred vision.	Discontinue. Call doctor right away.
• Constipation, nausea, tiredness, weakness, dizziness, skin rash, headache.	Continue. Call doctor when convenient.
Rare:	
• Muscle pain.	Discontinue. Call doctor right away.
• Impotence (lovastatin only).	Continue. Call doctor when convenient.
• Insomnia (lovastatin only).	Continue. Call doctor when convenient.

WARNINGS & PRECAUTIONS

Don't take if:
You are allergic to lovastatin.

Before you start, consult your doctor:
- If you take immunosuppressive drugs, particularly following a heart transplant.
- If you have low blood pressure.
- If you have hormone abnormalities
- If you have an active infection.
- If you have active liver disease.
- If you have a seizure disorder.
- If you have had a recent major accident.

Over age 60:
Likely to be more sensitive to drug.

Pregnancy:
Consult doctor. Risk category X (see page xxii).

Breast-feeding:
Discontinue nursing until you finish medicine. Consult doctor for advice on maintaining milk supply.

Infants & children:
Not recommended for children.

Prolonged use:
Talk to your doctor about the need for follow-up medical examinations or laboratory studies to check liver function, serum cholesterol, eyes.

Skin & sunlight:
No problems expected.

Driving, piloting or hazardous work:
No special problems expected.

Discontinuing:
Don't discontinue without consulting doctor. Dose may require gradual reduction if you have taken drug for a long time. Doses of other drugs may also require adjustment.

Others:
- Request liver function tests and eye examinations before beginning this medicine and repeat every 2 to 6 months.
- Advise any doctor or dentist whom you consult that you take this medicine.

POSSIBLE INTERACTION WITH OTHER DRUGS

GENERIC NAME OR DRUG CLASS	COMBINED EFFECT
Cholestyramine	With fluvastatin—Decreased effect of fluvastatin if taken at same time.
Cyclosporine	Increased risk of heart and kidney problems.
Digoxin	Increased digoxin effect.
Erythromycins*	Increased risk of heart and kidney problems.
Gemfibrozil	Increased risk of heart and kidney problems and muscle inflammation.
Immunosuppressants*	Increased risk of heart or kidney problems.
Niacin	Increased risk of heart and kidney problems.

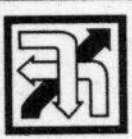

POSSIBLE INTERACTION WITH OTHER SUBSTANCES

INTERACTS WITH	COMBINED EFFECT
Alcohol:	None expected.
Beverages:	None expected.
Cocaine:	None expected.
Foods:	None expected.
Marijuana:	None expected.
Tobacco:	None expected.

***See Glossary**

HYDRALAZINE

BRAND NAMES

Apresoline
Novo-Hylazin

BASIC INFORMATION

Habit forming? No
Prescription needed? Yes
Available as generic? Yes
Drug class: Antihypertensive

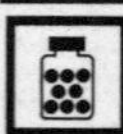

USES

Treatment for high blood pressure and congestive heart failure.

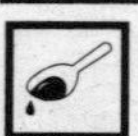

DOSAGE & USAGE INFORMATION

How to take:
Tablet—Swallow with liquid. If you can't swallow whole, crumble tablet and take with liquid or food.

When to take:
At the same time each day.

If you forget a dose:
Take as soon as you remember up to 2 hours late. If more than 2 hours, wait for next scheduled dose (don't double this dose).

What drug does:
Relaxes and expands blood vessel walls, lowering blood pressure.

Time lapse before drug works:
Regular use for several weeks may be necessary to determine drug's effectiveness.

Continued next column

OVERDOSE

SYMPTOMS:
Rapid and weak heartbeat, fainting, extreme weakness, cold and sweaty skin, flushing.
WHAT TO DO:

- **Dial 911 (emergency) or 0 (operator) for an ambulance or medical help. Then give first aid immediately.**
- **If patient is unconscious and not breathing, give mouth-to-mouth breathing. If there is no heartbeat, use cardiac massage and mouth-to-mouth breathing (CPR). Don't try to make patient vomit. If you can't get help quickly, take patient to nearest emergency facility.**
- **See emergency information on inside covers.**

Don't take with:

- Nonprescription drugs containing alcohol without consulting doctor.
- Any other medicine without consulting your doctor or pharmacist.

POSSIBLE ADVERSE REACTIONS OR SIDE EFFECTS

SYMPTOMS	WHAT TO DO
Life-threatening: In case of overdose, see previous column.	
Common:	
• Nausea or vomiting, rapid or irregular heartbeat.	Discontinue. Call doctor right away.
• Headache, diarrhea, appetite loss, painful or difficult urination.	Continue. Tell doctor at next visit.
Infrequent:	
• Hives or rash, flushed face, sore throat, fever, chest pain, swelling of lymph glands, skin blisters, swelling in feet or legs, joint pain.	Discontinue. Call doctor right away.
• Confusion, dizziness, anxiety, depression, joint pain, general discomfort or weakness, fever, muscle pain, chest pain.	Continue. Call doctor when convenient.
• Watery eyes and irritation, constipation.	Continue. Tell doctor at next visit.
Rare:	
• Weakness and faintness when arising from bed or chair, jaundice.	Discontinue. Call doctor right away.
• Numbness or tingling in hands or feet, nasal congestion, impotence.	Continue. Call doctor when convenient.

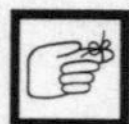

WARNINGS & PRECAUTIONS

Don't take if:

- You are allergic to hydralazine or tartrazine dye.
- You have history of coronary artery disease or rheumatic heart disease.

Before you start, consult your doctor:

- If you feel pain in chest, neck or arms on physical exertion.
- If you have had lupus.
- If you have had a stroke.

- If you have had kidney disease or impaired kidney function.
- If you will have surgery within 2 months, including dental surgery, requiring general or spinal anesthesia.

Over age 60:
Adverse reactions and side effects may be more frequent and severe than in younger persons.

Pregnancy:
Decide with your doctor if drug benefits justify risk to unborn child. Risk category C (see page xxii).

Breast-feeding:
Drug filters into milk. May harm child. Avoid.

Infants & children:
Not recommended.

Prolonged use:
- May cause lupus (arthritis-like illness).
- Possible psychosis.
- May cause numbness, tingling in hands or feet.
- Talk to your doctor about the need for follow-up medical examinations or laboratory studies to check blood pressure, complete blood counts (white blood cell count, platelet count, red blood cell count, hemoglobin, hematocrit), ANA titers*.

Skin & sunlight:
No problems expected.

Driving, piloting or hazardous work:
Don't drive or pilot aircraft until you learn how medicine affects you. Don't work around dangerous machinery. Don't climb ladders or work in high places. Danger increases if you drink alcohol or take medicine affecting alertness and reflexes, such as antihistamines, tranquilizers, sedatives, pain medicine, narcotics and mind-altering drugs.

Discontinuing:
Don't discontinue without doctor's advice until you complete prescribed dose, even though symptoms diminish or disappear.

Others:
- Vitamin B-6 diet supplement may be advisable. Consult doctor.
- Some products contain tartrazine dye. Avoid, especially if you are allergic to aspirin.
- May interfere with the accuracy of some medical tests.

POSSIBLE INTERACTION WITH OTHER DRUGS

GENERIC NAME OR DRUG CLASS	COMBINED EFFECT
Amphetamines*	Decreased hydralazine effect.
Antihypertensives, other*	Increased anti-hypertensive effect.
Anti-inflammatory drugs, nonsteroidal (NSAIDs)*	Decreased effect of hydralazine.
Carteolol	Increased anti-hypertensive effect.
Diazoxide & other anti-hypertensive drugs	Increased anti-hypertensive effect.
Didanosine	Increased risk of peripheral neuropathy.
Diuretics, oral*	Increased effects of both drugs. When monitored carefully, combination may be beneficial in controlling hypertension.
Guanfacine	Increased effects of both drugs.
Lisinopril	Increased anti-hypertensive effect. Dosage of each may require adjustment.
Monoamine oxidase (MAO) inhibitors*	Increased hydralazine effect.
Nicardipine	Blood pressure drop. Dosages may require adjustment.
Nimodipine	Dangerous blood pressure drop.

Continued on page 942

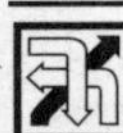

POSSIBLE INTERACTION WITH OTHER SUBSTANCES

INTERACTS WITH	COMBINED EFFECT
Alcohol:	May lower blood pressure excessively. Use extreme caution.
Beverages:	None expected.
Cocaine:	Increased risk of heart block and high blood pressure.
Foods:	Increased hydralazine absorption.
Marijuana:	Weakness on standing.
Tobacco:	Possible angina attacks.

HYDRALAZINE & HYDROCHLOROTHIAZIDE

BRAND NAMES

Apresazide
Aprozide
Hydra-zide

BASIC INFORMATION

Habit forming? No
Prescription needed? Yes
Available as generic? Yes
Drug class: Antihypertensive, diuretic

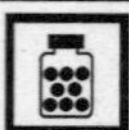

USES

- Controls, but doesn't cure, high blood pressure.
- Reduces fluid retention (edema).

DOSAGE & USAGE INFORMATION

How to take:
Tablet or capsule—Swallow with liquid. If you can't swallow whole, crumble tablet or open capsule and take with liquid or food.

When to take:
At the same time each day.

If you forget a dose:
Take as soon as you remember up to 2 hours late. If more than 2 hours, wait for next scheduled dose (don't double this dose).

Continued next column

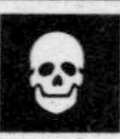

OVERDOSE

SYMPTOMS:
Cramps, drowsiness, weak pulse, rapid and weak heartbeat, fainting, extreme weakness, cold and sweaty skin, coma.
WHAT TO DO:

- **Dial 911 (emergency) or 0 (operator) for an ambulance or medical help. Then give first aid immediately.**
- **If patient is unconscious and not breathing, give mouth-to-mouth breathing. If there is no heartbeat, use cardiac massage and mouth-to-mouth breathing (CPR). Don't try to make patient vomit. If you can't get help quickly, take patient to nearest emergency facility.**
- **See emergency information on inside covers.**

What drug does:

- Forces sodium and water excretion, reducing body fluid.
- Relaxes and expands blood vessel walls, lowering blood pressure.
- Reduced body fluid and relaxed arteries lower blood pressure.

Time lapse before drug works:
Regular use for several weeks may be necessary to determine drug's effectiveness.

Don't take with:

- Nonprescription drugs containing alcohol without consulting doctor.
- Any other medicine without consulting your doctor or pharmacist.

POSSIBLE ADVERSE REACTIONS OR SIDE EFFECTS

SYMPTOMS	WHAT TO DO
Life-threatening:	
Chest pain, irregular and fast heartbeat, weak pulse.	Discontinue. Seek emergency treatment.
Common:	
• Nausea, vomiting.	Discontinue. Call doctor right away.
• Headache, diarrhea, appetite loss, frequent urination, dry mouth, thirst.	Continue. Call doctor when convenient.
Infrequent:	
• Rash; black, bloody or tarry stool; red or flushed face; sore throat, fever, mouth sores; constipation; lymph glands swelling; blurred vision; skin blisters; swelling in feet or legs.	Discontinue. Call doctor right away.
• Dizziness; confusion; watery eyes; weight gain or loss; joint, muscle or chest pain; depression; anxiety; fever.	Continue. Call doctor when convenient.
Rare:	
• Weakness and faintness when arising from bed or chair, jaundice.	Discontinue. Call doctor right away.
• Numbness or tingling in hands or feet, nasal congestion, impotence.	Continue. Call doctor when convenient.

HYDRALAZINE & HYDROCHLOROTHIAZIDE

WARNINGS & PRECAUTIONS

Don't take if:
- You are allergic to hydralazine, any thiazide diuretic drug or tartrazine dye.
- You have history of coronary artery disease or rheumatic heart disease.

Before you start, consult your doctor:
- If you feel pain in chest, neck or arms on physical exertion.
- If you are allergic to any sulfa drug.
- If you have had lupus or a stroke.
- If you have gout, liver, pancreas or kidney disorder.
- If you will have surgery within 2 months, including dental surgery, requiring general or spinal anesthesia.

Over age 60:
Adverse reactions and side effects may be more frequent and severe than in younger persons, especially dizziness and excessive potassium loss.

Pregnancy:
Decide with your doctor if drug benefits justify risk to unborn child. Risk category C (see page xxii).

Breast-feeding:
Drug passes into milk. Avoid drug or discontinue nursing until you finish medicine. Consult doctor for advice on maintaining milk supply.

Infants & children:
Not recommended.

Prolonged use:
- May cause lupus (arthritis-like illness).
- Possible psychosis.
- May cause numbness, tingling in hands or feet.
- Talk to your doctor about the need for follow-up medical examinations or laboratory studies to check blood pressure, complete blood counts (white blood cell count, platelet count, red blood cell count, hemoglobin, hematocrit), ANA titers*.

Skin & sunlight:
May cause rash or intensify sunburn in areas exposed to sun or sunlamp.

Driving, piloting or hazardous work:
Don't drive or pilot aircraft until you learn how medicine affects you. Don't work around dangerous machinery. Don't climb ladders or work in high places. Danger increases if you drink alcohol or take medicine affecting alertness and reflexes, such as antihistamines, tranquilizers, sedatives, pain medicine, narcotics and mind-altering drugs.

Discontinuing:
Don't discontinue without consulting doctor's advice until you complete prescribed dose, even though symptoms diminish or disappear.

Others:
- Vitamin B-6 diet supplement may be advisable. Consult doctor.
- Hot weather and fever may cause dehydration and drop in blood pressure. Dose may require temporary adjustment. Weigh daily and report any unexpected weight decreases to your doctor.
- May cause rise in uric acid, leading to gout.
- May cause blood sugar rise in diabetics.

POSSIBLE INTERACTION WITH OTHER DRUGS

GENERIC NAME OR DRUG CLASS	COMBINED EFFECT
Acebutolol	Decreased anti-hypertensive effect of acebutolol.
Allopurinol	Decreased allopurinol effect.
Amphetamines*	Decreased hydralazine effect.
Antidepressants, tricyclic*	Dangerous drop in blood pressure. Avoid combination unless under medical supervision.

Continued on page 942

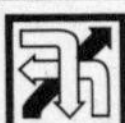

POSSIBLE INTERACTION WITH OTHER SUBSTANCES

INTERACTS WITH	COMBINED EFFECT
Alcohol:	May lower blood pressure excessively. Use extreme caution.
Beverages:	None expected.
Cocaine:	Dangerous blood pressure rise. Avoid.
Foods: Licorice.	Excessive potassium loss that causes dangerous heart rhythms.
Marijuana:	Weakness on standing. May increase blood pressure.
Tobacco:	Possible angina attacks.

***See Glossary**

HYDROCORTISONE (Cortisol)

BRAND NAMES

See complete list of brand names in the *Brand Name Directory*, page 909.

BASIC INFORMATION

Habit forming? No
Prescription needed? Yes
Available as generic? Yes
Drug class: Cortisone drug (adrenalcorticosteroid)

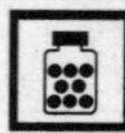

USES

- Reduces inflammation caused by many different medical problems.
- Treatment for some allergic diseases, blood disorders, kidney diseases, asthma and emphysema.
- Replaces corticosteroid deficiencies.

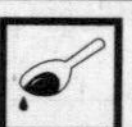

DOSAGE & USAGE INFORMATION

How to take:
- Tablet or liquid—Swallow with liquid or food to lessen stomach irritation. If you can't swallow whole, crumble tablet.
- Other forms—Follow label instructions.

When to take:
At the same times each day. Take once-a-day or once-every-other-day doses in mornings.

If you forget a dose:
- Several-doses-per-day prescription—Take as soon as you remember up to 2 hours late. If more than 2 hours, wait for next scheduled dose (don't double this dose).
- Once-a-day dose or less—Wait for next dose. Double this dose.

What drug does:
- Decreases inflammatory responses.
- Replaces cortisone in patients with adrenalin sufficiency.

Continued next column

OVERDOSE

SYMPTOMS:
Headache, convulsions, fluid retention, heart failure.
WHAT TO DO:
- **Dial 911 (emergency) or 0 (operator) for an ambulance or medical help. Then give first aid immediately.**
- **See emergency information on inside covers.**

Time lapse before drug works:
2 to 4 days.

Don't take with:
Any other medicine without consulting your doctor or pharmacist.

POSSIBLE ADVERSE REACTIONS OR SIDE EFFECTS

SYMPTOMS	WHAT TO DO
Life-threatening:	
Hives, rash, intense itching, faintness soon after a dose (anaphylaxis).	Seek emergency treatment immediately.
Common:	
Acne, poor wound healing, thirst, indigestion, nausea, vomiting.	Continue. Call doctor when convenient.
Infrequent:	
• Black, bloody or tarry stools.	Discontinue. Seek emergency treatment.
• Blurred vision; halos around lights; sore throat; fever; muscle cramps; swollen legs, feet.	Discontinue. Call doctor right away.
• Mood change, insomnia, fatigue, restlessness, frequent urination, weight gain, round face, weakness, irregular menstrual periods.	Continue. Tell doctor at next visit.
Rare:	
• Irregular heartbeat.	Discontinue. Seek emergency treatment.
• Rash, hallucinations, thrombophlebitis, pancreatitis, numbness or tingling in hands or feet, pancreatitis, convulsions.	Discontinue. Call doctor right away.

WARNINGS & PRECAUTIONS

Don't take if:
- You are allergic to any cortisone drug.
- You have tuberculosis or fungus infection.
- You have herpes infection of eyes, lips or genitals.

Before you start, consult your doctor:
- If you have had tuberculosis.
- If you have congestive heart failure.

- If you have diabetes, peptic ulcer, glaucoma, underactive thyroid, high blood pressure, myasthenia gravis, blood clots in legs or lungs.

Over age 60:
- Adverse reactions and side effects may be more frequent and severe than in younger persons.
- Likely to aggravate edema, diabetes or ulcers.
- Likely to cause cataracts and osteoporosis (softening of the bones).

Pregnancy:
Decide with your doctor if drug benefits justify risk to unborn child. Risk category C (see page xxii).

Breast-feeding:
Drug passes into milk. Avoid drug or discontinue nursing until you finish medicine. Consult doctor for advice on maintaining milk supply.

Infants & children:
Use only under medical supervision.

Prolonged use:
- Retards growth in children.
- Possible glaucoma, cataracts, diabetes, fragile bones and thin skin.
- Functional dependence.
- Talk to your doctor about the need for follow-up medical examinations or laboratory studies to check blood sugar, eyes, serum electrolytes, stools for blood.

Skin & sunlight:
No problems expected.

Driving, piloting or hazardous work:
No problems expected.

Discontinuing:
- Don't discontinue without doctor's advice until you complete prescribed dose, even though symptoms diminish or disappear.
- Drug affects your response to surgery, illness, injury or stress for 2 years after discontinuing. Tell anyone who takes medical care of you about the drug for up to 2 years after discontinuing.

Others:
- Avoid immunizations if possible.
- Your resistance to infection is less while taking this medicine.
- Those who have inactive or "cured" tuberculosis may be subjected to possible recurrence of active tuberculosis.
- Children who must take cortisone drugs may grow less well.

POSSIBLE INTERACTION WITH OTHER DRUGS

GENERIC NAME OR DRUG CLASS	COMBINED EFFECT
Amphotericin B	Potassium depletion.
Anticholinergics*	Possible glaucoma.
Anticoagulants, oral*	Decreased anticoagulant effect.
Anticonvulsants, hydantoin*	Decreased hydrocortisone effect.
Antidiabetics, oral*	Decreased antidiabetic effect.
Antihistamines*	Decreased hydrocortisone effect.
Anti-inflammatory drugs, nonsteroidal (NSAIDs)*	Increased risk of ulcers and increased hydrocortisone effect.
Aspirin	Increased hydrocortisone effect.
Attentuated virus vaccines*	Possible viral infection.
Barbiturates*	Decreased hydrocortisone effect. Oversedation.
Chloral hydrate	Decreased hydrocortisone effect.
Chlorthalidone	Potassium depletion.
Cholestyramine	Decreased hydrocortisone absorption effect.
Cholinergics*	Decreased cholinergic effect.
Colestipol	Decreased hydrocortisone absorption effect.
Contraceptives, oral*	Increased hydrocortisone effect.

Continued on page 943

POSSIBLE INTERACTION WITH OTHER SUBSTANCES

INTERACTS WITH	COMBINED EFFECT
Alcohol:	Risk of stomach ulcers.
Beverages:	No proven problems.
Cocaine:	Overstimulation. Avoid.
Foods:	No proven problems.
Marijuana:	Decreased immunity.
Tobacco:	Increased hydrocortisone effect. Possible toxicity.

*See Glossary

HYDROCORTISONE (Rectal)

BRAND NAMES

Anucort
Anusol-H.C.
Cort-Dome High Potency
Corticaine
Cortiment-10
Cortiment-40
Dermolate
Hemril-HC
Proctocort
Rectocort

BASIC INFORMATION

Habit forming? No
Prescription needed? Yes
Available as generic? Yes, for some
Drug class: Anti-inflammatory, steroidal (rectal); anesthetic (rectal)

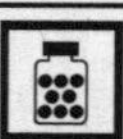

USES

In or around the rectum to relieve swelling, itching and pain for hemorrhoids (piles) and other rectal conditions. Frequently used after hemorrhoid surgery.

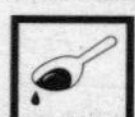

DOSAGE & USAGE INFORMATION

How to use:
- Follow instructions in package.
- Rectal cream or ointment—Apply to surface of rectum with fingers. Insert applicator into rectum no farther than halfway and apply inside. Wash applicator with warm soapy water or discard.
- Suppository—Remove wrapper and moisten with water. Lie on side. Push blunt end of suppository into rectum with finger. If suppository is too soft, run cold water over it or put in refrigerator for 15 to 45 minutes before using.
- Aerosol foam—Read patient instructions. Don't insert into rectum. Use the special applicator and wash carefully after using.

When to use:
Follow instructions in package or when needed.

Continued next column

OVERDOSE

SYMPTOMS:
None expected.
WHAT TO DO:
Not intended for internal use. If child accidentally swallows, call poison control center.

If you forget a dose:
Use as soon as you remember.

What drug does:
- Reduces inflammation.
- Relieves pain and itching.

Time lapse before drug works:
5 to 15 minutes.

Don't use with:
Other rectal medicines without consulting your doctor.

POSSIBLE ADVERSE REACTIONS OR SIDE EFFECTS

SYMPTOMS	WHAT TO DO
Life-threatening	
None expected.	
Common	
None expected.	
Infrequent	
• Nervousness, trembling, hives, rash, itch, inflammation or tenderness not present before application, slow heartbeat.	Discontinue. Call doctor right away.
• Dizziness, blurred vision, swollen feet.	Continue. Call doctor when convenient.
Rare	
• Blood in urine.	Discontinue. Call doctor right away.
• Increased or painful urination.	Continue. Call doctor when convenient.

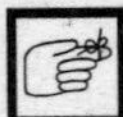

WARNINGS & PRECAUTIONS

Don't use if:
You are allergic to any topical anesthetic.

Before you start, consult your doctor:
- If you have skin infection at site of treatment.
- If you have had severe or extensive skin disorders such as eczema or psoriasis.
- If you have bleeding hemorrhoids.

Over age 60:
Adverse reactions and side effects may be more frequent and severe than in younger persons.

Pregnancy:
Decide with your doctor if drug benefits justify risk to unborn child. Risk category C (see page xxii).

Breast-feeding:
No problems expected. Consult doctor.

Infants & children:
Don't use without careful medical supervision. Too much may be absorbed into the blood stream and affect growth.

Prolonged use:
Possible excess absorption. Don't use longer than 3 days for any one problem.

Skin & sunlight:
No problems expected.

Driving, piloting or hazardous work:
No problems expected.

Discontinuing:
May be unnecessary to finish medicine. Follow doctor's instructions.

Others:
- Report any rectal bleeding to your doctor.
- Keep cool, but don't freeze.

POSSIBLE INTERACTION WITH OTHER DRUGS

GENERIC NAME OR DRUG CLASS	COMBINED EFFECT
Sulfa drugs*	Decreased anti-infective effect of sulfa drugs.

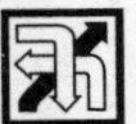

POSSIBLE INTERACTION WITH OTHER SUBSTANCES

INTERACTS WITH	COMBINED EFFECT
Alcohol:	None expected.
Beverages:	None expected.
Cocaine:	Possible nervous system toxicity. Avoid.
Foods:	None expected.
Marijuana:	None expected.
Tobacco:	None expected.

*See Glossary

HYDROXYCHLOROQUINE

BRAND NAMES

Plaquenil

BASIC INFORMATION

Habit forming? No
Prescription needed? Yes
Available as generic? No
Drug class: Antiprotozoal, antirheumatic

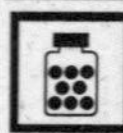

USES

- Treatment for protozoal infections, such as malaria and amebiasis.
- Treatment for some forms of arthritis and lupus.

DOSAGE & USAGE INFORMATION

How to take:
Tablet—Swallow with food or milk to lessen stomach irritation.

When to take:
- Depends on condition. Is adjusted during treatment.
- Malaria prevention—Begin taking medicine 2 weeks before entering areas where malaria is present.

If you forget a dose:
- 1 or more doses a day—Take as soon as you remember up to 2 hours late. If more than 2 hours, wait for next scheduled dose (don't double this dose).
- 1 dose weekly—Take as soon as possible, then return to regular dosing schedule.

What drug does:
- Inhibits parasite multiplication.
- Decreases inflammatory response in diseased joint.

Time lapse before drug works:
1 to 2 hours.

Continued next column

OVERDOSE

SYMPTOMS:
Severe breathing difficulty, drowsiness, faintness, headache, seizures.
WHAT TO DO:
- **Dial 911 (emergency) or 0 (operator) for an ambulance or medical help. Then give first aid immediately.**
- **See emergency information on inside covers.**

Don't take with:
Any other medicine without consulting your doctor or pharmacist.

POSSIBLE ADVERSE REACTIONS OR SIDE EFFECTS

SYMPTOMS	WHAT TO DO
Life-threatening:	
In case of overdose, see previous column.	
Common:	
Headache, appetite loss, abdominal pain.	Continue. Tell doctor at next visit.
Infrequent:	
• Blurred vision, changes in vision.	Discontinue. Call doctor right away.
• Rash or itch, diarrhea, nausea, vomiting, hair loss, blue-black skin or mouth, dizziness, nervousness.	Continue. Call doctor when convenient.
Rare:	
• Mood or mental changes, seizures, sore throat, fever, unusual bleeding or bruising, muscle weakness, convulsions.	Discontinue. Call doctor right away.
• Ringing or buzzing in ears, hearing loss.	Continue. Call doctor when convenient.

HYDROXYCHLOROQUINE

WARNINGS & PRECAUTIONS

Don't take if:
You are allergic to chloroquine or hydroxychloroquine.

Before you start, consult your doctor:
- If you plan to become pregnant within the medication period.
- If you have blood disease.
- If you have eye or vision problems.
- If you have a G6PD* deficiency.
- If you have liver disease.
- If you have nerve or brain disease (including seizure disorders).
- If you have porphyria.
- If you have psoriasis.
- If you have stomach or intestinal disease.
- If you drink more than 3 oz. of alcohol daily.

Over age 60:
Adverse reactions and side effects may be more frequent and severe than in younger persons.

Pregnancy:
Decide with your doctor if drug benefits justify risk to unborn child. Risk category C (see page xxii).

Breast-feeding:
Drug passes into milk. Avoid drug or discontinue nursing. Consult doctor for advice on maintaining milk supply.

Infants & children:
Not recommended. Dangerous.

Prolonged use:
- Permanent damage to the retina (back part of the eye) or nerve deafness.
- Talk to your doctor about the need for follow-up medical examinations or laboratory studies to check complete blood counts (white blood cell count, platelet count, red blood cell count, hemoglobin, hematocrit), eyes.

Skin & sunlight:
May cause rash or intensify sunburn in areas exposed to sun or sunlamp.

Driving, piloting or hazardous work:
Don't drive or pilot aircraft until you learn how medicine affects you. Don't work around dangerous machinery. Don't climb ladders or work in high places. Danger increases if you drink alcohol or take medicine affecting alertness and reflexes.

Discontinuing:
Don't discontinue without doctor's advice until you complete prescribed dose, even though symptoms diminish or disappear.

Others:
- Periodic physical and blood examinations recommended.
- If you are in a malaria area for a long time, you may need to change to another preventive drug every 2 years.

POSSIBLE INTERACTION WITH OTHER DRUGS

GENERIC NAME OR DRUG CLASS	COMBINED EFFECT
Estrogens*	Possible liver toxicity.
Gold compounds*	Risk of severe rash and itch.
Kaolin	Decreased absorption of hydroxychloroquine.
Magnesium trisilicate	Decreased absorption of hydroxychloroquine.
Penicillamine	Possible blood or kidney toxicity.

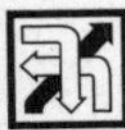

POSSIBLE INTERACTION WITH OTHER SUBSTANCES

INTERACTS WITH	COMBINED EFFECT
Alcohol:	Possible liver toxicity. Avoid.
Beverages:	None expected.
Cocaine:	None expected.
Foods:	None expected.
Marijuana:	None expected.
Tobacco:	None expected.

*See Glossary

HYDROXYUREA

BRAND NAMES

Hydrea

BASIC INFORMATION

Habit forming? No
Prescription needed? Yes
Available as generic? No
Drug class: Antineoplastic

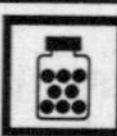

USES

- Treats head, neck, ovarian and cervical cancer.
- Treats leukemia, melanoma and polycythemia vera.

DOSAGE & USAGE INFORMATION

How to take:
Capsules—Swallow with liquid. If you can't swallow whole, open capsule and take with liquid or food. Instructions to take on empty stomach mean 1 hour before or 2 hours after eating.

When to take:
According to doctor's instructions.

If you forget a dose:
Skip this dose. Never double dose. Resume regular schedule.

What drug does:
Probably interferes with synthesis of DNA.

Time lapse before drug works:
2 hours.

Don't take with:
Any other medicines (including over-the-counter drugs such as cough and cold medicines, laxatives, antacids, diet pills, caffeine, nose drops or vitamins) without consulting your doctor.

OVERDOSE

SYMPTOMS:
Black, tarry stools; fainting; seizures.
WHAT TO DO:
- **Dial 911 (emergency) or 0 (operator) for an ambulance or medical help. Then give first aid immediately.**
- **See emergency information on inside covers.**

POSSIBLE ADVERSE REACTIONS OR SIDE EFFECTS

SYMPTOMS	WHAT TO DO
Life-threatening:	
In case of overdose, see previous column.	
Common:	
• Skin rash, fever, chills, cough, back pain.	Discontinue. Call doctor right away.
• Diarrhea, drowsiness, nausea, vomiting.	Continue. Call doctor when convenient.
Infrequent:	
Mouth sores, bruising, constipation, red skin.	Discontinue. Call doctor right away.
Rare:	
Confusion, hallucinations, headache, swollen feet.	Continue. Call doctor when convenient.

WARNINGS & PRECAUTIONS

Don't take if:
- You have chicken pox.
- You have shingles (herpes zoster).

Before you start, consult your doctor:
- If you have anemia.
- If you have gout.
- If you have an infection.
- If you have kidney disease.

Over age 60:
Adverse reactions and side effects may be more frequent and severe than in younger persons. You may need smaller doses for shorter periods of time.

Pregnancy:
Decide with your doctor if drug benefits justify risk to unborn child. Risk category C (see page xxii).

Breast-feeding:
Drug passes into milk. Avoid drug or discontinue nursing until you finish medicine. Consult doctor for advice on maintaining milk supply.

Infants & children:
Effect not documented. Consult your pediatrician.

Prolonged use:
Talk to your doctor about the need for follow-up medical examinations or laboratory studies to check kidney function, complete blood counts (white blood cell count, platelet count, red blood cell count, hemoglobin, hematocrit) and serum uric acid.

Skin & sunlight:
No problems expected.

Driving, piloting or hazardous work:
Avoid if you feel confused, drowsy or dizzy.

Discontinuing:
May still experience symptoms of bone marrow depression, such as: blood in stools, fever or chills, blood spots under the skin, back pain, hoarseness, bloody urine. If any of these occur, call your doctor right away.

Others:
- Advise any doctor or dentist whom you consult that you take this medicine.
- May affect results in some medical tests.

POSSIBLE INTERACTION WITH OTHER DRUGS

GENERIC NAME OR DRUG CLASS	COMBINED EFFECT
Bone marrow depressants, other*	Dangerous suppression of bone marrow activity.
Clozapine	Toxic effect on bone marrow.
Levamisole	Increased risk of bone marrow depression.
Probenecid	May require increased dosage to treat gout.
Sulfinpyrazone	May require increased dosage to treat gout.
Tiopronin	Increased risk of toxicity to bone marrow.
Vaccines, live or killed virus	Increased risk of side effects.

POSSIBLE INTERACTION WITH OTHER SUBSTANCES

INTERACTS WITH	COMBINED EFFECT
Alcohol:	No special problems expected.
Beverages:	No special problems expected.
Cocaine:	Increased confusion. Avoid.
Foods:	No special problems expected.
Marijuana:	Increased confusion. Avoid.
Tobacco:	No special problems expected.

*See Glossary

HYDROXYZINE

BRAND NAMES

See complete list of brand names in the *Brand Name Directory*, page 909.

BASIC INFORMATION

Habit forming? No
Prescription needed? Yes
Available as generic? Yes
Drug class: Tranquilizer, antihistamine

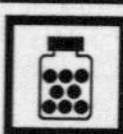

USES

- Treatment for anxiety, tension and agitation.
- Relieves itching from allergic reactions.

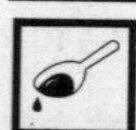

DOSAGE & USAGE INFORMATION

How to take:
- Tablet, syrup or capsule—Swallow with liquid. If you can't swallow whole, crumble tablet or open capsule and take with liquid or food.
- Liquid—If desired, dilute dose in beverage before swallowing.

When to take:
At the same times each day.

If you forget a dose:
Take as soon as you remember up to 2 hours late. If more than 2 hours, wait for next scheduled dose (don't double this dose).

What drug does:
May reduce activity in areas of the brain that influence emotional stability.

Time lapse before drug works:
15 to 30 minutes.

Don't take with:
- Nonprescription drugs without consulting doctor.
- Any other medicine without consulting your doctor or pharmacist.

OVERDOSE

SYMPTOMS:
Drowsiness, unsteadiness, agitation, purposeless movements, tremor, convulsions.
WHAT TO DO:
- **Dial 911 (emergency) or 0 (operator) for an ambulance or medical help. Then give first aid immediately.**
- **See emergency information on inside covers.**

POSSIBLE ADVERSE REACTIONS OR SIDE EFFECTS

SYMPTOMS	WHAT TO DO
Life-threatening: In case of overdose, see previous column.	
Common: Drowsiness, difficult urination, dry mouth.	Continue. Tell doctor at next visit.
Infrequent: Headache.	Continue. Tell doctor at next visit.
Rare: Tremor, rash.	Discontinue. Call doctor right away.

WARNINGS & PRECAUTIONS

Don't take if:
You are allergic to any antihistamine.

Before you start, consult your doctor:
- If you have epilepsy.
- If you will have surgery within 2 months, including dental surgery, requiring general or spinal anesthesia.

Over age 60:
- Adverse reactions and side effects may be more frequent and severe than in younger persons.
- Drug likely to increase urination difficulty caused by enlarged prostate gland.

Pregnancy:
Decide with your doctor if drug benefits justify risk to unborn child. Risk category C (see page xxii).

Breast-feeding:
Drug passes into milk. Avoid drug or discontinue nursing until you finish medicine. Consult doctor for advice on maintaining milk supply.

Infants & children:
Use only under medical supervision.

Prolonged use:
Tolerance develops and reduces effectiveness.

Skin & sunlight:
No problems expected.

Driving, piloting or hazardous work:
Don't drive or pilot aircraft until you learn how medicine affects you. Don't work around dangerous machinery. Don't climb ladders or work in high places. Danger increases if you drink alcohol or take medicine affecting alertness and reflexes, such as antihistamines, tranquilizers, sedatives, pain medicine, narcotics and mind-altering drugs.

Discontinuing:
Don't discontinue without consulting doctor. Dose may require gradual reduction if you have taken drug for a long time. Doses of other drugs may also require adjustment.

Others:
No problems expected.

POSSIBLE INTERACTION WITH OTHER DRUGS

GENERIC NAME OR DRUG CLASS	COMBINED EFFECT
Antidepressants, tricyclic*	Increased effect of both drugs.
Antihistamines*	Increased hydroxyzine effect.
Attapulgite	Decreased hydroxyzine effect.
Carteolol	Decreased antihistamine effect.
Central nervous system (CNS) depressants*	Greater depression of central nervous system.
Clozapine	Toxic effect on the central nervous system.
Dronabinol	Increased effects of both drugs. Avoid.
Ethinamate	Dangerous increased effects of ethinamate. Avoid combining.
Fluoxetine	Increased depressant effects of both drugs.
Guanfacine	May increase depressant effects of either drug.
Leucovorin	High alcohol content of leucovorin may cause adverse effects.
Methyprylon	Increased sedative effect, perhaps to dangerous level. Avoid.
Nabilone	Greater depression of central nervous system.
Narcotics*	Increased effect of both drugs.
Pain relievers*	Increased effect of both drugs.
Sedatives*	Increased effect of both drugs.
Sertraline	Increased depressive effects of both drugs.
Sleep inducers*	Increased effect of both drugs.
Sotalol	Increased antihistamine effect.
Tranquilizers*	Increased effect of both drugs.

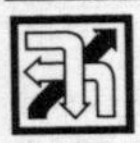

POSSIBLE INTERACTION WITH OTHER SUBSTANCES

INTERACTS WITH	COMBINED EFFECT
Alcohol:	Increased sedation and intoxication. Use with caution.
Beverages: Caffeine drinks.	Decreased tranquilizer effect of hydroxyzine.
Cocaine:	Decreased hydroxyzine effect. Avoid.
Foods:	None expected.
Marijuana:	None expected.
Tobacco:	None expected.

***See Glossary**

HYOSCYAMINE

BRAND NAMES

Anaspaz
Anaspaz PB
Atrohist Plus
Barbidonna
Barbidonna 2
Belladenal
Bellafoline
Cystospaz
Cystospaz-M
Gastrosed
Kinesed
Levsin
Levsin S/L
Levsinex
Levsinex Timecaps
Neoquess
Phenahist TR
Phenchlor SHA
Ru-Tuss
Stahist

BASIC INFORMATION

Habit forming? No
Prescription needed?
Low strength: No
High strength: Yes
Available as generic? No
Drug class: Antispasmodic, anticholinergic

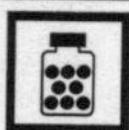

USES

Reduces spasms of digestive system, bladder and urethra.

DOSAGE & USAGE INFORMATION

How to take:

- Tablet or liquid—Swallow with liquid or food to lessen stomach irritation. You may chew or crush tablets.
- Extended-release capsules—Swallow each dose whole.
- Drops—Dilute dose in beverage before swallowing.

When to take:
30 minutes before meals (unless directed otherwise by doctor).

Continued next column

OVERDOSE

SYMPTOMS:
Dilated pupils, rapid pulse and breathing, dizziness, fever, hallucinations, confusion, slurred speech, agitation, flushed face, convulsions, coma.
WHAT TO DO:

- **Dial 911 (emergency) or 0 (operator) for an ambulance or medical help. Then give first aid immediately.**
- **See emergency information on inside covers.**

If you forget a dose:
Take as soon as you remember up to 2 hours late. If more than 2 hours, wait for next scheduled dose (don't double this dose).

What drug does:
Blocks nerve impulses at parasympathetic nerve endings, preventing muscle contractions and gland secretions of organs involved.

Time lapse before drug works:
15 to 30 minutes.

Don't take with:

- Antacids* or antidiarrheals*.
- Any other medicine without consulting your doctor or pharmacist.

POSSIBLE ADVERSE REACTIONS OR SIDE EFFECTS

SYMPTOMS	WHAT TO DO
Life-threatening: In case of overdose, see previous column.	
Common:	
• Confusion, delirium, rapid heartbeat.	Discontinue. Call doctor right away.
• Nausea, vomiting, decreased sweating.	Continue. Call doctor when convenient.
• Constipation.	Continue. Tell doctor at next visit.
• Dryness in ears, nose, throat, mouth.	No action necessary.
Infrequent:	
• Headache, painful or difficult urination, nasal congestion, altered taste.	Continue. Call doctor when convenient.
• Lightheadedness.	Discontinue. Call doctor right away.
Rare:	
Rash or hives, eye pain, blurred vision.	Discontinue. Call doctor right away.

WARNINGS & PRECAUTIONS

Don't take if:

- You are allergic to any anticholinergic.
- You have trouble with stomach bloating.
- You have difficulty emptying your bladder completely.
- You have narrow-angle glaucoma.
- You have severe ulcerative colitis.

HYOSCYAMINE

Before you start, consult your doctor:
- If you have open-angle glaucoma.
- If you have angina.
- If you have chronic bronchitis or asthma.
- If you have hiatal hernia.
- If you have liver, kidney or thyroid disease.
- If you have enlarged prostate.
- If you have myasthenia gravis.
- If you have peptic ulcer.
- If you will have surgery within 2 months, including dental surgery, requiring general or spinal anesthesia.

Over age 60:
Adverse reactions and side effects may be more frequent and severe than in younger persons.

Pregnancy:
Decide with your doctor if drug benefits justify risk to unborn child. Risk category C (see page xxii).

Breast-feeding:
Drug passes into milk and decreases milk flow. Avoid drug or discontinue nursing until you finish medicine. Consult doctor for advice on maintaining milk supply.

Infants & children:
Use only under medical supervision.

Prolonged use:
Chronic constipation, possible fecal impaction. Consult doctor immediately.

Skin & sunlight:
No problems expected.

Driving, piloting or hazardous work:
Use disqualifies you for piloting aircraft. Otherwise, no problems expected.

Discontinuing:
May be unnecessary to finish medicine. Follow doctor's instructions.

Others:
Advise any doctor or dentist whom you consult that you take this medicine.

POSSIBLE INTERACTION WITH OTHER DRUGS

GENERIC NAME OR DRUG CLASS	COMBINED EFFECT
Amantadine	Increased hyoscyamine effect.
Anticholinergics, other*	Increased hyoscyamine effect.
Antidepressants, tricyclic*	Increased hyoscyamine effect.
Antihistamines*	Increased hyoscyamine effect.
Cortisone drugs*	Increased internal eye pressure.
Haloperidol	Increased internal eye pressure.
Ketoconazole	Decreased ketoconazole effect.
Meperidine	Increased hyoscyamine effect.
Methylphenidate	Increased hyoscyamine effect.
Molindone	Increased anticholinergic effect
Monoamine oxidase (MAO) inhibitors*	Increased hyoscyamine effect..
Nizatidine	Increased nizatidine effect.
Orphenadrine	Increased hyoscyamine effect.
Phenothiazines*	Increased hyoscyamine effect.
Pilocarpine	Loss of pilocarpine effect in glaucoma treatment.
Sedatives* or central nervous system (CNS) depressants*	Increased sedative effect of both drugs.
Vitamin C	Decreased hyoscyamine effect. Avoid large doses of vitamin C.

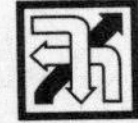

POSSIBLE INTERACTION WITH OTHER SUBSTANCES

INTERACTS WITH	COMBINED EFFECT
Alcohol:	None expected.
Beverages:	None expected.
Cocaine:	Excessively rapid heartbeat. Avoid.
Foods:	None expected.
Marijuana:	Drowsiness and dry mouth.
Tobacco:	None expected.

***See Glossary**

INDAPAMIDE

BRAND NAMES

Lozide
Lozol

BASIC INFORMATION

Habit forming? No
Prescription needed? Yes
Available as generic? No
Drug class: Antihypertensive, diuretic

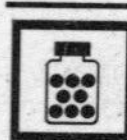

USES

- Controls, but doesn't cure, high blood pressure.
- Reduces fluid retention (edema) caused by conditions such as heart disorders.

DOSAGE & USAGE INFORMATION

How to take:
Tablet—Swallow with liquid or food to lessen stomach irritation.

When to take:
At the same times each day, usually at bedtime.

If you forget a dose:
Bedtime dose—If you forget your once-a-day bedtime dose, don't take it more than 3 hours late. Never double dose.

What drug does:
Forces kidney to excrete more sodium and causes excess salt and fluid to be excreted.

Time lapse before drug works:
2 hours for effect to begin. May require 1 to 4 weeks for full effects.

Continued next column.

OVERDOSE

SYMPTOMS:
Nausea, vomiting, diarrhea, very dry mouth, thirst, weakness, excessive fatigue, very rapid heart rate, weak pulse.
WHAT TO DO:
- **Dial 911 (emergency) or 0 (operator) for an ambulance or medical help. Then give first aid immediately.**
- **If patient is unconscious and not breathing, give mouth-to-mouth breathing. If there is no heartbeat, use cardiac massage and mouth-to-mouth breathing (CPR). Don't try to make patient vomit. If you can't get help quickly, take patient to nearest emergency facility.**
- **See emergency information on inside covers.**

Don't take with:
Any other medicine without consulting your doctor or pharmacist.

POSSIBLE ADVERSE REACTIONS OR SIDE EFFECTS

SYMPTOMS	WHAT TO DO
Life-threatening: In case of overdose, see previous column.	
Common:	
• Excessive tiredness or weakness, muscle cramps.	Discontinue. Call doctor right away.
• Frequent urination.	Continue. Tell doctor at next visit.
Infrequent: Insomnia, mood change, dizziness on changing position, headache, excessive thirst, diarrhea, appetite loss, nausea, dry mouth, decreased sex drive.	Continue. Call doctor when convenient.
Rare:	
• Weak pulse.	Discontinue. Seek emergency treatment.
• Itching, rash, hives, irregular heartbeat.	Discontinue. Call doctor right away.

WARNINGS & PRECAUTIONS

Don't take if:
- You are allergic to indapamide or to any sulfa drug or thiazide diuretic.*
- You have severe kidney disease.

Before you start, consult your doctor:
- If you have severe kidney disease.
- If you have diabetes.
- If you have gout.
- If you have liver disease.
- If you will have surgery within 2 months, including dental surgery, requiring general or spinal anesthesia.
- If you have lupus erythematosus.
- If you are pregnant or plan to become pregnant.

Over age 60:
Adverse reactions and side effects may be more frequent and severe than in younger persons.

Pregnancy:
Consult doctor. Risk category B (see page xxii).

Breast-feeding:
Unknown effect on child. Consult doctor.

Infants & children:
Use only under close medical supervision.

Prolonged use:
Request laboratory studies for blood sugar, BUN*, uric acid and serum electrolytes (potassium and sodium).

Skin & sunlight:
May cause rash or intensify sunburn in areas exposed to sun or sunlamp.

Driving, piloting or hazardous work:
Don't drive or pilot aircraft until you learn how medicine affects you. Don't work around dangerous machinery. Don't climb ladders or work in high places. Danger increases if you drink alcohol or take medicine affecting alertness and reflexes, such as antihistamines, tranquilizers, sedatives, pain medicine, narcotics and mind-altering drugs.

Discontinuing:
Don't discontinue without consulting doctor. Dose may require gradual reduction if you have taken drug for a long time. Doses of other drugs may also require adjustment.

Others:
No problems expected.

POSSIBLE INTERACTION WITH OTHER DRUGS

GENERIC NAME OR DRUG CLASS	COMBINED EFFECT
Allopurinol	Decreased allopurinol effect.
Amiodarone	Increased risk of heartbeat irregularity due to low potassium.
Amphotericin B	Increased potassium.
Angiotensin-converting enzyme (ACE) inhibitors*	Decreased blood pressure. Possible excessive potassium in blood.
Antidepressants, tricyclic*	Dangerous drop in blood pressure.
Antidiabetic agents, oral*	Increased blood sugar.
Antihypertensives, other*	Increased anti-hypertensive effect.
Barbiturates*	Increased indapamide effect.
Beta-adrenergic blocking agents*	Increased effect of indapamide.
Calcium supplements*	Increased calcium in blood.
Carteolol	Increased anti-hypertensive effect.
Cholestyramine	Decreased indapamide effect.
Colestipol	Decreased indapamide effect.
Cortisone drugs*	Excessive potassium loss that may cause dangerous heart rhythms.
Digitalis preparations*	Excessive potassium loss that may cause dangerous heart rhythms.
Diuretics, thiazide*	Increased effect of thiazide diuretics.
Indomethacin	Decreased indapamide effect.
Lithium	High risk of lithium toxicity.
Monoamine oxidase (MAO) inhibitors*	Increased indapamide effect.
Nicardipine	Dangerous blood pressure drop. Dosages may require adjustment.
Nimodipine	Dangerous blood pressure drop.

Continued on page 943

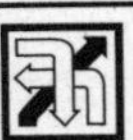

POSSIBLE INTERACTION WITH OTHER SUBSTANCES

INTERACTS WITH	COMBINED EFFECT
Alcohol:	Dangerous blood pressure drop. Avoid.
Beverages:	No problems expected.
Cocaine:	Increased risk of heart block and high blood pressure.
Foods: Licorice.	Excessive potassium loss that may cause dangerous heart rhythms.
Marijuana:	Reduced effectiveness of indapamide. Avoid.
Tobacco:	Reduced effectiveness of indapamide. Avoid.

*See Glossary

INSULIN

BRAND NAMES

See complete list of brand names in the *Brand Name Directory*, page 909.

BASIC INFORMATION

Habit forming? No
Prescription needed? No
Available as generic? Yes
Drug class: Antidiabetic

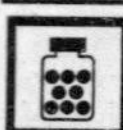

USES

Controls diabetes, a complex metabolic disorder, in which the body does not manufacture insulin.

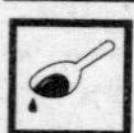

DOSAGE & USAGE INFORMATION

How to take:
Must be taken by injection under the skin. Use disposable, sterile needles. Rotate injection sites.

When to take:
At the same time each day.

If you forget a dose:
Take as soon as you remember. Wait at least 4 hours for next dose. Resume regular schedule.

What drug does:
Facilitates passage of blood sugar through cell membranes so sugar is usable.

Continued next column

OVERDOSE

SYMPTOMS:
Low blood sugar (hypoglycemia)—Anxiety; chills, cold sweats, pale skin; drowsiness; excess hunger; headache; nausea; nervousness; fast heartbeat; shakiness; unusual tiredness or weakness.
WHAT TO DO:

- **Eat some type of sugar immediately, such as orange juice, honey, sugar cubes, crackers, sandwich.**
- **If patient loses consciousness, give glucagon if you have it and know how to use it.**
- **Otherwise, dial 911 (emergency) or 0 (operator) for an ambulance or medical help. Then give first aid immediately.**
- **See emergency information on inside covers.**

Time lapse before drug works:
30 minutes to 8 hours, depending on type of insulin used.

Don't take with:
Any other medicine without consulting your doctor or pharmacist.

POSSIBLE ADVERSE REACTIONS OR SIDE EFFECTS

SYMPTOMS	WHAT TO DO
Life-threatening:	
Hives, rash, intense itching, faintness soon after a dose (anaphylaxis).	Seek emergency treatment immediately.
Common:	
Symptoms of low blood sugar—Nervousness, hunger (excessive), cold sweats, rapid pulse, anxiety, cold skin, chills, confusion, concentration loss, drowsiness, headache, nausea, weakness, shakiness, vision changes.	Seek emergency treatment.
Infrequent:	
• Hives.	Discontinue. Call doctor right away.
• Swelling, redness, itch at injection site.	Continue. Call doctor when convenient.
Rare:	
None expected.	

WARNINGS & PRECAUTIONS

Don't take if:

- Your diagnosis and dose schedule is not established.
- You don't know how to deal with overdose emergencies.

Before you start, consult your doctor:

- If you are allergic to insulin.
- If you take MAO inhibitors.
- If you have liver or kidney disease or low thyroid function.

Over age 60:
Guard against hypoglycemia. Repeated episodes can cause permanent confusion and abnormal behavior.

Pregnancy:
Adhere rigidly to diabetes treatment program. Risk category B (see page xxii).

Breast-feeding:
No problems expected. Consult doctor.

Infants & children:
Use only under medical supervision.

Prolonged use:
Talk to your doctor about the need for follow-up medical examinations or laboratory studies to check blood sugar, serum potassium, urine.

Skin & sunlight:
No problems expected.

Driving, piloting or hazardous work:
No problems expected after dose is established.

Discontinuing:
Don't discontinue without doctor's advice until you complete prescribed dose, even though symptoms diminish or disappear.

Others:
- Diet and exercise affect how much insulin you need. Work with your doctor to determine accurate dose.
- Notify your doctor if you skip a dose, overeat, have fever or infection.
- Notify doctor if you develop symptoms of high blood sugar: drowsiness, dry skin, orange fruit-like odor to breath, increased urination, appetite loss, unusual thirst.
- Never freeze insulin.
- May interfere with the accuracy of some medical tests.

POSSIBLE INTERACTION WITH OTHER DRUGS

GENERIC NAME OR DRUG CLASS	COMBINED EFFECT
Anticonvulsants, hydantoin*	Decreased insulin effect.
Antidiabetics, oral*	Increased antibiabetic effect.
Beta-adrenergic blocking agents*	Possible increased difficulty in regulating blood sugar levels.
Bismuth subsalicylate	Increased insulin effect. May require dosage adjustment.
Carteolol	Hypoglycemic effects may be prolonged.
Contraceptives, oral*	Decreased insulin effect.
Cortisone drugs*	Decreased insulin effect.
Diuretics, thiazide*	Decreased insulin effect.
Furosemide	Decreased insulin effect.
Monoamine oxidase (MAO) inhibitors*	Increased insulin effect.
Nicotine gum and other smoking deterrents	Increased insulin effect.
Oxyphenbutazone	Increased insulin effect.
Phenylbutazone	Increased insulin effect.
Salicylates*	Increased insulin effect.
Smoking deterrents	May require insulin dosage adjustment.
Sulfa drugs*	Increased insulin effect.
Tetracyclines*	Increased insulin effect.
Thyroid hormones*	Decreased insulin effect.

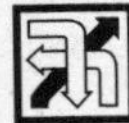

POSSIBLE INTERACTION WITH OTHER SUBSTANCES

INTERACTS WITH	COMBINED EFFECT
Alcohol:	Increased insulin effect. May cause hypoglycemia and brain damage.
Beverages:	None expected.
Cocaine:	May cause brain damage.
Foods:	None expected.
Marijuana:	Possible increase in blood sugar.
Tobacco:	Decreased insulin absorption.

***See Glossary**

IODINATED GLYCEROL

BRAND NAMES

Iophen-C Liquid
Iophen-DM
Tussi-Organidin DM Liquid
Tussi-Organidin Liquid
Tusso-DM

BASIC INFORMATION

Habit forming? No
Prescription needed? Yes
Available as generic? Yes
Drug class: Expectorant

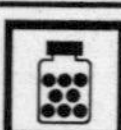

USES

Loosens mucus in bronchial tubes.

DOSAGE & USAGE INFORMATION

How to take:

- Tablets—Swallow with liquid. If you can't swallow whole, crumble tablet and take with liquid or food. Instructions to take on empty stomach mean 1 hour before or 2 hours after eating.
- Oral solution—Swallow with liquid to lessen stomach irritation.
- Elixir—Swallow with liquid.
- Drink a glass of water after each dose.

When to take:
Usually 4 times a day—approximately every 4 hours while awake.

If you forget a dose:
Take as soon as you remember up to 2 hours late. If more than 2 hours, wait for next scheduled dose (don't double this dose).

What drug does:
Increases secretions in bronchial tubes and makes them thinner, which aids in coughing them up.

Continued next column

OVERDOSE

SYMPTOMS:
None expected.
WHAT TO DO:
Overdose unlikely to threaten life. If person takes much larger amount than prescribed, call doctor, poison control center or hospital emergency room for instructions.

Time lapse before drug works:
None. Works immediately.

Don't take with:
Any other medicines (including over-the-counter drugs such as cough and cold medicines, laxatives, antacids, diet pills, caffeine, nose drops or vitamins) without consulting your doctor.

POSSIBLE ADVERSE REACTIONS OR SIDE EFFECTS

SYMPTOMS	WHAT TO DO
Life-threatening:	
Allergic reaction with fever, joint pain, hives, rash, swollen face.	Seek emergency treatment immediately.
Common:	
Diarrhea, nausea and vomiting, abdominal pain.	Continue. Call doctor when convenient.
Infrequent:	
Swollen glands below the ears.	Discontinue. Call doctor right away.
Rare:	
Iodism (burning mouth, headache, eye irritation, metallic taste, rash, sore teeth and gums).	Discontinue. Call doctor right away.

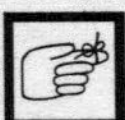

WARNINGS & PRECAUTIONS

Don't take if:
You are allergic to iodine or inorganic iodides.

Before you start, consult your doctor:
- If you have adolescent acne.
- If you have cystic fibrosis.
- If you have thyroid disease.

Over age 60:
No special problems expected.

Pregnancy:
Risk to unborn child outweighs drug benefits. Don't use. Risk category X (see page xxii).

Breast-feeding:
Drug passes into milk. Avoid drug or discontinue nursing until you finish medicine. Consult doctor for advice on maintaining milk supply.

Infants & children:
Effect not documented. Consult your doctor.

Prolonged use:
- May cause decreased thyroid function (hypothyroidism).
- Talk to your doctor about the need for follow-up medical examinations or laboratory studies to check thyroid function.

Skin & sunlight:
No problems expected.

Driving, piloting or hazardous work:
Avoid if you feel confused, drowsy or dizzy.

Discontinuing:
No special problems expected.

Others:
- Advise any doctor or dentist whom you consult that you take this medicine.
- May affect results in some medical tests.
- Do not use for prolonged periods of time.

POSSIBLE INTERACTION WITH OTHER DRUGS

GENERIC NAME OR DRUG CLASS	COMBINED EFFECT
Antithyroid drugs*	Increased likelihood of adversely affecting thyroid gland function.
Lithium	Increased likelihood of adversely affecting thyroid gland function.

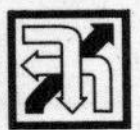

POSSIBLE INTERACTION WITH OTHER SUBSTANCES

INTERACTS WITH	COMBINED EFFECT
Alcohol:	Decreased iodinated glycerol effect.
Beverages:	No special problems expected.
Cocaine:	No special problems expected.
Foods:	No special problems expected.
Marijuana:	No special problems expected.
Tobacco:	No special problems expected.

***See Glossary**

IODOQUINOL

BRAND NAMES

Diiodohydroxyquin
Diodoquin
Diquinol
Yodoquinol
Yodoxin

BASIC INFORMATION

Habit forming? No
Prescription needed? Yes
Available as generic? Yes
Drug class: Antiprotozoal

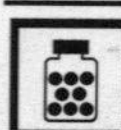

USES

Treatment for intestinal amebiasis and balantidiasis.

DOSAGE & USAGE INFORMATION

How to take:
Tablets—Mix with applesauce or chocolate syrup if unable to swallow tablets.

When to take:
Three times daily after meals for 20 days. Treatment may be repeated after 2 to 3 weeks.

If you forget a dose:
Take as soon as you remember up to 2 hours late. If more than 2 hours, wait for next scheduled dose (don't double this dose).

What drug does:
Kills amoeba (microscopic parasites) in intestinal tract.

Time lapse before drug works:
May require full course of treatment (20 days) to cure.

Don't take with:
Any other medication without consulting your doctor or pharmacist.

OVERDOSE

SYMPTOMS:

- **Prolonged dosing at high level may produce blurred vision, muscle pain, eye pain, numbness and tingling in hands or feet.**
- **Single overdosage unlikely to threaten life.**

WHAT TO DO:
If person takes much larger amount than prescribed, call doctor, poison control center or hospital emergency room for instructions.

POSSIBLE ADVERSE REACTIONS OR SIDE EFFECTS

SYMPTOMS	WHAT TO DO
Life-threatening:	
In case of overdose, see previous column.	
Common:	
Diarrhea, nausea, vomiting, abdominal pain.	Continue. Call doctor when convenient.
Infrequent:	
• Clumsiness, rash, hives, itching, blurred vision, muscle pain, numbness or tingling in hands or feet, chills, fever, weakness.	Discontinue. Call doctor right away.
• Swelling of neck. (thyroid gland)	Continue. Call doctor when convenient.
Rare:	
Dizziness, headache, rectal itching.	Continue. Call doctor when convenient.

WARNINGS & PRECAUTIONS

Don't take if:
You have kidney or liver disease.

Before you start, consult your doctor:
If you have optic atrophy thyroid disease.

Over age 60:
Adverse reactions and side effects may be more frequent and severe than in younger persons.

Pregnancy:
Decide with your doctor if drug benefits justify risk to unborn child. Risk category C (see page xxii).

Breast-feeding:
No proven problems, but avoid if possible. Discontinue nursing until you finish medicine. Consult doctor for advice on maintaining milk supply.

Infants & children:
Not recommended. Safety and dosage has not been established.

Prolonged use:
Not recommended.

Skin & sunlight:
No problems expected.

Driving, piloting or hazardous work:
No problems expected.

Discontinuing:
Don't discontinue without consulting doctor.

Others:
- Thyroid tests may be inaccurate for as long as 6 months after discontinuing iodoquinol treatment.
- May interfere with the accuracy of some medical tests.

POSSIBLE INTERACTION WITH OTHER DRUGS

GENERIC NAME OR DRUG CLASS	COMBINED EFFECT
None expected.	

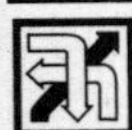

POSSIBLE INTERACTION WITH OTHER SUBSTANCES

INTERACTS WITH	COMBINED EFFECT
Alcohol:	None expected.
Beverages:	None expected.
Cocaine:	None expected.
Foods:	Taking with food may decrease gastrointestinal side effects.
Marijuana:	None expected.
Tobacco:	None expected.

*See Glossary

IPECAC

BRAND NAMES

Ipecac Syrup	Quelidrine Cough

BASIC INFORMATION

Habit forming? No
Prescription needed? No
Available as generic? Yes
Drug class: Emetic

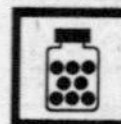

USES

- Used in emergencies to induce vomiting after medication overdose and in some instances of poisoning.
- Don't use if suspected substance to be vomited is strychnine or a corrosive such as lye, kerosene, gasoline, bleach, strong acid or cleaning fluid.

How to take:
- Call doctor, poison control center or emergency room before giving ipecac to any one.
- Don't give to an unconscious or semiconscious person.
- Syrup, undiluted—Carefully follow instructions on the bottle.
- Drink water immediately after taking ipecac.
- Place person in a head-down position to prevent aspiration of vomitus.

When to take:
- Upon discovery of accidental or intentional poisoning or overdose.
- May repeat in 30 minutes if vomiting doesn't occur with first ipecac dose.
- Don't give more than 2 doses.

If you forget a dose:
One-time use only.

Continued next column

OVERDOSE

SYMPTOMS:
Watery diarrhea, breathing difficulty, stiff muscles.
WHAT TO DO:
- **Dial 911 (emergency) or 0 (operator) for an ambulance or medical help. Then give first aid immediately.**
- **See emergency information on inside covers.**

What drug does:
Irritates stomach lining and stimulates the vomiting center in the brain.

Time lapse before drug works:
20 minutes.

Don't take with:
Any other medicines (including over-the-counter drugs such as cough and cold medicines, laxatives, antacids, diet pills, caffeine, nose drops or vitamins) without consulting your doctor.

POSSIBLE ADVERSE REACTIONS OR SIDE EFFECTS

SYMPTOMS	WHAT TO DO
Life-threatening:	
Heartbeat irregularity.	Seek emergency treatment immediately.
Common:	
None expected.	
Infrequent:	
None expected.	
Rare:	
None expected.	

WARNINGS & PRECAUTIONS

Don't take if:
You are drunk from any source.

Before you start, consult your doctor:
If you have heart disease (ipecac can be poisonous to a damaged heart).

Over age 60:
No special problems expected.

Pregnancy:
No studies done. Unknown effect. Consult doctor. Risk category C (see page xxii).

Breast-feeding:
Consult your doctor.

Infants & children:
Give only after consulting doctor or poison control center.

Prolonged use:
Not intended for long-term use.

Skin & sunlight:
No problems expected.

Driving, piloting or hazardous work:
Don't drive or pilot aircraft until you learn how medicine affects you. Don't work around dangerous machinery. Don't climb ladders or work in high places. Danger increases if you drink alcohol or take medicine affecting alertness and reflexes.

Discontinuing:
No special problems expected.

Others:
- If you are instructed to also use activated charcoal, don't use until after ipecac has induced vomiting.
- Don't give more than 2 doses to anyone.
- Don't use ipecac as a means of inducing vomiting to lose weight. It can be toxic to the heart and cause death as a result of chronic use.

POSSIBLE INTERACTION WITH OTHER DRUGS

GENERIC NAME OR DRUG CLASS	COMBINED EFFECT
Charcoal, activated	Improves treatment. If taken for the same overdose, charcoal should follow vomiting induced by ipecac.
Other medicines or herbs to cause vomiting	Decreased ipecac effect.

POSSIBLE INTERACTION WITH OTHER SUBSTANCES

INTERACTS WITH	COMBINED EFFECT
Alcohol:	Avoid. Vomiting while drunk can be dangerous.
Beverages:	
Carbonated.	Stomach distention. Avoid.
Milk.	Decreased ipecac effect.
Cocaine:	Avoid.
Foods:	No problems expected.
Marijuana:	Avoid. Aspiration of vomitus could be fatal.
Tobacco:	No problems expected.

IPRATROPIUM

BRAND NAMES

Apo-Ipravent
Atrovent
Kendral-Ipratropium

BASIC INFORMATION

Habit forming? No
Prescription needed? Yes
Available as generic? No
Drug class: Bronchodilator

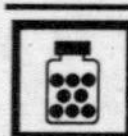

USES

- Treats asthma, bronchitis and emphysema.
- Should not be used alone for acute asthma attacks. May be used with inhalation forms of albuterol or fenoterol.

DOSAGE & USAGE INFORMATION

How to use:
- By inhalation. Follow printed instructions on package.
- Avoid contact with eyes.
- Allow 1 minute between inhalations.

When to take:
Follow your doctor's instructions.

If you forget a dose:
Take as soon as you remember up to 2 hours late. If more than 2 hours, wait for next scheduled dose (don't double this dose).

What drug does:
Dilates bronchial tubes by direct effect on them.

Time lapse before drug works:
None. Effect begins right away.

Don't take with:
Any other medicines (including over-the-counter drugs such as cough and cold medicines, laxatives, antacids, diet pills, caffeine, nose drops or vitamins) without consulting your doctor.

OVERDOSE

SYMPTOMS:
None likely.
WHAT TO DO:
Overdose unlikely to threaten life. If person takes much larger amount than prescribed, call doctor, poison control center or hospital emergency room for instructions.

POSSIBLE ADVERSE REACTIONS OR SIDE EFFECTS

SYMPTOMS	WHAT TO DO
Life-threatening:	
Pounding heartbeat.	Discontinue. Call doctor right away.
Common:	
Cough, headache, dizziness, nervousness, nausea.	Continue. Call doctor when convenient.
Infrequent:	
Blurred vision, difficult urination, stuffy nose, insomnia, tremors, weakness.	Continue. Call doctor when convenient.
Rare:	
Skin rash, ulcers on lips or in mouth, hives.	Discontinue. Call doctor right away.

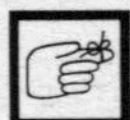

WARNINGS & PRECAUTIONS

Don't take if:
You are sensitive to belladonna or atropine.

Before you start, consult your doctor:
- If you have prostate trouble.
- If you have glaucoma.
- If you have severe dental problems.

Over age 60:
Adverse reactions and side effects may be more frequent and severe than in younger persons. You may need smaller doses for shorter periods of time.

Pregnancy:
Consult doctor. Risk category B (see page xxii).

Breast-feeding:
No special problems expected. Consult doctor.

Infants & children:
Effect not documented. Consult your pediatrician.

Prolonged use:
Decreases saliva flow and may increase cavities, gum disease, thrush and discomfort.

Skin & sunlight:
No problems expected.

Driving, piloting or hazardous work:
Avoid if you feel confused, drowsy or dizzy.

Discontinuing:
No special problems expected.

Others:
- Advise any doctor or dentist whom you consult that you take this medicine.
- Allow 5-minute intervals between ipratropium inhalations and inhalations of cromolyn, cortisone or other inhalant medicines.
- Check with doctor if this medicine doesn't bring relief within 30 minutes.

POSSIBLE INTERACTION WITH OTHER DRUGS

GENERIC NAME OR DRUG CLASS	COMBINED EFFECT
Anticholinergics*	Increased anticholinergic effect.
Cromolyn (inhalation form)	Wait 5 minutes before using cromolyn.

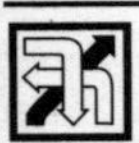

POSSIBLE INTERACTION WITH OTHER SUBSTANCES

INTERACTS WITH	COMBINED EFFECT
Alcohol:	No special problems expected.
Beverages:	No special problems expected.
Cocaine:	Excess central nervous system stimulation. Avoid.
Foods:	No special problems expected.
Marijuana:	Decreased ipratropium effect.
Tobacco:	Decreased ipratropium effect.

***See Glossary**

IRON SUPPLEMENTS

BRAND NAMES

See complete list of brand names in the *Brand Name Directory*, page 909.

BASIC INFORMATION

Habit forming? No
Prescription needed?
With folic acid: Yes
Without folic acid: No
Available as generic? Yes
Drug class: Mineral supplement (iron)

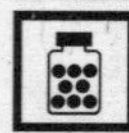

USES

Treatment for dietary iron deficiency or iron-deficiency anemia from other causes.

DOSAGE & USAGE INFORMATION

How to take:

- Tablet, capsule or syrup—Swallow with liquid or food to lessen stomach irritation. If you can't swallow whole, crumble tablet or open capsule and take with liquid or food. Place medicine far back on tongue to avoid staining teeth.
- Extended-release capsule—Swallow whole with liquid. Do not crush.
- Chewable tablets—Chew well before swallowing.
- Liquid—Dilute dose in beverage before swallowing and drink through a straw.

When to take:
1 hour before or 2 hours after eating.

If you forget a dose:
Take up to 2 hours late. If more than 2 hours, wait for next dose (don't double this dose).

Continued next column

OVERDOSE

SYMPTOMS:

- **Moderate overdose—Stomach pain, vomiting, diarrhea, black stools, lethargy.**
- **Serious overdose—Weakness and collapse; pallor, weak and rapid heartbeat; shallow breathing; convulsions and coma.**

WHAT TO DO:

- **Dial 911 (emergency) or 0 (operator) for an ambulance or medical help. Then give first aid immediately.**
- **See emergency information on inside covers.**

What drug does:
Stimulates bone marrow's production of hemoglobin (red blood cell pigment that carries oxygen to body cells).

Time lapse before drug works:
3 to 7 days. May require 3 weeks for maximum benefit.

Don't take with:

- Multiple vitamin and mineral supplements.
- Any other medicine without consulting your doctor or pharmacist.

POSSIBLE ADVERSE REACTIONS OR SIDE EFFECTS

SYMPTOMS	WHAT TO DO
Life-threatening:	
Weak, rapid heartbeat.	Seek emergency treatment immediately.
Always:	
Gray or black stool.	No action necessary.
Common:	
• Stained teeth with liquid iron.	No action necessary.
• Abdominal pain.	Continue. Call doctor when convenient.
Infrequent:	
• Constipation or diarrhea, heartburn, nausea, vomiting.	Discontinue. Call doctor right away.
• Fatigue, weakness.	Continue. Call doctor when convenient.
Rare:	
• Blue lips, fingernails, palms of hands; pale, clammy skin.	Discontinue. Seek emergency treatment.
• Throat pain on swallowing, pain, cramps, blood in stool.	Discontinue. Call doctor right away.
• Drowsiness.	Continue. Call doctor when convenient.

WARNINGS & PRECAUTIONS

Don't take if:

- You are allergic to any iron supplement or tartrazine dye.
- You take iron injections.
- You have acute hepatitis, hemosiderosis or hemochromatosis (conditions involving excess iron in body).
- You have hemolytic anemia.

Before you start, consult your doctor:
- If you plan to become pregnant while on medication.
- If you have had stomach surgery.
- If you have had peptic ulcer, enteritis or colitis.

Over age 60:
May cause hemochromatosis (iron storage disease) with bronze skin, liver damage, diabetes, heart problems and impotence.

Pregnancy:
Take only if your doctor advises. Risk category C (see page xxii).

Breast-feeding:
No problems expected. Take only if your doctor confirms you have a dietary deficiency or an iron-deficiency anemia.

Infants & children:
Use only under medical supervision. Overdose common and dangerous. Keep out of children's reach.

Prolonged use:
- May cause hemochromatosis (iron storage disease) with bronze skin, liver damage, diabetes, heart problems and impotence.
- Talk to your doctor about the need for follow-up medical examinations or laboratory studies to check complete blood counts (white blood cell count, platelet count, red blood cell count, hemoglobin, hematocrit), serum iron, total iron-binding capacity.

Skin & sunlight:
No problems expected.

Driving, piloting or hazardous work:
No problems expected.

Discontinuing:
May be unnecessary to finish medicine. Follow doctor's instructions.

Others:
- Liquid form stains teeth. Mix with water or juice to lessen the effect. Brush with baking soda or hydrogen peroxide to help remove stain.
- Some products contain tartrazine dye. Avoid, especially if you are allergic to aspirin.
- May interfere with the accuracy of some medical tests.

POSSIBLE INTERACTION WITH OTHER DRUGS

GENERIC NAME OR DRUG CLASS	COMBINED EFFECT
Acetohydroxamic acid	Decreased effects of both drugs.
Allopurinol	Possible excess iron storage in liver.
Antacids*	Poor iron absorption.
Chloramphenicol	Decreased effect of iron. Interferes with formation of red blood cells and hemoglobin.
Cholestyramine	Decreased iron effect.
Etidronate	Decreased etidronate effect. Take at least 2 hours after iron supplement.
Iron supplements, other*	Possible excess iron storage in liver.
Tetracyclines*	Decreased tetracycline effect. Take iron 3 hours before or 2 hours after taking tetracycline.
Vitamin E	Decreased iron and vitamin E effect.
Zinc supplements	Increased need for zinc.

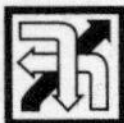

POSSIBLE INTERACTION WITH OTHER SUBSTANCES

INTERACTS WITH	COMBINED EFFECT
Alcohol:	Increased iron absorption. May cause organ damage. Avoid or use in moderation.
Beverages: Milk, tea.	Decreased iron effect.
Cocaine:	None expected.
Foods: Dairy foods, eggs, whole-grain bread and cereal.	Decreased iron effect.
Marijuana:	None expected.
Tobacco:	None expected.

***See Glossary**

ISOMETHEPTENE, DICHLORALPHENAZONE & ACETAMINOPHEN

BRAND NAMES

Amidrine
I.D.A.
Iso-Acetazone
Isocom
Midchlor
Midquin
Midrin
Migrapap
Migratine
Migrazone
Migrend
Migrex
Mitride

BASIC INFORMATION

Habit forming? No
Prescription needed? Yes
Available as generic? No
Drug class: Analgesic, sedative, vascular headache suppressant

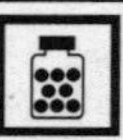

USES

Treatment of vascular (throbbing or migraine type) and tension headaches.

DOSAGE & USAGE INFORMATION

How to take:
Capsules—Take with fluid. Usual dose—2 capsules at start, then 1 every hour until fully relieved. Don't exceed 5 capsules in 12 hours.

When to take:
At first sign of headache.

If you forget a dose:
Use as soon as you remember.

What drug does:
Causes blood vessels in head to constrict or become narrower. Acetaminophen relieves pain by effects on hypothalamus—the part of the brain that helps regulate body heat and receives body's pain messages.

Time lapse before drug works:
30-60 minutes.

Continued next column

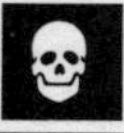

OVERDOSE

SYMPTOMS:
Stomach upsets, irritability, sweating, severe diarrhea, convulsions, coma.
WHAT TO DO:
- **Dial 911 (emergency) or 0 (operator) for an ambulance or medical help. Then give first aid immediately.**
- **See emergency information on inside covers.**

Don't take with:
- Any medicine that will decrease mental alertness or reflexes, such as alcohol, other mind-altering drugs, cough/cold medicines, antihistamines, allergy medicine, sedatives, tranquilizers (sleeping pills or "downers") barbiturates, seizure medicine, narcotics, other prescription medicine for pain, muscle relaxants, anesthetics.
- See Interaction column and consult doctor.

POSSIBLE ADVERSE REACTIONS OR SIDE EFFECTS

SYMPTOMS	WHAT TO DO
Life-threatening:	
In case of overdose, see previous column.	
Common:	
Dizziness, drowsiness.	Continue. Call doctor when convenient.
Infrequent:	
Diarrhea, vomiting, nausea, abdominal cramps, upper abdominal pain.	Discontinue. Call doctor right away.
Rare:	
Rash; itchy skin; sore throat, fever, mouth sores; unusual bleeding or bruising; weakness; jaundice.	Discontinue. Call doctor right away.

WARNINGS & PRECAUTIONS

Don't take if:
- You are allergic to acetaminophen or any other component of this combination medicine.
- Your symptoms don't improve after 2 days use. Call your doctor.

Before you start, consult your doctor:
If you have kidney disease, liver damage, glaucoma, heart or blood vessel disorder, hypertension, alcoholism (active).

Over age 60:
Don't exceed recommended dose. You can't eliminate drug as efficiently as younger persons.

Pregnancy:
Decide with your doctor if drug benefits justify risk to unborn child. Risk category C (see page xxii).

Breast-feeding:
No proven harm to nursing infant. Consult doctor.

Infants & children:
Give under careful medical supervision only.

ISOMETHEPTENE, DICHLORALPHENAZONE & ACETAMINOPHEN

Prolonged use:

- May affect blood system and cause anemia. Limit use to 5 days for children 12 and under, and 10 days for adults.
- Talk to your doctor about the need for follow-up medical examinations or laboratory studies to check complete blood counts (white blood cell count, platelet count, red blood cell count, hemoglobin, hematocrit), liver function.

Skin & sunlight:
No problems expected.

Driving, piloting or hazardous work:
Avoid if you feel drowsy. Otherwise, no restrictions.

Discontinuing:
Discontinue in 2 days if symptoms don't improve.

Others:
No problems expected.

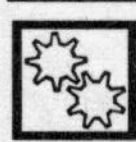

POSSIBLE INTERACTION WITH OTHER DRUGS

GENERIC NAME OR DRUG CLASS	COMBINED EFFECT
Anticoagulants, oral*	May increase anticoagulant effect. If combined frequently, prothrombin time should be monitored.
Anti-inflammatory drugs, nonsteroidal (NSAIDs)*	Long-term combined effect (3 years or longer) increases chance of damage to kidney, including malignancy.
Aspirin or other salicylates*	Long-term combined effect (3 years or longer) increases chance of damage to kidney, including malignancy.
Beta-adrenergic blocking agents*	Narrowed arteries in heart if taken in large doses.
Central nervous system (CNS) depressants*	Increased sedative effect.
Monoamine oxidase (MAO) inhibitors*	Sudden increase in blood pressure.
Phenacetin	Long-term combined effect (3 years or longer) increases chance of damage to kidney, including malignancy.
Phenobarbital	Quicker elimination and decreased effect of acetaminophen.
Tetracyclines* (effervescent granules or tablets)	May slow tetracycline absorption. Space doses 2 hours apart.
Zidovudine (AZT)	Increased toxic effect of zidovudine.

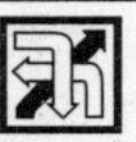

POSSIBLE INTERACTION WITH OTHER SUBSTANCES

INTERACTS WITH	COMBINED EFFECT
Alcohol:	Drowsiness. Toxicity to liver. Avoid.
Beverages:	None expected.
Cocaine:	None expected. However, cocaine may slow body's recovery. Avoid.
Foods:	None expected.
Marijuana:	Increased pain relief. However, marijuana may slow body's recovery. Avoid.
Tobacco:	May decrease medicine's effectiveness. Avoid.

*See Glossary

ISONIAZID

BRAND NAMES

INH
Isotamine
Laniazid
Nydrazid
PMS Isoniazid
Rifamate
Tubizid

BASIC INFORMATION

Habit forming? No
Prescription needed? Yes
Available as generic? Yes
Drug class: Antitubercular

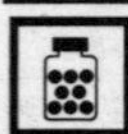

USES

Kills tuberculosis germs.

DOSAGE & USAGE INFORMATION

How to take:
- Tablet—Swallow with liquid to lessen stomach irritation.
- Syrup—Follow label directions.

When to take:
At the same time each day.

If you forget a dose:
Take as soon as you remember up to 12 hours late. If more than 12 hours, wait for next scheduled dose (don't double this dose).

What drug does:
Interferes with TB germ metabolism. Eventually destroys the germ.

Continued next column

OVERDOSE

SYMPTOMS:
Difficult breathing, convulsions, coma.
WHAT TO DO:
- **Dial 911 (emergency) or 0 (operator) for an ambulance or medical help. Then give first aid immediately.**
- **If patient is unconscious and not breathing, give mouth-to-mouth breathing. If there is no heartbeat, use cardiac massage and mouth-to-mouth breathing (CPR). Don't try to make patient vomit. If you can't get help quickly, take patient to nearest emergency facility.**
- **See emergency information on inside covers.**

Time lapse before drug works:
3 to 6 months. You may need to take drug as long as 2 years.

Don't take with:
Any other medication without consulting your doctor or pharmacist.

POSSIBLE ADVERSE REACTIONS OR SIDE EFFECTS

SYMPTOMS	WHAT TO DO
Life-threatening: In case of overdose, see previous column.	
Common:	
• Muscle pain and pain in joints, tingling or numbness in extremities, jaundice.	Discontinue. Call doctor right away.
• Confusion, unsteady walk.	Continue. Call doctor when convenient.
Infrequent:	
• Swollen glands, nausea, indigestion, diarrhea, vomiting, appetite loss.	Discontinue. Call doctor right away.
• Dizziness.	Continue. Call doctor when convenient.
Rare:	
• Rash, fever, impaired vision, anemia with fatigue, weakness, fever, sore throat, unusual bleeding or bruising.	Discontinue. Call doctor right away.
• Breast enlargement or discomfort.	Continue. Tell doctor at next visit.

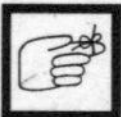

WARNINGS & PRECAUTIONS

Don't take if:
You are allergic to isoniazid.

Before you start, consult your doctor:
- If you plan to become pregnant within medication period.
- If you are allergic to athionamide, pyrazinamide or nicotinic acid.
- If you drink alcohol.
- If you have liver or kidney disease.
- If you have epilepsy, diabetes or lupus.

Over age 60:
Adverse reactions and side effects, especially jaundice, may be more frequent and severe than in younger persons. Kidneys may be less efficient.

Pregnancy:
Decide with your doctor if drug benefits justify risk to unborn child. Risk category C (see page xxii).

Breast-feeding:
Drug passes into milk. Avoid drug or discontinue nursing until you finish medicine. Consult doctor for advice on maintaining milk supply.

Infants & children:
Use only under medical supervision.

Prolonged use:
- Numbness and tingling of hands and feet.
- Talk to your doctor about the need for follow-up medical examinations or laboratory studies to check liver function, eyes.

Skin & sunlight:
No problems expected.

Driving, piloting or hazardous work:
Avoid if you feel dizzy. Otherwise, no problems expected.

Discontinuing:
Don't discontinue without doctor's advice until you complete prescribed dose, even though symptoms diminish or disappear.

Others:
- Diabetic patients may have false blood sugar tests.
- Periodic liver function tests and laboratory blood studies recommended.
- Prescription for vitamin B-6 (pyridoxine) recommended to prevent nerve damage.

POSSIBLE INTERACTION WITH OTHER DRUGS

GENERIC NAME OR DRUG CLASS	COMBINED EFFECT
Acetaminophen	Increased risk of liver damage.
Alfentanil	Prolonged duration of alfentanil effect (undesirable).
Antacids* (aluminum-containing)	Decreased absorption of isoniazid.
Anticholinergics*	May increase pressure within eyeball.
Anticoagulants, oral*	Increased anticoagulant effect.
Antidiabetics*	Increased anti-diabetic effect.
Antihypertensives*	Increased anti-hypertensive effect.
Carbamazepine	Increased risk of liver damage.
Cycloserine	Increased risk of central nervous system effects.
Didanosine	Increased risk of peripheral neuropathy.
Disulfiram	Increased effect of disulfiram.
Laxatives*	Decreased absorption and effect of isoniazid.
Hepatotoxics*	Increased risk of liver damage.
Ketoconazole	Increased risk of liver damage
Narcotics*	Increased narcotic effect.
Phenytoin	Increased phenytoin effect.
Pyridoxine (Vitamin B-6)	Decreased chance of nerve damage in extremities.
Rifampin	Increased isoniazid toxicity to liver.
Sedatives*	Increased sedative effect.
Stimulants*	Increased stimulant effect.

POSSIBLE INTERACTION WITH OTHER SUBSTANCES

INTERACTS WITH	COMBINED EFFECT
Alcohol:	Increased incidence of liver disease and seizures.
Beverages:	None expected.
Cocaine:	None expected.
Foods: Swiss or Cheshire cheese, fish.	Red or itching skin, fast heartbeat. Seek emergency treatment.
Marijuana:	No interactions expected, but marijuana may slow body's recovery.
Tobacco:	No interactions expected, but tobacco may slow body's recovery.

***See Glossary**

ISOPROTERENOL & PHENYLEPHRINE

BRAND NAMES

Duo-Medihaler
Isuprel-Neo Mistometer

BASIC INFORMATION

Habit forming? No
Prescription needed? Yes
Available as generic? No
Drug class: Sympathomimetic, bronchodilator

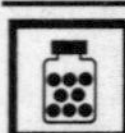

USES

- Temporary relief of congestion of nose, sinuses and throat caused by allergies, colds or sinusitis.
- Treatment for breathing difficulty from acute asthma, bronchitis and emphysema.

DOSAGE & USAGE INFORMATION

How to take:
Aerosol inhaler—Don't inhale more than twice per dose. Follow package instructions.

When to take:
As needed, no more often than every 4 hours.

If you forget a dose:
Take as soon as you remember. Wait 4 hours for next dose. Don't double this dose.

What drug does:
- Dilates constricted bronchial tubes, improving air flow.
- Stimulates heart muscle and dilates blood vessels.

Time lapse before drug works:
2 to 4 minutes.

Continued next column

OVERDOSE

SYMPTOMS:
Headache, blood pressure rise, slow and forceful pulse, nervousness, rapid or irregular heartbeat, fainting, sweating, tremor, vomiting, chest pain, convulsions, coma.
WHAT TO DO:
- **Dial 911 (emergency) or 0 (operator) for an ambulance or medical help. Then give first aid immediately.**
- **See emergency information on inside covers.**

Don't take with:
Nonprescription drugs for asthma, cough, cold, allergy, appetite suppressants, sleeping pills or drugs containing caffeine without consulting doctor.

POSSIBLE ADVERSE REACTIONS OR SIDE EFFECTS

SYMPTOMS	WHAT TO DO
Life-threatening:	
In case of overdose, see previous column.	
Common:	
• Insomnia, nervousness, restlessness.	Continue. Call doctor when convenient.
• Pink or red saliva or sputum.	No action necessary.
Infrequent:	
• Increased sweating.	Continue. Call doctor when convenient.
• Dizziness, headache, shakiness, weakness, red or flushed face, vomiting, nausea, pale skin.	Continue. Call doctor when convenient.
Rare:	
Tingling hands or feet, chest pain, irregular heartbeat.	Discontinue. Call doctor right away.

WARNINGS & PRECAUTIONS

Don't take if:
- You are allergic to any sympathomimetic*, including some diet pills.
- You have serious heart-rhythm disorder.
- You have taken a monoamine oxidase (MAO) inhibitor* in past 2 weeks.

Before you start, consult your doctor:
- If you have high blood pressure, heart disease, or take a digitalis preparation.
- If you have diabetes or overactive thyroid.
- If you are sensitive to sympathomimetics.
- If you use epinephrine.
- If your heartbeat is faster than 100 beats per minute.

Over age 60:
You may be more sensitive to drug's stimulant effects. Use with caution if you have hardening of the arteries.

Pregnancy:
Decide with your doctor if drug benefits justify risk to unborn child. Risk category C (see page xxii).

Breast-feeding:
Effect unknown. Consult doctor.

Infants & children:
Use only under close supervision.

Prolonged use:
- May cause functional dependence.
- Salivary glands may swell.

Skin & sunlight:
No problems expected.

Driving, piloting or hazardous work:
Use caution if you feel dizzy or nervous.

Discontinuing:
Discontinue if drug fails to provide relief after 2 or 3 days. Consult doctor.

Others:
No problems expected.

POSSIBLE INTERACTION WITH OTHER DRUGS

GENERIC NAME OR DRUG CLASS	COMBINED EFFECT
Acebutolol	Decreased effect of both drugs.
Amphetamines*	Increased nervousness.
Antiasthmatics*	Nervous stimulation.
Antidepressants*	Increased effect of both drugs.
Antihypertensives*	Increased anti-hypertensive effect.
Beta-adrenergic blocking agents*	Decreased effect of both drugs.
Digitalis	Increased risk of serious heart disturbances.
Ephedrine	Increased ephedrine effect.
Epinephrine	Increased chance of serious heart disturbances.
Ergoloid mesylates	Blood vessel restriction.
Ergonovine	Increased vasocon-striction.
Ergotamine	Blood vessel restriction.
Furazolidine	Sudden, severe increase in blood pressure.
Maprotiline	Increase risk of serious heart distrubances.
Methyldopa	Decreased methyldopa effect.
Monoamine oxidase (MAO) inhibitors*	Dangerous blood pressure rise.
Nitrates*	Possible decreased effect of both drugs.
Oxprenolol	Decreased effect of both drugs.
Sedatives*	Decreased sedative effect.
Sympathomimetics, other*	Increased effect of both drugs, especially harmful side effects.
Terazosin	Decreases effectiveness of terazosin.
Theophylline	Possible increased effect and toxicity of both drugs.
Tranquilizers*	Decreased tranquilizer effect.

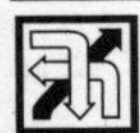

POSSIBLE INTERACTION WITH OTHER SUBSTANCES

INTERACTS WITH	COMBINED EFFECT
Alcohol:	Decreased isoproterenol effect.
Beverages:	
Caffeine drinks.	Overstimulation. Avoid.
Cocaine:	High risk of heartbeat irregularities and high blood pressure. Overstimulation of brain. Avoid.
Foods:	None expected.
Marijuana:	Increased antiasthmatic effect of isoproterenol.
Tobacco:	None expected.

*See Glossary

ISOTRETINOIN

BRAND NAMES

Accutane

Accutane Roche

BASIC INFORMATION

Habit forming? No
Prescription needed? Yes
Available as generic? No
Drug classification: Anti-acne

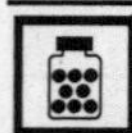

USES

- Decreases cystic acne formation in severe cases.
- Treats certain other skin disorders involving an overabundance of outer skin layer.

DOSAGE & USAGE INFORMATION

How to take:
Capsule—Swallow with liquid or food to lessen stomach irritation. If you can't swallow whole, open capsule and take with liquid or food.

When to take:
Twice a day. Follow prescription directions.

If you forget a dose:
Take as soon as you remember up to 2 hours late. If more than 2 hours, wait for next scheduled dose and double dose.

What drug does:
Reduces sebaceous gland activity and size.

Time lapse before drug works:
May require 15 to 20 weeks to experience full benefit.

Don't take with:
- Vitamin A or supplements containing Vitamin A.
- Any other medication without consulting your doctor or pharmacist.

OVERDOSE

SYMPTOMS:
None reported.
WHAT TO DO:
Overdose unlikely to threaten life. If person takes much larger amount than prescribed, call doctor, poison control center or hospital emergency room for instructions.

POSSIBLE ADVERSE REACTIONS OR SIDE EFFECTS

SYMPTOMS	WHAT TO DO
Life-threatening: None expected.	
Common:	
• Burning, red, itching eyes; lip scaling; burning pain; nosebleeds.	Discontinue. Call doctor right away.
• Itchy skin.	Continue. Call doctor when convenient.
• Dry mouth.	Continue. Tell doctor at next visit. (Suck ice or chew gum.)
Infrequent:	
• Rash, infection, nausea, vomiting.	Discontinue. Call doctor right away.
• Pain in muscles, bones, joints; hair thinning; tiredness.	Continue. Call doctor when convenient.
Rare:	
Abdominal pain, bleeding gums, blurred vision, diarrhea, headache, moodiness, vomiting, eye pain, rectal bleeding, yellow skin or eyes.	Discontinue. Call doctor right away.

WARNINGS & PRECAUTIONS

Don't take if:
- You are allergic to isotretinoin, etretinate, tretinoin or vitamin A derivatives.
- You are pregnant or plan pregnancy.
- *You are even able to bear children. Read, understand and follow the patient information enclosure with your prescription.*

Before you start, consult your doctor:
- If you have diabetes.
- If you or any member of family have high triglyceride levels in blood.

Over age 60:
Adverse reactions and side effects may be more frequent and severe than in younger persons.

Pregnancy:
Causes birth defects in fetus. Don't use. Risk category X (see page xxii).

Breast-feeding:
Effect unknown. Not recommended. Consult doctor.

Infants & children:
Not recommended.

Prolonged use:
- Possible damage to cornea.
- Talk to your doctor about the need for follow-up medical examinations or laboratory studies to check complete blood counts (white blood cell count, platelet count, red blood cell count, hemoglobin, hematocrit), liver function, blood lipids, blood sugar.

Skin & sunlight:
May cause rash or intensify sunburn in areas exposed to sun or sunlamp.

Driving, piloting or hazardous work:
Use caution if there is a decrease in your night vision or you are unable to see well. Consult doctor.

Discontinuing:
Single course of treatment is usually all that's needed. If second course required, wait 8 weeks after completing first course.

Others:
- Use only for severe cases of cystic acne that have not responded to less hazardous forms of acne treatment.
- May interfere with the accuracy of some medical tests.
- Don't donate blood for at least 30 days after discontinuing medicine.
- **If you are planning pregnancy or at risk of pregnancy, don't take this drug.**

POSSIBLE INTERACTION WITH OTHER DRUGS

GENERIC NAME OR DRUG CLASS	COMBINED EFFECT
Etretinate	Increased chance of toxicity of each drug.
Tetracyclines*	Increased risk of developing pseudotumor cerebri.*
Topical drugs or cosmetics	May interact with isotretinoin.
Tretinoin	Increased chance of toxicity.
Vitamin A	Additive toxic effect of each. Avoid.

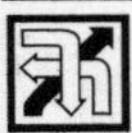

POSSIBLE INTERACTION WITH OTHER SUBSTANCES

INTERACTS WITH	COMBINED EFFECT
Alcohol:	Significant increase in triglycerides in blood. Avoid.
Beverages:	No problems expected.
Cocaine:	Increased chance of toxicity of isotretinoin. Avoid.
Foods:	No problems expected.
Marijuana:	Increased chance of toxicity of isotretinoin. Avoid.
Tobacco:	May decrease absorption of medicine. Avoid tobacco while in treatment.

***See Glossary**

ISOXSUPRINE

BRAND NAMES

Vasodilan Vasoprine

BASIC INFORMATION

Habit forming? No
Prescription needed? Yes
Available as generic? Yes
Drug class: Vasodilator

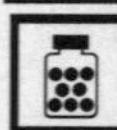

USES

- May improve poor blood circulation.
- Management of premature labor.
- Treatment for painful menstruation.

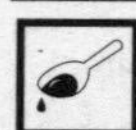

DOSAGE & USAGE INFORMATION

How to take:
Tablet—Swallow with liquid or food to lessen stomach irritation. If you can't swallow whole, crumble tablet and take with liquid or food.

When to take:
At the same times each day.

If you forget a dose:
Take as soon as you remember up to 2 hours late. If more than 2 hours, wait for next scheduled dose (don't double this dose).

What drug does:
Expands blood vessels, increasing flow and permitting distribution of oxygen and nutrients.

Time lapse before drug works:
1 hour.

Continued next column

OVERDOSE

SYMPTOMS:
Headache, dizziness, flush, vomiting, weakness, sweating, fainting, shortness of breath, coma.
WHAT TO DO:

- **Dial 911 (emergency) or 0 (operator) for an ambulance or medical help. Then give first aid immediately.**
- **If patient is unconscious and not breathing, give mouth-to-mouth breathing. If there is no heartbeat, use cardiac massage and mouth-to-mouth breathing (CPR). Don't try to make patient vomit. If you can't get help quickly, take patient to nearest emergency facility.**
- **See emergency information on inside covers.**

Don't take with:
Any other medication without consulting your doctor or pharmacist.

POSSIBLE ADVERSE REACTIONS OR SIDE EFFECTS

SYMPTOMS	WHAT TO DO
Life-threatening: In case of overdose, see previous column.	
Common: None expected.	
Infrequent: Nausea, vomiting.	Continue. Call doctor when convenient.
Rare: Rapid or irregular heartbeat, rash, chest pain, shortness of breath.	Discontinue. Call doctor right away.

WARNINGS & PRECAUTIONS

Don't take if:
- You are allergic to any vasodilator.
- You have any bleeding disease.

Before you start, consult your doctor:
- If you have high blood pressure, hardening of the arteries or heart disease.
- If you plan to become pregnant within medication period.
- If you have glaucoma.

Over age 60:
Adverse reactions and side effects may be more frequent and severe than in younger persons.

Pregnancy:
Decide with your doctor whether drug benefits justify risk to unborn child. Risk category C (see page xxii).

Breast-feeding:
No problems expected, but consult doctor.

Infants & children:
Not recommended.

Prolonged use:
Talk to your doctor about the need for follow-up medical examinations or laboratory studies.

Skin & sunlight:
No problems expected.

Driving, piloting or hazardous work:
Avoid if you feel dizzy or faint. Otherwise, no problems expected.

Discontinuing:
Don't discontinue without doctor's advice until you complete prescribed dose, even though symptoms diminish or disappear.

Others:
- Be cautious when arising from lying or sitting position, when climbing stairs, or if dizziness occurs.
- May interfere with the accuracy of some medical tests.

POSSIBLE INTERACTION WITH OTHER DRUGS

GENERIC NAME OR DRUG CLASS	COMBINED EFFECT
None significant.	

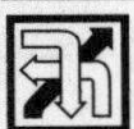

POSSIBLE INTERACTION WITH OTHER SUBSTANCES

INTERACTS WITH	COMBINED EFFECT
Alcohol:	None expected.
Beverages:	
Milk.	Decreased stomach irritation.
Cocaine:	Decreased blood circulation to extremities. Avoid.
Foods:	None expected.
Marijuana:	Rapid heartbeat.
Tobacco:	Decreased isoxsuprine effect; nicotine constricts blood vessels.

ITRACONAZOLE

BRAND NAMES

Sporanox

BASIC INFORMATION

Habit forming? No
Prescription needed? Yes
Available as generic? No
Drug class: Antifungal

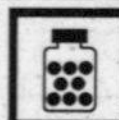

USES

Treatment for fungal infections including blastomycosis, histoplasmosis and others.

DOSAGE & USAGE INFORMATION

How to take:
Capsule—Swallow with liquid. Take at mealtime.

When to take:
At the same time each day.

If you forget a dose:

- For once-a-day dosage, take as soon as you remember up to 12 hours late. If more than 12 hours, wait for next scheduled dose (don't double this dose).
- For twice-a-day dosage, take as soon as you remember up to 2 hours late. If more than 2 hours, wait for next scheduled dose (don't double this dose).

What drug does:
Prevents fungi from growing and reproducing.

Time lapse before drug works:
May require several weeks or months, possibly years for some fungal infections.

Don't take with:

- Histamine H_2 receptor antagonists, antacids or didanosine. Take them at least 2 hours after any dose of itraconazole.
- Any other prescription or nonprescription drug without consulting your doctor.

OVERDOSE

SYMPTOMS:
None reported.
WHAT TO DO:
Overdose unlikely to threaten life. If person takes much larger amount than prescribed, call doctor, poison control center or hospital emergency room for instructions.

POSSIBLE ADVERSE REACTIONS OR SIDE EFFECTS

SYMPTOMS	WHAT TO DO
Life-threatening: None expected.	
Common: None expected.	
Infrequent:	
• Skin rash.	Discontinue. Call doctor right away.
• Abdominal pain, constipation or diarrhea, nausea, vomiting, appetite loss, headache.	Continue. Call doctor when convenient.
Rare: Yellow skin or eyes, pale stools, dark or amber urine, unusual tiredness or weakness.	Discontinue. Call doctor right away.

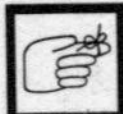

WARNINGS & PRECAUTIONS

Don't take if:
You are allergic to itraconazole, ketoconazole, fluconazole or miconazole.

Before you start, consult your doctor:
- If you have liver disease.
- If you have reduced stomach acidity (achlorhydria or hypochlorhydria).

Over age 60:
Adverse reactions and side effects may be more frequent and severe than in younger persons.

Pregnancy:
Decide with your doctor if drug benefits justify risk to unborn child. Risk category C (see page xxii).

Breast-feeding:
Drug passes into milk. Avoid drug or discontinue nursing until you finish medicine. Consult doctor for advice on maintaining milk supply.

Infants & children:
Give only under close medical supervision.

Prolonged use:
Request periodic liver function studies.

Skin & sunlight:
No problems expected.

Driving, piloting or hazardous work:
No problems expected.

Discontinuing:
May be unnecessary to finish medicine. Follow doctor's instructions.

Others:
- Advise any doctor or dentist whom you consult that you take this medicine.
- May affect the results in some medical tests.

POSSIBLE INTERACTION WITH OTHER DRUGS

GENERIC NAME OR DRUG CLASS	COMBINED EFFECT
Antacids*	Decreased itraconazole absorption.
Anticoagulants*, oral	Increased anticoagulant effect.
Antidiabetics*, oral	Increased risk of hypoglycemia.
Astemizole	Possible cardiac toxicity and death. Avoid combining.
Carbamazepine	Decreased itraconazole effect.
Cyclosporine	Possible toxic levels of cyclosporine.
Didanosine	Decreased itraconazole absorption.
Digoxin	Possible toxic levels of digoxin.
Histamine H_2 receptor antagonists	Decreased itraconazole absorption.
Isoniazid	Decreased anticoagulant effect.
Rifampin	Decreased itraconazole effect.
Phenytoin	Decreased itraconazole effect.
Terfenadine	Possible cardiac toxicity and death. Avoid combining.
Warfarin	Increased warfarin effect.

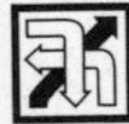

POSSIBLE INTERACTION WITH OTHER SUBSTANCES

INTERACTS WITH	COMBINED EFFECT
Alcohol:	None expected.
Beverages:	None expected.
Cocaine:	None expected.
Foods:	None expected.
Marijuana:	None expected.
Tobacco:	None expected.

*See Glossary

KANAMYCIN

BRAND NAMES

Kantrex

BASIC INFORMATION

Habit forming? No
Prescription needed? Yes
Available as generic? No
Drug class: Bowel preparation

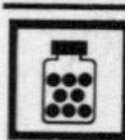

USES

- To cleanse bowel of bacteria prior to intestinal surgery.
- Treats hepatic coma.

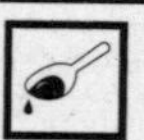

DOSAGE & USAGE INFORMATION

How to take:
Capsules—Swallow with liquid. If you can't swallow whole, open capsule and take with liquid or food. Instructions to take on empty stomach mean 1 hour before or 2 hours after eating.

When to take:
At the same time each day, according to instructions on prescription label.

If you forget a dose:
Take as soon as you remember up to 2 hours late. If more than 2 hours, wait for next scheduled dose (don't double this dose).

What drug does:
Kills susceptible bacteria in the intestines.

Time lapse before drug works:
15 to 30 minutes.

Don't take with:
Any other medication without consulting your doctor or pharmacist.

OVERDOSE

SYMPTOMS:
Clumsiness, dizziness, seizures, coma.
WHAT TO DO:
- **Dial 911 (emergency) or 0 (operator) for an ambulance or medical help. Then give first aid immediately.**
- **See emergency information on inside covers.**

POSSIBLE ADVERSE REACTIONS OR SIDE EFFECTS

SYMPTOMS	WHAT TO DO
Life-threatening: In case of overdose, see previous column.	
Common: Mouth irritation or soreness, nausea.	Continue. Call doctor when convenient.
Infrequent: Vomiting.	Discontinue. Call doctor right away.
Rare: Decreased urine, hearing loss, ringing in ears, clumsiness, unsteadiness, skin rash.	Discontinue. Call doctor right away.

WARNINGS & PRECAUTIONS

Don't take if:
- You are allergic to kanamycin.
- You can't tolerate any aminoglycoside.

Before you start, consult your doctor:
- If you have hearing difficulty.
- If you have intestinal obstruction.
- If you have severe kidney disease.
- If you have ulcerative colitis.

Over age 60:
Adverse reactions and side effects may be more frequent and severe than in younger persons. You may need smaller doses for shorter periods of time.

Pregnancy:
Consult doctor. Risk category D (see page xxii).

Breast-feeding:
No special problems expected. Consult doctor.

Infants & children:
Not recommended for prolonged use.

Prolonged use:
Not recommended for prolonged use.

Skin & sunlight:
No problems expected.

Driving, piloting or hazardous work:
Avoid if you feel confused, drowsy or dizzy.

Discontinuing:
Not recommended for prolonged use.

Others:
No problems expected.

POSSIBLE INTERACTION WITH OTHER DRUGS

GENERIC NAME OR DRUG CLASS	COMBINED EFFECT
None significant.	

POSSIBLE INTERACTION WITH OTHER SUBSTANCES

INTERACTS WITH	COMBINED EFFECT
Alcohol:	No special problems expected.
Beverages:	No special problems expected.
Cocaine:	No special problems expected.
Foods:	No special problems expected.
Marijuana:	No special problems expected.
Tobacco:	No special problems expected.

***See Glossary**

KAOLIN & PECTIN

BRAND NAMES

Donnagel-MB
Kao-Con
Kaotin
Kapectolin
K-C
K-P
K-Pek

BASIC INFORMATION

Habit forming? No
Prescription needed? No
Available as generic? Yes
Drug class: Antidiarrheal

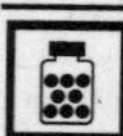

USES

Reduces intestinal cramps and diarrhea.

DOSAGE & USAGE INFORMATION

How to take:
Liquid—Swallow prescribed dosage (without diluting) after each loose bowel movement.

When to take:
After each loose bowel movement.

If you forget a dose:
Take when you remember.

What drug does:
Makes loose stools less watery, but may not prevent loss of fluids.

Time lapse before drug works:
15 to 30 minutes.

Don't take with:
Any other medication without consulting your doctor or pharmacist.

OVERDOSE

SYMPTOMS:
Fecal impaction.
WHAT TO DO:
Overdose unlikely to threaten life. If person takes much larger amount than prescribed, call doctor, poison control center or hospital emergency room for instructions.

POSSIBLE ADVERSE REACTIONS OR SIDE EFFECTS

SYMPTOMS	WHAT TO DO
Life-threatening: None expected.	
Common: None expected.	
Infrequent: None expected.	
Rare: Constipation (mild).	Continue. Call doctor when convenient.

WARNINGS & PRECAUTIONS

Don't take if:
You are allergic to kaolin or pectin.

Before you start, consult your doctor:
- If patient is child or infant.
- If you have any chronic medical problem with heart disease, peptic ulcer, asthma or others.
- If you have fever over 101F.

Over age 60:
Fluid loss caused by diarrhea, especially if taking other medicines, may lead to serious disability. Consult doctor.

Pregnancy:
Consult doctor. Risk category C (see page xxii).

Breast-feeding:
No problems expected.

Infants & children:
Fluid loss caused by diarrhea in infants and children can cause serious dehydration. Consult doctor before giving any medicine for diarrhea.

Prolonged use:
Not recommended.

Skin & sunlight:
No problems expected.

Driving, piloting or hazardous work:
No problems expected.

Discontinuing:
May be unnecessary to finish medicine. Follow doctor's instructions.

Others:
Consult doctor about fluids, diet and rest.

POSSIBLE INTERACTION WITH OTHER DRUGS

GENERIC NAME OR DRUG CLASS	COMBINED EFFECT
Digoxin	Decreases absorption of digoxin. Separate doses by at least 2 hours.
Lincomycins*	Decreases absorption of lincomycin. Separate doses by at least 2 hours.
All other oral medicines	May decrease absorption of other medicines. Separate doses by at least 2 hours.

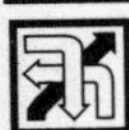

POSSIBLE INTERACTION WITH OTHER SUBSTANCES

INTERACTS WITH	COMBINED EFFECT
Alcohol:	Increased diarrhea. Prevents action of kaolin and pectin.
Beverages:	No problems expected.
Cocaine:	Aggravates underlying disease. Avoid.
Foods:	No problems expected.
Marijuana:	Aggravates underlying disease. Avoid.
Tobacco:	Aggravates underlying disease. Avoid.

***See Glossary**

KAOLIN, PECTIN, BELLADONNA & OPIUM

BRAND NAMES

Amogel PG
Donnagel-PG
Donnapectolin-PG
Kapectolin PG
Quiagel PG

BASIC INFORMATION

Habit forming? Yes
Prescription needed? Yes
Available as generic? No
Drug class: Narcotic, antidiarrheal, antispasmodic

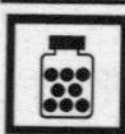

USES

Reduces intestinal cramps and diarrhea.

DOSAGE & USAGE INFORMATION

How to take:
Liquid—Swallow prescribed dosage (without diluting) after each loose bowel movement.

When to take:
As needed for diarrhea, no more often than every 4 hours.

If you forget a dose:
Take when you remember.

Continued next column

OVERDOSE

SYMPTOMS:
Fecal impaction, rapid pulse, dizziness, fever, hallucinations, confusion, slurred speech, agitation, flushed face, convulsions, deep sleep, slow breathing, slow pulse, warm skin, constricted pupils, coma.

WHAT TO DO:

- **Dial 911 (emergency) or 0 (operator) for an ambulance or medical help. Then give first aid immediately.**
- **If patient is unconscious and not breathing, give mouth-to-mouth breathing. If there is no heartbeat, use cardiac massage and mouth-to-mouth breathing (CPR). Don't try to make patient vomit. If you can't get help quickly, take patient to nearest emergency facility.**
- **See emergency information on inside covers.**

What drug does:

- Blocks nerve impulses at parasympathetic nerve endings, preventing muscle contractions and gland secretions of organs involved.
- Makes loose stools less watery, but may not prevent loss of fluids.
- Anesthetizes surface membranes of intestines and blocks nerve impulses.

Time lapse before drug works:
15 to 30 minutes.

Don't take with:
Any other medication without consulting your doctor or pharmacist.

POSSIBLE ADVERSE REACTIONS OR SIDE EFFECTS

SYMPTOMS	WHAT TO DO
Life-threatening:	
Unusually rapid heartbeat (over 100), difficult breathing, slow heartbeat (under 50/minute).	Discontinue. Seek emergency treatment.
Common (with large dosage):	
Weakness, increased sweating, red or flushed face, lightheadedness, headache, dry mouth, dry skin, drowsiness, dizziness, frequent urination, decreased sweating, constipation, confusion, tiredness.	Continue. Call doctor when convenient.
Infrequent:	
• Reduced taste sense, nervousness, eyes, sensitive to sunlight, blurred vision.	Discontinue. Call doctor right away.
• Diminished sex drive, memory loss.	Continue. Call doctor when convenient.
Rare:	
Bloating, abdominal cramps and vomiting, eye pain, hallucinations, shortness of breath, rash, itchy skin, slow heartbeat.	Discontinue. Call doctor right away.

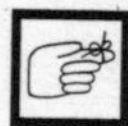

WARNINGS & PRECAUTIONS

Don't take if:

- You are allergic to any anticholinergic, narcotic, kaolin or pectin.
- You have trouble with stomach bloating, difficulty emptying your bladder completely, narrow-angle glaucoma, severe ulcerative colitis.

KAOLIN, PECTIN, BELLADONNA & OPIUM

Before you start, consult your doctor:
- If you have open-angle glaucoma, angina, chronic bronchitis or asthma, hiatal hernia, liver disease, enlarged prostate, myasthenia gravis, peptic ulcer, impaired liver or kidney function, fever over 101F, any chronic medical problem with heart disease, peptic ulcer, asthma or others.
- If patient is child or infant.
- If you will have surgery within 2 months, including dental surgery, requiring general or spinal anesthesia.

Over age 60:
- Adverse reactions and side effects may be more frequent and severe than in younger persons.
- More likely to be drowsy, dizzy, unsteady or constipated.
- Fluid loss caused by diarrhea, especially if taking other medicines, may lead to serious disability. Consult doctor.

Pregnancy:
Decide with your doctor if drug benefits justify risk to unborn child. Risk category C (see page xxii).

Breast-feeding:
Drug passes into milk. Avoid drug or discontinue nursing until you finish medicine. Consult doctor for advice on maintaining milk supply.

Infants & children:
Fluid loss caused by diarrhea in infants and children can cause serious dehydration. Consult doctor before giving any medicine for diarrhea.

Prolonged use:
- Causes psychological and physical dependence. Not recommended.
- Talk to your doctor about the need for follow-up medical examinations or laboratory studies to check liver function, kidney function.

Skin & sunlight:
May cause rash or intensify sunburn in areas exposed to sun or sunlamp.

Driving, piloting or hazardous work:
Don't drive or pilot aircraft until you learn how medicine affects you. Don't work around dangerous machinery. Don't climb ladders or work in high places. Danger increases if you drink alcohol or take medicine affecting alertness and reflexes, such as antihistamines, tranquilizers, sedatives, pain medicine, narcotics and mind-altering drugs.

Discontinuing:
May be unnecessary to finish medicine. Follow doctor's instructions.

Others:
- Great potential for abuse.
- Consult doctor about fluids, diet and rest.

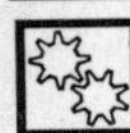

POSSIBLE INTERACTION WITH OTHER DRUGS

GENERIC NAME OR DRUG CLASS	COMBINED EFFECT
Amantadine	Increased belladonna effect.
Analgesics*	Increased analgesic effect.
Antidepressants*	Increased sedative effect.
Antihistamines*	Increased sedative effect.
Carteolol	Increased narcotic effect. Dangerous sedation.
Central nervous system (CNS) depressants*	Increased depressant effect of both.
Cortisone drugs*	Increased internal eye pressure.
Digoxin	Decreases absorption of digoxin. Separate doses by at least 2 hours.
Haloperidol	Increased internal eye pressure.

Continued on page 943

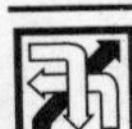

POSSIBLE INTERACTION WITH OTHER SUBSTANCES

INTERACTS WITH	COMBINED EFFECT
Alcohol:	Increases alcohol's intoxicating effect, increased diarrhea, prevents action of kaolin and pectin. Avoid.
Beverages:	No problems expected.
Cocaine:	Aggravates underlying disease. Avoid.
Foods:	No problems expected.
Marijuana:	Impairs physical and mental performance, aggravates underlying disease. Avoid.
Tobacco:	Aggravates underlying disease. Avoid.

***See Glossary**

KAOLIN, PECTIN & PAREGORIC

BRAND NAMES

Kapectolin with Paregoric

Parepectolin

BASIC INFORMATION

Habit forming? Yes
Prescription needed? Yes
Available as generic? No
Drug class: Narcotic, antidiarrheal, antispasmodic

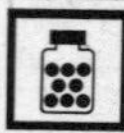

USES

- Reduces intestinal cramps and diarrhea.
- Relieves pain.

DOSAGE & USAGE INFORMATION

How to take:
Liquid—Swallow prescribed dosage (without diluting) after each loose bowel movement.

When to take:
After each loose bowel movement. No more often then every 4 hours.

If you forget a dose:
Take when you remember.

What drug does:
Makes loose stools less watery, but may not prevent loss of fluids.

Time lapse before drug works:
15 to 30 minutes.

Don't take with:
Any other medication without consulting your doctor or pharmacist.

OVERDOSE

SYMPTOMS:
Deep sleep; slow breathing; slow pulse; flushed, warm skin.
WHAT TO DO:
- **Dial 911 (emergency) or 0 (operator) for an ambulance or medical help. Then give first aid immediately.**
- **If patient is unconscious and not breathing, give mouth-to-mouth breathing. If there is no heartbeat, use cardiac massage and mouth-to-mouth breathing (CPR). Don't try to make patient vomit. If you can't get help quickly, take patient to nearest emergency facility.**
- **See emergency information on inside covers.**

POSSIBLE ADVERSE REACTIONS OR SIDE EFFECTS

SYMPTOMS	WHAT TO DO
Life-threatening:	
Unusually rapid heartbeat (over 100), difficult breathing, slow heartbeat (under 50/minute).	Discontinue. Seek emergency treatment.
Common (with large dosage):	
Weakness, increased sweating, red or flushed face, lightheadedness, headache, dry mouth, dry skin, drowsiness, dizziness, frequent urination, decreased sweating, constipation, confusion, tiredness.	Continue. Call doctor when convenient.
Infrequent:	
• Reduced taste sense, nervousness, eyes sensitive to sunlight, blurred vision.	Discontinue. Call doctor right away.
• Diminished sex drive, memory loss.	Continue. Call doctor when convenient.
Rare:	
Bloating, abdominal cramps and vomiting, eye pain, hallucinations, shortness of breath, rash, itchy skin, slow heartbeat.	Discontinue. Call doctor right away.

WARNINGS & PRECAUTIONS

Don't take if:
You are allergic to any narcotic, kaolin or pectin.

Before you start, consult your doctor:
- If you have impaired liver or kidney function, chronic medical problem with heart disease, peptic ulcer, asthma or others, fever over 101F.
- If patient is child or infant.
- If you will have surgery within 2 months, including dental surgery, requiring general or spinal anesthesia.

Over age 60:
Fluid loss caused by diarrhea, especially if taking other medicines, may lead to serious disability. Consult doctor.

Pregnancy:
Abuse by pregnant woman will result in addicted newborn. Withdrawal of newborn can be life-threatening. Risk category C (see page xxii).

Breast-feeding:
Drug filters into milk. May harm child. Avoid.

Infants & children:
Fluid loss caused by diarrhea in infants and children can cause serious dehydration. Consult doctor before giving any medicine for diarrhea.

Prolonged use:
- Causes psychological and physical dependence. Not recommended.
- Talk to your doctor about the need for follow-up medical examinations or laboratory studies to check liver function, kidney function.

Skin & sunlight:
May cause rash or intensify sunburn in areas exposed to sun or sunlamp.

Driving, piloting or hazardous work:
Don't drive or pilot aircraft until you learn how medicine affects you. Don't work around dangerous machinery. Don't climb ladders or work in high places. Danger increases if you drink alcohol or take medicine affecting alertness and reflexes, such as antihistamines, tranquilizers, sedatives, pain medicine, narcotics and mind-altering drugs.

Discontinuing:
May be unnecessary to finish medicine. Follow doctor's instructions.

Others:
Consult doctor about fluids, diet and rest.

POSSIBLE INTERACTION WITH OTHER DRUGS

GENERIC NAME OR DRUG CLASS	COMBINED EFFECT
Analgesics, other*	Increased analgesic effect.
Antidepressants*	Increased sedative effect.
Antihistamines*	Increased sedative effect.
Carteolol	Increased narcotic effect. Dangerous sedation.
Digoxin	Decreases absorption of digoxin. Separate doses by at least 2 hours.
Lincomycins*	Decreases absorption of lincomycin. Separate doses by at least 2 hours.
Mind-altering drugs*	Increased sedative effect.
Narcotics, other*	Increased narcotic effect.
Phenothiazines*	Increased phenothiazine effect.
Sedatives*	Increased sedative effect.
Sleep inducers*	Increased sedative effect.
Sotalol	Increased narcotic effect. Dangerous sedation.
Tranquilizers*	Increased sedative effect.
All other oral medicines	Decreases absorption of other medicines. Separate doses by at least 2 hours.

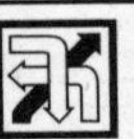

POSSIBLE INTERACTION WITH OTHER SUBSTANCES

INTERACTS WITH	COMBINED EFFECT
Alcohol:	Increases alcohol's intoxicating effect, increases diarrhea, prevents action of kaolin and pectin. Avoid.
Beverages:	No problems expected.
Cocaine:	Increases cocaine toxic effects, aggravates underlying disease. Avoid.
Foods:	No problems expected.
Marijuana:	Aggravates underlying disease. Avoid.
Tobacco:	Aggravates underlying disease. Avoid.

*See Glossary

KERATOLYTICS

BRAND NAMES

See complete list of brand names in the *Brand Name Directory*, page 909.

BASIC INFORMATION

Habit forming? No
Prescription needed? Yes, on some.
Available as generic? Yes
Drug class: Keratolytic, antiacne (topical), antiseborrheic

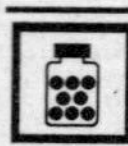

USES

Treatment for acne, psoriasis, ichthyosis, keratosis, folliculitis, flat warts, eczema, urticaria, calluses, corns, seborrheic dermatitis, dandruff.

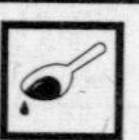

DOSAGE & USAGE INFORMATION

How to use:
Cream, gel, lotion, ointment, pads, plaster, shampoo, soap, topical solution, suspension—Always follow instructions on the label or use as directed by your doctor.

When to use:
At the same time each day or as needed.

If you forget an application:
Use as soon as you remember.

What drug does:
Keratolytics are drugs that soften, loosen and remove keratin (the tough outer layer of the skin).

Time lapse before drug works:
2 to 3 weeks. May require 6 weeks for maximum improvement.

Don't use with:
- Benzoyl peroxide. Apply 12 hours apart.
- Any other medicine without consulting your doctor or pharmacist.

OVERDOSE

SYMPTOMS:
None expected.
WHAT TO DO:
If person swallows drug, call doctor, poison control center or hospital emergency room for instructions.

POSSIBLE ADVERSE REACTIONS OR SIDE EFFECTS

SYMPTOMS	WHAT TO DO
Life-threatening: None expected.	
Common:	
• Pigment change in treated area, warmth or stinging, peeling.	Continue. Tell doctor at next visit.
• Sensitivity to wind or cold.	No action necessary.
Infrequent:	
Blistering, crusting, severe burning, swelling, skin irritation that begins after treatment.	Discontinue. Call doctor right away.
Rare:	
Symptoms of system toxicity (diarrhea, nausea, dizziness, headache, breathing difficulty, tiredness, weakness).	Discontinue. Call doctor right away.

WARNINGS & PRECAUTIONS

Don't take if:
- You are allergic to resorcinol or salicyclic acid.
- You are sunburned or windburned or have an open skin wound, skin irritation or infection.

Before you start, consult your doctor:
- If you have eczema.
- If you have diabetes mellitus.
- If you have peripheral vascular disease (blood vessel disease).

Over age 60:
No problems expected.

Pregnancy:
Risk factors vary for drugs in this group. See category list on page xxii and consult doctor.

Breast-feeding:
No problems expected. Consult doctor.

Infants & children:
Not recommended. Increased risk of toxicity.

Prolonged use:
No problems expected.

Skin & sunlight:
- May cause rash or intensify sunburn in areas exposed to sun or sunlamp.
- In some animal studies, tretinoin caused skin tumors to develop faster when treated area was exposed to ultraviolet light (sunlight or sunlamp). No proven similar effects in humans.

Driving, piloting or hazardous work:
No problems expected.

Discontinuing:
Follow your doctor's instructions or the directions on the label.

Others:
Acne may get worse before improvement starts in 2 or 3 weeks. Don't wash face more than 2 or 3 times daily.

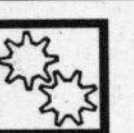

POSSIBLE INTERACTION WITH OTHER DRUGS

GENERIC NAME OR DRUG CLASS	COMBINED EFFECT
Anti-acne topical preparations (other)	Severe skin irritation.
Cosmetics (medicated)	Severe skin irritation.
Skin preparations with alcohol	Severe skin irritation.
Soaps or cleansers (abrasive)	Severe skin irritation.

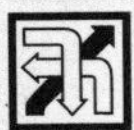

POSSIBLE INTERACTION WITH OTHER SUBSTANCES

INTERACTS WITH	COMBINED EFFECT
Alcohol:	None expected.
Beverages:	None expected.
Cocaine:	None expected.
Foods:	None expected.
Marijuana:	None expected.
Tobacco:	None expected.

***See Glossary**

KETOCONAZOLE

BRAND NAMES

Nizoral

BASIC INFORMATION

Habit forming? No
Prescription needed? Yes
Available as generic? No
Drug class: Antifungal

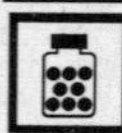

USES

Treatment of fungus infections susceptible to ketoconazole.

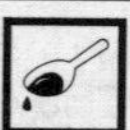

DOSAGE & USAGE INFORMATION

How to take:
Tablet or oral suspension—Swallow with liquid or food to lessen stomach irritation. If you can't swallow whole, crumble tablet and take with liquid or food.

When to take:
At same time once a day.

If you forget a dose:
Take as soon as you remember up to 2 hours late. If more than 2 hours, wait for next scheduled dose (don't double this dose).

What drug does:
Prevents fungi from growing and reproducing.

Time lapse before drug works:
8 to 10 months or longer.

Don't take with:
Any other medication without consulting your doctor or pharmacist.

OVERDOSE

SYMPTOMS:
Nausea, vomiting, diarrhea.
WHAT TO DO:
Overdose unlikely to threaten life. If person takes much larger amount than prescribed, call doctor, poison control center or hospital emergency room for instructions.

POSSIBLE ADVERSE REACTIONS OR SIDE EFFECTS

SYMPTOMS	WHAT TO DO
Life-threatening: None expected.	
Common: None expected.	
Infrequent: Nausea or vomiting, diarrhea.	Continue. Call doctor when convenient.
Rare:	
• Pale stools, abdominal pain, dark or amber urine, jaundice, rash or itchy skin.	Discontinue. Call doctor right away.
• Diminished sex drive in males, swollen breasts in males, tiredness, weakness, appetite loss, increased sensitivity to light, drowsiness, dizziness, headache, insomnia.	Continue. Call doctor when convenient.

WARNINGS & PRECAUTIONS

Don't take if:
You are allergic to ketoconazole.

Before you start, consult your doctor:
- If you have absence of stomach acid (achlorhydria).
- If you have liver disease.

Over age 60:
Adverse reactions and side effects may be more frequent and severe than in younger persons.

Pregnancy:
Decide with your doctor if drug benefits justify risk to unborn child. Risk category C (see page xxii).

Breast-feeding:
Drug passes into milk. Avoid drug or discontinue nursing until you finish medicine. Consult doctor for advice on maintaining milk supply.

Infants & children:
Only under close medical supervision.

Prolonged use:
Request liver-function studies.

Skin & sunlight:
Increased sensitivity to sunlight.

Driving, piloting or hazardous work:
Don't drive or pilot aircraft until you learn how medicine affects you. Don't work around dangerous machinery. Don't climb ladders or work in high places. Danger increases if you drink alcohol or take medicine affecting alertness and reflexes, such as antihistamines, tranquilizers, sedatives, pain medicine, narcotics and mind-altering drugs.

Discontinuing:
May be unnecessary to finish medicine. Follow doctor's instructions.

Others:
May interfere with some medical tests.

POSSIBLE INTERACTION WITH OTHER DRUGS

GENERIC NAME OR DRUG CLASS	COMBINED EFFECT
Antacids*	Decreased absorption of ketoconazole.
Anticoagulants, oral*	Increased anticoagulant effect.
Anticholinergics*	Decreased absorption of ketoconazole.
Astemizole	Heart problems. Never combine.
Atropine	Decreased absorption of ketoconazole.
Belladonna	Decreased absorption of ketoconazole.
Cimetidine	Decreased absorption of ketoconazole.
Clidinium	Decreased absorption of ketoconazole.
Cyclosporine	Increased risk of toxicity to kidney.
Didanosine	Reduced absorption of both drugs. Increased risk of pancreatitis.
Famotidine	Reduced absorption of ketoconazole. Take famatodine at least 2 hours after any dose of ketoconazole.
Glycopyrrolate	Decreased absorption of ketoconazole.
Hepatotoxic medications*	Increased risk of toxicity to kidney.
Histamine H_2 receptor antagonists	Decreased absorption of ketoconazole.
Hyoscyamine	Decreased absorption of ketoconazole.
Hypoglycemics, oral*	Increased effect of oral hypoglycemics.
Isoniazid	Decreased effect of ketoconazole.
Methscopolamine	Decreased absorption of ketoconazole.
Methylprednisolone	Increased effect of methylprednisolone.
Nizatidine	Decreased absorption of ketoconazole.
Omeprazole	Decreased absorption of ketoconazole.
Phenytoin	May alter effect of both drugs.
Propantheline	Decreased absorption of ketoconazole.
Ranitidine	Decreased absorption of ketoconazole.
Rifampin	Decreased effect of ketoconazole.
Scopolamine	Decreased absorption of ketoconazole.
Sodium bicarbonate	Decreased absorption of ketoconazole.
Terfenadine	Life-threatening heartbeat irregularity. Never combine.

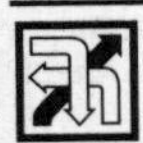

POSSIBLE INTERACTION WITH OTHER SUBSTANCES

INTERACTS WITH	COMBINED EFFECT
Alcohol:	Increased chance of liver damage and disulfiram reaction.*
Beverages:	No problems expected.
Cocaine:	Decreased ketoconazole effect. Avoid.
Foods:	No problems expected.
Marijuana:	Decreased ketoconazole effect. Avoid.
Tobacco:	Decreased ketoconazole effect. Avoid.

*See Glossary

LACTULOSE

BRAND NAMES

Cholac
Chronulac
Constilac
Duphalac
Enulose
Generlac
Portalac

BASIC INFORMATION

Habit forming? No
Prescription needed? No
Available as generic? Yes
Drug class: Laxative (hyperosmotic)

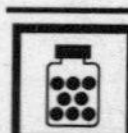

USES

- Constipation relief
- Treats brain changes caused by liver disease.

DOSAGE & USAGE INFORMATION

How to take:
Liquid—Dilute dose in beverage before swallowing.

When to take:
Usually once a day, preferably in the morning.

If you forget a dose:
Take as soon as you remember up to 8 hours before bedtime. If later, wait for next scheduled dose (don't double this dose). Don't take at bedtime.

What drug does:
Draws water into bowel from other body tissues. Causes distention through fluid accumulation, which promotes soft stool and accelerates bowel motion.

Time lapse before drug works:
30 minutes to 3 hours.

Don't take with:
Another medicine. Space 2 hours apart.

OVERDOSE

SYMPTOMS:
Fluid depletion, weakness, vomiting, fainting.
WHAT TO DO:
Overdose unlikely to threaten life. If person takes much larger amount than prescribed, call doctor, poison control center or hospital emergency room for instructions.

POSSIBLE ADVERSE REACTIONS OR SIDE EFFECTS

SYMPTOMS	WHAT TO DO
Life-threatening: None expected.	
Common: Increased thirst, cramps, nausea, diarrhea, gaseousness.	Continue. Tell doctor at next visit.
Infrequent: Irregular heartbeat, muscle cramps.	Discontinue. Call doctor right away.
Rare: Dizziness, confusion, fatigue, weakness.	Continue. Call doctor when convenient.

WARNINGS & PRECAUTIONS

Don't take if:
- You are allergic to any hyperosmotic laxative.
- You have symptoms of appendicitis, inflamed bowel or intestinal blockage.
- You have missed a bowel movement for only 1 or 2 days.

Before you start, consult your doctor:
- If you have congestive heart disease.
- If you have diabetes.
- If you have high blood pressure.
- If you have a colostomy or ileostomy.
- If you have kidney disease.
- If you have a laxative habit.
- If you have rectal bleeding.
- If you take another laxative.
- If you require a low-galactose diet.

Over age 60:
Adverse reactions and side effects may be more frequent and severe than in younger persons.

Pregnancy:
Avoid if possible. Consult doctor. Risk category B (see page xxii).

Breast-feeding:
No problems expected. Consult doctor.

Infants & children:
Use only under medical supervision.

Prolonged use:
Don't take for more than 1 week unless under a doctor's supervision. May cause laxative dependence.

Skin & sunlight:
No problems expected.

Driving, piloting or hazardous work:
No problems expected.

Discontinuing:
May be unnecessary to finish medicine. Follow doctor's instructions.

Others:
Don't take to "flush out" your system or as a "tonic."

POSSIBLE INTERACTION WITH OTHER DRUGS

GENERIC NAME OR DRUG CLASS	COMBINED EFFECT
Antacids*	Decreased lactulose effect.
Antibiotics*	Decreased lactulose effect.
Neomycin	Decreased lactulose effect.

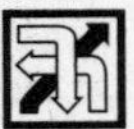

POSSIBLE INTERACTION WITH OTHER SUBSTANCES

INTERACTS WITH	COMBINED EFFECT
Alcohol:	None expected.
Beverages:	None expected.
Cocaine:	None expected.
Foods:	None expected.
Marijuana:	None expected.
Tobacco:	None expected.

***See Glossary**

LEUCOVORIN

BRAND NAMES

Citrocovorin Calcium
Citrovorum Factor
Folinic Acid
Wellcovorin

BASIC INFORMATION

Habit forming? No
Prescription needed? Yes
Available as generic? Yes
Drug class: Antianemic

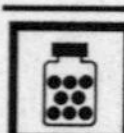

USES

- Antidote to folic acid antagonists.
- Treats anemia.

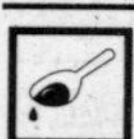

DOSAGE & USAGE INFORMATION

How to take:
Tablets—Swallow with liquid or food to lessen stomach irritation. If you can't swallow whole, crumble tablet and take with liquid or food.

When to take:
At the same time each day, according to instructions on prescription label.

If you forget a dose:
Take as soon as you remember up to 2 hours late. If more than 2 hours, wait for next scheduled dose (don't double this dose).

What drug does:
Favors development of DNA, RNA and protein synthesis.

Time lapse before drug works:
20 to 30 minutes.

Don't take with:
Any other medicine without consulting your doctor or pharmacist.

OVERDOSE

SYMPTOMS:
Unlikely to threaten life. If overdose is suspected, follow instructions below.
WHAT TO DO:
- **Dial 911 (emergency) or 0 (operator) for an ambulance or medical help. Then give first aid immediately.**
- **See emergency information on inside covers.**

POSSIBLE ADVERSE REACTIONS OR SIDE EFFECTS

SYMPTOMS	WHAT TO DO
Life-threatening: Wheezing.	Seek emergency treatment immediately.
Common: None expected.	
Infrequent: None expected.	
Rare: Skin rash, hives.	Discontinue. Call doctor right away.

WARNINGS & PRECAUTIONS

Don't take if:
- You have pernicious anemia.
- You have vitamin B-12 deficiency.

Before you start, consult your doctor:
- If you have acid urine, acites, dehydration.
- If you have kidney function impairment.

Over age 60:
Adverse reactions and side effects may be more frequent and severe than in younger persons. You may need smaller doses for shorter periods of time.

Pregnancy:
Recommended for the treatment of megaloblastic anemia caused by pregnancy. Decide with your doctor if drug benefits justify risk to unborn child. Risk category C (see page xxii).

Breast-feeding:
No problems expected. Consult doctor.

Infants & children:
May increase frequency of seizures. Avoid if possible.

Prolonged use:
No problems expected.

Skin & sunlight:
No problems expected.

Driving, piloting or hazardous work:
Don't drive or pilot aircraft until you learn how medicine affects you. Don't work around dangerous machinery. Don't climb ladders or work in high places. Danger increases if you drink alcohol or take medicine affecting alertness and reflexes.

Discontinuing:
Don't discontinue without consulting doctor. Dose may require gradual reduction if you have taken drug for a long time. Doses of other drugs may also require adjustment.

Others:
No problems expected.

POSSIBLE INTERACTION WITH OTHER DRUGS

GENERIC NAME OR DRUG CLASS	COMBINED EFFECT
Anticonvulsants, barbiturate and hydantoin*	Large doses of leucovorin may counteract the effects of these medicines.
Central nervous system (CNS) depressants*	High alcohol content of leucovorin may cause adverse effects.
Fluorouracil	Increased levels of fluorouracil.
Primidone	Large doses of leucovorin may counteract the effects of both drugs.

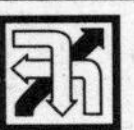

POSSIBLE INTERACTION WITH OTHER SUBSTANCES

INTERACTS WITH	COMBINED EFFECT
Alcohol:	Increased adverse reactions of both.
Beverages:	None expected.
Cocaine:	Increased adverse reactions of both drugs.
Foods:	None expected.
Marijuana:	Increased adverse reactions of both drugs.
Tobacco:	Increased adverse reactions of both.

*See Glossary

LEVAMISOLE

BRAND NAMES

Ergamisol

BASIC INFORMATION

Habit forming? No
Prescription needed? Yes
Available as generic? No
Drug class: Anticancer treatment adjunct

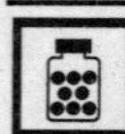

USES

- Treats colorectal cancer when used in combination with fluorouracil.
- Treats malignant melanoma after surgical removal when there is no evidence of spread to organs other than the skin.

DOSAGE & USAGE INFORMATION

How to take:
Tablet—Swallow with liquid or food to lessen stomach irritation. If you can't swallow whole, crumble tablet and take with liquid or food.

When to take:
At the same time each day, according to instructions on prescription label.

If you forget a dose:
Don't take until you notify your doctor.

What drug does:
Acts to help restore the immune system. May activate T-cell lymphocytes and other white cells. Also elevates mood.

Time lapse before drug works:
1-1/2 to 2 hours.

Don't take with:
Any other medicine without consulting your doctor or pharmacist.

OVERDOSE

SYMPTOMS:
None expected.
WHAT TO DO:
Overdose unlikely to threaten life. If person takes much larger amount than prescribed, call doctor, poison control center or hospital emergency room for instructions.

POSSIBLE ADVERSE REACTIONS OR SIDE EFFECTS

SYMPTOMS	WHAT TO DO
Life-threatening:	
Fever, muscle aches, headache, cough, hoarseness, sore throat, painful or difficult urination, low back or side pain.	Seek emergency treatment.
Common:	
• Diarrhea, metallic taste, nausea, joint or muscle pain, skin rash, insomnia, mental depression, nightmares, sleepiness or tiredness, increased dental problems.	Continue. Call doctor when convenient.
• Hair loss.	No action necessary.
Infrequent:	
Mouth, tongue and lip sores.	Call doctor right away.
Rare:	
Unsteady gait while walking; blurred vision; confusion; tremors; tingling or numbness in hands, feet or face; seizures; smacking and puckering of lips; uncontrolled tongue movements.	Call doctor right away.

WARNINGS & PRECAUTIONS

Don't take if:
You are allergic to levamisole.

Before you start, consult your doctor:
- If you take other drugs for cancer.
- If you have an active infection.
- If you have a seizure disorder.
- If you have allergies to other medications.

Over age 60:
No special problems expected.

Pregnancy:
Adequate studies not yet done. Consult your doctor. Risk category C (see page xxii).

Breast-feeding:
Effect unknown. Consult doctor.

Infants & children:
Effect not documented. Consult your doctor.

Prolonged use:
No special problems expected.

Skin & sunlight:
No special problems expected.

Driving, piloting or hazardous work:
No special problems expected.

Discontinuing:
Don't discontinue without consulting doctor. Dose may require gradual reduction if you have taken drug for a long time. Doses of other drugs may also require adjustment.

Others:
- Advise any doctor or dentist whom you consult that you take this medicine.
- Defer dental treatments until your blood count is normal. Pay particular attention to dental hygiene. You may be subject to additional risk of oral infection, delayed healing and bleeding.
- Avoid aspirin. May increase risk of internal bleeding.
- Avoid constipation. May increase risk of internal bleeding.

POSSIBLE INTERACTION WITH OTHER DRUGS

GENERIC NAME OR DRUG CLASS	COMBINED EFFECT
Anticoagulants*	Increased risk of bleeding.
Aspirin	Increased risk of bleeding.
Bone marrow depressants*	Increased risk of bone marrow depression.

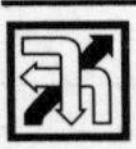

POSSIBLE INTERACTION WITH OTHER SUBSTANCES

INTERACTS WITH	COMBINED EFFECT
Alcohol:	Increased risk of gastritis and internal bleeding.
Beverages:	None expected.
Cocaine:	Increased risk of mental disturbances. Avoid.
Foods:	None expected.
Marijuana:	None expected.
Tobacco:	None expected.

LEVOCARNITINE

BRAND NAMES

Carnitor
L-Carnitine
VitaCarn

BASIC INFORMATION

Habit forming? No
Prescription needed? Yes
Available as generic? Yes
Drug class: Nutritional supplement

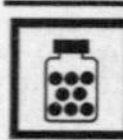

USES

Treats carnitine deficiency, a genetic impairment preventing normal utilization from diet.

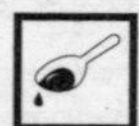

DOSAGE & USAGE INFORMATION

How to take:

- Oral solution—Take after meals with liquid to decrease stomach irritation.
- Tablets—Swallow with liquid or food to lessen stomach irritation. If you can't swallow whole, crumble tablet and take with liquid or food.
- Injection—Given by medical professional.

When to take:
Immediately following or during meals to reduce stomach irritation.

If you forget a dose:
Take as soon as you remember up to 2 hours late. If more than 2 hours, wait for next scheduled dose (don't double this dose).

What drug does:
Facilitates normal use of fat to produce energy. Dietary source is meat and milk.

Time lapse before drug works:
Immediate action.

Don't take with:
Any other medicine without consulting your doctor or pharmacist.

OVERDOSE

SYMPTOMS:
Severe muscle weakness.
WHAT TO DO:

- **Dial 911 (emergency) or 0 (operator) for an ambulance or medical help. Then give first aid immediately.**
- **See emergency information on inside covers.**

POSSIBLE ADVERSE REACTIONS OR SIDE EFFECTS

SYMPTOMS	WHAT TO DO
Life-threatening:	
None expected.	
Common:	
Changed body odor.	Continue. Call doctor when convenient.
Infrequent:	
Diarrhea, abdominal pain, nausea, vomiting.	Continue, but call doctor right away.
Rare:	
None expected.	

WARNINGS & PRECAUTIONS

Don't take if:
No contraindications.

Before you start, consult your doctor:
No documented reasons not to take.

Over age 60:
No problems expected.

Pregnancy:
No proven harm to unborn child, but avoid if possible. Consult doctor. Risk category B (see page xxii).

Breast-feeding:
No problems expected. Consult doctor.

Infants & children:
No problems expected. Deficiency can cause impaired growth and development.

Prolonged use:
Talk to your doctor about the need for follow-up medical examinations or laboratory studies to check triglycerides.

Skin & sunlight:
No problems expected.

Driving, piloting or hazardous work:
No problems expected.

Discontinuing:
Don't discontinue without consulting doctor. Dose may require gradual reduction if you have taken drug for a long time. Doses of other drugs may also require adjustment.

Others:
Health food store "vitamin B-T" contains dextro- and levo-carnitine which completely negates the effectiveness of levocarnitine (L-carnitine). Only the L-carnitine form is effective in levocarnitine deficiency.

POSSIBLE INTERACTION WITH OTHER DRUGS

GENERIC NAME OR DRUG CLASS	COMBINED EFFECT
Valproic acid	Decreased levocarnitine effect. Patients taking valproic acid may need to take the supplement levocarnitine.

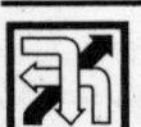

POSSIBLE INTERACTION WITH OTHER SUBSTANCES

INTERACTS WITH	COMBINED EFFECT
Alcohol:	None expected.
Beverages:	None expected.
Cocaine:	None expected.
Foods:	None expected.
Marijuana:	None expected.
Tobacco:	None expected.

LEVODOPA

BRAND NAMES

Dopar
Larodopa

BASIC INFORMATION

Habit forming? No
Prescription needed? Yes
Available as generic? Yes
Drug class: Antiparkinsonism

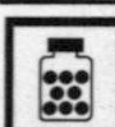

USES

Controls Parkinson's disease symptoms such as rigidity, tremor and unsteady gait.

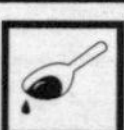

DOSAGE & USAGE INFORMATION

How to take:
Tablet or capsule—Swallow with liquid or food to lessen stomach irritation. If you can't swallow whole, crumble tablet or open capsule and take with liquid or food.

When to take:
At the same times each day.

If you forget a dose:
Take as soon as you remember up to 2 hours late. If more than 2 hours, wait for next scheduled dose (don't double this dose).

What drug does:
Restores chemical balance necessary for normal nerve impulses.

Continued next column

OVERDOSE

SYMPTOMS:
Muscle twitch, spastic eyelid closure, nausea, vomiting, diarrhea, irregular and rapid pulse, weakness, fainting, confusion, agitation, hallucination, coma.

WHAT TO DO:

- **Dial 911 (emergency) or 0 (operator) for an ambulance or medical help. Then give first aid immediately.**
- **If patient is unconscious and not breathing, give mouth-to-mouth breathing. If there is no heartbeat, use cardiac massage and mouth-to-mouth breathing (CPR). Don't try to make patient vomit. If you can't get help quickly, take patient to nearest emergency facility.**
- **See emergency information on inside covers.**

Time lapse before drug works:
2 to 3 weeks to improve; 6 weeks or longer for maximum benefit.

Don't take with:
Any other medication without consulting your doctor or pharmacist.

POSSIBLE ADVERSE REACTIONS OR SIDE EFFECTS

SYMPTOMS	WHAT TO DO
Life-threatening: In case of overdose, see previous column.	
Common:	
• Mood change, diarrhea, depression, anxiety.	Continue. Call doctor when convenient.
• Dry mouth, body odor.	No action necessary.
• Uncontrollable body movements.	Discontinue. Call doctor right away.
Infrequent:	
• Fainting, severe dizziness, headache, insomnia, nightmares, itchy skin, rash, nausea, vomiting, irregular heartbeat, eyelid spasm.	Discontinue. Call doctor right away.
• Flushed face, muscle twitching, discolored or dark urine, difficult urination, blurred vision, appetite loss.	Continue. Call doctor when convenient.
• Constipation, tiredness.	Continue. Tell doctor at next visit.
Rare:	
• High blood pressure.	Discontinue. Call doctor right away.
• Upper abdominal pain, anemia, increased sex drive.	Continue. Call doctor when convenient.

WARNINGS & PRECAUTIONS

Don't take if:

- You are allergic to levodopa or carbidopa.
- You have taken a monoamine oxidase (MAO) inhibitor* in past 2 weeks.
- You have glaucoma (narrow-angle type).

Before you start, consult your doctor:
- If you have diabetes or epilepsy.
- If you have had high blood pressure, heart or lung disease.
- If you have had liver or kidney disease.
- If you have a peptic ulcer.
- If you have malignant melanoma.
- If you will have surgery within 2 months, including dental surgery, requiring general or spinal anesthesia.

Over age 60:
Adverse reactions and side effects may be more frequent and severe than in younger persons.

Pregnancy:
Decide with your doctor if drug benefits justify risk to unborn child. Risk category C (see page xxii).

Breast-feeding:
Drug filters into milk. May harm child. Avoid.

Infants & children:
Not recommended.

Prolonged use:
- May lead to uncontrolled movements of head, face, mouth, tongue, arms or legs.
- Talk to your doctor about the need for follow-up medical examinations or laboratory studies to check complete blood counts (white blood cell count, platelet count, red blood cell count, hemoglobin, hematocrit), kidney function, liver function.

Skin & sunlight:
No problems expected.

Driving, piloting or hazardous work:
Don't drive or pilot aircraft until you learn how medicine affects you. Don't work around dangerous machinery. Don't climb ladders or work in high places. Danger increases if you drink alcohol or take medicine affecting alertness and reflexes, such as antihistamines, tranquilizers, sedatives, pain medicine, narcotics and mind-altering drugs.

Discontinuing:
Don't discontinue without doctor's advice until you complete prescribed dose, even though symptoms diminish or disappear.

Others:
Expect to start with small dose and increase gradually to lessen frequency and severity of adverse reactions.

POSSIBLE INTERACTION WITH OTHER DRUGS

GENERIC NAME OR DRUG CLASS	COMBINED EFFECT
Albuterol	Increased risk of heartbeat irregularity.
Antidepressants, tricyclic (TCA)*	Decreased blood pressure. Weakness and faintness when arising from bed or chair.
Anticonvulsants hydantoin*	Decreased levodopa effect.
Antihypertensives*	Decreased blood pressure and levodopa effect.
Antiparkinsonism drugs, other*	Increased levodopa effect.
Guanfacine	Increased effects of both drugs.
Haloperidol	Decreased levodopa effect.
MAO inhibitors*	Dangerous rise in blood pressure.
Methyldopa	Decreased levodopa effect.
Molindone	Decreased levodopa effect.
Papaverine	Decreased levodopa effect.
Phenothiazines*	Decreased levodopa effect.
Phenytoin	Decreased levodopa effect.
Pyridoxine (Vitamin B-6)	Decreased levodopa effect.
Rauwolfia alkaloids*	Decreased levodopa effect.
Selegiline	May require reduced dosage of levodopa.

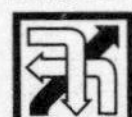

POSSIBLE INTERACTION WITH OTHER SUBSTANCES

INTERACTS WITH	COMBINED EFFECT
Alcohol:	None expected.
Beverages:	None expected.
Cocaine:	Increased risk of heartbeat irregularity.
Foods: High-protein diet.	Decreased levodopa effect.
Marijuana:	Increased fatigue, lethargy, fainting.
Tobacco:	None expected.

*See Glossary

LEVONORGESTREL

BRAND NAMES

Norplant

BASIC INFORMATION

Habit forming? No
Prescription needed? Yes
Available as generic? No
Drug class: Female sex hormone (progestin)

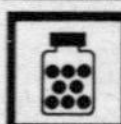

USES

Highly effective long-term reversible contraceptive method.

DOSAGE & USAGE INFORMATION

How to take:
Administered by means of implants consisting of six flexible closed capsules (about the size of matchsticks) that are inserted beneath the skin on the inside of the upper arm. Implantation is done by a health-care professional within seven days of the start of the last menstrual period. The drug slowly diffuses into the bloodstream, delivering a nearly constant level of levonorgestrel to the body for up to 5 years.

When to take:
Implanted when long-term (up to 5 years) contraception is desired.

If you forget a dose:
Not a concern.

What drug does:
Inhibits ovulation in some women so that eggs are not produced regularly. Causes the mucus of the cervix to thicken, preventing the sperm from reaching the egg if one is produced.

Time lapse before drug works:
24 hours

Don't take with:
Any other medicine without consulting your doctor or pharmacist.

OVERDOSE

SYMPTOMS:
None expected.

POSSIBLE ADVERSE REACTIONS OR SIDE EFFECTS

SYMPTOMS	WHAT TO DO
Life-threatening: None expected.	
Common: Increased, decreased, irregular or prolonged menstruation; spotting between periods.	Call doctor when convenient.
Infrequent: Headache, acne.	Call doctor when convenient.
Rare:	
• Severe bleeding, infection with pus at implant site, vaginal infection.	Call doctor right away.
• Swelling, numbness, discoloration or tenderness at implant site; breast discharge or tenderness; weight gain or loss; excess hair growth; hair loss from scalp; nausea; dizziness; muscle or abdominal pain; appetite changes; nervousness; depression.	Call doctor when convenient.

WARNINGS & PRECAUTIONS

Don't take if:
- You are allergic to any progestin hormone.
- You are or suspect you might be pregnant.
- You have liver disease or liver tumors.
- You have unexplained vaginal bleeding.
- You have breast cancer.
- You have now, or have a history of, blood clots in the legs, lungs or eyes.

Before you start, consult your doctor:
- If you have a condition that could be aggravated by fluid retention.
- If you have a history of depression or emotional disorders.

Over age 60:
Not recommended.

Pregnancy:
If pregnancy occurs, the capsules should be removed. Risk category X (see page xxii).

Breast-feeding:
Drug passes into milk. Consult your doctor about the advisability of breast-feeding.

Infants & children:
Not recommended.

Prolonged use:
- No problems expected.
- Capsules should be removed at end of five years. New capsules may be implanted if continuing contraception is desired.

Skin & sunlight:
No problems expected.

Driving, piloting or hazardous work:
No problems expected.

Discontinuing:
- Must be removed by a health-care professional.
- May be removed at your request at any time for any reason.
- Removal should be considered if you will be immobile for a long time due to illness or surgery.

Others:
- Review patient information booklet before you have Norplant implanted.
- May affect results of some medical tests.
- Does not protect against sexually transmitted diseases. For additional protection, couples may also use condoms and/or spermicidal agents.
- Fertility returns shortly after implants are removed, usually within two weeks.
- Have blood pressure checked by your doctor 3 months after implant.

POSSIBLE INTERACTION WITH OTHER DRUGS

GENERIC NAME OR DRUG CLASS	COMBINED EFFECT
Phenytoin	Decreased contraceptive effect.
Carbamazepine	Decreased contraceptive effect.
Barbiturates*	Decreased contraceptive effect.
Phenylbutazone	Decreased contraceptive effect.
Isoniazid	Decreased contraceptive effect.
Rifampin	Decreased contraceptive effect.

POSSIBLE INTERACTION WITH OTHER SUBSTANCES

INTERACTS WITH	COMBINED EFFECT
Alcohol:	None expected.
Beverages:	None expected.
Cocaine:	None expected.
Foods:	None expected.
Marijuana:	None expected.
Tobacco:	None expected, but consult doctor.

*See Glossary

LINCOMYCIN

BRAND NAMES

Lincocin

BASIC INFORMATION

Habit forming? No
Prescription needed? Yes
Available as generic? Yes
Drug class: Antibiotic (lincomycin)

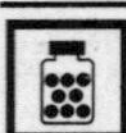

USES

Treatment of bacterial infections that are susceptible to lincomycin.

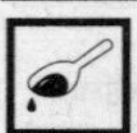

DOSAGE & USAGE INFORMATION

How to take:
Capsule—Swallow with liquid 1 hour before or 2 hours after eating. Drink 8 ounces of water with each dose.

When to take:
At the same times each day.

If you forget a dose:
Take as soon as you remember up to 2 hours late. If more than 2 hours, wait for next scheduled dose (don't double this dose).

What drug does:
Destroys susceptible bacteria. Does not kill viruses.

Time lapse before drug works:
3 to 5 days.

Don't take with:
Any other medication without consulting your doctor or pharmacist.

OVERDOSE

SYMPTOMS:
Severe nausea, vomiting, diarrhea.
WHAT TO DO:
Overdose unlikely to threaten life. If person takes much larger amount than prescribed, call doctor, poison control center or hospital emergency room for instructions.

POSSIBLE ADVERSE REACTIONS OR SIDE EFFECTS

SYMPTOMS	WHAT TO DO
Life-threatening:	
Hives, wheezing, faintness, itching, coma.	Seek emergency treatment.
Common:	
Bloating	Discontinue. Call doctor right away.
Infrequent:	
• Unusual thirst; vomiting; stomach cramps; severe and watery diarrhea with blood or mucus; painful, swollen joints; jaundice; fever; tiredness; weakness; weight loss.	Discontinue. Call doctor right away.
• Itch around groin, rectum or armpits; white patches in mouth; vaginal discharge, itching.	Continue. Call doctor when convenient.
Rare:	
Skin rash.	Discontinue. Call doctor right away.

WARNINGS & PRECAUTIONS

Don't take if:
- You are allergic to lincomycins.
- You have had ulcerative colitis.
- Prescribed for infant under 1 month old.

Before you start, consult your doctor:
- If you have had yeast infections of mouth, skin or vagina.
- If you will have surgery within 2 months, including dental surgery, requiring general or spinal anesthesia.
- If you have kidney or liver disease.
- If you have allergies of any kind.

Over age 60:
Adverse reactions and side effects may be more frequent and severe than in younger persons.

Pregnancy:
Decide with your doctor if drug benefits justify risk to unborn child. Risk category C (see page xxii).

Breast-feeding:
Drug passes into milk. Avoid drug or discontinue nursing until you finish medicine. Consult doctor for advice on maintaining milk supply.

Infants & children:
Don't give to infants younger than 1 month. Use for children only under medical supervision.

Prolonged use:
- Severe colitis with diarrhea and bleeding.
- You may become more susceptible to infections caused by germs not responsive to lincomycin.
- Talk to your doctor about the need for follow-up medical examinations or laboratory studies to check proctosigmoidoscopy.

Skin & sunlight:
No problems expected.

Driving, piloting or hazardous work:
No problems expected.

Discontinuing:
Don't discontinue without doctor's advice until you complete prescribed dose, even though symptoms diminish or disappear.

Others:
May interfere with the accuracy of some medical tests.

POSSIBLE INTERACTION WITH OTHER DRUGS

GENERIC NAME OR DRUG CLASS	COMBINED EFFECT
Antidiarrheal preparations*	Decreased lincomycin effect.
Attapulgite	May decrease effectiveness of lincomycin.
Chloramphenicol	Decreased lincomycin effect.
Erythromycins*	Decreased lincomycin effect.
Narcotics*	Increased risk of respiratory problems.

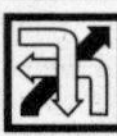

POSSIBLE INTERACTION WITH OTHER SUBSTANCES

INTERACTS WITH	COMBINED EFFECT
Alcohol:	None expected.
Beverages:	None expected.
Cocaine:	None expected.
Foods:	None expected.
Marijuana:	None expected.
Tobacco:	None expected.

***See Glossary**

LITHIUM

BRAND NAMES

Carbolith
Cibalith-S
Duralith
Eskalith
Eskalith CR
Lithane
Lithizine
Lithobid
Lithonate
Lithotabs

BASIC INFORMATION

Habit forming? No
Prescription needed? Yes
Available as generic? Yes
Drug class: Antidepressant

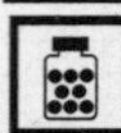

USES

- Normalizes mood and behavior in manic-depressive illness.
- Treats alcohol toxicity and addiction.
- Treats schizoid personality disorders.

DOSAGE & USAGE INFORMATION

How to take:
- Tablet or capsule—Swallow with liquid or food to lessen stomach irritation. If you can't swallow whole, crumble tablet or open capsule and take with liquid or food. Drink 2 or 3 quarts liquid per day.
- Extended-release tablets—Swallow each dose whole.
- Syrup—Take at mealtime. Follow with 8 oz. water.

When to take:
At the same times each day, preferably mealtime.

If you forget a dose:
Take as soon as you remember up to 2 hours late. If more than 2 hours, wait for next scheduled dose (don't double this dose).

Continued next column

OVERDOSE

SYMPTOMS:
Moderate overdose increases some side effects and may cause diarrhea, nausea. Large overdose may cause vomiting, muscle weakness, convulsions, stupor and coma.
WHAT TO DO:
- **Dial 911 (emergency) or 0 (operator) for an ambulance or medical help. Then give first aid immediately.**
- **See emergency information on inside covers.**

What drug does:
May correct chemical imbalance in brain's transmission of nerve impulses that influence mood and behavior.

Time lapse before drug works:
1 to 3 weeks. May require 3 months before depressive phase of illness improves.

Don't take with:
Any other medication without consulting your doctor or pharmacist.

POSSIBLE ADVERSE REACTIONS OR SIDE EFFECTS

SYMPTOMS	WHAT TO DO
Life-threatening:	
In case of overdose, see previous column.	
Common:	
• Dizziness, diarrhea, nausea, vomiting, shakiness, tremor.	Continue. Call doctor when convenient.
• Dry mouth, thirst, decreased sexual ability, increased urination, anorexia.	Continue. Tell doctor at next visit.
Infrequent:	
• Rash, stomach pain, fainting, heartbeat irregularities, shortness of breath, ear noises.	Discontinue. Call doctor right away.
• Swollen hands, feet; slurred speech; thyroid impairment (coldness, dry, puffy skin); muscle aches; headache; weight gain; fatigue; menstrual irregularities, acne-like eruptions.	Continue. Call doctor when convenient.
• Drowsiness, confusion, weakness.	Continue. Tell doctor at next visit.
Rare:	
• Blurred vision, eye pain.	Discontinue. Call doctor right away.
• Jerking of arms and legs, worsening of psoriasis, hair loss.	Continue. Call doctor when convenient.

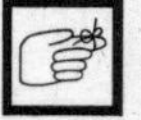

WARNINGS & PRECAUTIONS

Don't take if:
- You are allergic to lithium or tartrazine dye.
- You have kidney or heart disease.
- Patient is younger than 12.

Before you start, consult your doctor:
- About all medications you take.
- If you plan to become pregnant within medication period.

- If you have diabetes, low thyroid function, epilepsy or any significant medical problem.
- If you are on a low-salt diet or drink more than 4 cups of coffee per day.
- If you plan surgery within 2 months.

Over age 60:
Adverse reactions and side effects may be more frequent and severe than in younger persons.

Pregnancy:
Risk to unborn child outweighs drug benefits. Don't use. Risk category D (see page xxii).

Breast-feeding:
Drug passes into milk. Avoid drug or discontinue nursing until you finish medicine. Consult doctor for advice on maintaining milk supply.

Infants & children:
Don't give to children younger than 12.

Prolonged use:
- Enlarged thyroid with possible impaired function.
- Talk to your doctor about the need for follow-up medical examinations or laboratory studies to check lithium levels, ECG*, kidney function, thyroid, complete blood counts (white blood cell count, platelet count, red blood cell count, hemoglobin, hematocrit).

Skin & sunlight:
No problems expected.

Driving, piloting or hazardous work:
Don't drive or pilot aircraft until you learn how medicine affects you. Don't work around dangerous machinery. Don't climb ladders or work in high places. Danger increases if you drink alcohol or take medicine affecting alertness and reflexes.

Discontinuing:
Don't discontinue without consulting doctor. Dose may require gradual reduction if you have taken drug for a long time. Doses of other drugs may also require adjustment.

Others:
- Regular checkups, periodic blood tests, and tests of lithium levels and thyroid function recommended.
- Avoid exercise in hot weather and other activities that cause heavy sweating. This contributes to lithium poisoning.
- Some products contain tartrazine dye. Avoid, especially if allergic to aspirin.

POSSIBLE INTERACTION WITH OTHER DRUGS

GENERIC NAME OR DRUG CLASS	COMBINED EFFECT
Acetazolamide	Decreased lithium effect.
Antihistamines*	Possible excessive sedation.
Anti-inflammatory drugs, nonsteroidal (NSAIDs)*	Increased toxic effect of lithium.
Bupropion	Increased risk of major seizures.
Carbamazepine	Increased lithium effect.
Desmopressin	Possible decreased desmopressin effect.
Diazepam	Possible hypothermia.
Diclofenac	Possible increase in effect and toxicity.
Didanosine	Increased risk of peripheral neuropathy.
Diuretics*	Increased lithium effect.
Dronabinol	Increased effects of both drugs. Avoid.
Haloperidol	Increased toxicity of both drugs.
Indomethacin	Increased lithium effect.
Iodide salts	Increased lithium effects on thyroid function.

Continued on page 944

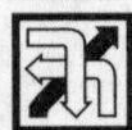

POSSIBLE INTERACTION WITH OTHER SUBSTANCES

INTERACTS WITH	COMBINED EFFECT
Alcohol:	Possible lithium poisoning.
Beverages: Caffeine drinks.	Decreased lithium effect.
Cocaine:	Possible psychosis.
Foods: Salt.	High intake could decrease lithium effect. Low intake could increase lithium effect. *Don't* restrict intake.
Marijuana:	Increased tremor and possible psychosis.
Tobacco:	None expected.

LOMUSTINE

BRAND NAMES

CeeNU
CCNU

BASIC INFORMATION

Habit forming? No
Prescription needed? Yes
Available as generic? No
Drug class: Antineoplastic

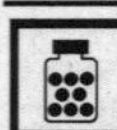

USES

- Treats brain cancer and Hodgkin's lymphoma.
- Sometimes used to treat breast, lung, skin and gastrointestinal cancer.

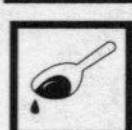

DOSAGE & USAGE INFORMATION

How to take:
Capsules—Swallow with liquid. If you can't swallow whole, open capsule and take with liquid or food. Instructions to take on empty stomach mean 1 hour before or 2 hours after eating. Note: There may be two or more different types of capsules in the container. This is not an error.

When to take:
According to doctor's instructions. Usual course of treatment requires single dosage repeated every 6 weeks.

If you forget a dose:
Take as soon as you remember. Don't ever double doses.

What drug does:
Interferes with growth of cancer cells.

Time lapse before drug works:
None. Works immediately.

Don't take with:
Any other medicines (including over-the-counter drugs such as cough and cold medicines, laxatives, antacids, diet pills, caffeine, nose drops or vitamins) without consulting your doctor

OVERDOSE

SYMPTOMS:
Decreased urine (kidney failure); high fever, chills (infection); bloody or black stools (bleeding).
WHAT TO DO:
- **Dial 911 (emergency) or 0 (operator) for an ambulance or medical help. Then give first aid immediately.**
- **See emergency information on inside covers.**

POSSIBLE ADVERSE REACTIONS OR SIDE EFFECTS

SYMPTOMS	WHAT TO DO
Life-threatening:	
In case of overdose, see previous column.	
Common:	
• Fever, chills, difficult urination, unusual bleeding.	Continue. Call doctor when convenient.
• Appetite loss, nausea, hair loss.	No action necessary.
Infrequent:	
• Anemia, confusion, slurred speech, mouth sores, skin rash.	Continue. Call doctor when convenient.
• Darkened skin.	No action necessary.
Rare:	
• Jaundice (yellow skin and eyes), cough.	Continue. Call doctor when convenient.
• Shortness of breath.	Discontinue. Call doctor right away.

WARNINGS & PRECAUTIONS

Don't take if:
- You have chicken pox.
- You have shingles (herpes zoster).

Before you start, consult your doctor:
- If you have an infection.
- If you have kidney disease.
- If you have had previous cancer chemotherapy or radiation treatment.

Over age 60:
Adverse reactions and side effects may be more frequent and severe than in younger persons. You may need smaller doses for shorter periods of time.

Pregnancy:
Risk to unborn child outweighs drug benefits. Don't use. Risk category D (see page xxii).

Breast-feeding:
Drug passes into milk. Avoid drug or discontinue nursing until you finish medicine. Consult doctor for advice on maintaining milk supply.

Infants & children:
Effect not documented. Consult your doctor.

Prolonged use:
Talk to your doctor about the need for follow-up medical examinations or laboratory studies to check kidney function, liver function and complete blood counts (white blood cell count, platelet count, red blood cell count, hemoglobin, hematocrit).

Skin & sunlight:
No problems expected.

Driving, piloting or hazardous work:
Don't drive or pilot aircraft until you learn how medicine affects you. Don't work around dangerous machinery. Don't climb ladders or work in high places. Danger increases if you drink alcohol or take medicine affecting alertness and reflexes.

Discontinuing:
Call doctor if any of these occur after discontinuing: black or tarry stools, bloody urine, hoarseness, bleeding or bruising, fever or chills.

Others:
- Advise any doctor or dentist whom you consult that you take this medicine.
- May affect results in some medical tests.
- Most adverse reactions and side effects are unavoidable.
- Avoid immunizations, if possible.
- Avoid persons with infections.
- Check with doctor about brushing or flossing teeth.
- Avoid contact sports.

POSSIBLE INTERACTION WITH OTHER DRUGS

GENERIC NAME OR DRUG CLASS	COMBINED EFFECT
Antineoplastic drugs, other*	Increased chance of drug toxicity.
Blood dyscrasia-causing medicines*	Adverse effect on bone marrow, causing decreased white cells and platelets.
Bone marrow depressants*, other	Increased risk of bone marrow depression.
Clozapine	Toxic effect on bone marrow.
Levamisole	Increased risk of bone marrow depression.
Tiopronin	Increased risk of toxicity to bone marrow.
Vaccines, live or killed virus	Increased chance of toxicity or reduced effectiveness of vaccine. Wait 3 to 12 months after lomustine treatment before getting vaccination.

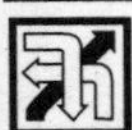

POSSIBLE INTERACTION WITH OTHER SUBSTANCES

INTERACTS WITH	COMBINED EFFECT
Alcohol:	Increased chance of liver damage.
Beverages:	No special problems expected.
Cocaine:	Increased chance of central nervous system toxicity.
Foods:	No special problems expected.
Marijuana:	No special problems expected.
Tobacco:	No special problems expected.

*See Glossary

LOPERAMIDE

BRAND NAMES

Imodium
Imodium A-D
Kaopectate II Caplets
Pepto Diarrhea Control

BASIC INFORMATION

Habit forming? No, unless taken in high doses for long periods.
Prescription needed? Yes, for some
Available as generic? Yes
Drug class: Antidiarrheal

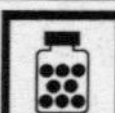

USES

Relieves diarrhea and reduces volume of discharge from ileostomies and colostomies.

DOSAGE & USAGE INFORMATION

How to take:

- Tablet or capsule—Swallow with food to lessen stomach irritation.
- Liquid—Follow label instructions and use marked dropper.

When to take:
No more often than directed on label.

If you forget a dose:
Take as soon as you remember up to 2 hours late. If more than 2 hours, wait for next scheduled dose (don't double this dose).

What drug does:
Blocks digestive tract's nerve supply, which reduces irritability and contractions in intestinal tract.

Time lapse before drug works:
1 to 2 hours.

Don't take with:
Any other medication without consulting your doctor or pharmacist.

OVERDOSE

SYMPTOMS:
Constipation, lethargy, drowsiness or unconsciousness.
WHAT TO DO:
Overdose unlikely to threaten life. If person takes much larger amount than prescribed, call doctor, poison control center or hospital emergency room for instructions.

POSSIBLE ADVERSE REACTIONS OR SIDE EFFECTS

SYMPTOMS	WHAT TO DO
Life-threatening:	
Unconsciousness.	Seek emergency treatment.
Common:	
None expected.	
Infrequent:	
• Rash.	Discontinue. Call doctor right away.
• Drowsiness, dizziness, dry mouth, bloating, constipation, appetite loss, abdominal pain.	Continue. Call doctor when convenient.
Rare:	
Unexplained fever, nausea, vomiting.	Discontinue. Call doctor right away.

WARNINGS & PRECAUTIONS

Don't take if:
- You have severe colitis.
- You have colitis resulting from antibiotic treatment or infection.
- You are allergic to loperamide.

Before you start, consult your doctor:
- If you are dehydrated from fluid loss caused by diarrhea.
- If you have liver disease.

Over age 60:
Adverse reactions and side effects may be more frequent and severe than in younger persons.

Pregnancy:
No proven harm. Avoid if possible. Consult doctor. Risk category B (see page xxii).

Breast-feeding:
No proven problems, but avoid if possible or discontinue nursing until you finish medicine. Consult doctor for advice on maintaining milk supply.

Infants & children:
Don't give to infants or toddlers. Use only under doctor's supervision for children older than 2.

Prolonged use:
Habit forming at high dose.

Skin & sunlight:
No problems expected.

Driving, piloting or hazardous work:
Don't drive or pilot aircraft until you learn how medicine affects you. Don't work around dangerous machinery. Don't climb ladders or work in high places. Danger increases if you drink alcohol or take medicine affecting alertness and reflexes.

Discontinuing:
- May be unnecessary to finish medicine. Follow doctor's instructions.
- After discontinuing, consult doctor if you experience muscle cramps, nausea, vomiting, trembling, stomach cramps or unusual sweating.

Others:
If acute diarrhea lasts longer than 48 hours, discontinue and call doctor. In chronic diarrhea, loperamide is unlikely to be effective if diarrhea doesn't improve in 10 days.

POSSIBLE INTERACTION WITH OTHER DRUGS

GENERIC NAME OR DRUG CLASS	COMBINED EFFECT
Narcotic analgesics	Increased risk of severe constipation.

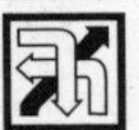

POSSIBLE INTERACTION WITH OTHER SUBSTANCES

INTERACTS WITH	COMBINED EFFECT
Alcohol:	Depressed brain function. Avoid.
Beverages:	None expected.
Cocaine:	Decreased loperamide effect.
Foods:	None expected.
Marijuana:	None expected.
Tobacco:	None expected.

LORACARBEF

BRAND NAMES

Lorabid

BASIC INFORMATION

Habit forming? No
Prescription needed? Yes
Available as generic? No
Drug class: Antibacterial (antibiotic)

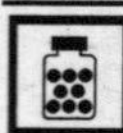

USES

Treatment for bacterial infections of the upper respiratory tract, lower respiratory tract, urinary tract, skin and skin structure.

DOSAGE & USAGE INFORMATION

How to take:

- Capsule—Swallow with liquid. If you can't swallow whole, open capsule and take with liquid. Instructions to take on an empty stomach mean 1 hour before or 2 hours after eating.
- Oral suspension—Follow label instructions for mixing the powder with water. Instructions to take on an empty stomach mean 1 hour before or 2 hours after eating.

When to take:
At the same times each day.

If you forget a dose:
Take as soon as you remember up to 2 hours late. If more than 2 hours, wait for next scheduled dose (don't double this dose).

What drug does:
Kills bacteria susceptible to loracarbef.

Time lapse before drug works:
May require several days to affect infection.

Don't take with:
Any other prescription or nonprescription drug without consulting your doctor.

OVERDOSE

SYMPTOMS:
Nausea, vomiting, diarrhea or abdominal cramps.
WHAT TO DO:
Overdose unlikely to threaten life. If person takes much larger amount than prescribed, call doctor, poison control center or hospital emergency room for instructions.

POSSIBLE ADVERSE REACTIONS OR SIDE EFFECTS

SYMPTOMS	WHAT TO DO
Life-threatening:	
Hives, rash, intense itching, faintness soon after a dose (anaphylaxis); difficulty in breathing.	Seek emergency treatment immediately.
Common:	
Abdominal pain, diarrhea, nausea and vomiting, loss of appetite	Continue. Call doctor when convenient.
Infrequent:	
Itching, skin rash.	Discontinue. Call doctor right away.
Rare:	
Dizziness, drowsiness, insomnia, nervousness, vaginal itching and discharge.	Continue. Call doctor when convenient.

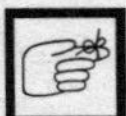

WARNINGS & PRECAUTIONS

Don't take if:
You are allergic to loracarbef, penicillins* or cephalosporins*.

Before you start, consult your doctor:
- If you have kidney disease.
- If you have a history of colitis.

Over age 60:
Adverse reactions and side effects may be more frequent and severe than in younger persons. You may need smaller doses for shorter periods of time.

Pregnancy:
Consult doctor. Risk category B (see page xxii).

Breast-feeding:
Effect not documented. Consult your doctor.

Infants & children:
Not recommended for patients under 6 months of age.

Prolonged use:
- Kills beneficial bacteria that protect body against other germs. Unchecked germs may cause secondary infections
- Talk to your doctor about the need for follow-up medical examinations or laboratory studies.

Skin & sunlight:
No problems expected.

Driving, piloting or hazardous work:
Avoid if you feel dizzy or drowsy. Otherwise, no problems expected.

Discontinuing:
Don't discontinue without doctor's advice until you complete prescribed dose, even though symptoms diminish or disappear.

Others:
- Advise any doctor or dentist whom you consult that you take this medicine.
- May affect the results in some medical tests.

POSSIBLE INTERACTION WITH OTHER DRUGS

GENERIC NAME OR DRUG CLASS	COMBINED EFFECT
Probenecid	Increased loracarbef effect.

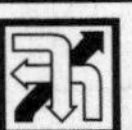

POSSIBLE INTERACTION WITH OTHER SUBSTANCES

INTERACTS WITH	COMBINED EFFECT
Alcohol:	None expected.
Beverages:	None expected.
Cocaine:	None expected.
Foods:	None expected.
Marijuana:	None expected.
Tobacco:	None expected.

LOXAPINE

BRAND NAMES

Loxapac
Loxitane
Loxitane C

BASIC INFORMATION

Habit forming? No
Prescription needed? Yes
Available as generic? Yes
Drug class: Tranquilizer, antidepressant

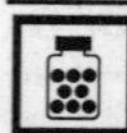

USES

- Treats serious mental illness.
- Treats anxiety and depression.

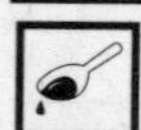

DOSAGE & USAGE INFORMATION

How to take:
- Oral solution—Take after meals with liquid to decrease stomach irritation.
- Tablets—Swallow with liquid or food to lessen stomach irritation. If you can't swallow whole, crumble tablet and take with liquid or food.
- Capsules—Swallow with liquid or food to lessen stomach irritation. If you can't swallow whole, open capsule and take with liquid or food.

When to take:
At the same time each day, according to instructions on prescription label.

If you forget a dose:
Take as soon as you remember up to 2 hours late. If more than 2 hours, wait for next scheduled dose (don't double this dose).

What drug does:
Probably blocks the effects of dopamine in the brain.

Time lapse before drug works:
1/2 to 3 hours.

Don't take with:
Any other medicine without consulting your doctor or pharmacist.

OVERDOSE

SYMPTOMS:
Dizziness, drowsiness, severe shortness of breath, muscle spasms, coma.
WHAT TO DO:
- **Dial 911 (emergency) or 0 (operator) for an ambulance or medical help. Then give first aid immediately.**
- **See emergency information on inside covers.**

POSSIBLE ADVERSE REACTIONS OR SIDE EFFECTS

SYMPTOMS	WHAT TO DO
Life-threatening:	
Severe shortness of breath, skin rash, heartbeat irregularities, profuse sweating, fever, convulsions (rare).	Seek emergency treatment immediately.
Common:	
• Increased dental problems because of dry mouth and less salivation.	Consult your dentist about a prevention program.
• Swallowing difficulty, expressionless face, stiff arms and legs, dizziness.	Discontinue. Call doctor right away.
Infrequent:	
• Chewing movements with lip smacking, loss of balance, shuffling walk, tremor of fingers and hands, uncontrolled tongue movements.	Discontinue. Call doctor right away.
• Constipation, difficult urination, blurred vision, confusion, loss of sex drive, headache, insomnia, menstrual irregularities, weight gain, light sensitivity, nausea.	Continue. Call doctor when convenient.
Rare:	
Rapid heartbeat, fever, sore throat, jaundice, unusual bleeding.	Discontinue. Call doctor right away.

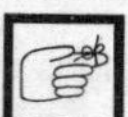

WARNINGS & PRECAUTIONS

Don't take if:
- You are an alcoholic.
- You have liver disease.

Before you start, consult your doctor:
- If you have a seizure disorder.
- If you have an enlarged prostate, glaucoma, Parkinson's disease, heart disease.

Over age 60:
Adverse reactions and side effects may be more frequent and severe than in younger persons. You may need smaller doses for shorter periods of time.

Pregnancy:
Decide with your doctor if drug benefits justify risk to unborn child. Risk category C (see page xxii).

Breast-feeding:
Drug may pass into milk. Avoid drug or discontinue nursing until you finish medicine. Consult doctor for advice on maintaining milk supply.

Infants & children:
Not recommended.

Prolonged use:
Talk to your doctor about the need for follow-up medical examinations or laboratory studies to check complete blood counts (white blood cell count, platelet count, red blood cell count, hemoglobin, hematocrit), liver function, eyes.

Skin & sunlight:
Increased sensitivity to sunlight.

Driving, piloting or hazardous work:
Don't drive or pilot aircraft until you learn how medicine affects you. Don't work around dangerous machinery. Don't climb ladders or work in high places. Danger increases if you drink alcohol or take medicine affecting alertness and reflexes.

Discontinuing:
- Don't discontinue without consulting doctor. Dose may require gradual reduction if you have taken drug for a long time. Doses of other drugs may also require adjustment.
- These symptoms may occur after medicine has been discontinued: dizziness; nausea; abdominal pain; uncontrolled movements of mouth, tongue and jaw.

Others:
Use careful oral hygiene.

POSSIBLE INTERACTION WITH OTHER DRUGS

GENERIC NAME OR DRUG CLASS	COMBINED EFFECT
Anticonvulsants*	Decreased effect of anticonvulsants.
Antidepressants, tricyclic*	May increase toxic effects of both drugs.
Bupropion	Increased risk of major seizures.
Central nervous system (CNS) depressants*	Increased sedative effect of both drugs.
Clozapine	Toxic effect on the central nervous system.
Epinephrine	Rapid heart rate and severe drop in blood pressure.
Ethinamate	Dangerous increased effects of ethinamate. Avoid combining.
Extrapyramidal reaction*-causing drugs	Increased risk of side effects.
Fluoxetine	Increased depressant effects of both drugs.
Guanadrel	Decreased effect of guanadrel.
Guanethidine	Decreased effect of guanethidine.
Guanfacine	Increased effect of both drugs.
Haloperidol	May increase toxic effects of both drugs.
Leucovorin	High alcohol content of leucovorin may cause adverse effects.
Methyldopa	May increase toxic effects of both drugs.
Methyprylon	Increased sedative effect, perhaps to dangerous level. Avoid.
Metoclopramide	May increase toxic effects of both drugs.
Metyrosine	May increase toxic effects of both drugs.
Molindone	May increase toxic effects of both drugs.
Nabilone	Greater depression of central nervous system.

Continued on page 944

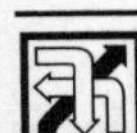

POSSIBLE INTERACTION WITH OTHER SUBSTANCES

INTERACTS WITH	COMBINED EFFECT
Alcohol:	May decrease effect of loxapine. Avoid.
Beverages:	None expected.
Cocaine:	May increase toxicity of both drugs. Avoid.
Foods:	None expected.
Marijuana:	May increase toxicity of both drugs. Avoid.
Tobacco:	May increase toxicity of both drugs. Avoid.

***See Glossary**

MAGNESIUM CITRATE

BRAND NAMES

Citrate of Magnesia
Citro-Mag
Citro-Nesia
Citroma

BASIC INFORMATION

Habit forming? No
Prescription needed? No
Available as generic? Yes
Drug class: Laxative (hyperosmotic)

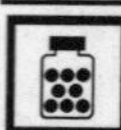

USES

Constipation relief.

DOSAGE & USAGE INFORMATION

How to take:
Liquid—Dilute dose in beverage before swallowing.

When to take:
Usually once a day, preferably in the morning.

If you forget a dose:
Take as soon as you remember up to 8 hours before bedtime. If later, wait for next scheduled dose (don't double this dose). Don't take at bedtime.

What drug does:
Draws water into bowel from other body tissues. Causes distention through fluid accumulation, which promotes soft stool and accelerates bowel motion.

Time lapse before drug works:
30 minutes to 3 hours.

Don't take with:
Any other medicine without consulting your doctor or pharmacist.

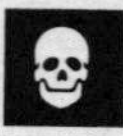

OVERDOSE

SYMPTOMS:
Fluid depletion, weakness, vomiting, fainting.
WHAT TO DO:

- **Dial 911 (emergency) or 0 (operator) for an ambulance or medical help. Then give first aid immediately.**
- **See emergency information on inside cover.**

POSSIBLE ADVERSE REACTIONS OR SIDE EFFECTS

SYMPTOMS	WHAT TO DO
Life-threatening:	
In case of overdose, see previous column.	
Common:	
None expected.	
Infrequent:	
• Irregular heartbeat.	Discontinue. Call doctor right away.
• Increased thirst, cramps, nausea, diarrhea, gaseousness.	Continue. Tell doctor at next visit.
Rare:	
Dizziness, confusion, tiredness or weakness.	Continue. Call doctor when convenient.

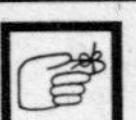

WARNINGS & PRECAUTIONS

Don't take if:
- You are allergic to any hyperosmotic laxative.
- You have symptoms of appendicitis, inflamed bowel or intestinal blockage.
- You have missed a bowel movement for only 1 or 2 days.

Before you start, consult your doctor:
- If you have congestive heart disease.
- If you have diabetes.
- If you have high blood pressure.
- If you have a colostomy or ileostomy.
- If you have kidney disease.
- If you have a laxative habit.
- If you have rectal bleeding.
- If you take another laxative.

Over age 60:
Adverse reactions and side effects may be more frequent and severe than in younger persons.

Pregnancy:
Salt content may cause fluid retention and swelling. Avoid if possible. Consult doctor. Risk category B (see page xxii).

Breast-feeding:
No problems expected. Consult doctor.

Infants & children:
Use only under medical supervision.

Prolonged use:
Don't take for more than 1 week unless under a doctor's supervision. May cause laxative dependence.

Skin & sunlight:
No problems expected.

Driving, piloting or hazardous work:
No problems expected.

Discontinuing:
May be unnecessary to finish medicine. Follow doctor's instructions.

Others:
- Don't take to "flush out" your system or as a "tonic."
- Don't take within 2 hours of taking another medicine.

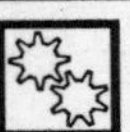

POSSIBLE INTERACTION WITH OTHER DRUGS

GENERIC NAME OR DRUG CLASS	COMBINED EFFECT
Anticoagulants*, oral	Decreased anticoagulant effect.
Antidepressants, tricyclic*	Decreased TCA effect.
Chlordiazepoxide	Decreased chlor-diazepoxide effect.
Chlorpromazine	Decreased chlor-promazine effect.
Ciprofloxacin	Decreased ciprofloxacin effect.
Clozapine	Toxic effect on the central nervous system.
Dicumarol	Decreased dicumarol effect.
Digitalis preparations*	Decreased digitalis effect.
Etidromate	Separate doses by 2 hours.
Isoniazid	Decreased isoniazid effect.
Mexiletine	May slow elimination of mexiletine and cause need to adjust dosage.
Propafenone	Increased effect of both drugs and increased risk of toxicity.
Tetracyclines*	Possible intestinal blockage.

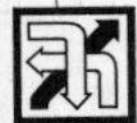

POSSIBLE INTERACTION WITH OTHER SUBSTANCES

INTERACTS WITH	COMBINED EFFECT
Alcohol:	None expected.
Beverages:	None expected.
Cocaine:	None expected.
Foods:	None expected.
Marijuana:	None expected.
Tobacco:	None expected.

***See Glossary**

MAGNESIUM SULFATE

BRAND NAMES

Bilagog
Epsom Salts

BASIC INFORMATION

Habit forming? No
Prescription needed? No
Available as generic? Yes
Drug class: Laxative (hyperosmotic)

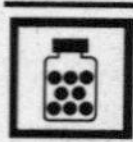

USES

Constipation relief.

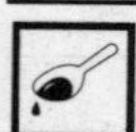

DOSAGE & USAGE INFORMATION

How to take:
- Tablet—Swallow with liquid.
- Powder or solid form—Dilute dose in beverage before swallowing. Solid form must be dissolved.

When to take:
Usually once a day, preferably in the morning.

If you forget a dose:
Take as soon as you remember up to 8 hours before bedtime. If later, wait for next scheduled dose (don't double this dose). Don't take at bedtime.

What drug does:
Draws water into bowel from other body tissues. Causes distention through fluid accumulation, which promotes soft stool and accelerates bowel motion.

Time lapse before drug works:
30 minutes to 3 hours.

Don't take with:
Any other medicine without consulting your doctor or pharmacist.

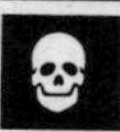

OVERDOSE

SYMPTOMS:
Fluid depletion, weakness, vomiting, fainting.
WHAT TO DO:
- **Dial 911 (emergency) or 0 (operator) for an ambulance or medical help. Then give first aid immediately.**
- **See emergency information on inside cover.**

POSSIBLE ADVERSE REACTIONS OR SIDE EFFECTS

SYMPTOMS	WHAT TO DO
Life-threatening: In case of overdose, see previous column.	
Common:	
Nausea.	Continue. Call doctor when convenient.
Infrequent:	
• Irregular heartbeat.	Discontinue. Call doctor right away.
• Increased thirst, cramps, diarrhea, gaseousness.	Continue. Tell doctor at next visit.
Rare:	
Dizziness, confusion, tiredness or weakness.	Continue. Call doctor when convenient.

WARNINGS & PRECAUTIONS

Don't take if:
- You are allergic to any hyperosmotic laxative.
- You have symptoms of appendicitis, inflamed bowel or intestinal blockage.
- You have missed a bowel movement for only 1 or 2 days.

Before you start, consult your doctor:
- If you have congestive heart disease.
- If you have diabetes.
- If you have high blood pressure.
- If you have a colostomy or ileostomy.
- If you have kidney disease.
- If you have a laxative habit.
- If you have rectal bleeding.
- If you take another laxative.

Over age 60:
Adverse reactions and side effects may be more frequent and severe than in younger persons.

Pregnancy:
Salt content may cause fluid retention and swelling. Avoid if possible. Consult doctor. Risk category B (see page xxii).

Breast-feeding:
No problems expected. Consult doctor.

Infants & children:
Use only under medical supervision.

Prolonged use:
Don't take for more than 1 week unless under a doctor's supervision. May cause laxative dependence.

Skin & sunlight:
No problems expected.

Driving, piloting or hazardous work:
No problems expected.

Discontinuing:
May be unnecessary to finish medicine. Follow doctor's instructions.

Others:
- Don't take to "flush out" your system or as a "tonic."
- Don't take within 2 hours of taking another medicine.

POSSIBLE INTERACTION WITH OTHER DRUGS

GENERIC NAME OR DRUG CLASS	COMBINED EFFECT
Anticoagulants*, oral	Decreased anticoagulant effect.
Antidepressants, tricyclic*	Decreased anti-depressant effect.
Chlordiazepoxide	Decreased chlor-diazepoxide effect.
Chlorpromazine	Decreased chlor-promazine effect.
Ciprofloxacin	Decreased ciprofloxacin effect.
Clozapine	Toxic effect on the central nervous system.
Dicumarol	Decreased dicumarol effect.
Digitalis preparations*	Decreased digitalis effect.
Etidronate	Separate doses by 2 hours.
Isoniazid	Decreased isoniazid effect.
Mexiletine	May slow elimination of mexiletine and cause need to adjust dosage.
Propafenone	Increased effect of both drugs and increased risk of toxicity.
Tetracyclines*	Possible intestinal blockage.

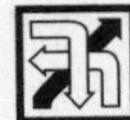

POSSIBLE INTERACTION WITH OTHER SUBSTANCES

INTERACTS WITH	COMBINED EFFECT
Alcohol:	None expected.
Beverages:	None expected.
Cocaine:	None expected.
Foods:	None expected.
Marijuana:	None expected.
Tobacco:	None expected.

MALT SOUP EXTRACT

BRAND NAMES

Maltsupex

BASIC INFORMATION

Habit forming? No
Prescription needed? No
Available as generic? Yes
Drug class: Laxative (bulk-forming)

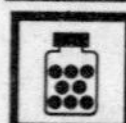

USES

Relieves constipation and prevents straining for bowel movement.

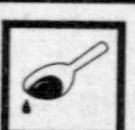

DOSAGE & USAGE INFORMATION

How to take:

- Liquid or powder—Dilute dose in 8 oz. cold water or fruit juice.
- Tablets—Swallow with 8 oz. cold liquid. Drink 6 to 8 glasses of water each day in addition to the one with each dose.

When to take:
At the same time each day, preferably morning.

If you forget a dose:
Take as soon as you remember. Resume regular schedule.

What drug does:
Absorbs water, stimulating the bowel to form a soft, bulky stool.

Time lapse before drug works:
May require 2 or 3 days to begin, then works in 12 to 24 hours.

Don't take with:

- Don't take within 2 hours of taking another medicine.
- Any other medicine without consulting your doctor or pharmacist.

OVERDOSE

SYMPTOMS:
Wheezing.
WHAT TO DO:
Overdose unlikely to threaten life. If person takes much larger amount than prescribed, call doctor, poison control center or hospital emergency room for instructions.

POSSIBLE ADVERSE REACTIONS OR SIDE EFFECTS

SYMPTOMS	WHAT TO DO
Life-threatening: None expected.	
Common: None expected.	
Infrequent: Swallowing difficulty, "lump in throat" sensation, nausea, vomiting, diarrhea.	Continue. Call doctor when convenient.
Rare: Itchy skin, rash, asthma, intestinal blockage.	Discontinue. Call doctor right away.

WARNINGS & PRECAUTIONS

Don't take if:
- You are allergic to any bulk-forming laxative.
- You have symptoms of appendicitis, inflamed bowel or intestinal blockage.
- You have missed a bowel movement for only 1 or 2 days.

Before you start, consult your doctor:
- If you have diabetes.
- If you have a laxative habit.
- If you have rectal bleeding.
- If you have difficulty swallowing.
- If you take other laxatives.

Over age 60:
Adverse reactions and side effects may be more frequent and severe than in younger persons.

Pregnancy:
Most bulk-forming laxatives contain sodium or sugars which may cause fluid retention. Risk factor not designated. Read categories on page xxii and consult doctor.

Breast-feeding:
No problems expected. Consult doctor.

Infants & children:
Use only under medical supervision.

Prolonged use:
Don't take for more than 1 week unless under a doctor's supervision. May cause laxative dependence.

Skin & sunlight:
No problems expected.

Driving, piloting or hazardous work:
No problems expected.

Discontinuing:
May be unnecessary to finish medicine. Follow doctor's instructions.

Others:
Don't take to "flush out" your system or as a "tonic."

POSSIBLE INTERACTION WITH OTHER DRUGS

GENERIC NAME OR DRUG CLASS	COMBINED EFFECT
Antibiotics*	Possible decreased antibiotic effect.
Digitalis preparations*	Decreased digitalis effect.
Salicylates* (including aspirin)	Decreased salicylate effect.

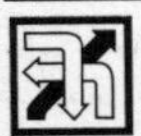

POSSIBLE INTERACTION WITH OTHER SUBSTANCES

INTERACTS WITH	COMBINED EFFECT
Alcohol:	None expected.
Beverages:	None expected.
Cocaine:	None expected.
Foods:	None expected.
Marijuana:	None expected.
Tobacco:	None expected.

***See Glossary**

MAPROTILINE

BRAND NAMES

Ludiomil

BASIC INFORMATION

Habit forming? No
Prescription needed? Yes
Available as generic? Yes
Drug class: Antidepressant

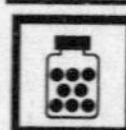

USES

- Treatment for depression or anxiety associated with depression.
- Used to treat some types of chronic pain.

DOSAGE & USAGE INFORMATION

How to take:
Tablet—Swallow with liquid.

When to take:
At the same time each day, usually bedtime.

If you forget a dose:
Bedtime dose—If you forget your once-a-day bedtime dose, don't take it more than 3 hours late. If more than 3 hours, wait for next scheduled dose. Don't double this dose.

What drug does:
Probably affects part of brain that controls messages between nerve cells.

Time lapse before drug works:
Begins in 1 to 2 weeks. May require 4 to 6 weeks for maximum benefit.

Continued next column

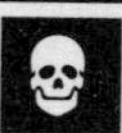

OVERDOSE

SYMPTOMS:
Respiratory failure, fever, cardiac arrhythmia, muscle stiffness, drowsiness, hallucinations, convulsions, coma.
WHAT TO DO:

- **Dial 911 (emergency) or 0 (operator) for an ambulance or medical help. Then give first aid immediately.**
- **If patient is unconscious and not breathing, give mouth-to-mouth breathing. If there is no heartbeat, use cardiac massage and mouth-to-mouth breathing (CPR). Don't try to make patient vomit. If you can't get help quickly, take patient to nearest emergency facility.**
- **See emergency information on inside covers.**

Don't take with:

- Nonprescription drugs without consulting doctor.
- See Interaction column and consult doctor.

POSSIBLE ADVERSE REACTIONS OR SIDE EFFECTS

SYMPTOMS	WHAT TO DO
Life-threatening:	
Seizures.	Seek emergency treatment immediately.
Common:	
• Tremor.	Discontinue. Call doctor right away.
• Headache, dry mouth or unpleasant taste, constipation or diarrhea, nausea, indigestion, fatigue, weakness, drowsiness, nervousness, anxiety, excessive sweating.	Continue. Call doctor when convenient.
• Insomnia, craving sweets.	Continue. Tell doctor at next visit.
Infrequent:	
• Convulsions.	Discontinue. Seek emergency treatment.
• Hallucinations, shakiness, dizziness, fainting, blurred vision, eye pain, vomiting, irregular heartbeat or slow pulse, inflamed tongue, abdominal pain, jaundice, hair loss, rash, chills, joint pain, palpitations, hiccups, vision changes.	Discontinue. Call doctor right away.
• Painful or difficult urination; fatigue; decreased sex drive; abnormal dreams; nasal congestion; back pain; muscle aches; frequent urination; painful, absent or irregular menstruation.	Continue. Call doctor when convenient.
Rare:	
Itchy skin; sore throat; jaundice; fever; involuntary movements of jaw, lips and tongue; nightmares; confusion; swollen breasts in men.	Discontinue. Call doctor right away.

WARNINGS & PRECAUTIONS

Don't take if:
- You are allergic to any tricyclic antidepressant.
- You drink alcohol.
- You have had a heart attack within 6 weeks.
- You have glaucoma.
- You have taken a monoamine oxidase (MAO) inhibitor* within 2 weeks.
- Patient is younger than 12.

Before you start, consult your doctor:
- If you will have surgery within 2 months, including dental surgery, requiring general or spinal anesthesia.
- If you have an enlarged prostate, heart disease or high blood pressure, stomach or intestinal problems, overactive thyroid, asthma, liver disease, schizophrenia, urinary retention, respiratory disorders, seizure disorders, diabetes, kidney disease.

Over age 60:
More likely to develop urination difficulty and side effects such as hallucinations, shakiness, dizziness, fainting, headache or insomnia.

Pregnancy:
Consult doctor. Risk category B (see page xxii).

Breast-feeding:
Drug passes into milk. Avoid drug or discontinue nursing until you finish medicine. Consult doctor for advice on maintaining milk supply.

Infants & children:
Don't give to children younger than 12.

Prolonged use:
Request blood cell counts, liver function studies, monitor blood pressure closely.

Skin & sunlight:
May cause rash or intensify sunburn in areas exposed to sun or sunlamp.

Driving, piloting or hazardous work:
Don't drive or pilot aircraft until you learn how medicine affects you. Don't work around dangerous machinery. Don't climb ladders or work in high places. Danger increases if you drink alcohol or take medicine affecting alertness and reflexes.

Discontinuing:
Don't discontinue without consulting doctor. Dose may require gradual reduction if you have taken drug for a long time. Doses of other drugs may also require adjustment.

Others:
No problems expected.

POSSIBLE INTERACTION WITH OTHER DRUGS

GENERIC NAME OR DRUG CLASS	COMBINED EFFECT
Anticholinergics*	Increased sedation.
Antihistamines*	Increased antihistamine effect.
Barbiturates*	Decreased anti-depressant effect.
Benzodiazepine	Increased sedation.
Central nervous system (CNS) depressants*	Increased sedation.
Cimetidine	Possible increased antidepressant effect and toxicity.
Clonidine	Decreased clonidine effect.
Clozapine	Toxic effect on the central nervous system.
Disulfiram	Delirium.
Diuretics, thiazide*	Increased maprotiline effect.
Ethchlorvynol	Delirium.
Ethinamate	Dangerous increased effects of ethinamate. Avoid combining.

Continued on page 944

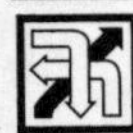

POSSIBLE INTERACTION WITH OTHER SUBSTANCES

INTERACTS WITH	COMBINED EFFECT
Alcohol: Beverages or medicines with alcohol.	Excessive intoxication. Avoid.
Beverages:	None expected.
Cocaine:	Excessive intoxication. Avoid.
Foods:	None expected.
Marijuana:	Excessive drowsiness. Avoid.
Tobacco:	May decrease absorption of maprotiline. Avoid.

***See Glossary**

MASOPROCOL

BRAND NAMES

Actinex

BASIC INFORMATION

Habit forming? No
Prescription needed? Yes
Available as generic? No
Drug class: Antineoplastic (topical)

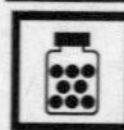

USES

Treats actinic keratoses (scaly, flat or slightly raised skin lesions).

DOSAGE & USAGE INFORMATION

How to take:
Cream–Wash and dry the skin where lesions are located. Massage cream into affected area. Wash hands immediately after use.

When to take:
Use at the same times each day.

If you forget a dose:
Apply as soon as you remember, then resume regular schedule.

What drug does:
Selectively destroys actively proliferating cells.

Time lapse before drug works:
1 to 2 months.

Don't take with:
Other topical prescription or nonprescription drugs without consulting your doctor.

OVERDOSE

SYMPTOMS:
None reported.
WHAT TO DO:
Not for internal use. If child accidently swallows, call poison control center.

POSSIBLE ADVERSE REACTIONS OR SIDE EFFECTS

SYMPTOMS	WHAT TO DO
Life-threatening: None expected.	
Common:	
• Skin reactions including itching, redness, dryness, flaking.	Continue. Call doctor when convenient.
• Temporary burning sensation right after application.	No action necessary.
Infrequent: Swelling, soreness, persistent burning in treated area.	Continue. Call doctor when convenient.
Rare: Bleeding, oozing, blistering skin.	Discontinue. Call doctor right away.

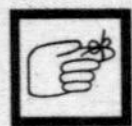

WARNINGS & PRECAUTIONS

Don't take if:
You are allergic to masoprocol.

Before you start, consult your doctor:
If you have a sulfite sensitivity.

Over age 60:
No problems expected.

Pregnancy:
Consult doctor. Risk category B (see page xxii).

Breast-feeding:
Effect not documented. Consult your doctor.

Infants & children:
Not used in this age group.

Prolonged use:
Effects of long-term use unknown.

Skin & sunlight:
Drug does not cause sensitivity to sunlight. However, keratoses are related to sun exposure, so avoid sunlight when possible.

Driving, piloting or hazardous work:
No problems expected.

Discontinuing:
No problems expected.

Others:
- If you accidently get masoprocol in your eye, promptly wash the eye with water.
- The cream may stain your clothing.
- Get doctor's approval before using cosmetics or make-up on the skin area you are treating.
- Leave the treated skin areas exposed. Don't cover them with a bandage or a dressing.

POSSIBLE INTERACTION WITH OTHER DRUGS

GENERIC NAME OR DRUG CLASS	COMBINED EFFECT
None significant.	

POSSIBLE INTERACTION WITH OTHER SUBSTANCES

INTERACTS WITH	COMBINED EFFECT
Alcohol:	None expected.
Beverages:	None expected.
Cocaine:	None expected.
Foods:	None expected.
Marijuana:	None expected.
Tobacco:	None expected.

MECAMYLAMINE

BRAND NAMES

Inversine

BASIC INFORMATION

Habit forming? No
Prescription needed? Yes
Available as generic? No
Drug class: Antihypertensive

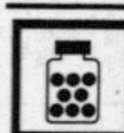

USES

Helps control, but doesn't cure, high blood pressure.

DOSAGE & USAGE INFORMATION

How to take:
Tablets—Swallow with liquid. If you can't swallow whole, crumble tablet and take with liquid or food. Instructions to take on empty stomach mean 1 hour before or 2 hours after eating.

When to take:
- At the same time each day, according to instructions on prescription label.
- Usually twice a day, every 8 or 12 hours apart. Follow label directions.

If you forget a dose:
Take as soon as you remember up to 2 hours late. If more than 2 hours, wait for next scheduled dose (don't double this dose).

What drug does:
Blocks transmission of electrical impulse where two nerve cells connect. Causes constricted blood vessels to relax.

Time lapse before drug works:
30 minutes to 2 hours.

Don't take with:
Any other medicines (including over-the-counter drugs such as cough and cold medicines, laxatives, antacids, diet pills, caffeine, nose drops or vitamins) without consulting your doctor.

OVERDOSE

SYMPTOMS:
Confusion, excitement, seizures, coma.
WHAT TO DO:
- **Dial 911 (emergency) or 0 (operator) for an ambulance or medical help. Then give first aid immediately.**
- **See emergency information on inside covers.**

POSSIBLE ADVERSE REACTIONS OR SIDE EFFECTS

SYMPTOMS	WHAT TO DO
Life-threatening:	
In case of overdose, see previous column.	
Common:	
Dizziness upon arising from chair or bed, blurred vision, decreased sex drive, dry mouth, enlarged pupils, constipation.	Continue. Call doctor when convenient.
Infrequent:	
• Confusion, depression, tremors, shortness of breath.	Discontinue. Call doctor right away.
• Difficult urination, tiredness.	Continue. Tell doctor at next visit.
Rare:	
Appetite loss, nausea and vomiting.	Continue. Tell doctor at next visit.

WARNINGS & PRECAUTIONS

Don't take if:
You are allergic to mecamylamine.

Before you start, consult your doctor:
- If you have heart disease.
- If you had a recent heart attack.
- If you have glaucoma or gout.
- If you have kidney disease.

Over age 60:
Adverse reactions and side effects may be more frequent and severe than in younger persons. You may need smaller doses for shorter periods of time.

Pregnancy:
Decide with your doctor if drug benefits justify risk to unborn child. Risk category C (see page xxii).

Breast-feeding:
Effect unknown. Consult doctor.

Infants & children:
Effect not documented. Consult your pediatrician.

Prolonged use:
Talk to your doctor about the need for follow-up medical examinations or laboratory studies to check blood pressure, kidney function and heart function.

Skin & sunlight:
No problems expected.

Driving, piloting or hazardous work:
Avoid if you feel confused, drowsy or dizzy.

Discontinuing:
Don't discontinue without consulting doctor. Dose may require gradual reduction if you have taken drug for a long time. Doses of other drugs may also require adjustment.

Others:
- Advise any doctor or dentist whom you consult that you take this medicine.
- May affect results in some medical tests.
- Get up slowly from chair or bed.
- Dosage may need to be adjusted for hot weather or heavy exercise.

POSSIBLE INTERACTION WITH OTHER DRUGS

GENERIC NAME OR DRUG CLASS	COMBINED EFFECT
Ambenonium	Swallowing difficulty.
Antacids*	Prolonged effect of mecamylamine.
Antibiotics*	Decreased antibiotic effect.
Alkalizers, urine*	Prolonged effect of mecamylamine.
Neostigmine	Swallowing difficulty.
Nimodipine	Dangerous blood pressure drop.
Pyridostigmine	Swallowing difficulty.
Sodium bicarbonate	Increased mecamylamine effect.
Sulfa drugs*	Decreased antibiotic effect.

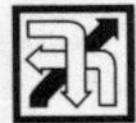

POSSIBLE INTERACTION WITH OTHER SUBSTANCES

INTERACTS WITH	COMBINED EFFECT
Alcohol:	Increased likelihood of fainting.
Beverages:	No special problems expected.
Cocaine:	Increased central nervous system stimulation. Avoid.
Foods: Food with high salt or sodium.	Decreased effectiveness of mecamylamine.
Marijuana:	Increased central nervous system stimulation. Avoid.
Tobacco:	No special problems expected.

***See Glossary**

MECHLORETHAMINE (Topical)

BRAND NAMES

Mustargen

BASIC INFORMATION

Habit forming? No
Prescription needed? Yes
Available as generic? No
Drug class: Antineoplastic (topical)

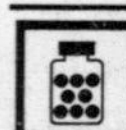

USES

- Treats mycosis fungoides.
- Treats other malignancies (by injection).

DOSAGE & USAGE INFORMATION

How to use:

- Solution—Mix according to doctor's instructions. Don't inhale vapors or powder.
- Shower and rinse before treatment.
- Use rubber gloves to apply over entire body.
- Avoid contact with eyes, nose and mouth.
- Ointment—Use according to doctor's instructions.

When to use:
Usually once a day.

If you forget a dose:
Notify your doctor.

What drug does:
Destroys cells that produce mycosis fungoides.

Time lapse before drug works:
None. Works immediately.

Don't use with:
Any other medicines (including over-the-counter drugs such as cough and cold medicines, laxatives, antacids, diet pills, caffeine, nose drops or vitamins) without consulting your doctor.

OVERDOSE

SYMPTOMS:
None expected for topical solutions.
WHAT TO DO:
Not intended for internal use. If child accidentally swallows, call poison control center.

POSSIBLE ADVERSE REACTIONS OR SIDE EFFECTS

SYMPTOMS	WHAT TO DO
Life-threatening:	
Immediate hives, shortness of breath.	Seek emergency treatment immediately.
Common:	
Darkening, dry skin.	Continue. Tell doctor at next visit.
Infrequent:	
Allergic reaction with rash, itching, hives.	Seek emergency treatment immediately.
Rare:	
None expected.	

WARNINGS & PRECAUTIONS

Don't use if:
You are allergic to mechlorethamine.

Before you start, consult your doctor:
- If you have chicken pox.
- If you have shingles (herpes zoster).
- If you have skin infection.

Over age 60:
No special problems expected.

Pregnancy:
Risk to unborn child outweighs drug benefits. Don't use. Risk category D (see page xxii).

Breast-feeding:
Drug may be absorbed and pass into milk. Avoid drug or discontinue nursing until you finish medicine. Consult doctor for advice on maintaining milk supply.

Infants & children:
Effect unknown. Consult doctor.

Prolonged use:
- Allergic or hypersensitive reactions more likely.
- Talk to your doctor about the need for follow-up medical examinations or laboratory studies to check liver function, complete blood counts (white blood cell count, platelet count, red blood cell count, hemoglobin, hematocrit) and hearing tests.

Skin & sunlight:
No problems expected.

Driving, piloting or hazardous work:
Don't drive or pilot aircraft until you learn how medicine affects you. Don't work around dangerous machinery. Don't climb ladders or work in high places. Danger increases if you drink alcohol or take medicine affecting alertness and reflexes.

Discontinuing:
No special problems expected.

Others:
- Advise any doctor or dentist whom you consult that you take this medicine.
- May affect results in some medical tests.
- Don't use if solution is discolored.

POSSIBLE INTERACTION WITH OTHER DRUGS

GENERIC NAME OR DRUG CLASS	COMBINED EFFECT
None significant.	

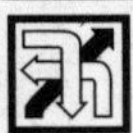

POSSIBLE INTERACTION WITH OTHER SUBSTANCES

INTERACTS WITH	COMBINED EFFECT
Alcohol:	None expected.
Beverages:	None expected.
Cocaine:	None expected.
Foods:	None expected.
Marijuana:	None expected.
Tobacco:	None expected.

MECLIZINE

BRAND NAMES

Antivert
Antivert/25
Antivert/50
Bonamine
Bonine
D-Vert 15
D-Vert 30
Meni-D
Ru-Vert-M

BASIC INFORMATION

Habit forming? No
Prescription needed?
U.S.: No, for some
Canada: Yes
Available as generic? Yes
Drug class: Antihistamine, antiemetic, anti-motion sickness

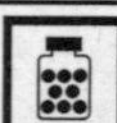

USES

- Prevents motion sickness.
- Treatment for vertigo.

DOSAGE & USAGE INFORMATION

How to take:
- Tablet or capsule—Swallow with liquid or food to lessen stomach irritation. If you can't swallow whole, crumble tablet or open capsule and take with liquid or food.
- Chewable tablet—May be chewed, swallowed whole or mixed with food.

When to take:
30 minutes to 1 hour before traveling or as directed by doctor.

If you forget a dose:
Take as soon as you remember. Wait 4 hours for next dose.

What drug does:
Reduces sensitivity of nerve endings in inner ear, blocking messages to brain's vomiting center.

Continued next column

OVERDOSE

SYMPTOMS:
Drowsiness, confusion, incoordination, stupor, coma, weak pulse, shallow breathing, hallucinations.
WHAT TO DO:
- **Dial 911 (emergency) or 0 (operator) for an ambulance or medical help. Then give first aid immediately.**
- **See emergency information on inside covers.**

Time lapse before drug works:
30 to 60 minutes.

Don't take with:
Any other medicine without consulting your doctor or pharmacist.

POSSIBLE ADVERSE REACTIONS OR SIDE EFFECTS

SYMPTOMS	WHAT TO DO
Life-threatening: In case of overdose, see previous column.	
Common: Drowsiness.	Continue. Tell doctor at next visit.
Infrequent:	
• Headache, diarrhea or constipation, fast heartbeat.	Continue. Call doctor when convenient.
• Dry mouth, nose, throat.	Continue. Tell doctor at next visit.
Rare:	
• Rash, hives.	Discontinue. Call doctor right away.
• Restlessness, excitement, insomnia, blurred vision, frequent and difficult urination, hallucinations.	Continue. Call doctor when convenient.
• Appetite loss, nausea.	Continue. Tell doctor at next visit.

WARNINGS & PRECAUTIONS

Don't take if:
- You are allergic to meclizine, buclizine or cyclizine.
- You have taken a monoamine oxidase (MAO) inhibitor* in the past 2 weeks.

Before you start, consult your doctor:
- If you have glaucoma.
- If you have prostate enlargement.
- If you have reacted badly to any antihistamine.

Over age 60:
Adverse reactions and side effects may be more frequent and severe than in younger persons, especially impaired urination from enlarged prostate gland.

Pregnancy:
Consult doctor. Risk category B (see page xxii).

Breast-feeding:
Drug passes into milk. Avoid drug or discontinue nursing until you finish medicine. Consult doctor for advice on maintaining milk supply.

Infants & children:
Safety not established. Avoid if under age 12.

Prolonged use:
No problems expected.

Skin & sunlight:
No problems expected.

Driving, piloting or hazardous work:
Don't fly aircraft. Don't drive until you learn how medicine affects you. Don't work around dangerous machinery. Don't climb ladders or work in high places. Danger increases if you drink alcohol or take medicine affecting alertness and reflexes, such as antihistamines, tranquilizers, sedatives, pain medicine, narcotics and mind-altering drugs.

Discontinuing:
No problems expected.

Others:
Some products contain tartrazine dye. Avoid, especially if you are allergic to aspirin.

POSSIBLE INTERACTION WITH OTHER DRUGS

GENERIC NAME OR DRUG CLASS	COMBINED EFFECT
Amphetamines*	May decrease drowsiness caused by meclizine.
Anticholinergics*	Increased effect of both drugs.
Antidepressants, tricyclic*	Increased effect of both drugs.
Carteolol	Decreased antihistamine effect.
Cisapride	Decreased meclizine effect.
Clozapine	Toxic effect on the central nervous system.
Dronabinol	Increases meclizine effect.
Ethinamate	Dangerous increased effects of ethinamate. Avoid combining.
Fluoxetine	Increased depressant effects of both drugs.
Guanfacine	May increase depressant effects of either drug.
Leucovorin	High alcohol content of leucovorin may cause adverse effects.
Methyprylon	Increased sedative effect, perhaps to dangerous level. Avoid.
Monoamine oxidase (MAO) inhibitors*	Increased meclizine effect.
Nabilone	Greater depression of central nervous system.
Narcotics*	Increased effect of both drugs.
Pain relievers*	Increased effect of both drugs.
Sedatives*	Increased effect of both drugs.
Sertraline	Increased depressive effects of both drugs.
Sleep inducers*	Increased effect of both drugs.
Sotalol	Increased antihistamine effect.
Tranquilizers*	Increased effect of both drugs.

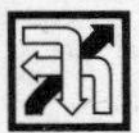

POSSIBLE INTERACTION WITH OTHER SUBSTANCES

INTERACTS WITH	COMBINED EFFECT
Alcohol:	Increased sedation. Avoid.
Beverages: Caffeine drinks.	May decrease drowsiness.
Cocaine:	None expected.
Foods:	None expected.
Marijuana:	Increased drowsiness, dry mouth.
Tobacco:	None expected.

MEFLOQUINE

BRAND NAMES

Lariam

BASIC INFORMATION

Habit forming? No
Prescription needed? Yes
Available as generic? No
Drug class: Antiprotozoal, antimalarial

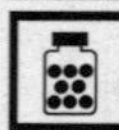

USES

- Treats malaria caused by *plasmodium falciparum* (either chloroquine-sensitive or chloroquine-resistant).
- Treats malaria caused by *plasmodium vivax.*
- Helps prevent malaria in people traveling into areas where malaria is prevalent.

DOSAGE & USAGE INFORMATION

How to take:
Tablet—Swallow with food, milk or 8 oz. of water to lessen stomach irritation.

When to take:
- Treatment—Usually given as 5 tablets in a single dose. Follow your doctor's instructions.
- Prevention—Start one week prior to traveling to an area where malaria is endemic. Continue during travel and for 4 weeks after return.

If you forget a dose:
Take as soon as you remember, then return to regular dosing schedule.

What drug does:
Exact mechanism unknown. Kills parasite in one of its developmental stages.

Continued next column

OVERDOSE

SYMPTOMS:
Seizures, heart rhythm disturbances.
WHAT TO DO:
- **Dial 911 (emergency) or 0 (operator) for an ambulance or medical help. Then give first aid immediately.**
- **Induce vomiting and see a doctor immediately because of the potential cardiotoxic effect. Treat vomiting or diarrhea with standard fluid therapy.**
- **See emergency information on inside covers.**

Time lapse before drug works:
7 to 24 hours.

Don't take with:
- Sulfadoxine and pyrimethamine combination (Fansidar).
- Any other medicines (including over-the-counter drugs such as cough and cold medicines, laxatives, antacids, diet pills, caffeine, nose drops or vitamins) without consulting your doctor.
- See Interaction column and consult doctor.

POSSIBLE ADVERSE REACTIONS OR SIDE EFFECTS

SYMPTOMS	WHAT TO DO
Life-threatening:	
Seizures.	Seek emergency treatment immediately.
Common:	
Dizziness, headache, insomnia, lightheadedness, abdominal pain, diarrhea, appetite loss, nausea or vomiting, visual disturbances.	Discontinue. Call doctor right away.
Infrequent:	
None expected.	
Rare:	
Slow heart rate, confusion, anxiety, depression, hallucinations, psychosis.	Discontinue. Call doctor right away.

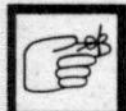

WARNINGS & PRECAUTIONS

Don't take if:
You are allergic to mefloquine, quinine, quinidine or related medications.

Before you start, consult your doctor:
- If you plan to become pregnant within the medication period or 2 months after.
- If you have heart trouble, especially heart block.
- If you have depression or other emotional problems.
- If you are giving this to a child under 40 pounds of body weight.
- If you have epilepsy or a seizure disorder.

Over age 60:
Adverse reactions and side effects may be more frequent and severe than in younger persons.

Pregnancy:
Not recommended. If traveling to an area where malaria is endemic, consult your doctor about prophylaxis. Risk category C (see page xxii).

Breast-feeding:
Mefloquine passes into mother's milk. Avoid drug or discontinue nursing.

Infants & children:
Not recommended for children under 2.

Prolonged use:
Not recommended.

Skin & sunlight:
No problems expected.

Driving, piloting or hazardous work:
Don't drive or pilot aircraft until you learn how medicine affects you. Don't work around dangerous machinery. Don't climb ladders or work in high places. Danger increases if you drink alcohol or take medicine affecting alertness and reflexes.

Discontinuing:
Don't discontinue without doctor's advice until you complete the prescribed dosage.

Others:
- Periodic physical (including eye) examinations and blood studies recommended.
- Resistance to mefloquine by some strains of malaria have been reported, so prevention and treatment of malaria may not be uniformly effective.

POSSIBLE INTERACTION WITH OTHER DRUGS

GENERIC NAME OR DRUG CLASS	COMBINED EFFECT
Antiseizure medications	Possible lowered seizure control.
Beta-adrenergic blocking agents*	Heartbeat irregularities or cardiac arrest. Avoid.
Calcium channel blockers*	Heartbeat irregularities.
Chloroquine	Increased chance of seizures. Avoid.
Divalproex	Increased risk of seizures.
Propranolol	Heartbeat irregularities.
Quinidine	Increased chance of seizures and heart rhythm disturbances.
Quinine	Increased chance of seizures and heart rhythm disturbances.
Typhoid vaccine (oral)	Concurrent use may decrease effectiveness of vaccine.
Valproic acid	Decreased valproic acid effect.

POSSIBLE INTERACTION WITH OTHER SUBSTANCES

INTERACTS WITH	COMBINED EFFECT
Alcohol:	Possible liver toxicity. Avoid.
Beverages: Any alcoholic beverage.	Possible liver toxicity. Avoid.
Cocaine:	No problems expected.
Foods:	No problems expected.
Marijuana:	No problems expected.
Tobacco:	No problems expected.

*See Glossary

MELPHALAN

BRAND NAMES

Alkeran	Phenylalanine
L-PAM	Mustard

BASIC INFORMATION

Habit forming? No
Prescription needed? Yes
Available as generic? No
Drug class: Antineoplastic

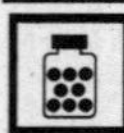

USES

- Treatment for some kinds of cancer.
- Suppresses immune response after organ transplantation and in immune disorders.

DOSAGE & USAGE INFORMATION

How to take:
Tablet—Swallow with liquid after light meal. Don't drink fluids with meals. Drink extra fluids between meals. Avoid sweet or fatty foods.

When to take:
At the same time each day.

If you forget a dose:
Take as soon as you remember. Don't ever double dose.

What drug does:
Inhibits abnormal cell reproduction. May suppress immune system.

Continued next column

OVERDOSE

SYMPTOMS:
Bleeding, chills, fever, collapse, stupor, seizure.
WHAT TO DO:

- **Dial 911 (emergency) or 0 (operator) for an ambulance or medical help. Then give first aid immediately.**
- **If patient is unconscious and not breathing, give mouth-to-mouth breathing. If there is no heartbeat, use cardiac massage and mouth-to-mouth breathing (CPR). Don't try to make patient vomit. If you can't get help quickly, take patient to nearest emergency facility.**
- **See emergency information on inside covers.**

Time lapse before drug works:
Up to 6 weeks for full effect.

Don't take with:
Any other medicine without consulting your doctor or pharmacist.

POSSIBLE ADVERSE REACTIONS OR SIDE EFFECTS

SYMPTOMS	WHAT TO DO
Life-threatening:	
In case of overdose, see previous column.	
Common:	
• Unusual bleeding or bruising, mouth sores with sore throat, chills and fever, black stools, sores in mouth and lips, menstrual irregularities, back pain.	Continue, but call doctor right away.
• Hair loss, joint pain.	Continue. Call doctor when convenient.
• Nausea, vomiting, diarrhea (unavoidable), tiredness, weakness.	Continue. Tell doctor at next visit.
Infrequent:	
• Skin rash.	Continue, but call doctor right away.
• Mental confusion, shortness of breath.	Continue. Call doctor when convenient.
• Cough.	Continue. Tell doctor at next visit.
Rare:	
Jaundice, swelling in feet or legs.	Continue, but call doctor right away.

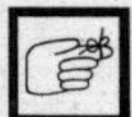

WARNINGS & PRECAUTIONS

Don't take if:
- You have had hypersensitivity to alkylating antineoplastic drugs.
- Your physician has not explained serious nature of your medical problem and risks of taking this medicine.

Before you start, consult your doctor:
- If you have gout.
- If you have had kidney stones.
- If you have active infection.
- If you have impaired kidney or liver function.
- If you have taken other antineoplastic drugs or had radiation treatment in last 3 weeks.
- If you have herpes zoster or chicken pox (or been exposed).

Over age 60:
Adverse reactions and side effects may be more frequent and severe than in younger persons.

Pregnancy:
Consult doctor. Risk category D (see page xxii).

Breast-feeding:
Safety not established. Consult doctor.

Infants & children:
Use only under special medical supervision at center experienced in anticancer drugs.

Prolonged use:
- Adverse reactions more likely the longer drug is required.
- Talk to your doctor about the need for follow-up medical examinations or laboratory studies to check complete blood counts (white blood cell count, platelet count, red blood cell count, hemoglobin, hematocrit), kidney function.

Skin & sunlight:
No problems expected.

Driving, piloting or hazardous work:
No problems expected.

Discontinuing:
Don't discontinue without doctor's advice until you complete prescribed dose, even though symptoms diminish or disappear. Some side effects may follow discontinuing. Report to doctor blurred vision, convulsions, confusion, persistent headache, fever or chills, blood in urine, unusual bleeding.

Others:
- May cause sterility.
- May increase chance of developing leukemia.

POSSIBLE INTERACTION WITH OTHER DRUGS

GENERIC NAME OR DRUG CLASS	COMBINED EFFECT
Antigout drugs*	Decreased antigout effect.
Antineoplastic drugs, other*	Increased effect of all drugs (may be beneficial).
Bone marrow depressants*	Increased risk of bone marrow toxicity.
Chloramphenicol	Increased likelihood of toxic effects of both drugs.
Clozapine	Toxic effect on bone marrow.
Lovastatin	Increased heart and kidney damage.
Probenecid	Increased likelihood of bone marrow toxicity.
Sulfinpyrazone	Increased likelihood of bone marrow toxicity.
Tiopronin	Increased risk of toxicity to bone marrow.
Vaccines, live or killed	Increased likelihood of toxicity or reduced effectiveness of vaccine.

POSSIBLE INTERACTION WITH OTHER SUBSTANCES

INTERACTS WITH	COMBINED EFFECT
Alcohol:	May increase chance of intestinal bleeding.
Beverages:	No problems expected.
Cocaine:	Increases chance of toxicity.
Foods:	Reduces irritation in stomach.
Marijuana:	No problems expected.
Tobacco:	Increases lung toxicity.

***See Glossary**

MEPROBAMATE

BRAND NAMES

See complete list of brand names in the *Brand Name Directory*, page 910.

BASIC INFORMATION

Habit forming? Yes
Prescription needed? Yes
Available as generic? Yes
Drug class: Tranquilizer, antianxiety drug

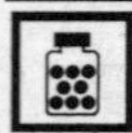

USES

Reduces mild anxiety, tension and insomnia.

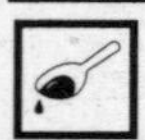

DOSAGE & USAGE INFORMATION

How to take:
- Tablet—Swallow with liquid.
- Extended-release capsules—Swallow each dose whole.

When to take:
At the same time each day.

If you forget a dose:
Take as soon as you remember up to 2 hours late. If more than 2 hours, wait for next scheduled dose (don't double this dose).

What drug does:
Sedates brain centers which control behavior and emotions.

Time lapse before drug works:
1 to 2 hours.

Don't take with:
- Nonprescription drugs containing alcohol or caffeine without consulting doctor.
- Any other medicine without consulting your doctor or pharmacist.

OVERDOSE

SYMPTOMS:
Dizziness, slurred speech, stagger, confusion, depressed breathing and heart function, stupor, coma.
WHAT TO DO:
- **Dial 911 (emergency) or 0 (operator) for an ambulance or medical help. Then give first aid immediately.**
- **See emergency information on inside covers.**

POSSIBLE ADVERSE REACTIONS OR SIDE EFFECTS

SYMPTOMS	WHAT TO DO
Life-threatening:	
Hives, rash, intense itching, faintness soon after a dose, wheezing (anaphylaxis).	Seek emergency treatment immediately.
Common:	
Dizziness, confusion, agitation, drowsiness, unsteadiness, fatigue, weakness.	Continue. Tell doctor at next visit.
Infrequent:	
• Rash, hives, itchy skin; change in vision; diarrhea, nausea or vomiting.	Discontinue. Call doctor right away.
• False sense of well-being, headache, slurred speech, blurred vision.	Continue. Call doctor when convenient.
Rare:	
Sore throat; fever; rapid, pounding, unusually slow or irregular heartbeat; difficult breathing; unusual bleeding or bruising.	Discontinue. Call doctor right away.

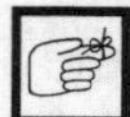

WARNINGS & PRECAUTIONS

Don't take if:
- You are allergic to meprobamate, tybamate, carbromal or carisoprodol.
- You have had porphyria.
- Patient is younger than 6.

Before you start, consult your doctor:
- If you have epilepsy.
- If you have impaired liver or kidney function.
- If you have tartrazine dye allergy.
- If you suffer from drug abuse or alcoholism, active or in remission.
- If you have porphyria.

Over age 60:
Adverse reactions and side effects may be more frequent and severe than in younger persons.

Pregnancy:
Risk to unborn child outweighs drug benefits. Don't use. Risk category D (see page xxii).

Breast-feeding:
Drug filters into milk. May cause sedation in child. Avoid.

Infants & children:
Not recommended.

Prolonged use:
- Habit forming.
- May impair blood cell production.

Skin & sunlight:
No problems expected.

Driving, piloting or hazardous work:
Don't drive or pilot aircraft until you learn how medicine affects you. Don't work around dangerous machinery. Don't climb ladders or work in high places. Danger increases if you drink alcohol or take medicine affecting alertness and reflexes, such as antihistamines, tranquilizers, sedatives, pain medicine, narcotics and mind-altering drugs.

Discontinuing:
Don't discontinue without consulting doctor. Dose may require gradual reduction if you have taken drug for a long time. Doses of other drugs may also require adjustment. Report to your doctor any unusual symptom that begins in the first week you discontinue this medicine. These symptoms may include convulsions, confusion, nightmares, insomnia.

Others:
No problems expected.

POSSIBLE INTERACTION WITH OTHER DRUGS

GENERIC NAME OR DRUG CLASS	COMBINED EFFECT
Addictive drugs*	Increased risk of addictive effect.
Antidepressants, tricyclic*	Increased anti-depressant effect.
Antihistamines*	Possible excessive sedation.
Monoamine oxidase (MAO) inhibitors*	Increased meprobamate effect.
Narcotics*	Increased narcotic effect.
Sedatives*	Increased sedative effect.
Sertraline	Increased depressive effects of both drugs.
Sleep inducers*	Increased effect of sleep inducer.
Tranquilizers*	Increased tranquilizer effect.

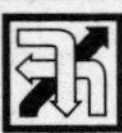

POSSIBLE INTERACTION WITH OTHER SUBSTANCES

INTERACTS WITH	COMBINED EFFECT
Alcohol:	Dangerous increased effect of meprobamate.
Beverages: Caffeine drinks.	Decreased calming effect of meprobamate.
Cocaine:	Decreased meprobamate effect.
Foods:	None expected.
Marijuana:	Increased sedative effect of meprobamate.
Tobacco:	None expected.

*See Glossary

MEPROBAMATE & ASPIRIN

BRAND NAMES

Epromate-M
Equagesic
Equazine-M
Heptogesic
Mepro Analgesic
Meprogese
Meprogesic
Meprogesic Q
Micrainin
Q-gesic
Tranquigesic

BASIC INFORMATION

Habit forming? Yes
Prescription needed? Yes
Available as generic? Yes
Drug class: Anti-inflammatory (nonsteroidal), analgesic, tranquilizer

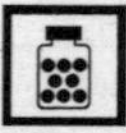

USES

- Reduces mild anxiety, tension and insomnia.
- Reduces pain, fever, inflammation.
- Relieves swelling, stiffness, joint pain.
- Antiplatelet effect.

DOSAGE & USAGE INFORMATION

How to take:
- Tablet—Swallow with liquid.
- Effervescent tablets—Dissolve in water.

When to take:
Pain, fever, inflammation—As needed, no more often than every 4 hours.

If you forget a dose:
Take as soon as you remember up to 2 hours late. If more than 2 hours, wait for next scheduled dose (don't double this dose).

What drug does:
- Sedates brain centers which control behavior and emotions.

Continued next column

OVERDOSE

SYMPTOMS:
Dizziness; slurred speech; stagger; depressed heart function; ringing in ears; nausea; vomiting; fever; deep, rapid breathing; hallucinations; convulsions; stupor; coma.
WHAT TO DO:
- **Dial 911 (emergency) or 0 (operator) for an ambulance or medical help. Then give first aid immediately.**
- **See emergency information on inside covers.**

- Affects hypothalamus, the part of the brain which regulates temperature by dilating small blood vessels in skin.
- Prevents clumping of platelets (small blood cells) so blood vessels remain open.
- Decreases prostaglandin effect.
- Suppresses body's pain messages.

Time lapse before drug works:
1 to 2 hours.

Don't take with:
- Tetracyclines.
- Nonprescription drugs containing alcohol or caffeine without consulting doctor.
- Any other medicine without consulting your doctor or pharmacist.

POSSIBLE ADVERSE REACTIONS OR SIDE EFFECTS

SYMPTOMS	WHAT TO DO
Life-threatening:	
Hives, rash, intense itching, faintness soon after a dose (anaphylaxis); difficulty breathing.	Seek emergency treatment immediately
Common:	
• Nausea, vomiting.	Discontinue. Call doctor right away.
• Dizziness, confusion, agitation, drowsiness, unsteadiness, fatigue, weakness, ears ringing, heartburn, indigestion, abdominal pain.	Continue. Call doctor when convenient.
Infrequent:	
Blurred vision, headache.	Continue. Call doctor when convenient.
Rare:	
• Black, bloody or tarry stool; vomiting blood or black material; blood in urine.	Discontinue. Seek emergency treatment.
• Rash, hives, itchy skin, change in vision, fever, jaundice, mental confusion.	Discontinue. Call doctor right away.

WARNINGS & PRECAUTIONS

Don't take if:
- You are allergic to meprobamate, tybamate, carbromal or carisoprodol.
- You are sensitive to aspirin.
- You have had porphyria.
- You have a peptic ulcer of stomach or duodenum or a bleeding disorder.
- Patient is younger than 6.

Before you start, consult your doctor:
- If you have epilepsy, impaired liver or kidney function, asthma or nasal polyps.
- If you are allergic to tartrazine.
- If you have had gout, stomach or duodenal ulcers.

Over age 60:
Adverse reactions and side effects may be more frequent and severe than in younger persons. More likely to cause hidden bleeding in stomach or intestines. Watch for dark stools.

Pregnancy:
Risk to unborn child outweighs drug benefits. Don't use.

Breast-feeding:
Drug passes into milk. Avoid drug or discontinue nursing until you finish medicine. Consult doctor for advice on maintaining milk supply.

Infants & children:
Not recommended.

Prolonged use:
- Habit forming.
- May impair blood cell production.
- Kidney damage. Periodic kidney function test recommended.

Skin & sunlight:
Aspirin combined with sunscreen may decrease sunburn.

Driving, piloting or hazardous work:
Don't drive or pilot aircraft until you learn how medicine affects you. Don't work around dangerous machinery. Don't climb ladders or work in high places. Danger increases if you drink alcohol or take medicine affecting alertness and reflexes, such as antihistamines, tranquilizers, sedatives, pain medicine, narcotics and mind-altering drugs.

Discontinuing:
Don't discontinue without consulting doctor. Dose may require gradual reduction if you have taken drug for a long time. Doses of other drugs may also require adjustment.

Others:
- Aspirin can complicate surgery; illness; pregnancy, labor and delivery.
- Urine tests for blood sugar may be inaccurate.

POSSIBLE INTERACTION WITH OTHER DRUGS

GENERIC NAME OR DRUG CLASS	COMBINED EFFECT
Acebutolol	Decreased anti-hypertensive effect of acebutolol.
Addictive drugs*	Increased risk of addictive effect.
Allopurinol	Decreased allopurinol effect.
Angiotensin-converting enzyme (ACE) inhibitors*	Decreased effect of ACE inhibitors.
Antacids*	Decreased aspirin effect.
Anticoagulants*	Increased anticoagulant effect. Abnormal bleeding.
Anticonvulsants*	Change in seizure pattern.
Antidepressants, tricyclic*	Increased anti-depressant effect.
Antidiabetics*, oral	Low blood sugar.
Anti-inflammatory drugs, nonsteroidal (NSAIDs)*	Risk of stomach bleeding and ulcers.
Aspirin, other	Likely aspirin toxicity.
Bumetanide	Possible aspirin toxicity.
Cortisone drugs*	Increased cortisone effect. Risk of ulcers and stomach bleeding.
Dronabinol	Increased effect of both drugs.

Continued on page 945

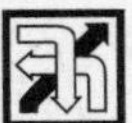

POSSIBLE INTERACTION WITH OTHER SUBSTANCES

INTERACTS WITH	COMBINED EFFECT
Alcohol:	Possible stomach irritation and bleeding. Dangerous increased effect of meprobamate. Avoid.
Beverages: Caffeine drinks.	Decreased calming effect of meprobamate.
Cocaine:	Decreased meprobamate effect.
Foods:	None expected.
Marijuana:	Possible increased pain relief, but marijuana may slow body's recovery. Avoid.
Tobacco:	None expected.

*See Glossary

MERCAPTOPURINE

BRAND NAMES

Purinethol | 6-MP

BASIC INFORMATION

Habit forming? No
Prescription needed? Yes
Available as generic? No
Drug class: Antineoplastic, immunosuppressant

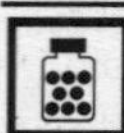

USES

- Treatment for some kinds of cancer.
- Treatment for regional enteritis and ulcerative colitis and other immune disorders.

DOSAGE & USAGE INFORMATION

How to take:
Tablet—Swallow with liquid.

When to take:
At the same time each day.

If you forget a dose:
Skip the missed dose. Don't double the next dose.

What drug does:
Inhibits abnormal cell reproduction.

Time lapse before drug works:
May require 6 weeks for maximum effect.

Don't take with:
Any other medicine without consulting your doctor or pharmacist.

OVERDOSE

SYMPTOMS:
Headache, stupor, seizures.
WHAT TO DO:

- **Dial 911 (emergency) or 0 (operator) for an ambulance or medical help. Then give first aid immediately.**
- **If patient is unconscious and not breathing, give mouth-to-mouth breathing. If there is no heartbeat, use cardiac massage and mouth-to-mouth breathing (CPR). Don't try to make patient vomit. If you can't get help quickly, take patient to nearest emergency facility.**
- **See emergency information on inside covers.**

POSSIBLE ADVERSE REACTIONS OR SIDE EFFECTS

SYMPTOMS	WHAT TO DO
Life-threatening: In case of overdose, see previous column.	
Common:	
• Black stools or bloody vomit.	Discontinue. Seek emergency treatment.
• Mouth sores, sore throat, unusual bleeding or bruising.	Discontinue. Call doctor right away.
• Abdominal pain, nausea, vomiting, weakness, tiredness.	Continue. Call doctor when convenient.
Infrequent:	
• Seizures.	Discontinue. Seek emergency treatment.
• Diarrhea, headache, confusion, blurred vision, shortness of breath, joint pain, blood in urine, jaundice, back pain, appetite loss, feet and leg swelling.	Discontinue. Call doctor right away.
• Cough.	Continue. Call doctor when convenient.
• Acne, boils, hair loss, itchy skin.	Continue. Tell doctor at next visit.
Rare:	
Fever and chills.	Discontinue. Call doctor right away.

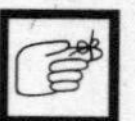

WARNINGS & PRECAUTIONS

Don't take if:
You are allergic to any antineoplastic.

Before you start, consult your doctor:

- If you are alcoholic.
- If you have blood, liver or kidney disease.
- If you have colitis or peptic ulcer.
- If you have gout.
- If you have an infection.
- If you plan to become pregnant within 3 months.

Over age 60:
Adverse reactions and side effects may be more frequent and severe than in younger persons.

Pregnancy:
Risk to unborn child outweighs drug benefits. Don't use. Risk category D (see page xxii).

Breast-feeding:
Avoid drug or discontinue nursing.

Infants & children:
Use only under special medical supervision.

Prolonged use:
- Adverse reactions more likely the longer drug is required.
- Talk to your doctor about the need for follow-up medical examinations or laboratory studies to check complete blood counts (white blood cell count, platelet count, red blood cell count, hemoglobin, hematocrit), liver function, kidney function, uric acid.

Skin & sunlight:
No problems expected.

Driving, piloting or hazardous work:
Avoid if you feel dizzy, drowsy or confused. Otherwise, no problems expected.

Discontinuing:
Don't discontinue without doctor's advice until you complete prescribed dose, even though symptoms diminish or disappear. Some side effects may follow discontinuing. Report to doctor blurred vision, convulsions, confusion, persistent headache, chills or fever, bloody urine or stools, back pain, jaundice.

Others:
- Drink more water than usual to cause frequent urination.
- Don't give this medicine to anyone else for any purpose. It is a strong drug that requires close medical supervision.
- Report for frequent medical follow-up and laboratory studies.

POSSIBLE INTERACTION WITH OTHER DRUGS

GENERIC NAME OR DRUG CLASS	COMBINED EFFECT
Acetaminophen	Increased likelihood of liver toxicity.
Allopurinol	Increased toxic effect of mercaptopurine.
Anticoagulants,* oral	May increase or decrease anticoagulant effect.
Antineoplastic drugs*, other	Increased effect of both (may be desirable) or increased toxicity of each.
Chloramphenicol	Increased toxicity of each.
Clozapine	Toxic effect on bone marrow.
Cyclosporine	May increase risk of infection.
Hepatotoxic drugs*	Increased risk of liver toxicity.
Immunosuppresants*, other	Increased risk of infections and neoplasms*.
Isoniazid	Increased risk of liver damage.
Levamisole	Increased risk of bone marrow depression.
Lovastatin	Increased heart and kidney damage.
Probenecid	Increased toxic effect of mercaptopurine.
Sulfinpyrazone	Increased toxic effect of mercaptopurine.
Tiopronin	Increased risk of toxicity to bone marrow.
Vaccines, live or killed	Increased risk of toxicity or reduced effectiveness of vaccine.

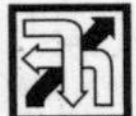

POSSIBLE INTERACTION WITH OTHER SUBSTANCES

INTERACTS WITH	COMBINED EFFECT
Alcohol:	May increase chance of intestinal bleeding.
Beverages:	No problems expected.
Cocaine:	Increased chance of toxicity.
Foods:	Reduced irritation in stomach.
Marijuana:	No problems expected.
Tobacco:	Increased lung toxicity.

MESALAMINE

BRAND NAMES

5-ASA
Asacol
Mesalazine
Pentasa
Rowasa
Salofalk

BASIC INFORMATION

Habit forming? No
Prescription needed? Yes
Available as generic? No
Drug class: Anti-inflammatory (nonsteroidal)

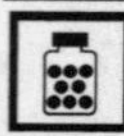

USES

- Treats ulcerative colitis.
- Reduces inflammatory conditions of the lower colon and rectum.

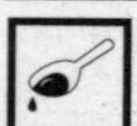

DOSAGE & USAGE INFORMATION

How to use:
- Rectal—Use as an enema. Insert the tip of the pre-packaged medicine container into the rectum. Squeeze container to empty contents. Retain in rectum all night or as long as possible.
- Delayed-release tablet or extended-release capsule—Swallow with liquid. Do not crush or chew tablet.

When to use:
- Rectal—Each night, preferably after a bowel movement. Continue for 3 to 6 weeks according to your doctor's instructions.
- Tablet—3 to 4 times a day or as directed by doctor.

If you forget a dose:
Take as soon as you remember up to 2 hours late. If more than 2 hours, wait for next scheduled dose (don't double this dose).

What drug does:
Decreases production of arachidonic acid forms which are increased in patients with chronic inflammatory bowel disease.

Time lapse before drug works:
3 to 21 days.

Continued next column

OVERDOSE

SYMPTOMS:
None expected.
WHAT TO DO:
No action needed.

Don't take with:
- Oral sulfasalazine concurrently. To do so may increase chances of kidney damage.
- Any other medicine without consulting your doctor or pharmacist.

POSSIBLE ADVERSE REACTIONS OR SIDE EFFECTS

SYMPTOMS	WHAT TO DO
Life-threatening:	
None expected.	
Common:	
None expected.	
Infrequent:	
None expected.	
Rare:	
• Abdominal pain, bloody diarrhea, fever, skin rash, anal irritation.	Discontinue. Call doctor right away.
• Gaseousness, nausea, headache, hair loss.	Continue. Call doctor when convenient.

WARNINGS & PRECAUTIONS

Don't take if:
You are allergic to salicylates* or any medication containing sulfasalazine (such as Azulfidine) or mesalamine.

Before you start, consult your doctor:
If you have had chronic kidney disease.

Over age 60:
More sensitive to drug. Aggravates symptoms of enlarged prostate. Causes impaired thinking, hallucinations, nightmares. Consult doctor about any of these.

Pregnancy:
Consult doctor. Risk category B (see page xxii).

Breast-feeding:
Effect unknown. Consult your doctor.

Infants & children:
Use for children only under doctor's supervision.

Prolonged use:
Talk to your doctor about the need for follow-up medical examinations or laboratory studies to check urine.

Skin & sunlight:
No problems expected.

Driving, piloting or hazardous work:
Don't drive or pilot aircraft until you learn how medicine affects you. Don't work around dangerous machinery. Don't climb ladders or work in high places. Danger increases if you drink alcohol or take medicine affecting alertness and reflexes.

Discontinuing:
Don't discontinue without consulting doctor. Dose may require gradual reduction if you have taken drug for a long time. Doses of other drugs may also require adjustment.

Others:
- Internal eye pressure should be measured regularly.
- Avoid becoming overheated.

POSSIBLE INTERACTION WITH OTHER DRUGS

GENERIC NAME OR DRUG CLASS	COMBINED EFFECT
None reported.	

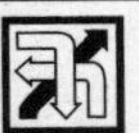

POSSIBLE INTERACTION WITH OTHER SUBSTANCES

INTERACTS WITH	COMBINED EFFECT
Alcohol:	None expected.
Beverages:	None expected.
Cocaine:	None expected.
Foods:	None expected.
Marijuana:	None expected.
Tobacco:	None expected.

***See Glossary**

METHENAMINE

BRAND NAMES

Hip-Rex
Hiprex
Mandelamine
Urex

BASIC INFORMATION

Habit forming? No
Prescription needed? Yes
Available as generic? Yes
Drug class: Anti-infective (urinary)

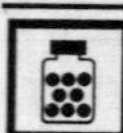

USES

Suppresses chronic urinary tract infections.

DOSAGE & USAGE INFORMATION

How to take:
- Tablet—Swallow with liquid or food to lessen stomach irritation. If you can't swallow whole, crumble tablet and take with liquid or food. If enteric-coated tablet, swallow whole.
- Liquid form—Use a measuring spoon to ensure correct dose.
- Granules—Dissolve dose in 4 oz. of water. Drink all the liquid.

When to take:
At the same times each day.

If you forget a dose:
Take as soon as you remember up to 8 hours late. If more than 8 hours, wait for next scheduled dose (don't double this dose).

What drug does:
A chemical reaction in the urine changes methenamine into formaldehyde, which destroys certain bacteria.

Continued next column

OVERDOSE

SYMPTOMS:
Bloody urine, weakness, deep breathing, stupor, coma.
WHAT TO DO:
- **Dial 911 (emergency) or 0 (operator) for an ambulance or medical help. Then give first aid immediately.**
- **See emergency information on inside covers.**

Time lapse before drug works:
Continual use for 3 to 6 months.

Don't take with:
Any other medicine without consulting your doctor or pharmacist.

POSSIBLE ADVERSE REACTIONS OR SIDE EFFECTS

SYMPTOMS	WHAT TO DO
Life-threatening: In case of overdose, see previous column.	
Common:	
• Rash.	Discontinue. Call doctor right away.
• Nausea, difficult urination.	Continue. Call doctor when convenient.
Infrequent:	
• Blood in urine.	Discontinue. Call doctor right away.
• Burning on urination, lower back pain.	Continue. Call doctor when convenient.
Rare: None expected.	

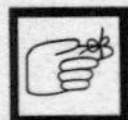

WARNINGS & PRECAUTIONS

Don't take if:

- You are allergic to methenamine.
- You have a severe impairment of kidney or liver function.
- Your urine cannot or should not be acidified (check with your doctor).

Before you start, consult your doctor:

- If you have had kidney or liver disease.
- If you plan to become pregnant within medication period.
- If you have had gout.

Over age 60:
Don't exceed recommended dose.

Pregnancy:
Decide with your doctor if drug benefits justify risk to unborn child. Risk category C (see page xxii).

Breast-feeding:
Drug passes into milk in small amounts. Consult doctor.

Infants & children:
Use only under medical supervision.

Prolonged use:
No problems expected.

Skin & sunlight:
No problems expected.

Driving, piloting or hazardous work:
No problems expected.

Discontinuing:
Don't discontinue without doctor's advice until you complete prescribed dose, even though symptoms diminish or disappear.

Others:
Requires an acid urine to be effective. Eat more protein foods, cranberries, cranberry juice with vitamin C, plums, prunes.

POSSIBLE INTERACTION WITH OTHER DRUGS

GENERIC NAME OR DRUG CLASS	COMBINED EFFECT
Antacids*	Decreased methenamine effect.
Carbonic anhydrase inhibitors*	Decreased methenamine effect.
Citrates*	Decreases effects of methenamine.
Diuretics, thiazide*	Decreased urine acidity.
Sodium bicarbonate	Decreased methenamine effect.
Sulfadoxine and pyrimethamine	Increased risk of kidney toxicity.
Sulfa drugs*	Possible kidney damage.

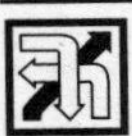

POSSIBLE INTERACTION WITH OTHER SUBSTANCES

INTERACTS WITH	COMBINED EFFECT
Alcohol:	Possible brain depression. Avoid or use with caution.
Beverages: Milk and other dairy products.	Decreased methenamine effect.
Cocaine:	None expected.
Foods: Citrus, cranberries, plums, prunes.	Increased methenamine effect.
Marijuana:	Drowsiness, muscle weakness or blood pressure drop.
Tobacco:	None expected.

*See Glossary

METHOTREXATE

BRAND NAMES

Amethopterin
Folex
Folex PFS
Mexate
Mexate AQ
Rheumatrex

BASIC INFORMATION

Habit forming? No
Prescription needed? Yes
Available as generic? Yes
Drug class: Antimetabolite, antipsoriatic

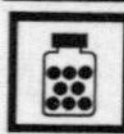

USES

- Treatment for some kinds of cancer.
- Treatment for psoriasis in patients with severe problems.
- Treatment for severe rheumatoid arthritis.

DOSAGE & USAGE INFORMATION

How to take:
Tablet—Swallow with liquid.

When to take:
At the same time each day.

If you forget a dose:
Skip the missed dose. Don't double the next dose.

What drug does:
Inhibits abnormal cell reproduction.

Time lapse before drug works:
May require 6 weeks for maximum effect.

Don't take with:
Any other medicine without consulting your doctor or pharmacist.

OVERDOSE

SYMPTOMS:
Headache, stupor, seizures.
WHAT TO DO:
- **Dial 911 (emergency) or 0 (operator) for an ambulance or medical help. Then give first aid immediately.**
- **If patient is unconscious and not breathing, give mouth-to-mouth breathing. If there is no heartbeat, use cardiac massage and mouth-to-mouth breathing (CPR). Don't try to make patient vomit. If you can't get help quickly, take patient to nearest emergency facility.**
- **See emergency information on inside covers.**

POSSIBLE ADVERSE REACTIONS OR SIDE EFFECTS

SYMPTOMS	WHAT TO DO
Life-threatening:	
Hives, rash, intense itching, faintness soon after a dose (anaphylaxis).	Seek emergency treatment immediately.
Common:	
• Black stools or bloody vomit.	Discontinue. Seek emergency treatment.
• Sore throat, fever, mouth sores; chills; unusual bleeding or bruising.	Discontinue. Call doctor right away.
• Abdominal pain, nausea, vomiting.	Continue. Call doctor when convenient.
Infrequent:	
• Seizures.	Discontinue. Seek emergency treatment.
• Dizziness when standing after sitting or lying, drowsiness, headache, confusion, blurred vision, shortness of breath, joint pain, blood in urine, jaundice, diarrhea, red skin, back pain.	Discontinue. Call doctor right away.
• Cough, rash, sexual difficulties in males.	Continue. Call doctor when convenient.
• Acne, boils, hair loss, itchy skin.	Continue. Tell doctor at next visit.
Rare:	
• Convulsions.	Seek emergency treatment.
• Painful urination.	Discontinue. Seek emergency treatment.

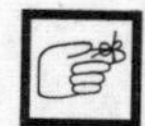

WARNINGS & PRECAUTIONS

Don't take if:
You are allergic to any antimetabolite.

Before you start, consult your doctor:
- If you are alcoholic.
- If you have blood, liver or kidney disease.
- If you have colitis or peptic ulcer.
- If you have gout.
- If you have an infection.
- If you plan to become pregnant within 3 months.

Over age 60:
Adverse reactions and side effects may be more frequent and severe than in younger persons.

Pregnancy:
- Psoriasis—Risk to unborn child outweighs drug benefits. Don't use.
- Cancer—Consult doctor.
- Risk category X (see page xxii).

Breast-feeding:
Drug passes into milk. Avoid drug or discontinue nursing.

Infants & children:
Use only under special medical supervision.

Prolonged use:
- Adverse reactions more likely the longer drug is required.
- Talk to your doctor about the need for follow-up medical examinations or laboratory studies to check liver function, kidney function, complete blood counts (white blood cell count, platelet count, red blood cell count, hemoglobin, hematocrit).

Skin & sunlight:
Increased sensitivity to sunlight.

Driving, piloting or hazardous work:
Avoid if you feel dizzy, drowsy or confused. Otherwise, no problems expected.

Discontinuing:
Don't discontinue without doctor's advice until you complete prescribed dose, even though symptoms diminish or disappear. Some side effects may follow discontinuing. Report to doctor blurred vision, convulsions, confusion, persistent headache.

Others:
- Drink more water than usual to cause frequent urination.
- Don't give this medicine to anyone else for any purpose. It is a strong drug that requires close medical supervision.
- Report for frequent medical follow-up and laboratory studies.

POSSIBLE INTERACTION WITH OTHER DRUGS

GENERIC NAME OR DRUG CLASS	COMBINED EFFECT
Anticoagulants,* oral	Increased anti-coagulant effect.
Anticonvulsants,* hydantoin	Possible methotrexate toxicity.
Antigout drugs*	Decreased antigout effect. Toxic levels of methotrexate.
Anti-inflammatory drugs, nonsteroidal (NSAIDs)*	Possible increased methotrexate toxicity.
Asparaginase	Decreased methotrexate effect.
Bone marrow depressants*, other	Increased risk of bone marrow depression.
Clozapine	Toxic effect on bone marrow.
Diclofenac	May increase toxicity.
Etretinate	Increased chance of toxicity to liver.
Fluorouracil	Decreased methotrexate effect.
Folic acid	Possible decreased methotrexate effect.
Isoniazid	Increased risk of liver damage.
Leukovorin calcium	Decreased methotrexate toxicity.
Levamisole	Increased risk of bone marrow depression.
Oxyphenbutazone	Possible methotrexate toxicity.
Penicillins*	Increased risk of methotrexate toxicity.
Phenylbutazone	Possible methotrexate toxicity.

Continued on page 946

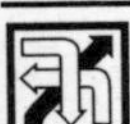

POSSIBLE INTERACTION WITH OTHER SUBSTANCES

INTERACTS WITH	COMBINED EFFECT
Alcohol:	Likely liver damage. Avoid.
Beverages:	Extra fluid intake decreases chance of methotrexate toxicity.
Cocaine:	Increased chance of methotrexate adverse reactions. Avoid.
Foods:	None expected.
Marijuana:	None expected.
Tobacco:	None expected.

*See Glossary

METHYLCELLULOSE

BRAND NAMES

Cellothyl
Citrucel
Cologel

BASIC INFORMATION

Habit forming? No
Prescription needed? No
Available as generic? Yes
Drug class: Laxative (bulk-forming)

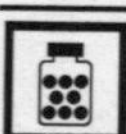

USES

Relieves constipation and prevents straining for bowel movement.

DOSAGE & USAGE INFORMATION

How to take:
Tablet, liquid, powder, flakes, granules—Dilute dose in 8 oz. cold water or fruit juice. Drink 6 to 8 glasses of water each day in addition to the one with each dose.

When to take:
At the same time each day, preferably morning.

If you forget a dose:
Take as soon as you remember. Resume regular schedule.

What drug does:
Absorbs water, stimulating the bowel to form a soft, bulky stool.

Time lapse before drug works:
May require 2 or 3 days to begin, then works in 12 to 24 hours.

Don't take with:
- Any other medicine without consulting your doctor or pharmacist.
- Don't take within 2 hours of taking another medicine. Laxative interferes with medicine absorption.

OVERDOSE

SYMPTOMS:
None expected.
WHAT TO DO:
Overdose unlikely to threaten life. If person takes much larger amount than prescribed, call doctor, poison control center or hospital emergency room for instructions.

POSSIBLE ADVERSE REACTIONS OR SIDE EFFECTS

SYMPTOMS	WHAT TO DO
Life-threatening: None expected.	
Common: None expected.	
Infrequent: Swallowing difficulty, "lump in throat" sensation, nausea, vomiting, diarrhea.	Continue. Call doctor when convenient.
Rare: Itchy skin, rash, intestinal blockage, asthma.	Discontinue. Call doctor right away.

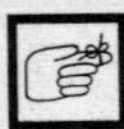

WARNINGS & PRECAUTIONS

Don't take if:
- You are allergic to any bulk-forming laxative.
- You have symptoms of appendicitis, inflamed bowel or intestinal blockage.
- You have missed a bowel movement for only 1 or 2 days.

Before you start, consult your doctor:
- If you have diabetes.
- If you have a laxative habit.
- If you have rectal bleeding.
- If you have difficulty swallowing.
- If you take other laxatives.

Over age 60:
Adverse reactions and side effects may be more frequent and severe than in younger persons.

Pregnancy:
Most bulk-forming laxatives contain sodium or sugars which may cause fluid retention. Avoid if possible. Consult doctor. Risk category C (see page xxii).

Breast-feeding:
No problems expected. Consult doctor.

Infants & children:
Use only under medical supervision.

Prolonged use:
Don't take for more than 1 week unless under a doctor's supervision. May cause laxative dependence.

Skin & sunlight:
No problems expected.

Driving, piloting or hazardous work:
No problems expected.

Discontinuing:
May be unnecessary to finish medicine. Follow doctor's instructions.

Others:
- Don't take to "flush out" your system or as a "tonic."
- Swelling of the throat or esophagus may occur if drug is not taken with an adequate amount of water.

POSSIBLE INTERACTION WITH OTHER DRUGS

GENERIC NAME OR DRUG CLASS	COMBINED EFFECT
Digitalis preparations*	Decreased digitalis effect.
Salicylates* (including aspirin)	Decreased salicylate effect.

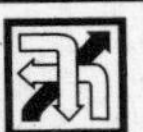

POSSIBLE INTERACTION WITH OTHER SUBSTANCES

INTERACTS WITH	COMBINED EFFECT
Alcohol:	None expected.
Beverages:	None expected.
Cocaine:	None expected.
Foods:	None expected.
Marijuana:	None expected.
Tobacco:	None expected.

***See Glossary**

METHYLDOPA

BRAND NAMES

Aldomet
Apo-Methyldopa
Dopamet
Novomedopa
Nu-Medopa

BASIC INFORMATION

Habit forming? No
Prescription needed? Yes
Available as generic? Yes
Drug class: Antihypertensive

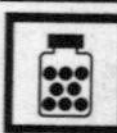

USES

Reduces high blood pressure.

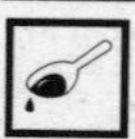

DOSAGE & USAGE INFORMATION

How to take:
Liquid or tablet—Swallow with liquid. If you can't swallow whole, crumble tablet and take with liquid or food.

When to take:
At the same times each day.

If you forget a dose:
Take as soon as you remember up to 2 hours late. If more than 2 hours, wait for next scheduled dose (don't double this dose).

What drug does:
Relaxes walls of small arteries to decrease blood pressure.

Time lapse before drug works:
Continual use for 2 to 4 weeks may be necessary to determine effectiveness.

Continued next column

OVERDOSE

SYMPTOMS:
Drowsiness; exhaustion; stupor; confusion; slow, weak pulse.
WHAT TO DO:

- **Dial 911 (emergency) or 0 (operator) for an ambulance or medical help. Then give first aid immediately.**
- **If patient is unconscious and not breathing, give mouth-to-mouth breathing. If there is no heartbeat, use cardiac massage and mouth-to-mouth breathing (CPR). Don't try to make patient vomit. If you can't get help quickly, take patient to nearest emergency facility.**
- **See emergency information on inside covers.**

Don't take with:
Any other medicine without consulting your doctor or pharmacist.

POSSIBLE ADVERSE REACTIONS OR SIDE EFFECTS

SYMPTOMS	WHAT TO DO
Life-threatening:	
In case of overdose, see previous column.	
Common:	
Depression, sedation, nightmares, headache, drowsiness, weakness, stuffy nose, dry mouth, fluid retention, swollen feet or legs.	Continue. Call doctor when convenient.
Infrequent:	
• Fast heartbeat, fainting.	Discontinue. Call doctor right away.
• Insomnia, nausea, vomiting, diarrhea, constipation, foot and hand numbness and tingling.	Continue. Call doctor when convenient.
• Swollen breasts, diminished sex drive.	Continue. Tell doctor at next visit.
Rare:	
Rash, jaundice, dark urine, chills, breathing difficulty, unexplained fever, sore or "black" tongue, severe abdominal pain, decreased mental activity and memory impairment, facial paralysis, slow heartbeat, chest pain, swollen abdomen.	Discontinue. Call doctor right away.

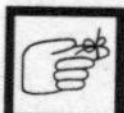

WARNINGS & PRECAUTIONS

Don't take if:
You will have surgery within 2 months, including dental surgery, requiring general or spinal anesthesia.

Before you start, consult your doctor:
If you have liver disease.

Over age 60:

- Increased susceptibility to dizziness, unsteadiness, fainting, falling.
- Drug can produce or intensify Parkinson's disease.

Pregnancy:
No proven problems. Consult doctor. Risk category B (see page xxii).

Breast-feeding:
No proven problems. Consult doctor.

Infants & children:
Not used.

Prolonged use:
- May cause anemia.
- Severe edema (fluid retention).
- Talk to your doctor about the need for follow-up medical examinations or laboratory studies to check complete blood counts (white blood cell count, platelet count, red blood cell count, hemoglobin, hematocrit), blood pressure, liver function.

Skin & sunlight:
No problems expected.

Driving, piloting or hazardous work:
Don't drive or pilot aircraft until you learn how medicine affects you. Don't work around dangerous machinery. Don't climb ladders or work in high places. Danger increases if you drink alcohol or take medicine affecting alertness and reflexes, such as antihistamines, tranquilizers, sedatives, pain medicine, narcotics and mind-altering drugs.

Discontinuing:
Don't discontinue without consulting doctor. Dose may require gradual reduction if you have taken drug for a long time. Doses of other drugs may also require adjustment.

Others:
Avoid heavy exercise, exertion, sweating.

POSSIBLE INTERACTION WITH OTHER DRUGS

GENERIC NAME OR DRUG CLASS	COMBINED EFFECT
Amphetamines*	Decreased methyldopa effect.
Angiotensin-converting enzyme (ACE) inhibitors*	Possible excessive potassium in blood.
Anticoagulants*, oral	Increased anti-coagulant effect.
Antidepressants, tricyclic*	Dangerous blood pressure rise. Decreased methyldopa effect.
Antihypertensives*	Increased anti-hypertensive effect.
Carteolol	Increased anti-hypertensive effect.
Clozapine	Toxic effect on the central nervous system.
Dapsone	Increased risk of adverse effect on blood cells.
Didanosine	Increased risk of pancreatitis.
Digitalis preparations*	Excessively slow heartbeat.
Diuretics, thiazide*	Increased methyldopa effect.
Ethinamate	Dangerous increased effects of ethinamate. Avoid combining.
Fluoxetine	Increased depressant effects of both drugs.
Guanfacine	May increase depressant effects of either drug.
Haloperidol	Increased sedation. Possibly dementia.
Isoniazid	Increased risk of liver damage.
Leucovorin	High alcohol content of leucovorin may cause adverse effects.
Levodopa	Increased effect of both drugs.
Loxapine	May increase toxic effects of both drugs.
Methyprylon	Increased sedative effect, perhaps to dangerous level. Avoid.

Continued on page 946

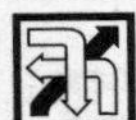

POSSIBLE INTERACTION WITH OTHER SUBSTANCES

INTERACTS WITH	COMBINED EFFECT
Alcohol:	Increased sedation. Excessive blood pressure drop. Avoid.
Beverages:	None expected.
Cocaine:	Increased risk of heart block and high blood pressure.
Foods:	None expected.
Marijuana:	Possible fainting.
Tobacco:	Possible increased blood pressure.

***See Glossary**

METHYLDOPA & THIAZIDE DIURETICS

BRAND AND GENERIC NAMES

Aldoclor
Aldoril
METHYLDOPA & CHLOROTHIAZIDE
METHYLDOPA & HYDROCHLOROTHIAZIDE
Novodoparil
PMS Dopazide

BASIC INFORMATION

Habit forming? No
Prescription needed? Yes
Available as generic? Yes
Drug class: Antihypertensive, diuretic (thiazide)

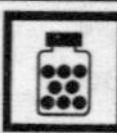

USES

- Controls, but doesn't cure, high blood pressure.
- Reduces fluid retention (edema).

DOSAGE & USAGE INFORMATION

How to take:
Tablet—Swallow with liquid. If you can't swallow whole, crumble tablet and take with liquid or food.

When to take:
At the same times each day.

If you forget a dose:
Take as soon as you remember up to 2 hours late. If more than 2 hours, wait for next scheduled dose (don't double this dose).

Continued next column

OVERDOSE

SYMPTOMS:
Drowsiness; exhaustion; cramps; weakness; stupor; confusion; slow, weak pulse; coma.

WHAT TO DO:
- **Dial 911 (emergency) or 0 (operator) for an ambulance or medical help. Then give first aid immediately.**
- **If patient is unconscious and not breathing, give mouth-to-mouth breathing. If there is no heartbeat, use cardiac massage and mouth-to-mouth breathing (CPR). Don't try to make patient vomit. If you can't get help quickly, take patient to nearest emergency facility.**
- **See emergency information on inside covers.**

What drug does:
- Relaxes walls of small arteries to decrease blood pressure.
- Forces sodium and water excretion, reducing body fluid.
- Reduced body fluid and relaxed arteries lower blood pressure.

Time lapse before drug works:
Continual use for 2 to 4 weeks may be necessary to determine effectiveness.

Don't take with:
- Nonprescription drugs without consulting doctor.
- Any other medicine without consulting your doctor or pharmacist.

POSSIBLE ADVERSE REACTIONS OR SIDE EFFECTS

SYMPTOMS	WHAT TO DO
Life-threatening:	
Irregular heartbeat, weak pulse.	Discontinue. Seek emergency treatment.
Common:	
Depression, nightmares, drowsiness, weakness, stuffy nose, dry mouth, swollen feet and ankles, dizziness, sedation, increased thirst, muscle cramps.	Continue. Call doctor when convenient.
Infrequent:	
• Fast heartbeat, change in vision, abdominal pain, nervousness.	Discontinue. Call doctor right away.
• Insomnia, nausea, vomiting, diarrhea, headache, constipation.	Continue. Call doctor when convenient.
Rare:	
Rash, jaundice, dark urine, chills, breathing difficulty, hives, sore throat, fever, mouth sores, sore or "black" tongue, severe abdominal pain, decreased mental activity, memory impairment, facial paralysis, slow heartbeat, chest pain.	Discontinue. Call doctor right away.

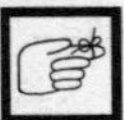

WARNINGS & PRECAUTIONS

Don't take if:
- You are allergic to any thiazide diuretic drug.
- You will have surgery within 2 months, including dental surgery, requiring general or spinal anesthesia.

Before you start, consult your doctor:
- If you are allergic to any sulfa drug.
- If you have gout, liver, pancreas or kidney disorder.

Over age 60:
- Increased susceptibility to dizziness, unsteadiness, fainting, falling.
- Drug can produce or intensify Parkinson's disease.

Pregnancy:
Decide with your doctor if drug benefits justify risk to unborn child. Risk category C (see page xxii).

Breast-feeding:
Drug passes into milk. Avoid drug or discontinue nursing until you finish medicine. Consult doctor for advice on maintaining milk supply.

Infants & children:
Not recommended.

Prolonged use:
- May cause anemia.
- Severe edema (fluid retention).
- Talk to your doctor about the need for follow-up medical examinations or laboratory studies to check complete blood counts (white blood cell count, platelet count, red blood cell count, hemoglobin, hematocrit), blood pressure, liver function.

Skin & sunlight:
May cause rash or intensify sunburn in areas exposed to sun or sunlamp.

Driving, piloting or hazardous work:
Don't drive or pilot aircraft until you learn how medicine affects you. Don't work around dangerous machinery. Don't climb ladders or work in high places. Danger increases if you drink alcohol or take medicine affecting alertness and reflexes, such as antihistamines, tranquilizers, sedatives, pain medicine, narcotics and mind-altering drugs.

Discontinuing:
Don't discontinue without consulting doctor. Dose may require gradual reduction if you have taken drug for a long time. Doses of other drugs may also require adjustment.

Others:
- Hot weather and fever may cause dehydration and drop in blood pressure. Dose may require temporary adjustment. Weigh daily and report any unexpected weight decreases to your doctor.
- May cause rise in uric acid, leading to gout.
- May cause blood sugar rise in diabetics.
- Avoid heavy exercise, exertion, sweating.

POSSIBLE INTERACTION WITH OTHER DRUGS

GENERIC NAME OR DRUG CLASS	COMBINED EFFECT
Acebutolol	Increased antihypertensive effect. Dosages of both drugs may require adjustments.
Allopurinol	Decreased allopurinol effect.
Amphetamines*	Decreased methyldopa effect.
Angiotensin-converting enzyme (ACE) inhibitors*	Possible excessive potassium in blood.
Anticoagulants*, oral	Increased anti-coagulant effect.
Antidepressants, tricyclic*	Dangerous changes in blood pressure. Avoid combination unless under medical supervision.

Continued on page 946

POSSIBLE INTERACTION WITH OTHER SUBSTANCES

INTERACTS WITH	COMBINED EFFECT
Alcohol:	Increased sedation. Excessive blood pressure drop. Avoid.
Beverages:	None expected.
Cocaine:	Increased risk of heart block and high blood pressure.
Foods: Licorice.	Excessive potassium loss that causes dangerous heart rhythms.
Marijuana:	May increase blood pressure.
Tobacco:	Possible increased blood pressure.

***See Glossary**

METHYLERGONOVINE

BRAND NAMES

Methergine
Methylergometrine

BASIC INFORMATION

Habit forming? No
Prescription needed? Yes
Available as generic? No
Drug class: Ergot preparation (uterine stimulant)

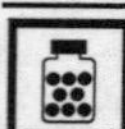

USES

Retards excessive post-delivery bleeding.

DOSAGE & USAGE INFORMATION

How to take:
Tablet—Swallow with liquid or food to lessen stomach irritation.

When to take:
At the same times each day.

If you forget a dose:
Don't take missed dose and don't double next one. Wait for next scheduled dose.

What drug does:
Causes smooth muscle cells of uterine wall to contract and surround bleeding blood vessels of relaxed uterus.

Time lapse before drug works:
Tablets—20 to 30 minutes.

Don't take with:
Any other medicine without consulting your doctor or pharmacist.

OVERDOSE

SYMPTOMS:
Vomiting, diarrhea, weak pulse, low blood pressure, dyspnea, angina, convulsions.
WHAT TO DO:

- **Dial 911 (emergency) or 0 (operator) for an ambulance or medical help. Then give first aid immediately.**
- **If patient is unconscious and not breathing, give mouth-to-mouth breathing. If there is no heartbeat, use cardiac massage and mouth-to-mouth breathing (CPR). Don't try to make patient vomit. If you can't get help quickly, take patient to nearest emergency facility.**
- **See emergency information on inside covers.**

POSSIBLE ADVERSE REACTIONS OR SIDE EFFECTS

SYMPTOMS	WHAT TO DO
Life-threatening: In case of overdose, see previous column.	
Common: Nausea, vomiting, severe lower abdominal menstrual-like cramps.	Discontinue. Call doctor right away.
Infrequent: • Confusion, ringing in ears, diarrhea, muscle cramps.	Discontinue. Call doctor right away.
• Unusual sweating.	Continue. Call doctor when convenient.
Rare: Sudden, severe headache; shortness of breath; chest pain; numb, cold hands and feet.	Discontinue. Seek emergency treatment.

WARNINGS & PRECAUTIONS

Don't take if:
You are allergic to any ergot preparation.

Before you start, consult your doctor:
- If you have coronary artery or blood vessel disease.
- If you have liver or kidney disease.
- If you have high blood pressure.
- If you have postpartum infection.

Over age 60:
Not recommended.

Pregnancy:
Consult doctor. Risk category C (see page xxii).

Breast-feeding:
Drug passes into milk. Avoid drug or discontinue nursing until you finish medicine. Consult doctor for advice on maintaining milk supply.

Infants & children:
Not recommended.

Prolonged use:
Talk to your doctor about the need for follow-up medical examinations or laboratory studies to check blood pressure, ECG*.

Skin & sunlight:
No problems expected.

Driving, piloting or hazardous work:
No problems expected.

Discontinuing:
May be unnecessary to finish medicine. Follow doctor's instructions.

Others:
Drug should be used for short time only following childbirth or miscarriage.

POSSIBLE INTERACTION WITH OTHER DRUGS

GENERIC NAME OR DRUG CLASS	COMBINED EFFECT
Antianginals*	Possible vasospasm (peripheral and cardiac)
Ergot preparations*, other	Increased methylergonovine effect.

POSSIBLE INTERACTION WITH OTHER SUBSTANCES

INTERACTS WITH	COMBINED EFFECT
Alcohol:	None expected.
Beverages:	None expected.
Cocaine:	None expected.
Foods:	None expected.
Marijuana:	None expected.
Tobacco:	Decreased methylergonovine effect. Don't smoke.

*See Glossary

METHYLPHENIDATE

BRAND NAMES

PMS-Methylphenidate
Ritalin
Ritalin SR

BASIC INFORMATION

Habit forming? Yes
Prescription needed? Yes
Available as generic? Yes
Drug class: Sympathomimetic

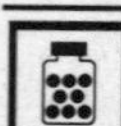

USES

- Treatment for hyperactive children.
- Treatment for narcolepsy (uncontrollable attacks of sleepiness).

DOSAGE & USAGE INFORMATION

How to take:
- Tablet—Swallow with liquid or food to lessen stomach irritation. If you can't swallow whole, crumble tablet and take with liquid or small amount of food.
- Extended-release tablet—Swallow whole with liquid.

When to take:
At the same times each day, preferably on an empty stomach.

If you forget a dose:
Take as soon as you remember up to 2 hours late. If more than 2 hours, wait for next scheduled dose (don't double this dose).

Continued next column

OVERDOSE

SYMPTOMS:
Rapid heartbeat, fever, confusion, vomiting, agitation, hallucinations, convulsions, coma.
WHAT TO DO:
- **Dial 911 (emergency) or 0 (operator) for an ambulance or medical help. Then give first aid immediately.**
- **If patient is unconscious and not breathing, give mouth-to-mouth breathing. If there is no heartbeat, use cardiac massage and mouth-to-mouth breathing (CPR). Don't try to make patient vomit. If you can't get help quickly, take patient to nearest emergency facility.**
- **See emergency information on inside covers.**

What drug does:
Stimulates brain to improve alertness, concentration and attention span. Calms the hyperactive child.

Time lapse before drug works:
- 1 month or more for maximum effect on child.
- 30 minutes to stimulate adults.

Don't take with:
Any other medicine without consulting your doctor or pharmacist.

POSSIBLE ADVERSE REACTIONS OR SIDE EFFECTS

SYMPTOMS	WHAT TO DO
Life-threatening:	
In case of overdose, see previous column.	
Common:	
• Mood change.	Continue. Call doctor when convenient.
• Nervousness, insomnia, dizziness, headache, appetite loss.	Continue. Tell doctor at next visit.
Infrequent:	
• Rash or hives; chest pain; fast, irregular heartbeat; unusual bruising; joint pain; psychosis; uncontrollable movements; unexplained fever.	Discontinue. Call doctor right away.
• Nausea, abdominal pain.	Continue. Call doctor when convenient.
Rare:	
• Blurred vision, sore throat, red spots under skin, convulsions.	Discontinue. Call doctor right away.
• Unusual tiredness.	Continue. Call doctor when convenient.

WARNINGS & PRECAUTIONS

Don't take if:
- You are allergic to methylphenidate.
- You have glaucoma.
- Patient is younger than 6.

Before you start, consult your doctor:
- If you have epilepsy.
- If you have high blood pressure.
- If you take MAO inhibitors.

Over age 60:
Adverse reactions and side effects may be more frequent and severe than in younger persons.

Pregnancy:
Decide with your doctor if drug benefits justify risk to unborn child. Risk category C (see page xxii).

Breast-feeding:
No proven problems. Consult doctor.

Infants & children:
Use only under medical supervision for children 6 or older.

Prolonged use:
- Rare possibility of physical growth retardation.
- Talk to your doctor about the need for follow-up medical examinations or laboratory studies to check blood pressure, complete blood counts (white blood cell count, platelet count, red blood cell count, hemoglobin, hematocrit), growth charts.

Skin & sunlight:
No problems expected.

Driving, piloting or hazardous work:
No problems expected.

Discontinuing:
Don't discontinue abruptly. Don't discontinue without doctor's advice until you complete prescribed dose, even though symptoms diminish or disappear. Report to your doctor any new symptoms of depression, unusual behavior, unusual weakness or tiredness.

Others:
Dose must be carefully adjusted by doctor.

POSSIBLE INTERACTION WITH OTHER DRUGS

GENERIC NAME OR DRUG CLASS	COMBINED EFFECT
Acebutolol	Decreased effects of both drugs.
Anticholinergics*	Increased anticholinergic effect.
Anticoagulants*, oral	Increased anti-coagulant effect.
Anticonvulsants*	Increased anticonvulsant effect.
Antidepressants, tricyclic*	Increased anti-depressant effect. Decreased methylphenidate effect.
Antihypertensives*	Decreased antihypertensive effect.
Central nervous system (CNS) stimulants*	Overstimulation.
Cisapride	Decreased methyl-phenidate effect.
Dextrothyroxine	Increased methylphenidate effect.
Guanadrel	Decreased guanadrel effect.
Guanethidine	Decreased guanethidine effect.
Minoxidil	Decreased minoxidil effect.
Monoamine oxidase (MAO) inhibitors*	Dangerous rise in blood pressure.
Nitrates*	Possible decreased effects of both drugs.
Oxprenolol	Decreased effects of both drugs.
Oxyphenbutazone	Increased oxyphenbutazone effect.
Phenylbutazone	Increased phenyl-butazone effect.
Pimozide	May mask the cause of tics.
Terazosin	Decreased effective-ness of terazosin.

POSSIBLE INTERACTION WITH OTHER SUBSTANCES

INTERACTS WITH	COMBINED EFFECT
Alcohol:	None expected.
Beverages: Caffeine drinks.	May raise blood pressure.
Cocaine:	High risk of heart-beat irregularities and high blood pressure.
Foods: Foods containing tyramine*.	May raise blood pressure.
Marijuana:	None expected.
Tobacco:	None expected.

*See Glossary

METHYLPREDNISOLONE

BRAND NAMES

See complete list of brand names in the *Brand Name Directory*, page 911.

BASIC INFORMATION

Habit forming? No
Prescription needed? Yes
Available as generic? Yes
Drug class: Cortisone drug (adrenal corticosteroid)

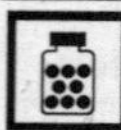

USES

- Reduces inflammation caused by many different medical problems.
- Treatment for some allergic diseases, blood disorders, kidney diseases, asthma and emphysema.
- Reduces corticosteroid deficiencies.

DOSAGE & USAGE INFORMATION

How to take:
- Tablet—Swallow with liquid or food to lessen stomach irritation. If you can't swallow whole, crumble tablet and take with liquid or food.
- Injection—Take under doctor's supervision.

When to take:
At the same times each day. Take once-a-day or once-every-other-day doses in mornings.

If you forget a dose:
- Several-doses-per-day prescription—Take as soon as you remember up to 2 hours late. If more than 2 hours, wait for next scheduled dose (don't double this dose).
- Once-a-day dose or less—Wait for next dose. Double this dose.

What drug does:
Decreases inflammatory responses.

Time lapse before drug works:
2 to 4 days.

Continued next column

OVERDOSE

SYMPTOMS:
Headache, convulsions, heart failure.
WHAT TO DO:
- **Dial 911 (emergency) or 0 (operator) for an ambulance or medical help. Then give first aid immediately.**
- **See emergency information on inside covers.**

Don't take with:
Any other medicine without consulting your doctor or pharmacist.

POSSIBLE ADVERSE REACTIONS OR SIDE EFFECTS

SYMPTOMS	WHAT TO DO
Life-threatening:	
Hives, rash, intense itching, faintness soon after a dose (anaphylaxis).	Seek emergency treatment immediately.
Common:	
Acne, poor wound healing, thirst, indigestion, nausea, vomiting, constipation, gaseousness, unpleasant taste, diarrhea, headache, cough, dizziness, hoarseness, appetite gain or loss.	Continue. Call doctor when convenient.
Infrequent:	
• Black, bloody or tarry stools; various infections; swallowing difficulty.	Discontinue. Seek emergency treatment.
• Blurred vision, halos around lights, sore throat, fever, muscle cramps, swollen legs or feet.	Discontinue. Call doctor right away.
• Mood change, insomnia, fatigue, restlessness, frequent urination, weight gain, round face, weakness, irregular menstrual periods, dry mouth, euphoria, nosebleeds.	Continue. Call doctor when convenient.
Rare:	
• Irregular heartbeat.	Discontinue. Seek emergency treatment.
• Rash, numbness or tingling in hands or feet, pancreatitis, thrombophlebitis, hallucinations, convulsions.	Discontinue. Call doctor right away.

METHYLPREDNISOLONE

WARNINGS & PRECAUTIONS

Don't take if:
- You are allergic to any cortisone drug.
- You have tuberculosis or fungus infection.
- You have herpes infection of eyes, lips or genitals.
- You have bone disease, thyroid disease, colitis, peptic ulcer, diabetes, myasthenia gravis, liver or kidney disease, diverticulitis, glaucoma, heart disease.

Before you start, consult your doctor:
- If you have had tuberculosis.
- If you have congestive heart failure.
- If you have diabetes, peptic ulcer, glaucoma, underactive thyroid, high blood pressure, myasthenia gravis, blood clots in legs or lungs.

Over age 60:
Adverse reactions and side effects may be more frequent and severe than in younger persons. Likely to aggravate edema, diabetes or ulcers. Likely to cause cataracts and osteoporosis (softening of the bones).

Pregnancy:
Decide with your doctor if drug benefits justify risk to unborn child. Risk category C (see page xxii).

Breast-feeding:
Drug passes into milk. Avoid drug or discontinue nursing until you finish medicine. Consult doctor for advice on maintaining milk supply.

Infants & children:
Use only under medical supervision.

Prolonged use:
- Retards growth in children.
- Possible glaucoma, cataracts, diabetes, fragile bones and thin skin.
- Functional dependence.
- Talk to your doctor about the need for follow-up medical examinations or laboratory studies to check blood pressure, serum electrolytes, stools for blood.

Skin & sunlight:
No problems expected.

Driving, piloting or hazardous work:
No problems expected.

Discontinuing:
- Don't discontinue without doctor's advice until you complete prescribed dose, even though symptoms diminish or disappear.
- Drug affects your response to surgery, illness, injury or stress for 2 years after discontinuing. Tell anyone who takes medical care of you within 2 years about drug.

Others:
- Avoid immunizations if possible.
- Your resistance to infection is less while taking this drug.
- Advise any doctor or dentist whom you consult that you take this medicine.
- Those who have inactive or "cured" tuberculosis may be subjected to a possible recurrence of active tuberculosis.
- Children who must take cortisone drugs may grow less well.

POSSIBLE INTERACTION WITH OTHER DRUGS

GENERIC NAME OR DRUG CLASS	COMBINED EFFECT
Amphotericin B	Potassium depletion.
Anticholinergics*	Possible glaucoma.
Anticoagulants*, oral	Decreased anti-coagulant effect.
Anticonvulsants*, hydantoin	Decreased methyl-prednisolone effect.
Antidiabetics*, oral	Decreased anti-diabetic effect.
Antihistamines*	Decreased methyl-prednisolone effect.
Anti-inflammatory drugs*nonsteroidal	Increased risk of ulcers and methyl-prednisolone effect.
Aspirin	Increased methyl-prednisolone effect.
Attentuated virus vaccines*	Possible viral infection.

Continued on page 947

POSSIBLE INTERACTION WITH OTHER SUBSTANCES

INTERACTS WITH	COMBINED EFFECT
Alcohol:	Risk of stomach ulcers.
Beverages:	No proven problems.
Cocaine:	Overstimulation. Avoid.
Foods:	No proven problems.
Marijuana:	Decreased immunity.
Tobacco:	Increased methyl-prednisolone effect. Possible toxicity.

METHYPRYLON

BRAND NAMES

Noludar

BASIC INFORMATION

Habit forming? Yes
Prescription needed? Yes
Available as generic? No
Drug class: Sedative (hypnotic)

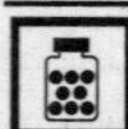

USES

Treats insomnia.

DOSAGE & USAGE INFORMATION

How to take:
Capsules or tablets—Swallow with liquid or food to lessen stomach irritation. If you can't swallow whole, open capsule and take with liquid or food.

When to take:
At bedtime.

If you forget a dose:
Take as soon as you remember up to 2 hours late. If more than 2 hours, wait for next scheduled dose (don't double this dose).

What drug does:
Increases threshold of arousal centers in the midbrain.

Time lapse before drug works:
Within 45 minutes.

Don't take with:
- Any other medicine that will affect alertness or reflexes.
- Any other medicine without consulting your doctor or pharmacist.

OVERDOSE

SYMPTOMS:
Confusion, difficulty breathing, slow heartbeat, staggering, severe weakness, convulsions, coma.
WHAT TO DO:
- **Dial 911 (emergency) or 0 (operator) for an ambulance or medical help. Then give first aid immediately.**
- **See emergency information on inside covers.**

POSSIBLE ADVERSE REACTIONS OR SIDE EFFECTS

SYMPTOMS	WHAT TO DO
Life-threatening:	
Coma.	Seek emergency treatment immediately.
Common:	
Dizziness, headache, daytime drowsiness.	Continue. Call doctor when convenient.
Infrequent:	
Diarrhea, nausea, vomiting, skin rash, unusual excitement, blurred vision, constipation.	Discontinue. Call doctor right away.
Rare:	
Mouth ulcers, unusual bleeding or bruising, depression, fever.	Discontinue. Call doctor right away.

WARNINGS & PRECAUTIONS

Don't take if:
You have a history of drug abuse.

Before you start, consult your doctor:
- If you have liver disease.
- If you have intermittent porphyria.
- If you have significant kidney disease.

Over age 60:
Adverse reactions and side effects may be more frequent and severe than in younger persons. You may need smaller doses for shorter periods of time.

Pregnancy:
Consult doctor. Risk category B (see page xxii).

Breast-feeding:
Effect unknown. Consult doctor.

Infants & children:
Not recommended. Avoid.

Prolonged use:
- Not intended for prolonged use.
- Talk to your doctor about the need for follow-up medical examinations or laboratory studies to check complete blood counts (white blood cell count, platelet count, red blood cell count, hemoglobin, hematocrit).

Skin & sunlight:
No problems expected.

Driving, piloting or hazardous work:
Don't drive or pilot aircraft until you learn how medicine affects you. Don't work around dangerous machinery. Don't climb ladders or work in high places. Danger increases if you drink alcohol or take medicine affecting alertness and reflexes.

Discontinuing:
These symptoms may occur after medicine has been discontinued: confusion, seizures, hallucinations, increased dreaming, vomiting, nightmares, restlessness, trembling, insomnia, weakness.

Others:
No problems expected.

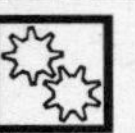

POSSIBLE INTERACTION WITH OTHER DRUGS

GENERIC NAME OR DRUG CLASS	COMBINED EFFECT
Addictive drugs*, other	Increased risk of habituation.
Central nervous system (CNS) depressants*	Increased sedative effect, perhaps to dangerous level. Avoid.
Clozapine	Toxic effect on the central nervous system.
Ethinamate	Dangerous increased effects of ethinamate. Avoid combining.
Fluoxetine	Increased depressant effects of both drugs.
Guanfacine	May increase depressant effects of either drug.
Leucovorin	High alcohol content of leucovorin may cause adverse effects.
Nabilone	Greater depression of central nervous system.
Sertraline	Increased depressive effects of both drugs.

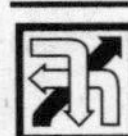

POSSIBLE INTERACTION WITH OTHER SUBSTANCES

INTERACTS WITH	COMBINED EFFECT
Alcohol:	Excess sedation. Avoid.
Beverages: Caffeine drinks.	Decreased methyprylon effect. Avoid.
Cocaine:	Decreased methyprylon effect.
Foods:	None expected.
Marijuana:	Decreased methyprylon effect.
Tobacco:	None expected.

*See Glossary

METHYSERGIDE

BRAND NAMES

Sansert

BASIC INFORMATION

Habit forming? Yes
Prescription needed? Yes
Available as generic? No
Drug class: Vasoconstrictor

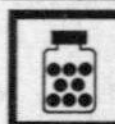

USES

Prevents migraine and other recurring vascular headaches. Not for acute attack.

DOSAGE & USAGE INFORMATION

How to take:
Tablet—Swallow with liquid or with food to lessen stomach irritation. If you can't swallow whole, crumble tablet and take with liquid or food.

When to take:
At the same times each day.

If you forget a dose:
Don't take missed dose. Wait for next scheduled dose (don't double this dose).

What drug does:
Blocks the action of serotonin, a chemical that constricts blood vessels.

Time lapse before drug works:
About 3 weeks.

Don't take with:
Any other medicine without consulting your doctor or pharmacist.

OVERDOSE

SYMPTOMS:
Nausea, vomiting, abdominal pain, severe diarrhea, lack of coordination, extreme thirst.
WHAT TO DO:
Overdose unlikely to threaten life. If person takes much larger amount than prescribed, call doctor, poison control center or hospital emergency room for instructions.

POSSIBLE ADVERSE REACTIONS OR SIDE EFFECTS

SYMPTOMS	WHAT TO DO
Life-threatening: In case of overdose, see previous column.	
Common:	
• Itchy skin.	Discontinue. Call doctor right away.
• Nausea, vomiting, diarrhea, numbness or tingling of extremities, leg weakness, abdominal pain.	Continue. Call doctor when convenient.
• Drowsiness, constipation.	Continue. Tell doctor at next visit.
Infrequent:	
• Anxiety, agitation, hallucinations, unusually fast or slow heartbeat, dizziness.	Discontinue. Call doctor right away.
• Change in vision, nightmares, insomnia.	Continue. Call doctor when convenient.
Rare:	
• Extreme thirst, chest pain, shortness of breath, fever, pale or swollen extremities, leg cramps, lower back pain, side or groin pain, appetite loss, joint and muscle pain, rash, facial flush.	Discontinue. Call doctor right away.
• Painful or difficult urination.	Continue. Call doctor when convenient.
• Weight change, hair loss.	Continue. Tell doctor at next visit.

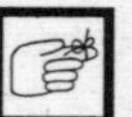

WARNINGS & PRECAUTIONS

Don't take if:

- You are allergic to any antiserotonin*.
- You plan to become pregnant within medication period.
- You have an infection.
- You have a heart or blood vessel disease.
- You have a chronic lung disease.
- You have a collagen (connective tissue) disorder.
- You have impaired liver or kidney function.

Before you start, consult your doctor:
- If you have been allergic to any ergot preparation.
- If you have had a peptic ulcer.

Over age 60:
Adverse reactions and side effects may be more frequent and severe than in younger persons.

Pregnancy:
Consult doctor. Risk category X (see page xxii).

Breast-feeding:
Drug probably passes into milk. Avoid drug or discontinue nursing until you finish medicine. Consult doctor for advice on maintaining milk supply.

Infants & children:
Not recommended.

Prolonged use:
- May cause fibrosis, a condition in which scar tissue is deposited on heart valves, in lung tissue, blood vessels and internal organs. After 6 months, decrease dose over 2 to 3 weeks. Then discontinue for at least 2 months for re-evaluation.
- Talk to your doctor about the need for follow-up medical examinations or laboratory studies to check retroperitoneal imaging*.

Skin & sunlight:
No problems expected.

Driving, piloting or hazardous work:
Avoid if you feel drowsy or dizzy. Otherwise, no problems expected.

Discontinuing:
- Don't discontinue without consulting doctor. Dose may require gradual reduction if you have taken drug for a long time. Doses of other drugs may also require adjustment.
- Probably should discontinue drug if you don't improve after 3 weeks use.

Others:
- Periodic laboratory tests for liver function and blood counts recommended.
- Potential for abuse.
- Some products contain tartrazine dye. Avoid, especially if you are allergic to aspirin.

POSSIBLE INTERACTION WITH OTHER DRUGS

GENERIC NAME OR DRUG CLASS	COMBINED EFFECT
Ergot preparations*	Unpredictable increased or decreased effect of either drug.
Narcotics*	Decreased narcotic effect.

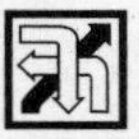

POSSIBLE INTERACTION WITH OTHER SUBSTANCES

INTERACTS WITH	COMBINED EFFECT
Alcohol:	None expected. However, alcohol may trigger a migraine headache.
Beverages: Caffeine drinks.	Decreased methysergide effect.
Cocaine:	May make headache worse.
Foods:	None expected. Avoid foods to which you are allergic.
Marijuana:	No proven problems.
Tobacco:	Blood vessel constriction. Makes headache worse.

*See Glossary

METOCLOPRAMIDE

BRAND NAMES

Apo-Metoclop	Octamide
Clopra	Octamide PFS
Emex	Reclomide
Maxeran	Reglan

BASIC INFORMATION

Habit forming? No
Prescription needed? Yes
Available as generic? Yes
Drug class: Antiemetic, dopaminergic blocker

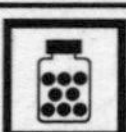

USES

- Relieves nausea and vomiting caused by chemotherapy and drug-related postoperative factors.
- Relieves symptoms of esophagitis and stomach swelling in people with diabetes.

DOSAGE & USAGE INFORMATION

How to take:
Tablet or syrup—Swallow with liquid or food to lessen stomach irritation.

When to take:
30 minutes before symptoms expected, up to 4 times a day.

If you forget a dose:
Take as soon as you remember up to 2 hours late. If more than 2 hours, wait for next scheduled dose (don't double this dose).

Continued next column

OVERDOSE

SYMPTOMS:
Severe drowsiness, muscle spasms, mental confusion, trembling, seizure, coma.
WHAT TO DO:
- **Dial 911 (emergency) or 0 (operator) for an ambulance or medical help. Then give first aid immediately.**
- **If patient is unconscious and not breathing, give mouth-to-mouth breathing. If there is no heartbeat, use cardiac massage and mouth-to-mouth breathing (CPR). Don't try to make patient vomit. If you can't get help quickly, take patient to nearest emergency facility.**
- **See emergency information on inside covers.**

What drug does:
- Prevents smooth muscle in stomach from relaxing.
- Affects vomiting center in brain.

Time lapse before drug works:
30 to 60 minutes.

Don't take with:
Any other medicine without consulting your doctor or pharmacist.

POSSIBLE ADVERSE REACTIONS OR SIDE EFFECTS

SYMPTOMS	WHAT TO DO
Life-threatening: In case of overdose, see previous column.	
Common:	
Drowsiness, restlessness.	Continue. Call doctor when convenient.
Frequent	
Rash.	Continue. Call doctor when convenient.
Infrequent:	
• Wheezing, shortness of breath.	Discontinue. Call doctor right away.
• Dizziness; headache; insomnia; tender, swollen breasts; increased milk flow, menstrual changes; decreased sex drive.	Continue. Call doctor when convenient.
Rare:	
• Abnormal, involuntary movements of jaw, lips and tongue; depression; Parkinson's syndrome*.	Discontinue. Call doctor right away.
• Constipation, nausea, diarrhea, dry mouth.	Continue. Call doctor when convenient.

WARNINGS & PRECAUTIONS

Don't take if:
You are allergic to procaine, procainamide or metoclopramide.

Before you start, consult your doctor:
- If you have Parkinson's disease.
- If you have liver or kidney disease.
- If you have epilepsy.
- If you have bleeding from gastrointestinal tract or intestinal obstruction.
- If you will have surgery within 2 months, including dental surgery, requiring general or spinal anesthesia.

Over age 60:
Adverse reactions and side effects may be more frequent and severe than in younger persons.

Pregnancy:
No proven harm to unborn child. Avoid if possible. Consult doctor. Risk category B (see page xxii).

Breast-feeding:
Unknown effect. Consult doctor.

Infants & children:
Adverse reactions more likely to occur than in adults.

Prolonged use:
Adverse reactions including muscle spasms and trembling hands more likely to occur.

Skin & sunlight:
No problems expected.

Driving, piloting or hazardous work:
Don't drive or pilot aircraft until you learn how medicine affects you. Don't work around dangerous machinery. Don't climb ladders or work in high places. Danger increases if you drink alcohol or take medicine affecting alertness and reflexes, such as antihistamines, tranquilizers, sedatives, pain medicine, narcotics and mind-altering drugs.

Discontinuing:
May be unnecessary to finish medicine. Follow doctor's instructions.

Others:
No problems expected.

POSSIBLE INTERACTION WITH OTHER DRUGS

GENERIC NAME OR DRUG CLASS	COMBINED EFFECT
Acetaminophen	Increased absorption of acetaminophen.
Anticholinergics*	Decreased metoclopramide effect.
Aspirin	Increased absorption of aspirin.
Bromocriptine	Decreased bromocriptine effect.
Butyophenone	Increased chance of muscle spasm and trembling.
Central nervous system (CNS) depressants*	Excess sedation.
Clozapine	Toxic effect on the central nervous system.
Digitalis preparations*	Decreased absorption of digitalis.
Ethinamate	Dangerous increased effects of ethinamate. Avoid combining.
Fluoxetine	Increased depressant effects of both drugs.
Guanfacine	May increase depressant effects of either drug.
Insulin	Unpredictable changes in blood glucose. Dosages may require adjustment.
Leucovorin	High alcohol content of leucovorin may cause adverse effects.
Levodopa	Increased absorption of levodopa.
Lithium	Increased absorption of lithium.
Loxapine	May increase toxic effects of both drugs.
Methyprylon	Increased sedative effect, perhaps to dangerous level. Avoid.
Nabilone	Greater depression of central nervous system.

Continued on page 948

POSSIBLE INTERACTION WITH OTHER SUBSTANCES

INTERACTS WITH	COMBINED EFFECT
Alcohol:	Excess sedation. Avoid.
Beverages:	
Coffee.	Decreased metoclopramide effect.
Cocaine:	Decreased metoclopramide effect.
Foods:	No problems expected.
Marijuana:	Decreased metoclopramide effect.
Tobacco:	Decreased metoclopramide effect.

*See Glossary

METRONIDAZOLE

BRAND NAMES

Apo-Metronidazole
Flagyl
Flagyl I.V.
Flagyl I.V. RTU
Metizol
Metric 21
Metrogel
Metrogel-Vaginal
Metro I.V.
Neo-Metric
Novonidazol
PMS Metronidazole
Protostat
Satric
Trikacide

BASIC INFORMATION

Habit forming? No
Prescription needed? Yes
Available as generic? Yes
Drug class: Antiprotozoal, antibacterial

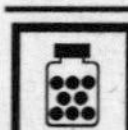

USES

- Treatment for infections susceptible to metronidazole, such as trichomoniasis and amebiasis.
- Treatment for bacterial infections.
- Topical—Treats acne rosacea (adult acne).
- Vaginal—Treats vaginal infections.

DOSAGE & USAGE INFORMATION

How to take:
- Tablet—Swallow with liquid or food to lessen stomach irritation. If you can't swallow whole, crumble tablet and take with liquid or food.
- Topical gel—Apply thin layer to involved area.

When to take:
- At the same times each day.
- Gel—Apply twice a day.

If you forget a dose:
Take as soon as you remember up to 2 hours late. If more than 2 hours, wait for next scheduled dose (don't double this dose).

What drug does:
Kills organisms causing the infection.

Continued next column

OVERDOSE

SYMPTOMS:
Weakness, nausea, vomiting, diarrhea, confusion, seizures.
WHAT TO DO:
Overdose unlikely to threaten life. If person takes much larger amount than prescribed, call doctor, poison control center or hospital emergency room for instructions.

Time lapse before drug works:
Begins in 1 hour. May require regular use for 10 days to cure infection.

Don't take with:
- Nonprescription medicines containing alcohol.
- Any other medicine without consulting your doctor or pharmacist.

POSSIBLE ADVERSE REACTIONS OR SIDE EFFECTS

SYMPTOMS	WHAT TO DO
Life-threatening: In case of overdose, see previous column.	
Common:	
• Appetite loss, nausea, abdominal pain, diarrhea, vomiting.	Discontinue. Call doctor right away.
• Unpleasant taste.	Continue. Tell doctor at next visit.
Infrequent:	
• Dizziness; headache; rash; hives; skin redness; itchy skin; mouth irritation, soreness or infection; sore throat; fever.	Discontinue. Call doctor right away.
• Vaginal irritation, discharge, dryness; fatigue; weakness.	Continue. Call doctor when convenient.
• Constipation.	Continue. Tell doctor at next visit.
Rare:	
• Mood change; unsteadiness; numbness, tingling, weakness or pain in hands or feet.	Discontinue. Call doctor right away.
• Metallic taste.	Continue. Call doctor when convenient.

WARNINGS & PRECAUTIONS

Don't take if:
- You are allergic to metronidazole.
- You have had a blood cell or bone marrow disorder.

Before you start, consult your doctor:
- If you plan to become pregnant within medication period.
- If you have a brain or nervous system disorder.
- If you have liver or heart disease.
- If you drink alcohol.

Over age 60:
Adverse reactions and side effects may be more frequent and severe than in younger persons.

Pregnancy:
Consult doctor. Risk category B (see page xxii).

Breast-feeding:
Drug passes into milk. Avoid drug or discontinue nursing until you finish medicine. Consult doctor for advice on maintaining milk supply.

Infants & children:
Use in children for amoeba infection only under close medical supervision.

Prolonged use:
Talk to your doctor about the need for follow-up medical examinations or laboratory studies to check for giardiasis in stools.

Skin & sunlight:
No problems expected.

Driving, piloting or hazardous work:
Avoid if you feel dizzy or unsteady. Otherwise, no problems expected.

Discontinuing:
Don't discontinue without doctor's advice until you complete prescribed dose, even though symptoms diminish or disappear.

Others:
Avoid alcohol 12 hours before and *at least* 24 hours after treatment period with metronidazole.

POSSIBLE INTERACTION WITH OTHER DRUGS

GENERIC NAME OR DRUG CLASS	COMBINED EFFECT
Anticoagulants*, oral	Increased anti-coagulant effect. Possible bleeding or bruising.
Cimetidine	Prolongs increased serum levels.
Didanosine	Increased risk of peripheral neuropathy.
Disulfiram	Disulfiram reaction*. Avoid.
Nizatidine	Increased effect and toxicity of metoprolol.
Oxytetracycline	Decreased metronidazole effect.
Phenobarbital	Decreased metron-idazole effect.
Phenytoin	Decreased metron-idazole effect.

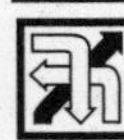

POSSIBLE INTERACTION WITH OTHER SUBSTANCES

INTERACTS WITH	COMBINED EFFECT
Alcohol:	Possible disulfiram reaction*. Avoid alcohol in *any* form or amount.
Beverages:	None expected.
Cocaine:	Decreased metron-idazole effect. Avoid.
Foods:	None expected.
Marijuana:	None expected.
Tobacco:	None expected.

***See Glossary**

METYRAPONE

BRAND NAMES

Metopirone

BASIC INFORMATION

Habit forming? No
Prescription needed? Yes
Available as generic? No
Drug class: Antiadrenal

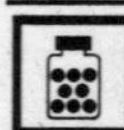

USES

- To diagnose the function of the pituitary gland.
- Treats Cushing's disease, a disorder characterized by higher than normal concentrations of cortisol (one of the hormones secreted by the adrenal glands) in the blood.

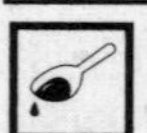

DOSAGE & USAGE INFORMATION

How to take:

- For medical testing purposes—Take the prescribed number of tablets with milk or food on the day before the scheduled test. On the day of the test, blood and urine studies will show the amount of hormones in your blood. Results of the test will help establish your diagnosis.
- For treatment of Cushing's syndrome—Swallow tablet with liquid. If you can't swallow whole, crumble tablet and take with liquid or food.

When to take:

- For medical testing—Take the prescribed number of tablets on the day before the scheduled test.
- For treatment of Cushing's disease—Take total daily amount in divided doses. Follow prescription directions carefully.

Continued next column

OVERDOSE

SYMPTOMS:
Nausea (severe), vomiting, diarrhea, abdominal pain, sudden weakness, irregular heartbeat.
WHAT TO DO:

- **Dial 911 (emergency) or 0 (operator) for an ambulance or medical help. Then give first aid immediately.**
- **See emergency information on inside covers.**

If you forget a dose:
Take as soon as you remember up to 2 hours late. If more than 2 hours, wait for next scheduled dose (don't double this dose).

What drug does:
Prevents one of the chemical reactions in the production of cortisol by the adrenal glands.

Time lapse before drug works:
Approximately 1 hour.

Don't take with:
Cortisone*-like medicines for 48 hours prior to testing.

POSSIBLE ADVERSE REACTIONS OR SIDE EFFECTS

SYMPTOMS	WHAT TO DO?
Life-threatening:	
In case of overdose, see previous column.	
Common:	
Dizziness, headache, nausea.	Continue. Call doctor when convenient.
Infrequent:	
Drowsiness.	Continue. Call doctor when convenient.
Rare:	
Hair loss or excess growth, decreased appetite, confusion, acne (may begin or may worsen if already present).	Continue. Call doctor when convenient.

WARNINGS & PRECAUTIONS

Don't take if:

- You have adrenal insufficiency (Addison's disease).
- You have decreased pituitary function.

Before you start, consult your doctor:

- If you are allergic to metyrapone.
- If you have porphyria.

Over age 60:
No special problems expected.

Pregnancy:
Safety not established. Take only under careful supervision of medical professional. Risk category C (see page xxii).

Breast-feeding:
Drug may pass into milk, although controlled studies in humans have not been performed. Since the possibility exists, avoid nursing until you finish the medicine.

Infants & children:
No special problems expected.

Prolonged use:
No special problems expected.

Skin & sunlight:
No special problems expected.

Driving, piloting or hazardous work:
Don't drive or pilot aircraft until you learn how medicine affects you. Don't work around dangerous machinery. Don't climb ladders or work in high places. Danger increases if you drink alcohol or take medicine affecting alertness and reflexes.

Discontinuing:
No special problems expected.

Others:
Advise any doctor or dentist whom you consult that you take this medicine.

POSSIBLE INTERACTION WITH OTHER DRUGS

GENERIC NAME OR DRUG CLASS	COMBINED EFFECT
Antidiabetics, oral*	Increased risk of adverse reactions.
Contraceptives, oral*	Possible inaccurate test results.
Estrogens*	Possible inaccurate test results.
Insulin	Increased risk of adverse reactions.
Phenytoin	Possible inaccurate test results.

POSSIBLE INTERACTION WITH OTHER SUBSTANCES

INTERACTS WITH	COMBINED EFFECT
Alcohol:	None expected.
Beverages:	None expected.
Cocaine:	None expected.
Foods:	Increased appetite and absorption of nutrients, causing difficulty with weight control.
Marijuana:	None expected.
Tobacco:	None expected.

METYROSINE

BRAND NAMES

Demser

BASIC INFORMATION

Habit forming? No
Prescription needed? Yes
Available as generic? No
Drug class: Antihypertensive

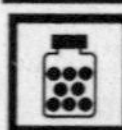

USES

- Treatment of pheochromocytoma* (adrenal gland tumor) that causes high blood pressure.
- Preoperative medication for removal of the tumor.

DOSAGE & USAGE INFORMATION

How to take:
Capsules—Swallow with liquid. If you can't swallow whole, open capsule and take with liquid or food. Instructions to take on empty stomach mean 1 hour before or 2 hours after eating.

When to take:
- Usually 4 times a day, approximately 6 hours apart.
- If used before surgery, take for at least 5 to 7 days.

If you forget a dose:
Take as soon as you remember up to 2 hours late. If more than 2 hours, wait for next scheduled dose (don't double this dose).

What drug does:
Reduces blood pressure in patients with pheochromocytoma* by reducing synthesis of catecholamines*.

Time lapse before drug works:
2 to 3 days.

Continued next column

OVERDOSE

SYMPTOMS:
Confusion, sudden shortness of breath, hallucinations, seizures, coma.
WHAT TO DO:
- **Dial 911 (emergency) or 0 (operator) for an ambulance or medical help. Then give first aid immediately.**
- **See emergency information on inside covers.**

Don't take with:
Any other medicines (including over-the-counter drugs such as cough and cold medicines, laxatives, antacids, diet pills, caffeine, nose drops or vitamins) without consulting your doctor.

POSSIBLE ADVERSE REACTIONS OR SIDE EFFECTS

SYMPTOMS	WHAT TO DO
Life-threatening:	
In case of overdose, see previous column.	
Common:	
• Severe diarrhea, tremors, drooling, speech difficulties.	Continue. Call doctor when convenient.
• Drowsiness.	Continue. Tell doctor at next visit.
Infrequent:	
Skin rash, sexual difficulties in males.	Continue. Call doctor when convenient.
Rare:	
• Shortness of breath, itching, bloody urine, muscle spasms, swollen feet.	Discontinue. Call doctor right away.
• Depression.	Continue. Call doctor when convenient.

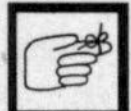

WARNINGS & PRECAUTIONS

Don't take if:
You are allergic to metyrosine.

Before you start, consult your doctor:
- If you have liver disease.
- If you have mental depression.
- If you have Parkinson's disease.
- If you have kidney disease.

Over age 60:
Adverse reactions and side effects may be more frequent and severe than in younger persons. You may need smaller doses for shorter periods of time.

Pregnancy:
Decide with your doctor if drug benefits justify risk to unborn child. Risk category C (see page xxii).

Breast-feeding:
Not recommended. Consult doctor.

Infants & children:
No proven problems.

Prolonged use:
Talk to your doctor about the need for follow-up medical examinations or laboratory studies to check blood pressure, heart function, ECG*, kidney function and urinary catecholamine measurements.

Skin & sunlight:
No problems expected.

Driving, piloting or hazardous work:
Don't drive or pilot aircraft until you learn how medicine affects you. Don't work around dangerous machinery. Don't climb ladders or work in high places. Danger increases if you drink alcohol or take medicine affecting alertness and reflexes.

Discontinuing:
May experience increased energy and insomnia for a short period (2 to 7 days).

Others:
- Advise any doctor or dentist whom you consult that you take this medicine.
- May affect results in some medical tests.

POSSIBLE INTERACTION WITH OTHER DRUGS

GENERIC NAME OR DRUG CLASS	COMBINED EFFECT
Antidepressants, tricyclic*	Increased sedative effect of each.
Central nervous system (CNS) depressants*	Increased sedative effect.
Clozapine	Toxic effect on the central nervous system.
Phenothiazines*	Increased likelihood of toxic symptoms of each.
Sertraline	Increased depressive effects of both drugs.
Trimeprazine	Increased likelihood of toxic symptoms of each.

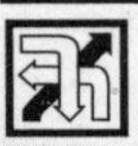

POSSIBLE INTERACTION WITH OTHER SUBSTANCES

INTERACTS WITH	COMBINED EFFECT
Alcohol:	May cause Parkinson's*-like disorder. Don't mix.
Beverages:	No special problems expected.
Cocaine:	No special problems expected.
Foods:	No special problems expected.
Marijuana:	No special problems expected.
Tobacco:	No special problems expected.

MEXILETINE

BRAND NAMES

Mexitil

BASIC INFORMATION

Habit forming? No
Prescription needed? Yes
Available as generic? No
Drug class: Antiarrhythmic

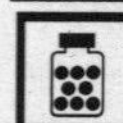

USES

Stabilizes irregular heartbeat.

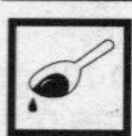

DOSAGE & USAGE INFORMATION

How to take:
Capsules—Swallow whole with food, milk or antacid to lessen stomach irritation.

When to take:
At the same times each day as directed by your doctor.

If you forget a dose:
Take as soon as you remember up to 4 hours late. If more than 4 hours, wait for next scheduled dose (don't double this dose).

What drug does:
Blocks the fast sodium channel in heart tissue.

Time lapse before drug works:
30 minutes to 2 hours.

Don't take with:
Any other medicine without consulting your doctor or pharmacist.

OVERDOSE

SYMPTOMS:
Nausea, vomiting, seizures, convulsions, cardiac arrest.
WHAT TO DO:

- **Dial 911 (emergency) or 0 (operator) for an ambulance or medical help. Then give first aid immediately.**
- **See emergency information on inside covers.**

POSSIBLE ADVERSE REACTIONS OR SIDE EFFECTS

SYMPTOMS	WHAT TO DO
Life-threatening:	
Chest pain, shortness of breath, irregular or fast heartbeat.	Discontinue. Seek emergency treatment.
Common:	
Dizziness, anxiety, shakiness, unsteadiness when walking, heartburn, nausea, vomiting.	Discontinue. Call doctor right away.
Infrequent:	
• Sore throat, fever, mouth sores; blurred vision; confusion; constipation; diarrhea; headache; numbness or tingling in hands or feet; ringing in ears; unexplained bleeding or bruising; rash; slurred speech; insomnia; weakness; difficult swallowing.	Discontinue. Call doctor right away.
• Loss of taste.	Continue. Call doctor when convenient.
Rare:	
• Seizures.	Discontinue. Seek emergency treatment.
• Hallucinations, psychosis, memory loss, difficult breathing, swollen feet and ankles, hiccups, jaundice.	Discontinue. Call doctor right away.
• Hair loss, impotence.	Continue. Call doctor when convenient.

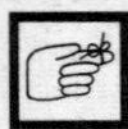

WARNINGS & PRECAUTIONS

Don't take if:
If you are allergic to mexiletine, lidocaine or tocainide.

Before you start, consult your doctor:
- If you have had liver or kidney disease or impaired kidney function.
- If you have had lupus.
- If you have a history of seizures.
- If you will have surgery within 2 months, including dental surgery, requiring general or spinal anesthesia.
- If you have heart disease or low blood pressure.

Over age 60:
Adverse reactions and side effects may be more frequent and severe than in younger persons. Ask doctor about smaller doses.

Pregnancy:
Decide with your doctor if drug benefits justify risk to unborn child. Risk category C (see page xxii).

Breast-feeding:
Drug passes into milk. Avoid drug or discontinue nursing until you finish medicine. Consult doctor for advice on maintaining milk supply.

Infants & children:
Use only under close medical supervision.

Prolonged use:
- May cause lupus*-like illness.
- Talk to your doctor about the need for follow-up medical examinations or laboratory studies to check ECG*, liver function.

Skin & sunlight:
No problems expected.

Driving, piloting or hazardous work:
Use caution if you feel dizzy or weak. Otherwise, no problems expected.

Discontinuing:
Don't discontinue without consulting doctor. Dose may require gradual reduction if you have taken drug for a long time. Doses of other drugs may also require adjustment.

Others:
No problems expected.

POSSIBLE INTERACTION WITH OTHER DRUGS

GENERIC NAME OR DRUG CLASS	COMBINED EFFECT
Cimetidine	Increased mexiletine effect and toxicity.
Encainide	Increased effect of toxicity on the heart muscle.
Nicardipine	Possible increased effect and toxicity of each drug.
Phenobarbital	Decreased mexiletine effect.
Phenytoin	Decreased mexiletine effect.
Propafenone	Increased effect of both drugs and increased risk of toxicity.
Rifampin	Decreased mexiletine effect.
Urinary acidifiers* (ammonium chloride, ascorbic acid, potassium or sodium phosphate)	May decrease effectiveness of medicine.
Urinary alkalizers* (acetazolamide, antacids with calcium or magnesium, citric acid, dichlorphenamide, methazolamide, potassium citrate, sodium bicarbonate, sodium citrate)	May slow elimination of mexiletine and cause need to adjust dosage.

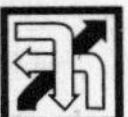

POSSIBLE INTERACTION WITH OTHER SUBSTANCES

INTERACTS WITH	COMBINED EFFECT
Alcohol:	Causes irregular effectiveness of mexiletine. Avoid.
Beverages: Caffeine drinks, iced drinks.	Irregular heartbeat.
Cocaine:	Decreased mexiletine effect.
Foods:	None expected.
Marijuana:	Irregular heartbeat. Avoid.
Tobacco:	Dangerous combination. May lead to liver problems and reduce excretion of mexiletine.

MINERAL OIL

BRAND NAMES

Agarol
Agoral
Agoral Marshmallow
Agoral Plain
Agoral Raspberry
Fleet Enema Mineral Oil
Haley's M-O
Kondremul
Kondremul with Cascara
Kondremul with Phenolphthalein
Kondremul Plain
Lansoyl
Liqui-Doss
Magnolax
Milkinol
Neo-Cultol
Nujol
Petrogalar Plain
Phenolphthalein Petrogalar
Zymenol

BASIC INFORMATION

Habit forming? Yes
Prescription needed? No
Available as generic? Yes
Drug class: Laxative (lubricant)

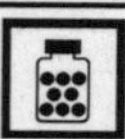

USES

Treats the temporary symptoms of constipation.

DOSAGE & USAGE INFORMATION

How to take:
Follow package instructions.

When to take:
According to instructions provided.

If you forget a dose:
No set dosage schedule. Use only when needed.

What drug does:
Coats the stool and the surface of the intestine with lubricant to make the passage of the stool easier.

Time lapse before drug works:
6 to 8 hours.

Don't take with:
Other drugs without talking to your doctor or pharmacist.

OVERDOSE

SYMPTOMS:
Loose stools.
WHAT TO DO:
Overdose unlikely to threaten life. If person takes much larger amount than prescribed, call doctor, poison control center or hospital emergency room for instructions.

POSSIBLE ADVERSE REACTIONS OR SIDE EFFECTS

SYMPTOMS	WHAT TO DO
Life-threatening: None expected.	
Common: Skin irritation around rectum.	Continue. Call doctor when convenient.
Infrequent: None expected.	
Rare: Abdominal pain.	Discontinue. Call doctor right away.

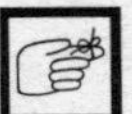

WARNINGS & PRECAUTIONS

Don't take if:
- You have abdominal pain, bloating or suspected appendicitis.
- You have undiagnosed rectal bleeding.

Before you start, consult your doctor:
- If you have difficulty swallowing.
- If you are bed-ridden.

Over age 60:
More susceptible to adverse effects.

Pregnancy:
Decide with your doctor if drug benefits justify risk to unborn child. Risk category C (see page xxii).

Breast-feeding:
No problems expected, but consult doctor.

Infants & children:
Use only under close medical supervision, particularly up to 6 years of age.

Prolonged use:
- Not intended for prolonged use. May interfere with absorption of essential nutrients.
- Don't take for longer than 1 week unless under a doctor's supervision. May cause laxative dependence.

Skin & sunlight:
No special problems expected.

Driving, piloting or hazardous work:
No special problems expected.

Discontinuing:
May be unnecessary to finish medicine. Follow doctor's instructions.

Others:
- May affect results of some medical tests.
- Don't take to "flush out" your system or as a tonic.

POSSIBLE INTERACTION WITH OTHER DRUGS

GENERIC NAME OR DRUG CLASS	COMBINED EFFECT
Anticoagulants, oral*	Decreased absorption of anticoagulants.
Contraceptives, oral*	Decreased effect of contraceptive drug.
Digitalis preparations*	Decreased effect of digitalis.
Laxatives*, stool-softening	May cause tumor-like deposits in tissues.
Medications, other	Decreased absorption of many medicines taken with mineral oil.
Vitamins A, D, E and K	Decreased absorption of vitamins.

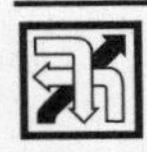

POSSIBLE INTERACTION WITH OTHER SUBSTANCES

INTERACTS WITH	COMBINED EFFECT
Alcohol:	No proven problems.
Beverages:	No proven problems.
Cocaine:	No proven problems.
Foods:	Decreased absorption of foods and fat-soluble vitamins (A, D, E and K).
Marijuana:	No proven problems.
Tobacco:	Possible increased laxative effect.

***See Glossary**

MINOXIDIL

BRAND NAMES

Loniten

BASIC INFORMATION

Habit forming? No
Prescription needed? Yes
Available as generic? Yes
Drug class: Antihypertensive

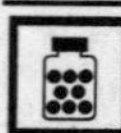

USES

- Treatment for high blood pressure in conjunction with other drugs, such as beta-adrenergic blockers and diuretics.
- Treatment for congestive heart failure.
- Can stimulate hair growth.

DOSAGE & USAGE INFORMATION

How to take:
Tablet—Swallow with liquid. If you can't swallow whole, crumble tablet and take with liquid or food.

When to take:
At the same time each day, according to instructions on prescription label.

If you forget a dose:
Take as soon as you remember up to 2 hours late. If more than 2 hours, wait for next scheduled dose (don't double this dose).

What drug does:
Relaxes small blood vessels (arterioles) so blood can pass through more easily.

Time lapse before drug works:
2 to 3 hours for effect to begin; 3 to 7 days of continuous use may be necessary for maximum blood pressure response.

Don't take with:
Any other medicine without consulting your doctor or pharmacist.

OVERDOSE

SYMPTOMS:
Low blood pressure, fainting, chest pain, shortness of breath, coma.
WHAT TO DO:

- **Dial 911 (emergency) or 0 (operator) for an ambulance or medical help. Then give first aid immediately.**
- **See emergency information on inside covers.**

POSSIBLE ADVERSE REACTIONS OR SIDE EFFECTS

SYMPTOMS	WHAT TO DO
Life-threatening: In case of overdose, see previous column.	
Common:	
• Excessive hair growth, flushed skin or redness.	Continue. Call doctor when convenient.
• Bloating.	Discontinue. Call doctor right away.
Infrequent:	
• Chest pain, irregular or slow heartbeat, shortness of breath, swollen feet or legs, rapid weight gain.	Discontinue. Call doctor right away.
• Numbness of hands, feet or face; headache; tender breasts; darkening of skin.	Continue. Call doctor when convenient.
Rare:	
Rash.	Discontinue. Call doctor right away.

WARNINGS & PRECAUTIONS

Don't take if:
You are allergic to minoxidil.

Before you start, consult your doctor:
- If you have had recent stroke or heart attack or angina pectoris in past 3 weeks.
- If you have impaired kidney function.
- If you have pheochromocytoma*

Over age 60:
Adverse reactions and side effects may be more frequent and severe than in younger persons.

Pregnancy:
Decide with your doctor if drug benefits justify risk to unborn child. Risk category C (see page xxii).

Breast-feeding:
Human studies not available. Avoid if possible. Consult doctor.

Infants & children:
Not recommended. Safety and dosage have not been established.

Prolonged use:
Request periodic blood examinations that include potassium levels.

Skin & sunlight:
No problems expected.

Driving, piloting or hazardous work:
Avoid if you become dizzy or faint. Otherwise, no problems expected.

Discontinuing:
Don't discontinue without consulting doctor. Dose may require gradual reduction if you have taken drug for a long time. Doses of other drugs may also require adjustment.

Others:
- Check pulse regularly. If it exceeds 20 or more beats per minute over your normal rate, consult doctor immediately.
- Check blood pressure frequently.

POSSIBLE INTERACTION WITH OTHER DRUGS

GENERIC NAME OR DRUG CLASS	COMBINED EFFECT
Anesthesia	Drastic blood pressure drop.
Antihypertensives*, other	Dosage adjustments may be necessary to keep blood pressure at desired level.
Carteolol	Increased anti-hypertensive effect.
Diuretics*	Dosage adjustments may be necessary to keep blood pressure at desired level.
Estrogens*	May increase blood pressure.
Guanadrel	Weakness and faintness when arising from bed or chair.
Guanethidine	Weakness and faintness when arising from bed or chair.
Lisinopril	Increased anti-hypertensive effect. Dosage of each may require adjustment.
Nicardipine	Blood pressure drop. Dosages may require adjustment.
Nimodipine	Dangerous blood pressure drop.
Nitrates*	Drastic blood pressure drop.
Sotalol	Increased anti-hypertensive effect.
Sympathomimetics*	Possible decreased minoxidil effect.
Terazosin	Decreased effective-ness of terazosin.

POSSIBLE INTERACTION WITH OTHER SUBSTANCES

INTERACTS WITH	COMBINED EFFECT
Alcohol:	Possible excessive blood pressure drop.
Beverages:	None expected.
Cocaine:	Increased risk of heart block and high blood pressure.
Foods: Salt substitutes.	Possible excessive potassium levels in blood.
Marijuana:	Increased dizziness.
Tobacco:	May decrease minoxidil effect. Avoid.

***See Glossary**

MINOXIDIL (Topical)

BRAND NAMES

Rogaine

BASIC INFORMATION

Habit forming? No
Prescription needed? Yes
Available as generic? No
Drug class: Hair growth stimulant

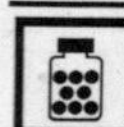

USES

Hair loss on scalp from male and female pattern baldness (alopecia androgenetica).

DOSAGE & USAGE INFORMATION

How to use:
Topical solution

- Apply only to dry hair and scalp. With the provided applicator, apply the amount prescribed to the scalp area being treated. Begin in center of the treated area.
- Wash hands immediately after use.
- Don't use a blow dryer.
- If you are using at bedtime, wait 30 minutes after applying before retiring.

When to use:
Twice a day or as directed.

If you forget a dose:
Use as soon as you remember. No need to ever double the dose.

What drug does:
Stimulates hair growth by possibly dilating small blood capillaries, thereby providing more blood to hair follicles.

Time lapse before drug works:
Varies with individuals.

Don't use with:
Any other medicine without consulting your doctor or pharmacist

OVERDOSE

SYMPTOMS:
None expected.
WHAT TO DO:
Not for internal use. If child accidentally swallows, call poison control center.

POSSIBLE ADVERSE REACTIONS OR SIDE EFFECTS

SYMPTOMS	WHAT TO DO
Life-threatening	
Fast, irregular heartbeat (rare; represents too much absorbed into body).	Discontinue. Seek emergency treatment.
Common	
None expected.	
Infrequent	
Itching scalp; flaking, reddened skin.	Continue. Call doctor when convenient.
Rare	
Burning scalp, skin rash, swollen face, headache, dizziness or fainting, hands and feet numb or tingling, rapid weight gain.	Discontinue. Call doctor right away.

WARNINGS & PRECAUTIONS

Don't use if:
You are allergic to minoxidil.

Before you start, consult your doctor:
- If you are allergic to anything.
- If you have heart disease or high blood pressure.
- If you have skin irritation or abrasion or severe sunburn (systemic absorption may be increased).

Over age 60:
No problems expected.

Pregnancy:
Decide with your doctor if drug benefits justify risk to unborn child. Risk category C (see page xxii).

Breast-feeding:
Don't use.

Infants & children:
Don't use.

Prolonged use:
No problems expected.

Skin & sunlight:
No problems expected.

Driving, piloting or hazardous work:
No problems expected.

Discontinuing:
No problems expected.

Others:
- Keep away from eyes, nose and mouth. Flush with plain water if accident occurs.
- New hair will drop out when you stop using minoxidil.
- Keep solution cool, but don't freeze.

POSSIBLE INTERACTION WITH OTHER DRUGS

GENERIC NAME OR DRUG CLASS	COMBINED EFFECT
Adrenocorticoids*, topical	May cause undesirable absorption of minoxidil.
Minoxidil, oral	Increased risk of toxicity.
Petrolatum, topical	May cause undesirable absorption of minoxidil.
Retinoids*, topical	May cause undesirable absorption of minoxidil.

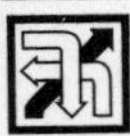

POSSIBLE INTERACTION WITH OTHER SUBSTANCES

INTERACTS WITH	COMBINED EFFECT
Alcohol:	None expected.
Beverages:	None expected.
Cocaine:	None expected.
Foods:	None expected.
Marijuana:	None expected.
Tobacco:	None expected.

*See Glossary

MISOPROSTOL

BRAND NAMES

Cytotec

BASIC INFORMATION

Habit forming? No
Prescription needed? Yes
Available as generic? No
Drug class: Antiulcer

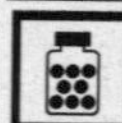

USES

Prevents development of stomach ulcers in persons taking nonsteroidal anti-inflammatory drugs (NSAIDs), including aspirin.

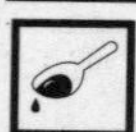

DOSAGE & USAGE INFORMATION

How to take:
Tablets—Swallow with liquid. If you can't swallow whole, crumble tablet and take with liquid or food. Instructions to take on empty stomach mean 1 hour before or 2 hours after eating.

When to take:
Usually 4 times a day while awake, with or after meals and at bedtime.

If you forget a dose:
Take as soon as you remember up to 2 hours late. If more than 2 hours, wait for next scheduled dose (don't double this dose).

What drug does:
- Improves defense against peptic ulcers by strengthening natural defenses of the stomach lining.
- Decreases stomach acid production.

Time lapse before drug works:
10 to 15 minutes.

Don't take with:
Any other medicines (including over-the-counter drugs such as cough and cold medicines, laxatives, antacids, diet pills, caffeine, nose drops or vitamins) without consulting your doctor or pharmacist.

OVERDOSE

SYMPTOMS:
None expected.
WHAT TO DO:
Overdose unlikely to threaten life. If person takes much larger amount than prescribed, call doctor, poison control center or hospital emergency room for instructions.

POSSIBLE ADVERSE REACTIONS OR SIDE EFFECTS

SYMPTOMS	WHAT TO DO
Life-threatening: None expected.	
Common: Abdominal pain, diarrhea.	Discontinue. Call doctor right away.
Infrequent:	
• Nausea or vomiting.	Continue. Call doctor when convenient.
• Constipation, headache.	Continue. Tell doctor at next visit.
Rare:	
• Gaseousness.	Continue. Tell doctor at next visit.
• Vaginal bleeding	Discontinue. Call doctor right away.

WARNINGS & PRECAUTIONS

Don't take if:
- You are allergic to any prostaglandin*.
- You are pregnant or of child-bearing age.

Before you start, consult your doctor:
- If you have epilepsy.
- If you have heart disease.
- If you have blood vessel disease of any kind.

Over age 60:
No special problems expected.

Pregnancy:
- Risk to unborn child outweighs drug benefits. Don't use.
- May also lead to serious complications in pregnant women, including excessive bleeding and future infertility.
- Risk category X (see page xxii).

Breast-feeding:
Drug passes into milk. Avoid drug or discontinue nursing until you finish medicine. Consult doctor for advice on maintaining milk supply.

Infants & children:
Not recommended for children under 18.

Prolonged use:
Talk to your doctor about the need for follow-up medical examinations or laboratory studies to check gastric analysis.

Skin & sunlight:
No problems expected.

Driving, piloting or hazardous work:
Avoid if you feel confused, drowsy or dizzy.

Discontinuing:
No special problems expected.

Others:
Advise any doctor or dentist whom you consult that you take this medicine.

POSSIBLE INTERACTION WITH OTHER DRUGS

GENERIC NAME OR DRUG CLASS	COMBINED EFFECT
Antacids*, magnesium-containing	Severe diarrhea.

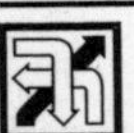

POSSIBLE INTERACTION WITH OTHER SUBSTANCES

INTERACTS WITH	COMBINED EFFECT
Alcohol:	Decreases misoprostol effect. Avoid.
Beverages: Caffeine-containing.	Decreases misoprostol effect. Avoid.
Cocaine:	Decreases misoprostol effect. Avoid.
Foods:	No special problems expected.
Marijuana:	Decreases misoprostol effect. Avoid.
Tobacco:	Decreases misoprostol effect. Avoid.

*See Glossary

MITOTANE

BRAND NAMES

Lysodren
o,p´-DDD

BASIC INFORMATION

Habit forming? No
Prescription needed? Yes
Available as generic? No
Drug class: Antineoplastic, antiadrenal

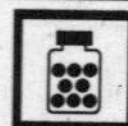

USES

- Treatment for some kinds of cancer.
- Treatment of Cushing's disease.

DOSAGE & USAGE INFORMATION

How to take:
Tablet—Take with liquid after light meal. Don't drink fluid with meals. Drink extra fluids between meals. Avoid sweet and fatty foods.

When to take:
At the same time each day.

If you forget a dose:
Take as soon as you remember. Don't ever double dose.

What drug does:
Suppresses adrenal cortex to prevent manufacture of excess cortisone.

Time lapse before drug works:
2 to 3 weeks for full effect.

Don't take with:
Any other medicine without consulting your doctor or pharmacist.

OVERDOSE

SYMPTOMS:
Headache, vomiting blood, stupor, seizure.
WHAT TO DO:

- **Dial 911 (emergency) or 0 (operator) for an ambulance or medical help. Then give first aid immediately.**
- **If patient is unconscious and not breathing, give mouth-to-mouth breathing. If there is no heartbeat, use cardiac massage and mouth-to-mouth breathing (CPR). Don't try to make patient vomit. If you can't get help quickly, take patient to nearest emergency facility.**
- **See emergency information on inside covers.**

POSSIBLE ADVERSE REACTIONS OR SIDE EFFECTS

SYMPTOMS	WHAT TO DO
Life-threatening:	
In case of overdose, see previous column.	
Common:	
• Darkened skin, appetite loss, nausea, vomiting.	Continue. Call doctor when convenient.
• Mental depression, drowsiness.	Continue. Tell doctor at next visit.
Infrequent:	
• Fever, chills, sore throat.	Discontinue. Seek emergency treatment.
• Unusual bleeding or bruising, difficult breathing.	Discontinue. Call doctor right away.
• Rash, hair loss, blurred vision, seeing double, cough, tiredness, weakness, dizziness when standing after sitting or lying down.	Continue. Call doctor when convenient.
Rare:	
Blood in urine.	Continue. Call doctor when convenient.

WARNINGS & PRECAUTIONS

Don't take if:
You are allergic to mitotane corticosteroids* or any antineoplastic drug.

Before you start, consult your doctor:

- If you have liver disease.
- If you have infection.

Over age 60:
Adverse reactions and side effects may be more frequent and severe than in younger persons.

Pregnancy:
Decide with your doctor whether drug benefits justify risk to unborn child. Risk category C (see page xxii).

Breast-feeding:
Unknown if drug passes into milk. Consult doctor.

Infants & children:
Use only under care of medical supervisors who are experienced in administering anticancer drugs.

Prolonged use:
Adverse reactions more likely the longer drug is required.

Skin & sunlight:
No problems expected.

Driving, piloting or hazardous work:
No problems expected.

Discontinuing:
- Don't discontinue without consulting doctor. Dose may require gradual reduction if you have taken drug for a long time. Doses of other drugs may also require adjustment.
- Some side effects may follow discontinuing. Report any new symptoms.

Others:
No problems expected.

POSSIBLE INTERACTION WITH OTHER DRUGS

GENERIC NAME OR DRUG CLASS	COMBINED EFFECT
Antidepressants*	Increased central nervous system depression.
Antihistamines*	Increased central nervous system depression.
Central nervous system (CNS) depressants*	Increased sedation.
Corticosteroids*	Decreased effect of corticosteroid.
Phenytoin	Possible increased metabolism.
Spironolactone	Decreased mitotane effect.
Warfarin	Decreased warfarin effect.

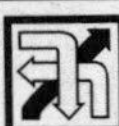

POSSIBLE INTERACTION WITH OTHER SUBSTANCES

INTERACTS WITH	COMBINED EFFECT
Alcohol:	Increased depression. Avoid.
Beverages:	No problems expected.
Cocaine:	Increased toxicity. Avoid.
Foods:	Reduced irritation in stomach.
Marijuana:	No problems expected.
Tobacco:	Increased possibility of lung toxicity.

*See Glossary

MOLINDONE

BRAND NAMES

Moban | Moban Concentrate

BASIC INFORMATION

Habit forming? No
Prescription needed? Yes
Available as generic? No
Drug class: Antipsychotic

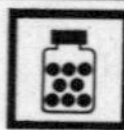

USES

Treats severe emotional, mental or nervous problems.

DOSAGE & USAGE INFORMATION

How to take:
Tablet or solution—Swallow with liquid or food to lessen stomach irritation. If you can't swallow tablet whole, crumble and take with food or liquid.

When to take:
Follow instructions on prescription label or side of package. Doses should be evenly spaced. For example, 4 times a day means every 6 hours.

If you forget a dose:
Take as soon as you remember up to 2 hours late. If more than 2 hours, wait for next scheduled dose (don't double this dose).

What drug does:
Corrects an imbalance in nerve impulses from the brain.

Time lapse before drug works:
4 to 6 weeks.

Don't take with:
- Antacid or medicine for diarrhea.
- Nonprescription drugs for cough, cold or allergy.
- See Interaction column and consult doctor.

OVERDOSE

SYMPTOMS:
Stupor, convulsions, coma.
WHAT TO DO:
- **Dial 911 (emergency) or 0 (operator) for an ambulance or medical help. Then give first aid immediately.**
- **See emergency information on inside covers.**

POSSIBLE ADVERSE REACTIONS OR SIDE EFFECTS

SYMPTOMS	WHAT TO DO
Life-threatening:	
Uncontrolled muscle movements of tongue, face and other muscles (neuroleptic malignant syndrome, rare); unsteady gait; difficult breathing; fever; muscle stiffness.	Discontinue. Seek emergency treatment.
Common:	
• Muscle spasms of face and neck, unsteady gait.	Discontinue. Seek emergency treatment.
• Restlessness, tremor, drowsiness, swallowing difficulty.	Discontinue. Call doctor right away.
• Decreased sweating, dry mouth, runny nose, constipation, headache.	Continue. Call doctor when convenient.
Infrequent:	
• Fainting.	Discontinue. Seek emergency treatment.
• Rash.	Discontinue. Call doctor right away.
• Frequent urination, diminished sex drive, swollen breasts, menstrual irregularities, depression.	Continue. Call doctor when convenient.
Rare:	
Change in vision, sore throat, fever, jaundice, abdominal pain, confusion.	Discontinue. Call doctor right away.

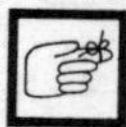

WARNINGS & PRECAUTIONS

Don't take if:
- You are allergic to any phenothiazine.
- You have a blood or bone marrow disease.

Before you start, consult your doctor:
- If you will have surgery within 2 months, including dental surgery, requiring general or spinal anesthesia.
- If you have asthma, emphysema or other lung disorder, glaucoma, prostate trouble.
- If you take nonprescription ulcer medicine, asthma medicine or amphetamines.

Over age 60:
Adverse reactions and side effects may be more frequent and severe than in younger persons. More likely to develop involuntary movement of jaws, lips, tongue, chewing. Report this to your doctor immediately. Early treatment can help.

Pregnancy:
Decide with your doctor if drug benefits justify risk to unborn child. Risk category C (see page xxii).

Breast-feeding:
Safety not established. Consult doctor.

Infants & children:
Don't give to children younger than 2.

Prolonged use:
- May lead to tardive dyskinesia (involuntary movement of jaws, lips, tongue, chewing).
- Talk to your doctor about the need for follow-up medical examinations or laboratory studies to check kidney function, eyes.

Skin & sunlight:
May cause rash or intensify sunburn in areas exposed to sun or sunlamp. Skin may remain sensitive for 3 months after discontinuing.

Driving, piloting or hazardous work:
Don't drive or pilot aircraft until you learn how medicine affects you. Don't work around dangerous machinery. Don't climb ladders or work in high places. Danger increases if you drink alcohol or take medicine affecting alertness and reflexes.

Discontinuing:
- Nervous and mental disorders—Don't discontinue without doctor's advice until you complete prescribed dose, even though symptoms diminish or disappear.
- Notify your doctor if any of the following occurs: uncontrollable movements of tongue, arms and legs; lip smacking.

Others:
No problems expected.

POSSIBLE INTERACTION WITH OTHER DRUGS

GENERIC NAME OR DRUG CLASS	COMBINED EFFECT
Anticholinergics*	Increased anticholinergic effect.
Antidepressants, tricyclic*	Increased molindone effect.
Antihistamines*	Increased antihistamine effect.
Appetite suppressants*	Decreased appetite suppressant effect.
Bupropion	Increased risk of major seizures.
Carteolol	Increased tranquilizer effect.
Clozapine	Toxic effect on the central nervous system.
Dronabinol	Increased effects of both drugs. Avoid.
Ethinamate	Dangerous increased effects of ethinamate. Avoid combining.
Extrapyramidal reaction-causing medications*	Increased frequency and severity of extrapyramidal effects.
Fluoxetine	Increased depressant effects of both drugs.
Guanethidine	Decreased guanethidine effect.
Guanfacine	May increase depressant effects of either drug.
Leucovorin	High alcohol content of leucovorin may cause adverse effects.
Levodopa	Decreased levodopa effect.
Loxapine	May increase toxic effects of both drugs.
Methyprylon	Increased sedative effect, perhaps to dangerous level. Avoid.
Mind-altering drugs*	Increased effect of mind-altering drugs.

Continued on page 948

***See Glossary**

POSSIBLE INTERACTION WITH OTHER SUBSTANCES

INTERACTS WITH	COMBINED EFFECT
Alcohol:	Dangerous oversedation.
Beverages:	None expected.
Cocaine:	Decreased molindone effect. Avoid.
Foods:	None expected.
Marijuana:	Drowsiness. May increase antinausea effect.
Tobacco:	None expected.

MONOAMINE OXIDASE (MAO) INHIBITORS

BRAND AND GENERIC NAMES

ISOCARBOXAZID	Parnate
Marplan	PHENELZINE
Nardil	TRANYLCYPROMINE

BASIC INFORMATION

Habit forming? No
Prescription needed? Yes
Available as generic? No
Drug class: MAO (monoamine oxidase) inhibitor, antidepressant

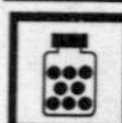

USES

- Treatment for depression and panic disorder.
- Prevention of vascular or tension headaches.

DOSAGE & USAGE INFORMATION

How to take:
Tablet—Swallow with liquid. If you can't swallow whole, crumble tablet and take with liquid or food.

When to take:
At the same times each day.

If you forget a dose:
Take as soon as you remember up to 2 hours late. If more than 2 hours, wait for next scheduled dose (don't double this dose).

What drug does:
Inhibits nerve transmissions in brain that may cause depression.

Time lapse before drug works:
4 to 6 weeks for maximum effect.

Continued next column

OVERDOSE

SYMPTOMS:
Restlessness, agitation, excitement, fever, confusion, dizziness, heartbeat irregularities, hallucinations, sweating, breathing difficulties, insomnia, irritability, convulsions, coma.
WHAT TO DO:
- **Dial 911 (emergency) or 0 (operator) for an ambulance or medical help. Then give first aid immediately.**
- **See emergency information on inside covers.**

Don't take with:
- Nonprescription diet pills, nose drops, medicine for asthma, cough, cold or allergy, or medicine containing caffeine or alcohol.
- Foods containing tyramine*.
- Any other medicine without consulting your doctor or pharmacist.

POSSIBLE ADVERSE REACTIONS OR SIDE EFFECTS

SYMPTOMS	WHAT TO DO
Life-threatening:	
In case of overdose, see previous column.	
Common:	
• Fatigue, weakness.	Continue. Call doctor when convenient.
• Dizziness when changing position, restlessness, tremors, dry mouth, constipation, difficult urination, blurred vision, "sweet tooth."	Continue. Tell doctor at next visit.
Infrequent:	
• Fainting, enlarged pupils.	Discontinue.Seek emergency treatment.
• Severe headache, chest pain.	Discontinue. Call doctor right away.
• Hallucinations, insomnia, nightmares, diarrhea, rapid or pounding heartbeat, swollen feet or legs, joint pain.	Continue. Call doctor when convenient.
• Diminished sex drive.	Continue. Tell doctor at next visit.
Rare:	
Rash, nausea, vomiting, stiff neck, jaundice, fever, increased sweating, dark urine, slurred speech.	Discontinue. Call doctor right away.

WARNINGS & PRECAUTIONS

Don't take if:
- You are allergic to any MAO inhibitor.
- You have heart disease, congestive heart failure, heart rhythm irregularities or high blood pressure.
- You have liver or kidney disease.

Before you start, consult your doctor:
- If you are alcoholic.
- If you have had a stroke.
- If you have diabetes, epilepsy, asthma, overactive thyroid, schizophrenia, Parkinson's disease, adrenal gland tumor.

- If you will have surgery within 2 months, including dental surgery, requiring general or spinal anesthesia.

Over age 60:
Not recommended.

Pregnancy:
Decide with your doctor if drug benefits justify risk to unborn child. Risk category C (see page xxii).

Breast-feeding:
Safety not established. Consult doctor.

Infants & children:
Not recommended. Consult doctor.

Prolonged use:
- May be toxic to liver.
- Talk to your doctor about the need for follow-up medical examinations or laboratory studies to check blood pressure, liver function.

Skin & sunlight:
May cause rash or intensify sunburn in areas exposed to sun or sunlamp.

Driving, piloting or hazardous work:
Don't drive or pilot aircraft until you learn how medicine affects you. Don't work around dangerous machinery. Don't climb ladders or work in high places. Danger increases if you drink alcohol or take medicine affecting alertness and reflexes.

Discontinuing:
- Don't discontinue without doctor's advice until you complete prescribed dose, even though symptoms diminish or disappear.
- Follow precautions regarding foods, drinks and other medicines for 2 weeks after discontinuing.
- Adverse symtoms caused by this medicine may occur even after discontinuation. If you develop any of the symptoms listed under Overdose, notify your doctor immediately.

Others:
- May affect blood sugar levels in patients with diabetes.
- Fever may indicate that MAO inhibitor dose requires adjustment.

POSSIBLE INTERACTION WITH OTHER DRUGS

GENERIC NAME OR DRUG CLASS	COMBINED EFFECT
Amphetamines*	Blood pressure rise to life-threatening level.
Anticholinergics*	Increased anticholinergic effect.
Anticonvulsants*	Changed seizure pattern.
Antidepressants, tricyclic*	Blood pressure rise to life-threatening level. Possible fever, convulsions, delirium.
Antidiabetics*, oral and insulin	Excessively low blood sugar.
Antihypertensives*	Excessively low blood pressure.
Beta-adrenergic blocking agents*	Possible blood pressure rise if MAO inhibitor is discontinued after simultaneous use with acebutolol.
Bupropion	Increased risk of bupropion toxicity.
Buspirone	Very high blood pressure.
Caffeine	Irregular heartbeat or high blood pressure.
Carbamazepine	Fever, seizures. Avoid.
Central nervous system (CNS) depressants*	Excessive depressant action.

Continued on page 948

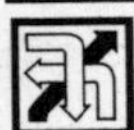

POSSIBLE INTERACTION WITH OTHER SUBSTANCES

INTERACTS WITH	COMBINED EFFECT
Alcohol:	Increased sedation to dangerous level.
Beverages:	
Caffeine drinks.	Irregular heartbeat or high blood pressure.
Drinks containing tyramine*.	Blood pressure rise to life-threatening level.
Cocaine:	Overstimulation. Possibly fatal.
Foods:	
Foods containing tyramine*.	Blood pressure rise to life-threatening level.
Marijuana:	Overstimulation. Avoid.
Tobacco:	No proven problems.

***See Glossary**

MORICIZINE

BRAND NAMES

Ethmozine

BASIC INFORMATION

Habit forming? No
Prescription needed? Yes
Available as generic? No
Drug class: Antiarrhythmic

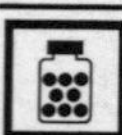

USES

Treats severe heartbeat irregularities, primarily life-threatening ventricular tachycardia.

DOSAGE & USAGE INFORMATION

How to take:
Tablets—As directed, by mouth with water.

When to take:
When directed. The first dose of this medicine is usually given in an emergency room or in the hospital under continuous monitoring.

If you forget a dose:
Take as soon as you remember up to 4 hours late. If more than 4 hours, wait for next scheduled dose (don't double this dose).

What drug does:
Affects the electrical conduction system inside the heart.

Time lapse before drug works:
Promptly, but may require up to 2 hours for full effect.

Don't take with:
Any other medicine without consulting your doctor or pharmacist.

OVERDOSE

SYMPTOMS:
Fainting, chest pain, vomiting, lethargy, coma.
WHAT TO DO:

- **Dial 911 (emergency) or 0 (operator) for an ambulance or medical help. Then give first aid immediately.**
- **See emergency information on inside covers.**

POSSIBLE ADVERSE REACTIONS OR SIDE EFFECTS

SYMPTOMS	WHAT TO DO
Life-threatening: In case of overdose, see previous column.	
Common: Dizziness.	Continue. Call doctor when convenient.
Infrequent: Chest pain; blurred vision; diarrhea; dry mouth; headache; numbness and tingling in arms, legs; nausea; abdominal pain.	Discontinue. Call doctor right away.
Rare: Sudden high fever.	Discontinue. Call doctor right away.

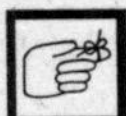

WARNINGS & PRECAUTIONS

Don't take if:
- You have pre-existing heart block.
- You have right bundle branch block.
- You are allergic to moricizine.

Before you start, consult your doctor:
- If you take any other prescription or nonprescription medicine.
- If you have liver or kidney disease.
- If you have any heart problems.

Over age 60:
No age-related adverse effects expected.

Pregnancy:
Consult doctor. Risk category B (see page xxii).

Breast-feeding:
Drug may pass into milk. Consult doctor.

Infants & children:
No special problems expected.

Prolonged use:
No special problems expected.

Skin & sunlight:
No special problems expected.

Driving, piloting or hazardous work:
Don't drive or pilot aircraft until you learn how medicine affects you. Don't work around dangerous machinery. Don't climb ladders or work in high places. Danger increases if you drink alcohol or take medicine affecting alertness and reflexes.

Discontinuing:
No special problems expected.

Others:
The first dose of this medication is usually given while the patient is being closely monitored in an intensive care setting with cardiac monitoring or in an emergency room.

POSSIBLE INTERACTION WITH OTHER DRUGS

GENERIC NAME OR DRUG CLASS	COMBINED EFFECT
Antiarrhythmics*, other	Possible increased effects of both drugs.
Cimetidine	Increased concentration of cimetidine in the blood.
Theophylline	Decreased effect of theophylline.

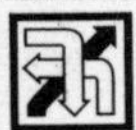

POSSIBLE INTERACTION WITH OTHER SUBSTANCES

INTERACTS WITH	COMBINED EFFECT
Alcohol:	Avoid.
Beverages:	None expected.
Cocaine:	Increased irregular heartbeat. Avoid.
Foods:	None expected.
Marijuana:	Possible increased irregular heartbeat. Avoid.
Tobacco:	Possible increased irregular heartbeat. Avoid.

***See Glossary**

MUSCLE RELAXANTS, SKELETAL

BRAND AND GENERIC NAMES

Carbacot	Rela
CARISOPRODOL	Robamol
CHLORPHENESIN	Robaxin
CHLORZOXAZONE	Robaxisal
Delaxin	Robomol
Marbaxin	Skelaxin
Maolate	Skelex
METAXALONE	Sodol
METHOCARBAMOL	Soma
Paraflex	Soprodol
Parafon Forte	Soridol

BASIC INFORMATION

Habit forming? Possibly
Prescription needed? Yes
Available as generic? Yes, for some.
Drug class: Muscle relaxant

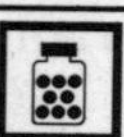

USES

Adjunctive treatment to rest, analgesics and physical therapy for muscle spasms.

DOSAGE & USAGE INFORMATION

How to take:
- Tablets—Swallow with liquid. If you can't swallow whole, crumble tablet and take with liquid or food. Instructions to take on empty stomach mean 1 hour before or 2 hours after eating.
- Extended-release tablets—Swallow whole with liquid. Don't crumble tablet.

When to take:
As needed, no more often than every 4 hours.

If you forget a dose:
Take as soon as you remember. Wait 4 hours for next dose (don't double this dose).

Continued next column

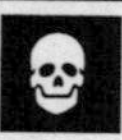

OVERDOSE

SYMPTOMS:
Nausea, vomiting, diarrhea, convulsions, headache. May progress to severe weakness, difficult breathing, sensation of paralysis, coma.

WHAT TO DO:
- **Dial 911 (emergency) or 0 (operator) for an ambulance or medical help. Then give first aid immediately.**
- **See emergency information on inside covers.**

What drug does:
Blocks body's pain messages to brain. Also causes sedation.

Time lapse before drug works:
30 to 60 minutes.

Don't take with:
Any other medicine without consulting your doctor or pharmacist.

POSSIBLE ADVERSE REACTIONS OR SIDE EFFECTS

SYMPTOMS	WHAT TO DO
Life-threatening:	
Hives, rash, intense itching, faintness soon after a dose (anaphylaxis); extreme weakness, transient paralysis, temporary vision loss.	Seek emergency treatment immediately.
Common:	
• Drowsiness, dizziness.	Continue. Call doctor when convenient.
• Orange or red-purple urine.	No action necessary.
Infrequent:	
• Agitation, constipation or diarrhea, nausea, cramps, vomiting, wheezing, shortness of breath, headache, depression, muscle weakness, trembling, insomnia, uncontrolled eye movements, fainting.	Discontinue. Call doctor right away.
• Blurred vision.	Continue. Call Doctor when convenient.
Rare:	
• Black, tarry or bloody stool; convulsions.	Discontinue. Seek emergency treatment.
• Rash, hives, or itch; sore throat; fever; jaundice; tiredness; weakness; hiccups.	Discontinue. Call doctor right away.

WARNINGS & PRECAUTIONS

Don't take if:
- You are allergic to any skeletal muscle relaxant.
- You have porphyria.

Before you start, consult your doctor:
- If you have had liver or kidney disease.
- If you plan pregnancy within medication period.
- If you are allergic to tartrazine dye.
- If you suffer from depression.

Over age 60:
Adverse reactions and side effects may be more frequent and severe than in younger persons.

Pregnancy:
Safety not proven. Avoid if possible. Consult doctor. Risk category C (see page xxii).

Breast-feeding:
Drug may pass into milk. Avoid drug or discontinue nursing until you finish medicine. Consult doctor for advice on maintaining milk supply.

Infants & children:
Not recommended.

Prolonged use:
- Talk to your doctor about the need for follow-up medical examinations or laboratory studies to check liver function, kidney function, complete blood counts (white blood cell count, platelet count, red blood cell count, hemoglobin, hematocrit).
- Safety beyond 8 weeks of treatment not established.

Skin & sunlight:
No problems expected.

Driving, piloting or hazardous work:
Don't drive or pilot aircraft until you learn how medicine affects you. Don't work around dangerous machinery. Don't climb ladders or work in high places. Danger increases if you drink alcohol or take medicine affecting alertness and reflexes, such as antihistamines, tranquilizers, sedatives, pain medicine, narcotics and mind-altering drugs.

Discontinuing:
Don't discontinue without doctor's advice until you complete prescribed dose, even though symptoms diminish or disappear.

Others:
- May affect results in some medical tests.
- Advise any doctor or dentist whom you consult that you take this medicine.

POSSIBLE INTERACTION WITH OTHER DRUGS

GENERIC NAME OR DRUG CLASS	COMBINED EFFECT
Antidepressants*	Increased sedation.
Antihistamines*	Increased sedation.
Clozapine	Toxic effect on the central nervous system.
Central nervous system (CNS) depressants*	Increased depressive effects of both drugs.
Dronabinol	Increased effect of dronabinol on central nervous system. Avoid combination.
Mind-altering drugs*	Increased sedation.
Muscle relaxants*, others	Increased sedation.
Narcotics*	Increased sedation.
Sedatives*	Increased sedation.
Sertraline	Increased depressive effects of both drugs.
Sleep inducers*	Increased sedation.
Tranquilizers*	Increased sedation.

POSSIBLE INTERACTION WITH OTHER SUBSTANCES

INTERACTS WITH	COMBINED EFFECT
Alcohol:	Increased sedation.
Beverages:	None expected.
Cocaine:	Lack of coordination, increased sedation.
Foods:	None expected.
Marijuana:	Lack of coordination, drowsiness, fainting.
Tobacco:	None expected.

*See Glossary

NABILONE

BRAND NAMES

Cesamet

BASIC INFORMATION

Habit forming? No
Prescription needed? Yes
Available as generic? No
Drug class: Antiemetic

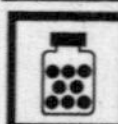

USES

- Treats nausea and vomiting.
- Prevents nausea and vomiting in patients receiving cancer chemotherapy.

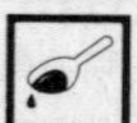

DOSAGE & USAGE INFORMATION

How to take:
Capsule—Swallow with liquid. If you can't swallow whole, open capsule and take with liquid or food.

When to take:
At the same times each day, according to instructions on prescription label.

If you forget a dose:
Take as soon as you remember up to 2 hours late. If more than 2 hours, wait for next scheduled dose (don't double this dose).

What drug does:
Chemically related to marijuana, it probably regulates the vomiting control center in the brain.

Continued next column

OVERDOSE

SYMPTOMS:
Mood changes; confusion and delusions; hallucinations; mental depression; nervousness; breathing difficulty; fast, slow or pounding heartbeat; fainting.
WHAT TO DO:
- **Dial 911 (emergency) or 0 (operator) for an ambulance or medical help. Then give first aid immediately.**
- **If patient is unconscious and not breathing, give mouth-to-mouth breathing. If there is no heartbeat, use cardiac massage and mouth-to-mouth breathing (CPR). Don't try to make patient vomit. If you can't get help quickly, take patient to nearest emergency facility.**
- **See emergency information on inside covers.**

Time lapse before drug works:
2 hours.

Don't take with:
Alcohol or any drug that depresses the central nervous system. See Central Nervous System (CNS) Depressants in the Glossary.

POSSIBLE ADVERSE REACTIONS OR SIDE EFFECTS

SYMPTOMS	WHAT TO DO
Life-threatening:	
Mood changes; fainting; hallucinations; fast, slow or pounding heartbeat; confusion and delusions; mental depression; nervousness; breathing difficulty.	Seek emergency treatment.
Common:	
Dry mouth.	Continue. Call doctor when convenient.
Infrequent:	
Clumsiness, mental changes, drowsiness, headache, false sense of well-being.	Discontinue. Call doctor right away.
Rare:	
Blurred vision, dizziness on standing, appetite loss, muscle pain.	Discontinue. Call doctor right away.

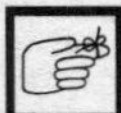

WARNINGS & PRECAUTIONS

Don't take if:
- You are allergic to nabilone or marijuana.
- You have schizophrenic, manic or depressive states.

Before you start, consult your doctor:
- If you have abused drugs or are dependent on them, including alcohol.
- If you have had high blood pressure or heart disease.
- If you have had impaired liver function.

Over age 60:
Adverse reactions and side effects may be more frequent and severe than in younger persons. You may need smaller doses for shorter periods of time.

Pregnancy:
Decide with your doctor whether drug benefits justify risk to unborn child. Risk category C (see page xxii).

Breast-feeding:
Drug passes into milk. Avoid drug or discontinue nursing until you finish medicine. Consult doctor for advice on maintaining milk supply.

Infants & children:
Not recommended for children 18 and younger. Use only under doctor's supervision.

Prolonged use:
- Avoid prolonged use. This medicine is intended to be used only during a cycle of cancer chemotherapy.
- Talk to your doctor about the need for follow-up medical examinations or laboratory studies to check blood pressure, heart function.

Skin & sunlight:
No problems expected.

Driving, piloting or hazardous work:
Don't drive or pilot aircraft until you learn how medicine affects you. Don't work around dangerous machinery. Don't climb ladders or work in high places. Danger increases if you drink alcohol or take medicine affecting alertness and reflexes.

Discontinuing:
No problems expected.

Others:
- Blood pressure should be measured regularly.
- Learn to count and recognize changes in your pulse.
- Get up from bed or chair slowly to avoid fainting.

POSSIBLE INTERACTION WITH OTHER DRUGS

GENERIC NAME OR DRUG CLASS	COMBINED EFFECT
Apomorphine	Decreased effect of apomorphine.
Central nervous system (CNS) depressants*, other	Greater depression of the central nervous system.

POSSIBLE INTERACTION WITH OTHER SUBSTANCES

INTERACTS WITH	COMBINED EFFECT
Alcohol:	Dangerous depression of the central nervous system. Avoid.
Beverages:	None expected.
Cocaine:	Decreased nabilone effect. Avoid.
Foods:	None expected.
Marijuana:	None expected.
Tobacco:	None expected.

*See Glossary

NAFARELIN

BRAND NAMES

Synarel

BASIC INFORMATION

Habit forming? No
Prescription needed? Yes
Available as generic? No
Drug class: Gonadotropin inhibitor

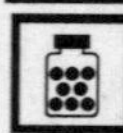

USES

- Treatment for endometriosis to relieve pain and reduce scattered implants of endometrial tissue.
- Treatment for central precocious puberty.

DOSAGE & USAGE INFORMATION

How to take:
Nasal spray—Follow instructions on package insert provided with your medicine.

When to take:
As directed by your doctor. Usually two times a day.

If you forget a dose:
Take as soon as you remember. Don't double this dose.

What drug does:
Reduces estrogen production by ovaries.

Time lapse before drug works:
May require 6 months for full effect.

Don't take with:
- Birth control pills.
- Nasal sprays to decongest the membranes in the nose.
- Any other medicine without consulting your doctor or pharmacist.

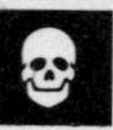

OVERDOSE

SYMPTOMS:
None expected.
WHAT TO DO:
Overdose unlikely to threaten life. If person takes much larger amount than prescribed, call doctor, poison control center or hospital emergency room for instructions.

POSSIBLE ADVERSE REACTIONS OR SIDE EFFECTS

SYMPTOMS	WHAT TO DO
Life-threatening: None expected.	
Common: Hot flashes.	No action necessary.
Infrequent: Decreased sexual desire, vaginal dryness, headache, acne, swelling of hands and feet, reduction of breast size, weight gain, itchy scalp with flaking, muscle ache, nasal irritation.	Continue. Call doctor when convenient.
Rare: Insomnia, depression, weight loss.	Continue. Call doctor when convenient.

WARNINGS & PRECAUTIONS

Don't take if:
- You become pregnant.
- You have breast cancer.
- You are allergic to any of the ingredients in nafarelin.
- You have undiagnosed abnormal vaginal bleeding.

Before you start, consult your doctor:
- If you take birth control pills.
- If you have diabetes.
- If you have heart disease.
- If you have epilepsy.
- If you have kidney disease.
- If you have liver disease.
- If you have migraine headaches.
- If you need to use topical nasal decongestants.

Over age 60:
Adverse reactions and side effects may be more frequent and severe than in younger persons.

Pregnancy:
Risk to unborn child outweighs drug benefits. Don't use. Stop if you get pregnant. Consult doctor. Risk category X (see page xxii).

Breast-feeding:
Unknown whether medicine filters into milk. Consult doctor.

Infants & children:
Not recommended.

Prolonged use:
- Full effect requires prolonged use. Don't discontinue without consulting doctor.
- Talk to your doctor about the need for mammogram, follow-up medical examinations or laboratory studies to check liver function.

Skin & sunlight:
No special problems expected.

Driving, piloting or hazardous work:
No special problems expected.

Discontinuing:
Don't discontinue without consulting doctor. Menstrual periods may be absent for 2 to 3 months after discontinuation.

Others:
- May alter blood sugar levels in diabetic persons.
- Interferes with accuracy of laboratory tests to study pituitary gonadotropic and gonadal functions.
- Experience with nafarelin has been limited to women 18 years of age and older.
- Bone density decreases during treatment phase, but recovers following treatment.

POSSIBLE INTERACTION WITH OTHER DRUGS

GENERIC NAME OR DRUG CLASS	COMBINED EFFECT
Decongestant nasal sprays*	Decreased absorption of nafarelin.

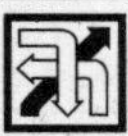

POSSIBLE INTERACTION WITH OTHER SUBSTANCES

INTERACTS WITH	COMBINED EFFECT
Alcohol:	Excessive nervous system depression. Avoid.
Beverages: Caffeine drinks.	Rapid, irregular heartbeat. Avoid.
Cocaine:	May interfere with expected action of nafarelin. Avoid.
Foods:	None expected.
Marijuana:	May interfere with expected action of nafarelin. Avoid.
Tobacco:	Rapid, irregular heartbeat; increased leg cramps. Avoid.

***See Glossary**

NALIDIXIC ACID

BRAND NAMES

NegGram

BASIC INFORMATION

Habit forming? No
Prescription needed? Yes
Available as generic? Yes
Drug class: Antimicrobial

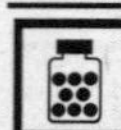

USES

Treatment for urinary tract infections.

DOSAGE & USAGE INFORMATION

How to take:

- Tablet—Swallow with food or milk to lessen stomach irritation. If you can't swallow whole, crumble tablet and take with liquid or food.
- Liquid—Take with liquid or food.

When to take:
At the same times each day.

If you forget a dose:
Take as soon as you remember up to 2 hours late. If more than 2 hours, wait for next scheduled dose (don't double this dose).

What drug does:
Destroys bacteria susceptible to nalidixic acid.

Time lapse before drug works:
1 to 2 weeks.

Don't take with:
Any other medicine without consulting your doctor or pharmacist.

OVERDOSE

SYMPTOMS:
Lethargy, stomach upset, behavioral changes, hyperglycemia, psychosis, convulsions and stupor.
WHAT TO DO:

- **Dial 911 (emergency) or 0 (operator) for an ambulance or medical help. Then give first aid immediately.**
- **If patient is unconscious and not breathing, give mouth-to-mouth breathing. If there is no heartbeat, use cardiac massage and mouth-to-mouth breathing (CPR). Don't try to make patient vomit. If you can't get help quickly, take patient to nearest emergency facility.**
- **See emergency information on inside covers.**

POSSIBLE ADVERSE REACTIONS OR SIDE EFFECTS

SYMPTOMS	WHAT TO DO
Life-threatening:	
Hives, rash, intense itching, faintness soon after a dose (anaphylaxis).	Seek emergency treatment immediately.
Common:	
Rash; itchy skin; decreased, blurred or double vision; halos around lights or excess brightness; changes in color vision; nausea; vomiting; diarrhea.	Discontinue. Call doctor right away.
Infrequent:	
• Dizziness, drowsiness, sensitivity to sun, headache.	Continue. Call doctor when convenient.
• Dark urine, hallucinations, mood changes.	Discontinue. Call doctor right away.
Rare:	
Paleness, sore throat or fever, severe abdominal pain, pale stool, unusual bleeding or bruising, jaundice, fatigue, weakness, seizures, psychosis, joint pain, numbness or tingling in hands or feet.	Discontinue. Call doctor right away.

WARNINGS & PRECAUTIONS

Don't take if:
- You are allergic to nalidixic acid.
- You have a seizure disorder (epilepsy, convulsions).

Before you start, consult your doctor:
- If you plan to become pregnant within medication period.
- If you have or have had kidney or liver disease.
- If you have impaired circulation of the brain (hardened arteries).
- If you have Parkinson's disease.
- If you have diabetes (drug may affect urine sugar tests).

Over age 60:
Adverse reactions and side effects may be more frequent and severe than in younger persons.

Pregnancy:
Consult doctor. Risk category B (see page xxii).

Breast-feeding:
Drug passes into milk. Avoid drug or discontinue nursing until you finish medicine. Consult doctor for advice on maintaining milk supply.

Infants & children:
Not recommended.

Prolonged use:
Talk to your doctor about the need for follow-up medical examinations or laboratory studies to check complete blood counts (white blood cell count, platelet count, red blood cell count, hemoglobin, hematocrit), liver function, kidney function.

Skin & sunlight:
May cause rash or intensify sunburn in areas exposed to sun or sunlamp.

Driving, piloting or hazardous work:
Avoid if you feel drowsy, dizzy or have vision problems. Otherwise, no problems expected.

Discontinuing:
Don't discontinue without consulting doctor. Dose may require gradual reduction if you have taken drug for a long time. Doses of other drugs may also require adjustment.

Others:
Periodic blood counts and liver and kidney function tests recommended.

POSSIBLE INTERACTION WITH OTHER DRUGS

GENERIC NAME OR DRUG CLASS	COMBINED EFFECT
Antacids*	Decreased absorption of nalidixic acid.
Anticoagulants*, oral	Increased anticoagulant effect.
Calcium supplements*	Decreased effect of nalidixic acid.
Nitrofurantoin	Decreased effect of nalidixic acid.
Probenecid	Decreased effect of nalidixic acid.
Vitamin C (in large doses)	Increased effect of nalidixic acid.

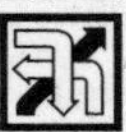

POSSIBLE INTERACTION WITH OTHER SUBSTANCES

INTERACTS WITH	COMBINED EFFECT
Alcohol:	Impaired alertness, judgment and coordination.
Beverages:	None expected.
Cocaine:	Impaired judgment and coordination.
Foods:	None expected.
Marijuana:	Impaired alertness, judgment and coordination.
Tobacco:	None expected.

*See Glossary

NALTREXONE

BRAND NAMES

Trexan

BASIC INFORMATION

Habit forming? No
Prescription needed? Yes
Available as generic? No
Drug class: Narcotic antagonist

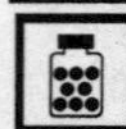

USES

- Treats detoxified former narcotics addicts. It helps maintain a drug-free state.
- May be used to treat alcoholism (in conjunction with counseling).

DOSAGE & USAGE INFORMATION

How to take:
- *Don't take at all until detoxification has been accomplished.*
- Tablets—Swallow with liquid or food to lessen stomach irritation. If you can't swallow whole, crumble tablet and take with liquid or food.

When to take:
At the same time every day or every other day as directed.

If you forget a dose:
Follow detailed instructions from the one who prescribed for you.

What drug does:
Binds to opioid receptors in the central nervous system and prohibits the effects of narcotic drugs.

Time lapse before drug works:
1 hour.

Don't take with:
- Narcotics.
- Any other medicine without consulting your doctor or pharmacist.

OVERDOSE

SYMPTOMS:
Seizures, coma.
WHAT TO DO:
- **Dial 911 (emergency) or 0 (operator) for an ambulance or medical help. Then give first aid immediately.**
- **See emergency information on inside covers.**

POSSIBLE ADVERSE REACTIONS OR SIDE EFFECTS

SYMPTOMS	WHAT TO DO
Life-threatening:	
Hallucinations, very fast heartbeat, fainting, breathing difficulties.	Seek emergency treatment immediately.
Common:	
Skin rash, chills, constipation, appetite loss, irritability, insomnia, anxiety, headache, nausea, vomiting.	Continue. Call doctor when convenient.
Infrequent:	
• Nosebleeds, joint pain.	Discontinue. Call doctor right away.
• Abdominal pain, blurred vision, confusion, earache, fever, hallucinations, depression, diarrhea, common cold symptoms.	Continue. Call doctor when convenient.
Rare:	
• Pain, tenderness or color change in feet.	Discontinue. Call doctor right away.
• Ringing in ears, swollen glands, decreased sex drive.	Continue. Call doctor when convenient.

WARNINGS & PRECAUTIONS

Don't take if:

- You don't have close medical supervision.
- You are currently dependent on drugs.
- You have severe liver disease.

Before you start, consult your doctor:
If you have mild liver disease.

Over age 60:
Adverse reactions and side effects may be more frequent and severe than in younger persons. You may need smaller doses for shorter periods of time.

Pregnancy:
Decide with your doctor whether drug benefits justify risk to unborn child. Risk category C (see page xxii).

Breast-feeding:
Safety not established. Consult doctor.

Infants & children:
Not recommended.

Prolonged use:

- Not recommended.
- Talk to your doctor about the need for follow-up medical examinations or laboratory studies to check kidney function.

Skin & sunlight:
No problems expected.

Driving, piloting or hazardous work:
Don't drive or pilot aircraft until you learn how medicine affects you. Don't work around dangerous machinery. Don't climb ladders or work in high places. Danger increases if you drink alcohol or take medicine affecting alertness and reflexes.

Discontinuing:
Don't discontinue without consulting doctor. Dose may require gradual reduction if you have taken drug for a long time. Doses of other drugs may also require adjustment.

Others:

- Probably not effective in treating people addicted to substances other than opium or morphine derivatives.
- Must be given under close supervision by people experienced in using naltrexone to treat addicts.
- Attempting to use narcotics to overcome effects of naltrexone may lead to coma and death.
- Withdraw several days prior to expected surgery.

POSSIBLE INTERACTION WITH OTHER DRUGS

GENERIC NAME OR DRUG CLASS	COMBINED EFFECT
Narcotic medicines* (butorphenal, codeine, heroin, hydrocodone, hydromorphone, levorphanol, morphine, nalbuphine, opium, oxycodone, oxymorphone, paregoric, pentazocine, propoxyphene)	Precipitates withdrawal symptoms. May lead to cardiac arrest, coma and death.
Isoniazid	Increased risk of liver damage.

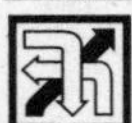

POSSIBLE INTERACTION WITH OTHER SUBSTANCES

INTERACTS WITH	COMBINED EFFECT
Alcohol:	Unpredictable effects. Avoid.
Beverages:	None expected.
Cocaine:	Unpredictable effects. Avoid.
Foods:	None expected.
Marijuana:	Unpredictable effects. Avoid.
Tobacco:	None expected.

***See Glossary**

NARCOTIC & ACETAMINOPHEN

BRAND AND GENERIC NAMES

See complete list of brand and generic names in the *Brand Name Directory*, page 911.

BASIC INFORMATION

Habit forming? Yes
Prescription needed? Yes
Available as generic? Yes
Drug class: Narcotic, analgesic, fever reducer

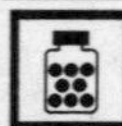

USES

Relieves pain.

DOSAGE & USAGE INFORMATION

How to take:

- Tablet or capsule—Swallow with liquid. If you can't swallow whole, crumble tablet or open capsule and take with liquid or food.
- Drops or liquid—Dilute dose in beverage before swallowing.

When to take:
When needed. No more often than every 4 hours.

If you forget a dose:
Take as soon as you remember. Wait 4 hours for next dose.

Continued next column

OVERDOSE

SYMPTOMS:
Stomach upset; irritability; sweating, convulsions; deep sleep; slow breathing; slow pulse; flushed, warm skin; constricted pupils; coma.
WHAT TO DO:

- **Dial 911 (emergency) or 0 (operator) for an ambulance or medical help. Then give first aid immediately.**
- **If patient is unconscious and not breathing, give mouth-to-mouth breathing. If there is no heartbeat, use cardiac massage and mouth-to-mouth breathing (CPR). Don't try to make patient vomit. If you can't get help quickly, take patient to nearest emergency facility.**
- **See emergency information on inside covers.**

What drug does:

- May affect hypothalamus—the part of the brain that helps regulate body heat and receives body's pain messages.
- Blocks pain messages to brain and spinal cord.
- Reduces sensitivity of brain's cough control center.

Time lapse before drug works:
15 to 30 minutes. May last 4 hours.

Don't take with:

- Other drugs with acetaminophen. Too much acetaminophen can damage liver and kidneys.
- Any other medicine without consulting your doctor or pharmacist.

POSSIBLE ADVERSE REACTIONS OR SIDE EFFECTS

SYMPTOMS	WHAT TO DO
Life-threatening:	
Irregular or slow heartbeat, difficult breathing, wheezing.	Discontinue. Seek emergency treatment.
Common:	
Dizziness, agitation, tiredness, dry mouth, headache.	Continue. Call doctor when convenient.
Infrequent:	
Abdominal pain, constipation, vomiting, confusion, pinpoint eye pupils, hallucinations, flushed face, face swelling, uncontrolled muscle movements, jaundice, nightmares, insomnia.	Discontinue. Call doctor right away.
Rare:	
• Itchy skin; rash; sore throat, fever, mouth sores; bruising and bleeding increased; painful or difficult urination; blood in urine; blurred vision.	Discontinue. Call doctor right away.
• Depression.	Continue. Call doctor when convenient.

WARNINGS & PRECAUTIONS

Don't take if:
- You are allergic to any narcotic or acetaminophen.
- Your symptoms don't improve after 2 days use. Call your doctor.

Before you start, consult your doctor:
- If you have bronchial asthma, kidney disease or liver damage.
- If you will have surgery within 2 months, including dental surgery, requiring general or spinal anesthesia.

Over age 60:
More likely to be drowsy, dizzy, unsteady or constipated. Don't exceed recommended dose. You can't eliminate drug as efficiently as younger persons. Use only if absolutely necessary.

Pregnancy:
Risk factors vary for drugs in this group. See category list on page xxii and consult doctor.

Breast-feeding:
Drug filters into milk. May harm child. Avoid.

Infants & children:
Not recommended.

Prolonged use:
- Causes psychological and physical dependence (addiction).
- May affect blood stream and cause anemia. Limit use to 5 days for children 12 and under, 10 days for adults.

Skin & sunlight:
No problems expected.

Driving, piloting or hazardous work:
Don't drive or pilot aircraft until you learn how medicine affects you. Don't work around dangerous machinery. Don't climb ladders or work in high places. Danger increases if you drink alcohol or take medicine affecting alertness and reflexes, such as antihistamines, tranquilizers, sedatives, pain medicine, narcotics and mind-altering drugs.

Discontinuing:
Discontinue in 2 days if symptoms don't improve. Report to your doctor any symptoms that develop after discontinuing such as gooseflesh, irritability, insomnia, yawning, weakness, large eye pupils.

Others:
No problems expected.

POSSIBLE INTERACTION WITH OTHER DRUGS

GENERIC NAME OR DRUG CLASS	COMBINED EFFECT
Analgesics*, other	Increased analgesic effect.
Anticoagulants*, other	May increase anticoagulant effect. Prothrombin times should be monitored.
Anticholinergics*	Increased anticholinergic effect.
Antidepressants*	Increased sedative effect.
Antihistamines*	Increased sedative effect.
Carteolol	Increased narcotic effect. Dangerous sedation.
Mind-altering drugs*	Increased sedative effect.
Narcotics*, other	Increased narcotic effect.
Nitrates*	Excessive blood pressure drop.
Phenobarbital and other barbiturates*	Quicker elimination and decreased effect of acetaminophen.

Continued on page 949

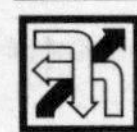

POSSIBLE INTERACTION WITH OTHER SUBSTANCES

INTERACTS WITH	COMBINED EFFECT
Alcohol:	Increased intoxicating effect of alcohol. Long-term use may cause toxic effect in liver. Avoid.
Beverages:	None expected.
Cocaine:	Increased toxic effects of cocaine. Avoid.
Foods:	None expected.
Marijuana:	Impaired physical and mental performance. Avoid.
Tobacco:	None expected.

*See Glossary

NARCOTIC ANALGESICS

BRAND AND GENERIC NAMES

See complete list of brand and generic names in the *Brand Name Directory*, page 911.

BASIC INFORMATION

Habit forming? Yes
Prescription needed? Yes
Available as generic? Yes
Drug class: Narcotic

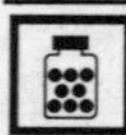

USES

Relieves pain and diarrhea; suppresses cough.

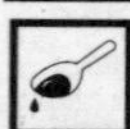

DOSAGE & USAGE INFORMATION

How to take:

- Tablet, capsule or extended-release tablet—Swallow with liquid. If you can't swallow whole, crumble tablet or open capsule and take with liquid or food.
- Drops or liquid—Dilute dose in beverage before swallowing.
- Transdermal—follow instructions on prescription.
- Nasal—Follow package instructions.

When to take:
When needed. No more often than every 4 hours.

If you forget a dose:
Take as soon as you remember. Wait 4 hours for next dose.

Continued next column

OVERDOSE

SYMPTOMS:
Deep sleep, slow breathing; slow pulse; respiratory arrest; flushed, warm skin; seizures; constricted pupils.
WHAT TO DO:

- **Dial 911 (emergency) or 0 (operator) for an ambulance or medical help. Then give first aid immediately.**
- **If patient is unconscious and not breathing, give mouth-to-mouth breathing. If there is no heartbeat, use cardiac massage and mouth-to-mouth breathing (CPR). Don't try to make patient vomit. If you can't get help quickly, take patient to nearest emergency facility.**
- **See emergency information on inside covers.**

What drug does:

- Blocks pain messages to brain and spinal cord.
- Reduces sensitivity of brain's cough control center.

Time lapse before drug works:
30 minutes.

Don't take with:
Any other medicine without consulting your doctor or pharmacist.

POSSIBLE ADVERSE REACTIONS OR SIDE EFFECTS

SYMPTOMS	WHAT TO DO
Life-threatening:	
Hives, rash, intense itching, faintness soon after a dose (anaphylaxis); seizures; restlessness (severe); slow heartbeat; breathing difficulty.	Seek emergency treatment immediately.
Common:	
Dizziness, flushed face, difficult urination, unusual tiredness.	Continue. Call doctor when convenient.
Infrequent:	
• Severe constipation, abdominal pain, vomiting, nausea.	Discontinue. Call doctor right away.
• Dry mouth, headache, appetite loss, nightmares, decreased sex drive.	Continue. Call doctor when convenient.
Rare:	
• Hives, rash, itchy skin, face swelling, slow heartbeat, irregular breathing, hallucinations, jaundice, disorientation, fainting.	Discontinue. Call doctor right away.
• Depression, blurred vision, decreased mental performance, anxiety, insomnia, weakness and faintness when arising from bed or chair, euphoria, ears ringing.	Continue. Call doctor when convenient.

WARNINGS & PRECAUTIONS

Don't take if:

- You are allergic to any narcotic.
- Diarrhea is due to toxic effect of drugs or poisons.

Before you start, consult your doctor:
- If you have impaired liver or kidney function.
- If you will have surgery within 2 months, including dental surgery, requiring general or spinal anesthesia.
- If you have asthma.

Over age 60:
More likely to be drowsy, dizzy, unsteady or constipated. Use only if absolutely necessary.

Pregnancy:
Risk factors vary for drugs in this group. See category list on page xxii and consult doctor.

Breast-feeding:
Drug filters into milk. May harm child. Avoid.

Infants & children:
Not recommended.

Prolonged use:
Causes psychological and physical dependence (addiction).

Skin & sunlight:
May cause rash or intensify sunburn in areas exposed to sun or sunlamp.

Driving, piloting or hazardous work:
Don't drive or pilot aircraft until you learn how medicine affects you. Don't work around dangerous machinery. Don't climb ladders or work in high places. Danger increases if you drink alcohol or take medicine affecting alertness and reflexes, such as antihistamines, tranquilizers, sedatives, pain medicine, narcotics and mind-altering drugs.

Discontinuing:
May be unnecessary to finish medicine. Follow doctor's instructions. Notify doctor of any withdrawal symptoms such as gooseflesh, irritability, insomnia, yawning, weakness, large eye pupils.

Others:
Some products contain tartrazine dye. Avoid, especially if you are allergic to aspirin.

POSSIBLE INTERACTION WITH OTHER DRUGS

GENERIC NAME OR DRUG CLASS	COMBINED EFFECT
Analgesics*, other	Increased analgesic effect.
Anticoagulants*, oral	Possible increased anticoagulant effect.
Anticholinergics*	Increased anticholinergic effect.
Antidepressants*	Increased sedative effect.
Antihistamines*	Increased sedative effect.
Anti-inflammatory drugs, nonsteroidal (NSAIDs)*	Increased narcotic effect.
Butorphanol	Possibly precipitates withdrawal with chronic narcotic use.
Carbamazepine	Increased carbamazepine effect possible with propoxyphene.
Carteolol	Increased narcotic effect. Dangerous sedation.
Cimetidine	Possible increased narcotic effect and toxicity.
Clozapine	Toxic effect on the central nervous system.
Ethinamate	Dangerous increased effects of ethinamate. Avoid combining.
Fluoxetine	Increased depressant effects of both drugs.
Guanfacine	May increase depressant effects of either drug.
Leucovorin	High alcohol content of leucovorin may cause adverse effects.
Methyprylon	Increased sedative effect, perhaps to dangerous level. Avoid.

Continued on page 949

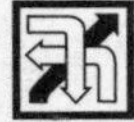

POSSIBLE INTERACTION WITH OTHER SUBSTANCES

INTERACTS WITH	COMBINED EFFECT
Alcohol:	Increased intoxicating effect of alcohol. Avoid.
Beverages:	None expected.
Cocaine:	Increased toxic effects of cocaine. Avoid.
Foods:	None expected.
Marijuana:	Impaired physical and mental performance. Avoid.
Tobacco:	None expected.

***See Glossary**

NARCOTIC & ASPIRIN

BRAND AND GENERIC NAMES

See complete list of brand and generic names in the *Brand Name Directory*, page 912.

BASIC INFORMATION

Habit forming? Yes
Prescription needed? Yes
Available as generic? Yes
Drug class: Narcotic, analgesic, anti-inflammatory (nonsteroidal)

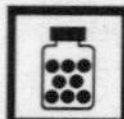

USES

Reduces pain, fever, inflammation.

DOSAGE & USAGE INFORMATION

How to take:
Tablet or capsule—Swallow with liquid. If you can't swallow whole, crumble tablet or open capsule and take with liquid or food.

When to take:
When needed. No more often than every 4 hours.

If you forget a dose:
Take as soon as you remember. Wait 4 hours for next dose.

Continued next column

OVERDOSE

SYMPTOMS:
Ringing in ears; nausea; vomiting; dizziness; fever; deep sleep; slow breathing; slow pulse; flushed, warm skin; constricted pupils; hallucinations; convulsions; coma.
WHAT TO DO:
- **Dial 911 (emergency) or 0 (operator) for an ambulance or medical help. Then give first aid immediately.**
- **If patient is unconscious and not breathing, give mouth-to-mouth breathing. If there is no heartbeat, use cardiac massage and mouth-to-mouth breathing (CPR). Don't try to make patient vomit. If you can't get help quickly, take patient to nearest emergency facility.**
- **See emergency information on inside covers.**

What drug does:
- Affects hypothalamus, the part of the brain which regulates temperature by dilating small blood vessels in skin.
- Prevents clumping of platelets (small blood cells) so blood vessels remain open.
- Decreases prostaglandin effect.
- Suppresses body's pain messages.
- Reduces sensitivity of brain's cough control center.

Time lapse before drug works:
30 minutes.

Don't take with:
- Tetracyclines. Space doses 1 hour apart.
- Any other medicine without consulting your doctor or pharmacist.

POSSIBLE ADVERSE REACTIONS OR SIDE EFFECTS

SYMPTOMS	WHAT TO DO
Life-threatening:	
• Hives, rash, intense itching, faintness soon after a dose (anaphylaxis); difficulty breathing.	Seek emergency treatment immediately.
• Lump (caused by blood clot in vein) or pain over blood vessel; cold hands, feet; seizures; pin-point pupils.	Discontinue. Seek emergency treatment.
Common:	
• Headache (severe), slow heartbeat, excitement, vomiting of blood.	Discontinue. Call doctor right away.
• Dizziness, red or flushed face, ringing in ears, unusual tiredness, frequent urination, heartburn, indigestion, fever, hallucinations, constipation.	Continue. Call doctor when convenient.
Infrequent:	
Abdominal pain or cramps, vomiting.	Discontinue. Call doctor right away.
Rare:	
• Change in vision; black, bloody or tarry stool; blood in urine; jaundice; mental confusion; irregular breathing; face swelling.	Discontinue. Call doctor right away.
• Depression, blurred vision.	Continue. Call doctor when convenient.

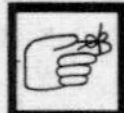

WARNINGS & PRECAUTIONS

Don't take if:
- You are allergic to any narcotic or subject to any substance abuse.
- You have a peptic ulcer of stomach or duodenum or a bleeding disorder.

Before you start, consult your doctor:
- If you have impaired liver or kidney function, asthma or nasal polyps.
- If you have had stomach or duodenal ulcers, gout.
- If you will have surgery within 2 months, including dental surgery, requiring general or spinal anesthesia.

Over age 60:
- More likely to be drowsy, dizzy, unsteady or constipated. Use only if absolutely necessary.
- More likely to cause hidden bleeding in stomach or intestines. Watch for dark stools.

Pregnancy:
Risk factors vary for drugs in this group. See category list on page xxii and consult doctor.

Breast-feeding:
Drug passes into milk and may harm child. Avoid drug or discontinue nursing until you finish medicine. Consult doctor for advice on maintaining milk supply.

Infants & children:
Not recommended.

Prolonged use:
- Causes psychological and physical dependence (addiction).
- Kidney damage. Periodic kidney function test recommended.

Skin & sunlight:
May cause rash or intensify sunburn in areas exposed to sun or sunlamp.

Driving, piloting or hazardous work:
Don't drive or pilot aircraft until you learn how medicine affects you. Don't work around dangerous machinery. Don't climb ladders or work in high places. Danger increases if you drink alcohol or take medicine affecting alertness and reflexes, such as antihistamines, tranquilizers, sedatives, pain medicine, narcotics and mind-altering drugs.

Discontinuing:
May be unnecessary to finish medicine. Follow doctor's instructions. Notify doctor of any withdrawal symptoms such as gooseflesh, irritability, insomnia, yawning, weakness, large eye pupils.

Others:
- Aspirin can complicate surgery; illness; pregnancy, labor and delivery.
- Urine tests for blood sugar may be inaccurate.

POSSIBLE INTERACTION WITH OTHER DRUGS

GENERIC NAME OR DRUG CLASS	COMBINED EFFECT
Acebutolol	Decreased antihypertensive effect of acebutolol.
Allopurinol	Decreased allopurinol effect.
Angiotensin-converting enzyme (ACE) inhibitors*	Decreased effect of ACE inhibitor.
Antacids*	Decreased aspirin effect.
Anticoagulants*, oral	Increased anticoagulant effect. Abnormal bleeding.
Antidepressants*	Increased sedative effect.
Antidiabetics*, oral	Low blood sugar.
Aspirin, other	Likely aspirin toxicity.
Anti-inflammatory drugs, nonsteroidal (NSAIDs)*	Risk of stomach bleeding and ulcers.
Bumetanide	Possible aspirin toxicity.
Carteolol	Increased narcotic effect. Dangerous sedation.

Continued on page 950

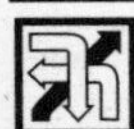

POSSIBLE INTERACTION WITH OTHER SUBSTANCES

INTERACTS WITH	COMBINED EFFECT
Alcohol:	Possible stomach irritation and bleeding. Increased intoxicating effect of alcohol. Avoid.
Beverages:	None expected.
Cocaine:	Decreased cocaine toxic effects. Avoid.
Foods:	None expected.
Marijuana:	Impaired physical and mental performance. Avoid.
Tobacco:	None expected.

*See Glossary

NATAMYCIN (Ophthalmic)

BRAND NAMES

Natacyn
Pimaricin

BASIC INFORMATION

Habit forming? No
Prescription needed? Yes
Available as generic? No
Drug class: Antifungal (ophthalmic).

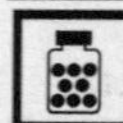

USES

Treats fungus infections of the eye.

DOSAGE & USAGE INFORMATION

How to use:
Eye drops

- Wash hands.
- Apply pressure to inside corner of eye with middle finger.
- Tilt head backward. Pull lower lid away from eye with index finger of the same hand.
- Drop eye drops into pouch and close eye. Don't blink.
- Continue pressure for 1 minute after placing medicine in eye.
- Keep eyes closed for 1 to 2 minutes.
- Don't touch applicator tip to any surface (including the eye). If you accidentally touch tip, clean with warm soap and water.
- Keep container tightly closed.
- Keep drops cool, but don't freeze.
- Wash hands immediately after using.

When to use:
As directed. Usually 1 drop in eye every 1 or 2 hours for 3 or 4 days, then every 3 to 4 hours.

If you forget a dose:
Use as soon as you remember.

What drug does:
Changes cell membrane of fungus causing loss of essential constituents of fungus cell.

Continued next column

OVERDOSE

SYMPTOMS:
None expected.
WHAT TO DO:
Not intended for internal use. If child accidentally swallows, call poison control center.

Time lapse before drug works:
Starts to work immediately. May require 2 weeks or more to cure infection.

Don't use with:
Other eye drops without consulting your eye doctor.

POSSIBLE ADVERSE REACTIONS OR SIDE EFFECTS

SYMPTOMS	WHAT TO DO
Life-threatening: None expected.	
Common: None expected.	
Infrequent:	
Eye irritation not present before using natamycin.	Discontinue. Call doctor right away.
Rare: None expected.	

WARNINGS & PRECAUTIONS

Don't use if:
You are allergic to natamycin or any antifungal medicine*.

Before you start, consult your doctor:
If you have allergies to any substance.

Over age 60:
No problems expected.

Pregnancy:
Decide with your doctor if drug benefits justify risk to unborn child. Risk category C (see page xxii).

Breast-feeding:
No problems expected, but check with doctor.

Infants & children:
No problems expected.

Prolonged use:
May cause eye irritation.

Skin & sunlight:
No problems expected.

Driving, piloting or hazardous work:
No problems expected.

Discontinuing:
Don't discontinue without consulting your eye doctor.

Others:
- Keep eye drops cool, but don't freeze.
- Notify doctor if condition doesn't improve within 1 week.

POSSIBLE INTERACTION WITH OTHER DRUGS

GENERIC NAME OR DRUG CLASS	COMBINED EFFECT
Clinically significant interactions with oral or injected medicines unlikely.	

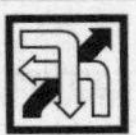

POSSIBLE INTERACTION WITH OTHER SUBSTANCES

INTERACTS WITH	COMBINED EFFECT
Alcohol:	None expected.
Beverages:	None expected.
Cocaine:	None expected.
Foods:	None expected.
Marijuana:	None expected.
Tobacco:	None expected.

***See Glossary**

NEDOCROMIL

BRAND NAMES

Tilade

BASIC INFORMATION

Habit forming? No
Prescription needed? Yes
Available as generic? No
Drug class: Antiasthmatic (anti-inflammatory)

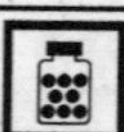

USES

For maintenance treatment of mild to moderate asthma. Not used to treat an active asthma attack.

DOSAGE & USAGE INFORMATION

How to take:
Inhaler–Follow instructions on the metered-dose inhaler pack.

When to take:
At the same times each day. Initial treatment is usually 2 inhalations 4 times a day. After symptoms subside, dosage may be reduced by your doctor.

If you forget a dose:
Take as soon as you remember up to 2 hours late. If more than 2 hours, wait for next scheduled dose (don't double this dose).

What drug does:
Inhibits inflammatory cells associated with asthma. Inhibits reflex reactions to irritants and to exercise and cold.

Time lapse before drug works:
2 to 4 days, but may require several weeks to achieve maximum effectiveness.

Don't take with:
Any other prescription or nonprescription drug without consulting your doctor.

OVERDOSE

SYMPTOMS:
None expected.
WHAT TO DO:
Overdose unlikely to threaten life. If person takes much larger amount than prescribed, call doctor, poison control center or hospital emergency room for instructions.

POSSIBLE ADVERSE REACTIONS OR SIDE EFFECTS

SYMPTOMS	WHAT TO DO
Life-threatening:	
None expected.	
Common:	
Unpleasant taste.	No action necessary.
Infrequent:	
• Headache, nausea, throat irritation, cough.	Continue. Call doctor when convenient.
• Increased broncho-spasm (increased wheezing, tightness in chest, difficulty in breathing).	Discontinue. Call doctor right away.
Rare:	
None expected.	

WARNINGS & PRECAUTIONS

Don't take if:
You are allergic to nedocromil.

Before you start, consult your doctor:
No problems expected.

Over age 60:
No problems expected.

Pregnancy:
Decide with your doctor if drug benefits outweigh risks to unborn child. Risk category C (see page xxii).

Breast-feeding:
Not known if drug passes into milk. Consult with your doctor.

Infants & children:
Give only under close medical supervision, especially to children younger than age 12.

Prolonged use:
No problems expected.

Skin & sunlight:
No problems expected.

Driving, piloting or hazardous work:
No problems expected.

Discontinuing:
No problems expected. Don't discontinue abruptly without talking to your doctor.

Others:
- Advise any doctor or dentist whom you consult that you take this medicine.
- May affect the results in some medical tests.

POSSIBLE INTERACTION WITH OTHER DRUGS

GENERIC NAME OR DRUG CLASS	COMBINED EFFECT
None expected.	

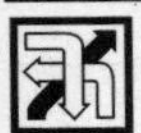

POSSIBLE INTERACTION WITH OTHER SUBSTANCES

INTERACTS WITH	COMBINED EFFECT
Alcohol:	None expected.
Beverages:	None expected.
Cocaine:	None expected.
Foods:	None expected.
Marijuana:	None expected.
Tobacco:	None expected.

NEOMYCIN (Oral)

BRAND NAMES

Mycifradin

BASIC INFORMATION

Habit forming? No
Prescription needed? Yes
Available as generic? Yes
Drug class: Antibiotic

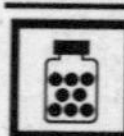

USES

- Clears intestinal tract of germs prior to surgery.
- Treats some causes of diarrhea.
- Lowers blood cholesterol.
- Lessens symptoms of hepatic coma.

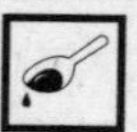

DOSAGE & USAGE INFORMATION

How to take:
Tablet—Swallow with liquid or food to lessen stomach irritation. If you can't swallow whole, crumble tablet and take with liquid or food.

When to take:
According to directions on prescription.

If you forget a dose:
Take as soon as you remember up to 2 hours late. If more than 2 hours, wait for next scheduled dose (don't double this dose).

What drug does:
Kills germs susceptible to neomycin.

Time lapse before drug works:
2 to 3 days.

Continued next column

OVERDOSE

SYMPTOMS:
Loss of hearing, difficulty breathing, respiratory paralysis.
WHAT TO DO:

- **Dial 911 (emergency) or 0 (operator) for an ambulance or medical help. Then give first aid immediately.**
- **If patient is unconscious and not breathing, give mouth-to-mouth breathing. If there is no heartbeat, use cardiac massage and mouth-to-mouth breathing (CPR). Don't try to make patient vomit. If you can't get help quickly, take patient to nearest emergency facility.**
- **See emergency information on inside covers.**

Don't take with:
Any other medicine without consulting your doctor or pharmacist.

POSSIBLE ADVERSE REACTIONS OR SIDE EFFECTS

SYMPTOMS	WHAT TO DO
Life-threatening: In case of overdose, see previous column.	
Common: Sore mouth or rectum, nausea, vomiting.	Continue. Call doctor when convenient.
Infrequent: None expected.	
Rare: Clumsiness, dizziness, rash, hearing loss, ringing or noises in ear, frothy stools, gaseousness, decreased frequency of urination, diarrhea.	Discontinue. Call doctor right away.

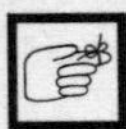

WARNINGS & PRECAUTIONS

Don't take if:
You are allergic to neomycin or any aminoglycoside*.

Before you start, consult your doctor:
- If you will have surgery within 2 months, including dental surgery, requiring general or spinal anesthesia.
- If you have hearing loss or loss of balance secondary to 8th cranial nerve disease.
- If you have intestinal obstruction.
- If you have myasthenia gravis, Parkinson's disease, kidney disease, ulcers in intestines.

Over age 60:
Adverse reactions and side effects may be more frequent and severe than in younger persons.

Pregnancy:
Risk to unborn child outweighs drug benefits. Don't use. Risk category D (see page xxii).

Breast-feeding:
Avoid if possible. Effect unknown. Consult doctor.

Infants & children:
Give only under close medical supervision.

Prolonged use:
- Adverse effects more likely.
- Talk to your doctor about the need for follow-up medical examinations or laboratory studies to check hearing, kidney function.

Skin & sunlight:
No problems expected.

Driving, piloting or hazardous work:
No problems expected.

Discontinuing:
May be unnecessary to finish medicine. Follow doctor's instructions.

Others:
No problems expected.

POSSIBLE INTERACTION WITH OTHER DRUGS

GENERIC NAME OR DRUG CLASS	COMBINED EFFECT
Aminoglycosides*	Increased chance of toxic effect on hearing, kidneys, muscles.
Beta carotene	Decreased absorption of beta carotene.
Capreomycin	Increased chance of toxic effects on hearing, kidneys.
Cephalothin	Increased chance of toxic effect on kidneys.
Cisplatin	Increased chance of toxic effects on hearing, kidneys.
Ethacrynic acid	Increased chance of toxic effects on hearing, kidneys.
Furosemide	Increased chance of toxic effects on hearing, kidneys.
Mercaptomerin	Increased chance of toxic effects on hearing, kidneys.
Penicillins*	Decreased antibiotic effect.
Tiopronin	Increased risk of toxicity to kidneys.
Vancomycin	Increased chance of toxic effects on hearing, kidneys.

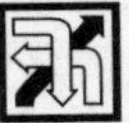

POSSIBLE INTERACTION WITH OTHER SUBSTANCES

INTERACTS WITH	COMBINED EFFECT
Alcohol:	Increased chance of toxicity. Avoid.
Beverages:	No problems expected.
Cocaine:	Increased chance of toxicity. Avoid.
Foods:	No problems expected.
Marijuana:	Increased chance of toxicity. Avoid.
Tobacco:	No problems expected.

***See Glossary**

NEOMYCIN (Topical)

BRAND NAMES

Myciguent

BASIC INFORMATION

Habit forming? No
Prescription needed? No
Available as generic? Yes
Drug class: Antibacterial (topical)

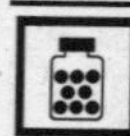

USES

Treats skin infections that may accompany burns, superficial boils, insect bites or stings, skin ulcers, minor surgical wounds.

DOSAGE & USAGE INFORMATION

How to take:

- Cream, lotion, ointment—Bathe and dry area before use. Apply small amount and rub gently.
- May cover with gauze or bandage if desired.

When to take:
3 or 4 times daily, or as directed by doctor.

If you forget a dose:
Use as soon as you remember.

What drug does:
Kills susceptible bacteria by interfering with bacterial DNA and RNA.

Time lapse before drug works:
Begins first day. May require treatment for a week or longer to cure infection.

Don't take with:
Any other medicine without consulting your doctor or pharmacist.

OVERDOSE

SYMPTOMS:
None expected.
WHAT TO DO:

- **Not for internal use. If child accidentally swallows, call poison control center.**
- **Dial 911 (emergency) or 0 (operator) for an ambulance or medical help. Then give first aid immediately.**
- **See emergency information on inside covers.**

POSSIBLE ADVERSE REACTIONS OR SIDE EFFECTS

SYMPTOMS	WHAT TO DO
Life-threatening: None expected.	
Common: None expected.	
Infrequent: Itching, swollen, red skin.	Discontinue. Call doctor right away.
Rare: None expected.	

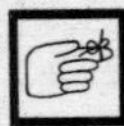

WARNINGS & PRECAUTIONS

Don't take if:
You are allergic to neomycin or any topical medicine.

Before you start, consult your doctor:
If any lesions on the skin are open sores.

Over age 60:
No problems expected.

Pregnancy:
Consult doctor. Risk category C (see page xxii).

Breast-feeding:
No problems expected, but check with doctor.

Infants & children:
No problems expected, but check with doctor.

Prolonged use:
No problems expected, but check with doctor.

Skin & sunlight:
No problems expected, but check with doctor.

Driving, piloting or hazardous work:
No problems expected, but check with doctor.

Discontinuing:
No problems expected, but check with doctor.

Others:
- Heat and moisture in bathroom medicine cabinet can cause breakdown of medicine. Store someplace else.
- Keep medicine cool, but don't freeze.

POSSIBLE INTERACTION WITH OTHER DRUGS

GENERIC NAME OR DRUG CLASS	COMBINED EFFECT
Any other topical medication	Hypersensitivity reactions more likely to occur.

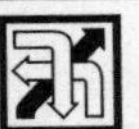

POSSIBLE INTERACTION WITH OTHER SUBSTANCES

INTERACTS WITH	COMBINED EFFECT
Alcohol:	None expected.
Beverages:	None expected.
Cocaine:	None expected.
Foods:	None expected.
Marijuana:	None expected.
Tobacco:	None expected.

***See Glossary**

NEOSTIGMINE

BRAND NAMES

Prostigmin

BASIC INFORMATION

Habit forming? No
Prescription needed? Yes
Available as generic? Yes
Drug class: Cholinergic, antimyasthenic

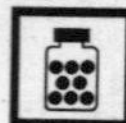

USES

- Diagnosis and treatment of myasthenia gravis.
- Treatment of urinary retention and abdominal distention.
- Antidote to adverse effects of muscle relaxants used in surgery.

DOSAGE & USAGE INFORMATION

How to take:
Tablet—Swallow with liquid or food to lessen stomach irritation.

When to take:
As directed, usually 3 or 4 times a day.

If you forget a dose:
Take as soon as you remember up to 2 hours late. If more than 2 hours, wait for next scheduled dose (don't double this dose).

What drug does:
Inhibits the chemical activity of an enzyme (cholinesterase) so nerve impulses can cross the junction of nerves and muscles.

Continued in next column

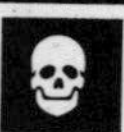

OVERDOSE

SYMPTOMS:
Muscle weakness or paralysis, cramps, twitching or clumsiness; severe diarrhea, nausea, vomiting, stomach cramps or pain; breathing difficulty; confusion, irritability, nervousness, restlessness, fear; unusually slow heartbeat; seizures; blurred vision; extreme fatigue.
WHAT TO DO:
- **Dial 911 (emergency) or 0 (operator) for an ambulance or medical help. Then give first aid immediately.**
- **See emergency information on inside covers.**

Time lapse before drug works:
3 hours.

Don't take with:
Any other medicine without consulting your doctor or pharmacist.

POSSIBLE ADVERSE REACTIONS OR SIDE EFFECTS

SYMPTOMS	WHAT TO DO
Life-threatening:	
In case of overdose, see previous column.	
Common:	
• Mild diarrhea, nausea, vomiting, stomach cramps or pain.	Discontinue. Call doctor right away.
• Excess saliva, unusual sweating.	Continue. Call doctor when convenient.
Infrequent:	
• Confusion, irritability.	Discontinue. Seek emergency treatment.
• Constricted pupils, watery eyes, lung congestion, frequent urge to urinate.	Continue. Call doctor when convenient.
Rare:	
Bronchospasm, slow heartbeat, weakness.	Discontinue. Call doctor right away.

WARNINGS & PRECAUTIONS

Don't take if:
- You are allergic to any cholinergic* or bromide.
- You take mecamylamine.

Before you start, consult your doctor:
- If you plan to become pregnant within medication period.
- If you have bronchial asthma.
- If you have heartbeat irregularities.
- If you have urinary obstruction or urinary tract infection.

Over age 60:
Adverse reactions and side effects may be more frequent and severe than in younger persons.

Pregnancy:
Decide with your doctor if drug benefits justify risk to unborn child. Risk category C (see page xxii).

Breast-feeding:
Effect unknown. Consult doctor.

Infants & children:
Not recommended.

Prolonged use:
Medication may lose effectiveness. Discontinuing for a few days may restore effect.

Skin & sunlight:
No problems expected.

Driving, piloting or hazardous work:
Don't drive or pilot aircraft until you learn how medicine affects you. Don't work around dangerous machinery. Don't climb ladders or work in high places. Danger increases if you drink alcohol or take medicine affecting alertness and reflexes, such as antihistamines, tranquilizers, sedatives, pain medicine, narcotics and mind-altering drugs.

Discontinuing:
Don't discontinue without doctor's advice until you complete prescribed dose, even though symptoms diminish or disappear.

Others:
No problems expected.

POSSIBLE INTERACTION WITH OTHER DRUGS

GENERIC NAME OR DRUG CLASS	COMBINED EFFECT
Anesthetics, local or general*	Decreased neostigmine effect.
Antiarrhythmics*	Decreased neostigmine effect.
Anticholinergics*	Decreased neostigmine effect. May mask severe side effects.
Cholinergics*, other	Reduced intestinal tract function. Possible brain and nervous system toxicity.
Cholinesterase inhibitors*	Increased risk of toxicity.
Guanadrel	Decreased neostigmine effect.
Guanethridine	Decreased neostigmine effect.
Mecamylamine	Decreased neostigmine effect.
Nitrates*	Decreased neostigmine effect.
Procainamide	Decreased neostigmine effect.
Quinidine	Decreased neostigmine effect.
Trimethaphan	Decreased neostigmine effect.

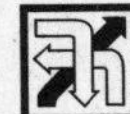

POSSIBLE INTERACTION WITH OTHER SUBSTANCES

INTERACTS WITH	COMBINED EFFECT
Alcohol:	No proven problems with small doses.
Beverages:	None expected.
Cocaine:	Decreased neostigmine effect. Avoid.
Foods:	None expected.
Marijuana:	No proven problems.
Tobacco:	No proven problems.

***See Glossary**

NIACIN (Vitamin B-3, Nicotinic Acid)

BRAND AND GENERIC NAMES

Endur-Acin
Nia-Bid
Niac
Niacels
Niacin
Niacor
Nico-400
Nicobid
Nicolar
NICOTINAMIDE
Nicotinex
Nicotinyl alcohol
Papulex
Roniacol
Ronigen
Rycotin
Slo-Niacin
Span-Niacin
Tega-Span
Tri-B3
VITAMIN B-3

There are numerous other multiple vitamin-mineral supplements available. Check labels.

BASIC INFORMATION

Habit forming? No
Prescription needed?
Tablets: No
Liquid, capsules: Yes
Available as generic? Yes
Drug class: Vitamin supplement, vasodilator, antihyperlipidemic

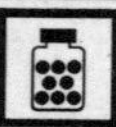

USES

- Replacement for niacin lost due to inadequate diet.
- Treatment for vertigo (dizziness) and ringing in ears.
- Prevention of premenstrual headache.
- Reduction of blood levels of cholesterol and triglycerides.
- Treatment for pellagra.

DOSAGE & USAGE INFORMATION

How to take:
- Tablet, capsule or liquid—Swallow with liquid or food to lessen stomach irritation.
- Extended-release tablets or capsules—Swallow each dose whole.

Continued next column

OVERDOSE

SYMPTOMS:
Body flush, nausea, vomiting, abdominal cramps, diarrhea, weakness, lightheadedness, fainting, sweating.
WHAT TO DO:
Overdose unlikely to threaten life. If person takes much larger amount than prescribed, call doctor, poison control center or hospital emergency room for instructions.

When to take:
At the same times each day.

If you forget a dose:
Take as soon as you remember. Wait 4 hours for next dose.

What drug does:
- Corrects niacin deficiency.
- Dilates blood vessels.
- In large doses, decreases cholesterol production.

Time lapse before drug works:
15 to 20 minutes.

Don't take with:
Any other medicine without consulting your doctor or pharmacist.

POSSIBLE ADVERSE REACTIONS OR SIDE EFFECTS

SYMPTOMS	WHAT TO DO
Life-threatening: None expected.	
Common: Dry skin.	Continue. Call doctor when convenient.
Infrequent: • Upper abdominal pain, diarrhea.	Discontinue. Call doctor right away.
• Headache, dizziness, faintness, temporary numbness and tingling in hands and feet.	Continue. Call doctor when convenient.
• "Hot" feeling, flush.	No action necessary.
Rare: Rash, itching, jaundice, double vision, weakness and faintness when arising from bed or chair.	Discontinue. Call doctor right away.

NIACIN (Vitamin B-3, Nicotinic Acid)

WARNINGS & PRECAUTIONS

Don't take if:
You are allergic to niacin or any niacin-containing vitamin mixtures.

Before you start, consult your doctor:
- If you have sensitivity to tartrazine dye.
- If you have diabetes.
- If you have gout.
- If you have gallbladder or liver disease.
- If you have impaired liver function.
- If you have active peptic ulcer.

Over age 60:
Response to drug cannot be predicted. Dose must be individualized.

Pregnancy:
Consult doctor. Risk category C (see page xxii).

Breast-feeding:
Studies inconclusive. Consult doctor.

Infants & children:
- Use only under supervision.
- Keep vitamin-mineral supplements out of children's reach.

Prolonged use:
- May cause impaired liver function.
- Talk to your doctor about the need for follow-up medical examinations or laboratory studies to check liver function, blood sugar.

Skin & sunlight:
No problems expected.

Driving, piloting or hazardous work:
Avoid if you feel dizzy or faint. Otherwise, no problems expected.

Discontinuing:
May be unnecessary to finish medicine. Follow doctor's instructions.

Others:
- A balanced diet should provide all the niacin a healthy person needs and make supplements unnecessary. Best sources are meat, eggs and dairy products.
- Store in original container in cool, dry, dark place. Bathroom medicine chest too moist.
- Obesity reduces effectiveness.
- Some nicotinic acid products contain tartrazine dye. Read labels carefully if sensitive to tartrazine.

POSSIBLE INTERACTION WITH OTHER DRUGS

GENERIC NAME OR DRUG CLASS	COMBINED EFFECT
Antidiabetics*	Decreased antidiabetic effect.
Beta-adrenergic blocking agents*	Excessively low blood pressure.
HMG-CoA reductase inhibitors*	Increased risk of heart or kidney problems.
Mecamylamine	Excessively low blood pressure.
Methyldopa	Excessively low blood pressure.
Probenecid	Decreased effect of probenecid.
Sulfinpyrazone	Decreased effect of sulfinpyrazone.

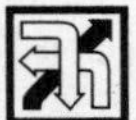

POSSIBLE INTERACTION WITH OTHER SUBSTANCES

INTERACTS WITH	COMBINED EFFECT
Alcohol:	Excessively low blood pressure. Use caution.
Beverages:	None expected.
Cocaine:	Increased flushing.
Foods:	None expected.
Marijuana:	None expected.
Tobacco:	Decreased niacin effect.

*See Glossary

NICOTINE (Skin Patch)

BRAND NAMES

Habitrol
Nicoderm
ProStep
Nicotrol

BASIC INFORMATION

Habit Forming? Yes
Prescription needed? Yes
Available as generic? No
Drug class: Antismoking agent

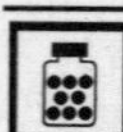

USES

As an aid to stop smoking, used in conjunction with a comprehensive behavioral smoking cessation program.

DOSAGE & USAGE INFORMATION

How to use:
Apply skin patch to clean, nonhairy site on the trunk or upper outer arm.

When to take:
Daily. Remove old patch and apply new patch to new location on the skin. Follow directions in the instruction packet that comes with the prescription.

If you forget a dose:
Remove old patch and apply new patch as soon as you remember, then return to regular schedule.

What drug does:
Delivers steady but gradually reduced supply of nicotine to the body for relief of smoking withdrawal symptoms. Reduces craving for cigarettes.

Time lapse before drug works:
2 to 4 hours.

Don't take with:
Any other medicine without consulting your doctor or pharmacist.

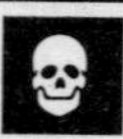

OVERDOSE

SYMPTOMS:
None expected.
WHAT TO DO:
Overdose unlikely to threaten life. If person uses much larger amount than prescribed, call doctor, poison control center or hospital emergency room for instruction.

POSSIBLE ADVERSE REACTIONS OR SIDE EFFECTS

SYMPTOMS	WHAT TO DO
Life-threatening: None expected.	
Common: Itching, redness, burning or skin rash at site of patch.	Continue. Call doctor when convenient.
Infrequent: Diarrhea, dizziness, indigestion, nervousness, strange dreams, muscle aches, constipation, sore throat, nausea, increased cough, pain, change in taste, excessive tiredness, change in menstruation, insomnia, headache.	Continue call doctor when convenient.
Rare: Mild chest pain, sinusitis, stomach pain, vomiting, dry mouth, numbness or tingling in hands or feet.	Continue. Call doctor when convenient.

WARNINGS & PRECAUTIONS

Don't take if:
You are allergic to nicotine or any of the components in the skin patch.

Before you start, consult your doctor:
- If you are pregnant.
- If you have a skin disorder (such as eczema).
- If you are using other skin patch medication.
- If you have cardiovascular or peripheral vascular disease.
- If you have liver or kidney disease.
- If you have hyperthyroidism, insulin-dependent diabetes, pheochromocytoma, peptic ulcer disease or high blood pressure.

Over age 60:
Adverse reactions and side effects may be more frequent and severe than in younger persons.

Pregnancy:
Tobacco smoke and nicotine are harmful to the fetus. The specific effects of nicotine from the skin patch are unknown. Discuss the risks of both with your doctor. Risk category D (see page xxii).

Breast-feeding:
Drug passes into breast milk. Avoid drug or discontinue nursing until you finish medicine. Consult doctor for advice on maintaining milk supply.

Infants & children:
Not recommended.

Prolonged use:
Use for longer than 3 months not recommended.

Skin & sunlight:
No problems expected.

Driving, piloting or hazardous work:
No problems expected.

Discontinuing:
- Adverse reactions and side effects related to nicotine withdrawal may continue for some time.
- Entire course of treatment should take 8 to 12 weeks, depending on the size of the initial dose.

Others:
- Advise any doctor or dentist whom you consult that you take this medicine.
- May affect results of some medical tests.
- Keep both the used and unused skin patches out of the reach of children and pets. Dispose of old patches according to package instructions.
- For full benefit from this treatment, stop cigarette smoking as soon as you begin treatment.

POSSIBLE INTERACTION WITH OTHER DRUGS

GENERIC NAME OR DRUG CLASS	COMBINED EFFECT
Acetaminophen	Increased effect of acetaminophen.
Beta-adrenergic blocking agents*	Increased effect of beta blocker.
Brochodilators, xanthine* (except dyphylline)	Increased broncho-dilator effect.
Caffeine-containing drugs	Increased effect of caffeine.
Imipramine	Increased effect of imipramine.
Insulin	May require insulin dosage adjustment.
Isoproterenol	Decreased effect of isoproterenol.
Labetalol	Increased effect of labetalol.
Oxazepam	Increased effect of oxazepam.
Pentazocine	Increased effect of pentazocine.
Phenylephrine	Decreased effect of phenylephrine.
Theophylline	Increased effect of theophylline.

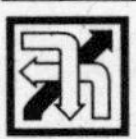

POSSIBLE INTERACTION WITH OTHER SUBSTANCES

INTERACTS WITH	COMBINED EFFECT
Alcohol:	Increased cardiac irritability. Avoid.
Beverages: Caffeine drinks.	Increased cardiac irritability. Avoid.
Cocaine:	Increased cardiac irritability. Avoid.
Foods:	No proven problems.
Marijuana:	Increased toxic effects. Avoid.
Tobacco:	Increased adverse effects of nicotine. Avoid.

*See Glossary

NICOTINE CHEWING GUM

BRAND NAMES

Nicorette

BASIC INFORMATION

Habit forming? Yes
Prescription needed? Yes
Available as generic? No
Drug class: Antismoking agent

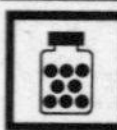

USES

Treats smoking addiction.

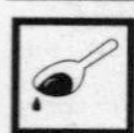

DOSAGE & USAGE INFORMATION

How to take:
Chewing gum tablets
- Chew gum pieces slowly for best effect.
- Follow detailed instructions on patient instruction sheet provided with prescription.

When to take:
Follow detailed instructions on patient instruction sheet provided with prescription.

If you forget a dose:
Follow detailed instructions on patient instruction sheet provided with prescription.

What drug does:
Satisfies physical craving for nicotine in addicted persons and avoids peaks in blood nicotine level resulting from smoking.

Time lapse before drug works:
30 minutes.

Don't take with:
- Any other medicine without consulting your doctor or pharmacist.
- Coffee, soda or fruit juice within 15 minutes prior to chewing gum. They interfere with nicotine absorption.

OVERDOSE

SYMPTOMS:
Vomiting, irregular heartbeat, mouth watering, abdominal pain, diarrhea, headache (severe), fainting, convulsions, coma.
WHAT TO DO:
- **Dial 911 (emergency) or 0 (operator) for an ambulance or medical help. Then give first aid immediately.**
- **See emergency information on inside cover.**

POSSIBLE ADVERSE REACTIONS OR SIDE EFFECTS

SYMPTOMS	WHAT TO DO
Life-threatening: In case of overdose, see previous column.	
Frequent:	
Increased irritability causing heartbeat irregularity.	Continue. Call doctor when convenient.
Common:	
• Injury to loose teeth, jaw muscle ache.	Continue. Call doctor when convenient.
• Belching, mouth irritation or tingling, excessive salivation.	Continue. Tell doctor at next visit.
Infrequent:	
• Nausea and vomiting, abdominal pain.	Discontinue. Call doctor right away.
• Lightheadedness, headache, hiccups, constipation, coughing, dry mouth, appetite loss.	Continue. Call doctor when convenient.
Rare:	
Insomnia.	Continue. Tell doctor at next visit.

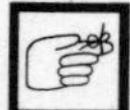

WARNINGS & PRECAUTIONS

Don't take if:
- You are a nonsmoker.
- You are pregnant or intend to become pregnant.
- You recently suffered a heart attack.

Before you start, consult your doctor:
- If you have coronary artery disease.
- If you have active temperomandibular joint disease.
- If you have severe angina.
- If you have peptic ulcer.

Over age 60:
Adverse reactions and side effects may be more frequent and severe than in younger persons.

Pregnancy:
Risk to unborn child outweighs drug benefits. Don't use. Risk category X (see page xxii).

Breast-feeding:
Drug passes into milk. Avoid drug or discontinue nursing until you finish medicine. Consult doctor for advice on maintaining milk supply.

Infants & children:
Don't use.

Prolonged use:
May cause addiction and greater likelihood of toxicity.

Skin & sunlight:
No problems expected.

Driving, piloting or hazardous work:
No problems expected.

Discontinuing:
May be unnecessary to finish medicine. Follow doctor's instructions.

Others:
- Children are very susceptible to toxic effects of nicotine; low doses can be fatal.
- Can cause tooth fillings to be pulled out.

POSSIBLE INTERACTION WITH OTHER DRUGS

GENERIC NAME OR DRUG CLASS	COMBINED EFFECT
Beta-adrenergic blocking agents*	Decreased blood pressure (slight).
Brochodilators, xanthine* (except dyphylline)	Excessive absorption of bronchodilator.
Caffeine	Increased effect of caffeine.
Cortisone drugs*	Increased cortisone circulating in blood.
Furosemide	Increased effect of furosemide.
Glutethimide	Increased absorption of glutethimide.
Imipramine	Increased effect of imipramine.
Insulin	Excessive insulin absorption. Dosage adjustment required.
Pentazocine	Increased effect of pentazocine.
Phenacetin	Increased effect of phenacetin.
Propoxyphene	Decreased blood level of propoxyphene.
Propranolol	Excessive absorption of propranolol.
Theophylline	Increased effect of theophylline.

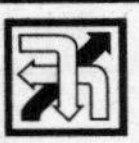

POSSIBLE INTERACTION WITH OTHER SUBSTANCES

INTERACTS WITH	COMBINED EFFECT
Alcohol:	Increased cardiac irritability. Avoid.
Beverages:	
Caffeine.	Increased cardiac irritability. Avoid any beverage with caffeine.
Cocaine:	Increased cardiac irritability. Avoid.
Foods:	No problems expected.
Marijuana:	Increased toxic effects. Avoid.
Tobacco:	Increased toxic effects. Avoid.

*See Glossary

NIMODIPINE

BRAND NAMES

Nimotop

BASIC INFORMATION

Habit Forming? No
Prescription needed? Yes
Available as generic? No
Drug class: Calcium channel blocker

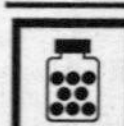

USES

Helps repair the damage caused by a ruptured blood vessel in the head (also called ruptured aneurysm or subarachnoid hemorrhage).
Note: Unlike other calcium channel blockers, nimodipine is not used for angina or high blood pressure.

DOSAGE & USAGE INFORMATION

How to take:
Capsule—Swallow with liquid.

When to take:
Results are best if you begin taking within 96 hours after bleeding into the brain begins. Continue taking for 21 days or as directed by your physician.

If you forget a dose:
Take as soon as you remember up to 2 hours late. If more than 2 hours, wait for next scheduled dose (don't double this dose).

What drug does:
This is a calcium channel blocking drug that crosses easily from blood vessels into the brain, where it prevents spasms of the brain's arteries.

Continued next column

OVERDOSE

SYMPTOMS:
Unusally fast or unusually slow heartbeat, loss of consciousness, cardiac arrest.
WHAT TO DO:

- **Dial 911 (emergency) or 0 (operator) for an ambulance or medical help. Then give first aid immediately.**
- **If patient is unconscious and not breathing, give mouth-to-mouth breathing. If there is no heartbeat, use cardiac massage and mouth-to-mouth breathing (CPR). Don't try to make patient vomit. If you can't get help quickly, take patient to nearest emergency facility.**
- **See emergency information on inside covers.**

Time lapse before drug works:
1 to 2 hours.

Don't take with:
Any other medicine without consulting your doctor or pharmacist.

POSSIBLE ADVERSE REACTIONS OR SIDE EFFECTS

SYMPTOMS	WHAT TO DO
Life-threatening: In case of overdose, see previous column.	
Common:	
Tiredness, flushing, swelling of feet, ankles and abdomen.	Continue. Tell doctor at next visit.
Infrequent:	
• Unusually fast or unusually slow heartbeat, wheezing, cough, shortness of breath.	Discontinue. Call doctor right away.
• Dizziness; numbness or tingling in hands or feet; difficult urination.	Continue. Call doctor when convenient.
• Nausea, constipation.	Continue. Tell doctor at next visit.
Rare:	
• Transient blindness, increased angina.	Discontinue. Seek emergency treatment.
• Fainting, chest pain, fever, rash, jaundice, depression, psychosis.	Discontinue. Call doctor right away.
• Pain and swelling in joints, hair loss, vivid dreams.	Continue. Call doctor when convenient.
• Headache.	Continue. Tell doctor at next visit.

WARNINGS & PRECAUTIONS

Don't take if:

- You are allergic to any calcium channel blocking drug*.
- You have very low blood pressure.

Before you start, consult your doctor:

- If you have kidney or liver disease.
- If you have high blood pressure.
- If you have heart disease other than coronary artery disease.

Over age 60:
Adverse reactions and side effects may be more frequent and severe than in younger persons.

Pregnancy:
Decide with your doctor if drug benefits justify risk to unborn child. Risk category C (see page xxii).

Breast-feeding:
Safety not established. Avoid if possible. Consult doctor.

Infants & children:
Not recommended.

Prolonged use:
Talk to your doctor about the need for follow-up medical examinations or laboratory studies to check blood pressure, liver function, kidney function, ECG*.

Skin & sunlight:
Increased sensitivity to sunlight.

Driving, piloting or hazardous work:
Avoid if you feel dizzy. Otherwise, no problems expected.

Discontinuing:
Don't discontinue without doctor's advice until you complete prescribed dose, even though symptoms diminish or disappear.

Others:
- Learn to check your own pulse rate. If it drops to 50 beats per minute or lower, don't take nimodipine until you consult your doctor.
- Drug may lower blood sugar level if daily dose is more than 60 mg.

POSSIBLE INTERACTION WITH OTHER DRUGS

GENERIC NAME OR DRUG CLASS	COMBINED EFFECT
Angiotensin-converting enzyme (ACE) inhibitors*	Possible excessive potassium in blood. Dosages may need adjustment.
Antiarrhythmics*	Possible increased effect and toxicity of each drug.
Anticoagulants*, oral	Possible increased anticoagulant effect.
Anticonvulsants, hydantoin*	Increased anti-convulsant effect.
Antihypertensives*	Blood pressure changes. Dosage may need adjustment.
Beta-adrenergic blocking agents* (oral or ophthalmic)	Possible irregular heartbeat. May worsen congestive heart failure.
Betaxolol eye drops	May cause increased effect of nimodipine on heart function.
Calcium (large doses)	Possible decreased nimodipine effect.
Carbamazepine	May increase carbamazepine effect and toxicity.
Cimetidine	Possible increased nimodipine effect and toxicity.
Cyclosporine	Increased cyclosporine toxicity.
Disopyramide	May cause dangerously slow, fast or irregular heartbeat.
Diuretics*	Dangerous blood pressure drop.
Levobutanol eye drops	May cause increased effect of nimodipine on heart function.
Lithium	Possible decreased lithium effect.
Nicardipine	Possible increased effect and toxicity of each drug.
Phenytoin	Possible decreased nimodipine effect.
Quinidine	Increased quinidine effect.
Rifampin	Decreased nimodipine effect.

Continued on page 951

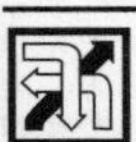

POSSIBLE INTERACTION WITH OTHER SUBSTANCES

INTERACTS WITH	COMBINED EFFECT
Alcohol:	Dangerously low blood pressure. Avoid.
Beverages:	None expected.
Cocaine:	Possible irregular heartbeat. Avoid.
Foods:	None expected.
Marijuana:	Possible irregular heartbeat. Avoid.
Tobacco:	Possible rapid heartbeat. Avoid.

***See Glossary**

NITRATES

BRAND AND GENERIC NAMES

See complete list of brand and generic names in the *Brand Name Directory*, page 912.

BASIC INFORMATION

Habit forming? No
Prescription needed? Yes
Available as generic? Yes
Drug class: Antianginal (nitrate)

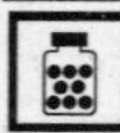

USES

- Reduces frequency and severity of angina attacks.
- Treats congestive heart failure.

DOSAGE & USAGE INFORMATION

How to take:

- Extended-release tablets or capsules—Swallow each dose whole with liquid.
- Chewable tablet—Chew tablet at earliest sign of angina, and hold in mouth for 2 minutes.
- Regular tablet or capsule—Swallow whole with liquid. Don't crush, chew or open.
- Buccal tablets (Nitrogard)—Allow to dissolve inside of mouth.
- Translingual spray (Nitrolingual)—Spray under tongue according to instructions enclosed with prescription.
- Ointment—Apply as directed.
- Patches—Apply to skin according to package instructions.
- Sublingual tablets—Place under tongue every 3 to 5 minutes at earliest sign of angina. If you don't have complete relief with 3 or 4 tablets, call doctor.

Continued next column

OVERDOSE

SYMPTOMS:
Dizziness; blue fingernails and lips; feeling of pressure in head, fever, fainting; shortness of breath; weak, fast heartbeat; convulsions.
WHAT TO DO:

- **Dial 911 (emergency) or 0 (operator) for an ambulance or medical help. Then give first aid immediately.**
- **See emergency information on inside covers.**

When to take:

- Swallowed tablets—Take at the same times each day, 1 or 2 hours after meals.
- Sublingual tablets or spray—At onset of angina.
- Ointment—Follow prescription directions.
- Patches—According to physician's instructions.

If you forget a dose:
Take as soon as you remember up to 2 hours late. If more than 2 hours, wait for next scheduled dose (don't double this dose).

What drug does:
Relaxes blood vessels, increasing blood flow to heart muscle.

Time lapse before drug works:

- Sublingual tablets and spray—1 to 3 minutes.
- Other forms—15 to 30 minutes. Will not stop an attack, but may prevent attacks.

Don't take with:
Any other medicine without consulting your doctor or pharmacist.

POSSIBLE ADVERSE REACTIONS OR SIDE EFFECTS

SYMPTOMS	WHAT TO DO
Life-threatening:	
In case of overdose, see previous column.	
Common:	
Headache, flushed face and neck, dry mouth, nausea, vomiting.	Continue. Tell doctor at next visit.
Infrequent:	
• Fainting, rapid heartbeat.	Discontinue. Call doctor right away.
• Restlessness, blurred vision, dizziness.	Continue. Call doctor when convenient.
Rare:	
• Rash.	Discontinue. Call doctor right away.
• Severe irritation, peeling.	Continue. Call doctor when convenient.

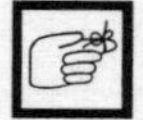

WARNINGS & PRECAUTIONS

Don't take if:
You are allergic to nitrates, including nitroglycerin.

Before you start, consult your doctor:

- If you are taking nonprescription drugs.
- If you plan to become pregnant within medication period.
- If you have glaucoma.

- If you have reacted badly to any vasodilator drug.
- If you drink alcoholic beverages or smoke marijuana.

Over age 60:
Adverse reactions and side effects may be more frequent and severe than in younger persons.

Pregnancy:
Decide with your doctor if drug benefits justify risk to unborn child. Risk category C (see page xxii).

Breast-feeding:
Effect unknown. Consult your doctor.

Infants & children:
Not recommended.

Prolonged use:
- Drug may become less effective and require higher doses.
- Talk to your doctor about the need for follow-up medical examinations or laboratory studies to check blood pressure, heart rate.

Skin & sunlight:
No problems expected.

Driving, piloting or hazardous work:
Don't drive or pilot aircraft until you learn how medicine affects you. Don't work around dangerous machinery. Don't climb ladders or work in high places. Danger increases if you drink alcohol or take medicine affecting alertness and reflexes.

Discontinuing:
Except for sublingual tablets, don't discontinue without doctor's advice until you complete prescribed dose, even though symptoms diminish or disappear.

Others:
- If discomfort is not caused by angina, nitrate medication will not bring relief. Call doctor if discomfort persists.
- Periodic urine and laboratory blood studies of white cell counts recommended if you take nitrates.
- Keep sublingual tablets in original container. Always carry them with you, but keep from body heat if possible.
- Sublingual tablets produce a burning, stinging sensation when placed under the tongue. Replace supply if no burning or stinging is noted.

POSSIBLE INTERACTION WITH OTHER DRUGS

GENERIC NAME OR DRUG CLASS	COMBINED EFFECT
Anticholinergics*	Increased internal eye pressure.
Antihypertensives*	Excessive blood pressure drop.
Beta-adrenergic blocking agents*	Excessive blood pressure drop.
Calcium channel blockers*	Decreased blood pressure.
Carteolol	Possible excessive blood pressure drop.
Guanfacine	Increased effects of both drugs.
Narcotics*	Excessive blood pressure drop.
Phenothiazines*	May decrease blood pressure.
Sympathomimetics*	Possible reduced effects of both medicines.

POSSIBLE INTERACTION WITH OTHER SUBSTANCES

INTERACTS WITH	COMBINED EFFECT
Alcohol:	Excessive blood pressure drop.
Beverages:	None expected.
Cocaine:	Reduced effectiveness of nitrates.
Foods:	None expected.
Marijuana:	Decreased nitrate effect.
Tobacco:	Decreased nitrate effect.

NITROFURANTOIN

BRAND NAMES

Apo-Nitrofurantoin
Cyantin
Furadantin
Furalan
Furaloid
Furan
Furanite
Furantoin
Furatine
Furaton
Macrobid
Macrodantin
Nephronex
Nifuran
Nitrex
Nitrofan
Nitrofor
Nitrofuracot
Novofuran
Ro-Antoin
Sarodant
Trantoin
Urotoin

BASIC INFORMATION

Habit forming? No
Prescription needed? Yes
Available as generic? Yes
Drug class: Antimicrobial, antibacterial

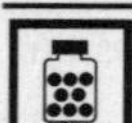

USES

Treatment for urinary tract infections.

DOSAGE & USAGE INFORMATION

How to take:

- Tablet or capsule—Swallow with food or milk to lessen stomach irritation. If you can't swallow whole, crumble tablet or open capsule and take with liquid or food.
- Extended-release capsule—Swallow with liquid. Do not open capsule.
- Liquid—Shake well and take with food. Use a measuring spoon to ensure accuracy.

When to take:
At the same times each day.

If you forget a dose:
Take as soon as you remember up to 2 hours late. If more than 2 hours, wait for next scheduled dose (don't double this dose).

Continued next column

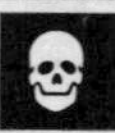

OVERDOSE

SYMPTOMS:
Nausea, vomiting, abdominal pain, diarrhea.
WHAT TO DO:
Overdose unlikely to threaten life. If person takes much larger amount than prescribed, call doctor, poison control center or hospital emergency room for instructions.

What drug does:
Prevents susceptible bacteria in the urinary tract from growing and multiplying.

Time lapse before drug works:
1 to 2 weeks.

Don't take with:
Any other medicine without consulting your doctor or pharmacist.

POSSIBLE ADVERSE REACTIONS OR SIDE EFFECTS

SYMPTOMS	WHAT TO DO
Life-threatening:	
Hives, rash, intense itching, faintness soon after a dose (anaphylaxis).	Seek emergency treatment immediately.
Common:	
• Diarrhea, appetite loss, nausea, vomiting, chest pain, cough, difficult breathing, chills or unexplained fever, abdominal pain.	Discontinue. Call doctor right away.
• Rusty-colored or brown urine.	No action necessary.
Infrequent:	
• Rash, itchy skin, numbness, tingling or burning of face or mouth, fatigue, weakness.	Discontinue. Call doctor right away.
• Dizziness, headache, drowsiness, paleness (in children), discolored teeth (from liquid form).	Continue. Call doctor when convenient.
Rare:	
Jaundice.	Discontinue. Call doctor right away.

WARNINGS & PRECAUTIONS

Don't take if:
- You are allergic to nitrofurantoin.
- You have impaired kidney function.
- You drink alcohol.

Before you start, consult your doctor:
- If you are prone to allergic reactions.
- If you are pregnant and within 2 weeks of delivery.
- If you have had kidney disease, lung disease, anemia, nerve damage, or G6PD* deficiency (a metabolic deficiency).
- If you have diabetes. Drug may affect urine sugar tests.

Over age 60:
Adverse reactions and side effects may be more frequent and severe than in younger persons.

Pregnancy:
Consult doctor. Risk category B (see page xxii).

Breast-feeding:
Drug passes into milk. Avoid drug or discontinue nursing until you finish medicine. Consult doctor for advice on maintaining milk supply.

Infants & children:
Don't give to infants younger than 1 month. Use only under medical supervision for older children.

Prolonged use:
- Chest pain, cough, shortness of breath.
- Talk to your doctor about the need for follow-up medical examinations or laboratory studies to check liver function, lung function.

Skin & sunlight:
No problems expected.

Driving, piloting or hazardous work:
Avoid if you feel dizzy or drowsy. Otherwise, no problems expected.

Discontinuing:
Don't discontinue without consulting doctor. Dose may require gradual reduction if you have taken drug for a long time. Doses of other drugs may also require adjustment.

Others:
Periodic blood counts, liver function tests, and chest x-rays recommended.

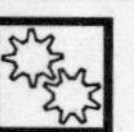

POSSIBLE INTERACTION WITH OTHER DRUGS

GENERIC NAME OR DRUG CLASS	COMBINED EFFECT
Didanosine	Increased risk of pancreatitis and peripheral neuropathy.
Hemolytics*, other	Increased risk of toxicity.
Nalidixic acid	Decreased nitrofurantoin effect.
Neurotoxic medicines*	Increased risk of damage to nerve cells.
Probenecid	Increased nitrofurantoin effect.
Sulfinpyrazone	Possible nitrofurantoin toxicity.

POSSIBLE INTERACTION WITH OTHER SUBSTANCES

INTERACTS WITH	COMBINED EFFECT
Alcohol:	Possible disulfiram reaction*. Avoid.
Beverages:	None expected.
Cocaine:	No proven problems.
Foods:	None expected.
Marijuana:	None expected.
Tobacco:	None expected.

***See Glossary**

NYLIDRIN

BRAND NAMES

Arlidin
Arlidin Forte
PMS Nylidrin

BASIC INFORMATION

Habit forming? No
Prescription needed? Yes
Available as generic? Yes
Drug class: Vasodilator

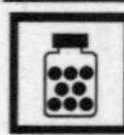

USES

- May improve circulation in extremities.
- Reduces dizziness caused by poor circulation in inner ear.

DOSAGE & USAGE INFORMATION

How to take:
Tablet—Swallow with liquid or food to lessen stomach irritation. If you can't swallow whole, crumble tablet and take with liquid or food.

When to take:
At the same times each day.

If you forget a dose:
Take as soon as you remember up to 2 hours late. If more than 2 hours, wait for next scheduled dose (don't double this dose).

What drug does:
Stimulates nerves that dilate blood vessels, increasing oxygen and nutrients.

Continued next column

OVERDOSE

SYMPTOMS:
Blood pressure drop; nausea, vomiting; rapid, irregular heartbeat, chest pain; blurred vision; metallic taste.
WHAT TO DO:
- **Dial 911 (emergency) or 0 (operator) for an ambulance or medical help. Then give first aid immediately.**
- **If patient is unconscious and not breathing, give mouth-to-mouth breathing. If there is no heartbeat, use cardiac massage and mouth-to-mouth breathing (CPR). Don't try to make patient vomit. If you can't get help quickly, take patient to nearest emergency facility.**
- **See emergency information on inside covers.**

Time lapse before drug works:
10 to 30 minutes.

Don't take with:
Any other medicine without consulting your doctor or pharmacist.

POSSIBLE ADVERSE REACTIONS OR SIDE EFFECTS

SYMPTOMS	WHAT TO DO
Life-threatening:	
In case of overdose, see previous column.	
Common:	
• Chest pain.	Discontinue. Call doctor right away.
• Blurred vision, fever, decreased or difficult urination.	Continue. Call doctor when convenient.
Infrequent:	
• Rapid or irregular heartbeat.	Discontinue. Call doctor right away.
• Dizziness, weakness, tiredness.	Continue. Call doctor when convenient.
Rare:	
• Shakiness, chills.	Discontinue. Call doctor right away.
• Headache, nausea, vomiting, flushed face, nervousness.	Continue. Call doctor when convenient.

WARNINGS & PRECAUTIONS

Don't take if:
- You are allergic to any vasodilator drugs.
- You have had a heart attack or stroke within 4 weeks.
- You have an active peptic ulcer.

Before you start, consult your doctor:
- If you have had heart disease, heart rhythm disorders (especially rapid heartbeat), a stroke or poor circulation to the brain.
- If you have glaucoma.
- If you have an overactive thyroid gland.
- If you plan to become pregnant within medication period.
- If you use tobacco.

Over age 60:
Adverse reactions and side effects may be more frequent and severe than in younger persons.

Pregnancy:
Decide with your doctor if drug benefits justify risk to unborn child. Risk category C (see page xxii).

Breast-feeding:
No proven problems. Consult doctor.

Infants & children:
Not recommended.

Prolonged use:
No problems expected.

Skin & sunlight:
No problems expected.

Driving, piloting or hazardous work:
Don't drive or pilot aircraft until you learn how medicine affects you. Don't work around dangerous machinery. Don't climb ladders or work in high places. Danger increases if you drink alcohol or take medicine affecting alertness and reflexes, such as antihistamines, tranquilizers, sedatives, pain medicine, narcotics and mind-altering drugs.

Discontinuing:
Don't discontinue without consulting doctor. If your condition worsens, contact your doctor immediately. Dose may require gradual reduction if you have taken drug for a long time. Doses of other drugs may also require adjustment.

Others:
No problems expected.

POSSIBLE INTERACTION WITH OTHER DRUGS

GENERIC NAME OR DRUG CLASS	COMBINED EFFECT
None significant.	

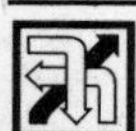

POSSIBLE INTERACTION WITH OTHER SUBSTANCES

INTERACTS WITH	COMBINED EFFECT
Alcohol:	Possible increased stomach acid secretion. Use with caution.
Beverages:	None expected.
Cocaine:	Increased adverse effects of nylidrin.
Foods:	None expected.
Marijuana:	None expected.
Tobacco:	Decreased nylidrin effect. Worsens circulation. Avoid.

NYSTATIN

BRAND NAMES

Dermacomb	Mykacet II
Myco II	Mytrex
Mycobiotic II	Nadostine
Mycogen II	Nilstat
Mycolog II	Nystaform
Mycostatin	Nystex
Myco-Triacet II	Tristatin II
Mykacet	

BASIC INFORMATION

Habit forming? No
Prescription needed? Yes
Available as generic? Yes
Drug class: Antifungal

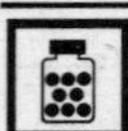

USES

Treatment of fungus infections of the mouth or vagina that are susceptible to nystatin.

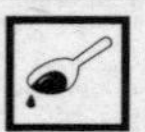

DOSAGE & USAGE INFORMATION

How to take:

- Tablet—Swallow with liquid. If you can't swallow whole, crumble tablet and take with liquid or food.
- Ointment, cream or lotion—Use as directed by doctor and label.
- Liquid—Take as directed. Instruction varies by preparation.
- Lozenges—Take as directed on label.

When to take:
At the same time each day.

If you forget a dose:
Take as soon as you remember up to 2 hours late. If more than 2 hours, wait for next scheduled dose (don't double this dose).

Continued next column

OVERDOSE

SYMPTOMS:
Mild overdose may cause nausea, vomiting, diarrhea.
WHAT TO DO:
Overdose unlikely to threaten life. If person takes much larger amount than prescribed, call doctor, poison control center or hospital emergency room for instructions.

What drug does:
Prevents growth and reproduction of fungus.

Time lapse before drug works:
Begins immediately. May require 3 weeks for maximum benefit, depending on location and severity of infection.

Don't take with:
Any other medicine without consulting your doctor or pharmacist.

POSSIBLE ADVERSE REACTIONS OR SIDE EFFECTS

SYMPTOMS	WHAT TO DO
Life-threatening: None expected.	
Common: (at high doses) Nausea, stomach pain, vomiting, diarrhea.	Discontinue. Call doctor right away.
Infrequent: Mild irritation, itch at application site.	Discontinue. Call doctor right away.
Rare: None expected.	

WARNINGS & PRECAUTIONS

Don't take if:
You are allergic to nystatin.

Before you start, consult your doctor:
If you plan to become pregnant within medication period.

Over age 60:
No problems expected.

Pregnancy:
No proven harm to unborn child. Avoid if possible. Consult doctor. Risk category B (see page xxii).

Breast-feeding:
No proven problems. Consult doctor.

Infants & children:
No problems expected.

Prolonged use:
No problems expected.

Skin & sunlight:
No problems expected.

Driving, piloting or hazardous work:
No problems expected.

Discontinuing:
Don't discontinue without doctor's advice until you complete prescribed dose, even though symptoms diminish or disappear.

Others:
No problems expected.

POSSIBLE INTERACTION WITH OTHER DRUGS

GENERIC NAME OR DRUG CLASS	COMBINED EFFECT
None reported.	

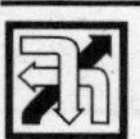

POSSIBLE INTERACTION WITH OTHER SUBSTANCES

INTERACTS WITH	COMBINED EFFECT
Alcohol:	None expected.
Beverages:	None expected.
Cocaine:	None expected.
Foods:	None expected.
Marijuana:	None expected.
Tobacco:	None expected.

OLSALAZINE

BRAND NAMES

Dipentum

BASIC INFORMATION

Habit forming? No
Prescription needed? Yes
Available as generic? No
Drug class: Inflammatory bowel disease suppressant

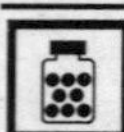

USES

To maintain remission of ulcerative colitis. Generally prescribed when intolerance to sulfasalazine exists.

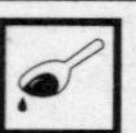

DOSAGE & USAGE INFORMATION

How to take:
Capsule—Swallow with liquid or food to lessen stomach irritation. If you can't swallow whole, open capsule and take with liquid or food.

When to take:
Usually twice a day, or as directed on prescription label.

If you forget a dose:
- Take as soon as possible.
- Skip if it is almost time for next dose.
- Don't double next dose.
- Notify your doctor if there are questions.

What drug does:
Inhibits prostaglandin production in the colon.

Time lapse before drug works:
1 hour.

Don't take with:
Any other medicine without consulting your doctor or pharmacist.

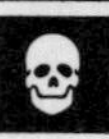

OVERDOSE

SYMPTOMS:
None expected.
WHAT TO DO:
Overdose unlikely to threaten life. If person takes much larger amount than prescribed, call doctor, poison control center or hospital emergency room for instructions.

POSSIBLE ADVERSE REACTIONS OR SIDE EFFECTS

SYMPTOMS	WHAT TO DO
Life-threatening:	
Fever, sore throat, paleness, unusual bleeding (representing effect on blood, a rare complication).	Seek emergency treatment.
Common:	
Diarrhea, appetite loss, nausea, vomiting.	Continue. Call doctor when convenient.
Infrequent:	
Mood changes, sleeplessness, headache.	Continue. Call doctor when convenient.
Rare:	
Skin eruption (acne-like), muscle aches.	Continue. Call doctor when convenient.

WARNINGS & PRECAUTIONS

Don't take if:
- You are allergic to aspirin or any other salicylate.
- You are allergic to mesalamine.

Before you start, consult your doctor:
- If you have kidney disease.
- If you are taking any other prescription or nonprescription medicine.

Over age 60:
No special problems expected.

Pregnancy:
Decide with your doctor if drug benefits justify risk to unborn child. Risk category C (see page xxii).

Breast-feeding:
Unknown effects. Consult doctor.

Infants & children:
Effect not documented. Consult your family doctor or pediatrician.

Prolonged use:
Follow through with full prescribed course of treatment.

Skin & sunlight:
No special problems expected.

Driving, piloting or hazardous work:
Don't drive or pilot aircraft until you learn how medicine affects you. Don't work around dangerous machinery. Don't climb ladders or work in high places. Danger increases if you drink alcohol or take medicine affecting alertness and reflexes.

Discontinuing:
Don't discontinue without consulting doctor. Dose may require gradual reduction if you have taken drug for a long time. Doses of other drugs may also require adjustment.

Others:
Request your doctor to check blood counts and kidney function on a regular basis.

POSSIBLE INTERACTION WITH OTHER DRUGS

GENERIC NAME OR DRUG CLASS	COMBINED EFFECT

None expected since olsalazine is not appreciably absorbed from the gastrointestinal tract into the bloodstream.

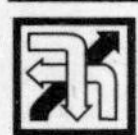

POSSIBLE INTERACTION WITH OTHER SUBSTANCES

INTERACTS WITH	COMBINED EFFECT
Alcohol:	Increased risk of gastrointestinal upset and/or bleeding.
Beverages: Highly spiced beverages.	Will irritate underlying condition that olsalazine treats.
Cocaine:	Avoid.
Foods: Highly spiced foods.	Will irritate underlying condition that olsalazine treats.
Marijuana:	Avoid.
Tobacco:	Will irritate underlying condition that olsalazine treats. Avoid.

OMEPRAZOLE

BRAND NAMES

Losec | Prilosec

BASIC INFORMATION

Habit forming? No
Prescription needed? Yes
Available as generic? No
Drug class: Antiulcer

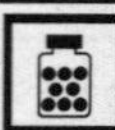

USES

- Treats gastroesophageal reflux (splashing of stomach acid from the stomach up onto the lower end of the esophagus).
- Treats peptic ulcer in the stomach and duodenum.
- Treats any disorder associated with excess production of stomach acid.

DOSAGE & USAGE INFORMATION

How to take:
- Capsules—Swallow whole. Do not crush, chew or break open.
- If directed by your doctor, it is permissible and sometimes helpful to take with antacid medicine to relieve upper abdominal pain. Antacids may be used more than once daily if needed.

When to take:
Once daily, immediately before a meal (preferably breakfast), unless otherwise directed by your doctor.

If you forget a dose:
Take as soon as you remember up to 2 hours late. If more than 2 hours, wait for next scheduled dose (don't double this dose).

What drug does:
Prevents secretion of stomach acid no matter what its original cause.

Continued next column

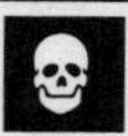

OVERDOSE

SYMPTOMS:
Severe drowsiness, seizures, breathing difficulty, decreased body temperature.
WHAT TO DO:
- **Dial 911 (emergency) or 0 (operator) for an ambulance or medical help. Then give first aid immediately.**
- **See emergency information on inside covers.**

Time lapse before drug works:
30 minutes to 1 hour.

Don't take with:
- Tobacco, excess caffeine or spicy diet.
- Any other medicine without consulting your doctor or pharmacist.

POSSIBLE ADVERSE REACTIONS OR SIDE EFFECTS

SYMPTOMS	WHAT TO DO
Life-threatening: In case of overdose, see previous column.	
Common: Abdominal pain, itching skin.	Discontinue. Call doctor right away.
Infrequent: Muscle pain; dizziness, headache, drowsiness; chest pain, diarrhea, gaseousness.	Discontinue. Call doctor right away.
Rare: Weakness or unusual tiredness, sore throat, fever sores on mouth, unusual bleeding or bruising, cloudy urine, difficult or painful urination, painful nocturnal erections in males.	Discontinue. Call doctor right away.

WARNINGS & PRECAUTIONS

Don't take if:
You are allergic to omeprazole.

Before you start, consult your doctor:
- If you are allergic to any other medicines, foods, preservatives or dyes.
- If you have liver disease now or a history of liver disease in the past.

Over age 60:
No special problems expected.

Pregnancy:
Decide with your doctor if drug benefits justify risk to unborn child. Risk category C (see page xxii).

Breast-feeding:
Safety not established. Best to avoid or discontinue nursing until you finish medicine. Consult doctor for advice on maintaining milk supply.

Infants & children:
Safety not established. Consult doctor.

Prolonged use:
May cause carcinoid tumors if taken for over 8 weeks.

Skin & sunlight:
No problems expected.

Driving, piloting or hazardous work:
Don't drive or pilot aircraft until you learn how medicine affects you. Don't work around dangerous machinery. Don't climb ladders or work in high places. Danger increases if you drink alcohol or take medicine affecting alertness and reflexes.

Discontinuing:
Don't discontinue without consulting doctor. Dose may require gradual reduction if you have taken drug for a long time. Doses of other drugs may also require adjustment.

Others:
- Treatment of ulcers usually requires 4 to 6 weeks, although symptoms may greatly improve in 1 or 2 weeks.
- May affect results of some medical tests.

POSSIBLE INTERACTION WITH OTHER DRUGS

GENERIC NAME OR DRUG CLASS	COMBINED EFFECT
Anticoagulants* (warfarin, coumadin, indandione derivatives)	Increased anticoagulant effect. May require dosage adjustment.
Diazepam	Delayed excretion and therefore increased concentration of diazepam.
Phenytoin	Delayed excretion and therefore increased concentration of omeprazole.

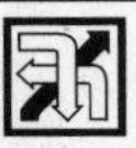

POSSIBLE INTERACTION WITH OTHER SUBSTANCES

INTERACTS WITH	COMBINED EFFECT
Alcohol:	Decreased omeprazole effect.
Beverages: Caffeine drinks.	Decreased omeprazole effect.
Cocaine:	None expected.
Foods: Spicy or highly seasoned.	Decreased omeprazole effect.
Marijuana:	None expected.
Tobacco:	Decreased omeprazole effect.

*See Glossary

ORPHENADRINE

BRAND NAMES

Banflex
Blanex
Disipal
Flexagin
Flexain
Flexoject
Flexon
K-Flex
Marflex
Myolin
Myotrol
Neocyten
Noradex
Norflex
O-Flex
Orflagen
Orfro
Orphenate
Tega-Flex

BASIC INFORMATION

Habit forming? Possibly
Prescription needed?
U.S.: Yes
Canada: No
Available as generic? Yes
Drug class: Muscle relaxant, anticholinergic, antihistamine, antiparkinsonism

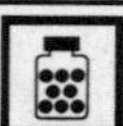

USES

- Reduces discomfort of muscle strain.
- Relieves symptoms of Parkinson's disease.
- Adjunctive treatment to rest, analgesics and physical therapy for muscle spasms.

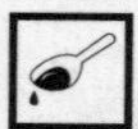

DOSAGE & USAGE INFORMATION

How to take:
- Tablet—Swallow with liquid. If you can't swallow whole, crumble tablet and take with liquid or food.
- Extended-release tablet—Swallow whole. Do not crumble.

When to take:
At the same times each day.

Continued next column

OVERDOSE

SYMPTOMS:
Fainting, confusion, blurred vision, difficulty swallowing, difficulty breathing, decreased urination, widely dilated pupils, rapid heart-beat, rapid pulse, paralysis, convulsions, coma.
WHAT TO DO:
- **Dial 911 (emergency) or 0 (operator) for an ambulance or medical help. Then give first aid immediately.**
- **See emergency information on inside covers.**

If you forget a dose:
Take as soon as you remember up to 6 hours late. If more than 6 hours, wait for next scheduled dose (don't double this dose).

What drug does:
Sedative and analgesic effects reduce spasm and pain in skeletal muscles.

Time lapse before drug works:
1 to 2 hours.

Don't take with:
Any other medicine without consulting your doctor or pharmacist.

POSSIBLE ADVERSE REACTIONS OR SIDE EFFECTS

SYMPTOMS	WHAT TO DO
Life-threatening:	
Extreme weakness; transient paralysis; temporary loss of vision; hives, rash, intense itching, faintness soon after a dose (anaphylaxis).	Seek emergency treatment immediately.
Common:	
None expected.	
Infrequent:	
• Weakness, headache, dizziness, agitation, drowsiness, tremor, confusion, rapid or pounding heartbeat, depression, hearing loss.	Discontinue. Call doctor right away.
• Dry mouth, nausea, vomiting, constipation, urinary hesitancy or retention, abdominal pain, muscle weakness.	Continue. Call doctor when convenient.
Rare:	
Rash, itchy skin, blurred vision, hallucinations.	Discontinue. Call doctor right away.

WARNINGS & PRECAUTIONS

Don't take if:
- You are allergic to orphenadrine.
- You are allergic to tartrazine dye.

Before you start, consult your doctor:
- If you have glaucoma.
- If you have myasthenia gravis.
- If you have difficulty emptying bladder.
- If you have had heart disease or heart rhythm disturbance.
- If you have had a peptic ulcer.
- If you have prostate enlargement.

Over age 60:
Adverse reactions and side effects may be more frequent and severe than in younger persons.

Pregnancy:
Decide with your doctor if drug benefits justify risk to unborn child. Risk category C (see page xxii).

Breast-feeding:
No proven problems. Consult doctor.

Infants & children:
Not recommended for children younger than 12.

Prolonged use:
- Increased internal eye pressure.
- Talk to your doctor about the need for follow-up medical examinations or laboratory studies to check complete blood counts (white blood cell count, platelet count, red blood cell count, hemoglobin, hematocrit), liver function, kidney function.

Skin & sunlight:
No problems expected.

Driving, piloting or hazardous work:
Don't drive or pilot aircraft until you learn how medicine affects you. Don't work around dangerous machinery. Don't climb ladders or work in high places. Danger increases if you drink alcohol or take medicine affecting alertness and reflexes, such as antihistamines, tranquilizers, sedatives, pain medicine, narcotics and mind-altering drugs.

Discontinuing:
May be unnecessary to finish medicine. Follow doctor's instructions.

Others:
No problems expected.

POSSIBLE INTERACTION WITH OTHER DRUGS

GENERIC NAME OR DRUG CLASS	COMBINED EFFECT
Anticholinergics*	Increased anticholinergic effect.
Antidepressants, tricyclic*	Increased sedation.
Antihistamines*	Increased sedation.
Attapulgite	Decreased orphenadrine effect.
Carteolol	Decreased antihistamine effect.
Chlorpromazine	Hypoglycemia (low blood sugar).
Cisapride	Decreased orphenadrine effect.
Contraceptives, oral*	Decreased contraceptive effect.
Griseofulvin	Decreased griseofulvin effect.
Levodopa	Increased levodopa effect. (Improves effectiveness in treating Parkinson's disease.)
Nabilone	Greater depression of central nervous system.
Nitrates*	Increased internal eye pressure.
Nizatidine	Increased nizatidine effect.
Phenylbutazone	Decreased phenylbutazone effect.
Potassium supplements*	Increased possibility of intestinal ulcers with oral potassium tablets.
Propoxyphene	Possible confusion, nervousness, tremors.

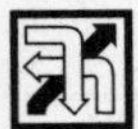

POSSIBLE INTERACTION WITH OTHER SUBSTANCES

INTERACTS WITH	COMBINED EFFECT
Alcohol:	Increased drowsiness. Avoid.
Beverages:	None expected.
Cocaine:	Decreased orphenadrine effect. Avoid.
Foods:	None expected.
Marijuana:	Increased drowsiness, mouth dryness, muscle weakness, fainting.
Tobacco:	None expected.

***See Glossary**

ORPHENADRINE, ASPIRIN & CAFFEINE

BRAND NAMES

Norgesic	**N3 Gesic**
Norgesic Forte	**N3 Gesic Forte**
Norphadrine	**Orphenagesic**
Norphadrine Forte	**Orphenagesic Forte**

BASIC INFORMATION

Habit forming? Yes
Prescription needed? Yes
Available as generic? No
Drug class: Stimulant, vasoconstrictor, muscle relaxant, analgesic, anti-inflammatory (nonsteroidal)

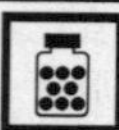

USES

- Reduces discomfort of muscle strain.
- Reduces pain, fever, inflammation.
- Relieves swelling, stiffness, joint pain.
- Treats drowsiness and fatigue.

DOSAGE & USAGE INFORMATION

How to take:
Tablet—Swallow with liquid. If you can't swallow whole, crumble and take with liquid or food.

When to take:
At the same times each day.

If you forget a dose:
Take as soon as you remember up to 2 hours late. If more than 2 hours, wait for next scheduled dose (don't double this dose).

What drug does:
- Sedative and analgesic effects reduce spasm and pain in skeletal muscles.
- Affects hypothalamus, the part of the brain which regulates temperature by dilating small blood vessels in skin.

Continued next column

OVERDOSE

SYMPTOMS:
Fainting, confusion, widely dilated pupils, rapid pulse, ringing in ears, nausea, vomiting, dizziness, fever, deep and rapid breathing, excitement, rapid heartbeat, hallucinations, coma.
WHAT TO DO:
- **Dial 911 (emergency) or 0 (operator) for an ambulance or medical help. Then give first aid immediately.**
- **See emergency information on inside covers.**

- Prevents clumping of platelets (small blood cells) so blood vessels remain open.
- Decreases prostaglandin effect.
- Suppresses body's pain messages.
- Constricts blood vessel walls.
- Stimulates central nervous system.

Time lapse before drug works:
1 hour.

Don't take with:
- Tetracyclines. Space doses 1 hour apart.
- Nonprescription drugs without consulting doctor.
- Any other medicine without consulting your doctor or pharmacist.

POSSIBLE ADVERSE REACTIONS OR SIDE EFFECTS

SYMPTOMS	WHAT TO DO
Life-threatening:	
Hives, rash, intense itching, wheezing, faintness soon after a dose (anaphylaxis), convulsions, fever.	Seek emergency treatment immediately.
Common:	
• Nausea, vomiting, abdominal cramps, nervousness, urgent urination, low blood sugar (hunger, anxiety, cold sweats, rapid pulse).	Discontinue. Call doctor right away.
• Ringing in ears, indigestion, heartburn, insomnia.	Continue. Call doctor when convenient.
Infrequent:	
• Weakness, headache, dizziness, drowsiness, agitation, tremor, confusion, irregular heartbeat, hearing loss, diarrhea, hallucinations.	Discontinue. Call doctor right away.
• Dry mouth, constipation.	Continue. Call doctor when convenient.
Rare:	
• Black or bloody vomit.	Discontinue. Seek emergency treatment.
• Change in vision; blurred vision; black, bloody or tarry stool; bloody urine; dilated pupils; uncontrolled movement of hands; sore throat; fever.	Discontinue. Call doctor right away.

ORPHENADRINE, ASPIRIN & CAFFEINE

WARNINGS & PRECAUTIONS

Don't take if:
- You need to restrict sodium in your diet. Buffered effervescent tablets and sodium salicylate are high in sodium.
- Aspirin has a strong vinegar-like odor, which means it has decomposed.
- You have a peptic ulcer of stomach or duodenum, a bleeding disorder, heart disease.
- You are allergic to any stimulant or orphenadrine.

Before you start, consult your doctor:
- If you have had stomach or duodenal ulcers, gout, heart disease or heart rhythm disturbance, peptic ulcer.
- If you have asthma, nasal polyps, irregular heartbeat, hypoglycemia (low blood sugar), epilepsy, glaucoma, myasthenia gravis, difficulty emptying bladder, prostate enlargement.

Over age 60:
- More likely to cause hidden bleeding in stomach or intestines. Watch for dark stools.
- Adverse reactions and side effects may be more frequent and severe than in younger persons.

Pregnancy:
Risk to unborn child outweighs drug benefits. Don't use. Risk category D (see page xxii).

Breast-feeding:
Drug passes into milk. Avoid drug or discontinue nursing until you finish medicine. Consult doctor for advice on maintaining milk supply.

Infants & children:
- Overdose frequent and severe. Keep bottles out of children's reach.
- Consult doctor before giving to persons under age 18 who have fever and discomfort of viral illness, especially chicken pox and influenza. Probably increases risk of Reye's syndrome.
- Not recommended for children younger than 12.

Prolonged use:
- Kidney damage. Periodic kidney function test recommended.
- Stomach ulcers more likely.
- Increased internal eye pressure.
- Talk to your doctor about the need for follow-up medical examinations or laboratory studies to check liver function, complete blood counts (white blood cell count, platelet count, red blood cell count, hemoglobin, hematocrit).

Skin & sunlight:
Aspirin combined with sunscreen may decrease sunburn.

Driving, piloting or hazardous work:
Don't drive or pilot aircraft until you learn how medicine affects you. Don't work around dangerous machinery. Don't climb ladders or work in high places. Danger increases if you drink alcohol or take medicine affecting alertness and reflexes, such as antihistamines, tranquilizers, sedatives, pain medicine, narcotics and mind-altering drugs.

Discontinuing:
- For chronic illness—Don't discontinue without doctor's advice until you complete prescribed dose, even though symptoms diminish or disappear.
- May be unnecessary to finish medicine if you take it for a short-term illness. Follow doctor's instructions.

Others:
- Aspirin can complicate surgery; illness; pregnancy, labor and delivery.
- For arthritis, don't change dose without consulting doctor.
- Urine tests for blood sugar may be inaccurate.
- May produce or aggravate fibrocystic breast disease in women.

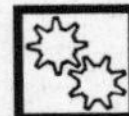

POSSIBLE INTERACTION WITH OTHER DRUGS

GENERIC NAME OR DRUG CLASS	COMBINED EFFECT
Acebutolol	Decreased antihypertensive effect of acebutolol.

Continued on page 951

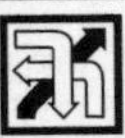

POSSIBLE INTERACTION WITH OTHER SUBSTANCES

INTERACTS WITH	COMBINED EFFECT
Alcohol:	Possible stomach irritation and bleeding, increased drowsiness. Avoid.
Beverages: Caffeine drinks.	Increased caffeine effect.
Cocaine:	Decreased orphenadrine effect. Overstimulation. Avoid.
Foods:	No proven problems.
Marijuana:	Increased effect of drugs. May lead to dangerous, rapid heartbeat. Increased dry mouth. Avoid.
Tobacco:	Increased heartbeat. Avoid.

***See Glossary**

OXTRIPHYLLINE & GUAIFENESIN

BRAND NAMES

Brondecon
Brondelate
Choledyl Expectorant

BASIC INFORMATION

Habit forming? No
Prescription needed? Yes
Available as generic? Yes
Drug class: Bronchodilator (xanthine), cough/cold preparation

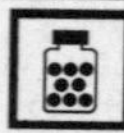

USES

- Treatment for bronchial asthma symptoms.
- Loosens mucus in respiratory passages from allergies and infections.

DOSAGE & USAGE INFORMATION

How to take:
Tablet or elixir—Swallow with liquid. If you can't swallow tablet whole, crumble and take with liquid or food.

When to take:
Most effective taken on empty stomach 1 hour before or 2 hours after eating. However, may take with food to lessen stomach upset.

If you forget a dose:
Take as soon as you remember up to 2 hours late. If more than 2 hours, wait for next scheduled dose (don't double this dose).

What drug does:
- Relaxes and expands bronchial tubes.
- Increases production of watery fluids to thin mucus so it can be coughed out or absorbed.

Time lapse before drug works:
15 to 30 minutes.

Don't take with:
- Any stimulant.
- Any other medicine without consulting your doctor or pharmacist.

OVERDOSE

SYMPTOMS:
Restlessness, irritability, confusion, delirium, convulsions, rapid pulse, nausea, vomiting, coma.
WHAT TO DO:
- **Dial 911 (emergency) or 0 (operator) for an ambulance or medical help. Then give first aid immediately.**
- **See emergency information on inside covers.**

POSSIBLE ADVERSE REACTIONS OR SIDE EFFECTS

SYMPTOMS	WHAT TO DO
Life-threatening:	
Difficult breathing, irregular or fast heartbeat.	Discontinue. Seek emergency treatment.
Common:	
Headache, irritability, nervousness, restlessness, insomnia, nausea, vomiting, abdominal pain, drowsiness.	Continue. Call doctor when convenient.
Infrequent:	
• Hives, rash, red or flushed face, diarrhea, heartburn, muscle twitching.	Discontinue. Call doctor right away.
• Dizziness, lightheadedness, appetite loss.	Continue. Call doctor when convenient.
Rare:	
None expected.	

WARNINGS & PRECAUTIONS

Don't take if:
- You are allergic to any cough or cold preparation containing guaifenesin or any bronchodilator.
- You have an active peptic ulcer.

Before you start, consult your doctor:
- If you have had impaired kidney or liver function.
- If you have gastritis, peptic ulcer, high blood pressure or heart disease.
- If you take medication for gout.

Over age 60:
Adverse reactions and side effects may be more frequent and severe than in younger persons. For drug to work, you must drink 8 to 10 glasses of fluid per day.

Pregnancy:
Decide with your doctor if drug benefits justify risk to unborn child. Risk category C (see page xxii).

Breast-feeding:
Drug passes into milk. Avoid drug or discontinue nursing until you finish medicine. Consult doctor for advice on maintaining milk supply.

Infants & children:
Use only under medical supervision.

Prolonged use:
- Stomach irritation.
- Talk to your doctor about the need for follow-up medical examinations or laboratory studies to check serum oxtriphylline levels, lung function.

Skin & sunlight:
No problems expected.

Driving, piloting or hazardous work:
Avoid if lightheaded or dizzy. Otherwise, no problems expected.

Discontinuing:
May be unnecessary to finish medicine. Follow doctor's instructions.

Others:
No problems expected.

POSSIBLE INTERACTION WITH OTHER DRUGS

GENERIC NAME OR DRUG CLASS	COMBINED EFFECT
Allopurinol	Decreased allopurinol effect.
Anticoagulants,* oral	Possible risk of bleeding.
Ephedrine	Increased effect of both drugs.
Epinephrine	Increased effect of both drugs.
Erythromycins*	Increased bronchodilator effect.
Furosemide	Increased furosemide effect.
Lincomycins*	Increased bronchodilator effect.
Lithium	Decreased lithium effect.
Probenecid	Decreased effect of both drugs.
Propranolol	Decreased bronchodilator effect.
Rauwolfia alkaloids*	Rapid heartbeat.
Sulfinpyrazone	Decreased sulfin pyrazone effect.
Troleandomycin	Increased bronchodilator effect.

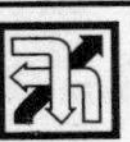

POSSIBLE INTERACTION WITH OTHER SUBSTANCES

INTERACTS WITH	COMBINED EFFECT
Alcohol:	None expected.
Beverages:	
Caffeine drinks.	Nervousness and insomnia.
Other.	You must drink 8 to 10 glasses of fluid per day for drug to work.
Cocaine:	Excess stimulation. Avoid.
Foods:	None expected.
Marijuana:	Slightly increased antiasthmatic effect of bronchodilator.
Tobacco:	Decreased bronchodilator effect and harmful for all conditions requiring bronchodilator treatment. Avoid.

*See Glossary

OXYBUTYNIN

BRAND NAMES

Ditropan

BASIC INFORMATION

Habit forming? No
Prescription needed? Yes
Available as generic? Yes
Drug class: Antispasmodic (urinary tract)

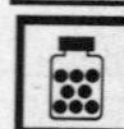

USES

Reduces spasms of urinary bladder and urethra that cause symptoms of frequent urination, urgency, night-time urination and incontinence.

DOSAGE & USAGE INFORMATION

How to take:
Tablets or syrup—Swallow with water.

When to take:
At the same time every day. Do not take with food unless instructed to do so by doctor.

If you forget a dose:
Take as soon as you remember up to 2 hours late. If more than 2 hours, wait for next scheduled dose. Don't double this dose.

What drug does:
Blocks nerve impulses at parasympathetic nerve endings, preventing muscle contractions and gland secretions of organs involved.

Time lapse before drug works:
30 minutes to 1 hour.

Don't take with:
Any other medicine without consulting your doctor or pharmacist.

OVERDOSE

SYMPTOMS:
Unsteadiness, confusion, dizziness, severe drowsiness, fast heartbeat, fever, red face, hallucinations, difficult breathing.
WHAT TO DO:
Overdose unlikely to threaten life. If person takes much larger amount than prescribed, call doctor, poison control center or hospital emergency room for instructions.

POSSIBLE ADVERSE REACTIONS OR SIDE EFFECTS

SYMPTOMS	WHAT TO DO
Life-threatening: In case of overdose, see previous column.	
Common: Constipation; decreased sweating; drowsiness; dryness of mouth, nose and throat.	Continue. Call doctor when convenient.
Infrequent: Difficult swallowing, decreased sexual ability, headache, difficult urination, sensitivity to light, nausea, vomiting, insomnia, tiredness.	Continue. Call doctor when convenient.
Rare: Skin rash, eye pain, blurred vision.	Discontinue. Call doctor right away.

WARNINGS & PRECAUTIONS

Don't take if:

- You are allergic to any anticholinergic.
- You have trouble with stomach bloating.
- You have difficulty emptying your bladder completely.
- You have narrow-angle glaucoma.
- You have severe ulcerative colitis.

Before you start, consult your doctor:

- If you have open-angle glaucoma.
- If you have angina or fast heartbeat.
- If you have chronic bronchitis or asthma.
- If you have hiatal hernia; liver, kidney or thyroid disease; enlarged prostate or myasthenia gravis.
- If you will have surgery within 2 months, including dental surgery, requiring general or spinal anesthesia.

Over age 60:
Adverse reactions and side effects may be more frequent and severe than in younger persons. You may require smaller doses for shorter periods of time.

Pregnancy:
No proven harm to unborn child, but avoid if possible. Consult doctor. Risk category B (see page xxii).

Breast-feeding:
Unknown effect. Consult doctor.

Infants & children:
Not recommended for children under 5.

Prolonged use:
Side effects more likely.

Skin & sunlight:
No special problems expected.

Driving, piloting or hazardous work:
Don't drive or pilot aircraft until you learn how medicine affects you. Don't work around dangerous machinery. Don't climb ladders or work in high places. Danger increases if you drink alcohol or take medicine affecting alertness and reflexes.

Discontinuing:
May be unnecessary to finish medicine. Follow doctor's instructions.

Others:
Advise any doctor or dentist whom you consult that you take this medicine.

POSSIBLE INTERACTION WITH OTHER DRUGS

GENERIC NAME OR DRUG CLASS	COMBINED EFFECT
Anticholinergics*	Increased effect of oxybutynin.
Central nervous system (CNS) depressants*	Increased sedative effect.

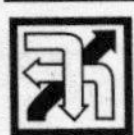

POSSIBLE INTERACTION WITH OTHER SUBSTANCES

INTERACTS WITH	COMBINED EFFECT
Alcohol:	Increased sedative effect.
Beverages:	None expected.
Cocaine:	Excessively rapid heartbeat. Avoid.
Foods:	None expected.
Marijuana:	Drowsiness and dry mouth.
Tobacco:	None expected.

*See Glossary

OXYMETAZOLINE (Nasal)

BRAND NAMES

See complete list of brand names in the *Brand Name Directory*, page 913.

BASIC INFORMATION

Habit forming? No
Prescription needed? No
Available as generic? Yes
Drug class: Sympathomimetic

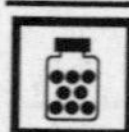

USES

Relieves congestion of nose, sinuses and throat from allergies and infections.

DOSAGE & USAGE INFORMATION

How to take:
Nasal solution, nasal spray—Use as directed on label. Avoid contamination. Don't use same container for more than 1 person.

When to take:
When needed, no more often than every 4 hours.

If you forget a dose:
Take as soon as you remember. Wait 4 hours for next dose.

What drug does:
Constricts walls of small arteries in nose, sinuses and eustachian tubes.

Time lapse before drug works:
5 to 30 minutes.

Continued next column

OVERDOSE

SYMPTOMS:
Headache, sweating, anxiety, agitation, rapid and irregular heartbeat (rare occurrence with systemic absorption).
WHAT TO DO:
- **Dial 911 (emergency) or 0 (operator) for an ambulance or medical help. Then give first aid immediately.**
- **If patient is unconscious and not breathing, give mouth-to-mouth breathing. If there is no heartbeat, use cardiac massage and mouth-to-mouth breathing (CPR). If you can't get help quickly, take patient to nearest emergency facility.**
- **See emergency information on inside covers.**

Don't take with:
- Nonprescription drugs for allergy, cough or cold without consulting doctor.
- Any other medicine without consulting your doctor or pharmacist.

POSSIBLE ADVERSE REACTIONS OR SIDE EFFECTS

SYMPTOMS	WHAT TO DO
Life-threatening: In case of overdose, see previous column.	
Common: None expected.	
Infrequent: Burning, dry or stinging nasal passages.	Continue. Call doctor when convenient.
Rare: Rebound congestion (increased runny or stuffy nose); headache, insomnia, nervousness (may occur with systemic absorption).	Discontinue. Call doctor right away.

WARNINGS & PRECAUTIONS

Don't take if:
You are allergic to any sympathomimetic nasal spray.

Before you start, consult your doctor:
- If you have heart disease or high blood pressure.
- If you have diabetes.
- If you have overactive thyroid.
- If you have taken MAO inhibitors in past 2 weeks.
- If you have glaucoma.

Over age 60:
Adverse reactions and side effects may be more frequent and severe than in younger persons.

Pregnancy:
Consult doctor. Risk category C (see page xxii).

Breast-feeding:
No proven problems. Consult doctor.

Infants & children:
Don't give to children younger than 2.

Prolonged use:
Drug may lose effectiveness, cause increased congestion (rebound effect*) and irritate nasal membranes.

Skin & sunlight:
No problems expected.

Driving, piloting or hazardous work:
No problems expected.

Discontinuing:
May be unnecessary to finish medicine. Follow doctor's instructions.

Others:
No problems expected.

POSSIBLE INTERACTION WITH OTHER DRUGS

GENERIC NAME OR DRUG CLASS	COMBINED EFFECT
Antidepressants, tricyclic*	Possible rise in blood pressure.
Butorphanol	Delays start of butorphanol effect.
Maprotiline	Possible increased blood pressure.

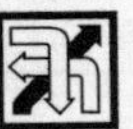

POSSIBLE INTERACTION WITH OTHER SUBSTANCES

INTERACTS WITH	COMBINED EFFECT
Alcohol:	None expected.
Beverages: Caffeine drinks.	Nervousness or insomnia.
Cocaine:	High risk of heart-beat irregularities and high blood pressure.
Foods:	None expected.
Marijuana:	Overstimulation. Avoid.
Tobacco:	None expected.

*See Glossary

PACLITAXEL

BRAND NAMES

Taxol

BASIC INFORMATION

Habit forming? No
Prescription needed? Yes
Available as generic? No
Drug class: Antineoplastic

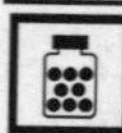

USES

Treats ovarian cancer, breast cancer and some lung cancers.

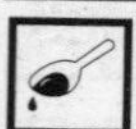

DOSAGE & USAGE INFORMATION

How to take:
Injection–Administered only by a doctor or under the supervision of a doctor.

When to take:
Your doctor will determine the schedule. Usually the drug is infused over a 24-hour period at 21-day intervals. Other drugs may be given prior to paclitaxel injection to help prevent adverse effects.

If you forget a dose:
Not a concern since drug is administered by a doctor.

What drug does:
Interferes with the growth of cancer cells, which are eventually destroyed.

Time lapse before drug works:
Results may not show for several weeks or months.

Don't take with:
- Any other prescription or nonprescription drug without consulting your doctor.
- See Interaction column and consult doctor.

OVERDOSE

SYMPTOMS:
None expected.
WHAT TO DO:
Overdose is unlikely. You will be monitored by medical personnel during the time of the infusion.

POSSIBLE ADVERSE REACTIONS OR SIDE EFFECTS

SYMPTOMS	WHAT TO DO
Life-threatening:	
Anaphylactic reaction soon after an injection (hives, rash, intense itching, faintness, breathing difficulty).	Emergency care will be provided.
Common:	
• Paleness, tiredness, flushing of face, skin rash or itching, shortness of breath, fever, chills, cough or hoarseness, back or side pain, difficult or painful urination, unusual bleeding or bruising, black or tarry stools, blood in stool or urine, pinpoint red spots on skin, bleeding gums, delayed wound healing.	Call doctor right away.
• Pain in joints or muscles; diarrhea; nausea and vomiting; numbness, burning or tingling in hands or feet.	Call doctor when convenient.
• Loss of hair (should regrow after treatment completed).	No action necessary.
Infrequent:	
Heart rhythm disturbances, chest pain.	Call doctor right away.
Rare:	
Pain or redness at injection site, mouth or lip sores.	Call doctor right away.

WARNINGS & PRECAUTIONS

Don't take if:
You are allergic to paclitaxel.

Before you start, consult your doctor:
- If you have an infection or any other medical problem.
- If you have or recently had chickenpox or herpes zoster (shingles).
- If you have heart problems.
- If you are pregnant or if you plan to become pregnant.
- If you have had radiation therapy or previously taken anticancer drugs.

Over age 60:
No problems expected.

Pregnancy:
Animal studies show fetal abnormalities and increased risk of abortion. Discuss with your doctor whether drug benefits justify risk to unborn child. Risk category D (see page xxii).

Breast-feeding:
Not known if drug passes into milk. Avoid drug or discontinue nursing until you finish medicine. Consult doctor for advice on maintaining milk supply.

Infants & children:
Safety and effectiveness of use in children not established.

Prolonged use:
Not recommended for long-term use.

Skin & sunlight:
No problems expected.

Driving, piloting or hazardous work:
Avoid if you feel side effects such as nausea and vomiting.

Discontinuing:
Your doctor will determine the schedule.

Others:
- Advise any doctor or dentist whom you consult that you take this medicine.
- May affect the results in some medical tests.
- Do not have any immunizations (vaccinations) without doctor's approval. Other household members should not take oral polio vaccine. It could pass the polio virus on to you. Avoid any contact with persons who have taken oral polio vaccine.
- Possible delayed effects (including some types of cancers) may occur months to years after use. Your doctor should discuss with you all risks involving this drug.
- You will have increased risk of infections. Take extra precautions (handwashing), and avoid people with infections. Avoid crowds if possible. Contact your doctor immediately if you develop signs or symptoms of infection.
- Use care in the use of toothbrushes, dental floss and toothpicks. Talk to your medical doctor before you have dental work done.
- Do not touch your eyes or the inside of your nose without carefully washing your hands first.
- Avoid activities (e.g., contact sports) that could cause bruising or injury.
- Avoid cutting yourself when using a safety razor, fingernail or toenail clippers.

POSSIBLE INTERACTION WITH OTHER DRUGS

GENERIC NAME OR DRUG CLASS	COMBINED EFFECT
Blood dyscrasia-causing medicines*	Increased risk of paclitaxel toxicity.
Bone marrow depressants,* (other)	Increased risk of paclitaxel toxicity.

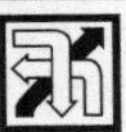

POSSIBLE INTERACTION WITH OTHER SUBSTANCES

INTERACTS WITH	COMBINED EFFECT
Alcohol:	None expected.
Beverages:	None expected.
Cocaine:	None expected.
Foods:	None expected.
Marijuana:	None expected.
Tobacco:	None expected.

*See Glossary

PANCREATIN, PEPSIN, BILE SALTS, HYOSCYAMINE, ATROPINE, SCOPOLAMINE & PHENOBARBITAL

BRAND NAMES

Donnazyme

BASIC INFORMATION

Habit forming? Yes
Prescription needed? Yes
Available as generic? No
Drug class: Digestant, sedative, anticholinergic

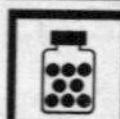

USES

- Replaces deficient digestive enzymes.
- Sometimes used to relieve indigestion.

DOSAGE & USAGE INFORMATION

How to take:
Tablet—Swallow with liquid or food to lessen stomach irritation. If you can't swallow whole, crumble tablet and take with food or liquid.

When to take:
With or after meals.

If you forget a dose:
Skip it and resume schedule. Don't double dose.

What drug does:
Blocks nerve impulses at parasympathetic nerve endings, preventing smooth muscle contraction and gland secretions.

Time lapse before drug works:
30 to 60 minutes.

Continued next column

OVERDOSE

SYMPTOMS:
Hallucinations, excitement, breathing difficulty, irregular heartbeat (too fast or too slow), fainting, collapse, coma.
WHAT TO DO:
- **Dial 911 (emergency) or 0 (operator) for an ambulance or medical help. Then give first aid immediately.**
- **See emergency information on inside covers.**

Don't take with:
- Any medicine that will decrease mental alertness or reflexes, such as alcohol, other mind-altering drugs, cough/cold medicines, antihistamines, allergy medicine, sedatives, tranquilizers (sleeping pills or "downers"), barbiturates, seizure medicine, narcotics, other prescription medicine for pain, muscle relaxants, anesthetics.
- See Interaction column and consult doctor.

POSSIBLE ADVERSE REACTIONS OR SIDE EFFECTS

SYMPTOMS	WHAT TO DO
Life-threatening: In case of overdose, see previous column.	
Common:	
• Constipation, decreased sweating, headache.	Discontinue. Call doctor right away.
• Drowsiness, dry mouth, frequent urination.	Continue. Call doctor when convenient.
Infrequent:	
• Blurred vision.	Discontinue. Call doctor right away.
• Diminished sex drive, swallowing difficulty, sensitivity to light, insomnia.	Continue. Call doctor when convenient.
Rare:	
• Jaundice; unusual bleeding or bruising; swollen feet and ankles; abdominal pain; sore throat, fever, mouth sores; rash; hives; vomiting; joint pain; eye pain; diarrhea; blood in urine.	Discontinue. Call doctor right away.
• Unusual tiredness.	Continue. Call doctor when convenient.

WARNINGS & PRECAUTIONS

Don't take if:
- You are allergic to any of the drugs in this combination.
- You have trouble with stomach bloating, difficulty emptying your bladder completely, narrow-angle glaucoma, severe ulcerative colitis, porphyria.

PANCREATIN, PEPSIN, BILE SALTS, HYOSCYAMINE, ATROPINE, SCOPOLAMINE & PHENOBARBITAL

Before you start, consult your doctor:
- If you have open-angle glaucoma, angina, chronic bronchitis or asthma, liver disease, hiatal hernia, enlarged prostate, myasthenia gravis, epilepsy, kidney or liver damage, anemia, chronic pain.
- If you will have surgery within 2 months, including dental surgery, requiring general or spinal anesthesia.

Over age 60:
Adverse reactions and side effects may be more frequent and severe than in younger persons

Pregnancy:
Decide with your doctor if drug benefits justify risk to unborn child. Risk category C (see page xxii).

Breast-feeding:
Drug passes into milk. Avoid drug or discontinue nursing until you finish medicine. Consult doctor for advice on maintaining milk supply.

Infants & children:
Use only under medical supervision.

Prolonged use:
- Chronic constipation, possible fecal impaction.
- May cause addiction, anemia, chronic intoxication.
- May lower body temperature, making exposure to cold temperatures hazardous.

Skin & sunlight:
May cause rash or intensify sunburn in areas exposed to sun or sunlamp.

Driving, piloting or hazardous work:
Don't drive or pilot aircraft until you learn how medicine affects you. Don't work around dangerous machinery. Don't climb ladders or work in high places. Danger increases if you drink alcohol or take medicine affecting alertness and reflexes, such as antihistamines, tranquilizers, sedatives, pain medicine, narcotics and mind-altering drugs.

Discontinuing:
- May be unnecessary to finish medicine. Follow doctor's instructions.
- If you develop withdrawal symptoms of hallucinations, agitation or sleeplessness after discontinuing, call doctor right away.

Others:
- Potential for abuse.
- Enzyme deficiencies probably better treated with identified separate substances rather than a mixture of components.

POSSIBLE INTERACTION WITH OTHER DRUGS

GENERIC NAME OR DRUG CLASS	COMBINED EFFECT
Amantadine	Increased atropine effect.
Antacids*	Decreased absorption of scopolamine.
Anticholinergics*, other	Increased anticholinergic effect.
Anticoagulants*, oral	Decreased anticoagulant effect.
Antidepressants, tricyclic*	Decreased antidepressant effect. Possible dangerous oversedation.
Antidiabetics*, oral	Increased phenobartital effect.
Antihistamines*	Increased atropine effect.
Anti-inflammatory drugs, nonsteroidal (NSAIDs)*	Decreased anti-inflammatory effects.
Aspirin	Decreased aspirin effect.

Continued on page 952

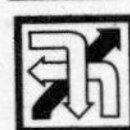

POSSIBLE INTERACTION WITH OTHER SUBSTANCES

INTERACTS WITH	COMBINED EFFECT
Alcohol:	Possible fatal oversedation. Avoid.
Beverages:	None expected.
Cocaine:	Excessively rapid heartbeat. Avoid.
Foods:	None expected.
Marijuana:	Excessive sedation, drowsiness and dry mouth.
Tobacco:	May increase stomach acidity, decreasing the effectiveness of the drug. Avoid.

***See Glossary**

PANCRELIPASE

BRAND NAMES

Cotazym
Cotazym E.C.S.
Cotazym-S
Cotazym-65B
Enzymase-16
Ilozyme
Ku-Zyme HP
Lipancreatin
Pancoate
Pancrease
Pancrease MT4
Pancrease MT10
Pancrease MT16
Protilase
Ultrase MT 12
Ultrase MT 20
Ultrase MT 24
Viokase
Zymase

BASIC INFORMATION

Habit forming? No
Prescription needed? Yes
Available as generic? Yes
Drug class: Enzyme (pancreatic)

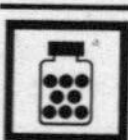

USES

- Replaces pancreatic enzyme lost due to surgery or disease.
- Treats fatty stools (steatorrhea).

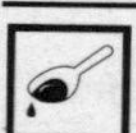

DOSAGE & USAGE INFORMATION

How to take:
- Tablets, capsules or delayed-release capsules—Swallow whole. Do not take with milk or milk products.
- Powder—Sprinkle on liquid or soft food.

When to take:
Before meals.

If you forget a dose:
Take as soon as you remember up to 2 hours late. If more than 2 hours, wait for next scheduled dose (don't double this dose).

What drug does:
Enhances digestion of proteins, carbohydrates and fats.

Time lapse before drug works:
30 minutes.

Don't take with:
Any other medicine without consulting your doctor or pharmacist.

OVERDOSE

SYMPTOMS:
Shortness of breath, wheezing, diarrhea.
WHAT TO DO:
Overdose unlikely to threaten life. If person takes much larger amount than prescribed, call doctor, poison control center or hospital emergency room for instructions.

POSSIBLE ADVERSE REACTIONS OR SIDE EFFECTS

SYMPTOMS	WHAT TO DO
Life-threatening: None expected.	
Common: None expected.	
Infrequent: Diarrhea, asthma.	Discontinue. Call doctor right away.
Rare: • Rash, hives, blood in urine, swollen feet or legs, abdominal cramps.	Discontinue. Call doctor right away.
• Nausea, joint pain.	Continue. Call doctor when convenient.

WARNINGS & PRECAUTIONS

Don't take if:
You are allergic to pancreatin, pancrelipase, or pork.

Before you start, consult your doctor:
If you take any other medicines.

Over age 60:
Adverse reactions and side effects may be more frequent and severe than in younger persons.

Pregnancy:
Decide with your doctor if drug benefits justify risk to unborn child. Risk category C (see page xxii).

Breast-feeding:
Drug may pass into milk. Avoid drug or discontinue nursing until you finish medicine. Consult doctor for advice on maintaining milk supply.

Infants & children:
Give under close medical supervision only.

Prolonged use:
No additional problems expected.

Skin & sunlight:
No problems expected.

Driving, piloting or hazardous work:
No problems expected.

Discontinuing:
Don't discontinue without consulting doctor. Dose may require gradual reduction if you have taken drug for a long time. Doses of other drugs may also require adjustment.

Others:
If you take powder form, avoid inhaling.

POSSIBLE INTERACTION WITH OTHER DRUGS

GENERIC NAME OR DRUG CLASS	COMBINED EFFECT
Calcium carbonate antacids*	Decreased effect of pancrelipase.
Iron supplements	Decreased iron absorption.
Magnesium hydroxide antacids*	Decreased effect of pancrelipase.

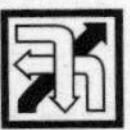

POSSIBLE INTERACTION WITH OTHER SUBSTANCES

INTERACTS WITH	COMBINED EFFECT
Alcohol:	Unknown.
Beverages: Milk.	Decreased effect of pancrelipase.
Cocaine:	Unknown.
Foods: Ice cream, milk products.	Decreased effect of pancrelipase.
Marijuana:	Decreased absorption of pancrelipase.
Tobacco:	Decreased absorption of pancrelipase.

PANTOTHENIC ACID (Vitamin B-5)

BRAND AND GENERIC NAMES

CALCIUM PANTOTHENATE
Dexol T.D.

An ingredient in numerous multiple vitamin-mineral supplements. Check labels.

BASIC INFORMATION

Habit forming? No
Prescription needed? No
Available as generic? Yes
Drug class: Vitamin supplement

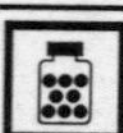

USES

Prevents and treats vitamin B-5 deficiency.

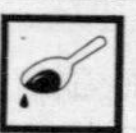

DOSAGE & USAGE INFORMATION

How to take:
Tablet—Swallow with liquid.

When to take:
At the same times each day.

If you forget a dose:
Take as soon as you remember, then resume regular schedule.

What drug does:
Acts as co-enzyme in carbohydrate, protein and fat metabolism.

Time lapse before drug works:
15 to 20 minutes.

Don't take with:
- Levodopa—Small amounts of pantothenic acid will nullify levodopa effect. Carbidopa-levodopa combination not affected by this interaction.
- Any other medicine without consulting your doctor or pharmacist.

OVERDOSE

SYMPTOMS:
None expected.
WHAT TO DO:
Overdose unlikely to threaten life.

POSSIBLE ADVERSE REACTIONS OR SIDE EFFECTS

SYMPTOMS	WHAT TO DO
Life-threatening: None expected.	
Common: Heartburn.	Discontinue. Seek emergency treatment.
Infrequent: Cramps.	Discontinue Call doctor right away.
Rare: Rash, hives, difficult breathing.	Discontinue. Seek emergency treatment.

PANTOTHENIC ACID (Vitamin B-5)

WARNINGS & PRECAUTIONS

Don't take if:
You are allergic to pantothenic acid.

Before you start, consult your doctor:
If you have hemophilia.

Over age 60:
No problems expected.

Pregnancy:
Risk factor not designated. See category list on page xxii and consult doctor.

Breast-feeding:
Don't exceed recommended dose. Consult doctor.

Infants & children:
Don't exceed recommended dose.

Prolonged use:
Large doses for more than 1 month may cause toxicity.

Skin & sunlight:
No problems expected.

Driving, piloting or hazardous work:
No problems expected.

Discontinuing:
No problems expected.

Others:
Regular pantothenic acid supplements are recommended if you take chloramphenicol, cycloserine, ethionamide, hydralazine, immunosuppressants*, isoniazid or penicillamine. These decrease pantothenic acid absorption and can cause anemia or tingling and numbness in hands and feet.

POSSIBLE INTERACTION WITH OTHER DRUGS

GENERIC NAME OR DRUG CLASS	COMBINED EFFECT
None significant.	

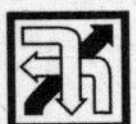

POSSIBLE INTERACTION WITH OTHER SUBSTANCES

INTERACTS WITH	COMBINED EFFECT
Alcohol:	None expected.
Beverages:	None expected.
Cocaine:	None expected.
Foods:	None expected.
Marijuana:	None expected.
Tobacco:	May decrease pantothenic acid absorption. Decreased pantothenic acid effect.

***See Glossary**

PAPAVERINE

BRAND NAMES

Cerespan
Genabid
Pavabid
Pavabid Plateau Caps
Pavacot
Pavagen
Pavarine
Pavased
Pavatine
Pavatym
Paverolan

BASIC INFORMATION

Habit forming? No
Prescription needed? Yes
Available as generic? Yes
Drug class: Vasodilator

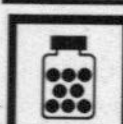

USES

- May improve circulation in the extremities or brain.
- Injected into penis to produce erections.

DOSAGE & USAGE INFORMATION

How to take:
- Tablet—Swallow with liquid or food to lessen stomach irritation. If you can't swallow whole, crumble tablet and take with liquid or food.
- Extended-release capsules—Swallow whole with liquid.
- Injections to penis—Follow doctor's instructions.

When to take:
At the same times each day.

If you forget a dose:
Take as soon as you remember up to 2 hours late. If more than 2 hours, wait for next scheduled dose (don't double this dose).

What drug does:
Relaxes and expands blood vessel walls, allowing better distribution of oxygen and nutrients.

Time lapse before drug works:
30 to 60 minutes.

Continued next column

OVERDOSE

SYMPTOMS:
Weakness, fainting, flush, sweating, stupor, irregular heartbeat.
WHAT TO DO:
- **Dial 911 (emergency) or 0 (operator) for an ambulance or medical help. Then give first aid immediately.**
- **See emergency information on inside covers.**

Don't take with:
- Nonprescription drugs without consulting doctor.
- Any other medicine without consulting your doctor or pharmacist.

POSSIBLE ADVERSE REACTIONS OR SIDE EFFECTS

SYMPTOMS	WHAT TO DO
Life-threatening: None expected.	
Common:	
• Drowsiness, dizziness, headache, flushed face, stomach irritation, indigestion, nausea, mild constipation.	Continue. Call doctor when convenient.
• Dry mouth, throat.	Continue. Tell doctor at next visit.
Infrequent: Rash, itchy skin, blurred or double vision, weakness, fast heartbeat.	Discontinue. Call doctor right away.
Rare: Jaundice.	Discontinue. Call doctor right away.

WARNINGS & PRECAUTIONS

Don't take if:
You are allergic to papaverine.

Before you start, consult your doctor:
- If you plan to become pregnant within medication period.
- If you have had a heart attack, heart disease, angina or stroke.
- If you have Parkinson's disease.

Over age 60:
Adverse reactions and side effects may be more frequent and severe than in younger persons.

Pregnancy:
Decide with your doctor if drug benefits justify risk to unborn child. Risk category C (see page xxii).

Breast-feeding:
Drug may filter into milk. May harm child. Avoid.

Infants & children:
Not recommended.

Prolonged use:
No problems expected.

Skin & sunlight:
No problems expected.

Driving, piloting or hazardous work:
Don't drive or pilot aircraft until you learn how medicine affects you. Don't work around dangerous machinery. Don't climb ladders or work in high places. Danger increases if you drink alcohol or take medicine affecting alertness and reflexes, such as antihistamines, tranquilizers, sedatives, pain medicine, narcotics and mind-altering drugs.

Discontinuing:
May be unnecessary to finish medicine. If drug does not help in 1 to 2 weeks, consult doctor about discontinuing.

Others:
- Periodic liver function tests recommended.
- Internal eye pressure measurements recommended if you have glaucoma.

POSSIBLE INTERACTION WITH OTHER DRUGS

GENERIC NAME OR DRUG CLASS	COMBINED EFFECT
Levodopa	Decreased levodopa effect.
Narcotics*	Increased sedation.
Pain relievers*	Increased sedation.
Pergolide	Decreased pergolide effect.
Sedatives*	Increased sedation.
Sympathomimetics*	Reversal of the effect of papaverine.
Tranquilizers*	Increased sedation.

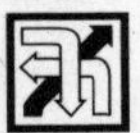

POSSIBLE INTERACTION WITH OTHER SUBSTANCES

INTERACTS WITH	COMBINED EFFECT
Alcohol:	None expected.
Beverages:	None expected.
Cocaine:	Decreased papaverine effect.
Foods:	None expected.
Marijuana:	None expected.
Tobacco:	Decrease in papaverine's dilation of blood vessels.

*See Glossary

PARALDEHYDE

BRAND NAMES

Paral

BASIC INFORMATION

Habit forming? Yes
Prescription needed? Yes
Available as generic? Yes
Drug class: Anticonvulsant

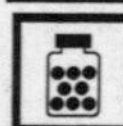

USES

- Treats convulsions.
- Treats toxic symptoms caused by drugs that may produce convulsions.

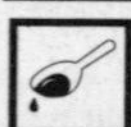

DOSAGE & USAGE INFORMATION

How to take:
- Follow doctor's instructions.
- May be given orally, rectally or by injection into a muscle.

When to take:
Follow doctor's instructions.

If you forget a dose:
Take as soon as you remember up to 2 hours late. If more than 2 hours, wait for next scheduled dose (don't double this dose).

What drug does:
Depresses central nervous system.

Time lapse before drug works:
- Oral—30 minutes to 1 hour.
- Rectal—2 to 3 hours.

Don't take with:
Any other medicines (including over-the-counter drugs such as cough and cold medicines, laxatives, antacids, diet pills, caffeine, nose drops or vitamins) without consulting your doctor.

OVERDOSE

SYMPTOMS:
Decreased urination, breathing difficulty, confusion, slow heartbeat, weakness.
WHAT TO DO:
- **Dial 911 (emergency) or 0 (operator) for an ambulance or medical help. Then give first aid immediately.**
- **See emergency information on inside covers.**

POSSIBLE ADVERSE REACTIONS OR SIDE EFFECTS

SYMPTOMS	WHAT TO DO
Life-threatening:	
In case of overdose, see previous column.	
Common:	
• Skin rash, jaundice (yellow skin and eyes).	Discontinue. Call doctor right away.
• Drowsiness, nausea, halitosis.	Continue. Call doctor when convenient.
Infrequent:	
Clumsiness, dizziness, headache.	Continue. Call doctor when convenient.
Rare:	
Abdominal cramps.	Continue. Call doctor when convenient.

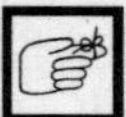

WARNINGS & PRECAUTIONS

Don't take if:
You know you are allergic to paraldehyde.

Before you start, consult your doctor:
- If you have chronic lung disease.
- If you have history of drug abuse.
- If you have liver disease.
- If you have peptic ulcer.
- If you have colitis.

Over age 60:
No special problems expected.

Pregnancy:
Decide with your doctor if drug benefits justify risk to unborn child. Risk category C (see page xxii).

Breast-feeding:
Effect not documented. Consult your doctor.

Infants & children:
No special problems expected.

Prolonged use:
- May be habit forming.
- Talk to your doctor about the need for follow-up medical examinations or laboratory studies to check liver function.

Skin & sunlight:
No problems expected.

Driving, piloting or hazardous work:
Avoid if you feel confused, drowsy or dizzy.

Discontinuing:
May develop withdrawal symptoms, such as: convulsions, hallucinations, sweating, muscle cramps, nausea or vomiting, trembling. If you experience any of these, notify your doctor right away.

Others:
- Advise any doctor or dentist whom you consult that you take this medicine.
- May affect results in some medical tests.
- Strong odor of paraldehyde on breath lasts for 24 hours.

POSSIBLE INTERACTION WITH OTHER DRUGS

GENERIC NAME OR DRUG CLASS	COMBINED EFFECT
Addictive drugs*	Increased risk of addiction.
Central nervous system (CNS) depressants*, other	Possible oversedation. Avoid simultaneous use.
Disulfiram	Increased paraldehyde effect. Avoid simultaneous use.
Sertraline	Increased depressive effects of both drugs.

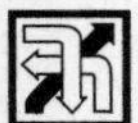

POSSIBLE INTERACTION WITH OTHER SUBSTANCES

INTERACTS WITH	COMBINED EFFECT
Alcohol:	Dangerous sedation. Avoid.
Beverages:	No special problems expected.
Cocaine:	No special problems expected.
Foods:	No special problems expected.
Marijuana:	No special problems expected.
Tobacco:	No special problems expected.

*See Glossary

PARAMETHASONE

BRAND NAMES

Haldrone

BASIC INFORMATION

Habit forming? No
Prescription needed? Yes
Available as generic? No
Drug class: Cortisone drug (adrenal corticosteroid)

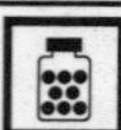

USES

- Reduces inflammation caused by many different medical problems.
- Treats some allergic diseases, blood disorders, kidney diseases, asthma and emphysema.
- Replaces corticosteroid deficiencies.

DOSAGE & USAGE INFORMATION

How to take:
Tablet—Swallow with liquid or food to lessen stomach irritation. If you can't swallow whole, crumble tablet and take with liquid or food.

When to take:
At the same times each day. Take once-a-day or once-every-other-day doses in mornings.

If you forget a dose:
- Several-doses-per-day prescription—Take as soon as you remember up to 2 hours late. If more than 2 hours, wait for next scheduled dose (don't double this dose).
- Once-a-day dose or less—Wait for next dose. Double this dose.

What drug does:
Decreases inflammatory responses.

Time lapse before drug works:
2 to 4 days.

Don't take with:
Any other medicine without consulting your doctor or pharmacist.

OVERDOSE

SYMPTOMS:
Headache, convulsions, heart failure.
WHAT TO DO:
- **Dial 911 (emergency) or 0 (operator) for an ambulance or medical help. Then give first aid immediately.**
- **Read additional emergency information on inside covers.**

POSSIBLE ADVERSE REACTIONS OR SIDE EFFECTS

SYMPTOMS	WHAT TO DO
Life-threatening:	
Rash, hives, intense itching, faintness soon after a dose (anaphylaxis).	Seek emergency treatment immediately.
Common:	
Acne, poor wound healing, indigestion, nausea, vomiting, thirst, constipation, gaseousness, unpleasant taste, diarrhea, headache, cough, dizziness, hoarseness, appetite gain or loss.	Continue. Call doctor when convenient.
Infrequent:	
• Black, bloody or tarry stool; various infections; swallowing difficulties.	Discontinue. Seek emergency treatment.
• Blurred vision, halos around lights, sore throat, fever, muscle cramps.	Discontinue. Call doctor right away.
• Mood change, fatigue, frequent urination, weight gain, round face, weakness, irregular menstrual periods, insomnia, restlessness, dry mouth, euphoria, nose bleeds.	Continue. Call doctor when convenient.
Rare:	
• Irregular heartbeat.	Discontinue. Seek emergency treatment.
• Rash, pancreatitis, numbness or tingling in hands or feet, thrombophlebitis, hallucinations, convulsions.	Discontinue. Call doctor right away.

WARNINGS & PRECAUTIONS

Don't take if:
- You are allergic to any cortisone drug.
- You have tuberculosis or fungus infection.
- You have herpes infection of eyes, lips or genitals.
- You have bone disease, thyroid disease, colitis, peptic ulcer, diabetes, myasthenia gravis, liver or kidney disease, diverticulitis, glaucoma, heart disease.

Before you start, consult your doctor:
- If you have had tuberculosis.
- If you have congestive heart failure, diabetes, peptic ulcer, glaucoma, underactive thyroid, high blood pressure, myasthenia gravis.
- If you have blood clots in legs or lungs.

Over age 60:
Adverse reactions and side effects may be more frequent and severe than in younger persons. Likely to aggravate edema, diabetes or ulcers. Likely to cause cataracts and osteoporosis (softening of the bones).

Pregnancy:
Decide with your doctor if drug benefits justify risk to unborn child. Risk category C (see page xxii).

Breast-feeding:
Drug passes into milk. Avoid drug or discontinue nursing until you finish medicine. Consult doctor for advice on maintaining milk supply.

Infants & children:
Use only under medical supervision.

Prolonged use:
- Retards growth in children.
- Possible glaucoma, cataracts, diabetes, fragile bones and thin skin.
- Functional dependence.
- Talk to your doctor about the need for follow-up medical examinations or laboratory studies to check blood pressure, serum electrolytes, stools for blood.

Skin & sunlight:
No problems expected.

Driving, piloting or hazardous work:
No problems expected.

Discontinuing:
- Don't discontinue without doctor's advice until you complete prescribed dose, even though symptoms diminish or disappear.
- Drug affects your response to surgery, illness, injury or stress for 2 years after discontinuing. Tell anyone who takes medical care of you within 2 years about drug.

Others:
- Avoid immunizations if possible.
- Your resistance to infection is less while taking this medicine.
- Advise any doctor or dentist whom you consult that you take this medicine.
- Those who have inactive or "cured" tuberculosis may be subjected to a possible recurrence of active tuberculosis.
- Children who must take cortisone drugs may grow less well.

POSSIBLE INTERACTION WITH OTHER DRUGS

GENERIC NAME OR DRUG CLASS	COMBINED EFFECT
Amphotericin B	Potassium depletion.
Anticholinergics*	Possible glaucoma.
Anticoagulants*, oral	Decreased anticoagulant effect.
Anticonvulsants*, hydantoin	Decreased paramethasone effect.
Antidiabetics*, oral	Decreased antidiabetic effect.
Antihistamines*	Decreased paramethasone effect.
Anti-inflammatory drugs, nonsteroidal (NSAIDs)*	Increased risk of ulcers and paramethasone effect.
Aspirin	Increased paramethasone effect.
Attenuated virus vaccines*	Possible viral infection.
Barbiturates*	Decreased paramethasone effect. Oversedation.
Chloral hydrate	Decreased paramethasone effect.
Chlorthalidone	Potassium depletion.
Cholestyramine	Decreased paramethasone absorption.
Cholinergics*	Decreased cholinergic effect.

Continued on page 953

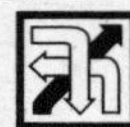

POSSIBLE INTERACTION WITH OTHER SUBSTANCES

INTERACTS WITH	COMBINED EFFECT
Alcohol:	Risk of stomach ulcers.
Beverages:	No proven problems.
Cocaine:	Overstimulation. Avoid.
Foods:	No proven problems.
Marijuana:	Decreased immunity.
Tobacco:	Increased paramethasone effect. Possible toxicity.

PARAGORIC

BRAND NAMES

Brown Mixture
Camphorated Opium Tincture
Laudanum
Opium Tincture

BASIC INFORMATION

Habit forming? Yes
Prescription needed? Yes
Available as generic? Yes
Drug class: Narcotic, antidiarrheal

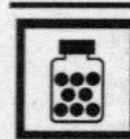

USES

Reduces intestinal cramps and diarrhea.

DOSAGE & USAGE INFORMATION

How to take:
Drops or liquid—Dilute dose in beverage before swallowing.

When to take:
As needed for diarrhea, no more often than every 4 hours.

If you forget a dose:
Take as soon as you remember. Wait 4 hours for next dose.

What drug does:
Anesthetizes surface membranes of intestines and blocks nerve impulses.

Time lapse before drug works:
2 to 6 hours.

Don't take with:
Any other medicine without consulting your doctor or pharmacist.

OVERDOSE

SYMPTOMS:
Deep sleep; slow breathing; slow pulse; flushed, warm skin; constricted pupils.
WHAT TO DO:

- **Dial 911 (emergency) or 0 (operator) for an ambulance or medical help. Then give first aid immediately.**
- **If patient is unconscious and not breathing, give mouth-to-mouth breathing. If there is no heartbeat, use cardiac massage and mouth-to-mouth breathing (CPR). Don't try to make patient vomit. If you can't get help quickly, take patient to nearest emergency facility.**
- **See emergency information on inside covers.**

POSSIBLE ADVERSE REACTIONS OR SIDE EFFECTS

SYMPTOMS	WHAT TO DO
Life-threatening: In case of overdose, see previous column.	
Common: Dizziness, flushed face, unusual tiredness, difficult urination.	Continue. Call doctor when convenient.
Infrequent: Severe constipation, abdominal pain, vomiting.	Discontinue. Call doctor right away.
Rare: • Hives, rash, itchy skin, slow heartbeat, irregular breathing.	Discontinue. Call doctor right away.
• Depression.	Continue. Call doctor when convenient.

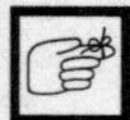

WARNINGS & PRECAUTIONS

Don't take if:
You are allergic to any narcotic*.

Before you start, consult your doctor:
If you have impaired liver or kidney function.

Over age 60:
More likely to be drowsy, dizzy, unsteady or constipated.

Pregnancy:
Risk factor varies with length of pregnancy. See category list on page xxii and consult doctor.

Breast-feeding:
Drug filters into milk. May depress infant. Avoid.

Infants & children:
Use only under medical supervision.

Prolonged use:
Causes psychological and physical dependence.

Skin & sunlight:
No problems expected.

Driving, piloting or hazardous work:
Don't drive or pilot aircraft until you learn how medicine affects you. Don't work around dangerous machinery. Don't climb ladders or work in high places. Danger increases if you drink alcohol or take medicine affecting alertness and reflexes, such as antihistamines, tranquilizers, sedatives, pain medicine, narcotics and mind-altering drugs.

Discontinuing:
May be unnecessary to finish medicine. Follow doctor's instructions.

Others:
Great potential for abuse.

POSSIBLE INTERACTION WITH OTHER DRUGS

GENERIC NAME OR DRUG CLASS	COMBINED EFFECT
Analgesics*	Increased analgesic effect.
Anticholinergics*	Increased risk of constipation.
Antidepressants*	Increased sedation.
Antidiarrheal preparations*	Increased sedative effect. Avoid.
Antihistamines*	Increased sedation.
Central nervous system (CNS) depressants*	Increased central nerve system depression.
Naloxone	Decreased paregoric effect.
Naltrexone	Decreased paregoric effect.
Narcotics*, other	Increased narcotic effect.

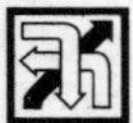

POSSIBLE INTERACTION WITH OTHER SUBSTANCES

INTERACTS WITH	COMBINED EFFECT
Alcohol:	Increases alcohol's intoxicating effect. Avoid.
Beverages:	None expected.
Cocaine:	None expected.
Foods:	None expected.
Marijuana:	Impairs physical and mental performance.
Tobacco:	None expected.

*See Glossary

PARAXETINE

BRAND NAMES

Paxil

BASIC INFORMATION

Habit forming? No
Prescription needed? Yes
Available as generic? No
Drug class: Antidepressant

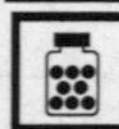

USES

Treats mental depression.

DOSAGE & USAGE INFORMATION

How to take:
Tablet–Swallow with liquid. May be taken with food to lessen gastric irritation.

When to take:
At the same time each day, usually in the morning.

If you forget a dose:
Take as soon as you remember up to 2 hours late. If more than 2 hours, wait for next scheduled dose (don't double this dose).

What drug does:
Helps brain maintain normal levels of serotonin, a chemical necessary for transmission of nerve impulses.

Time lapse before drug works:
1 to 4 weeks.

Don't take with:
- Any other prescription or nonprescription drug without consulting your doctor.
- See Interaction column and consult doctor.

OVERDOSE

SYMPTOMS:
Vomiting, severe drowsiness, heart rhythm disturbances, dilated pupils, severe mouth dryness.
WHAT TO DO:
- **Dial 911 (emergency) or 0 (operator) for an ambulance or medical help. Then give first aid immediately.**
- **See emergency information on inside covers.**

POSSIBLE ADVERSE REACTIONS OR SIDE EFFECTS

SYMPTOMS	WHAT TO DO
Life-threatening: In case of overdose, see previous column.	
Common: Weakness, sweating, nausea, sleepiness, dry mouth, dizziness, insomnia, tremor, male ejaculatory problems, male genital disorders, constipation, diarrhea, problems in urinating, vomiting.	Continue. Call doctor when convenient.
Infrequent: Anxiety, nervousness, decreased or increased appetite, decreased libido, heart palpitations, taste changes, weight loss or gain.	Continue. Call doctor when convenient.
Rare: Blurred vision.	Discontinue. Call doctor right away.

WARNINGS & PRECAUTIONS

Don't take if:

- You are allergic to paroxetine.
- You currently take (or have taken in the last 2 weeks) a monoamine oxidase (MAO) inhibitor*.

Before you start, consult your doctor:

- If you have a history of seizure disorders.
- If you have thoughts of suicide.
- If you have kidney or liver disease.
- If you have a history of drug abuse or mania.

Over age 60:
Adverse reactions and side effects may be more frequent and severe than in younger persons. You may need smaller dosages for shorter periods of time.

Pregnancy:
Consult doctor. Risk category B (see page xxii).

Breast-feeding:
Drug passes into milk. Avoid drug or discontinue nursing until you finish medicine. Consult doctor for advice on maintaining milk supply.

Infants & children:
Safety and effectiveness not yet determined.

Prolonged use:
No problems expected. Your doctor should periodically evaluate your response to the drug and adjust the dosage if necessary.

Skin & sunlight:
No problems expected.

Driving, piloting or hazardous work:
Don't drive or pilot aircraft until you learn how medicine affects you. Don't work around dangerous machinery. Don't climb ladders or work in high places. Danger increases if you drink alcohol or take other medicines affecting alertness and reflexes such as antihistamines, tranquilizers, sedatives, pain medicine, narcotics and mind-altering drugs.

Discontinuing:

- Don't discontinue without consulting doctor. Dose may require gradual reduction if you have taken drug for a long time. Doses of other drugs may also require adjustment.
- Consult doctor if the following symptoms appear after you discontinue the drug: Dizziness, lightheadedness, agitation, confusion, restlessness, vision changes, insomnia, headache, muscle aches, runny nose, unusual tiredness or weakness, nausea or vomiting.

Others:
Advise any doctor or dentist whom you consult that you take this medicine.

POSSIBLE INTERACTION WITH OTHER DRUGS

GENERIC NAME OR DRUG CLASS	COMBINED EFFECT
Antidepressants*, other	Increased effects of both drugs.
Cimetidine	Increased levels of paroxetine in blood.
Digoxin	Decreased digoxin effect.
Lithium	Unknown effect. Consult doctor.
Monoamine oxidase (MAO) inhibitors *	Can cause a life-threatening reaction. Avoid.
Phenytoin	Decreased effect of phenytoin.
Tryptophan	Increased likelihood of dizziness, headache, nausea, sweating. Avoid.
Warfarin	Increased risk of bleeding.

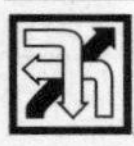

POSSIBLE INTERACTION WITH OTHER SUBSTANCES

INTERACTS WITH	COMBINED EFFECT
Alcohol:	Contributes to depression. Avoid.
Beverages:	None expected.
Cocaine:	Effects unknown. Avoid.
Foods:	None expected..
Marijuana:	Effects unknown. Avoid.
Tobacco:	None expected.

***See Glossary**

PEDICULISIDES (Topical)

BRAND AND GENERIC NAMES

A-200 Gel
A-200 Shampoo
Barc
Bio-Well
Blue
Derbac
Elimite Cream
GBH
G-well
Kwell
Kwellada
Kwildane
Lice-Enz Foam and Comb Lice Killing Shampoo Kit
Licetrol
LINDANE
MALATHION
Nix Creme Rinse
Ovide
PMS Lindane
PERMETHRIN
Prioderm
Pronto Lice Killing Shampoo Kit
PYRETHRINS AND PIPERONYL BUTOXIDE
Pyrinyl
R&C
RID
Scabene
Thionex
TISIT
TISIT Blue
Triple X

BASIC INFORMATION

Habit forming? No
Prescription needed? Yes
Available as generic? Yes, some
Drug class: Pediculiside, scabicide

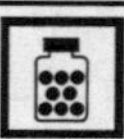

USES

- Treats scabies and lice infections of skin or scalp.
- Cream and lotion treats scabies.
- Shampoo treats lice infections.
- Carefully read patient instructions contained in package.

OVERDOSE

SYMPTOMS:
Rarely (toxic effects from too much absorbed through skin)—Vomiting, muscle cramps, dizziness, seizure, rapid heartbeat.
WHAT TO DO:
- **Not for internal use. If child accidentally swallows, call poison control center.**
- **Dial 911 (emergency) or 0 (operator) for an ambulance or medical help. Then give first aid immediately.**
- **See emergency information on inside covers.**

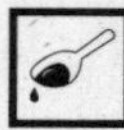

DOSAGE & USAGE INFORMATION

How to use:
- Follow package directions.
- Wear plastic gloves when you apply.
- Bathe before applying.
- Use in well-ventilated room.
- Use care not to apply more than directed.

When to use:
As directed on package.

If you forget a dose:
Use as soon as you remember.

What drug does:
Absorbed into bodies of lice and scabies organisms and stimulates their central nervous system causing convulsions and death. Does not affect humans in this way.

Time lapse before drug works:
Cream or lotion requires 8 to 12 hours contact with skin.

Don't use with:
Other medicines for scabies or lice.

POSSIBLE ADVERSE REACTIONS OR SIDE EFFECTS

SYMPTOMS	WHAT TO DO
Life-threatening	
None expected.	
Common	
None expected.	
Infrequent	
None expected.	
Rare	
Skin irritation or rash.	Discontinue. Call doctor right away.

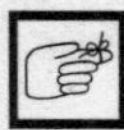

WARNINGS & PRECAUTIONS

Don't use if:
You are allergic to any medicine with lindane, pyrethrins or piperonyl butoxide.

Before you start, consult your doctor:
- If you are allergic to anything that touches your skin.
- If you are using any other medicines, creams, lotions or oils.

Over age 60:
Adverse reactions and side effects may be more frequent and severe than in younger persons. Ask doctor about smaller doses.

Pregnancy:
Risk factors vary for drugs in this group. See category list on page xxii and consult doctor.

Breast-feeding:
Effect unknown. Avoid if possible. Consult doctor.

Infants & children:
More likely to be toxic. Use only under close medical supervision.

Prolonged use:
Not recommended. Avoid.

Skin & sunlight:
No problems expected, but check with doctor.

Driving, piloting or hazardous work:
No problems expected, but check with doctor.

Discontinuing:
No problems expected, but check with doctor.

Others:
- Don't use on open sores or wounds.
- Put on freshly dry cleaned or washed clothing after treatment.
- After treatment, boil all bed sheets, covers and towels before using.
- Store items that can't be washed or cleaned in plastic bags for 2 weeks.
- Avoid inhaling or swallowing drug.
- Thoroughly clean house.
- Wash combs and hairbrushes in hot soapy water. Don't share with others.

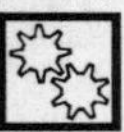

POSSIBLE INTERACTION WITH OTHER DRUGS

GENERIC NAME OR DRUG CLASS	COMBINED EFFECT
Antimyasthenics*	Excessive absorption and chance of toxicity (with malathion only).
Cholinesterase inhibitors*	Excessive absorption and chance of toxicity (with malathion only).

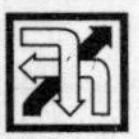

POSSIBLE INTERACTION WITH OTHER SUBSTANCES

INTERACTS WITH	COMBINED EFFECT
Alcohol:	None expected.
Beverages:	None expected.
Cocaine:	None expected.
Foods:	None expected.
Marijuana:	None expected.
Tobacco:	None expected.

***See Glossary**

PEMOLINE

BRAND NAMES

Cylert
Cylert Chewable

BASIC INFORMATION

Habit forming? Yes
Prescription needed? Yes
Available as generic? No
Drug class: Central nervous system stimulant

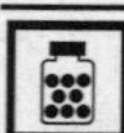

USES

- Decreases overactivity and lengthens attention span in hyperactive children.
- Treats minimal brain dysfunction.

DOSAGE & USAGE INFORMATION

How to take:
- Tablet—Swallow with liquid or food to lessen stomach irritation. If you can't swallow whole, crumble tablet and take with liquid or food.
- Chewable tablets—Chew well before swallowing.

When to take:
At the same times each day.

If you forget a dose:
Take as soon as you remember up to 2 hours late. If more than 2 hours, wait for next scheduled dose (don't double this dose).

What drug does:
Stimulates brain to improve alertness, concentration and attention span. Calms the hyperactive child.

Continued next column

OVERDOSE

SYMPTOMS:
Rapid heartbeat, hallucinations, fever, confusion, convulsions, coma.
WHAT TO DO:
- **Dial 911 (emergency) or 0 (operator) for an ambulance or medical help. Then give first aid immediately.**
- **If patient is unconscious and not breathing, give mouth-to-mouth breathing. If there is no heartbeat, use cardiac massage and mouth-to-mouth breathing (CPR). Don't try to make patient vomit. If you can't get help quickly, take patient to nearest emergency facility.**
- **See emergency information on inside covers.**

Time lapse before drug works:
- 1 month or more for maximum effect on child.
- 30 minutes to stimulate adults.

Don't take with:
Any other medicine without consulting your doctor or pharmacist.

POSSIBLE ADVERSE REACTIONS OR SIDE EFFECTS

SYMPTOMS	WHAT TO DO
Life-threatening: In case of overdose, see previous column.	
Common: Insomnia.	Continue. Call doctor when convenient.
Infrequent:	
• Irritability, depression dizziness, headache, drowsiness, unusual movement of eyes, rapid heartbeat.	Discontinue. Call doctor right away.
• Rash, unusual movements of tongue, appetite loss, abdominal pain, nausea, weight loss.	Continue. Call doctor when convenient.
Rare:	
• Seizures.	Discontinue. Seek emergency treatment.
• Abnormal muscular movements, jaundice, hallucinations.	Discontinue. Call doctor right away.

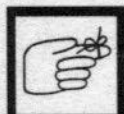

WARNINGS & PRECAUTIONS

Don't take if:
You are allergic to pemoline.

Before you start, consult your doctor:
- If you have liver disease.
- If you have kidney disease.
- If patient is younger than 6 years.
- If there is marked emotional instability.

Over age 60:
Adverse reactions and side effects may be more frequent and severe than in younger persons.

Pregnancy:
No proven harm to unborn child. Avoid if possible. Consult doctor. Risk category B (see page xxii).

Breast-feeding:
Effect unknown. Consult doctor.

Infants & children:
Use only under close medical supervision for children 6 or older.

Prolonged use:
- Rare possibility of physical growth retardation.
- Talk to your doctor about the need for follow-up medical examinations or laboratory studies to check liver function, growth charts.

Skin & sunlight:
No problems expected.

Driving, piloting or hazardous work:
Don't drive or pilot aircraft until you learn how medicine affects you. Don't work around dangerous machinery. Don't climb ladders or work in high places. Danger increases if you drink alcohol or take medicine affecting alertness and reflexes, such as antihistamines, tranquilizers, sedatives, pain medicine, narcotics and mind-altering drugs.

Discontinuing:
- Don't discontinue without consulting doctor. Dose may require gradual reduction if you have taken drug for a long time. Doses of other drugs may also require adjustment.
- If you notice any of the following symptoms after discontinuing, notify your doctor: mental depression (severe), tiredness or weakness.

Others:
Dose must be carefully adjusted by doctor.

POSSIBLE INTERACTION WITH OTHER DRUGS

GENERIC NAME OR DRUG CLASS	COMBINED EFFECT
Anticonvulsants*	Dosage adjustment for anticonvulsant may be necessary.
Central nervous system (CNS) stimulants*, other	May increase toxic effects of both drugs.

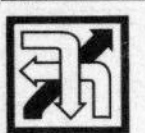

POSSIBLE INTERACTION WITH OTHER SUBSTANCES

INTERACTS WITH	COMBINED EFFECT
Alcohol:	More chance of depression. Avoid.
Beverages: Caffeine drinks.	May raise blood pressure. Avoid.
Cocaine:	Convulsions or excessive nervousness.
Foods:	No problems expected.
Marijuana:	Unknown.
Tobacco:	Unknown.

PENICILLAMINE

BRAND NAMES

Cuprimine Depen

BASIC INFORMATION

Habit forming? No
Prescription needed? Yes
Available as generic? No
Drug class: Chelating agent, antirheumatic, antidote (heavy metal)

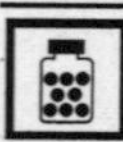

USES

- Treatment for rheumatoid arthritis.
- Prevention of kidney stones.
- Treatment for heavy metal poisoning.

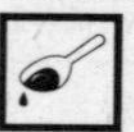

DOSAGE & USAGE INFORMATION

How to take:
Tablets or capsules—With liquid on an empty stomach 1 hour before or 2 hours after eating.

When to take:
At the same times each day.

If you forget a dose:
- 1 dose a day—Take as soon as you remember up to 12 hours late. If more than 12 hours, wait for next scheduled dose (don't double this dose).
- More than 1 dose a day—Take as soon as you remember up to 2 hours late. If more than 2 hours, wait for next scheduled dose (don't double this dose).

Continued next column

OVERDOSE

SYMPTOMS:
Ulcers, sores, convulsions, coughing up blood, coma.
WHAT TO DO:
- **Dial 911 (emergency) or 0 (operator) for an ambulance or medical help. Then give first aid immediately.**
- **See emergency information on inside covers.**

What drug does:
- Combines with heavy metals so kidney can excrete them.
- Combines with cysteine (amino acid found in many foods) to prevent cysteine kidney stones.
- May improve protective function of some white blood cells against rheumatoid arthritis.

Time lapse before drug works:
2 to 3 months.

Don't take with:
Any other medicine without consulting your doctor or pharmacist.

POSSIBLE ADVERSE REACTIONS OR SIDE EFFECTS

SYMPTOMS	WHAT TO DO
Life-threatening: In case of overdose, see previous column.	
Common: Rash, itchy skin, swollen lymph glands, appetite loss, nausea, diarrhea, vomiting, decreased taste.	Discontinue. Call doctor right away.
Infrequent: Sore throat, fever, unusual bruising, swollen feet or legs, bloody or cloudy urine, weight gain, fatigue, weakness, joint pain.	Discontinue. Call doctor right away.
Rare: Double or blurred vision; pain; ringing in ears; ulcers, sores, white spots in mouth; difficult breathing; coughing up blood; jaundice; abdominal pain; skin blisters; peeling skin.	Discontinue. Call doctor right away.

WARNINGS & PRECAUTIONS

Don't take if:
- You are allergic to penicillamine.
- You have severe anemia.

Before you start, consult your doctor:
- If you have kidney disease.
- If you are allergic to any pencillin antibiotic.

Over age 60:
More likely to damage blood cells and kidneys.

Pregnancy:
Decide with your doctor if drug benefits justify risk to unborn child. Risk category C (see page xxii).

Breast-feeding:
Safety not established. Consult doctor.

Infants & children:
Use only under medical supervision.

Prolonged use:
- May damage blood cells, kidney, liver.
- Talk to your doctor about the need for follow-up medical examinations or laboratory studies to check complete blood counts (white blood cell count, platelet count, red blood cell count, hemoglobin, hematocrit), kidney function, liver function.

Skin & sunlight:
No problems expected.

Driving, piloting or hazardous work:
No problems expected.

Discontinuing:
No problems expected.

Others:
Request laboratory studies on blood and urine every 2 weeks. Kidney and liver function studies recommended every 6 months.

POSSIBLE INTERACTION WITH OTHER DRUGS

GENERIC NAME OR DRUG CLASS	COMBINED EFFECT
Gold compounds*	Damage to blood cells and kidney.
Immuno-suppressants*	Damage to blood cells and kidney.
Iron supplements*	Decreased effect of penicillamine. Wait 2 hours between doses.
Pyridoxine (vitamin B-6)	Increased need for pyridoxine.

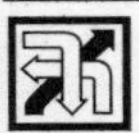

POSSIBLE INTERACTION WITH OTHER SUBSTANCES

INTERACTS WITH	COMBINED EFFECT
Alcohol:	Increased side effects of penicillamine.
Beverages:	None expected.
Cocaine:	Increased side effects of penicillamine.
Foods:	Possible decreased penicillamine effect due to decreased absorption.
Marijuana:	Increased side effects of penicillamine.
Tobacco:	None expected.

*See Glossary

PENICILLINS

BRAND AND GENERIC NAMES

See complete list of brand and generic names in the *Brand Name Directory*, page 913.

BASIC INFORMATION

Habit forming? No
Prescription needed? Yes
Available as generic? Yes
Drug class: Antibiotic (penicillin)

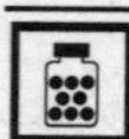

USES

Treatment of bacterial infections that are susceptible to penicillin, including lower respiratory tract infections, otitis media, sinusitis, skin and skin structure infections, urinary tract infections, gastrointestinal disorders, endocarditis, pharyngitis. Different penicillins treat different kinds of infections.

DOSAGE & USAGE INFORMATION

How to take:

- Tablet or capsule—Swallow with liquid on an empty stomach 1 hour before or 2 hours after eating. You may take amoxicillin, penicillin V, pivampicillin or pivmecillinam on a full stomach.
- Chewable tablet—Chew or crush before swallowing.
- Oral suspension—Measure each dose with an accurate measuring device (not a household teaspoon). Store according to instructions.

When to take:
Follow instructions on prescription label, or take as directed by doctor. The number of doses, the time between doses and the length of treatment will depend on the problem being treated.

If you forget a dose:
Take as soon as you remember, then continue regular schedule. If it is almost time for the next dose, wait for that dose (don't double that dose).

Continued next column

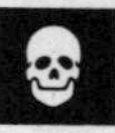

OVERDOSE

SYMPTOMS:
Severe diarrhea, nausea or vomiting.
WHAT TO DO:
Overdose unlikely to threaten life. If person takes much larger amount than prescribed, call doctor, poison control center or hospital emergency room for instructions.

What drug does:
Destroys susceptible bacteria. Does not kill viruses (e.g., colds or influenza), fungi or parasites.

Time lapse before drug works:
May be several days before medicine affects infection.

Don't take with:
Any other medicine without consulting your doctor or pharmacist.

POSSIBLE ADVERSE REACTIONS OR SIDE EFFECTS

SYMPTOMS	WHAT TO DO
Life-threatening:	
Hives, rash, intense itching, shortness of breath, faintness soon after a dose (anaphylaxis).	Seek emergency treatment immediately.
Common:	
Nausea, vomiting or diarrhea (all mild); sore mouth or tongue; white patches in mouth or on tongue; vaginal itching or discharge; stomach pain.	Continue. Call doctor when convenient.
Infrequent:	
None expected.	
Rare:	
Unexplained bleeding or bruising, weakness, sore throat, fever, severe abdominal cramps, diarrhea (watery and severe), convulsions.	Discontinue. Call doctor right away.

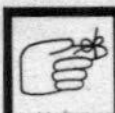

WARNINGS & PRECAUTIONS

Don't take if:
You are allergic to penicillins* or cephalosporins*. A life-threatening reaction may occur.

Before you start, consult your doctor:
- If you are allergic to any substance or drug.
- If you have mononucleosis.
- If you have congestive heart failure.
- If you have high blood pressure or any bleeding disorder.
- If you have cystic fibrosis.
- If you have kidney disease or a stomach or intestinal disorder.

Over age 60:
No special problems expected.

Pregnancy:
Consult doctor. Risk category B (see page xxii).

Breast-feeding:
Drug passes into milk. Child may become sensitive to penicillins and have allergic reactions to penicillin drugs. Discuss risks and benefits with your doctor.

Infants & children:
No special problems expected.

Prolonged use:
- You may become more susceptible to infections caused by germs not responsive to penicillins.
- Talk to your doctor about the need for follow-up medical examinations or laboratory studies.

Skin & sunlight:
No problems expected.

Driving, piloting or hazardous work:
Usually not dangerous. Most hazardous reactions likely to occur a few minutes after taking penicillin.

Discontinuing:
Don't discontinue without doctor's advice until you complete prescribed dose, even though symptoms diminish or disappear.

Others:
- Urine sugar test for diabetes may show false positive result.
- If your symptoms don't improve within a few days (or if they worsen), call your doctor.
- Don't take medicines for diarrhea without your doctor's approval.
- Birth control pills may not be effective. Use additional birth control methods.

POSSIBLE INTERACTION WITH OTHER DRUGS

GENERIC NAME OR DRUG CLASS	COMBINED EFFECT
Chloramphenicol	Decreased effect of both drugs.
Cholestyramine	May decrease penicillin effect.
Colestipol	May decrease penicillin effect.
Contraceptives, oral*	Impaired contraceptive efficiency.
Erythromycins*	Decreased effect of both drugs.
Methotrexate	Increased risk of methotrexate toxicity.
Probenecid	Increased effect of all penicillins.
Sodium benzoate & sodium phenylacetate	May reduce effect of sodium benzoate & sodium phenylacetate.
Tetracyclines*	Decreased effect of both drugs.

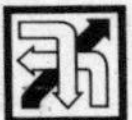

POSSIBLE INTERACTION WITH OTHER SUBSTANCES

INTERACTS WITH	COMBINED EFFECT
Alcohol:	Occasional stomach irritation.
Beverages:	None expected.
Cocaine:	No proven problems.
Foods: Acidic fruits or juices, aged cheese, wines, syrups (if taken with penicillin G).	Decreased antibiotic effect.
Marijuana:	No proven problems.
Tobacco:	None expected.

*See Glossary

PENICILLINS & BETA-LACTAMASE INHIBITORS

BRAND AND GENERIC NAMES

AMOXICILLIN & CLAVULANATE	**Augmentin** **Clavulin**

BASIC INFORMATION

Habit forming? No
Prescription needed? Yes
Available as generic? No
Drug class: Antibiotic (penicillin)

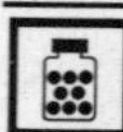

USES

Treatment of bacterial infections that are susceptible to penicillin and beta-lactamase inhibitors, including lower respiratory tract infections, otitis media, sinusitis, skin and skin structure infections, urinary tract infections.

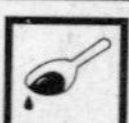

DOSAGE & USAGE INFORMATION

How to take:

- Tablet—Swallow with liquid on a full or empty stomach. Taking with food may lessen any stomach irritation.
- Chewable tablet—Chew or crush before swallowing.
- Oral suspension—Measure each dose with an accurate measuring device (not a household teaspoon).

When to take:
Follow instructions on prescription label, or take as directed by doctor. Normally the drug is taken every 8 hours for 7 to 10 days.

If you forget a dose:
Take as soon as you remember, then continue regular schedule. If it is almost time for the next dose, wait for that dose (don't double it).

Continued next column

OVERDOSE

SYMPTOMS:
Severe diarrhea, nausea or vomiting.
WHAT TO DO:
Overdose unlikely to threaten life. If person takes much larger amount than prescribed, call doctor, poison control center or hospital emergency room for instructions.

What drug does:
Destroys susceptible bacteria. Does not kill viruses, fungi or parasites. Beta-lactamase inhibitors increase penicillin's effectiveness by inactivating beta-lactamase (a substance in the body which destroys the penicillin).

Time lapse before drug works:
May be several days before medicine affects infection.

Don't take with:
Any other medicine without consulting your doctor or pharmacist.

POSSIBLE ADVERSE REACTIONS OR SIDE EFFECTS

SYMPTOMS	WHAT TO DO
Life-threatening:	
Hives, rash, intense itching, shortness of breath, faintness soon after a dose (anaphylaxis).	Seek emergency treatment immediately.
Common:	
Nausea, vomiting or diarrhea (all mild); sore mouth or tongue; white patches in mouth or on tongue; vaginal itching or discharge; stomach pain.	Continue. Call doctor when convenient.
Infrequent:	
None expected.	
Rare:	
Unexplained bleeding or bruising, weakness, sore throat, fever, severe abdominal cramps, diarrhea (watery and severe), convulsions.	Discontinue. Call doctor right away.

PENICILLINS & BETA-LACTAMASE INHIBITORS

WARNINGS & PRECAUTIONS

Don't take if:
You are allergic to penicillins or cephalosporins. Life-threatening reaction may occur.

Before you start, consult your doctor:
- If you are allergic to any substance or drug.
- If you have mononucleosis.
- If you have congestive heart failure.
- If you have high blood pressure or any bleeding disorder.
- If you have cystic fibrosis.
- If you have kidney disease or a stomach or intestinal disorder.

Over age 60:
No special problems expected.

Pregnancy:
Consult doctor. Risk category B (see page xxii).

Breast-feeding:
Drug passes into milk. Child may become sensitive to penicillins and have allergic reactions to penicillin drugs. Avoid penicillin or discontinue nursing until you finish medicine. Consult doctor for advice on maintaining milk supply.

Infants & children:
No special problems expected.

Prolonged use:
- You may become more susceptible to infections caused by germs not responsive to penicillins.
- Talk to your doctor about the need for follow-up medical examinations or laboratory studies to check SGPT*, SGOT*.

Skin & sunlight:
No problems expected.

Driving, piloting or hazardous work:
Usually not dangerous. Most hazardous reactions likely to occur a few minutes after taking.

Discontinuing:
Don't discontinue without doctor's advice until you complete prescribed dose, even though symptoms diminish or disappear.

Others:
- Urine sugar test for diabetes may show false positive result.
- If your symptoms don't improve within a few days (or if they worsen), call your doctor.
- Don't take for diarrhea without your doctor's approval.
- Birth control pills may not be effective. Use additional birth control methods.

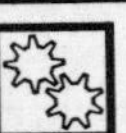

POSSIBLE INTERACTION WITH OTHER DRUGS

GENERIC NAME OR DRUG CLASS	COMBINED EFFECT
Chloramphenicol	Decreased effect of both drugs.
Cholestyramine	May decrease penicillin effect.
Colestipol	May decrease penicillin effect.
Contraceptives, oral*	Impaired contraceptive efficiency.
Erythromycins*	Decreased effect of both drugs.
Methotrexate	Increased risk of methotrexate toxicity.
Probenecid	Increased effect of all penicillins.
Sodium benzoate & sodium phenylacetate	May reduce effect of sodium benzoate & sodium phenylacetate.
Tetracyclines*	Decreased effect of both drugs.

POSSIBLE INTERACTION WITH OTHER SUBSTANCES

INTERACTS WITH	COMBINED EFFECT
Alcohol:	Occasional stomach irritation.
Beverages:	None expected.
Cocaine:	No proven problems.
Foods:	None expected.
Marijuana:	No proven problems.
Tobacco:	None expected.

***See Glossary**

PENTAMIDINE

BRAND NAMES

NebuPent
Pentacarinat
Pneumopent

BASIC INFORMATION

Habit forming? No
Prescription needed? Yes
Available as generic? No
Drug class: Antiprotozoal

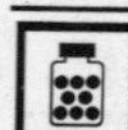

USES

- Treats pneumocystis carinii, which is common in AIDS patients.
- Treats some tropical diseases such as leishmaniasis, African sleeping sickness and others.

DOSAGE & USAGE INFORMATION

How to take:
Inhalation—Follow package instructions.

When to take:
According to doctor's instructions.

If you forget a dose:
Not likely to happen.

What drug does:
Interferes with RNA and DNA of infecting organisms.

Time lapse before drug works:
30 minutes to 1 hour.

Don't take with:
Any other medicines (including over-the-counter drugs such as cough and cold medicines, laxatives, antacids, diet pills, caffeine, nose drops or vitamins) without consulting your doctor.

OVERDOSE

SYMPTOMS:
None expected.
WHAT TO DO:
Overdose unlikely to threaten life. If person takes much larger amount than prescribed, call doctor, poison control center or hospital emergency room for instructions.

POSSIBLE ADVERSE REACTIONS OR SIDE EFFECTS

SYMPTOMS	WHAT TO DO
Life-threatening:	
Unconsciousness, rapid pulse, cold sweats.	Seek emergency treatment immediately.
Common:	
Chest pain or congestion; wheezing; coughing; difficulty in breathing; skin rash; pain, dryness or sensation of lump in throat.	Discontinue. Call doctor right away.
Infrequent:	
• Abdomen or back pain, nausea, vomiting, anxiety, cold sweats, chills, headache, appetite changes, decreased urination, unusual tiredness.	Discontinue. Call doctor right away.
• Bitter or metallic taste.	No action necessary.
Rare:	
None expected.	

WARNINGS & PRECAUTIONS

Don't take if:
You know you are allergic to pentamidine.

Before you start, consult your doctor:
If you have asthma.

Over age 60:
Adverse reactions and side effects may be more frequent and severe than in younger persons. You may need smaller doses for shorter periods of time.

Pregnancy:
Decide with your doctor if drug benefits justify risk to unborn child. Risk category C (see page xxii).

Breast-feeding:
Unknown effects. Not recommended. Consult doctor.

Infants & children:
Unknown effects. Consult doctor.

Prolonged use:
Talk to your doctor about the need for follow-up medical examinations or laboratory studies to check blood sugar; blood pressure; kidney, liver and heart function; complete blood counts (white blood cell count, platelet count, red blood cell count, hemoglobin, hematocrit); ECG* and serum calcium.

Skin & sunlight:
No problems expected.

Driving, piloting or hazardous work:
Avoid if you feel confused, drowsy or dizzy.

Discontinuing:
No special problems expected.

Others:
- Advise any doctor or dentist whom you consult that you take this medicine.
- May affect results in some medical tests.
- Avoid exposure to people who have infectious diseases.
- To help decrease bitter taste in mouth, dissolve a hard candy after taking medicine.
- Consult your doctor for additional information on the injectable form of this drug.

POSSIBLE INTERACTION WITH OTHER DRUGS

GENERIC NAME OR DRUG CLASS	COMBINED EFFECT
None reported with inhalation form of drug.	

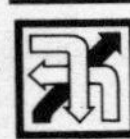

POSSIBLE INTERACTION WITH OTHER SUBSTANCES

INTERACTS WITH	COMBINED EFFECT
Alcohol:	Increased likelihood of adverse reactions. Avoid.
Beverages:	No special problems expected.
Cocaine:	Increased likelihood of adverse reactions. Avoid.
Foods:	No special problems expected.
Marijuana:	Increased likelihood of adverse reactions. Avoid.
Tobacco:	Increased likelihood of adverse reactions. Avoid.

***See Glossary**

PENTOXIFYLLINE

BRAND NAMES

Trental

BASIC INFORMATION

Habit forming? No
Prescription needed? Yes
Available as generic? No
Drug class: Hemorrheologic agent

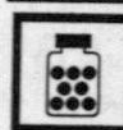

USES

Reduces pain in legs caused by poor circulation.

DOSAGE & USAGE INFORMATION

How to take:
Extended-release tablets—Swallow whole with water and food.

When to take:
At mealtimes. Taking with food decreases the likelihood of irritating the stomach to cause nausea.

If you forget a dose:
Take as soon as you remember up to 3 hours late. If more than 3 hours, wait for next scheduled dose (don't double this dose).

What drug does:
- Reduces "stickiness" of red blood cells and improves flexibility of the red cells.
- Improves blood flow through blood vessels.

Time lapse before drug works:
1 hour. Several weeks for full effect on circulation.

Don't take with:
- Tobacco or medicines to treat hypertension.
- Any other medicine without consulting your doctor or pharmacist.

OVERDOSE

SYMPTOMS:
Drowsiness, flushed face, fainting, nervousness, convulsions, coma.
WHAT TO DO:
- **Dial 911 (emergency) or 0 (operator) for an ambulance or medical help. Then give first aid immediately.**
- **See emergency information on inside covers.**

POSSIBLE ADVERSE REACTIONS OR SIDE EFFECTS

SYMPTOMS	WHAT TO DO
Life-threatening:	
Chest pain, irregular heartbeat.	Discontinue. Seek emergency treatment.
Common:	
None expected.	
Infrequent:	
• Dizziness, headache, nausea, vomiting. low blood pressure, nosebleed, swollen feet and ankles, viral-like syndrome, nasal congestion, laryngitis, rash, itchy skin, blurred vision, abdominal pain.	Discontinue. Call doctor right away.
• Insomnia, nervousness, red eyes.	Continue. Call doctor when convenient.
Rare:	
None expected.	

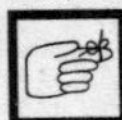

WARNINGS & PRECAUTIONS

Don't take if:
You are allergic to pentoxifylline.

Before you start, consult your doctor:
- If you are allergic to caffeine, theophylline, theobromine, aminophyllin, dyphyllin, oxtriphylline, theobromine.
- If you have angina.
- If you have liver or kidney disease.

Over age 60:
Adverse reactions and side effects may be more frequent and severe than in younger persons. Ask doctor about smaller doses.

Pregnancy:
Decide with your doctor if drug benefits justify risk to unborn child. Risk category C (see page xxii).

Breast-feeding:
Drug passes into milk. Avoid drug or discontinue nursing until you finish medicine. Consult doctor for advice on maintaining milk supply.

Infants & children:
Not recommended.

Prolonged use:
No problems expected.

Skin & sunlight:
No problems expected.

Driving, piloting or hazardous work:
Wait to see if drug causes drowsiness or dizziness. If none, no problems expected.

Discontinuing:
No problems expected.

Others:
Don't smoke.

POSSIBLE INTERACTION WITH OTHER DRUGS

GENERIC NAME OR DRUG CLASS	COMBINED EFFECT
Anticoagulants*, oral	Possible decreased effect of anticoagulant.
Antihypertensives*	Possible increased effect of hypertensive medication.

POSSIBLE INTERACTION WITH OTHER SUBSTANCES

INTERACTS WITH	COMBINED EFFECT
Alcohol:	Unknown. Best to avoid.
Beverages: Coffee, tea or other caffeine-containing beverages.	May decrease effectiveness of pentoxifylline.
Cocaine:	Reduced effect of pentoxifylline.
Foods:	None expected.
Marijuana:	Decreased effect of pentoxifylline.
Tobacco:	Decreased effect of pentoxifylline. Avoid.

*See Glossary

PERGOLIDE

BRAND NAMES

Permax

BASIC INFORMATION

Habit forming? No
Prescription needed? Yes
Available as generic? No
Drug class: Antidyskinetic

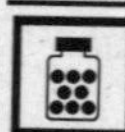

USES

Treats Parkinson's disease when used together with levodopa or carbidopa.

DOSAGE & USAGE INFORMATION

How to take:
Tablets—Swallow with liquid. If you can't swallow whole, crumble tablet and take with liquid or food. Instructions to take on empty stomach mean 1 hour before or 2 hours after eating.

When to take:
Follow doctor's instructions. Usually 3 times a day.

If you forget a dose:
Take as soon as you remember up to 2 hours late. If more than 2 hours, wait for next scheduled dose (don't double this dose).

What drug does:

- Stimulates dopamine receptors in the central nervous system to make them more active.
- Lowers the required dosage of carbidopa and levodopa.

Time lapse before drug works:
Not documented.

Don't take with:
Any other medicines (including over-the-counter drugs such as cough and cold medicines, laxatives, antacids, diet pills, caffeine, nose drops or vitamins) without consulting your doctor or pharmacist.

OVERDOSE

SYMPTOMS:
None expected.
WHAT TO DO:
Overdose unlikely to threaten life. If person takes much larger amount than prescribed, call doctor, poison control center or hospital emergency room for instructions.

POSSIBLE ADVERSE REACTIONS OR SIDE EFFECTS

SYMPTOMS	WHAT TO DO
Life-threatening:	
Seizures, chest pain, shortness of breath.	Seek emergency treatment immediately.
Common:	
• Confusion; hallucinations; painful urination; unusual movements of face, head, hands and tongue.	Discontinue. Seek emergency treatment.
• Abdominal pain, constipation, dizziness, nasal stuffiness.	Continue. Call doctor when convenient.
Infrequent:	
Chills, diarrhea, dry mouth, appetite loss, facial swelling, increased sex drive.	Continue. Call doctor when convenient.
Rare:	
Weakness, vision changes, fainting, increased sweating, nausea and vomiting.	Discontinue. Seek emergency treatment.

WARNINGS & PRECAUTIONS

Don't take if:
You are allergic to pergolide or any ergot preparation*.

Before you start, consult your doctor:
- If you have heartbeat irregularities.
- If you have hallucinations.

Over age 60:
No special problems expected.

Pregnancy:
Consult doctor. Risk category B (see page xxii).

Breast-feeding:
Not recommended. Pergolide can prevent lactation. Consult doctor.

Infants & children:
Effect not documented. Consult your doctor.

Prolonged use:
Request frequent blood pressure checks.

Skin & sunlight:
No problems expected.

Driving, piloting or hazardous work:
Don't drive or pilot aircraft until you learn how medicine affects you. Don't work around dangerous machinery. Don't climb ladders or work in high places. Danger increases if you drink alcohol or take medicine affecting alertness and reflexes.

Discontinuing:
No special problems expected.

Others:
- Advise any doctor or dentist whom you consult that you take this medicine.
- May affect results in some medical tests.

POSSIBLE INTERACTION WITH OTHER DRUGS

GENERIC NAME OR DRUG CLASS	COMBINED EFFECT
Chlorprothixene	Decreased pergolide effect.
Droperidol	Decreased pergolide effect.
Flupenthixol	Decreased pergolide effect.
Haloperidol	Decreased pergolide effect.
Hypotension-causing drugs*	Increased hypotension effect.
Loxapine	Decreased pergolide effect.
Methyldopa	Decreased pergolide effect.
Metoclopropamide	Decreased pergolide effect.
Molindone	Decreased pergolide effect.
Papaverine	Decreased pergolide effect.
Phenothiazines*	Decreased pergolide effect.
Reserpine	Decreased pergolide effect.
Sertraline	Increased depressive effects of both drugs.
Thiothixene	Decreased pergolide effect.

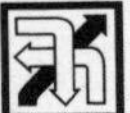

POSSIBLE INTERACTION WITH OTHER SUBSTANCES

INTERACTS WITH	COMBINED EFFECT
Alcohol:	Increased likelihood of adverse reactions. Avoid.
Beverages:	No special problems expected.
Cocaine:	Increased likelihood of adverse reactions. Avoid.
Foods:	No special problems expected.
Marijuana:	Increased likelihood of adverse reactions. Avoid.
Tobacco:	No special problems expected.

*See Glossary

PERPHENAZINE & AMITRIPTYLINE

BRAND NAMES

Elavil Plus
Etrafon
PMS Levazine
Triavil

BASIC INFORMATION

Habit forming? No
Prescription needed? Yes
Available as generic? Yes
Drug class: Tranquilizer (phenothiazine), antidepressant, antipsychotic

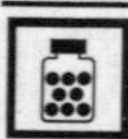

USES

- Decreases nausea, vomiting, hiccups.
- Gradually relieves, but doesn't cure, symptoms of depression, anxiety, agitation.
- Pain relief (sometimes).

DOSAGE & USAGE INFORMATION

How to take:
Tablet or liquid—Swallow with liquid.

When to take:
At the same time each day.

If you forget a dose:
Bedtime dose—If you forget your once-a-day bedtime dose, don't take it more than 3 hours late. If more than 3 hours, wait for next scheduled dose (don't double this dose).

Continued next column

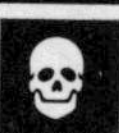

OVERDOSE

SYMPTOMS:
Stupor, convulsions, hallucinations, coma.
WHAT TO DO:
- **Dial 911 (emergency) or 0 (operator) for an ambulance or medical help. Then give first aid immediately.**
- **If patient is unconscious and not breathing, give mouth-to-mouth breathing. If there is no heartbeat, use cardiac massage and mouth-to-mouth breathing (CPR). Don't try to make patient vomit. If you can't get help quickly, take patient to nearest emergency facility.**
- **See emergency information on inside covers.**

What drug does:
- Suppresses brain's vomiting center.
- Suppresses brain centers that control abnormal emotions and behavior.
- Probably affects part of brain that controls messages between nerve cells.

Time lapse before drug works:
- Nausea and vomiting—1 hour or less.
- Nervous and mental disorders—4 to 6 weeks.
- Begins in 1 to 2 weeks. May require 4 to 6 weeks for maximum benefit.

Don't take with:
- Antacid or medicine for diarrhea.
- Any other medicine without consulting your doctor or pharmacist.

POSSIBLE ADVERSE REACTIONS OR SIDE EFFECTS

SYMPTOMS	WHAT TO DO
Life-threatening:	
Seizures; irregular heartbeat; weak pulse; fainting; muscle spasms; uncontrolled muscle movements of tongue, face and other muscles (neuroleptic malignant syndrome*).	Discontinue. Seek emergency treatment.
Common:	
• Headache, nausea, vomiting, irregular heartbeat, drowsiness.	Discontinue. Call doctor right away.
• Insomnia, dry mouth, "sweet tooth," decreased sweating, runny nose, constipation.	Continue. Call doctor when convenient.
Infrequent:	
• Hallucinations, dizziness, tremor, blurred vision, eye pain, inflamed tongue, joint pain, back pain, hiccups.	Discontinue. Call doctor right away.
• Frequent urination, diminished sex drive, breast swelling, menstrual irregularities, nasal congestion.	Continue. Call doctor when convenient.
Rare:	
• Rash; itchy skin; jaundice; change in vision; sore throat, fever, mouth sores; abdominal pain.	Discontinue. Call doctor right away.
• Fatigue, weakness.	Continue. Call doctor when convenient.

PERPHENAZINE & AMITRIPTYLINE

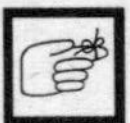

WARNINGS & PRECAUTIONS

Don't take if:
- You are allergic to any phenothiazine, tricyclic antidepressant.
- You have a blood or bone marrow disease, glaucoma, prostate trouble.
- You drink alcohol.
- You have had a heart attack within 6 weeks.
- You have taken MAO inhibitors within 2 weeks.
- Patient is younger than 12.

Before you start, consult your doctor:
- If you have asthma, emphysema or other lung disorder.
- If you have an enlarged prostate, heart disease, high blood pressure, stomach or intestinal problems, overactive thyroid, liver disease.
- If you take nonprescription ulcer medicine, asthma medicine or amphetamines.
- If you will have surgery within 2 months, including dental surgery, requiring general or spinal anesthesia.

Over age 60:
Adverse reactions and side effects may be more frequent and severe than in younger persons. More likely to develop involuntary movement of jaws, lips, tongue; chewing; difficult urination. Report this to your doctor immediately. Early treatment can help.

Pregnancy:
Risk to unborn child outweighs drug benefits. Don't use. Risk category D (see page xxii).

Breast-feeding:
Drug passes into milk. Avoid drug or discontinue nursing until you finish medicine. Consult doctor for advice on maintaining milk supply.

Infants & children:
Don't give to children younger than 12.

Prolonged use:
May lead to tardive dyskinesia (involuntary movement of jaws, lips, tongue; chewing).

Skin & sunlight:
May cause rash or intensify sunburn in areas exposed to sun or sunlamp. Skin may remain sensitive for 3 months after discontinuing.

Driving, piloting or hazardous work:
Don't drive or pilot aircraft until you learn how medicine affects you. Don't work around dangerous machinery. Don't climb ladders or work in high places. Danger increases if you drink alcohol or take medicine affecting alertness and reflexes, such as antihistamines, tranquilizers, sedatives, pain medicine, narcotics and mind-altering drugs.

Discontinuing:
- Nervous and mental disorders—Don't discontinue without doctor's advice until you complete prescribed dose, even though symptoms diminish or disappear.
- Dose may require gradual reduction if you have taken drug for a long time. Doses of other drugs may also require adjustment.

Others:
No problems expected.

POSSIBLE INTERACTION WITH OTHER DRUGS

GENERIC NAME OR DRUG CLASS	COMBINED EFFECT
Anticholinergics*	Increased anti-cholinergic effect, increased sedation.
Anticoagulants*, oral	Increased anticoagulant effect.
Antihistamines*	Increased antihistamine effect.
Appetite suppressants*	Decreased appetite suppressant effect.
Barbiturates*	Decreased anti-depressant effect. Increased sedation.
Cimetidine	Possible increased effect and toxicity of perphenazine and amitriptyline.
Clonidine	Possible decreased clonidine effect.

Continued on page 953

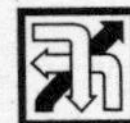

POSSIBLE INTERACTION WITH OTHER SUBSTANCES

INTERACTS WITH	COMBINED EFFECT
Alcohol: Beverages or medicines with alcohol.	Excessive intoxication. Avoid.
Beverages: Coffee.	Reduced effectiveness.
Cocaine:	Excessive intoxication. Avoid.
Foods:	None expected.
Marijuana:	Excessive drowsiness. Avoid.
Tobacco:	None expected.

***See Glossary**

PHENAZOPYRIDINE

BRAND NAMES

Azo-Cheragan
Azo-Gantrisin
Azo-Standard
Baridium
Eridium
Geridium
Phen-Azo
Phenazodine
Pyrazodine
Pyridiate
Pyridium
Pyronium
Urodine
Urogesic
Viridium

BASIC INFORMATION

Habit forming? No
Prescription needed? Yes
Available as generic? Yes
Drug class: Analgesic (urinary)

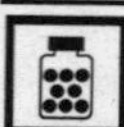

USES

Relieves pain of lower urinary tract irritation, as in cystitis, urethritis or prostatitis. Relieves symptoms only. Phenazopyridine alone does not cure infections.

DOSAGE & USAGE INFORMATION

How to take:
Tablet—Swallow with liquid or food to lessen stomach irritation.

When to take:
At the same times each day.

If you forget a dose:
Take as soon as you remember up to 2 hours late. If more than 2 hours, wait for next scheduled dose (don't double this dose).

What drug does:
Anesthetizes lower urinary tract. Relieves pain, burning, pressure and urgency to urinate.

Time lapse before drug works:
1 to 2 hours.

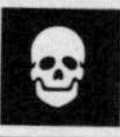

OVERDOSE

SYMPTOMS:
Shortness of breath, weakness.
WHAT TO DO:
Overdose unlikely to threaten life. If person takes much larger amount than prescribed, call doctor, poison control center or hospital emergency room for instructions.

Don't take with:
Any other medicine without consulting your doctor or pharmacist.

POSSIBLE ADVERSE REACTIONS OR SIDE EFFECTS

SYMPTOMS	WHAT TO DO
Life-threatening:	
In case of overdose, see previous column.	
Common:	
Red-orange urine.	No action necessary.
Infrequent:	
Indigestion, fatigue, weakness, dizziness, abdominal pain.	Continue. Call doctor when convenient.
Rare:	
• Rash, jaundice, bluish skin color.	Discontinue. Call doctor right away.
• Headache.	Continue. Call doctor when convenient.

PHENAZOPYRIDINE

WARNINGS & PRECAUTIONS

Don't take if:
- You have hepatitis.
- You are allergic to any urinary analgesic.

Before you start, consult your doctor:
If you have kidney or liver disease.

Over age 60:
Adverse reactions and side effects may be more frequent and severe than in younger persons.

Pregnancy:
No proven harm to unborn child. Avoid if possible. Consult doctor. Risk category B (see page xxii).

Breast-feeding:
Effect unknown. Consult doctor.

Infants & children:
Not recommended.

Prolonged use:
- Orange or yellow skin.
- Anemia. Occasional blood studies recommended.

Skin & sunlight:
No problems expected.

Driving, piloting or hazardous work:
No problems expected.

Discontinuing:
May be unnecessary to finish medicine. Follow doctor's instructions.

Others:
No problems expected.

POSSIBLE INTERACTION WITH OTHER DRUGS

GENERIC NAME OR DRUG CLASS	COMBINED EFFECT
None significant.	

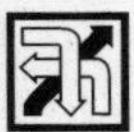

POSSIBLE INTERACTION WITH OTHER SUBSTANCES

INTERACTS WITH	COMBINED EFFECT
Alcohol:	None expected.
Beverages:	None expected.
Cocaine:	None expected.
Foods:	None expected.
Marijuana:	None expected.
Tobacco:	None expected.

PHENOLPHTHALEIN

BRAND NAMES

Agoral
Agoral Marshmallow
Agoral Raspberry
Alophen
Caroid Laxative
Colax
Correctol
Dialose Plus
Disolan
Doxidan
Espotabs
Evac-U-Gen
Evac-U-Lax
Ex-Lax Pills
Ex-Lax Maximum Relief Formula
Extra Gentle Ex-Lax
Feen-A-Mint
Feen-A-Mint Gum
Feen-A-Mint Pills
Kondremul with Phenolphthalein
Medilax
Modane
Phenolax
Phenolphthalein Petrogalar
Phillips' Gelcaps
Phillips' Laxcaps
Trilax

BASIC INFORMATION

Habit forming? No
Prescription needed? No
Available as generic? Yes
Drug class: Laxative (stimulant)

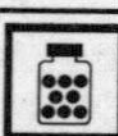

USES

Constipation relief.

DOSAGE & USAGE INFORMATION

How to take:

- Tablet or wafer—Swallow with liquid. If you can't swallow whole, chew or crumble and take with liquid or food.
- Liquid—Drink 6 to 8 glasses of water each day, in addition to one taken with each dose.
- Chewable tablets—Chew thoroughly before swallowing.

When to take:
Usually at bedtime with a snack, unless directed otherwise.

Continued next column

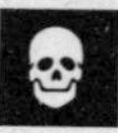

OVERDOSE

SYMPTOMS:
Vomiting, electrolyte depletion.
WHAT TO DO:

- **Dial 911 (emergency) or 0 (operator) for an ambulance or medical help. Then give first aid immediately.**
- **See emergency information on inside cover.**

If you forget a dose:
Take as soon as you remember.

What drug does:
Acts on smooth muscles of intestine wall to cause vigorous bowel movement.

Time lapse before drug works:
6 to 10 hours.

Don't take with:

- Any other medicine without consulting your doctor or pharmacist.
- Don't take within 2 hours of taking another medicine. Laxative interferes with medicine absorption.

POSSIBLE ADVERSE REACTIONS OR SIDE EFFECTS

SYMPTOMS	WHAT TO DO
Life-threatening:	
In case of overdose, see previous column.	
Common:	
• Rectal irritation.	Continue. Call doctor when convenient.
• Pink to orange urine.	No action necessary.
Infrequent:	
• Dangerous potassium loss (thirst, weakness, heartbeat irregularity, paralysis, and diarrhea).	Discontinue. Call doctor right away.
• Belching, cramps, nausea.	Continue. Call doctor when convenient.
Rare:	
Irritability, confusion, headache, rash, difficult breathing, irregular heartbeat, muscle cramps, unusual tiredness or weakness, burning on urination.	Discontinue. Call doctor right away.

WARNINGS & PRECAUTIONS

Don't take if:
- You have symptoms of appendicitis, inflamed bowel or intestinal blockage.
- You are allergic to a stimulant laxative.
- You have missed a bowel movement for only 1 or 2 days.

Before you start, consult your doctor:
- If you have a colostomy or ileostomy.
- If you have congestive heart disease.
- If you have diabetes.
- If you have high blood pressure.
- If you have a laxative habit.
- If you have rectal bleeding.
- If you take other laxatives.

Over age 60:
Adverse reactions and side effects may be more frequent and severe than in younger persons.

Pregnancy:
Decide with your doctor if drug benefits justify risk to unborn child. Risk category C (see page xxii).

Breast-feeding:
Drug passes into milk. Avoid drug or discontinue nursing until you finish medicine. Consult doctor for advice on maintaining milk supply.

Infants & children:
Use only under medical supervision.

Prolonged use:
Don't take for more than 1 week unless under a doctor's supervision. May cause laxative dependence.

Skin & sunlight:
No problems expected.

Driving, piloting or hazardous work:
No problems expected.

Discontinuing:
May be unnecessary to finish medicine. Follow doctor's instructions.

Others:
Don't take to "flush out" your system or as a "tonic."

POSSIBLE INTERACTION WITH OTHER DRUGS

GENERIC NAME OR DRUG CLASS	COMBINED EFFECT
Antacids*	Tablet coating may dissolve too rapidly, irritating stomach or bowel.
Antihypertensives*	May cause dangerous low potassium level.
Digitalis preparations*	Increased digitalis toxicity due to decreased serum potassium level.
Diuretics*	May cause dangerous low potassium level.

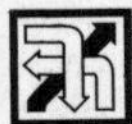

POSSIBLE INTERACTION WITH OTHER SUBSTANCES

INTERACTS WITH	COMBINED EFFECT
Alcohol:	None expected.
Beverages: Milk.	Tablet coating may dissolve too rapidly, irritating stomach or bowel.
Cocaine:	None expected.
Foods:	None expected.
Marijuana:	None expected.
Tobacco:	None expected.

*See Glossary

PHENOTHIAZINES

BRAND AND GENERIC NAMES

See complete list of brand and generic names in the *Brand Names Directory*, page 913.

BASIC INFORMATION

Habit forming? No
Prescription needed? Yes
Available as generic? Yes, for some.
Drug class: Tranquilizer, antiemetic (phenothiazine)

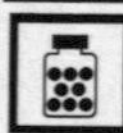

USES

- Stops nausea, vomiting, hiccups.
- Reduces anxiety, agitation.

DOSAGE & USAGE INFORMATION

How to take:
- Tablet or extended-release capsule—Swallow with liquid or food to lessen stomach irritation.
- Suppositories—Remove wrapper and moisten suppository with water. Gently insert into rectum, large end first.
- Drops or liquid—Dilute dose in beverage.

When to take:
- Nervous and mental disorders—Take at the same times each day.
- Nausea and vomiting—Take as needed, no more often than every 4 hours.

If you forget a dose:
- Nervous and mental disorders—Take up to 2 hours late. If more than 2 hours, wait for next scheduled dose (don't double this dose).
- Nausea and vomiting—Take as soon as you remember. Wait 4 hours for next dose.

What drug does:
- Suppresses brain's vomiting center.
- Suppresses brain centers that control abnormal emotions and behavior.

Continued next column

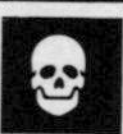

OVERDOSE

SYMPTOMS:
Stupor, convulsions, coma.
WHAT TO DO:
- **Dial 911 (emergency) or 0 (operator) for an ambulance or medical help. Then give first aid immediately.**
- **See emergency information on inside covers.**

Time lapse before drug works:
- Nausea and vomiting—1 hour or less.
- Nervous and mental disorders—4 to 6 weeks.

Don't take with:
- Antacid or medicine for diarrhea.
- Nonprescription drug for cough, cold or allergy.
- Any other medicine without consulting your doctor or pharmacist.

POSSIBLE ADVERSE REACTIONS OR SIDE EFFECTS

SYMPTOMS	WHAT TO DO
Life-threatening:	
Uncontrolled muscle movements of tongue, face and other muscles (neuroleptic malignant syndrome, rare).	Discontinue. Seek emergency treatment.
Common:	
• Muscle spasms of face and neck, unsteady gait.	Discontinue. Seek emergency treatment.
• Restlessness, tremor, drowsiness, blurred vision, lip smacking, worm-like movements of tongue.	Discontinue. Call doctor right away.
• Decreased sweating, dry mouth, stuffy nose, constipation.	Continue. Call doctor when convenient.
Infrequent:	
• Fainting.	Discontinue. Seek emergency treatment.
• Rash.	Discontinue. Call doctor right away.
• Difficult urination, decreased sex drive, swollen breasts, menstrual irregularities, dizziness.	Continue. Call doctor when convenient.
Rare:	
Vision changes, sore throat, fever, jaundice, abdominal pain, confusion, hot dry skin, prolonged penile erections.	Discontinue. Call doctor right away.

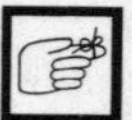

WARNINGS & PRECAUTIONS

Don't take if:
- You are allergic to any phenothiazine.
- You have a blood or bone marrow disease.

Before you start, consult your doctor:
- If you will have surgery within 2 months, including dental surgery, requiring general or spinal anesthesia.

- If you have asthma, emphysema or other lung disorder; glaucoma; or prostate trouble.
- If you take nonprescription ulcer medicine, asthma medicine or amphetamines.

Over age 60:
Adverse reactions and side effects may be more frequent and severe than in younger persons. More likely to develop involuntary movement of jaws, lips, tongue; chewing. Report this to your doctor immediately. Early treatment can help.

Pregnancy:
Risk factors vary for drugs in this group. See category list on page xxii and consult doctor.

Breast-feeding:
Drug passes into milk. Avoid drug or discontinue nursing until you finish medicine. Consult doctor for advice on maintaining milk supply.

Infants & children:
Don't give to children younger than 2.

Prolonged use:
- May lead to tardive dyskinesia (involuntary movement of jaws, lips, tongue; chewing).
- Talk to your doctor about the need for follow-up medical examinations or laboratory studies to check complete blood counts (white blood cell count, platelet count, red blood cell count, hemoglobin, hematocrit), blood pressure, liver function, eyes.

Skin & sunlight:
May cause rash or intensify sunburn in areas exposed to sun or sunlamp. Skin may remain sensitive for 3 months after discontinuing.

Driving, piloting or hazardous work:
Don't drive or pilot aircraft until you learn how medicine affects you. Don't work around dangerous machinery. Don't climb ladders or work in high places. Danger increases if you drink alcohol or take medicine affecting alertness and reflexes.

Discontinuing:
- Nervous and mental disorders—Don't discontinue without doctor's advice until you complete prescribed dose, even though symptoms diminish or disappear.
- Nausea and vomiting—May be unnecessary to finish medicine. Follow doctor's instructions.

Others:
- No problems expected.
- Advise any doctor or dentist whom you consult that you take this medicine.

POSSIBLE INTERACTION WITH OTHER DRUGS

GENERIC NAME OR DRUG CLASS	COMBINED EFFECT
Anticholinergics*	Increased anticholinergic effect.
Antidepressants, tricyclic*	Increased phenothiazine effect.
Antihistamines*	Increased antihistamine effect.
Antihypertensives*	Severe low blood pressure.
Antithyroid agents*	Increased risk of blood disorders.
Appetite suppressants*	Decreased appetite suppressant effect.
Bupropion	Increased risk of major seizures.
Calcium supplements*	Decreased phenothiazine effect.
Clozapine	Toxic effect on the central nervous system.
Dronabinol	Increased effects of both drugs. Avoid.
Guanethidine	Increased guanethidine effect.
Isoniazid	Increased risk of liver damage.
Levodopa	Decreased levodopa effect.
Lithium	Decreased lithium effect.
Mind-altering drugs*	Increased effect of mind-altering drug.
Metrizamide	Increased seizures.
Metyrosine	Increased likelihood of toxic symptoms of each.

Continued on page 954

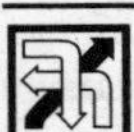

POSSIBLE INTERACTION WITH OTHER SUBSTANCES

INTERACTS WITH	COMBINED EFFECT
Alcohol:	Dangerous oversedation. Avoid
Beverages:	None expected.
Cocaine:	Decreased phenothiazine effect. Avoid.
Foods:	None expected.
Marijuana:	Drowsiness. May increase antinausea effect.
Tobacco:	None expected.

*See Glossary

PHENYLEPHRINE

BRAND NAMES

See complete list of brand names in the *Brand Name Directory*, page 914.

BASIC INFORMATION

Habit forming? No
Prescription needed? No
Available as generic? Yes
Drug class: Sympathomimetic

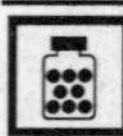

USES

- Temporary relief of congestion of nose, sinuses and throat caused by allergies, colds or sinusitis.
- Treats congestion of eustachian tubes caused by middle ear infections.

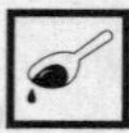

DOSAGE & USAGE INFORMATION

How to take:
According to package directions.

When to take:
As needed, no more often than every 4 hours.

If you forget a dose:
Take when you remember. Wait 4 hours for next dose. Never double a dose.

What drug does:
Contracts blood vessel walls of nose, sinus and throat tissues, enlarging airways.

Time lapse before drug works:
5 to 30 minutes.

Don't take with:
- Nonprescription drugs for asthma, cough, cold, allergy, appetite suppressants, sleeping pills or drugs containing caffeine without consulting doctor.
- See Interaction column and consult doctor.

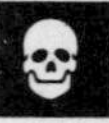

OVERDOSE

SYMPTOMS:
Headache, heart palpitations, vomiting, blood pressure rise, slow and forceful pulse.
WHAT TO DO:
- **Dial 911 (emergency) or 0 (operator) for an ambulance or medical help. Then give first aid immediately.**
- **See emergency information on inside covers.**

POSSIBLE ADVERSE REACTIONS OR SIDE EFFECTS

SYMPTOMS	WHAT TO DO
Life-threatening:	
In case of overdose, see previous column.	
Common:	
• Fast or pounding heartbeat.	Discontinue. Call doctor right away.
• Headache or dizziness; shakiness; insomnia; burning, dryness, stinging inside nose; nervousness.	Continue. Call doctor when convenient.
Infrequent:	
Paleness.	Continue. Call doctor when convenient.
Rare:	
Unusual sweating.	Discontinue. Call doctor right away.

WARNINGS & PRECAUTIONS

Don't take if:
You are allergic to any sympathomimetic.

Before you start, consult your doctor:
- If you have high blood pressure.
- If you have heart disease.
- If you have diabetes.
- If you have overactive thyroid.
- If you have taken MAO inhibitors in past 2 weeks.

Over age 60:
Adverse reactions and side effects may be more frequent and severe than in younger persons.

Pregnancy:
Decide with your doctor if drug benefits justify risk to unborn child. Risk category C (see page xxii).

Breast-feeding:
Drug passes into milk. Avoid drug or discontinue nursing until you finish medicine. Consult doctor for advice on maintaining milk supply.

Infants & children:
Use only under close supervision.

Prolonged use:
- Rebound* congestion and chemical irritation of nasal membranes.
- May cause functional dependence.
- Talk to your doctor about the need for follow-up medical examinations or laboratory studies to check blood pressure, ECG*.

Skin & sunlight:
No problems expected.

Driving, piloting or hazardous work:
No problems expected.

Discontinuing:
May be unnecessary to finish medicine. Follow doctor's instructions.

Others:
No problems expected.

POSSIBLE INTERACTION WITH OTHER DRUGS

GENERIC NAME OR DRUG CLASS	COMBINED EFFECT
Alpha-adrenergic blocking agents*	Increased risk of low blood pressure.
Amphetamines*	Increased nervousness.
Antiasthmatics*	Nervous stimulation.
Antidepressants, tricyclic*	Increased phenylephrine effect.
Antihypertensives*	Decreased anti-hypertensive effect.
Beta-adrenergic blocking agents*	Decreased effect of both drugs.
Digitalis preparations*	Decreased digitalis effect.
Doxapam	Decreased effect of both drugs.
Ergoloid mesylates*	Increased risk of vascular problems and gangrene. Avoid.
Ergotamine	Increased risk of vascular problems and gangrene. Avoid.
Furazolidine	Sudden, severe increase in blood pressure.
Guanadrel	Decreased effect of both drugs.
Methyldopa	Possible increased blood pressure.
Monoamine oxidase (MAO) inhibitors*	Dangerous blood pressure rise.
Nicotine	Decreased phenylephrine effect.
Nitrates*	Possible decreased effects of both drugs.
Oxprenolol	Decreased effects of both drugs.
Phenothiazines*	Possible increased phenylephrine toxicity. Possible decreased phenylephrine effect.
Rauwolfia	Decreased rauwolfia effect.
Sedatives*	Decreased sedative effect.
Sympathomimetics*, other	Increased stimulant effect.
Tranquilizers*	Decreased tranquilizer effect.

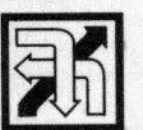

POSSIBLE INTERACTION WITH OTHER SUBSTANCES

INTERACTS WITH	COMBINED EFFECT
Alcohol:	None expected.
Beverages: Caffeine drinks.	Excess brain stimulation.
Cocaine:	Excess brain stimulation.
Foods:	None expected.
Marijuana:	None expected.
Tobacco:	None expected.

*See Glossary

PHENYLEPHRINE (Ophthalmic)

BRAND NAMES

Ak-Dilate
Ak-Nefrin
Dilatair
I-Phrine
Isopto Frin
Minims Phenylephrine
Mydfrin
Neo-Synephrine
Ocugestrin
Ocu-Phrin
Prefrin Liquifilm
Relief Eye Drops for Red Eyes
Spersaphrine

BASIC INFORMATION

Habit forming? No
Prescription needed? Yes, some strengths
Available as generic? No
Drug class: Mydriatic, decongestant

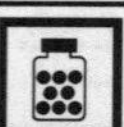

USES

- High-concentration drops—Dilates pupils.
- Low-concentration drops (available without prescription)—Relieves minor eye irritations caused by colds, hay fever, dust, wind, swimming, sun, smog, hard contact lenses, eye strain, smoke.

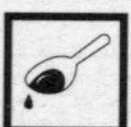

DOSAGE & USAGE INFORMATION

How to use:
Eye drops
- Wash hands.
- Apply pressure to inside corner of eye with middle finger.
- Continue pressure for 1 minute after placing medicine in eye.
- Tilt head backward. Pull lower lid away from eye with index finger of the same hand.
- Drop eye drops into pouch and close eye. Don't blink.
- Keep eyes closed for 1 to 2 minutes.
- Don't touch applicator tip to any surface (including the eye). If you accidentally touch tip, clean with warm soap and water.
- Keep container tightly closed.
- Keep cool, but don't freeze.
- Wash hands immediately after using.

Continued next column

OVERDOSE

SYMPTOMS:
None expected.
WHAT TO DO:
Not intended for internal use. If child accidentally swallows, call poison control center.

When to use:
As directed on label.

If you forget a dose:
Use as soon as you remember.

What drug does:
Acts on small blood vessels to make them constrict.

Time lapse before drug works:
15 to 90 minutes.

Don't use with:
- Other eye drops or ointment without consulting your eye doctor.
- Antidepressants*, guanadrel, guanethidine, maprotiline, pargyline, any monoamine oxidase (MAO) inhibitor*.

POSSIBLE ADVERSE REACTIONS OR SIDE EFFECTS

SYMPTOMS	WHAT TO DO
Life-threatening	
None expected, unless you use much more than directed.	Discontinue. Call doctor right away.
Common	
None expected.	
Infrequent	
None expected, unless you use much more than directed. If too much is used—Burning or stinging eyes, headache, watery eyes, eye irritation not present before.	Continue. Call doctor when convenient.
Rare	
None expected, unless you use much more than directed. If too much gets absorbed—Paleness, dizziness, tremor, increased sweating, irregular or fast heartbeat.	Discontinue. Call doctor right away.

PHENYLEPHRINE (Ophthalmic)

WARNINGS & PRECAUTIONS

Don't use if:
- You are allergic to phenylephrine.
- You have glaucoma.

Before you start, consult your doctor:
- If you have heart disease with irregular heartbeat, high blood pressure, diabetes.
- If you take antidepressants*, guanadrel, guanethidine, maprotiline, pargyline, any monoamine oxidase (MAO) inhibitor*.

Over age 60:
Adverse reactions and side effects may be more frequent and severe than in younger persons. Ask doctor about smaller doses.

Pregnancy:
Decide with your doctor if drug benefits justify risk to unborn child. Risk category C (see page xxii).

Breast-feeding:
Safety not established. Consult doctor.

Infants & children:
Use only under close medical supervision.

Prolonged use:
Avoid if possible.

Skin & sunlight:
Sometimes causes increased sensitivity to sunlight.

Driving, piloting or hazardous work:
No problems expected.

Discontinuing:
No problems expected.

Others:
- Keep cool, but don't freeze.
- Consult doctor if condition doesn't improve in 3 to 4 days.

POSSIBLE INTERACTION WITH OTHER DRUGS

GENERIC NAME OR DRUG CLASS	COMBINED EFFECT
Clinically significant interactions with oral or injected medicines unlikely.	

POSSIBLE INTERACTION WITH OTHER SUBSTANCES

INTERACTS WITH	COMBINED EFFECT
Alcohol:	None expected.
Beverages:	None expected.
Cocaine:	None expected.
Foods:	None expected.
Marijuana:	None expected.
Tobacco:	None expected.

*See Glossary

PHENYLPROPANOLAMINE

BRAND NAMES

See complete list of brand names in the *Brand Name Directory*, page 914.

BASIC INFORMATION

Habit forming? No
Prescription needed?
High strength: Yes
Low strength: No
Available as generic? Yes
Drug class: Sympathomimetic

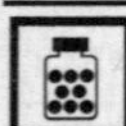

USES

- Relieves bronchial asthma.
- Decreases congestion of breathing passages.
- Suppresses allergic reactions.
- Decreases appetite. Used for obesity.
- Treatment for urinary incontinence.

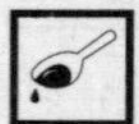

DOSAGE & USAGE INFORMATION

How to take:
- Tablet—Swallow with liquid. You may chew or crush tablet.
- Extended-release capsules—Swallow each dose whole.

When to take:
As needed, no more often than every 4 hours.

If you forget a dose:
Take up to 2 hours late. If more than 2 hours, wait for next dose (don't double this dose).

What drug does:
- Prevents cells from releasing allergy-causing chemicals (histamines).
- Relaxes muscles of bronchial tubes.
- Decreases blood vessel size and blood flow, thus causing decongestion.

Time lapse before drug works:
30 to 60 minutes.

Continued next column

OVERDOSE

SYMPTOMS:
Severe anxiety, confusion, delirium, muscle tremors, rapid and irregular pulse.
WHAT TO DO:
- **Dial 911 (emergency) or 0 (operator) for an ambulance or medical help. Then give first aid immediately.**
- **See emergency information on inside covers.**

Don't take with:
- Nonprescription drugs for cough, cold, allergy or asthma without consulting doctor.
- See Interaction column and consult doctor.

POSSIBLE ADVERSE REACTIONS OR SIDE EFFECTS

SYMPTOMS	WHAT TO DO
Life-threatening:	
In case of overdose, see previous column.	
Common:	
• Rapid heartbeat.	Discontinue. Call doctor right away.
• Nervousness, headache, paleness.	Continue. Call doctor when convenient.
• Insomnia.	Continue. Tell doctor at next visit.
Infrequent:	
• Irregular heartbeat.	Discontinue. Call doctor right away.
• Dizziness, appetite loss, nausea, vomiting, difficult urination, nightmares, weakness.	Continue. Call doctor when convenient.
Rare:	
Tightness in chest.	Discontinue. Call doctor right away.

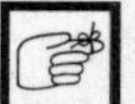

WARNINGS & PRECAUTIONS

Don't take if:
You are allergic to any sympathomimetic drug*.

Before you start, consult your doctor:
- If you have high blood pressure, diabetes, overactive thyroid gland, difficulty urinating.
- If you have taken any MAO inhibitors in past 2 weeks.
- If you have taken digitalis preparations in the last 7 days.
- If you will have surgery within 2 months, including dental surgery, requiring general or spinal anesthesia.
- If you take any other over-the-counter medicine.

Over age 60:
More likely to develop high blood pressure, heart rhythm disturbances and angina and to feel drug's stimulant effects.

Pregnancy:
Decide with your doctor if drug benefits justify risk to unborn child. Risk category C (see page xxii).

Breast-feeding:
Safety not established. Consult doctor.

Infants & children:
Don't give to children under 6 years old.

Prolonged use:
- Excessive doses—Rare toxic psychosis.
- Men with enlarged prostate gland may have more urination difficulty.
- Talk to your doctor about the need for follow-up medical examinations or laboratory studies.

Skin & sunlight:
No known problems.

Driving, piloting or hazardous work:
No restrictions unless you feel dizzy.

Discontinuing:
May be unnecessary to finish medicine. Follow doctor's instructions.

Others:
No problems expected.

POSSIBLE INTERACTION WITH OTHER DRUGS

GENERIC NAME OR DRUG CLASS	COMBINED EFFECT
Anesthetics, general*	Increased phenylpropanolamine effect.
Antidepressants, tricyclic*	Increased phenylpropanolamine effect. Excessive stimulation of heart and blood pressure.
Antihypertensives*	Decreased antihypertensive effect.
Beta-adrenergic blocking agents*	Decreased effect of both drugs.
Central nervous system (CNS) stimulants*	Increased CNS stimulation.
Digitalis preparations*	Serious heart rhythm disturbances.
Epinephrine	Increased epinephrine effect.
Ergot preparations*	Serious blood pressure rise.
Guanethidine	Decreased effect of both drugs.
Guanadrel	Decreased effect of both drugs.
Methyldopa	Possible increased blood pressure.
Monoamine oxidase (MAO) inhibitors*	Increased pheny propanolamine effect. Dangerous blood pressure rise.
Nitrates*	Possible decreased effects of both drugs.
Phenothiazines*	Possible increased phenypropanolamine toxicity. Possible decreased phenylpropanolamine effect.
Rauwolfia	Decreased rauwolfia effect.
Sympathomimetics*	Increased phenypropanolamine effect.
Terazosin	Decreased effectiveness of terazosin.

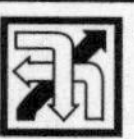

POSSIBLE INTERACTION WITH OTHER SUBSTANCES

INTERACTS WITH	COMBINED EFFECT
Alcohol:	Increased sedation.
Beverages: Caffeine drinks.	Nervousness or insomnia.
Cocaine:	High risk of heartbeat irregularities and high blood pressure.
Foods:	None expected.
Marijuana:	Rapid heartbeat, possible heart rhythm disturbance. Avoid.
Tobacco:	None expected.

***See Glossary**

PILOCARPINE

BRAND NAMES

Adsorbocarpine	Pilokair
Akarpine	Pilopine HS
Almocarpine	Piloptic
I-Pilocarpine	Pilostat
Isopto Carpine	P.V. Carpine
Minims Pilocarpine	P.V. Carpine Liquifilm
Miocarpine	Salagen
Ocu-Carpine	Spectro-Pilo
Ocusert Pilo	Spersacarpine
Pilocar	

BASIC INFORMATION

Habit forming? No
Prescription needed?
U.S.: Yes
Canada: No
Available as generic? Yes
Drug class: Antiglaucoma

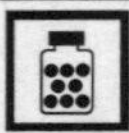

USES

Treatment for glaucoma.

DOSAGE & USAGE INFORMATION

How to take:

- Drops—Apply to eyes. Close eyes for 1 or 2 minutes to absorb medicine.
- Eye system—Follow label directions.
- Gel—Follow label directions.

Continued next column

OVERDOSE

SYMPTOMS:
If swallowed—Nausea, vomiting, diarrhea, forceful urination, profuse sweating, rapid pulse, breathing difficulty, loss of consciousness.
WHAT TO DO:

- **Dial 911 (emergency) or 0 (operator) for an ambulance or medical help. Then give first aid immediately.**
- **If patient is unconscious and not breathing, give mouth-to-mouth breathing. If there is no heartbeat, use cardiac massage and mouth-to-mouth breathing (CPR). Don't try to make patient vomit. If you can't get help quickly, take patient to nearest emergency facility.**
- **See emergency information on inside covers.**

When to use:
As directed on label.

If you forget a dose:
Apply as soon as possible, then return to prescribed schedule. Don't double dose.

What drug does:
Reduces internal eye pressure.

Time lapse before drug works:
15 to 30 minutes.

Don't take with:
Any other medicine without consulting your doctor or pharmacist.

POSSIBLE ADVERSE REACTIONS OR SIDE EFFECTS

SYMPTOMS	WHAT TO DO
Life-threatening: In case of overdose, see previous column.	
Common: Pain, blurred or altered vision.	Continue. Call doctor when convenient.
Infrequent: • Headache, eye irritation or twitching, nausea, vomiting, diarrhea, difficult breathing, muscle tremors.	Discontinue. Call doctor right away.
• Profuse sweating, unusual saliva flow.	Continue. Call doctor when convenient.
Rare: None expected.	

WARNINGS & PRECAUTIONS

Don't take if:
You are allergic to pilocarpine.

Before you start, consult your doctor:
- If you take sedatives, sleeping pills, tranquilizers, antidepressants, antihistamines, narcotics or mind-altering drugs.
- If you have asthma.
- If you have conjunctivitis (pink eye).

Over age 60:
Adverse reactions and side effects may be more frequent and severe than in younger persons.

Pregnancy:
Decide with your doctor if drug benefits justify risk to unborn child. Risk category C (see page xxii).

Breast-feeding:
Effect unknown. Consult doctor.

Infants & children:
Not recommended.

Prolonged use:
- You may develop tolerance for drug, making it ineffective.
- Talk to your doctor about the need for follow-up medical examinations to check eye pressure.

Skin & sunlight:
No problems expected.

Driving, piloting or hazardous work:
Don't drive or pilot aircraft until you learn how medicine affects you. Don't work around dangerous machinery. Don't climb ladders or work in high places. Danger increases if you drink alcohol or take medicine affecting alertness and reflexes, such as antihistamines, tranquilizers, sedatives, pain medicine, narcotics and mind-altering drugs.

Discontinuing:
Doctor may discontinue and substitute another drug to keep treatment effective.

Others:
- Can provoke asthma attack in susceptible individuals.
- Drops may impair vision for 2 to 3 hours.

POSSIBLE INTERACTION WITH OTHER DRUGS

GENERIC NAME OR DRUG CLASS	COMBINED EFFECT
Belladonna (ophthalmic)	Decreased pilocarpine effect.
Cyclopentolate	Decreased pilocarpine effect.

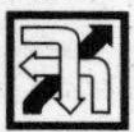

POSSIBLE INTERACTION WITH OTHER SUBSTANCES

INTERACTS WITH	COMBINED EFFECT
Alcohol:	May prolong alcohol's effect on brain.
Beverages:	None expected.
Cocaine:	Decreased pilocarpine effect. Avoid.
Foods:	None expected.
Marijuana (if prescribed):	Used once or twice weekly—May help lower internal eye pressure.
Tobacco:	None expected.

PODOPHYLLUM (Topical)

BRAND NAMES

Podofin

BASIC INFORMATION

Habit forming? No
Prescription needed? Yes
Available as generic? No
Drug class: Cytotoxic (topical)

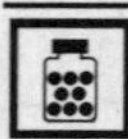

USES

Treats venereal warts *(condylomata acuminata)*.

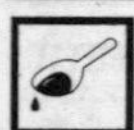

DOSAGE & USAGE INFORMATION

How to use:

- Apply petroleum jelly on normal skin surrounding warts.
- With a glass applicator or cotton swab, carefully apply podophyllum to the warts.
- Wash hands immediately after application.
- Allow to remain on warts for 1 to 6 hours after application, then remove with soap and water.

When to use:
Follow doctor's instructions. Usually at 1-week intervals.

If you forget a dose:
Apply it as soon as you remember, then return to regular schedule.

What drug does:
Kills cells and erodes tissue.

Time lapse before drug works:
Up to 4 weeks.

Don't use with:
Any other medicines (including over-the-counter drugs such as cough and cold medicines, laxatives, antacids, diet pills, caffeine, nose drops or vitamins) without consulting your doctor.

OVERDOSE

SYMPTOMS:
The following symptoms occur when the body absorbs too much podophyllum: Seizures, painful urination, breathing difficulty, dizziness, heartbeat irregularity, numbness and tingling of hands and feet, abdominal pain, excitement, irritability.
WHAT TO DO:

- **Dial 911 (emergency) or 0 (operator) for an ambulance or medical help. Then give first aid immediately.**
- **See emergency information on inside covers.**

POSSIBLE ADVERSE REACTIONS OR SIDE EFFECTS

SYMPTOMS	WHAT TO DO
Life-threatening:	
In case of overdose, see previous column.	
Common:	
Burning, red skin.	Discontinue. Call doctor right away.
Infrequent:	
Skin rash, hallucinations, diarrhea, nausea and vomiting, unusual bleeding.	Discontinue. Call doctor right away.
Rare:	
In case of overdose, see previous column.	

WARNINGS & PRECAUTIONS

Don't use if:
Warts are crumbled and bleeding.

Before you start, consult your doctor:
If you have used podophyllum before.

Over age 60:
No special problems expected.

Pregnancy:
Risk to unborn child outweighs drug benefits. Don't use. Risk factor not designated, but see category list on page xxii.

Breast-feeding:
Drug passes into milk. Avoid drug or discontinue nursing until you finish medicine. Consult doctor for advice on maintaining milk supply.

Infants & children:
No special problems expected.

Prolonged use:
Increased chance of adverse reactions.

Skin & sunlight:
No problems expected.

Driving, piloting or hazardous work:
Avoid if you feel confused, drowsy or dizzy.

Discontinuing:
No special problems expected.

Others:
- Advise any doctor or dentist whom you consult that you take this medicine.
- Keep away from eyes, nose and mouth.
- Don't use on moles or birthmarks.
- Don't use near heat or open flame.

POSSIBLE INTERACTION WITH OTHER DRUGS

GENERIC NAME OR DRUG CLASS	COMBINED EFFECT
None significant.	

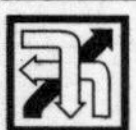

POSSIBLE INTERACTION WITH OTHER SUBSTANCES

INTERACTS WITH	COMBINED EFFECT
Alcohol:	Increased chance of central nervous system stimulation. Avoid.
Beverages:	No special problems expected.
Cocaine:	Increased chance of central nervous system stimulation. Avoid.
Foods:	No special problems expected.
Marijuana:	Increased chance of central nervous system stimulation. Avoid.
Tobacco:	Podophyllum is flammable. Don't use while smoking.

POLOXAMER 188

BRAND NAMES

Alaxin
Poloxalkol

BASIC INFORMATION

Habit forming? No
Prescription needed? No
Available as generic? Yes
Drug class: Laxative (emollient)

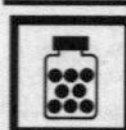

USES

Constipation relief.

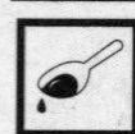

DOSAGE & USAGE INFORMATION

How to take:
Capsule—Swallow with liquid. Don't open capsules.

When to take:
At the same time each day, preferably bedtime.

If you forget a dose:
Take as soon as you remember. Wait 12 hours for next dose, then return to regular schedule.

What drug does:
Makes stool hold fluid so it is easier to pass.

Time lapse before drug works:
2 to 3 days of continual use.

Don't take with:
- Other medicines at same time. Wait 2 hours.
- Any other medicine without consulting your doctor or pharmacist.

OVERDOSE

SYMPTOMS:
Appetite loss, nausea, vomiting, diarrhea.
WHAT TO DO:
Overdose unlikely to threaten life. If person takes much larger amount than prescribed, call doctor, poison control center or hospital emergency room for instructions.

POSSIBLE ADVERSE REACTIONS OR SIDE EFFECTS

SYMPTOMS	WHAT TO DO
Life-threatening: None expected.	
Common: None expected.	
Infrequent: Throat irritation (liquid only), intestinal and abdominal cramps.	Continue. Call doctor when convenient.
Rare: Rash.	Discontinue. Call doctor right away.

WARNINGS & PRECAUTIONS

Don't take if:

- You are allergic to any emollient laxative.
- You have abdominal pain and fever that might be appendicitis.

Before you start, consult your doctor:

- If you are taking other laxatives.
- To be sure constipation isn't a sign of a serious disorder.

Over age 60:
You must drink 6 to 8 glasses of fluid every 24 hours for drug to work.

Pregnancy:
Risk factor not designated, but see category list on page xxii.

Breast-feeding:
No problems expected. Consult doctor.

Infants & children:
No problems expected.

Prolonged use:
Avoid. Overuse of laxatives may damage intestine lining.

Skin & sunlight:
No problems expected.

Driving, piloting or hazardous work:
No problems expected.

Discontinuing:
May be unnecessary to finish medicine. Follow doctor's instructions.

Others:
No problems expected.

POSSIBLE INTERACTION WITH OTHER DRUGS

GENERIC NAME OR DRUG CLASS	COMBINED EFFECT
Danthron	Possible liver damage.
Digitalis preparations*	Toxic absorption of digitalis.
Mineral oil	Increased mineral oil absorption into bloodstream. Avoid.
Phenolphthalein	Increased phenolphthalein absorption. Possible toxicity.

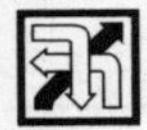

POSSIBLE INTERACTION WITH OTHER SUBSTANCES

INTERACTS WITH	COMBINED EFFECT
Alcohol:	None expected.
Beverages:	None expected.
Cocaine:	None expected.
Foods:	None expected.
Marijuana:	None expected.
Tobacco:	None expected.

*See Glossary

POLYCARBOPHIL CALCIUM

BRAND NAMES

Equalactin
FiberCon
Mitrolan

BASIC INFORMATION

Habit forming? No
Prescription needed? No
Available as generic? Yes
Drug class: Laxative (bulk-forming), antidiarrheal

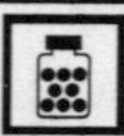

USES

- Relieves constipation and prevents straining for bowel movement.
- Stops diarrhea.

DOSAGE & USAGE INFORMATION

How to take:
- Tablets (laxative)—Swallow with 8 oz. cold liquid. Drink 6 to 8 glasses of water each day in addition to the one with each dose.
- Tablets (diarrhea)—Follow package instructions.
- Chewable tablets—Chew well before swallowing.

When to take:
At the same times each day.

If you forget a dose:
Take as soon as you remember, then resume regular schedule.

What drug does:
Absorbs water, stimulating the bowel to form a soft, bulky stool and decreasing watery diarrhea.

Time lapse before drug works:
May require 2 or 3 days to begin, then works in 12 to 24 hours.

Don't take with:
- Any other medicine without consulting your doctor or pharmacist.
- Don't take within 2 hours of taking another medicine.

OVERDOSE

SYMPTOMS:
None expected.
WHAT TO DO:
Overdose unlikely to threaten life. If person takes much larger amount than prescribed, call doctor, poison control center or hospital emergency room for instructions.

POSSIBLE ADVERSE REACTIONS OR SIDE EFFECTS

SYMPTOMS	WHAT TO DO
Life-threatening: None expected.	
Common: None expected.	
Infrequent: Swallowing difficulty, "lump in throat" sensation, nausea, vomiting, diarrhea.	Continue. Call doctor when convenient.
Rare: Itchy skin, rash, intestinal blockage, asthma.	Discontinue. Call doctor right away.

WARNINGS & PRECAUTIONS

Don't take if:
- You are allergic to any bulk-forming laxative.
- You have symptoms of appendicitis, inflamed bowel or intestinal blockage.
- You have missed a bowel movement for only 1 or 2 days.

Before you start, consult your doctor:
- If you have diabetes.
- If you have a laxative habit.
- If you have rectal bleeding.
- If you have difficulty swallowing.
- If you take other laxatives.

Over age 60:
Adverse reactions and side effects may be more frequent and severe than in younger persons.

Pregnancy:
Most bulk-forming laxatives contain sodium or sugars which may cause fluid retention. Avoid if possible. Consult doctor. Risk factor not designated, but see category list on page xxii.

Breast-feeding:
No problems expected. Consult doctor.

Infants & children:
Use only under medical supervision.

Prolonged use:
Don't take for more than 1 week unless under a doctor's supervision. May cause laxative dependence.

Skin & sunlight:
No problems expected.

Driving, piloting or hazardous work:
No problems expected.

Discontinuing:
May be unnecessary to finish medicine. Follow doctor's instructions.

Others:
- Don't take to "flush out" your system or as a "tonic."
- Blockage of the throat or esophagus may occur if drug is not taken with an adequate amount of water.

POSSIBLE INTERACTION WITH OTHER DRUGS

GENERIC NAME OR DRUG CLASS	COMBINED EFFECT
Digitalis preparations*	Decreased digitalis effect.
Salicylates* (including aspirin)	Decreased salicylate effect.
Tetracyclines*	Decreased tetracycline effect.

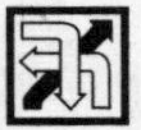

POSSIBLE INTERACTION WITH OTHER SUBSTANCES

INTERACTS WITH	COMBINED EFFECT
Alcohol:	None expected.
Beverages:	None expected.
Cocaine:	None expected.
Foods:	None expected.
Marijuana:	None expected.
Tobacco:	None expected.

***See Glossary**

POTASSIUM IODIDE

BRAND NAMES

Pima	KI
Thyro-Block	SSKI

BASIC INFORMATION

Habit forming? No
Prescription needed? Yes
Available as generic? Yes
Drug class: Antihyperthyroid

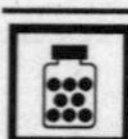

USES

- Treats overactive thyroid disease.
- Treats iodine deficiency.
- Formerly used to decrease thickness of bronchial secretions.

DOSAGE & USAGE INFORMATION

How to take:
Tablets or syrup—Take in full glass of water, fruit juice, milk or broth.

When to take:
- Take after meals and at bedtime with food or milk.
- Follow your doctor's instructions.

If you forget a dose:
Take as soon as you remember up to 2 hours late. If more than 2 hours, wait for next scheduled dose (don't double this dose).

What drug does:
Decreases release of thyroid hormone.

Time lapse before drug works:
Approximately 10 days.

Don't take with:
Any other medicines (including over-the-counter drugs such as cough and cold medicines, laxatives, antacids, diet pills, caffeine, nose drops or vitamins) without consulting your doctor.

OVERDOSE

SYMPTOMS:
None expected.
WHAT TO DO:
Overdose unlikely to threaten life. If person takes much larger amount than prescribed, call doctor, poison control center or hospital emergency room for instructions.

POSSIBLE ADVERSE REACTIONS OR SIDE EFFECTS

SYMPTOMS	WHAT TO DO
Life-threatening:	
Black or tarry stools.	Discontinue. Seek emergency treatment.
Common:	
• Skin rash, swollen salivary glands.	Discontinue. Call doctor right away.
• Diarrhea, nausea, abdominal pain.	Continue. Call doctor when convenient.
Infrequent:	
Burning mouth, severe headache, increased salivation.	Discontinue. Call doctor right away.
Rare:	
Confusion, fever, heartbeat irregularities, numbness and tingling of feet and hands, swollen neck, unusual tiredness.	Discontinue. Call doctor right away.

WARNINGS & PRECAUTIONS

Don't take if:
You are intolerant of or allergic to potassium iodide.

Before you start, consult your doctor:
If you have kidney disease.

Over age 60:
No special problems expected.

Pregnancy:
Risk to unborn child outweighs drug benefits. Don't use. Risk category D (see page xxii).

Breast-feeding:
Drug passes into milk. Avoid drug or discontinue nursing until you finish medicine. Consult doctor for advice on maintaining milk supply.

Infants & children:
Avoid.

Prolonged use:
- Talk to your doctor about the need for follow-up medical examinations or laboratory studies to check serum potassium levels.
- If burning mouth, headache or salivation occur, discontinue and call doctor.

Skin & sunlight:
No problems expected.

Driving, piloting or hazardous work:
Avoid if you feel confused, drowsy or dizzy.

Discontinuing:
No special problems expected.

Others:
- Advise any doctor or dentist whom you consult that you take this medicine.
- Don't use if solution turns yellow.

POSSIBLE INTERACTION WITH OTHER DRUGS

GENERIC NAME OR DRUG CLASS	COMBINED EFFECT
Angiotensin-converting enzyme (ACE) inhibitors*	May raise potassium in blood to toxic levels.
Antithyroid drugs*	Excessive effect of antithyroid drugs.
Diuretics, potassium-sparing	May raise potassium in blood to toxic levels.
Lithium	Increased chance of producing a thyroid goiter.

POSSIBLE INTERACTION WITH OTHER SUBSTANCES

INTERACTS WITH	COMBINED EFFECT
Alcohol:	No special problems expected.
Beverages:	No special problems expected.
Cocaine:	No special problems expected.
Foods: Foods high in iodine.	Too much iodine in blood.
Marijuana:	No special problems expected.
Tobacco:	No special problems expected.

***See Glossary**

POTASSIUM PHOSPHATES

BRAND NAMES

K-Phos Original
Neutra-Phos K

BASIC INFORMATION

Habit forming? No
Prescription needed? Yes, for some
Available as generic? Yes, for some
Drug class: Electrolyte replenisher

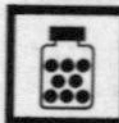

USES

- Provides supplement of phosphorus for people with diseases which decrease phosphorus absorption from food.
- Treatment of hypercalcemia due to cancer.

DOSAGE & USAGE INFORMATION

How to take:

- Tablets—Dissolve tablets in 3/4 to 1 glass of water. Let tablets soak 2 to 5 minutes, then stir to completely dissolve.
- Oral solution—Follow directions on label.

When to take:
After meals or with food to prevent or lessen stomach irritation or loose stools.

If you forget a dose:
Take within 1 hour then return to original schedule. If later than 1 hour, skip dose. Don't double dose.

What drug does:

- Provides supplemental phosphates.
- Makes uric acid.

Time lapse before drug works:
30-60 minutes.

Don't take with:
Any other medicine without consulting your doctor or pharmacist.

OVERDOSE

SYMPTOMS:
Irregular heartbeat, blood pressure drop with weakness, coma, cardiac arrest.
WHAT TO DO:

- **Dial 911 (emergency) or 0 (operator) for an ambulance or medical help. Then give first aid immediately.**
- **See emergency information on inside covers.**

POSSIBLE ADVERSE REACTIONS OR SIDE EFFECTS

SYMPTOMS	WHAT TO DO
Life-threatening:	
Irregular heartbeat, shortness of breath, seizures.	Discontinue. Seek emergency treatment.
Common:	
Muscle cramps.	Discontinue. Call doctor right away.
Infrequent:	
Bone and joint pain, numbness or tingling in hands or feet, unusual tiredness, weakness, diarrhea, nausea, abdominal pain, vomiting, confusion, headache, dizziness.	Discontinue. Call doctor right away.
Rare:	
Foot and leg swelling.	Discontinue. Call doctor right away.

WARNINGS & PRECAUTIONS

Don't take if:
You have had allergic reaction to potassium, sodium or phosphates; severe kidney disease; severe burns.

Before you start, consult your doctor:
If you have heart problems, adrenalin sufficiency, liver disease, high blood pressure, pregnancy, hypoparathyroidism, chronic kidney disease, osteomalacia, pancreatitis, rickets.

Over age 60:
Adverse reactions and side effects may be more frequent and severe than in younger persons. Ask doctor about smaller doses.

Pregnancy:
Decide with your doctor if drug benefits justify risk to unborn child. Risk category C (see page xxii).

Breast-feeding:
Effect unknown. Consult doctor.

Infants & children:
Use only under medical supervision.

Prolonged use:
Monitor ECG*, serum calcium, phosphorus and potassium levels.

Skin & sunlight:
No problems expected.

Driving, piloting or hazardous work:
Avoid if medicine causes dizziness or confusion.

Discontinuing:
Don't discontinue without consulting doctor. Dose may require gradual reduction if you have taken drug for a long time. Doses of other drugs may also require adjustment.

Others:
Protect liquid medicine from freezing.

POSSIBLE INTERACTION WITH OTHER DRUGS

GENERIC NAME OR DRUG CLASS	COMBINED EFFECT
Angiotensin-converting enzyme (ACE) inhibitors*	Level of potassium in blood too high.
Antacids*	May decrease potassium absorption.
Calcium	Decreased potassium effect.
Cortisone drugs*	Increased fluid retention.
Digitalis preparations*	Level of potassium in blood too high.
Diuretics* (amiloride, spironolactone, triamterene)	Level of potassium in blood too high.
Male hormones*	Fluid retention.
Potassium supplements*	Level of potassium in blood too high.
Vitamin D (calcifidiol and calcitriol)	Level of phosphorus in blood too high.

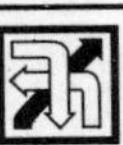

POSSIBLE INTERACTION WITH OTHER SUBSTANCES

INTERACTS WITH	COMBINED EFFECT
Alcohol:	None expected.
Beverages: Salty drinks such as tomato juice, commercial thirst quenchers, salt substitutes.	Increased fluid retention.
Cocaine:	May cause irregular heartbeat.
Foods: Salty foods such as canned soups, potato chips, TV dinners, hot dogs, pickles.	Increased fluid retention.
Marijuana:	May cause irregular heartbeat.
Tobacco:	May aggravate irregular heartbeat.

*See Glossary

POTASSIUM & SODIUM PHOSPHATES

BRAND AND GENERIC NAMES

DIBASIC POTASSIUM & SODIUM PHOSPHATES	MONOBASIC POTASSIUM & SODIUM PHOSPHATES
K-Phos M.F.	Neutra-Phos
K-Phos Neutral	Uro-KP-Neutral
K-Phos 2	

BASIC INFORMATION

Habit forming? No
Prescription needed? Yes
Available as generic? Yes
Drug class: Electrolyte replenisher

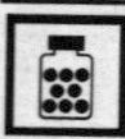

USES

- Provides supplement of phosphorus for people with diseases which decrease phosphorus absorption from food.
- Treatment of hypercalcemia due to cancer.

DOSAGE & USAGE INFORMATION

How to take:
- Tablets or capsules—Dissolve tablets or open capsules in 3/4 to 1 glass of water. Let tablets soak 2 to 5 minutes, then stir to completely dissolve.
- Oral solution—Take after meals with liquid to decrease stomach irritation.

When to take:
After meals or with food to prevent or lessen stomach irritation or loose stools.

If you forget a dose:
Take within 1 hour, then return to original schedule. If later than 1 hour, skip dose. Don't double dose.

Continued next column

OVERDOSE

SYMPTOMS:
Irregular heartbeat, blood pressure drop with weakness, coma, cardiac arrest.
WHAT TO DO:
- **Dial 911 (emergency) or 0 (operator) for an ambulance or medical help. Then give first aid immediately.**
- **See emergency information on inside covers.**

What drug does:
- Provides supplemental phosphates.
- Makes uric acid.

Time lapse before drug works:
30-60 minutes.

Don't take with:
Any other medicine without consulting your doctor or pharmacist.

POSSIBLE ADVERSE REACTIONS OR SIDE EFFECTS

SYMPTOMS	WHAT TO DO
Life-threatening:	
Irregular heartbeat, difficult breathing, anxiety, weak legs, seizures.	Discontinue. Seek emergency treatment.
Common:	
None expected.	
Infrequent:	
Numbness or tingling in hands or feet, diarrhea, nausea, abdominal pain, vomiting, headache, dizziness, muscle cramps, swollen feet and ankles, thirst, weakness.	Discontinue. Call doctor right away.
Rare:	
Confusion.	Discontinue. Call doctor right away.

POTASSIUM & SODIUM PHOSPHATES

WARNINGS & PRECAUTIONS

Don't take if:
You have had allergic reaction to potassium, sodium or phosphates; severe kidney disease; severe burns.

Before you start, consult your doctor:
If you have heart problems, adrenalin sufficiency, liver disease, high blood pressure, pregnancy, hypoparathyroidism, chronic kidney disease, osteomalacia, pancreatitis, rickets.

Over age 60:
Adverse reactions and side effects may be more frequent and severe than in younger persons. Ask doctor about smaller doses.

Pregnancy:
Decide with your doctor if drug benefits justify risk to unborn child. Risk category C (see page xxii).

Breast-feeding:
Effect unknown. Consult doctor.

Infants & children:
Use only under medical supervision.

Prolonged use:
Monitor ECG*, serum calcium, phosphorus and potassium levels.

Skin & sunlight:
No problems expected.

Driving, piloting or hazardous work:
Avoid if medicine causes dizziness or confusion.

Discontinuing:
Don't discontinue without consulting doctor. Dose may require gradual reduction if you have taken drug for a long time. Doses of other drugs may also require adjustment.

Others:
Protect liquid medicine from freezing.

POSSIBLE INTERACTION WITH OTHER DRUGS

GENERIC NAME OR DRUG CLASS	COMBINED EFFECT
Angiotensin-converting enzyme (ACE) inhibitors*	Level of potassium in blood too high.
Antacids*	May decrease potassium absorption.
Calcium	Decreased potassium effect.
Cortisone drugs*	Increased fluid retention.
Digitalis preparations*	Level of potassium in blood too high.
Diuretics* (amiloride, spironolactone, triamterene)	Level of potassium in blood too high.
Male hormones*	Fluid retention.
Potassium supplements*	Level of potassium in blood too high.
Vitamin D (calcifidiol and calcitriol)	Level of phosphorus in blood too high.

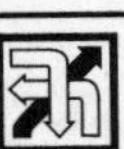

POSSIBLE INTERACTION WITH OTHER SUBSTANCES

INTERACTS WITH	COMBINED EFFECT
Alcohol:	None expected.
Beverages: Salty drinks such as tomato juice, commercial thirst quenchers, salt substitutes.	Increased fluid retention.
Cocaine:	May cause irregular heartbeat.
Foods: Salty foods such as canned soups, potato chips, TV dinners, hot dogs, pickles.	Increased fluid retention.
Marijuana:	May cause irregular heartbeat.
Tobacco:	May aggravate irregular heartbeat.

*See Glossary

POTASSIUM SUPPLEMENTS

BRAND AND GENERIC NAMES

See complete list of brand and generic names in the *Brand Name Directory*, page 916.

BASIC INFORMATION

Habit forming? No
Prescription needed? Yes
Available as generic? Yes
Drug class: Mineral supplement (potassium)

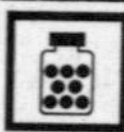

USES

- Treatment for potassium deficiency due to diuretics, cortisone or digitalis medicines.
- Treatment for low potassium associated with some illnesses.

DOSAGE & USAGE INFORMATION

How to take:
- Tablet or capsule—Swallow with liquid or food to lessen stomach irritation. You may chew or crush tablet.
- Extended-release tablets or capsules—Swallow each dose whole with liquid.
- Effervescent tablets, granules, powder or liquid—Dilute dose in water.

When to take:
At the same time each day, preferably with food or immediately after meals.

If you forget a dose:
Take as soon as you remember. Don't double next dose.

What drug does:
Preserves or restores normal function of nerve cells, heart and skeletal muscle cells and kidneys, as well as stomach juice secretions.

Continued next column

OVERDOSE

SYMPTOMS:
Paralysis of arms and legs, irregular heartbeat, blood pressure drop, convulsions, coma, cardiac arrest.
WHAT TO DO:
- **Dial 911 (emergency) or 0 (operator) for an ambulance or medical help. Then give first aid immediately.**
- **See emergency information on inside covers.**

Time lapse before drug works:
1 to 2 hours. Full benefit may require 12 to 24 hours.

Don't take with:
Any other medicine without consulting your doctor or pharmacist.

POSSIBLE ADVERSE REACTIONS OR SIDE EFFECTS

SYMPTOMS	WHAT TO DO
Life-threatening: In case of overdose, see previous column.	
Common: None expected.	
Infrequent: Diarrhea, nausea, vomiting, skin rash, abdominal pain.	Continue. Call doctor when convenient.
Rare: • Confusion; irregular heartbeat; difficult breathing; unusual fatigue; weakness; heaviness of legs; hemorrhage, perforation with enteric-coated tablets (rarely with wax matrix tablets); esophageal ulceration with tablets; bloody stools.	Discontinue. Call doctor right away.
• Numbness or tingling in hands or feet, anxiety.	Continue. Call doctor when convenient.

WARNINGS & PRECAUTIONS

Don't take if:
- You are allergic to any potassium supplement.
- You have acute or chronic kidney disease.

Before you start, consult your doctor:
- If you have Addison's disease or familial periodic paralysis.
- If you have heart disease.
- If you have intestinal blockage.
- If you have a stomach ulcer.
- If you use diuretics.
- If you use heart medicine.
- If you use laxatives or have chronic diarrhea.
- If you use salt substitutes or low-salt milk.

Over age 60:
Observe dose schedule strictly. Potassium balance is critical. Deviation above or below normal can have serious results.

Pregnancy:
Decide with your doctor if drug benefits justify risk to unborn child. Risk category C (see page xxii).

Breast-feeding:
Studies inconclusive on harm to infant. Consult doctor.

Infants & children:
Use only under doctor's supervision.

Prolonged use:
- Slows absorption of vitamin B-12. May cause anemia.
- Request frequent lab tests to monitor potassium levels in blood, especially if you take digitalis preparations.

Skin & sunlight:
No problems expected.

Driving, piloting or hazardous work:
No problems expected.

Discontinuing:
Don't discontinue without consulting doctor. Dose may require gradual reduction if you have taken drug for a long time. Doses of other drugs may also require adjustment.

Others:
- Overdose or underdose serious. Frequent EKGs and laboratory blood studies to measure serum electrolytes and kidney function recommended.
- Prolonged diarrhea may call for increased dosage of potassium.
- Serious injury may necessitate temporary decrease in potassium.
- Some products contain tartrazine dye. Avoid, especially if you are allergic to aspirin.

POSSIBLE INTERACTION WITH OTHER DRUGS

GENERIC NAME OR DRUG CLASS	COMBINED EFFECT
Amiloride	Dangerous rise in blood potassium.
Angiotensin-converting enzyme (ACE) inhibitors*	Possible increased potassium effect.
Anticholinergics, other*	Increased possibility of intestinal ulcers, which sometimes occur with oral potassium tablets.
Anti-inflammatory drugs, nonsteroidal (NSAIDs)*	Increased risk of stomach irritation.
Beta-adrenergic blocking agents*	Increased potassium levels.
Cortisone medicines*	Decreased effect of potassium.
Digitalis preparations*	Possible irregular heartbeat.
Diuretics, thiazide or loop*	Decreased potassium effect.
Laxatives*	Possible decreased potassium effect.
Potassium-containing drugs*	Increased potassium levels.
Spironolactone	Dangerous rise in blood potassium.
Triamterene	Dangerous rise in blood potassium.
Vitamin B-12	Extended-release tablets may decrease vitamin B-12 absorption and increase vitamin B-12 requirements.

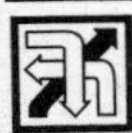

POSSIBLE INTERACTION WITH OTHER SUBSTANCES

INTERACTS WITH	COMBINED EFFECT
Alcohol:	None expected.
Beverages:	
• Salty drinks such as tomato juice, commercial thirst quenchers.	Increased fluid retention.
• Low-salt milk or salt substitutes.	Increased potassium levels.
Cocaine:	May cause irregular heartbeat.
Foods: Salty foods. retention.	Increased fluid
Marijuana:	May cause irregular heartbeat.
Tobacco:	None expected.

*See Glossary

PRAZOSIN

BRAND NAMES

Minipress

BASIC INFORMATION

Habit forming? No
Prescription needed? Yes
Available as generic? Yes
Drug class: Antihypertensive

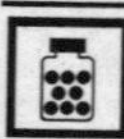

USES

- Treatment for high blood pressure.
- May relieve congestive heart failure.
- Treatment for Raynaud's disease.

DOSAGE & USAGE INFORMATION

How to take:
Tablet or capsule—Swallow with liquid. If you can't swallow whole, crumble tablet or open capsule and take with liquid or food.

When to take:
At the same times each day.

If you forget a dose:
Take as soon as you remember up to 2 hours late. If more than 2 hours, wait for next scheduled dose (don't double this dose).

What drug does:
Expands and relaxes blood vessel walls to lower blood pressure.

Time lapse before drug works:
30 minutes.

Don't take with:
Any other medicine without consulting your doctor or pharmacist.

OVERDOSE

SYMPTOMS:
Extreme weakness; loss of consciousness; cold, sweaty skin; weak, rapid pulse; coma.
WHAT TO DO:

- **Dial 911 (emergency) or 0 (operator) for an ambulance or medical help. Then give first aid immediately.**
- **If patient is unconscious and not breathing, give mouth-to-mouth breathing. If there is no heartbeat, use cardiac massage and mouth-to-mouth breathing (CPR). Don't try to make patient vomit. If you can't get help quickly, take patient to nearest emergency facility.**
- **See emergency information on inside covers.**

POSSIBLE ADVERSE REACTIONS OR SIDE EFFECTS

SYMPTOMS	WHAT TO DO
Life-threatening:	
In case of overdose, see previous column.	
Common:	
• Rapid heartbeat.	Discontinue. Call doctor right away.
• Vivid dreams, drowsiness, dizziness.	Continue. Call doctor when convenient.
Infrequent:	
• Rash or itchy skin, blurred vision, shortness of breath, difficult breathing, chest pain.	Discontinue. Call doctor right away.
• Appetite loss, constipation or diarrhea, abdominal pain, nausea, vomiting, fluid retention, joint or muscle aches, weakness and faintness when arising from bed or chair.	Continue. Call doctor when convenient.
• Headache, irritability, depression, dry mouth, stuffy nose, increased urination.	Continue. Tell doctor at next visit.
Rare:	
Decreased sexual function, numbness or tingling in hands or feet.	Continue. Call doctor when convenient.

WARNINGS & PRECAUTIONS

Don't take if:
- You are allergic to prazosin.
- You are depressed.
- You will have surgery within 2 months, including dental surgery, requiring general or spinal anesthesia.

Before you start, consult your doctor:
- If you experience lightheadedness or fainting with other antihypertensive drugs*.
- If you are easily depressed.
- If you have impaired brain circulation or have had a stroke.
- If you have coronary heart disease (with or without angina).
- If you have kidney disease or impaired liver function.

Over age 60:
Begin with no more than 1 mg per day for first 3 days. Increases should be gradual and supervised by your doctor. Don't stand while taking. Sudden changes in position may cause falls. Sit or lie down promptly if you feel dizzy. If you have impaired brain circulation or coronary heart disease, excessive lowering of blood pressure should be avoided. Report problems to your doctor immediately.

Pregnancy:
Decide with your doctor if drug benefits justify risk to unborn child. Risk category C (see page xxii).

Breast-feeding:
No proven problems. Consult doctor.

Infants & children:
Not recommended.

Prolonged use:
Talk to your doctor about the need for follow-up medical examinations or laboratory studies.

Skin & sunlight:
No problems expected.

Driving, piloting or hazardous work:
Don't drive or pilot aircraft until you learn how medicine affects you. Don't work around dangerous machinery. Don't climb ladders or work in high places.

Discontinuing:
Don't discontinue without doctor's advice until you complete prescribed dose, even though symptoms diminish or disappear.

Others:
First dose likely to cause fainting. Take it at night and get out of bed slowly next morning.

POSSIBLE INTERACTION WITH OTHER DRUGS

GENERIC NAME OR DRUG CLASS	COMBINED EFFECT
Amphetamines*	Decreased effect of prazosin.
Antihypertensives*, other*	Increased anti-hypertensive effect. Dosages may require adjustments.
Anti-inflammatory drugs, nonsteroidal (NSAIDs)*	Decreased effect of prazosin.
Estrogens*	Decreased effect of prazosin.
Hypotension-causing drugs*	Increased hypotension effect.
Sympathomimetics*	Decreased effect of prazosin.

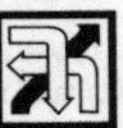

POSSIBLE INTERACTION WITH OTHER SUBSTANCES

INTERACTS WITH	COMBINED EFFECT
Alcohol:	Excessive blood pressure drop.
Beverages:	None expected.
Cocaine:	Increased risk of heart block and high blood pressure.
Foods:	None expected.
Marijuana:	Possible fainting. Avoid.
Tobacco:	Possible spasm of coronary arteries. Avoid.

PRAZOSIN & POLYTHIAZIDE

BRAND NAMES

Minizide

BASIC INFORMATION

Habit forming? No
Prescription needed? Yes
Available as generic? No
Drug class: Antihypertensive, diuretic (thiazide)

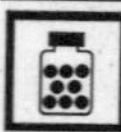

USES

- Controls, but doesn't cure, high blood pressure.
- Reduces fluid retention (edema) caused by conditions such as heart disorders and liver disease.
- Treats Raynaud's disease.

DOSAGE & USAGE INFORMATION

How to take:
Capsule—Swallow with 8 ounces of liquid. If you can't swallow whole, open capsule and take with liquid or food. Don't exceed dose.

When to take:
At the same times each day.

If you forget a dose:
Take as soon as you remember up to 2 hours late. If more than 2 hours, wait for next scheduled dose (don't double this dose).

Continued next column

OVERDOSE

SYMPTOMS:
Extreme weakness; loss of consciousness; cold, sweaty skin; weak, rapid pulse; cramps; weakness; drowsiness; coma.
WHAT TO DO:

- **Dial 911 (emergency) or 0 (operator) for an ambulance or medical help. Then give first aid immediately.**
- **If patient is unconscious and not breathing, give mouth-to-mouth breathing. If there is no heartbeat, use cardiac massage and mouth-to-mouth breathing (CPR). Don't try to make patient vomit. If you can't get help quickly, take patient to nearest emergency facility.**
- **See emergency information on inside covers.**

What drug does:

- Expands and relaxes blood vessel walls to lower blood pressure.
- Forces sodium and water excretion, reducing body fluid.
- Relaxes muscle cells of small arteries.
- Reduced body fluid and relaxed arteries lower blood pressure.

Time lapse before drug works:
4 to 6 hours. May require several weeks to lower blood pressure.

Don't take with:

- Nonprescription drugs without consulting doctor.
- See Interaction column and consult doctor.

POSSIBLE ADVERSE REACTIONS OR SIDE EFFECTS

SYMPTOMS	WHAT TO DO
Life-threatening:	
Irregular heartbeat, weak pulse, fast heartbeat, difficult breathing, chest pain.	Discontinue. Seek emergency treatment.
Common:	
Nightmares, vivid dreams, drowsiness, dizziness, dry mouth, stuffy nose.	Continue. Call doctor when convenient.
Infrequent:	
• Blurred vision, abdominal pain, nausea, vomiting, difficult breathing.	Discontinue. Call doctor right away.
• Mood change, headache, dry mouth, muscle pain, urgent urination, weakness, tiredness, weight gain or loss, runny nose, joint or muscle pain, agitation, depression, rash, appetite loss, weakness and faintness when arising from bed or chair, constipation.	Continue. Call doctor when convenient.
Rare:	
• Sore throat, fever, mouth sores; jaundice.	Discontinue. Call doctor right away.
• Diminished sex drive, numbness or tingling in hands or feet.	Continue. Call doctor when convenient.

WARNINGS & PRECAUTIONS

Don't take if:
- You are allergic to any thiazide diuretic drug or prazosin.
- You are depressed.
- You will have surgery within 2 months, including dental surgery, requiring general or spinal anesthesia.

Before you start, consult your doctor:
- If you are allergic to any sulfa drug.
- If you have gout or impaired circulation in brain or have had a stroke, coronary heart disease (with or without angina), kidney disease or impaired liver function.
- If you experience lightheadedness or fainting with other antihypertensive drugs.
- If you are easily depressed.

Over age 60:
- Adverse reactions and side effects may be more frequent and severe than in younger persons, especially dizziness and excessive potassium loss.
- Don't stand while taking. Sudden changes in position may cause falls. Sit or lie down promptly if you feel dizzy. If you have impaired circulation in brain or coronary heart disease, excessive lowering of blood pressure should be avoided. Report problems to your doctor immediately.

Pregnancy:
Decide with your doctor if drug benefits justify risk to unborn child. Risk category C (see page xxii).

Breast-feeding:
Drug passes into milk. Avoid drug or discontinue nursing until you finish medicine. Consult doctor for advice on maintaining milk supply.

Infants & children:
Not recommended.

Prolonged use:
- You may need medicine to treat high blood pressure for the rest of your life.
- Talk to your doctor about the need for follow-up medical examinations or laboratory studies.

Skin & sunlight:
May cause rash or intensify sunburn in areas exposed to sun or sunlamp.

Driving, piloting or hazardous work:
Don't drive or pilot aircraft until you learn how medicine affects you. Don't work around dangerous machinery. Don't climb ladders or work in high places. Danger increases if you drink alcohol or take medicine affecting alertness and reflexes, such as antihistamines, tranquilizers, sedatives, pain medicine, narcotics and mind-altering drugs.

Discontinuing:
Don't discontinue without consulting doctor.

Others:
- First dose likely to cause fainting. Take it at night and get out of bed slowly next morning.
- Hot weather and fever may cause dehydration and drop in blood pressure. Dose may require temporary adjustment. Weigh daily and report any unexpected weight decreases to your doctor.
- May cause rise in uric acid, leading to gout.
- May cause blood sugar rise in diabetics.

POSSIBLE INTERACTION WITH OTHER DRUGS

GENERIC NAME OR DRUG CLASS	COMBINED EFFECT
Acebutolol	Increased anti-hypertensive effect. Dosages may require adjustments.
Allopurinol	Decreased allopurinol effect.
Amphetamines*	Decreased prazosin effect.
Amphotericin B	Increased potassium.
Angiotensin-converting enzyme (ACE) inhibitors*	Decreased blood pressure.

Continued on page 954

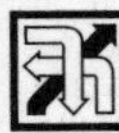

POSSIBLE INTERACTION WITH OTHER SUBSTANCES

INTERACTS WITH	COMBINED EFFECT
Alcohol:	Dangerous blood pressure drop. Avoid.
Beverages:	None expected.
Cocaine:	Increased risk of heart block and high blood pressure.
Foods: Licorice.	Excessive potassium loss that causes dangerous heart rhythms.
Marijuana:	Possible fainting, increased blood pressure. Avoid.
Tobacco:	Possible spasm of coronary arteries. Avoid.

*See Glossary

PREDNISOLONE

BRAND NAMES

See complete list of brand names in the *Brand Name Directory*, page 916.

BASIC INFORMATION

Habit forming? No
Prescription needed? Yes
Available as generic? Yes
Drug class: Cortisone drug (adrenal corticosteroid)

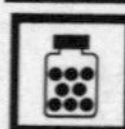

USES

- Reduces inflammation caused by many different medical problems.
- Treatment for some allergic diseases, blood disorders, kidney diseases, asthma and emphysema.
- Replaces corticosteroid lost due to deficiencies.

DOSAGE & USAGE INFORMATION

How to take:
Tablet or liquid—Swallow with liquid or food to lessen stomach irritation. If you can't swallow whole, crumble tablet and take with liquid or food.

When to take:
At the same times each day. Take once-a-day or once-every-other-day doses in mornings.

If you forget a dose:
- Several-doses-per-day prescription—Take as soon as you remember up to 2 hours late. If more than 2 hours, wait for next scheduled dose (don't double this dose).
- Once-a-day dose or less—Wait for next dose. Double this dose.

What drug does:
Decreases inflammatory responses.

Time lapse before drug works:
2 to 4 days.

Continued next column

OVERDOSE

SYMPTOMS:
Headache, convulsions, heart failure.
WHAT TO DO:
- **Dial 911 (emergency) or 0 (operator) for an ambulance or medical help. Then give first aid immediately.**
- **See emergency information on inside covers.**

Don't take with:
Any other medicine without consulting your doctor or pharmacist.

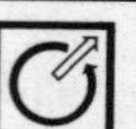

POSSIBLE ADVERSE REACTIONS OR SIDE EFFECTS

SYMPTOMS	WHAT TO DO
Life-threatening: Hives, rash, intense itching, faintness soon after a dose (anaphylaxis).	Seek emergency treatment immediately.
Common: Acne, poor wound healing, thirst, indigestion, nausea, vomiting, constipation, gaseousness, unpleasant taste, diarrhea, headache, cough, dizziness, hoarseness, appetite gain or loss.	Continue. Call doctor when convenient.
Infrequent:	
• Black, bloody or tarry stool; various infections; swallowing difficulties.	Discontinue. Seek emergency treatment.
• Blurred vision, halos around lights, sore throat, fever, muscle cramps, swollen legs or feet.	Discontinue. Call doctor right away.
• Mood change, fatigue, insomnia, weakness, restlessness, frequent urination, weight gain, round face, irregular menstrual periods, dry mouth, euphoria, nosebleeds.	Continue. Call doctor when convenient.
Rare:	
• Irregular heartbeat.	Discontinue. Seek emergency treatment.
• Rash, numbness or tingling of hands or feet, pancreatitis, hallucinations, thrombophlebitis, convulsions.	Discontinue. Call doctor right away.

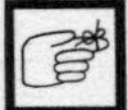

WARNINGS & PRECAUTIONS

Don't take if:
- You are allergic to any cortisone drug*.
- You have tuberculosis or fungus infection.
- You have herpes infection of eyes, lips or genitals.
- You have bone disease, thyroid disease, colitis, peptic ulcer, diabetes, myasthenia gravis, liver or kidney disease, diverticulitis, glaucoma, heart disease.

Before you start, consult your doctor:
- If you have had tuberculosis.
- If you have congestive heart failure, diabetes, peptic ulcer, glaucoma, underactive thyroid, high blood pressure, myasthenia gravis, blood clots in legs or lungs.

Over age 60:
Adverse reactions and side effects may be more frequent and severe than in younger persons. Likely to aggravate edema, diabetes or ulcers. Likely to cause cataracts and osteoporosis (softening of the bones).

Pregnancy:
Decide with your doctor if drug benefits justify risk to unborn child. Risk category C (see page xxii).

Breast-feeding:
Drug passes into milk. Avoid drug or discontinue nursing until you finish medicine. Consult doctor for advice on maintaining milk supply.

Infants & children:
Use only under medical supervision.

Prolonged use:
- Retards growth in children.
- Possible glaucoma, cataracts, diabetes, fragile bones and thin skin.
- Functional dependence.
- Talk to your doctor about the need for follow-up medical examinations or laboratory studies to check blood pressure, serum electrolytes, stools for blood.

Skin & sunlight:
No problems expected.

Driving, piloting or hazardous work:
No problems expected.

Discontinuing:
- Don't discontinue without doctor's advice until you complete prescribed dose, even though symptoms diminish or disappear.
- Drug affects your response to surgery, illness, injury or stress for 2 years after discontinuing. Tell anyone who takes medical care of you within 2 years about drug.

Others:
- Avoid immunizations if possible.
- Your resistance to infection is less while taking this medicine.
- Advise any doctor or dentist whom you consult that you take this medicine.
- Those who have inactive or "cured" tuberculosis may be subjected to a possible recurrence of active tuberculosis.
- Children who must take cortisone drugs may grow less well.

POSSIBLE INTERACTION WITH OTHER DRUGS

GENERIC NAME OR DRUG CLASS	COMBINED EFFECT
Amphotericin B	Potassium depletion.
Anticholinergics*	Possible glaucoma.
Anticoagulants*, oral	Decreased anticoagulant effect.
Anticonvulsants, hydantoin*	Decreased prednisolone effect.
Antidiabetics*, oral	Decreased antidiabetic effect.
Antihistamines*	Decreased prednisolone effect.
Anti-inflammatory drugs, nonsteroidal (NSAIDs)*	Increased risk of ulcers, increased prednisolone effect.
Aspirin	Increased prednisolone effect.
Attenuated virus vaccines*	Possible viral infection.
Barbiturates*	Decreased prednisolone effect. Oversedation.

Continued on page 955

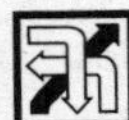

POSSIBLE INTERACTION WITH OTHER SUBSTANCES

INTERACTS WITH	COMBINED EFFECT
Alcohol:	Risk of stomach ulcers.
Beverages:	No proven problems.
Cocaine:	Overstimulation. Avoid.
Foods:	No proven problems.
Marijuana:	Decreased immunity.
Tobacco:	Increased prednisolone effect. Possible toxicity.

***See Glossary**

PREDNISONE

BRAND NAMES

Apo-Prednisone
Deltasone
Liquid-Pred
Meticorten
Orasone
Prednicen-M
Prednisone Intensol
Sterapred
Winpred

BASIC INFORMATION

Habit forming? No
Prescription needed? Yes
Available as generic? Yes
Drug class: Cortisone drug (adrenal corticosteroid)

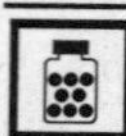

USES

- Reduces inflammation caused by many different medical problems.
- Treatment for some allergic diseases, blood disorders, kidney diseases, asthma and emphysema.
- Replaces corticosteroid lost due to deficiencies.

DOSAGE & USAGE INFORMATION

How to take:
Tablet or liquid—Swallow with liquid or food to lessen stomach irritation. If you can't swallow whole, crumble tablet.

When to take:
At the same times each day. Take once-a-day or once-every-other-day doses in mornings.

If you forget a dose:
- Several-doses-per-day prescription—Take as soon as you remember up to 2 hours late. If more than 2 hours, wait for next scheduled dose (don't double this dose).
- Once-a-day dose or less—Wait for next dose. Double this dose.

What drug does:
Decreases inflammatory responses.

Continued next column

OVERDOSE

SYMPTOMS:
Headache, convulsions, heart failure.
WHAT TO DO:
- **Dial 911 (emergency) or 0 (operator) for an ambulance or medical help. Then give first aid immediately.**
- **See emergency information on inside covers.**

Time lapse before drug works:
2 to 4 days.

Don't take with:
Any other medicine without consulting your doctor or pharmacist.

POSSIBLE ADVERSE REACTIONS OR SIDE EFFECTS

SYMPTOMS	WHAT TO DO
Life-threatening:	
Hives, rash, intense itching, faintness soon after a dose (anaphylaxis).	Seek emergency treatment immediately.
Common:	
Acne, poor wound healing, thirst, indigestion, nausea, vomiting, constipation, gaseousness, unpleasant taste, diarrhea, headache, cough, dizziness, hoarseness, appetite gain or loss.	Continue. Call doctor when convenient.
Infrequent:	
• Black, bloody or tarry stool; various infections; swallowing difficulties.	Discontinue. Seek emergency treatment.
• Blurred vision, halos around lights, sore throat, fever, muscle cramps, swollen legs or feet.	Discontinue. Call doctor right away.
• Mood change, fatigue, insomnia, weakness, restlessness, frequent urination, weight gain, round face, irregular menstrual periods, dry mouth, euphoria, nosebleeds.	Continue. Call doctor when convenient.
Rare:	
• Irregular heartbeat.	Discontinue. Seek emergency treatment.
• Skin rash, fever, joint pain, acute psychosis, hair loss, pancreatitis, numbness or tingling in hands or feet, convulsions, thrombophlebitis, hallucinations.	Discontinue. Call doctor right away.

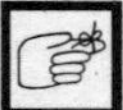

WARNINGS & PRECAUTIONS

Don't take if:
- You are allergic to any cortisone drug*.
- You have tuberculosis or fungus infection.
- You have herpes infection of eyes, lips or genitals.
- You have bone disease, thyroid disease, colitis, peptic ulcer, diabetes, myasthenia gravis, liver or kidney disease, diverticulitis, glaucoma, heart disease.

Before you start, consult your doctor:
- If you have had tuberculosis.
- If you have congestive heart failure.
- If you have diabetes.
- If you have peptic ulcer.
- If you have glaucoma.
- If you have underactive thyroid.
- If you have high blood pressure.
- If you have myasthenia gravis.
- If you have blood clots in legs or lungs.

Over age 60:
Adverse reactions and side effects may be more frequent and severe than in younger persons. Likely to aggravate edema, diabetes or ulcers. Likely to cause cataracts and osteoporosis (softening of the bones).

Pregnancy:
Decide with your doctor if drug benefits justify risk to unborn child. Risk category C (see page xxii).

Breast-feeding:
Drug passes into milk. Avoid drug or discontinue nursing until you finish medicine. Consult doctor for advice on maintaining milk supply.

Infants & children:
Use only under medical supervision.

Prolonged use:
- Retards growth in children.
- Possible glaucoma, cataracts, diabetes, fragile bones and thin skin.
- Functional dependence.
- Talk to your doctor about the need for follow-up medical examinations or laboratory studies to check blood pressure, serum electrolytes, stools for blood.

Skin & sunlight:
No problems expected.

Driving, piloting or hazardous work:
No problems expected.

Discontinuing:
- Don't discontinue without doctor's advice until you complete prescribed dose, even though symptoms diminish or disappear.
- Drug affects your response to surgery, illness, injury or stress for 2 years after discontinuing. Tell anyone who takes medical care of you within 2 years about drug.

Others:
- Avoid immunizations if possible.
- Your resistance to infection is less while taking this medicine.
- Advise any doctor or dentist whom you consult that you take this medicine.
- Those who have inactive or "cured" tuberculosis may be subjected to a possible recurrence of active tuberculosis.
- Children who must take cortisone drugs may grow less well.

POSSIBLE INTERACTION WITH OTHER DRUGS

GENERIC NAME OR DRUG CLASS	COMBINED EFFECT
Amphotericin B	Potassium depletion.
Anticholinergics*	Possible glaucoma.
Anticoagulants*, oral	Decreased anti-coagulant effect.
Anticonvulsants, hydantoin*	Decreased prednisone effect.
Antidiabetics*, oral	Decreased anti-diabetic effect.
Antihistamines*	Decreased prednisone effect.
Anti-inflammatory drugs, nonsteroidal (NSAIDs)*	Increased risk of ulcers, increased prednisone effect.
Aspirin	Increased prednisone effect.
Attenuated virus vaccines*	Possible viral infection.

Continued on page 955

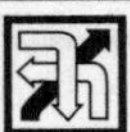

POSSIBLE INTERACTION WITH OTHER SUBSTANCES

INTERACTS WITH	COMBINED EFFECT
Alcohol:	Risk of stomach ulcers.
Beverages:	No proven problems.
Cocaine:	Overstimulation. Avoid.
Foods:	No proven problems.
Marijuana:	Decreased immunity.
Tobacco:	Increased predni-sone effect. Possible toxicity.

***See Glossary**

PRIMAQUINE

GENERIC NAME

PRIMAQUINE

BASIC INFORMATION

Habit forming? No
Prescription needed? Yes
Available as generic? Yes
Drug class: Antiprotozoal (antimalarial)

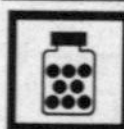

USES

- Treats some forms of malaria.
- Prevents relapses of some forms of malaria.
- Treats pneumocystis carinii pneumonia (used in combination with clindamycin).

DOSAGE & USAGE INFORMATION

How to take:
Tablets—Take with meals or antacids to minimize stomach irritation.

When to take:
At the same time each day, according to instructions on prescription label.

If you forget a dose:
Take as soon as you remember up to 2 hours late. If more than 2 hours, wait for next scheduled dose. Don't double this dose.

What drug does:
Alters the properties of DNA in malaria organisms to prevent them from multiplying.

Time lapse before drug works:
2 to 3 hours.

Don't take with:
Any other medicine without consulting your doctor or pharmacist.

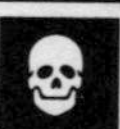

OVERDOSE

SYMPTOMS:
None expected.
WHAT TO DO:
Overdose unlikely to threaten life. If person takes much larger amount than prescribed, call doctor, poison control center or hospital emergency room for instructions.

POSSIBLE ADVERSE REACTIONS OR SIDE EFFECTS

SYMPTOMS	WHAT TO DO
Life-threatening: None expected.	
Common: None expected.	
Infrequent: Dark urine; back, leg or stomach pain; appetite loss; pale skin; fever.	Discontinue. Call doctor right away.
Rare: Blue fingernails, lips and skin; dizziness; difficult breathing; extraordinary tiredness; sore throat; fever.	Discontinue. Call doctor right away.

WARNINGS & PRECAUTIONS

Don't take if:
- You have G6PD* deficiency.
- You are hypersensitive to primaquine.

Before you start, consult your doctor:
If you are Black, Oriental, Asian or of Mediterranean origin.

Over age 60:
No special problems expected.

Pregnancy:
Decide with your doctor if drug benefits justify risk to unborn child. Risk category C (see page xxii).

Breast-feeding:
Effect unknown. Consult doctor.

Infants & children:
No special problems expected.

Prolonged use:
No special problems expected.

Skin & sunlight:
No special problems expected.

Driving, piloting or hazardous work:
No special problems expected.

Discontinuing:
No special problems expected.

Others:
- If you are Black, Asian, Oriental or of Mediterranean origin, insist on a test for G6PD* deficiency before taking this medicine.
- Advise any doctor or dentist whom you consult that you take this medicine.

POSSIBLE INTERACTION WITH OTHER DRUGS

GENERIC NAME OR DRUG CLASS	COMBINED EFFECT
Hemolytics*, other	Increased risk of serious side effects affecting the blood.
Quinacrine	Increased toxic effects of primaquine.

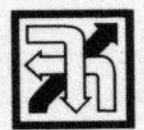

POSSIBLE INTERACTION WITH OTHER SUBSTANCES

INTERACTS WITH	COMBINED EFFECT
Alcohol:	Possible liver toxicity. Avoid.
Beverages:	None expected.
Cocaine:	None expected.
Foods:	None expected.
Marijuana:	None expected.
Tobacco:	None expected.

*See Glossary

PRIMIDONE

BRAND NAMES

Apo-Primidone
Myidone
Mysoline
PMS Primadone
Sertan

BASIC INFORMATION

Habit forming? No
Prescription needed? Yes
Available as generic? Yes
Drug class: Anticonvulsant

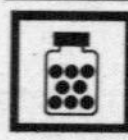

USES

Prevents some forms of epileptic seizures.

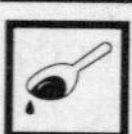

DOSAGE & USAGE INFORMATION

How to take:
- Tablet—Swallow with liquid. If you can't swallow whole, crumble tablet and take with liquid or food.
- Liquid—If desired, dilute dose in beverage before swallowing.

When to take:
Daily in regularly spaced doses, according to doctor's prescription.

If you forget a dose:
Take as soon as you remember up to 2 hours late. If more than 2 hours, wait for next scheduled dose (don't double this dose).

What drug does:
Probably inhibits repetitious spread of impulses along nerve pathways.

Continued next column

OVERDOSE

SYMPTOMS:
Slow, shallow breathing; weak, rapid pulse; confusion, deep sleep, coma.
WHAT TO DO:
- **Dial 911 (emergency) or 0 (operator) for an ambulance or medical help. Then give first aid immediately.**
- **If patient is unconscious and not breathing, give mouth-to-mouth breathing. If there is no heartbeat, use cardiac massage and mouth-to-mouth breathing (CPR). Don't try to make patient vomit. If you can't get help quickly, take patient to nearest emergency facility.**
- **See emergency information on inside covers.**

Time lapse before drug works:
2 to 3 weeks.

Don't take with:
Any other medicine without consulting your doctor or pharmacist.

POSSIBLE ADVERSE REACTIONS OR SIDE EFFECTS

SYMPTOMS	WHAT TO DO
Life-threatening: In case of overdose, see previous column.	
Common:	
• Difficult breathing.	Discontinue. Call doctor right away.
• Confusion, change in vision.	Continue. Call doctor when convenient.
• Clumsiness, dizziness, drowsiness.	Continue. Tell doctor at next visit.
Infrequent:	
• Unusual excitement, particularly in children; nausea; vomiting.	Discontinue. Call doctor right away.
• Headache, fatigue, weakness.	Continue. Call doctor when convenient.
Rare:	
• Rash or hives, appetite loss, acute psychosis, hair loss, fever, joint pain.	Discontinue. Call doctor right away.
• Swollen eyelids or legs.	Continue. Call doctor when convenient.
• Decreased sexual ability.	Continue. Tell doctor at next visit.

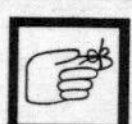

WARNINGS & PRECAUTIONS

Don't take if:
- You are allergic to any barbiturate.
- You have had porphyria.

Before you start, consult your doctor:
- If you have had liver, kidney or lung disease or asthma.
- If you have lupus.

Over age 60:
Adverse reactions and side effects may be more frequent and severe than in younger persons.

Pregnancy:
Consult doctor. Risk category D (see page xxii).

Breast-feeding:
Drug filters into milk. May harm child. Avoid. Consult doctor.

Infants & children:
Use only under medical supervision.

Prolonged use:
- Enlarged lymph and thyroid glands.
- Anemia.
- Rickets in children and osteomalacia (insufficient calcium to bones) in adults.
- Talk to your doctor about the need for follow-up medical examinations or laboratory studies to check complete blood counts (white blood cell count, platelet count, red blood cell count, hemoglobin, hematocrit), liver function, kidney function.

Skin & sunlight:
None expected.

Driving, piloting or hazardous work:
Don't drive or pilot aircraft until you learn how medicine affects you. Don't work around dangerous machinery. Don't climb ladders or work in high places. Danger increases if you drink alcohol or take medicine affecting alertness and reflexes.

Discontinuing:
Don't discontinue abruptly or without doctor's advice until you complete prescribed dose, even though symptoms diminish or disappear.

Others:
- Tell doctor if you become ill or injured and must interrupt dose schedule.
- Periodic laboratory blood tests of drug level recommended.

POSSIBLE INTERACTION WITH OTHER DRUGS

GENERIC NAME OR DRUG CLASS	COMBINED EFFECT
Anticoagulants*, oral	Decreased primidone effect.
Anticonvulsants*, other	Changed seizure pattern.
Antidepressants*	Increased antidepressant effect.
Antihistamines*	Increased sedation effect of primidone.
Aspirin	Decreased aspirin effect.
Carbamazepine	Unpredictable increase or decrease of primidone effect.
Carbonic anhydrase inhibitors*	Possible decreased primidone effect.
Central nervous system (CNS) depressants*	Increased CNS depressant effects.
Contraceptives, oral*	Decreased contraceptive effect.
Cortisone drugs*	Decreased cortisone effect.
Cyclosporine	Decreased cyclosporine effect.
Digitalis preparations*	Decreased digitalis effect.
Disulfiram	Possible increased primidone effect.
Estrogens*	Decreased estrogen effect.
Griseofulvin	Possible decreased griseofulvin effect.
Isoniazid	Decreased primidone effect.
Leucovorin (large dose)	May counteract anticonvulsant effect of primidone.
Loxapine	Decreased anticonvulsant effect of primidone.
Metronidazole	Possible decreased metronidazole effect.
Mind-altering drugs*	Increased effect of mind-altering drug.
Monoamine oxidase (MAO) inhibitors*	Increased sedation effect of primidone.
Nabilone	Greater depression of central nervous system.

Continued on page 956

POSSIBLE INTERACTION WITH OTHER SUBSTANCES

INTERACTS WITH	COMBINED EFFECT
Alcohol:	Dangerous sedative effect. Avoid.
Beverages:	None expected.
Cocaine:	Decreased primidone effect.
Foods:	Possible need for more vitamin D.
Marijuana:	Decreased anticonvulsant effect of primidone. Drowsiness, unsteadiness.
Tobacco:	None expected.

***See Glossary**

PROBENECID

BRAND NAMES

Benemid
Benuryl
Probalan

BASIC INFORMATION

Habit forming? No
Prescription needed? Yes
Available as generic? Yes
Drug class: Antigout

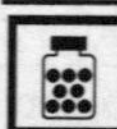

USES

- Treats chronic gout.
- Increases blood levels of penicillins and cephalosporins.

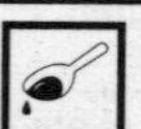

DOSAGE & USAGE INFORMATION

How to take:
Tablet—Swallow with liquid or food to lessen stomach irritation. If you can't swallow whole, crumble tablet and take with liquid or food.

When to take:
At the same time each day.

If you forget a dose:
Take as soon as you remember up to 12 hours late. If more than 12 hours, wait for next scheduled dose (don't double this dose).

What drug does:
- Forces kidneys to excrete uric acid.
- Reduces amount of penicillin excreted in urine.

Time lapse before drug works:
May require several months of regular use to prevent acute gout.

Don't take with:
- Nonprescription drugs containing aspirin or caffeine.
- Any other medicine without consulting your doctor or pharmacist.

OVERDOSE

SYMPTOMS:
Breathing difficulty, severe nervous agitation, vomiting, seizures, convulsions, delirium, coma.
WHAT TO DO:
- **Dial 911 (emergency) or 0 (operator) for an ambulance or medical help. Then give first aid immediately.**
- **See emergency information on inside covers.**

POSSIBLE ADVERSE REACTIONS OR SIDE EFFECTS

SYMPTOMS	WHAT TO DO
Life-threatening:	
In case of overdose, see previous column.	
Common:	
Headache, appetite loss, nausea, vomiting.	Continue. Call doctor when convenient.
Infrequent:	
• Blood in urine, low back pain. worsening gout.	Discontinue. Call doctor right away.
• Dizziness, flushed face, itchy skin.	Continue. Call doctor when convenient.
• Painful or frequent urination, sore gums.	Continue. Tell doctor at next visit.
Rare:	
Sore throat, fever and chills; difficult breathing; unusual bleeding or bruising; red, painful joint; jaundice; foot, leg or face swelling.	Discontinue. Call doctor right away.

WARNINGS & PRECAUTIONS

Don't take if:
- You are allergic to any uricosuric*.
- You have acute gout.
- Patient is younger than 2.

Before you start, consult your doctor:
- If you have had kidney stones or kidney disease.
- If you have a peptic ulcer.
- If you have bone marrow or blood cell disease.
- If you are undergoing chemotherapy for cancer.

Over age 60:
Adverse reactions and side effects may be more frequent and severe than in younger persons.

Pregnancy:
Consult doctor. Risk category B (see page xxii).

Breast-feeding:
Effect unknown. Consult doctor.

Infants & children:
Not recommended.

Prolonged use:
- Possible kidney damage.
- Talk to your doctor about the need for follow-up medical examinations or laboratory studies to check serum uric acid, urine uric acid.

Skin & sunlight:
No problems expected.

Driving, piloting or hazardous work:
Avoid if you feel dizzy. Otherwise, no problems expected.

Discontinuing:
Don't discontinue without consulting doctor. Dose may require gradual reduction if you have taken drug for a long time. Doses of other drugs may also require adjustment.

Others:
If signs of gout attack develop while taking medicine, consult doctor.

POSSIBLE INTERACTION WITH OTHER DRUGS

GENERIC NAME OR DRUG CLASS	COMBINED EFFECT
Allopurinol	Increased effect of each drug.
Anticoagulants*, oral	Increased anti-coagulant effect.
Anti-inflammatory drugs, nonsteroidal (NSAIDs)*	Increased toxic risk.
Aspirin	Decreased probenecid effect.
Bismuth subsalicylate	Decreased probenecid effect.
Cefixime	Increased cefixime effect.
Cephalosporins*	Increased cephalosporin effect.
Ciprofloxacin	May cause kidney dysfunction.
Dapsone	Increased dapsone effect. Increased toxicity.
Diclofenac	Increased diclofenac effect.
Diuretics, thiazide*	Decreased probenecid effect.
Hypoglycemics, oral*	Increased hypo-glycemic effect.
Indomethacin	Increased adverse effects of indomethacin.
Ketoprofen	Increased risk of ketoprofen toxicity.
Loracarbef	Increased loracarbef effect.
Methotrexate	Increased methotrexate toxicity.
Nitrofurantoin	Incresed effect of nitrofurantoin.
Para-aminosalicylic acid	Increased effect of para-aminosalicylic acid.
Penicillins*	Enhanced penicillin effect.
Pyrazinamide	Decreased probenecid effect.
Salicylates*	Decreased probenecid effect.
Sodium benzoate & sodium phenylacetate	May reduce effect of sodium benzoate & sodium phenylacetate.
Sulfa drugs*	Slows elimination. May cause harmful accumulation of sulfa.
Thioguanine	More likelihood of toxicity of both drugs.
Zidovudine	Increased zidovudine toxicity risk.

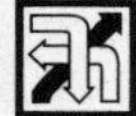

POSSIBLE INTERACTION WITH OTHER SUBSTANCES

INTERACTS WITH	COMBINED EFFECT
Alcohol:	Decreased probenecid effect.
Beverages: Caffeine drinks.	Loss of probenecid effectiveness.
Cocaine:	None expected.
Foods:	None expected.
Marijuana:	Daily use—Decreased probenecid effect.
Tobacco:	None expected.

*See Glossary

PROBENECID & COLCHICINE

BRAND NAMES

Col Benemid
Col-Probenecid
Proben-C

BASIC INFORMATION

Habit forming? No
Prescription needed? Yes
Available as generic? Yes
Drug class: Antigout

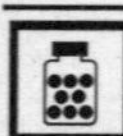

USES

- Increases blood levels of penicillins and cephalosporins.
- Relieves joint pain, inflammation, swelling from gout.
- Also used for familial Mediterranean fever, dermatitis herpetiformis.

DOSAGE & USAGE INFORMATION

How to take:
Tablet—Swallow with liquid or food to lessen stomach irritation. If you can't swallow whole, crumble tablet and take with liquid or food.

When to take:
At the same time each day.

If you forget a dose:
Take as soon as you remember up to 12 hours late. If more than 12 hours, wait for next scheduled dose (don't double this dose).

What drug does:
- Forces kidneys to excrete uric acid.
- Reduces amount of penicillin excreted in urine.
- Decreases acidity of joint tissues and prevents deposits of uric acid crystals.

Time lapse before drug works:
12 to 48 hours.

Continued next column

OVERDOSE

SYMPTOMS:
Breathing difficulty, severe nervous agitation, convulsions, bloody urine, diarrhea, vomiting, muscle weakness, fever, stupor, seizures, delirium, coma.
WHAT TO DO:
- **Dial 911 (emergency) or 0 (operator) for an ambulance or medical help. Then give first aid immediately.**
- **See emergency information on inside covers.**

Don't take with:
- Nonprescription drugs containing aspirin or caffeine.
- Any other medicine without consulting your doctor or pharmacist.

POSSIBLE ADVERSE REACTIONS OR SIDE EFFECTS

SYMPTOMS	WHAT TO DO
Life-threatening:	
Blood in urine; convulsions; severe muscle weakness; difficult breathing; burning feeling of stomach, throat or skin; worsening gout.	Discontinue. Seek emergency treatment.
Common:	
Diarrhea, headache, abdominal pain.	Discontinue. Call doctor right away.
Infrequent:	
• Back pain; painful, difficult urination.	Discontinue. Call doctor right away.
• Dizziness, red or flushed face, urgent urination, sore gums, hair loss.	Continue. Call doctor when convenient.
Rare:	
Sudden decrease in urine output; nausea; vomiting; mood change; fever; chills; diarrhea; jaundice; numbness or tingling in hands or feet; rash; sore throat, fever, mouth sores; swollen face, feet and ankles; unexplained bleeding or bruising; weight gain or loss; low white or red blood cells.	Discontinue. Call doctor right away.

WARNINGS & PRECAUTIONS

Don't take if:
You are allergic to any uricosuric* or colchicine.

Before you start, consult your doctor:
- If you have had kidney stones, kidney disease, heart or liver disease, peptic ulcers or ulcerative colitis.
- If you have bone marrow or blood cell disease.
- If you will have surgery within 2 months, including dental surgery, requiring general or spinal anesthesia.
- If you are undergoing chemotherapy for cancer.

Over age 60:
Adverse reactions and side effects may be more frequent and severe than in younger persons. Colchicine has a narrow margin of safety for people in this age group.

Pregnancy:
Risk factor varies with length of pregnancy. See category list on page xxii and consult doctor.

Breast-feeding:
No problems expected, but consult doctor.

Infants & children:
Not recommended.

Prolonged use:
- Possible kidney damage.
- Permanent hair loss.
- Anemia. Request blood counts.
- Numbness or tingling in hands and feet.
- Talk to your doctor about the need for follow-up medical examinations or laboratory studies to check serum uric acid, urine uric acid.

Skin & sunlight:
No problems expected.

Driving, piloting or hazardous work:
Don't drive or pilot aircraft until you learn how medicine affects you. Don't work around dangerous machinery. Don't climb ladders or work in high places. Danger increases if you drink alcohol or take medicine affecting alertness and reflexes, such as antihistamines, tranquilizers, sedatives, pain medicine, narcotics and mind-altering drugs.

Discontinuing:
- May be unnecessary to finish medicine. Follow doctor's instructions.
- Stop taking if severe digestive upsets occur before symptoms are relieved.

Others:
- If signs of gout attack develop while taking medicine, consult doctor.
- Limit each course of treatment to 8 mg. Don't exceed 3 mg per 24 hours.
- May decrease sperm count in males.

POSSIBLE INTERACTION WITH OTHER DRUGS

GENERIC NAME OR DRUG CLASS	COMBINED EFFECT
Acetohexamide	Increased aceto-hexamide effect.
Allopurinol	Increased effect of each drug.
Anticoagulants*, oral	Irregular effect on anticoagulation, sometimes increased, sometimes decreased. Follow prothrombin times.
Antidepressants*	Oversedation.
Antihistamines*	Oversedation.
Antihypertensives*	Decreased anti-hypertensive effect.
Anti-inflammatory drugs, nonsteroidal (NSAIDs)*	Increased toxic risk.
Appetite suppressants*	Increased appetite suppressant effect.
Bismuth subsalicylate	Decreased probenecid effect.
Cefixime	Increased cefixime effect.
Cephalosporins*	Increased cephalosporin effect.
Dapsone	Increased dapsone effect. Increased toxicity.
Diclofenac	Increased diclofenac effect.
Diuretics, thiazide*	Decreased probenecid effect.
Indomethacin	Increased adverse effects of indomethacin.

Continued on page 956

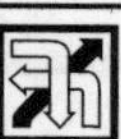

POSSIBLE INTERACTION WITH OTHER SUBSTANCES

INTERACTS WITH	COMBINED EFFECT
Alcohol:	Decreased probenecid effect.
Beverages:	
Caffeine drinks.	Loss of probenecid effectiveness.
Herbal teas.	Increased colchicine effect. Avoid.
Cocaine:	Overstimulation. Avoid.
Foods:	No proven problems.
Marijuana:	Decreased colchicine and probenecid effect.
Tobacco:	No proven problems.

*See Glossary

PROBUCOL

BRAND NAMES

Lorelco

BASIC INFORMATION

Habit forming? No
Prescription needed? Yes
Available as generic? No
Drug class: Antihyperlipidemic

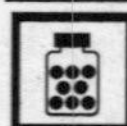

USES

Lowers cholesterol level in blood in persons with type IIa hyperlipoproteinemia.

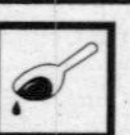

DOSAGE & USAGE INFORMATION

How to take:
Tablet—Swallow with liquid. If you can't swallow whole, crumble tablet and take with liquid or food.

When to take:
With morning and evening meals.

If you forget a dose:
Take as soon as you remember up to 2 hours late. If more than 2 hours, wait for next scheduled dose (don't double this dose).

What drug does:
Reduces serum cholesterol without reducing liver cholesterol.

Time lapse before drug works:
3 to 4 months.

Don't take with:
Other medicines or vitamins. Separate by 1 to 2 hours.

OVERDOSE

SYMPTOMS:
None reported.
WHAT TO DO:
Overdose unlikely to threaten life. If person takes much larger amount than prescribed, call doctor, poison control center or hospital emergency room for instructions.

POSSIBLE ADVERSE REACTIONS OR SIDE EFFECTS

SYMPTOMS	WHAT TO DO
Life-threatening: None expected.	
Common: Bloating, diarrhea, nausea, vomiting, abdominal pain, flatus.	Continue. Call doctor when convenient.
Infrequent:	
• Dizziness, headache.	Discontinue. Call doctor right away.
• Numbness or tingling in feet, toes, fingers, face.	Continue. Call doctor when convenient.
Rare:	
• Swelling of hands, face, feet, mouth.	Discontinue. Seek emergency treatment.
• Rash.	Discontinue. Call doctor right away.

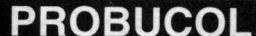

WARNINGS & PRECAUTIONS

Don't take if:
You are allergic to probucol.

Before you start, consult your doctor:
- If you have liver disease such as cirrhosis.
- If you have heartbeat irregularity.
- If you have congestive heart failure that is not under control.
- If you have gallstones.

Over age 60:
Adverse reactions and side effects may be more frequent and severe than in younger persons.

Pregnancy:
No proven problems. Avoid if possible. Continue using birth control methods for 6 months after discontinuing medicine. Consult doctor. Risk category B (see page xxii).

Breast-feeding:
Not recommended. Animal studies show drug passes into milk. Studies not available for human beings. Consult doctor.

Infants & children:
Not recommended. Safety and dosage have not been established.

Prolonged use:
Request serum cholesterol and serum triglyceride laboratory studies every 2 to 4 months.

Skin & sunlight:
No problems expected.

Driving, piloting or hazardous work:
If medicine does not cause dizziness, no problems expected.

Discontinuing:
Don't discontinue without consulting doctor. Dose may require gradual reduction if you have taken drug for a long time. Doses of other drugs may also require adjustment.

Others:
- Medicine works best in conjunction with low-fat, low-cholesterol diet and an active, regular exercise program.
- May affect results in some medical tests.

POSSIBLE INTERACTION WITH OTHER DRUGS

GENERIC NAME OR DRUG CLASS	COMBINED EFFECT
Chenodiol	Decreased chenodiol effect.
Clofibrate	Combination no more effective than one drug only, so don't take both.
Ursodiol	Decreased ursodiol effect.

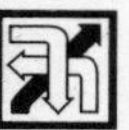

POSSIBLE INTERACTION WITH OTHER SUBSTANCES

INTERACTS WITH	COMBINED EFFECT
Alcohol:	May aggravate liver problems. Avoid.
Beverages:	None expected.
Cocaine:	None expected.
Foods:	None expected.
Marijuana:	None expected.
Tobacco:	None expected.

PROCAINAMIDE

BRAND NAMES

Procan SR
Promine
Pronestyl
Pronestyl SR

BASIC INFORMATION

Habit forming? No
Prescription needed? Yes
Available as generic? Yes
Drug class: Antiarrhythmic

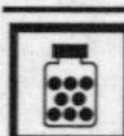

USES

Stabilizes irregular heartbeat.

DOSAGE & USAGE INFORMATION

How to take:
- Tablet or capsule—Swallow with liquid.
- Extended-release tablets—Swallow each dose whole. Do not crush them.

When to take:
Best taken on empty stomach, 1 hour before or 2 hours after meals. If necessary, may be taken with food or milk to lessen stomach upset.

If you forget a dose:
Take as soon as you remember up to 2 hours late (4 hours for extended-release tablets). If more than 2 hours, wait for next scheduled dose (don't double this dose).

What drug does:
Slows activity of pacemaker (rhythm control center of heart) and delays transmission of electrical impulses.

Time lapse before drug works:
30 to 60 minutes.

Don't take with:
Any other medicine without consulting your doctor or pharmacist.

OVERDOSE

SYMPTOMS:
Fast and irregular heartbeat, confusion, stupor, decreased blood pressure, fainting, cardiac arrest.
WHAT TO DO:
- **Dial 911 (emergency) or 0 (operator) for an ambulance or medical help. Then give first aid immediately.**
- **See emergency information on inside covers.**

POSSIBLE ADVERSE REACTIONS OR SIDE EFFECTS

SYMPTOMS	WHAT TO DO
Life-threatening:	
Hives, rash, intense itching, faintness soon after dose (anaphylaxis); convulsions.	Seek emergency treatment immediately.
Common:	
Diarrhea, appetite loss, nausea, vomiting, bitter taste.	Continue. Call doctor when convenient.
Infrequent:	
• Joint pain, painful breathing.	Discontinue. Call doctor right away.
• Dizziness.	Continue. Call doctor when convenient.
Rare:	
• Hallucinations, depression, confusion, psychosis, itchy skin, rash, sore throat, fever, jaundice, unusual bleeding or bruising.	Discontinue. Call doctor right away.
• Headache, fatigue.	Continue. Call doctor when convenient.

WARNINGS & PRECAUTIONS

Don't take if:
- You are allergic to procainamide.
- You have myasthenia gravis.

Before you start, consult your doctor:
- If you are allergic to local anesthetics that end in "caine."
- If you have had liver or kidney disease or impaired kidney function.
- If you have had lupus.
- If you take digitalis preparations*.
- If you will have surgery within 2 months, including dental surgery, requiring general or spinal anesthesia.

Over age 60:
Adverse reactions and side effects may be more frequent and severe than in younger persons.

Pregnancy:
Decide with your doctor if drug benefits justify risk to unborn child. Risk category C (see page xxii).

Breast-feeding:
No proven problems. Consult doctor.

Infants & children:
Not recommended.

Prolonged use:
- May cause lupus*-like illness.
- Talk to your doctor about the need for follow-up medical examinations or laboratory studies to check ANA titers*, blood pressure, complete blood counts (white blood cell count, platelet count, red blood cell count, hemoglobin, hematocrit).

Skin & sunlight:
No problems expected.

Driving, piloting or hazardous work:
Use caution if you feel dizzy or weak. Otherwise, no problems expected.

Discontinuing:
Don't discontinue without doctor's advice until you complete prescribed dose, even though symptoms diminish or disappear.

Others:
- Some products contain tartrazine dye. Avoid, especially if you are allergic to aspirin.
- May affect results of some medical tests.

POSSIBLE INTERACTION WITH OTHER DRUGS

GENERIC NAME OR DRUG CLASS	COMBINED EFFECT
Acetazolamide	Increased procainamide effect.
Ambenonium	Decreased ambenonium effect.
Aminoglycosides*	Possible severe muscle weakness, impaired breathing.
Antiarrhythmics*, other	Increased likelihood of adverse reactions with either drug. Possible increased effect of both drugs.
Anticholinergics*	Increased anticholinergic effect.
Antihypertensives*	Increased antihypertensive effect.
Antimyasthenics*	Decreased antimyasthenic effect.
Cimetidine	Increased procainamide effect.
Cisapride	Decreased procainamide effect.

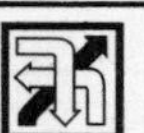

POSSIBLE INTERACTION WITH OTHER SUBSTANCES

INTERACTS WITH	COMBINED EFFECT
Alcohol:	None expected.
Beverages: Caffeine drinks, iced drinks.	Irregular heartbeat.
Cocaine:	Decreased procainamide effect.
Foods:	None expected.
Marijuana:	None expected.
Tobacco:	Decreased procainamide effect.

*See Glossary

PROCARBAZINE

BRAND NAMES

Matulane | Natulan

BASIC INFORMATION

Habit forming? No
Prescription needed? Yes
Available as generic? No
Drug class: Antineoplastic

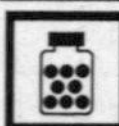

USES

Treatment for some kinds of cancer.

DOSAGE & USAGE INFORMATION

How to take:
Capsule—Swallow with liquid after light meal. Don't drink fluids with meals. Drink extra fluids between meals. Avoid sweet or fatty foods.

When to take:
At the same time each day.

If you forget a dose:
Take as soon as you remember. Don't double dose ever.

What drug does:
Inhibits abnormal cell reproduction. Procarbazine is an alkylating agent* and an MAO inhibitor.

Time lapse before drug works:
Up to 6 weeks for full effect.

Don't take with:
Any other medicine without consulting your doctor or pharmacist.

OVERDOSE

SYMPTOMS:
Restlessness, agitation, fever, convulsions, bleeding.
WHAT TO DO:
- **Dial 911 (emergency) or 0 (operator) for an ambulance or medical help. Then give first aid immediately.**
- **If patient is unconscious and not breathing, give mouth-to-mouth breathing. If there is no heartbeat, use cardiac massage and mouth-to-mouth breathing (CPR). Don't try to make patient vomit. If you can't get help quickly, take patient to nearest emergency facility.**
- **See emergency information on inside covers.**

POSSIBLE ADVERSE REACTIONS OR SIDE EFFECTS

SYMPTOMS	WHAT TO DO
Life-threatening: In case of overdose, see previous column.	
Common:	
• Nausea, vomiting, decreased urination, numbness or tingling in hands or feet, hair loss, rapid or pounding heartbeat, shortness of breath.	Discontinue. Call doctor right away.
• Fatigue, weakness, confusion.	Continue. Call doctor when convenient.
• Dizziness when changing position, dry mouth, inflamed tongue, constipation, difficult urination.	Continue. Tell doctor at next visit.
Infrequent:	
• Fainting.	Discontinue. Seek emergency treatment.
• Severe headache; abnormal bleeding or bruising; muscle, joint or chest pain, enlarged eye pupils; black, tarry stools; bloody urine.	Discontinue. Call doctor right away.
• Hallucinations, insomnia, nightmares, diarrhea, swollen feet or legs, nervousness, eyes sensitive to light, cough or hoarseness, mouth sores depression.	Continue. Call doctor when convenient.
• Diminished sex drive.	Continue. Tell doctor at next visit.
Rare:	
Rash, stiff neck, jaundice, fever, sore throat, vomiting blood, wheezing.	Discontinue. Call doctor right away.

WARNINGS & PRECAUTIONS

Don't take if:
- You are allergic to any MAO inhibitor.
- You have heart disease, congestive heart failure, heart rhythm irregularities or high blood pressure.
- You have liver or kidney disease.

Before you start, consult your doctor:
- If you are alcoholic.
- If you have asthma.
- If you have had a stroke.

- If you have diabetes or epilepsy.
- If you have overactive thyroid.
- If you have schizophrenia.
- If you have Parkinson's disease.
- If you have adrenal gland tumor.
- If you will have surgery within 2 months, including dental surgery, requiring general or spinal anesthesia.

Over age 60:
Not recommended.

Pregnancy:
Consult doctor. Risk category D (see page xxii).

Breast-feeding:
Safety not established. Consult doctor.

Infants & children:
Not recommended.

Prolonged use:
- May be toxic to liver.
- Talk to your doctor about the need for follow-up medical examinations or laboratory studies to check complete blood counts (white blood cell count, platelet count, red blood cell count, hemoglobin, hematocrit), bone marrow, kidney function.

Skin & sunlight:
May cause rash or intensify sunburn in areas exposed to sun or sunlamp.

Driving, piloting or hazardous work:
Don't drive or pilot aircraft until you learn how medicine affects you. Don't work around dangerous machinery. Don't climb ladders or work in high places. Danger increases if you drink alcohol or take medicine affecting alertness and reflexes.

Discontinuing:
- Don't discontinue without doctor's advice until you complete prescribed dose, even though symptoms diminish or disappear.
- Follow precautions regarding foods, drinks and other medicines for 2 weeks after discontinuing.

Others:
- May affect blood sugar levels in patients with diabetes.
- Advise any doctor or dentist whom you consult that you take this drug.

POSSIBLE INTERACTION WITH OTHER DRUGS

GENERIC NAME OR DRUG CLASS	COMBINED EFFECT
Amphetamines*	Blood pressure rise to life-threatening level.
Anticonvulsants*, oral	Changed seizure pattern.
Antidepressants, tricyclic*	Blood pressure rise to life-threatening level.
Antidiabetics*, oral and insulin	Excessively low blood sugar.
Antihistamines*	Increased sedation.
Barbiturates*	Increased sedation.
Bone marrow depressants*	Increased toxicity to bone marrow.
Buspirone	Elevated blood pressure.
Caffeine	Irregular heartbeat or high blood pressure.
Carbamazepine	Fever, seizures. Avoid.
Central nervous system (CNS) depressants*	Increased CNS depression.
Clozapine	Toxic effect on bone marrow and central nervous system.
Cyclobenzaprine	Fever, seizures. Avoid.
Dextromethorphan	Fever, hypertension.

Continued on page 956

POSSIBLE INTERACTION WITH OTHER SUBSTANCES

INTERACTS WITH	COMBINED EFFECT
Alcohol:	Increased sedation to dangerous level. Disulfiram-like reaction*.
Beverages:	
Caffeine drinks.	Irregular heartbeat or high blood pressure.
Drinks containing tyramine*.	Blood pressure rise to life-threatening level.
Cocaine:	Overstimulation. Possibly fatal.
Foods:	
Foods containing tyramine*.	Blood pressure rise to life-threatening level.
Marijuana:	Overstimulation. Avoid.
Tobacco:	No proven problems.

*See Glossary

PROGESTINS

BRAND AND GENERIC NAMES

See complete list of brand and generic names in the *Brand Names Directory*, page 916.

BASIC INFORMATION

Habit forming? No
Prescription needed? Yes
Available as generic? Yes, for some.
Drug class: Female sex hormone (progestin)

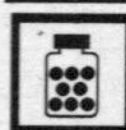

USES

- Treatment for menstrual or uterine disorders caused by progestin imbalance.
- Contraceptive (when combined with estrogens in birth control pills).
- Treatment for cancer of breast and uterus.
- Treatment for toxic sleep apnea.
- Treatment for female hormone imbalance.
- Treatment for weight loss.

DOSAGE & USAGE INFORMATION

How to take:
- Tablet—Swallow with liquid or food to lessen stomach irritation. You may crumble tablet.
- Injection—Under doctor's supervision.
- Oral suspension—Follow package instructions.

When to take:
At the same time each day.

If you forget a dose:
- Treatment for menstrual disorders—Take up to 2 hours late. If more than 2 hours, wait for next dose (don't double this dose).
- Contraceptive—Consult your doctor. You may need to use another birth control method until next period.

Continued next column

OVERDOSE

SYMPTOMS:
Nausea, vomiting, fluid retention, breast discomfort or enlargement, vaginal bleeding.
WHAT TO DO:
Overdose unlikely to threaten life. If person takes much larger amount than prescribed, call doctor, poison control center or hospital emergency room for instructions.

What drug does:
- Creates a uterine lining similar to that of pregnancy that prevents bleeding.
- Suppresses a pituitary gland hormone responsible for ovulation.
- Stimulates cervical mucus, which stops sperm penetration and prevents pregnancy.

Time lapse before drug works:
- Menstrual disorders—24 to 48 hours.
- Contraception—3 weeks.
- Cancer—May require 2 to 3 months regular use for maximum benefit.

Don't take with:
Any other medicine without consulting your doctor or pharmacist.

POSSIBLE ADVERSE REACTIONS OR SIDE EFFECTS

SYMPTOMS	WHAT TO DO
Life-threatening:	
Blood clot in leg, brain or lung; hives, rash, intense itching, faintness soon after a dose (anaphylaxis).	Seek emergency treatment immediately.
Common:	
Appetite or weight changes, swollen feet or ankles, unusual tiredness or weakness, menstrual cycle changes.	Continue. Tell doctor at next visit.
Infrequent:	
• Prolonged vaginal bleeding, pain in calf.	Discontinue. Call doctor right away.
• Depression.	Continue. Call doctor when convenient.
• Acne, increased facial or body hair, nausea, tender breasts, headache, enlarged clitoris.	Continue. Tell doctor at next visit.
Rare:	
• Rash, stomach or side pain, jaundice, fever, vision changes.	Discontinue. Call doctor right away.
• Amenorrhea, hair loss, insomnia, brown skin spots, voice change.	Continue. Call doctor when convenient.

WARNINGS & PRECAUTIONS

Don't take if:
- You are allergic to any progestin hormone.
- You may be pregnant.
- You have liver or gallbladder disease.
- You have had thrombophlebitis, embolism or stroke.
- You have unexplained vaginal bleeding.
- You have had breast or uterine cancer.

Before you start, consult your doctor:
- If you have heart or kidney disease.
- If you have diabetes.
- If you have a seizure disorder.
- If you suffer migraines.
- If you are easily depressed.

Over age 60:
No special problems expected.

Pregnancy:
Risk factors vary for drugs in this group. See category list on page xxii and consult doctor.

Breast-feeding:
Drug passes into milk. Avoid drug or discontinue nursing until you finish medicine. Consult doctor for advice on maintaining milk supply.

Infants & children:
Use only for female children under medical supervision.

Prolonged use:
No problems expected.

Skin & sunlight:
No problems expected.

Driving, piloting or hazardous work:
No problems expected.

Discontinuing:
Consult doctor. This medicine stays in the body and causes fetal abnormalities. Wait at least 3 months before becoming pregnant.

Others:
- Patients with diabetes must be monitored closely.
- Symptoms of blood clot in leg, brain or lung are: chest, groin, leg pain; sudden, severe headache; loss of coordination; vision change; shortness of breath; slurred speech.
- May affect results in some medical tests.
- Advise any doctor or dentist whom you consult that you take this medicine.

POSSIBLE INTERACTION WITH OTHER DRUGS

GENERIC NAME OR DRUG CLASS	COMBINED EFFECT
Bromocriptine	Decreased bromocriptine effect.
Hypoglycemics, oral*	Decreased oral hypoglycemic effect.
Insulin	Decreased insulin effect.
Phenobarbital	Decreased progestin effect.
Phenothiazines*	Increased phenothiazine effect.
Phenylbutazone	Decreased progestin effect.
Rifampin	Decreased contraceptive effect.

POSSIBLE INTERACTION WITH OTHER SUBSTANCES

INTERACTS WITH	COMBINED EFFECT
Alcohol:	None expected.
Beverages:	None expected.
Cocaine:	Decreased progestin effect.
Foods: Salt.	Fluid retention.
Marijuana:	Possible menstrual irregularities or bleeding between periods.
Tobacco: All forms.	Possible blood clots in lung, brain, legs. Avoid.

*See Glossary

PROPAFENONE

BRAND NAMES

Rhythmol

BASIC INFORMATION

Habit forming? No
Prescription needed? Yes
Available as generic? No
Drug class: Antiarrhythmic

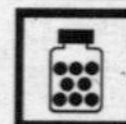

USES

Treats severe heartbeat irregularities (life-threatening ventricular rhythm disturbances).

DOSAGE & USAGE INFORMATION

How to take:
Tablet—Swallow with liquid or food to lessen stomach irritation. If you can't swallow whole, crumble tablet and take with liquid or food.

When to take:
At the same time each day, according to instructions on prescription label.

If you forget a dose:
Take as soon as you remember up to 2 hours late. If more than 2 hours, wait for next scheduled dose. Don't double this dose.

What drug does:
Slows electrical activity in the heart to decrease the excitability of the heart muscle.

Time lapse before drug works:
3-1/2 hours to 1 week for full effect. Begins working almost immediately.

Don't take with:
Any other medicine (including nonprescription drugs such as cough and cold medicines, nose drops, vitamins, laxatives, antacids, diet pills, or caffeine) without consulting your doctor or pharmacist.

OVERDOSE

SYMPTOMS:
Very rapid heart rate that is also irregular.
WHAT TO DO:
Overdose unlikely to threaten life. If person takes much larger amount than prescribed, call doctor, poison control center or hospital emergency room for instructions.

POSSIBLE ADVERSE REACTIONS OR SIDE EFFECTS

SYMPTOMS	WHAT TO DO
Life-threatening:	
Severe chest pain, severe shortness of breath	Seek emergency treatment.
Common:	
• Faster or more irregular heartbeat.	Discontinue. Call doctor right away.
• Taste change, dizziness.	Continue. Call doctor when convenient.
Infrequent:	
• Blurred vision, skin rash.	Discontinue. Call doctor right away.
• Constipation, diarrhea.	Continue. Call doctor when convenient.
• Dry mouth, nausea.	Continue. Tell doctor at next visit.
Rare:	
Fever, chills, trembling, joint pain, slow heartbeat.	Discontinue. Call doctor right away.

WARNINGS & PRECAUTIONS

Don't take if:
You are allergic to propafenone.

Before you start, consult your doctor:
- If you have asthma or bronchospasm.
- If you have congestive heart failure.
- If you have liver disease or kidney disease.
- If you have a recent history of heart attack.
- If you have a pacemaker.

Over age 60:
More likely to have decreased kidney function and require dosage modification.

Pregnancy:
Decide with your doctor if drug benefits justify risk to unborn child. Risk category C (see page xxii).

Breast-feeding:
No proven problems. Consult doctor.

Infants & children:
Safety and efficacy not established.

Prolonged use:
Don't discontinue without consulting doctor. Dose may require gradual reduction if you have taken drug for a long time. Dosages of other drugs may also require adjustment.

Skin & sunlight:
No special problems expected.

Driving, piloting or hazardous work:
Don't drive or pilot aircraft until you learn how medicine affects you. Don't work around dangerous machinery. Don't climb ladders or work in high places. Danger increases if you drink alcohol or take medicine affecting alertness and reflexes.

Discontinuing:
Don't discontinue without consulting doctor. Dose may require gradual reduction if you have taken drug for a long time. Doses of other drugs may also require adjustment.

Others:
- Advise any doctor or dentist whom you consult that you take this medicine, especially if you are to be anesthetized.
- Report changes in symptoms to your doctor and return for periodic visits to check progress.
- Carry or wear a medical I.D. card or bracelet.

POSSIBLE INTERACTION WITH OTHER DRUGS

GENERIC NAME OR DRUG CLASS	COMBINED EFFECT
Anesthetics, local (e.g., prior to dental procedures)	May increase risk of side effects.
Antiarrhythmics*, other	Increased risk of adverse reactions.
Beta-adrenergic blocking agents*	Increased beta blocker effect.
Digitalis preparations*	Increased digitalis absorption. May require decreased dosage of digitalis preparation.
Warfarin	Increased warfarin effect.

POSSIBLE INTERACTION WITH OTHER SUBSTANCES

INTERACTS WITH	COMBINED EFFECT
Alcohol:	Unpredictable effect on heartbeat. Avoid.
Beverages: Caffeine drinks.	Increased heartbeat irregularity. Avoid.
Cocaine:	Increased heartbeat irregularity. Avoid.
Foods:	None expected.
Marijuana:	Increased heartbeat irregularity. Avoid.
Tobacco:	Increased heartbeat irregularity. Avoid.

*See Glossary

PROPANTHELINE

BRAND NAMES

Pro-Banthine   Propanthel

BASIC INFORMATION

Habit forming? No
Prescription needed?
High strength: Yes
Low strength: No
Available as generic? Yes
Drug class: Antispasmodic, anticholinergic

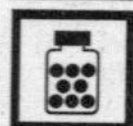

USES

- Reduces spasms of digestive system, bladder and urethra.
- Treats peptic ulcers.

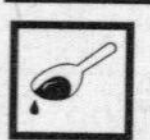

DOSAGE & USAGE INFORMATION

How to take:
Tablet—Swallow with liquid or food to lessen stomach irritation.

When to take:
30 minutes before meals (unless directed otherwise by doctor).

If you forget a dose:
Take as soon as you remember up to 2 hours late. If more than 2 hours, wait for next scheduled dose (don't double this dose).

What drug does:
Blocks nerve impulses at parasympathetic nerve endings, preventing muscle contractions and gland secretions of organs involved.

Time lapse before drug works:
15 to 30 minutes.

Don't take with:
Any other medicine without consulting your doctor or pharmacist.

OVERDOSE

SYMPTOMS:
Dilated pupils, blurred vision, rapid pulse and breathing, dizziness, fever, hallucinations, confusion, slurred speech, agitation, flushed face, convulsions, coma.
WHAT TO DO:
- **Dial 911 (emergency) or 0 (operator) for an ambulance or medical help. Then give first aid immediately.**
- **See emergency information on inside covers.**

POSSIBLE ADVERSE REACTIONS OR SIDE EFFECTS

SYMPTOMS	WHAT TO DO
Life-threatening:	
Hives, rash, intense itching, faintness soon after a dose (anaphylaxis).	Seek emergency treatment immediately.
Common:	
• Confusion, delirium, rapid heartbeat.	Discontinue. Call doctor right away.
• Nausea, vomiting, decreased sweating.	Continue. Call doctor when convenient.
• Constipation, loss of taste.	Continue. Tell doctor at next visit.
• Dry ears, nose, throat, mouth.	No action necessary.
Infrequent:	
• Headache, difficult urination, nasal congestion, altered taste, impotence.	Continue. Call doctor when convenient.
• Lightheadedness.	Discontinue. Call doctor right away.
Rare:	
Rash or hives, eye pain, blurred vision.	Discontinue. Call doctor right away.

WARNINGS & PRECAUTIONS

Don't take if:
- You are allergic to any anticholinergic.
- You have trouble with stomach bloating.
- You have difficulty emptying your bladder completely.
- You have narrow-angle glaucoma.
- You have severe ulcerative colitis.

Before you start, consult your doctor:
- If you have open-angle glaucoma.
- If you have angina.
- If you have chronic bronchitis or asthma.
- If you have hiatal hernia.
- If you have liver, kidney or thyroid disease.
- If you have enlarged prostate.
- If you have myasthenia gravis.
- If you have peptic ulcer.
- If you will have surgery within 2 months, including dental surgery, requiring general or spinal anesthesia.

Over age 60:
Adverse reactions and side effects may be more frequent and severe than in younger persons.

Pregnancy:
Decide with your doctor whether drug benefits justify risk to unborn child. Risk category C (see page xxii).

Breast-feeding:
Drug passes into milk and decreases milk flow. Avoid drug or discontinue nursing until you finish medicine. Consult doctor for advice on maintaining milk supply.

Infants & children:
Use only under medical supervision.

Prolonged use:
Chronic constipation, possible fecal impaction. Consult doctor immediately.

Skin & sunlight:
No problems expected.

Driving, piloting or hazardous work:
Use disqualifies you for piloting aircraft. Otherwise, no problems expected.

Discontinuing:
May be unnecessary to finish medicine. Follow doctor's instructions.

Others:
Advise any doctor or dentist whom you consult that you take this medicine.

POSSIBLE INTERACTION WITH OTHER DRUGS

GENERIC NAME OR DRUG CLASS	COMBINED EFFECT
Amantadine	Increased propantheline effect.
Antacids*	Decreased propantheline effect.
Anticholinergics*, other	Increased propantheline effect.
Antidepressants, tricyclic*	Increased propantheline effect. Increased sedation.
Antidiarrhea preparations*	Reduced propantheline effect.
Antihistamines*	Increased propantheline effect.
Attapulgite	Decreased propantheline effect.
Buclizine	Increased propantheline effect.
Cortisone drugs*	Increased internal eye pressure.
Digitalis preparations*	Possible decreased absorption of digitalis.
Haloperidol	Increased internal eye pressure.
Ketoconazole	Decreased ketoconazole effect.
Meperidine	Increased propantheline effect.
Methylphenidate	Increased propantheline effect.
Molindone	Increased anti-cholinergic effect.
Monoamine oxidase (MAO) inhibitors*	Increased propantheline effect.
Nitrates*	Increased internal eye pressure.
Nizatidine	Increased nizatidine effect.
Orphenadrine	Increased propantheline effect.
Phenothiazines*	Increased propantheline effect.
Pilocarpine	Loss of pilocarpine effect in glaucoma treatment.
Potassium supplements*	Increased possibility of intestinal ulcers with oral potassium tablets.
Quinidine	Increased propantheline effect.
Sedatives* or central nervous system (CNS) depressants*	Increased sedative effect of both drugs.
Terfenadine	Possible increased propantheline effect.
Vitamin C	Decreased propantheline effect. Avoid large doses of vitamin C.

POSSIBLE INTERACTION WITH OTHER SUBSTANCES

INTERACTS WITH	COMBINED EFFECT
Alcohol:	None expected.
Beverages:	None expected.
Cocaine:	Excessively rapid heartbeat. Avoid.
Foods:	None expected.
Marijuana:	Drowsiness and dry mouth.
Tobacco:	None expected.

*See Glossary

PROTECTANT (Ophthalmic)

BRAND AND GENERIC NAMES

Gonak
Goniosol
HYDROXYPROPYL CELLULOSE
HYDROXYPROPYL METHYL-CELLULOSE
Isopto Alkaline
Isopto Plain
Isopto Tears
Just Tears
Lacril (ophthalmic)
Lacrisert
Moisture Drops
Tearisol
Tears Naturale
Tears Renewed
Ultra Tears

BASIC INFORMATION

Habit forming? No
Prescription needed? Yes
Available as generic? Yes, for some
Drug class: Protectant (ophthalmic), artificial tears

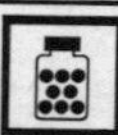

USES

- Relieves eye dryness and irritation caused by inadequate flow of tears.
- Moistens contact lenses and artificial eyes.

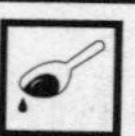

DOSAGE & USAGE INFORMATION

How to use:
Eye drops
- Wash hands.
- Apply pressure to inside corner of eye with middle finger.
- Continue pressure for 1 minute after placing medicine in eye.
- Tilt head backward. Pull lower lid away from eye with index finger of the same hand.
- Drop eye drops into pouch and close eye. Don't blink.
- Keep eyes closed for 1 to 2 minutes.
- Don't touch applicator tip to any surface (including the eye). If you accidentally touch tip, clean with warm soap and water.
- Keep container tightly closed.
- Keep cool, but don't freeze.
- Wash hands immediately after using.

Continued next column

OVERDOSE

SYMPTOMS:
None expected.
WHAT TO DO:
Not intended for internal use. If child accidentally swallows, call poison control center.

When to use:
As directed. Usually every 3 or 4 hours.

If you forget a dose:
Use as soon as you remember.

What drug does:
- Stabilizes and thickens tear film.
- Lubricates and protects eye.

Time lapse before drug works:
2 to 10 minutes.

Don't use with:
Other eye drops without consulting your doctor.

POSSIBLE ADVERSE REACTIONS OR SIDE EFFECTS

SYMPTOMS	WHAT TO DO
Life-threatening	
None expected.	
Common	
None expected.	
Infrequent	
Eye irritation not present before using artificial tears.	Discontinue. Call doctor right away.
Rare	
None expected.	

WARNINGS & PRECAUTIONS

Don't use if:
You are allergic to any artificial tears.

Before you start, consult your doctor:
If you use any other eye drops.

Over age 60:
No problems expected.

Pregnancy:
Risk factor not designated. See category list on page xxii and consult doctor.

Breast-feeding:
No problems expected, but check with doctor.

Infants & children:
Don't use.

Prolonged use:
Don't use for more than 3 or 4 days.

Skin & sunlight:
No problems expected.

Driving, piloting or hazardous work:
No problems expected.

Discontinuing:
May not need all the medicine in container. If symptoms disappear, stop using.

Others:
- Keep cool, but don't freeze.
- Check with your doctor if eye irritation continues or becomes worse.

POSSIBLE INTERACTION WITH OTHER DRUGS

GENERIC NAME OR DRUG CLASS	COMBINED EFFECT

Clinically significant interactions with oral or injected medicines unlikely.

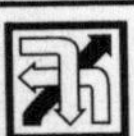

POSSIBLE INTERACTION WITH OTHER SUBSTANCES

INTERACTS WITH	COMBINED EFFECT
Alcohol:	None expected.
Beverages:	None expected.
Cocaine:	None expected.
Foods:	None expected.
Marijuana:	None expected.
Tobacco:	None expected.

***See Glossary**

PSEUDOEPHEDRINE

BRAND NAMES

See complete list of brand names in the *Brand Name Directory*, page 916.

BASIC INFORMATION

Habit forming? No
Prescription needed?
U.S.: High strength—Yes
Low strength—No
Canada: No
Available as generic? Yes
Drug class: Sympathomimetic, decongestant

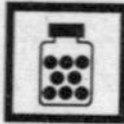

USES

Reduces congestion of nose, sinuses, eustachian tubes and throat from allergies and infections.

DOSAGE & USAGE INFORMATION

How to take:

- Tablet or capsule—Swallow with liquid. You may chew or crush tablet or open capsule.
- Extended-release tablet or capsule—Swallow each dose whole.
- Syrup—Take as directed on label.
- Drops—Place directly on tongue and swallow.
- Oral solution—Take as direced on label.

When to take:

- At the same times each day.
- To prevent insomnia, take last dose of day a few hours before bedtime.

If you forget a dose:
Take up to 2 hours late. If more than 2 hours, wait for next dose (don't double this dose).

What drug does:
Decreases blood volume in nasal tissues, shrinking tissues and enlarging airways.

Continued next column

OVERDOSE

SYMPTOMS:
Nervousness, restlessness, headache, rapid or irregular heartbeat, sweating, nausea, vomiting, anxiety, confusion, delirium, muscle tremors, convulsions, hallucinations.
WHAT TO DO:

- **Dial 911 (emergency) or 0 (operator) for an ambulance or medical help. Then give first aid immediately.**
- **See emergency information on inside covers.**

Time lapse before drug works:
15 to 20 minutes.

Don't take with:

- Nonprescription drugs with caffeine without consulting doctor.
- Any other medicine without consulting your doctor or pharmacist.

POSSIBLE ADVERSE REACTIONS OR SIDE EFFECTS

SYMPTOMS	WHAT TO DO
Life-threatening: In case of overdose, see previous column.	
Common: Agitation, insomnia.	Continue. Tell doctor at next visit.
Infrequent:	
• Nausea or vomiting, irregular or slow heartbeat, difficult breathing, unusually fast or pounding heartbeat, painful or difficult urination, increased sweating, trembling.	Discontinue. Call doctor right away.
• Dizziness, headache, shakiness, weakness.	Continue. Call doctor when convenient.
• Paleness.	Continue. Tell doctor at next visit.
Rare: Hallucinations, seizures.	Discontinue. Seek emergency treatment.

WARNINGS & PRECAUTIONS

Don't take if:
You are allergic to any sympathomimetic drug.

Before you start, consult your doctor:
- If you have overactive thyroid or diabetes.
- If you have taken any monoamine oxidase (MAO) inhibitor* in past 2 weeks.
- If you take digitalis preparations or have high blood pressure or heart disease.
- If you will have surgery within 2 months, including dental surgery, requiring general or spinal anesthesia.
- If you have urination difficulty.

Over age 60:
Adverse reactions and side effects may be more frequent and severe than in younger persons.

Pregnancy:
No proven harm to unborn child. Avoid if possible. Consult doctor. Risk category B (see page xxii).

Breast-feeding:
Drug passes into milk. Avoid drug or discontinue nursing until you finish medicine. Consult doctor for advice on maintaining milk supply.

Infants & children:
Keep dose low or avoid.

Prolonged use:
No proven problems.

Skin & sunlight:
No problems expected.

Driving, piloting or hazardous work:
Avoid if you feel dizzy. Otherwise, no problems expected.

Discontinuing:
May be unnecessary to finish medicine. Follow doctor's instructions.

Others:
No problems expected.

POSSIBLE INTERACTION WITH OTHER DRUGS

GENERIC NAME OR DRUG CLASS	COMBINED EFFECT
Antihypertensives*	Decreased anti-hypertensive effect.
Beta-adrenergic blocking agents*	Decreased effect of both drugs.
Calcium supplements*	Increased pseudo-ephedrine effect.
Digitalis preparations*	Irregular heartbeat.
Epinephrine	Increased epinephrine effect. Excessive heart stimulation and blood pressure increase.
Ergot preparations*	Serious blood pressure rise.
Guanadrel	Decreased effect of both drugs.
Guanethidine	Decreased effect of both drugs.
Methyldopa	Possible increased blood pressure.
Monoamine oxidase (MAO) inhibitors*	Increased pseudo-ephedrine effect.
Nitrates*	Possible decreased effects of both drugs.
Phenothiazines*	Possible increased pseudoephedrine toxicity. Possible decreased pseudo-ephedrine effect.
Rauwolfia	Decreased rauwolfia effect.
Sympathomimetics*, other	Increased pseudo-ephedrine effect.
Terazosin	Decreased effective-ness of terazosin.

POSSIBLE INTERACTION WITH OTHER SUBSTANCES

INTERACTS WITH	COMBINED EFFECT
Alcohol:	None expected.
Beverages: Caffeine drinks.	Nervousness or insomnia.
Cocaine:	High risk of heart-beat irregularities and high blood pressure.
Foods:	None expected.
Marijuana:	Rapid heartbeat.
Tobacco:	None expected.

***See Glossary**

PSORALENS

BRAND AND GENERIC NAMES

METHOXSALEN
Methoxsalen Lotion (Topical)
Oxsoralen
Oxsoralen-Ultra
Oxsoralen (Topical)
TRIOXSALEN
Trisoralen
UltraMOP

BASIC INFORMATION

Habit forming? No
Prescription needed? Yes
Available as generic? No
Drug class: Repigmenting agent (psoralen)

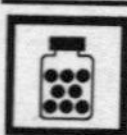

USES

- Repigmenting skin affected with vitiligo (absence of skin pigment).
- Treatment for psoriasis, when other treatments haven't helped.
- Treatment for mycosis fungoides.

DOSAGE & USAGE INFORMATION

How to take or apply:
- Tablet or capsule—Swallow with liquid or food to lessen stomach irritation.
- Topical—As directed by doctor.

When to take or apply:
2 to 4 hours before exposure to sunlight or sunlamp.

If you forget a dose:
Take as soon as you remember. Delay sun exposure for at least 2 hours after taking.

What drug does:
Helps pigment cells when used in conjunction with ultraviolet light.

Time lapse before drug works:
- For vitiligo, 6 to 9 months.
- For psoriasis, 10 weeks or longer.
- For tanning, 3 to 4 days.

Don't take with:
Any other medicine which causes skin sensitivity to sun. Ask pharmacist.

OVERDOSE

SYMPTOMS:
Blistering skin, swelling feet and legs.
WHAT TO DO:
Overdose unlikely to threaten life. If person takes much larger amount than prescribed, call doctor, poison control center or hospital emergency room for instructions.

POSSIBLE ADVERSE REACTIONS OR SIDE EFFECTS

SYMPTOMS	WHAT TO DO
Life-threatening: None expected.	
Common:	
• Increased skin sensitivity to sun.	Always protect from overexposure.
• Increased eye sensitivity to sunlight.	Always protect with wrap-around sunglasses.
• Nausea.	Continue. Call doctor when convenient.
Infrequent:	
• Skin red and sore.	Discontinue. Call doctor right away.
• Dizziness, headache, depression, leg cramps, insomnia.	Continue. Call doctor when convenient.
Rare:	
Hepatitis with jaundice, blistering and peeling.	Discontinue. Call doctor right away.

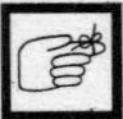

WARNINGS & PRECAUTIONS

Don't take if:
- You are allergic to any other psoralen.
- You are unwilling or unable to remain under close medical supervision.

Before you start, consult your doctor:
- If you have heart or liver disease.
- If you have allergy to sunlight.
- If you have cataracts.
- If you have albinism.
- If you have lupus erythematosis, porphyria, chronic infection, skin cancer or peptic ulcer.
- If you will have surgery within 2 months, including dental surgery, requiring general or spinal anesthesia.
- If you have skin cancer.

Over age 60:
Adverse reactions and side effects may be more frequent and severe than in younger persons.

Pregnancy:
Risk factors vary for drugs in this group. See category list on page xxii and consult doctor.

Breast-feeding:
Drug may pass into milk. Avoid drug or discontinue nursing until you finish medicine. Consult doctor for advice on maintaining milk supply.

Infants & children:
Not recommended.

Prolonged use:
- Increased chance of toxic effects.
- Talk to your doctor about the need for follow-up medical examinations or laboratory studies to check ANA titers*, complete blood counts (white blood cell count, platelet count, red blood cell count, hemoglobin, hematocrit), liver function, kidney function, eyes.

Skin & sunlight:
Too much can burn skin. Cover skin for 24 hours before and 8 hours following treatments.

Driving, piloting or hazardous work:
No problems expected. Protect eyes and skin from bright light.

Discontinuing:
Skin may remain sensitive for some time after treatment stops. Use extra protection from sun.

Others:
- Use sunblock on lips.
- Don't use just to make skin tan.
- Don't use hard gelatin capsules interchangeably with soft gelatin capsules.

POSSIBLE INTERACTION WITH OTHER DRUGS

GENERIC NAME OR DRUG CLASS	COMBINED EFFECT
Photosensitizing medications*	Greatly increased likelihood of extreme sensitivity to sunlight.

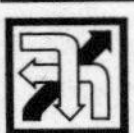

POSSIBLE INTERACTION WITH OTHER SUBSTANCES

INTERACTS WITH	COMBINED EFFECT
Alcohol:	May increase chance of liver toxicity.
Beverages: Lime drinks.	Avoid—toxic.
Cocaine:	Increased chance of toxicity. Avoid.
Foods: Those containing furocoumarin (limes, parsley, figs, parsnips, carrots, celery, mustard).	May cause toxic reaction to psoralens.
Marijuana:	Increased chance of toxicity. Avoid.
Tobacco:	May cause uneven absorption of medicine. Avoid.

*See Glossary

PSYLLIUM

BRAND NAMES

See complete list of brand names in the *Brand Name Directory*, page 918.

BASIC INFORMATION

Habit forming? No
Prescription needed? No
Available as generic? Yes
Drug class: Laxative (bulk-forming)

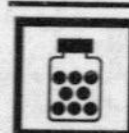

USES

Relieves constipation and prevents straining for bowel movement.

DOSAGE & USAGE INFORMATION

How to take:

- Powder or granules—Dilute dose in 8 oz. cold water or fruit juice.
- Wafers or chewable pieces—Chew and swallow with liquid.

When to take:
At the same time each day, preferably morning.

If you forget a dose:
Take as soon as you remember, then resume regular schedule.

What drug does:
Absorbs water, stimulating the bowel to form a soft, bulky stool.

Time lapse before drug works:
May require 2 or 3 days to begin, then works in 12 to 24 hours.

Don't take with:

- Any other medicine without consulting your doctor or pharmacist.
- Don't take within 2 hours of taking another medicine.

OVERDOSE

SYMPTOMS:
None expected.
WHAT TO DO:
Overdose unlikely to threaten life. If person takes much larger amount than prescribed, call doctor, poison control center or hospital emergency room for instructions.

POSSIBLE ADVERSE REACTIONS OR SIDE EFFECTS

SYMPTOMS	WHAT TO DO
Life-threatening	
None expected.	
Common:	
None expected.	
Infrequent:	
Swallowing difficulty, "lump in throat" sensation.	Continue. Call doctor when convenient.
Rare:	
Rash, itchy skin, asthma.	Discontinue. Call doctor right away.

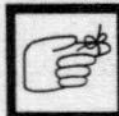

WARNINGS & PRECAUTIONS

Don't take if:
- You are allergic to any bulk-forming laxative.
- You have symptoms of appendicitis, inflamed bowel or intestinal blockage.
- You have missed a bowel movement for only 1 or 2 days.

Before you start, consult your doctor:
- If you have diabetes.
- If you have kidney disease.
- If you have a laxative habit.
- If you have rectal bleeding.
- If you have difficulty swallowing.
- If you take other laxatives.

Over age 60:
Adverse reactions and side effects may be more frequent and severe than in younger persons.

Pregnancy:
Most bulk-forming laxatives contain sodium or sugars which may cause fluid retention. Avoid if possible. Consult doctor. Risk category C (see page xxii).

Breast-feeding:
No problems expected. Consult doctor.

Infants & children:
Use only under medical supervision.

Prolonged use:
Don't take for more than 1 week unless under a doctor's supervision. May cause laxative dependence.

Skin & sunlight:
No problems expected.

Driving, piloting or hazardous work:
No problems expected.

Discontinuing:
May be unnecessary to finish medicine. Follow doctor's instructions.

Others:
- Don't take to "flush out" your system, or as a "tonic."
- Blockage of the throat or esophagus may occur if drug is not taken with an adequate amount of water.

POSSIBLE INTERACTION WITH OTHER DRUGS

GENERIC NAME OR DRUG CLASS	COMBINED EFFECT
Digitalis preparations*	Decreased digitalis effect.
Salicylates* (including aspirin)	Decreased salicylate effect.

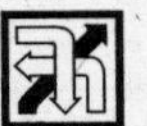

POSSIBLE INTERACTION WITH OTHER SUBSTANCES

INTERACTS WITH	COMBINED EFFECT
Alcohol:	None expected.
Beverages:	None expected.
Cocaine:	None expected.
Foods:	None expected.
Marijuana:	None expected.
Tobacco:	None expected.

***See Glossary**

PYRIDOSTIGMINE

BRAND NAMES

Mestinon
Mestinon Timespans
Regonol

BASIC INFORMATION

Habit forming? No
Prescription needed? Yes
Available as generic? No
Drug class: Cholinergic, antimyasthenic

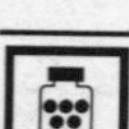

USES

- Diagnosis and treatment of myasthenia gravis.
- Treatment of urinary retention and abdominal distention.
- Antidote to adverse effects of muscle relaxants used in surgery.

DOSAGE & USAGE INFORMATION

How to take:
- Tablet or syrup—Swallow with liquid or food to lessen stomach irritation.
- Extended-release tablets—Swallow each dose whole. If you take regular tablets, you may chew or crush them.

When to take:
As directed, usually 3 or 4 times a day.

If you forget a dose:
Take as soon as you remember up to 2 hours late. If more than 2 hours, wait for next scheduled dose (don't double this dose).

What drug does:
Inhibits the chemical activity of an enzyme (cholinesterase) so nerve impulses can cross the junction of nerves and muscles.

Continued next column

OVERDOSE

SYMPTOMS:
Muscle weakness or paralysis, cramps, twitching or clumsiness; severe diarrhea, nausea, vomiting, stomach cramps or pain; breathing difficulty; confusion, irritability, nervousness, restlessness, fear; unusually slow heartbeat; seizures; blurred vision; extreme fatigue.
WHAT TO DO:
- **Dial 911 (emergency) or 0 (operator) for an ambulance or medical help. Then give first aid immediately.**
- **See emergency information on inside covers.**

Time lapse before drug works:
3 hours.

Don't take with:
Any other medicine without consulting your doctor or pharmacist.

POSSIBLE ADVERSE REACTIONS OR SIDE EFFECTS

SYMPTOMS	WHAT TO DO
Life-threatening:	
In case of overdose, see previous column.	
Common:	
• Mild diarrhea, nausea, vomiting, stomach cramps or pain.	Discontinue. Call doctor right away.
• Excess saliva, unusual sweating.	Continue. Call doctor when convenient.
Infrequent:	
• Confusion, irritability.	Discontinue. Seek emergency treatment.
• Constricted pupils, watery eyes, lung congestion, frequent urge to urinate.	Continue. Call doctor when convenient.
Rare:	
Bronchospasm, slow heartbeat, weakness.	Discontinue. Call doctor right away.

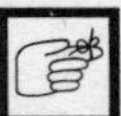

WARNINGS & PRECAUTIONS

Don't take if:
- You are allergic to any cholinergic* or bromide.
- You take mecamylamine.

Before you start, consult your doctor:
- If you plan to become pregnant within medication period.
- If you have bronchial asthma.
- If you have heartbeat irregularities.
- If you have urinary obstruction or urinary tract infection.

Over age 60:
Adverse reactions and side effects may be more frequent and severe than in younger persons.

Pregnancy:
Decide with your doctor if drug benefits justify risk to unborn child. Risk category C (see page xxii).

Breast-feeding:
Drug passes into milk. Avoid drug or discontinue nursing until you finish medicine. Consult doctor for advice on maintaining milk supply.

Infants & children:
Not recommended.

Prolonged use:
Medication may lose effectiveness. Discontinuing for a few days may restore effect.

Skin & sunlight:
No problems expected.

Driving, piloting or hazardous work:
Don't drive or pilot aircraft until you learn how medicine affects you. Don't work around dangerous machinery. Don't climb ladders or work in high places. Danger increases if you drink alcohol or take medicine affecting alertness and reflexes, such as antihistamines, tranquilizers, sedatives, pain medicine, narcotics and mind-altering drugs.

Discontinuing:
Don't discontinue without doctor's advice until you complete prescribed dose, even though symptoms diminish or disappear.

Others:
No problems expected.

POSSIBLE INTERACTION WITH OTHER DRUGS

GENERIC NAME OR DRUG CLASS	COMBINED EFFECT
Anesthetics, local or general*	Decreased pyridostigmine effect.
Antiarrhythmics*	Decreased pyridostigmine effect.
Anticholinergics*	Decreased pyridostigmine effect. May mask severe side effects.
Cholinergics*, other	Reduced intestinal tract function. Possible brain and nervous system toxicity.
Guanadrel	Decreased pyridostigmine effect.
Guanethidine	Decreased pyridostigmine effect.
Mecamylamine	Decreased pyridostigmine effect.
Procainamide	Decreased pyridostigmine effect.
Quinidine	Decreased pyridostigmine effect.

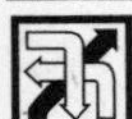

POSSIBLE INTERACTION WITH OTHER SUBSTANCES

INTERACTS WITH	COMBINED EFFECT
Alcohol:	No proven problems with small doses.
Beverages:	None expected.
Cocaine:	Decreased pyridostigmine effect. Avoid.
Foods:	None expected.
Marijuana:	No proven problems.
Tobacco:	No proven problems.

*See Glossary

PYRIDOXINE (Vitamin B-6)

BRAND NAMES

Beesix
Hexa-Betalin
Pyroxine
Rodex
Vitabec 6

Numerous other multiple vitamin-mineral supplements. Check labels.

BASIC INFORMATION

Habit forming? No
Prescription needed?
High strength: Yes
Low strength: No
Available as generic? Yes
Drug class: Vitamin supplement

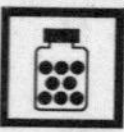

USES

- Prevention and treatment of pyridoxine deficiency.
- Treatment of some forms of anemia.
- Treatment of INH (isonicotinic acid hydrozide), cycloserine poisoning.

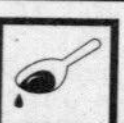

DOSAGE & USAGE INFORMATION

How to take:
- Tablets—Swallow with liquid.
- Extended-release capsules—Swallow each dose whole with liquid.

When to take:
At the same times each day.

If you forget a dose:
Take as soon as you remember, then resume regular schedule.

What drug does:
Acts as co-enzyme in carbohydrate, protein and fat metabolism.

Time lapse before drug works:
15 to 20 minutes.

Don't take with:
- Levodopa—Small amounts of pyridoxine will nullify levodopa effect. Carbidopa-levodopa combination not affected by this interaction.
- Any other medicine without consulting your doctor or pharmacist.

OVERDOSE

SYMPTOMS:
None expected.
WHAT TO DO:
Overdose unlikely to threaten life.

POSSIBLE ADVERSE REACTIONS OR SIDE EFFECTS

SYMPTOMS	WHAT TO DO
Life-threatening: None expected.	
Common: None expected.	
Infrequent: Nausea, headache.	Discontinue. Call doctor right away.
Rare: Numbness or tingling in hands or feet (large doses).	Discontinue. Call doctor right away.

PYRIDOXINE (Vitamin B-6)

WARNINGS & PRECAUTIONS

Don't take if:
You are allergic to pyridoxine.

Before you start, consult your doctor:
If you are pregnant or breast-feeding.

Over age 60:
No problems expected.

Pregnancy:
Don't exceed recommended dose. Consult doctor. Risk category A (see page xxii).

Breast-feeding:
Don't exceed recommended dose. Consult doctor.

Infants & children:
Don't exceed recommended dose.

Prolonged use:
Large doses for more than 1 month may cause toxicity.

Skin & sunlight:
No problems expected.

Driving, piloting or hazardous work:
No problems expected.

Discontinuing:
No problems expected.

Others:
Regular pyridoxine supplements recommended if you take chloramphenicol, cycloserine, ethionamide, hydralazine, immunosuppressants, isoniazid or penicillamine. These decrease pyridoxine absorption and can cause anemia or tingling and numbness in hands and feet.

POSSIBLE INTERACTION WITH OTHER DRUGS

GENERIC NAME OR DRUG CLASS	COMBINED EFFECT
Contraceptives, oral*	Decreased pyridoxine effect.
Cycloserine	Decreased pyridoxine effect.
Estrogens*	Decreased pyridoxine effect.
Ethionamide	Decreased pyridoxine effect.
Hydralazine	Decreased pyridoxine effect.
Hypnotics, barbiturates*	Decreased hypnotic effect.
Immuno-suppressants*	Decreased pyridoxine effect.
Isoniazid	Decreased pyridoxine effect.
Levodopa	Decreased levodopa effect.
Penicillamine	Decreased pyridoxine effect.
Phenobarbital	Possible decreased phenobarbital effect.
Phenytoin	Decreased phenytoin effect.

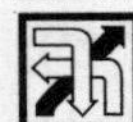

POSSIBLE INTERACTION WITH OTHER SUBSTANCES

INTERACTS WITH	COMBINED EFFECT
Alcohol:	None expected.
Beverages:	None expected.
Cocaine:	None expected.
Foods:	None expected.
Marijuana:	None expected.
Tobacco:	May decrease pyridoxine absorption. Decreased pyridoxine effect.

*See Glossary

QUINACRINE

BRAND NAMES

Atabrine

BASIC INFORMATION

Habit forming? No
Prescription needed? Yes
Available as generic? Yes
Drug class: Antiprotozoal

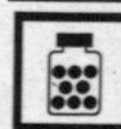

USES

- Treats disease caused by the intestinal parasite *Giardia lamblia.*
- Treats mild to moderate discoid lupus erythematosus.

DOSAGE & USAGE INFORMATION

How to take:
Tablets—Swallow with full glass of water, tea or fruit juice. If you can't swallow whole, crumble tablet and mix with jam or chocolate syrup.

When to take:
After meals.

If you forget a dose:
Take as soon as you remember up to 2 hours late. If more than 2 hours, wait for next scheduled dose (don't double this dose).

What drug does:
Destroys *Gardia lamblia* parasites in the gastrointestinal system.

Continued next column

OVERDOSE

SYMPTOMS:
Severe abdominal cramps, convulsions, severe diarrhea, fainting, irregular heartbeat, restlessness.

WHAT TO DO:
- **Dial 911 (emergency) or 0 (operator) for an ambulance or medical help. Then give first aid immediately.**
- **If patient is unconscious and not breathing, give mouth-to-mouth breathing. If there is no heartbeat, use cardiac massage and mouth-to-mouth breathing (CPR). Don't try to make patient vomit. If you can't get help quickly, take patient to nearest emergency facility.**
- **See emergency information on inside covers.**

Time lapse before drug works:
1 day.

Don't take with:
Any other medicine without consulting your doctor or pharmacist.

POSSIBLE ADVERSE REACTIONS OR SIDE EFFECTS

SYMPTOMS	WHAT TO DO
Life-threatening: In case of overdose, see previous column.	
Common:	
• Dizziness, nausea, headache.	Discontinue. Call doctor right away.
• Yellow eyes, skin, urine (due to dye-like characteristics of quinacrine).	Report to doctor, but no action necessary.
Infrequent:	
• Mild abdominal cramps; mild diarrhea; appetite loss; skin rash, itching or peeling.	Discontinue. Call doctor right away.
• Mood changes.	Continue. Call doctor when convenient.
Rare:	
Hallucinations, nightmares.	Discontinue. Call doctor right away.

WARNINGS & PRECAUTIONS

Don't take if:
You are allergic to quinacrine.

Before you start, consult your doctor:
- If you have porphyria.
- If you have had psoriasis.
- If you have a history of severe mental disorders.
- If you are on a low-salt, low-sugar or other special diet.

Over age 60:
No special problems.

Pregnancy:
Decide with your doctor whether drug benefits justify risk to unborn child. Treatment best begun after child has been delivered. Risk category C (see page xxii).

Breast-feeding:
Effect unknown. Consult doctor.

Infants & children:
Children tolerate quinacrine poorly. Quinacrine may cause vomiting due to bitter taste. Try crushing tablets in jam, honey or chocolate syrup.

Prolonged use:
- Can cause eye problems, liver disease, aplastic anemia. Don't use for more than 5 days.
- Talk to your doctor about the need for follow-up medical examinations or laboratory studies to check stools for giardiasis.

Skin & sunlight:
No problems expected.

Driving, piloting or hazardous work:
Don't drive or pilot aircraft until you learn how medicine affects you. Don't work around dangerous machinery. Don't climb ladders or work in high places. Danger increases if you drink alcohol or take medicine affecting alertness and reflexes, such as antihistamines, tranquilizers, sedatives, pain medicine, narcotics and mind-altering drugs.

Discontinuing:
Don't discontinue before 5 days without consulting doctor.

Others:
Request 3 stool exams several days apart.

POSSIBLE INTERACTION WITH OTHER DRUGS

GENERIC NAME OR DRUG CLASS	COMBINED EFFECT
Primaquine	Decreased effect of primaquine.

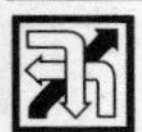

POSSIBLE INTERACTION WITH OTHER SUBSTANCES

INTERACTS WITH	COMBINED EFFECT
Alcohol:	Increased adverse effects of both. Avoid.
Beverages:	No special problems expected.
Cocaine:	No special problems expected.
Foods:	No special problems expected.
Marijuana:	No special problems expected.
Tobacco:	No special problems expected.

*See Glossary

QUINIDINE

BRAND NAMES

Apo-Quinidine
Cardioquin
Cin-Quin
Duraquin
Novoquinidin
Quinaglute Dura-Tabs
Quinalan
Quinate
Quinidex Extentabs
Quinora

BASIC INFORMATION

Habit forming? No
Prescription needed?
U.S.: Yes
Canada: No
Available as generic? Yes
Drug class: Antiarrhythmic

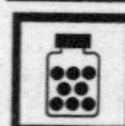

USES

- Corrects heart rhythm disorders.
- May be used in treatment of malaria.

DOSAGE & USAGE INFORMATION

How to take:
- Tablet or capsule—Swallow with liquid or food to lessen stomach irritation.
- Extended-release tablets—Swallow each dose whole. Don't crush them.

When to take:
At the same times each day.

If you forget a dose:
Take as soon as you remember up to 2 hours late. If more than 2 hours, wait for next scheduled dose (don't double this dose).

Continued next column

OVERDOSE

SYMPTOMS:
Confusion, severe blood pressure drop, lethargy, breathing difficulty, fainting, seizures, coma.
WHAT TO DO:
- **Dial 911 (emergency) or 0 (operator) for an ambulance or medical help. Then give first aid immediately.**
- **If patient is unconscious and not breathing, give mouth-to-mouth breathing. If there is no heartbeat, use cardiac massage and mouth-to-mouth breathing (CPR). Don't try to make patient vomit. If you can't get help quickly, take patient to nearest emergency facility.**
- **See emergency information on inside covers.**

What drug does:
Delays nerve impulses to the heart to regulate heartbeat.

Time lapse before drug works:
2 to 4 hours.

Don't take with:
Any other medicine without consulting your doctor or pharmacist.

POSSIBLE ADVERSE REACTIONS OR SIDE EFFECTS

SYMPTOMS	WHAT TO DO
Life-threatening:	
Hives, rash, intense itching, faintness soon after a dose (anaphylaxis); wheezing.	Seek emergency treatment immediately.
Common:	
Bitter taste, diarrhea, nausea, vomiting, appetite loss, abdominal pain.	Discontinue. Call doctor right away.
Infrequent:	
• Dizziness, lightheadedness, fainting, headache, confusion, rash, change in vision, difficult breathing, rapid heartbeat.	Discontinue. Call doctor right away.
• Ringing in ears.	Continue. Call doctor when convenient.
Rare:	
• Unusual bleeding or bruising, difficulty or pain on swallowing, fever, joint pain, jaundice, hepatitis.	Discontinue. Call doctor right away.
• Weakness.	Continue. Call doctor when convenient.

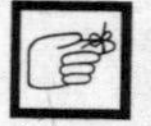

WARNINGS & PRECAUTIONS

Don't take if:
- You are allergic to quinidine.
- You have an active infection.

Before you start, consult your doctor:
About any drug you take, including nonprescription drugs.

Over age 60:
Adverse reactions and side effects may be more frequent and severe than in younger persons.

Pregnancy:
Decide with your doctor if drug benefits justify risk to unborn child. Risk category C (see page xxii).

Breast-feeding:
Drug filters into milk. May harm child. Consult doctor.

Infants & children:
No problems expected.

Prolonged use:
Talk to your doctor about the need for follow-up medical examinations or laboratory studies to check complete blood counts (white blood cell count, platelet count, red blood cell count, hemoglobin, hematocrit), liver function, kidney function, serum potassium levels, ECG*.

Skin & sunlight:
No problems expected.

Driving, piloting or hazardous work:
Don't drive or pilot aircraft until you learn how medicine affects you. Don't work around dangerous machinery. Don't climb ladders or work in high places. Danger increases if you drink alcohol or take medicine affecting alertness and reflexes, such as antihistamines, tranquilizers, sedatives, pain medicine, narcotics and mind-altering drugs.

Discontinuing:
Don't discontinue without doctor's advice until you complete prescribed dose, even though symptoms diminish or disappear.

Others:
No problems expected.

POSSIBLE INTERACTION WITH OTHER DRUGS

GENERIC NAME OR DRUG CLASS	COMBINED EFFECT
Alkalizers, urinary*	Slows quinidine elimination, increasing its effect and toxicity.
Antiarrhythmics*	May increase or decrease effect or toxicity of quinidine.
Anticholinergics*	Increased anti-cholinergic effect.
Anticoagulants*, oral	Possible increased anticoagulant effect.
Antihypertensives*	Increased anti-hypertensive effect.
Beta-adrenergic blocking agents*	May slow heartbeat excessively.
Cholinergics*	Decreased cholinergic effect.
Cimetidine	Increased quinidine effect.
Cisapride	Decreased quinidine effect.
Dapsone	Increased risk of adverse effect on blood cells.
Digitalis preparations*	May slow heartbeat excessively. Dose adjustments may be needed.
Encainide	Increased effect of toxicity on heart muscle.
Flecainide	Possible irregular heartbeat.
Guanfacine	Increased effect of both medicines.
Nicardipine	Possible increased effect and toxicity of each drug.
Nifedipine	Possible decreased quinidine effect.
Nimodipine	Increased quinidine effect.
Phenobarbital	Decreased quinidine effect.
Phenothiazines*	Possible increased quinidine effect.
Phenytoin	Decreased quinidine effect.
Pimozide	Increased risk of heartbeat irregularities.
Propafenone	Increased effect of both drugs and increased risk of toxicity.

Continued on page 957

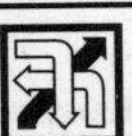

POSSIBLE INTERACTION WITH OTHER SUBSTANCES

INTERACTS WITH	COMBINED EFFECT
Alcohol:	None expected.
Beverages: Caffeine drinks.	Causes rapid heart-beat. Use sparingly.
Cocaine:	Irregular heartbeat. Avoid.
Foods:	None expected.
Marijuana:	Can cause fainting.
Tobacco:	Irregular heartbeat. Avoid.

***See Glossary**

QUININE

BRAND NAMES

Legatrin
NovoQuinine
Quin-260
Quin-amino
Quinamm
Quindan
Quiphile
Q-Vel

BASIC INFORMATION

Habit forming? No
Prescription needed?
High strength: Yes
Low strength: No
Available as generic? Yes
Drug class: Antiprotozoal

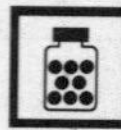

USES

- Treatment or prevention of malaria.
- Relief of muscle cramps.

DOSAGE & USAGE INFORMATION

How to take:
Tablet or capsule—Swallow with liquid or food to lessen stomach irritation.

When to take:
- Prevention—At the same time each day, usually at bedtime.
- Treatment—At the same times each day in evenly spaced doses.

If you forget a dose:
- Prevention—Take as soon as you remember up to 12 hours late. If more than 12 hours, wait for next scheduled dose (don't double this dose).
- Treatment—Take as soon as you remember up to 2 hours late. If more than 2 hours, wait for next scheduled dose (don't double this dose).

Continued next column

OVERDOSE

SYMPTOMS:
Severe impairment of vision and hearing; severe nausea, vomiting, diarrhea; shallow breathing, fast heartbeat; apprehension, confusion, delirium.
WHAT TO DO:
Dial 911 (emergency) or 0 (operator) for an ambulance or medical help. Then give first aid immediately.

What drug does:
- Reduces contractions of skeletal muscles.
- Increases blood flow.
- Interferes with genes in malaria micro-organisms.

Time lapse before drug works:
May require several days or weeks for maximum effect.

Don't take with:
Any other medicine without consulting your doctor or pharmacist.

POSSIBLE ADVERSE REACTIONS OR SIDE EFFECTS

SYMPTOMS	WHAT TO DO
Life-threatening: In case of overdose, see previous column.	
Common:	
• Blurred vision or change in vision, eyes sensitive to light.	Discontinue. Call doctor right away.
• Dizziness, headache, abdominal discomfort, mild nausea, vomiting, diarrhea.	Continue. Call doctor when convenient.
• Ringing or buzzing in ears, impaired hearing.	Continue. Tell doctor at next visit.
Infrequent: Rash, hives, itchy skin, difficult breathing.	Discontinue. Call doctor right away.
Rare: Sore throat, fever, unusual bleeding or bruising, unusual tiredness or weakness, angina.	Discontinue. Call doctor right away.

WARNINGS & PRECAUTIONS

Don't take if:
You are allergic to quinine or quinidine.

Before you start, consult your doctor:
- If you plan to become pregnant within medication period.
- If you have asthma.
- If you have eye disease, hearing problems or ringing in the ears.
- If you have heart disease.
- If you have myasthenia gravis.

Over age 60:
Adverse reactions and side effects may be more frequent and severe than in younger persons.

Pregnancy:
Risk to unborn child outweighs drug benefits. Don't use. Risk category X (see page xxii).

Breast-feeding:
Drug filters into milk. May harm child. Consult doctor.

Infants & children:
Use only under medical supervision.

Prolonged use:
May develop headache, blurred vision, nausea, temporary hearing loss, but seldom need to discontinue because of these symptoms.

Skin & sunlight:
Increased sensitivity to sunlight.

Driving, piloting or hazardous work:
Avoid if you feel dizzy or have blurred vision. Otherwise, no problems expected.

Discontinuing:
Don't discontinue without doctor's advice until you complete prescribed dose, even though symptoms diminish or disappear.

Others:
Don't confuse with quinidine, a medicine for heart rhythm problems.

POSSIBLE INTERACTION WITH OTHER DRUGS

GENERIC NAME OR DRUG CLASS	COMBINED EFFECT
Alkalizers*, urinary	Possible toxic effects of quinine.
Antacids* (with aluminum hydroxide)	Decreased quinine effect.
Anticoagulants*, oral	Increased anti-coagulant effect.
Dapsone	Increased risk of adverse effect on blood cells.
Digitalis	Possible increased digitalis effect.
Digoxin	Possible increased digoxin effect.
Mefloquine	Increased risk of heartbeat irregularities.
Quinidine	Possible toxic effects of quinine.

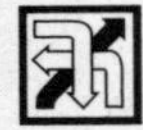

POSSIBLE INTERACTION WITH OTHER SUBSTANCES

INTERACTS WITH	COMBINED EFFECT
Alcohol:	No proven problems.
Beverages:	None expected.
Cocaine:	No proven problems.
Foods:	None expected.
Marijuana:	No proven problems.
Tobacco:	None expected.

*See Glossary

RADIO-PHARMACEUTICALS

BRAND NAMES

See complete list of brand names in the *Brand Name Directory*, page 918.

BASIC INFORMATION

Habit forming? No
Prescription needed? Yes
Available as generic? Yes
Drug class: Radio-pharmaceuticals

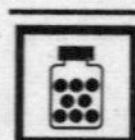

USES

To help establish an accurate diagnosis for many medical problems, such as pernicious anemia, malabsorption, iron metabolism, cancer, abscess, infection, cerebrospinal fluid flow, blood volume, kidney diseases, lung diseases, pancreas diseases, red blood cell disorders, spleen diseases, thyroid diseases, thyroid cancer, brain diseases or tumor, bladder diseases, eye tumors, liver diseases, heart diseases, bone diseases, bone marrow diseases.

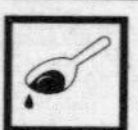

DOSAGE & USAGE INFORMATION

How to take:
- As directed by nuclear medicine specialist. Most are given intravenously by the doctor, but some are taken by mouth.
- Drink lots of liquids and urinate often after test to decrease possible radiation effect on the kidneys and urinary bladder.

When to take:
According to individual instructions.

If you forget a dose:
Take as soon as you remember.

What drug does:
Very small quantities of radioactive substances concentrate in various organs of the body and become measurable. Pictures or readings of the organ or system under study become possible.

Time lapse before drug works:
Varies between products.

Don't take with:
Any other medicine without consulting doctor.

OVERDOSE

SYMPTOMS:
None expected.

POSSIBLE ADVERSE REACTIONS OR SIDE EFFECTS

SYMPTOMS	WHAT TO DO
Life-threatening:	
Hives, rash, intense itching, faintness soon after a dose (anaphylaxis).	Seek emergency treatment immediately.
Common:	
Appetite loss.	Call doctor when convenient.
Infrequent:	
Drowsiness; fast heartbeat; swollen feet, ankles, hands or throat; abdominal pain; rash; hives; nausea; vomiting, headache; red or flushed face; fever; fainting.	Call doctor right away.
Rare:	
Constipation, coughing, sneezing, runny nose, wheezing.	Call doctor right away.

WARNINGS & PRECAUTIONS

Don't take if:
You are allergic to the prescribed drug.

Before you start, consult your doctor:
- If you have had allergic reactions to human serum albumin.
- If you are allergic to anything.

Over age 60:
Adverse reactions and side effects may be more frequent and severe than in younger persons. Ask doctor about smaller doses.

Pregnancy:
Avoid during pregnancy if possible. Consult doctor. Risk category C (see page xxii).

Breast-feeding:
Drug passes into milk. Avoid drug or discontinue nursing until you finish medicine. Consult doctor for advice on maintaining milk supply.

Infants & children:
No problems expected.

Prolonged use:
Not intended for prolonged use.

Skin & sunlight:
No problems expected.

Driving, piloting or hazardous work:
No problems expected.

Discontinuing:
No problems expected.

Others:
Some of these agents may accumulate in the urinary bladder. To decrease chance of excessive radiation, drink 8 oz. of fluid every hour for 10 to 12 hours following the test, unless otherwise specified by your doctor.

POSSIBLE INTERACTION WITH OTHER DRUGS

GENERIC NAME OR DRUG CLASS	COMBINED EFFECT
None expected.	

POSSIBLE INTERACTION WITH OTHER SUBSTANCES

INTERACTS WITH	COMBINED EFFECT
Alcohol:	None expected.
Beverages:	None expected.
Cocaine:	None expected.
Foods:	None expected.
Marijuana:	None expected.
Tobacco:	None expected.

***See Glossary**

RAUWOLFIA ALKALOIDS

BRAND AND GENERIC NAMES

See complete list of brand and generic names in the *Brand Name Directory*, page 919.

BASIC INFORMATION

Habit forming? No
Prescription needed? Yes
Available as generic? Yes
Drug class: Antihypertensive, tranquilizer (rauwolfia alkaloid)

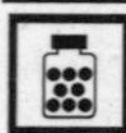

USES

- Treatment for high blood pressure.
- Tranquilizer for mental and emotional disturbances.

DOSAGE & USAGE INFORMATION

How to take:
Tablet or timed-release capsule—Swallow with liquid or food to lessen stomach irritation. If you can't swallow whole, crumble tablet or open capsule and take with liquid or food.

When to take:
At the same times each day.

If you forget a dose:
Take as soon as you remember up to 2 hours late. If more than 2 hours, wait for next scheduled dose (don't double this dose).

What drug does:
- Interferes with nerve impulses and relaxes blood vessel muscles, reducing blood pressure.
- Suppresses brain centers that control emotions.

Time lapse before drug works:
3 weeks continual use required to determine effectiveness.

Continued next column

OVERDOSE

SYMPTOMS:
Drowsiness; slow, weak pulse; slow, shallow breathing; diarrhea; coma; flush; low body temperature; pinpoint pupils.
WHAT TO DO:
- **Dial 911 (emergency) or 0 (operator) for an ambulance or medical help. Then give first aid immediately.**
- **See emergency information on inside covers.**

Don't take with:
Any other medicine without consulting your doctor or pharmacist.

POSSIBLE ADVERSE REACTIONS OR SIDE EFFECTS

SYMPTOMS	WHAT TO DO
Life-threatening: In case of overdose, see previous column.	
Common:	
• Depression, dizziness.	Continue. Call doctor when convenient.
• Headache, faintness, drowsiness, lethargy, red eyes, stuffy nose, impotence, diminished sex drive, diarrhea, dry mouth.	Continue. Tell doctor at next visit.
Infrequent:	
• Black stool; bloody vomit; chest pain; shortness of breath; irregular or slow heartbeat; stiffness in muscles, bones, joints.	Discontinue. Call doctor right away.
• Trembling hands, foot and leg swelling.	Continue. Call doctor when convenient.
Rare:	
• Rash or itchy skin, sore throat, fever, abdominal pain, nausea, vomiting, unusual bleeding or bruising, jaundice.	Discontinue. Call doctor right away.
• Painful urination, nightmares.	Continue. Call doctor when convenient.

WARNINGS & PRECAUTIONS

Don't take if:
- You are allergic to any rauwolfia alkaloid.
- You are depressed.
- You have active peptic ulcer.
- You have ulcerative colitis.

Before you start, consult your doctor:
- If you have been depressed.
- If you have had peptic ulcer, ulcerative colitis or gallstones.
- If you have epilepsy.
- If you will have surgery within 2 months, including dental surgery, requiring general or spinal anesthesia.

Over age 60:
Adverse reactions and side effects may be more frequent and severe than in younger persons.

Pregnancy:
Decide with your doctor whether drug benefits justify risk to unborn child. Risk category C (see page xxii).

Breast-feeding:
Drug passes into milk. Avoid drug or discontinue nursing until you finish medicine. Consult doctor for advice on maintaining milk supply.

Infants & children:
Not recommended.

Prolonged use:
- Causes cancer in laboratory animals. Consult your doctor if you have a family or personal history of cancer.
- Talk to your doctor about the need for follow-up medical examinations or laboratory studies.

Skin & sunlight:
No problems expected.

Driving, piloting or hazardous work:
Avoid if you feel drowsy, dizzy or faint. Otherwise, no problems expected.

Discontinuing:
Don't discontinue without consulting doctor. Dose may require gradual reduction if you have taken drug for a long time. Doses of other drugs may also require adjustment.

Others:
Consult your doctor if you do isometric exercises. These raise blood pressure. Drug may intensify blood pressure rise.

POSSIBLE INTERACTION WITH OTHER DRUGS

GENERIC NAME OR DRUG CLASS	COMBINED EFFECT
Anticoagulants*, oral	Unpredictable increased or decreased effect of anticoagulant.
Anticonvulsants*	Serious change in seizure pattern.
Antidepressants*	Increased anti-depressant effect.
Antihistamines*	Increased anti-histamine effect.
Antihypertensives*, other	Increased rauwolfia effect.
Aspirin	Decreased aspirin effect.
Beta-adrenergic blocking agents*	Increased rauwolfia alkaloid effect. Excessive sedation.
Carteolol	Increased anti-hypertensive effect.
Central nervous system (CNS) depressants*	Increased CNS depression.
Clozapine	Toxic effect on the central nervous system.
Digitalis preparations*	Possible irregular heartbeat.
Dronabinol	Increased effects of both drugs. Avoid.
Ethinamate	Dangerous increased effects of ethinamate. Avoid combining.
Fluoxetine	Increased depressant effects of both drugs.
Guanfacine	May increase depressant effects of either medicine.
Leucovorin	High alcohol content of leucovorin may cause adverse effects.
Levodopa	Decreased levodopa effect.

Continued on page 957

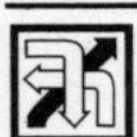

POSSIBLE INTERACTION WITH OTHER SUBSTANCES

INTERACTS WITH	COMBINED EFFECT
Alcohol:	Increased intoxication. Use with extreme caution.
Beverages: Carbonated drinks.	Decreased rauwolfia alkaloid effect.
Cocaine:	Increased risk of heart block and high blood pressure.
Foods: Spicy foods.	Possible digestive upset.
Marijuana:	Occasional use—Mild drowsiness. Daily use—Moderate drowsiness, low blood pressure, depression.
Tobacco:	No problems expected.

*See Glossary

RAUWOLFIA & THIAZIDE DIURETICS

BRAND AND GENERIC NAMES

See complete list of brand and generic names in the *Brand Name Directory*, page 919.

BASIC INFORMATION

Habit forming? No
Prescription needed? Yes
Available as generic? Yes
Drug class: Antihypertensive, diuretic, tranquilizer

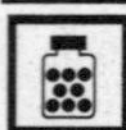

USES

- Controls, but doesn't cure, high blood pressure.
- Reduces fluid retention (edema).

DOSAGE & USAGE INFORMATION

How to take:
Tablet—Swallow with liquid. If you can't swallow whole, crumble tablet and take with liquid or food.

When to take:
At the same time each day.

If you forget a dose:
Take as soon as you remember up to 2 hours late. If more than 2 hours, wait for next scheduled dose (don't double this dose).

What drug does:
- Forces sodium and water excretion, reducing body fluid. Reduced body fluid and relaxed arteries lower blood pressure.
- Interferes with nerve impulses and relaxes blood vessel muscles, reducing blood pressure.
- Suppresses brain centers that control emotion.

Continued next column

OVERDOSE

SYMPTOMS:
Cramps; weakness; drowsiness; pinpoint pupils; slow, weak pulse; slow, shallow breathing; diarrhea; flush; low body temperature; coma.
WHAT TO DO:
- **Dial 911 (emergency) or 0 (operator) for an ambulance or medical help. Then give first aid immediately.**
- **See emergency information on inside covers.**

Time lapse before drug works:
3 weeks continual use required to determine effectiveness.

Don't take with:
Any other prescription or nonprescription drugs without consulting your doctor or pharmacist.

POSSIBLE ADVERSE REACTIONS OR SIDE EFFECTS

SYMPTOMS	WHAT TO DO
Life-threatening:	
Irregular heartbeat, weak pulse, hives, black stool, bloody vomit.	Discontinue. Seek emergency treatment.
Common:	
Lethargy, drowsiness, tremor, depression, red eyes, runny nose, diarrhea, dry mouth.	Continue. Call doctor when convenient.
Infrequent:	
• Blurred vision, abdominal pain, nausea, vomiting, irregular heartbeat, joint pain.	Discontinue. Call doctor right away.
• Dizziness, mood change, headache, dry mouth, weakness, tiredness, weight gain or loss, foot and leg swelling.	Continue. Call doctor when convenient.
Rare:	
• Sore throat, fever, mouth sores; jaundice; unexplained bleeding or bruising.	Discontinue. Call doctor right away.
• Rash, painful or difficult urination, tremor, impotence, nightmares.	Continue. Call doctor when convenient.

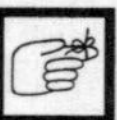

WARNINGS & PRECAUTIONS

Don't take if:
- You are allergic to any thiazide diuretic drug or any rauwolfia alkaloid.
- You are depressed.
- You have active peptic ulcer or ulcerative colitis.

Before you start, consult your doctor:
- If you are allergic to any sulfa drug*.
- If you have gout, liver, pancreas or kidney disorder, epilepsy.
- If you have had peptic ulcer, ulcerative colitis or gallstones.
- If you have been depressed.

- If you will have surgery within 2 months, including dental surgery, requiring general or spinal anesthesia.

Over age 60:
Adverse reactions and side effects may be more frequent and severe than in younger persons, especially dizziness and excessive potassium loss.

Pregnancy:
Risk factors vary for drugs in this group. See category list on page xxii and consult doctor.

Breast-feeding:
Drug passes into milk. Avoid drug or discontinue nursing until you finish medicine. Consult doctor for advice on maintaining milk supply.

Infants & children:
Not recommended.

Prolonged use:
- You may need medicine to treat high blood pressure for the rest of your life.
- Causes cancer in laboratory animals. Consult your doctor if you have a family or personal history of cancer.
- Talk to your doctor about the need for follow-up medical examinations or laboratory studies to check blood pressure.

Skin & sunlight:
May cause rash or intensify sunburn in areas exposed to sun or sunlamp.

Driving, piloting or hazardous work:
Don't drive or pilot aircraft until you learn how medicine affects you. Don't work around dangerous machinery. Don't climb ladders or work in high places. Danger increases if you drink alcohol or take medicine affecting alertness and reflexes, such as antihistamines, tranquilizers, sedatives, pain medicine, narcotics and mind-altering drugs.

Discontinuing:
Don't discontinue without consulting doctor. Dose may require gradual reduction if you have taken drug for a long time. Doses of other drugs may also require adjustment.

Others:
- Hot weather and fever may cause dehydration and drop in blood pressure. Dose may require temporary adjustment. Weigh daily and report any unexpected weight decreases to your doctor.
- May cause rise in uric acid, leading to gout.
- May cause blood sugar rise in diabetics.
- Consult your doctor if you do isometric exercises. These raise blood pressure. Drug may intensify blood pressure rise.

POSSIBLE INTERACTION WITH OTHER DRUGS

GENERIC NAME OR DRUG CLASS	COMBINED EFFECT
Anticoagulants*, oral	Unpredictable increased or decreased effect of anticoagulant.
Anticonvulsants*	Serious change in seizure pattern.
Antidepressants, tricyclic*	Dangerous drop in blood pressure. Avoid combination unless under medical supervision.
Antihistamines*	Increased antihistamine effect.
Antihypertensives*	Increased rauwolfia effect.
Aspirin	Decreased aspirin effect.

Continued on page 958

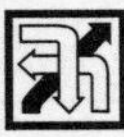

POSSIBLE INTERACTION WITH OTHER SUBSTANCES

INTERACTS WITH	COMBINED EFFECT
Alcohol:	Increased intoxication. Dangerous blood pressure drop. Avoid.
Beverages: Carbonated drinks.	Decreased rauwolfia effect.
Cocaine:	Increased risk of heart block and high blood pressure.
Foods: Spicy foods.	Possible digestive upset.
Licorice.	Excessive potassium loss that causes dangerous heart rhythms.
Marijuana:	Occasional use—Mild drowsiness. Daily use—Moderate drowsiness, low blood pressure, depression.
Tobacco:	No proven problems.

*See Glossary

RESERPINE, HYDRALAZINE & HYDROCHLOROTHIAZIDE

BRAND NAMES

Cam-Ap-Es
Cherapas
Ser-A-Gen
Seralazide
Ser-Ap-Es
Serpazide
Tri-Hydroserpine
Unipres

BASIC INFORMATION

Habit forming? No
Prescription needed? Yes
Available as generic? Yes
Drug class: Antihypertensive

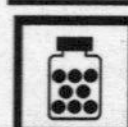

USES

- Treatment for high blood pressure and congestive heart failure.
- Reduces fluid retention (edema).

DOSAGE & USAGE INFORMATION

How to take:
Tablet—Swallow with liquid. If you can't swallow whole, crumble and take with liquid or food.

When to take:
At the same times each day.

If you forget a dose:
Take as soon as you remember up to 2 hours late. If more than 2 hours, wait for next scheduled dose (don't double this dose).

What drug does:
- Interferes with nerve impulses and relaxes blood vessels, reducing blood pressure.
- Suppresses brain centers that control emotions.
- Forces sodium and water excretion, reducing body fluid. Reduced body fluid and relaxed arteries lower blood pressure.

Continued next column

OVERDOSE

SYMPTOMS:
Drowsiness; slow, shallow breathing; pinpoint pupils; diarrhea; flush; low body temperature; rapid, weak heartbeat; fainting; extreme weakness; cold, sweaty skin; cramps, coma.

WHAT TO DO:
- **Dial 911 (emergency) or 0 (operator) for an ambulance or medical help. Then give first aid immediately.**
- **See emergency information on inside covers.**

Time lapse before drug works:
Regular use for several weeks may be necessary to determine drug's effectiveness.

Don't take with:
- Nonprescription drugs containing alcohol without consulting doctor.
- Any other medicine without consulting your doctor or pharmacist.

POSSIBLE ADVERSE REACTIONS OR SIDE EFFECTS

SYMPTOMS	WHAT TO DO
Life-threatening:	
Rapid or irregular heartbeat, weak pulse, fainting, black stool, black or bloody vomit, chest pain.	Discontinue. Seek emergency treatment.
Common:	
• Nausea, vomiting.	Discontinue. Call doctor right away.
• Headache, diarrhea, drowsiness, runny nose, appetite loss.	Continue. Call doctor when convenient.
Infrequent:	
• Blurred vision, chest pain, abdominal pain, rash, hives, joint pain.	Discontinue. Call doctor right away.
• Dizziness; mood change; headache; dry mouth; weakness; tiredness; weight gain or loss; eyes red, watery, irritated; confusion; constipation; red or flushed face; joint stiffness; depression; anxiety; foot and leg swelling.	Continue. Call doctor when convenient.
Rare:	
• Jaundice; unexplained bleeding or bruising; sore throat, fever, mouth sores; weakness and faintness when arising from bed or chair.	Discontinue. Call doctor right away.
• Numbness, tingling, burning feeling in feet and hands; nasal congestion; impotence; nightmares.	Continue. Call doctor when convenient.

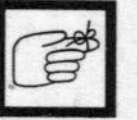

WARNINGS & PRECAUTIONS

Don't take if:
- You are allergic to any rauwolfia alkaloid, hydralazine, any thiazide diuretic drug*, or tartrazine dye.

- You are depressed.
- You have active peptic ulcer, ulcerative colitis, history of coronary artery disease or rheumatic heart disease.

Before you start, consult your doctor:
- If you have been depressed.
- If you have had peptic ulcer, ulcerative colitis, gallstones, kidney disease or impaired kidney function, lupus or a stroke.
- If you have epilepsy, gout; liver, pancreas or kidney disorder.
- If you feel pain in chest, neck or arms on physical exertion.
- If you are allergic to any sulfa drug*.
- If you will have surgery within 2 months, including dental surgery, requiring general or spinal anesthesia.

Over age 60:
Adverse reactions and side effects may be more frequent and severe than in younger persons, especially dizziness and excessive potassium loss.

Pregnancy:
Decide with your doctor if drug benefits justify risk to unborn child. Risk category C (see page xxii).

Breast-feeding:
Drug passes into milk. Avoid drug or discontinue nursing until you finish medicine. Consult doctor.

Infants & children:
Not recommended.

Prolonged use:
- Causes cancer in laboratory animals. Consult your doctor if you have a family or personal history of cancer.
- Possible psychosis.
- May cause lupus; numbness, tingling in hands or feet.
- Talk to your doctor about the need for follow-up medical examinations or laboratory studies.

Skin & sunlight:
May cause rash or intensify sunburn in areas exposed to sun or sunlamp.

Driving, piloting or hazardous work:
Don't drive or pilot aircraft until you learn how medicine affects you. Don't work around dangerous machinery. Don't climb ladders or work in high places. Danger increases if you drink alcohol or take medicine affecting alertness and reflexes.

Discontinuing:
Don't discontinue without consulting doctor. Dose may require gradual reduction if you have taken drug for a long time. Doses of other drugs may also require adjustment.

Others:
- Consult your doctor if you do isometric exercises. These raise blood pressure. Drug may intensify blood pressure rise.
- Vitamin B-6 supplement may be advisable. Consult doctor.
- Hot weather and fever may cause dehydration and drop in blood pressure. Dose may require temporary adjustment. Weigh daily and report any unexpected weight decreases to your doctor.
- May cause rise in uric acid, leading to gout.
- May cause blood sugar rise in diabetics.
- Some products contain tartrazine dye. Avoid, especially if you are allergic to aspirin.

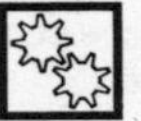

POSSIBLE INTERACTION WITH OTHER DRUGS

GENERIC NAME OR DRUG CLASS	COMBINED EFFECT
Acebutolol	Possible increased effects of drugs.

Continued on page 958

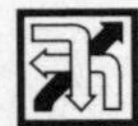

POSSIBLE INTERACTION WITH OTHER SUBSTANCES

INTERACTS WITH	COMBINED EFFECT
Alcohol:	Increased intoxication. Avoid.
Beverages: Carbonated drinks.	Decreased rauwolfia alkaloids effect.
Cocaine:	Dangerous blood pressure rise. Avoid.
Foods: Spicy foods.	Possible digestive upset.
Licorice.	Excessive potassium loss that causes dangerous heart rhythms.
Marijuana:	Weakness on standing. May increase blood pressure. Occasional use—Mild drowsiness. Daily use—Moderate drowsiness, low blood pressure, depression.
Tobacco:	Possible angina attacks.

*See Glossary

RIBAVIRIN

BRAND NAMES

Tribavirin
Virazid
Virazole

BASIC INFORMATION

Habit forming? No
Prescription needed? Yes
Available as generic? No
Drug class: Antiviral

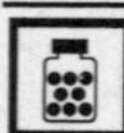

USES

- Treats severe viral pneumonia.
- Treats respiratory syncytial virus (RSV) infections in hospitalized infants or children.
- Treats influenza A and B with some success.
- Does not treat other viruses such as the common cold.

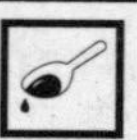

DOSAGE & USAGE INFORMATION

How to take:
By inhalation of a fine mist through mouth. Requires a special sprayer attached to oxygen mask, face mask for infants or hood.

When to take:
As ordered by your doctor.

If you forget a dose:
Use as soon as you remember.

What drug does:
Kills virus or prevents its growth.

Time lapse before drug works:
Begins working in 1 hour. May require treatment for 12 to 18 hours per day for 3 to 7 days.

Don't take with:
Any other medicine without consulting your doctor or pharmacist.

OVERDOSE

SYMPTOMS:
None expected.
WHAT TO DO:
Overdose unlikely to threaten life. If person takes much larger amount than prescribed, call doctor, poison control center or hospital emergency room for instructions.

POSSIBLE ADVERSE REACTIONS OR SIDE EFFECTS

SYMPTOMS	WHAT TO DO
Life-threatening: None expected.	
Common: None expected.	
Infrequent:	
• Unusual tireness or weakness.	Discontinue. Call doctor right away.
• Headache, insomnia, appetite loss, nausea.	Continue. Call doctor when convenient.
Rare:	
Skin irritation or rash.	Continue. Call doctor when convenient.

WARNINGS & PRECAUTIONS

Don't take if:
You are allergic to ribavirin.

Before you start, consult your doctor:
- If you are now on low-salt, low-sugar or any special diet.
- If you have severe anemia.

Over age 60:
Adverse reactions and side effects may be more frequent and severe than in younger persons. Ask doctor about smaller doses.

Pregnancy:
Risk to unborn child outweighs drug benefits. Don't use. Risk category X (see page xxii).

Breast-feeding:
Drug may pass into milk. Avoid drug or discontinue nursing until you finish medicine. Consult doctor for advice on maintaining milk supply.

Infants & children:
Use only under close medical supervision.

Prolonged use:
No problems expected.

Skin & sunlight:
Increased sensitivity to light.

Driving, piloting or hazardous work:
Don't drive or pilot aircraft until you learn how medicine affects you. Don't work around dangerous machinery. Don't climb ladders or work in high places. Danger increases if you drink alcohol or take medicine affecting alertness and reflexes, such as antihistamines, tranquilizers, sedatives, pain medicine, narcotics and mind-altering drugs.

Discontinuing:
Don't discontinue without consulting doctor. Dose may require gradual reduction if you have taken drug for a long time. Doses of other drugs may also require adjustment.

Others:
- Ribavirin is indicated for use in treatment of severe viral pneumonia caused by repiratory syncytial virus (RSV) in hospitalized infants and young children.
- Health care workers exposed to ribavirin may experience headache; eye itching, redness or swelling.
- Female health care workers who are pregnant or may become pregnant should avoid exposure to drug.

POSSIBLE INTERACTION WITH OTHER DRUGS

GENERIC NAME OR DRUG CLASS	COMBINED EFFECT
Zidovudine	Decreased effect of ribavirin and zidovudine.

POSSIBLE INTERACTION WITH OTHER SUBSTANCES

INTERACTS WITH	COMBINED EFFECT
Alcohol:	None expected.
Beverages:	None expected.
Cocaine:	None expected.
Foods:	None expected.
Marijuana:	None expected.
Tobacco:	None expected.

RIBOFLAVIN (Vitamin B-2)

BRAND NAMES

Many multivitamin preparations. Check labels.

BASIC INFORMATION

Habit forming? No
Prescription needed? No
Available as generic? Yes
Drug class: Vitamin supplement

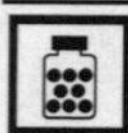

USES

- Dietary supplement to ensure normal growth and health.
- Dietary supplement to treat symptoms caused by deficiency of B-2: sores in mouth, eyes sensitive to light, itching and peeling skin.

DOSAGE & USAGE INFORMATION

How to take:
Tablet—Swallow with liquid or food to lessen stomach irritation. If you can't swallow whole, crumble tablet and take with liquid or food.

When to take:
At the same times each day.

If you forget a dose:
Take as soon as you remember. Resume regular schedule. Don't double dose.

What drug does:
Promotes normal growth and health.

Time lapse before drug works:
Requires continual intake.

Don't take with:
Any other medicine without consulting your doctor or pharmacist.

OVERDOSE

SYMPTOMS:
Dark urine, nausea, vomiting.
WHAT TO DO:
Overdose unlikely to threaten life. If person takes much larger amount than prescribed, call doctor, poison control center or hospital emergency room for instructions.

POSSIBLE ADVERSE REACTIONS OR SIDE EFFECTS

SYMPTOMS	WHAT TO DO
Life-threatening:	
None expected.	
Common:	
Urine yellow in color.	No action necessary.
Infrequent:	
None expected.	
Rare:	
None expected.	

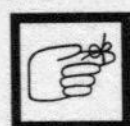

WARNINGS & PRECAUTIONS

Don't take if:
- You are allergic to any B vitamin.
- You have chronic kidney failure.

Before you start, consult your doctor:
If you are pregnant or plan pregnancy.

Over age 60:
No problems expected.

Pregnancy:
Take within recommended guidelines. Consult doctor. Risk category A (see page xxii).

Breast-feeding:
Take within recommended guidelines. Consult doctor.

Infants & children:
Consult doctor.

Prolonged use:
No problems expected.

Skin & sunlight:
No problems expected.

Driving, piloting or hazardous work:
No problems expected.

Discontinuing:
No problems expected.

Others:
A balanced diet should provide all the vitamin B-2 a healthy person needs and make supplements unnecessary during periods of good health. Best sources are milk, meats and green leafy vegetables.

POSSIBLE INTERACTION WITH OTHER DRUGS

GENERIC NAME OR DRUG CLASS	COMBINED EFFECT
Anticholinergics*	Possible increased riboflavin absorption.
Antidepressants, tricyclic*	Decreased riboflavin effect.
Phenothiazines*	Decreased riboflavin effect.
Probenecid	Decreased riboflavin effect.

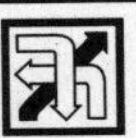

POSSIBLE INTERACTION WITH OTHER SUBSTANCES

INTERACTS WITH	COMBINED EFFECT
Alcohol:	Prevents uptake and absorption of vitamin B-2.
Beverages:	No problems expected.
Cocaine:	No problems expected.
Foods:	No problems expected.
Marijuana:	No problems expected.
Tobacco:	Prevents absorption of vitamin B-2 and other vitamins and nutrients.

*See Glossary

RIFAMPIN

BRAND NAMES

Rifadin
Rifamate
Rifampicin
Rimactane
Rofact

BASIC INFORMATION

Habit forming? No
Prescription needed? Yes
Available as generic? No
Drug class: Antibiotic (rifamycin)

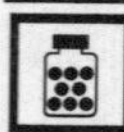

USES

Treatment for tuberculosis and other infections. Requires daily use for 1 to 2 years.

DOSAGE & USAGE INFORMATION

How to take:
Capsule—Swallow with liquid. If you can't swallow whole, open capsule and take with liquid or small amount of food. For child, mix with small amount of applesauce or jelly.

When to take:
1 hour before or 2 hours after a meal.

If you forget a dose:
Take as soon as you remember up to 2 hours late. If more than 2 hours, wait for next scheduled dose (don't double this dose).

What drug does:
Prevents multiplication of tuberculosis germs.

Time lapse before drug works:
Usually 2 weeks. May require 1 to 2 years without missed doses for maximum benefit.

Continued next column

OVERDOSE

SYMPTOMS:
Slow, shallow breathing; weak, rapid pulse; cold, sweaty skin; coma.
WHAT TO DO:
- **Dial 911 (emergency) or 0 (operator) for an ambulance or medical help. Then give first aid immediately.**
- **If patient is unconscious and not breathing, give mouth-to-mouth breathing. If there is no heartbeat, use cardiac massage and mouth-to-mouth breathing (CPR). Don't try to make patient vomit. If you can't get help quickly, take patient to nearest emergency facility.**
- **See emergency information on inside covers.**

Don't take with:
Any other medicine without consulting your doctor or pharmacist.

POSSIBLE ADVERSE REACTIONS OR SIDE EFFECTS

SYMPTOMS	WHAT TO DO
Life-threatening: In case of overdose, see previous column.	
Common: Diarrhea; reddish urine, stool, saliva, sweat and tears.	Continue. Call doctor when convenient.
Infrequent:	
• Rash; flushed, itchy skin of face and scalp; blurred vision; difficult breathing; nausea, vomiting; abdominal cramps.	Discontinue. Call doctor right away.
• Dizziness, unsteady gait, confusion, muscle or bone pain, heartburn, flatulence, chills.	Continue. Call doctor when convenient.
• Headache, fever.	Continue. Tell doctor at next visit.
Rare:	
• Sore throat, mouth or tongue; jaundice.	Discontinue. Call doctor right away.
• Appetite loss, less urination.	Continue. Call doctor when convenient.

WARNINGS & PRECAUTIONS

Don't take if:
- You are allergic to rifampin.
- You wear soft contact lenses.

Before you start, consult your doctor:
If you are alcoholic or have liver disease.

Over age 60:
Adverse reactions and side effects may be more frequent and severe than in younger persons.

Pregnancy:
Decide with your doctor if drug benefits justify risk to unborn child. Risk category C (see page xxii).

Breast-feeding:
Effect unknown. Consult doctor.

Infants & children:
Use only under medical supervision.

Prolonged use:
- You may become more susceptible to infections caused by germs not responsive to rifampin.
- Talk to your doctor about the need for follow-up medical examinations or laboratory studies to check liver function.

Skin & sunlight:
No problems expected.

Driving, piloting or hazardous work:
Don't drive or pilot aircraft until you learn how medicine affects you. Don't work around dangerous machinery. Don't climb ladders or work in high places. Danger increases if you drink alcohol or take medicine affecting alertness and reflexes, such as antihistamines, tranquilizers, sedatives, pain medicine, narcotics and mind-altering drugs.

Discontinuing:
Don't discontinue without doctor's advice until you complete prescribed dose, even though symptoms diminish or disappear.

Others:
Reddish tears may discolor soft contact lenses.

POSSIBLE INTERACTION WITH OTHER DRUGS

GENERIC NAME OR DRUG CLASS	COMBINED EFFECT
Anticoagulants*, oral	Decreased anti-coagulant effect.
Antidiabetics*, oral	Decreased antidiabetic effect.
Barbiturates*	Decreased barbiturate effect.
Chloramphenicol	Decreased effect of both drugs.
Clozapine	Toxic effect on bone marrow.
Contraceptives, oral*	Decreased contra-ceptive effect.
Cortisone drugs*	Decreased effect of cortisone drug.
Cyclosporine	Decreased effect of both drugs.
Dapsone	Decreased dapsone effect.
Digitalis preparations*	Decreased digitoxin effect.
Disopyramide	Decreased disopyramide effect.
Estrogens* (including contraceptive pills)	Decreased effect of both drugs.
Flecainide	Possible decreased blood cell production in bone marrow.
Fluconazole	Decreased fluconazole effect.
Hepatotoxics*	Increased risk of liver toxicity.
Isoniazid	Possible toxicity to liver.
Itraconazole	Decreased itraconazole effect.
Ketoconazole	Decreased ketoconazole effect.
Methadone	Decreased methadone effect.
Mexiletine	Decreased mexiletine effect.
Nicardipine	Decreased nicardipine effect.
Nimodipine	Decreased nimodipine effect.
Para-aminosalicylic acid	Decreased rifampin effect.
Phenytoin	Decreased phenytoin effect.
Probenecid	Possible toxicity to liver.
Quinidine	Decreased effect of both drugs.
Theophyllines*	Decreased theophylline effect.
Tiopronin	Increased risk of toxicity to bone marrow and kidneys.
Tocainide	Possible decreased blood cell production in bone marrow.
Trimethoprim	Decreased trimethoprim effect.
Verapamil	Decreased verapamil effect.

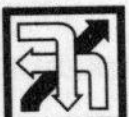

POSSIBLE INTERACTION WITH OTHER SUBSTANCES

INTERACTS WITH	COMBINED EFFECT
Alcohol:	Possible toxicity to liver.
Beverages:	None expected.
Cocaine:	No proven problems.
Foods:	None expected.
Marijuana:	No proven problems.
Tobacco:	None expected.

***See Glossary**

RISPERIDONE

BRAND NAMES

Risperdal

BASIC INFORMATION

Habit forming? No
Prescription needed? Yes
Available as generic? No
Drug class: Antipsychotic

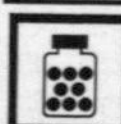

USES

Treats nervous, mental and emotional conditions. Helps in managing the signs and symptoms of schizophrenia.

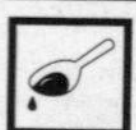

DOSAGE & USAGE INFORMATION

How to take:
Tablet—Swallow with liquid. May be taken with or without food.

When to take:
At the same times each day. The prescribed dosage will gradually be increased over the first few days of use.

If you forget a dose:
Take as soon as you remember. If it is almost time for the next dose, wait for the next scheduled dose (don't double this dose).

What drug does:
The exact mechanism is unknown. It appears to block certain nerve impulses between nerve cells.

Time lapse before drug works:
One to 7 days. A further increase in the dosage amount may be necessary to relieve symptoms for some patients.

Don't take with:
Any other medication without consulting your doctor.

OVERDOSE

SYMPTOMS:
Extreme drowsiness, rapid heartbeat, faintness, convulsions, excessive sweating, difficulty in breathing, loss of muscular control.
WHAT TO DO:
- **Dial 911 (emergency) or 0 (operator) for an ambulance or medical help. Then give first aid immediately.**
- **See emergency information on inside covers.**

POSSIBLE ADVERSE REACTIONS OR SIDE EFFECTS

SYMPTOMS	WHAT TO DO
Life-threatening:	
Rapid or irregular heartbeat, high fever, extreme sweating, trouble breathing, loss of bladder control, convulsions (seizures), severe muscle stiffness, excessive tiredness or weakness (all rare).	Call doctor right away or seek emergency help.
Common:	
• Difficulty in swallowing or speaking, unusual sweating, stiffness or spasms of neck and back muscles, stiffness or weakness in arms or legs, anxiety, trembling hands, pale skin, unusual tiredness, nervousness, irritability, masklike face, walking or balancing problems.	Continue, but call doctor right away.
• Stomach pain, gas, insomnia, dizziness or lightheadedness when arising from a sitting or lying position, cough, stuffy nose, nausea or vomiting, headache, constipation, sleepiness.	Continue. Tell doctor at next visit.
Infrequent:	
• Chest pain, fainting, trouble breathing, lightheadedness, vision changes.	Continue, but call doctor right away.
• Joint pain, low fever, decreased sexual interest, impotence, rash or skin problems, sore throat, increased mouth watering, toothache.	Continue. Call doctor when convenient.
Rare:	
Lip smacking; cheek puffing; uncontrolled tongue movements; uncontrollable movements of head, neck, arms or legs.	Continue, but call doctor right away.

WARNINGS & PRECAUTIONS

Don't take if:
You are allergic to risperidone.

Before you start, consult your doctor:
- If you have liver or kidney disease.
- If you are allergic to any other medications.
- If you have a history of seizures.

Over age 60:
Adverse reactions and side effects may be more severe than in younger persons. A lower starting dosage is usually recommended until a response is determined.

Pregnancy:
Decide with your doctor if drug benefits justify any possible risk to unborn child. Risk category C (see page xxii).

Breast-feeding:
It is unknown if drug passes into milk. Avoid nursing until you finish medicine. Consult doctor for advice on maintaining milk supply.

Infants & children:
Safety in children under age 12 has not been established. Use only under close medical supervision.

Prolonged use:
Consult with your doctor on a regular basis while taking this drug to check your progress or to discuss any increase or changes in side effects and the need for continued treatment.

Skin & sunlight:
May cause sensitivity to sunlight. Avoid excess sun exposure until you determine how you react.

Driving, piloting or hazardous work:
Don't drive or pilot aircraft until you learn how medicine affects you. Don't work around dangerous machinery. Don't climb ladders or work in high places. Danger increases if you drink alcohol or take medicine affecting alertness and reflexes.

Discontinuing:
Don't discontinue this drug without consulting doctor. Dosage may require a gradual reduction before stopping.

Others:
- Get up slowly from a sitting or lying position to avoid any dizziness, faintness or lightheadedness.
- Advise any doctor or dentist whom you consult that you take this medicine.
- Take medicine only as directed. Do not increase or reduce dosage without doctor's approval.

POSSIBLE INTERACTION WITH OTHER DRUGS

GENERIC NAME OR DRUG CLASS	COMBINED EFFECT
Antihypertensives*	Increased antihypertensive effect.
Clozapine	Increased risperidone effect.
Central nervous system (CNS) depressants*, other	Increased sedative effect.

POSSIBLE INTERACTION WITH OTHER SUBSTANCES

INTERACTS WITH	COMBINED EFFECT
Alcohol:	Increased sedative affect. Avoid.
Beverages:	None expected.
Cocaine:	Effect not known. Best to avoid.
Foods:	None expected.
Marijuana:	Effect not known. Best to avoid.
Tobacco:	None expected.

*See Glossary

RITODRINE

BRAND NAMES

Yutopar

BASIC INFORMATION

Habit forming? No
Prescription needed? Yes
Available as generic? Yes
Drug class: Labor inhibitor, beta-adrenergic stimulator

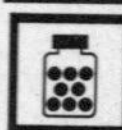

USES

Halts premature labor in pregnancies of 20 or more weeks.

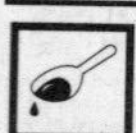

DOSAGE & USAGE INFORMATION

How to take:
Tablet—Swallow with liquid or food to lessen stomach irritation. If you can't swallow whole, crumble tablet and take with liquid or food.

When to take:
Every 4 to 6 hours until term.

If you forget a dose:
Take as soon as you remember up to 2 hours late. If more than 2 hours, wait for next scheduled dose (don't double this dose).

What drug does:
Inhibits contractions of uterus (womb).

Time lapse before drug works:
30 to 60 minutes (oral form). Faster intravenously.

Don't take with:
Any other medicine without consulting your doctor or pharmacist.

OVERDOSE

SYMPTOMS:
Rapid, irregular heartbeat to 120 or more; shortness of breath.
WHAT TO DO:

- **Dial 911 (emergency) or 0 (operator) for an ambulance or medical help. Then give first aid immediately.**
- **If patient is unconscious and not breathing, give mouth-to-mouth breathing. If there is no heartbeat, use cardiac massage and mouth-to-mouth breathing (CPR). Don't try to make patient vomit. If you can't get help quickly, take patient to nearest emergency facility.**
- **See emergency information on inside covers.**

POSSIBLE ADVERSE REACTIONS OR SIDE EFFECTS

SYMPTOMS	WHAT TO DO
Life-threatening:	
Hives, rash, intense itching, faintness soon after a dose (anaphylaxis).	Seek emergency treatment immediately.
Common:	
Irregular heartbeat, fast heartbeat.	Discontinue. Call doctor right away.
Infrequent:	
• Shortness of breath.	Discontinue. Call doctor right away.
• Nervousness, trembling, headache, nausea, vomiting.	Continue. Call doctor when convenient.
Rare:	
Rash, angina, jaundice.	Discontinue. Call doctor right away.

WARNINGS & PRECAUTIONS

Don't take if:
- You have heart disease.
- You have eclampsia.
- You have lung congestion.
- You have infection in the uterus.
- You have an overactive thyroid.
- You have a bleeding disorder.

Before you start, consult your doctor:
- If you have asthma.
- If you have diabetes.
- If you have high blood pressure.
- If you have pre-eclampsia.

Over age 60:
Not used.

Pregnancy:
Ritodrine crosses placenta, but animal studies show that it doesn't affect fetuses. Benefits versus risks must be assessed by you and your doctor. Risk category B (see page xxii).

Breast-feeding:
Not applicable.

Infants & children:
Not used.

Prolonged use:
Talk to your doctor about the need for follow-up medical examinations or laboratory studies to check blood sugar, ECG*, fluid and electrolytes.

Skin & sunlight:
No problems expected.

Driving, piloting or hazardous work:
Don't drive or pilot aircraft until you learn how medicine affects you. Don't work around dangerous machinery. Don't climb ladders or work in high places. Danger increases if you drink alcohol or take medicine affecting alertness and reflexes, such as antihistamines, tranquilizers, sedatives, pain medicine, narcotics and mind-altering drugs.

Discontinuing:
Don't discontinue without consulting doctor. Dose may require gradual reduction if you have taken drug for a long time. Doses of other drugs may also require adjustment.

Others:
No problems expected.

POSSIBLE INTERACTION WITH OTHER DRUGS

GENERIC NAME OR DRUG CLASS	COMBINED EFFECT
Adrenal corticosteroids*	Increased chance of fluid in lungs of mother. Avoid.
Anesthetics, general*	Possible cardiac arrhythmias or hypotension.
Beta-adrenergic blocking agents*	Decreased effect of ritodrine.
Diazoxide	Possible cardiac arrhythmias or hypotension.
Magnesium sulfate	Possible cardiac arrhythmias or hypotension.
Meperidine	Possible cardiac arrhythmias or hypotension.
Sympathomimetics*	Increased side effects of both.

POSSIBLE INTERACTION WITH OTHER SUBSTANCES

INTERACTS WITH	COMBINED EFFECT
Alcohol:	Increased adverse effects. Avoid.
Beverages:	No problems expected.
Cocaine:	Injury to fetus. Avoid.
Foods:	No problems expected.
Marijuana:	Injury to fetus. Avoid.
Tobacco:	Injury to fetus. Avoid.

SALICYLATES

BRAND AND GENERIC NAMES

See complete list of brand and generic names in the *Brand Name Directory*, page 919.

BASIC INFORMATION

Habit forming? No
Prescription needed? For some
Available as generic? Yes
Drug class: Analgesic, anti-inflammatory (nonsteroidal)

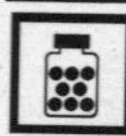

USES

- Reduces pain, fever, inflammation.
- Relieves swelling, stiffness, joint pain of arthritis or rheumatism.
- Decreases risk of myocardial infarction in unstable angina (aspirin only).

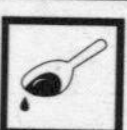

DOSAGE & USAGE INFORMATION

How to take:
- Tablet or capsule—Swallow with liquid.
- Extended-release tablets—Swallow each dose whole.
- Suppositories—Remove wrapper and moisten suppository with water. Gently insert into rectum, large end first.

When to take:
Pain, fever, inflammation—As needed, no more often than every 4 hours.

If you forget a dose:
- Pain, fever—Take as soon as you remember. Wait 4 hours for next dose.
- Arthritis—Take as soon as you remember up to 2 hours late. Return to regular schedule.

What drug does:
- Affects hypothalamus, the part of the brain that regulates temperature by dilating small blood vessels in skin.

Continued next column

- Prevents clumping of platelets (small blood cells) so blood vessels remain open.
- Decreases prostaglandin effect.
- Suppresses body's pain messages.

Time lapse before drug works:
30 minutes for pain, fever, arthritis.

Don't take with:
- Tetracyclines. Space doses 1 hour apart.
- Any other medicine without consulting your doctor or pharmacist.

OVERDOSE

SYMPTOMS:
Ringing in ears; nausea; vomiting; dizziness; fever; deep, rapid breathing; hallucinations; convulsions; coma.
WHAT TO DO:
- **Dial 911 (emergency) or 0 (operator) for an ambulance or medical help. Then give first aid immediately.**
- **See emergency information on inside covers.**

POSSIBLE ADVERSE REACTIONS OR SIDE EFFECTS

SYMPTOMS	WHAT TO DO
Life-threatening:	
Hives, rash, intense itching, faintness soon after a dose (anaphylaxis); black or bloody vomit; blood in urine.	Seek emergency treatment immediately.
Common:	
• Nausea, vomiting, abdominal pain.	Discontinue. Seek emergency treatment.
• Heartburn, indigestion.	Continue. Call doctor when convenient.
• Ringing in ears.	Continue. Tell doctor at next visit.
Infrequent:	
None expected.	
Rare:	
• Black stools, unexplained fever.	Discontinue. Seek emergency treatment.
• Rash, hives, itchy skin, diminished vision, shortness of breath, wheezing, jaundice.	Discontinue. Call doctor right away.
• Drowsiness, headache.	Continue. Call doctor when convenient.

WARNINGS & PRECAUTIONS

Don't take if:
- You need to restrict sodium in your diet. Buffered effervescent tablets and sodium salicylate are high in sodium.
- Salicylates have a strong vinegar-like odor, which means they have decomposed.
- You have a peptic ulcer of stomach or duodenum.
- You have a bleeding disorder.

Before you start, consult your doctor:
- If you have had stomach or duodenal ulcers.
- If you have had gout.
- If you have asthma or nasal polyps.

Over age 60:
More likely to cause hidden bleeding in stomach or intestines. Watch for dark stools.

Pregnancy:
Risk factors vary for drugs in this group. See category list on page xxii and consult doctor.

Breast-feeding:
Drug passes into milk. Avoid drug or discontinue nursing until you finish medicine. Consult doctor for advice on maintaining milk supply.

Infants & children:
- Overdose frequent and severe. Keep bottles out of children's reach.
- Consult doctor before giving to persons under age 18 who have fever and discomfort of viral illness, especially chicken pox and influenza. Probably increases risk of Reye's syndrome.

Prolonged use:
- Kidney damage. Periodic kidney function test recommended.
- Talk to your doctor about the need for follow-up medical examinations or laboratory studies to check liver function.

Skin & sunlight:
Aspirin combined with sunscreen may decrease sunburn.

Driving, piloting or hazardous work:
No restrictions unless you feel drowsy.

Discontinuing:
For chronic illness—Don't discontinue without doctor's advice until you complete prescribed dose, even though symptoms diminish or disappear.

Others:
- Salicylates can complicate surgery, pregnancy, labor and delivery, and illness.
- For arthritis—Don't change dose without consulting doctor.
- Urine tests for blood sugar may be inaccurate.

POSSIBLE INTERACTION WITH OTHER DRUGS

GENERIC NAME OR DRUG CLASS	COMBINED EFFECT
Acetaminophen	Increased risk of kidney damage (with high, prolonged dose of each).
Allopurinol	Decreased allopurinol effect.
Angiotensin-converting enzyme (ACE) inhibitors*	Decreased ACE inhibitor effect.
Antacids*	Decreased salicylate effect.
Anticoagulants*, oral	Increased anti-coagulant effect. Abnormal bleeding.
Antidiabetics*, oral	Low blood sugar.
Anti-inflammatory drugs, nonsteroidal (NSAIDs)*	Risk of stomach bleeding and ulcers
Aspirin, other	Likely salicylate toxicity.
Beta-adrenergic blocking agents*	Decreased anti-hypertensive effect.
Bismuth subsalicylate	Increased risk of salicylate toxicity.
Bumetanide	Decreased diuretic effect.
Calcium supplements*	Increased salicylate effect.
Carteolol	Decreased anti-hypertensive effect of carteolol.
Cortisone drugs*	Increased cortisone effect. Risk of ulcers and stomach bleeding.
Ethacrynic acid	Decreased diuretic effect.
Furosemide	Possible salicylate toxicity.
Gold compounds*	Increased likelihood of kidney damage.
Indomethacin	Risk of stomach bleeding and ulcers.

Continued on page 959

POSSIBLE INTERACTION WITH OTHER SUBSTANCES

INTERACTS WITH	COMBINED EFFECT
Alcohol:	Possible stomach irritation and bleeding. Avoid.
Beverages:	None expected.
Cocaine:	None expected.
Foods:	None expected.
Marijuana:	Possible increased pain relief, but marijuana may slow body's recovery. Avoid.
Tobacco:	None expected.

***See Glossary**

SCOPOLAMINE (Hyoscine)

BRAND NAMES

See complete list of brand names in the *Brand Name Directory*, page 919.

BASIC INFORMATION

Habit forming? No
Prescription needed?
High strength: Yes
Low strength: No
Available as generic? Yes
Drug class: Antispasmodic, anticholinergic

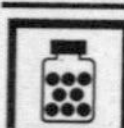

USES

- Reduces spasms of digestive system, bladder and urethra.
- Relieves painful menstruation.
- Prevents motion sickness.

DOSAGE & USAGE INFORMATION

How to take:
- Tablet or capsule—Swallow with liquid or food to lessen stomach irritation.
- Drops—Dilute dose in beverage.
- Skin discs—Clean application site. Change application sites with each dose.

When to take:
- Motion sickness—Apply disc 30 minutes before departure.
- Other uses—Take 30 minutes before meals (unless directed otherwise by doctor).

If you forget a dose:
Take up to 2 hours late. If more than 2 hours, wait for next dose (don't double this dose).

What drug does:
Blocks nerve impulses at parasympathetic nerve endings, preventing muscle contractions and gland secretions of organs involved.

Continued next column

OVERDOSE

SYMPTOMS:
Dilated pupils, blurred vision, rapid pulse and breathing, dizziness, fever, hallucinations, confusion, slurred speech, agitation, flushed face, convulsions, coma.
WHAT TO DO:
- **Dial 911 (emergency) or 0 (operator) for an ambulance or medical help. Then give first aid immediately.**
- **See emergency information on inside covers.**

Time lapse before drug works:
15 to 30 minutes.

Don't take with:
Any other medicine without consulting your doctor or pharmacist.

POSSIBLE ADVERSE REACTIONS OR SIDE EFFECTS

SYMPTOMS	WHAT TO DO
Life-threatening:	
Hives, rash, intense itching, faintness soon after a dose (anaphylaxis).	Seek emergency treatment immediately.
Common:	
• Confusion, delirium, rapid heartbeat.	Discontinue. Call doctor right away.
• Nausea, vomiting, decreased sweating.	Continue. Call doctor when convenient.
• Constipation, loss of taste.	Continue. Tell doctor at next visit.
• Dryness in ears, nose, throat, mouth.	No action necessary.
Infrequent:	
• Headache, difficult urination, nasal congestion, altered taste.	Continue. Call doctor when convenient.
• Lightheadedness.	Discontinue. Call doctor right away.
Rare:	
Rash or hives, eye pain, blurred vision.	Discontinue. Call doctor right away.

WARNINGS & PRECAUTIONS

Don't take if:
- You are allergic to any anticholinergic.
- You have trouble with stomach bloating.
- You have difficulty emptying your bladder completely.
- You have narrow-angle glaucoma.
- You have severe ulcerative colitis.

Before you start, consult your doctor:
- If you have open-angle glaucoma, angina, chronic bronchitis or asthma, hiatal hernia, liver disease, enlarged prostate, myasthenia gravis, peptic ulcer, kidney or thyroid disease.
- If you will have surgery within 2 months, including dental surgery, requiring general or spinal anesthesia.

Over age 60:
Adverse reactions and side effects may be more frequent and severe than in younger persons.

Pregnancy:
Decide with your doctor whether drug benefits justify risk to unborn child. Risk category C (see page xxii).

Breast-feeding:
Drug passes into milk and decreases milk flow. Avoid drug or discontinue nursing until you finish medicine. Consult doctor for advice on maintaining milk supply.

Infants & children:
Use only under medical supervision.

Prolonged use:
Chronic constipation, possible fecal impaction. Consult doctor immediately.

Skin & sunlight:
No problems expected.

Driving, piloting or hazardous work:
Use disqualifies you for piloting aircraft. Don't drive until you learn how medicine affects you. Don't work around dangerous machinery. Don't climb ladders or work in high places.

Discontinuing:
May be unnecessary to finish medicine. Follow doctor's instructions.

Others:
Advise any doctor or dentist whom you consult that you take this medicine.

POSSIBLE INTERACTION WITH OTHER DRUGS

GENERIC NAME OR DRUG CLASS	COMBINED EFFECT
Amantadine	Increased scopolamine effect.
Antacids*	Decreased scopolamine effect.
Anticholinergics*, other	Increased scopolamine effect.
Antidepressants, tricyclic*	Increased scopolamine effect. Increased sedation.
Antidiarrheals*	Decreased scopolamine effect.
Antihistamines*	Increased scopolamine effect.
Attapulgite	Decreased scopolamine effect.
Buclizine	Increased scopolamine effect.
Clozapine	Toxic effect on the central nervous system.
Cortisone drugs*	Increased internal eye pressure.
Digitalis preparations*	Possible decreased absorption of scopolamine.
Encainide	Increased effect of toxicity on heart muscle.
Ethinamate	Dangerous increased effects of ethinamate. Avoid combining.
Fluoxetine	Increased depressant effects of both drugs.
Guanfacine	May increase depressant effects of either medicine.
Haloperidol	Increased internal eye pressure.
Ketoconazole	Decreased keto-conazole effect.
Leucovorin	High alcohol content of leucovorin may cause adverse effects.
Meperidine	Increased scopolamine effect.
Methylphenidate	Increased scopolamine effect.
Methyprylon	May increase seda-tive effect to danger-ous level. Avoid.
Molindone	Increased anti-cholinergic effect.
Monoamine oxidase (MAO) inhibitors*	Increased scopolamine effect.
Nabilone	Greater depression of central nervous system.
Nitrates*	Increased internal eye pressure.

Continued on page 960

POSSIBLE INTERACTION WITH OTHER SUBSTANCES

INTERACTS WITH	COMBINED EFFECT
Alcohol:	None expected.
Beverages:	None expected.
Cocaine:	Excessively rapid heartbeat. Avoid.
Foods:	None expected.
Marijuana:	Drowsiness, dry mouth.
Tobacco:	None expected.

*See Glossary

SELEGILINE

BRAND NAMES

Eldepryl
Jumex
Jumexal
Juprenil
Movergan
Procythol
SD Deprenyl

BASIC INFORMATION

All the information in this chart applies only when selegiline is given with other drugs that treat Parkinson's disease.

Habit forming? No
Prescription needed? Yes
Available as generic? No
Drug class: Antidyskinetic

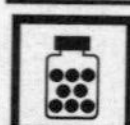

USES

- Treats Parkinson's disease *(paralysis agitans)* when given with levodopa or the combination of levodopa and carbidopa.
- Treats mental depression when taken alone.

DOSAGE & USAGE INFORMATION

How to take:
Tablets—Swallow with liquid. If you can't swallow whole, crumble tablet and take with liquid or food.

Continued next column

OVERDOSE

SYMPTOMS:
Mouth-opening difficulty; neck and heel muscle spasm; sweating; irregular, fast heartbeat; reflexes hyperactive; cold or clammy skin; chest pain; agitation; fainting; seizures; coma. Symptoms can develop 12 to 48 hours after ingestion.
WHAT TO DO:
- **Dial 911 (emergency) or 0 (operator) for an ambulance or medical help. Then give first aid immediately.**
- **If patient is unconsciousness and not breathing, give mouth-to-mouth breathing. If there is no heartbeat, use cardiac massage and mouth-to-mouth breathing (CPR). Don't try to make patient vomit. If you can't get help quickly, take patient to nearest emergency facility.**
- **See emergency information on inside covers.**

When to take:
Usually taken at breakfast and lunch to minimize nausea or insomnia. Don't take after mid-afternoon.

If you forget a dose:
Take as soon as you remember up to 2 hours late. If more than 2 hours, wait for next scheduled dose (don't double this dose).

What drug does:
Inhibits action of monoamine oxidase Type B (MAO B), a major chemical enzyme in the brain. Doses higher than recommended can cause high blood pressure.

Time lapse before drug works:
2 hours.

Don't take with:
- Any foods containing tyramine, such as cheese; wine; beer; nonalcoholic beer; liqueurs; yeast extracts; bean pods; pickled or smoked fish, meat, chicken, turkey or other poultry; fermented sausage (summer sausage, salami, pepperoni); bologna; overripe fruit; caffeine.
- Any other medicines (including over-the-counter drugs such as cough and cold medicines, laxatives, antacids, diet pills, nose drops or vitamins) without consulting your doctor.
- Study Interaction column.

POSSIBLE ADVERSE REACTIONS OR SIDE EFFECTS

SYMPTOMS	WHAT TO DO
Life-threatening:	
• In case of overdose, see previous column.	
• Severe chest pain, enlarged pupils, heartbeat irregularities, severe nausea and vomiting, stiff neck.	Seek emergency treatment.
Common:	
• Mood changes, unusual or uncontrolled body movements, hallucinations, headache, lip smacking, difficult urination.	Discontinue. Call doctor right away.
• Abdominal pain, dizziness, dry mouth, insomnia, mild nausea.	Continue. Call doctor when convenient.
Infrequent:	
• Chest pain, heartbeat irregularities, wheezing, swollen feet, speech difficulty, bloody or black stools.	Discontinue. Seek emergency treatment.

• Constipation; anxiety; tiredness; eyelid spasm; unpleasant taste; blurred vision; leg pain; ringing ears; chills; skin rash; burning lips or mouth; drowsiness; frequent, decreased urination.	Continue. Call doctor when convenient.
Rare:	
Weight loss, heartburn, jaw clenching or teeth gnashing, impaired memory, uncontrolled body movements.	Continue. Call doctor when convenient.

WARNINGS & PRECAUTIONS

Don't take if:
You are allergic to selegiline.

Before you start, consult your doctor:
If you have a past medical history of peptic ulcer, profound dementia, severe psychosis, tardive dyskinesia, excessive tremor.

Over age 60:
Adverse reactions and side effects may be more frequent and severe than in younger persons. You may need smaller doses for shorter periods of time.

Pregnancy:
Decide with your doctor if drug benefits justify risk to unborn child. Risk category C (see page xxii).

Breast-feeding:
Unknown if drug passes into milk. Consult doctor.

Infants & children:
Not recommended.

Prolonged use:
Talk to your doctor about the need for follow-up medical examinations or laboratory studies to check complete blood counts (white blood cell count, platelet count, red blood cell count, hemoglobin, hematocrit), stomach x-rays.

Skin & sunlight:
Increased sensitivity to ultraviolet rays from sun or sunlamps. Avoid overexposure.

Driving, piloting or hazardous work:
Don't drive or pilot aircraft until you learn how medicine affects you. Don't work around dangerous machinery. Don't climb ladders or work in high places. Danger increases if you drink alcohol or take medicine affecting alertness and reflexes.

Discontinuing:
No special problems expected.

Others:
- Avoid sudden rises from lying-down or sitting positions.
- Advise any doctor or dentist whom you consult that you take this medicine.
- May affect results in some medical tests.

POSSIBLE INTERACTION WITH OTHER DRUGS

GENERIC NAME OR DRUG CLASS	COMBINED EFFECT
Caffeine (high doses)	Can cause same symptoms as tyramine-containing foods*. (See "Don't Take With" information block on previous page.)
Fluoxetine	Increased risk of mental status changes.
Levodopa	Increased risk of adverse reactions.
Meperdine	Possibly severe drop in blood pressure. Avoid.
Narcotics*	Severe toxic reaction leading to seizures, coma, and/or death.

Continued on page 960

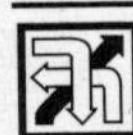

POSSIBLE INTERACTION WITH OTHER SUBSTANCES

INTERACTS WITH	COMBINED EFFECT
Alcohol:	Can cause severe toxicity. Avoid.
Beverages: Drinks containing large quantities of caffeine.	Can cause severe toxicity. Avoid.
Cocaine:	High blood pressure, rapid heartbeat. Avoid.
Foods: Tyramine-containing*. (See "Don't Take With" information block on previous page.)	Severe toxicity, perhaps leading to death. *Carefully* avoid.
Marijuana:	Rapid heart rate. Avoid.
Tobacco:	Rapid heart rate. Avoid.

*See Glossary

SENNAS

BRAND AND GENERIC NAMES

Black-Draught Lax Senna
Fletcher's Castoria
Gentlax
Gentle Nature
Glysennid
Nytilax
Prodiem
Prompt
Senexon
SENNA
SENNOSIDES A & B
Senokot
Senokot-S
Senolax
X-Prep Liquid

BASIC INFORMATION

Habit forming? No
Prescription needed? No
Available as generic? Yes
Drug class: Laxative (stimulant)

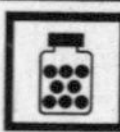

USES

Constipation relief.

DOSAGE & USAGE INFORMATION

How to take:
- Tablet—Swallow with liquid. If you can't swallow whole, chew or crumble tablet and take with liquid or food.
- Liquid, granules—Drink 6 to 8 glasses of water each day, in addition to one taken with each dose.
- Suppositories—Remove wrapper and moisten suppository with water. Gently insert larger end into rectum. Push well into rectum with finger.

When to take:
Usually at bedtime with a snack, unless directed otherwise.

If you forget a dose:
Take as soon as you remember.

What drug does:
Acts on smooth muscles of intestine wall to cause vigorous bowel movement.

Continued next column

OVERDOSE

SYMPTOMS:
Vomiting, electrolyte depletion.
WHAT TO DO:
Overdose unlikely to threaten life. If person takes much larger amount than prescribed, call doctor, poison control center or hospital emergency room for instructions.

Time lapse before drug works:
6 to 10 hours.

Don't take with:
- See Interaction column and consult doctor.
- Don't take within 2 hours of taking another medicine. Laxative interferes with medicine absorption.

POSSIBLE ADVERSE REACTIONS OR SIDE EFFECTS

SYMPTOMS	WHAT TO DO
Life-threatening: None expected.	
Common:	
• Rectal irritation.	Continue. Call doctor when convenient.
• Yellow-brown or red-violet urine.	No action necessary.
Infrequent:	
• Dangerous potassium loss (thirst, weakness, heartbeat irregularity, paralysis, nausea and diarrhea).	Discontinue. Call doctor right away.
• Belching, cramps, nausea.	Continue. Call doctor when convenient.
Rare:	
• Irritability, headache, confusion, rash, difficult breathing, irregular heartbeat, muscle cramps, unusual tiredness or weakness.	Discontinue. Call doctor right away.
• Burning on urination.	Continue. Call doctor when convenient.

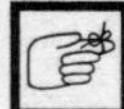

WARNINGS & PRECAUTIONS

Don't take if:
- You have symptoms of appendicitis, inflamed bowel or intestinal blockage.
- You are allergic to a stimulant laxative*.
- You have missed a bowel movement for only 1 or 2 days.

Before you start, consult your doctor:
- If you have a colostomy or ileostomy.
- If you have congestive heart disease.
- If you have diabetes.
- If you have high blood pressure.
- If you have a laxative habit.
- If you have rectal bleeding.
- If you take other laxatives.

Over age 60:
Adverse reactions and side effects may be more frequent and severe than in younger persons.

Pregnancy:
Consult doctor for advice about laxative use. Risk category C (see page xxii).

Breast-feeding:
May pass into breast milk. Consult doctor.

Infants & children:
Use only under medical supervision.

Prolonged use:
Don't take for more than 1 week unless under a doctor's supervision. May cause laxative dependence.

Skin & sunlight:
No problems expected.

Driving, piloting or hazardous work:
No problems expected.

Discontinuing:
May be unnecessary to finish medicine. Follow doctor's instructions.

Others:
- Don't take to "flush out" your system or as a "tonic."
- May cause urine to get discolored. No action necessary.

POSSIBLE INTERACTION WITH OTHER DRUGS

GENERIC NAME OR DRUG CLASS	COMBINED EFFECT
Antihypertensives*	May cause dangerous low potassium level.
Digitalis preparations*	Increased digitalis toxicity.
Diuretics*, potassium sparing	May cause dangerous low potassium level.
Salicylates	Decreased salicylate effect. Take drugs 2 hours apart.

POSSIBLE INTERACTION WITH OTHER SUBSTANCES

INTERACTS WITH	COMBINED EFFECT
Alcohol:	None expected.
Beverages:	None expected.
Cocaine:	None expected.
Foods:	None expected.
Marijuana:	None expected.
Tobacco:	None expected.

*See Glossary

SERTRALINE

BRAND NAMES

Zoloft

BASIC INFORMATION

Habit forming? No
Prescription needed? Yes
Available as generic? No
Drug class: Antidepressant

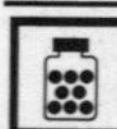

USES

Treats mental depression.

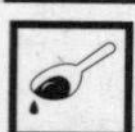

DOSAGE & USAGE INFORMATION

How to take:
Tablets—Swallow with liquid. If you can't swallow whole, crumble tablet and take with liquid or food.

When to take:
Once daily, either in the morning or in the evening.

If you forget a dose:
Take as soon as you remember up to 2 hours late. If more than 2 hours, wait for next scheduled dose (don't double this dose).

What drug does:
Inhibits uptake of serotonin in the central nervous system, preventing depression.

Time lapse before drug works:
1 to 4 weeks.

Don't take with:
- Any monoamine oxidase (MAO) inhibitor* (or within 14 days of discontinuing an MAO inhibitor). To do so may cause serious or even fatal reactions.
- Any other nonprescription drugs without consulting your doctor.

OVERDOSE

SYMPTOMS:
Seizures, agitation, violent vomiting.
WHAT TO DO:
- **Dial 911 (emergency) or 0 (operator) for an ambulance or medical help. Then give first aid immediately.**
- **See emergency information on inside covers.**

POSSIBLE ADVERSE REACTIONS OR SIDE EFFECTS

SYMPTOMS	WHAT TO DO
Life-threatening: In case of overdose, see previous column.	
Common:	
Weight loss, dry mouth, sweating, headache, insomnia.	Continue. Call doctor when convenient.
Infrequent:	
• Nausea, diarrhea, tremor, fatigue.	Continue. Call doctor when convenient.
• Palpitations, dizziness.	Discontinue. Call doctor right away.
Rare:	
Mania, chest pain, skin rash.	Discontinue. Call doctor right away.

WARNINGS & PRECAUTIONS

Don't take if:
- You have epilepsy.
- You have an allergy to sertraline.

Before you start, consult your doctor:
If you have severe liver or kidney disease.

Over age 60:
Adverse reactions may be more frequent and severe than in younger persons. You may need smaller doses for shorter periods of time.

Pregnancy:
Don't take unless essential. Consult doctor. Risk category B (see page xxii).

Breast-feeding:
Unknown effects. Consult doctor.

Infants & children:
Not recommended.

Prolonged use:
No special problems expected.

Skin & sunlight:
No special problems expected.

Driving, piloting or hazardous work:
Don't drive or pilot aircraft until you learn how the medicine affects you. Don't work around dangerous machinery. Don't climb ladders or work in high places.

Discontinuing:
Don't discontinue without consulting doctor. Dose may require gradual reduction if you have taken drug for a long time. Doses of other drugs may also require adjustment.

Others:
- Advise any doctor or dentist whom you consult that you take this medicine.
- May affect results of some medical tests.

POSSIBLE INTERACTION WITH OTHER DRUGS

GENERIC NAME OR DRUG CLASS	COMBINED EFFECT
Central nervous system (CNS) depressants*	Increased depressive effects of both drugs.
Digitoxin	Increased risk of adverse effects of both drugs.
Lithium	May increase risk of side effects.
Monoamine oxidase (MAO) inhibitors*	Increased risk of adverse effects. May lead to convulsions and hypertensive crisis. Let 4 days elapse between taking the 2 drugs.
Selegiline	Increased risk of adverse effects. May lead to convulsions and hypertensive crisis. Let 4 days elapse between taking the 2 drugs.

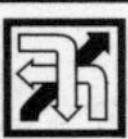

POSSIBLE INTERACTION WITH OTHER SUBSTANCES

INTERACTS WITH	COMBINED EFFECT
Alcohol:	May increase depression.
Beverages:	No proven problems.
Cocaine:	Decreased effect of sertraline.
Foods:	No proven problems.
Marijuana:	Decreased effect of sertraline.
Tobacco:	No proven problems.

***See Glossary**

SIMETHICONE

BRAND NAMES

Di-Gel
Extra Stength Gas-X
Gas-X
Gas Relief
Gelusil
Maximum Strength Gas Relief
Maximum Strength Phazyme
Mygel
Mylanta Gas
Mylicon
Mylicon-80
Mylicon-125
Ovol
Ovol-40
Ovol-80
Phazyme
Phazyme 95
Phazyme 55
Riopan Plus

BASIC INFORMATION

Habit forming? No
Prescription needed? No
Available as generic? Yes, for some
Drug class: Antiflatulent

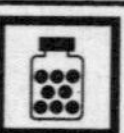

USES

- Treatment for retention of abdominal gas.
- Used prior to x-ray of abdomen to reduce gas shadows.

DOSAGE & USAGE INFORMATION

How to take:
- Tablet or capsule—Swallow with liquid.
- Liquid—Dissolve in water. Drink complete dose.
- Chewable tablets—Chew completely. Don't swallow whole.

When to take:
After meals and at bedtime.

If you forget a dose:
Take when remembered if needed.

What drug does:
Reduces surface tension of gas bubbles in stomach.

Time lapse before drug works:
10 minutes.

Don't take with:
Any other medicine without consulting your doctor or pharmacist.

OVERDOSE

SYMPTOMS:
None expected.
WHAT TO DO:
Overdose unlikely to threaten life.

POSSIBLE ADVERSE REACTIONS OR SIDE EFFECTS

SYMPTOMS **WHAT TO DO**

Life-threatening:
None expected.

Common:
None expected.

Infrequent:
None expected.

Rare:
None expected.

WARNINGS & PRECAUTIONS

Don't take if:
You are allergic to simethicone.

Before you start, consult your doctor:
No problems expected.

Over age 60:
No problems expected.

Pregnancy:
Consult doctor. Risk category C (see page xxii).

Breast-feeding:
No problems expected. Consult doctor.

Infants & children:
Not recommended.

Prolonged use:
No problems expected.

Skin & sunlight:
No problems expected.

Driving, piloting or hazardous work:
No problems expected.

Discontinuing:
May be unnecessary to finish medicine. Discontinue when symptoms disappear.

Others:
No problems expected.

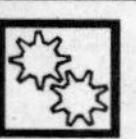

POSSIBLE INTERACTION WITH OTHER DRUGS

GENERIC NAME OR DRUG CLASS	COMBINED EFFECT
None significant.	

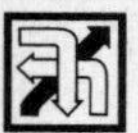

POSSIBLE INTERACTION WITH OTHER SUBSTANCES

INTERACTS WITH	COMBINED EFFECT
Alcohol:	None expected.
Beverages:	None expected.
Cocaine:	None expected.
Foods:	None expected.
Marijuana:	None expected.
Tobacco:	None expected.

SODIUM BICARBONATE

BRAND NAMES

Arm & Hammer Pure Baking Soda
Bell/ans
Citrocarbonate
Soda Mint

BASIC INFORMATION

Habit forming? No
Prescription needed? No
Available as generic? Yes
Drug class: Alkalizer, antacid

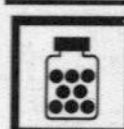

USES

- Treats metobolic acidosis.
- Alkalinizes urine to reduce uric acid kidney stones.
- Treats hyperacidity of the stomach that is present with indigestion, gastroesophageal reflux and peptic ulcer disease.

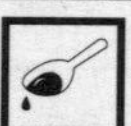

DOSAGE & USAGE INFORMATION

How to take:

- Tablets—Swallow with liquid. If you can't swallow whole, crumble tablet and take with liquid or food.
- Powder—Mix in a glass of water and drink.
- Effervescent sodium bicarbonate—Mix in a glass of cold water and drink.

When to take:

- For hyperacidity—1 to 3 hours after meals.
- For kidney stones—According to prescription instructions.

If you forget a dose:
Take as soon as you remember up to 2 hours late. If more than 2 hours, wait for next scheduled dose (don't double this dose).

What drug does:

- Buffers acid in the stomach.
- Increases excretion of bicarbonate in the urine to help dissolve uric acid stones.

Continued next column

OVERDOSE

SYMPTOMS:
Excessive swelling of feet and lower legs.
WHAT TO DO:
Overdose unlikely to threaten life. If person takes much larger amount than prescribed, call doctor, poison control center or hospital emergency room for instructions.

Time lapse before drug works:
Works immediately, but the duration of effect is short.

Don't take with:

- Nonprescription drugs without consulting doctor.
- See Interaction column and consult doctor.

POSSIBLE ADVERSE REACTIONS OR SIDE EFFECTS

SYMPTOMS	WHAT TO DO
Life-threatening: None expected.	
Common: None expected.	
Infrequent:	
• Stomach cramps that continue.	Discontinue. Call doctor right away.
• Nausea, headache, appetite loss (with long-term use).	Continue. Call doctor when convenient.
Rare:	
Muscle pain or twitching, nervousness, breathing difficulty, mild swelling of feet or lower legs (with large doses).	Discontinue. Call doctor right away.

WARNINGS & PRECAUTIONS

Don't take if:
You are allergic to sodium bicarbonate.

Before you start, consult your doctor:
If you have heart disease, kidney disease or toxemia of pregnancy.

Over age 60:
Adverse reactions and side effects may be more frequent and severe than in younger persons.

Pregnancy:
May cause weight gain and swelling of feet and ankles. Avoid if you have high blood pressure. Consult doctor. Risk category C (see page xxii).

Breast-feeding:
No problems expected, but consult doctor.

Infants & children:
Not recommended. Safety and dosage have not been established.

Prolonged use:
Don't use for longer than prescribed or recommended. May cause sodium overload.

Skin & sunlight:
No special problems expected.

Driving, piloting or hazardous work:
No special problems expected.

Discontinuing:
May be unnecessary to finish medicine. Follow doctor's instructions.

Others:
- Heat and moisture in bathroom medicine cabinet can cause breakdown of medicine. Store someplace else.
- May interfere with the accuracy of some medical tests (especially acidosis and urinalysis tests).

POSSIBLE INTERACTION WITH OTHER DRUGS

GENERIC NAME OR DRUG CLASS	COMBINED EFFECT
Adrenocorticoids*	Sodium overload.
Cortisone	Sodium overload.
Ketoconazole	Decreased absorption of ketoconazole.
Mecamylamine	Increased mecamylamine effect.
Methenamine	Decreased methenamine effect.
Tetracyclines*	Greatly reduced absorption of tetracyclines.
Any other medicine	Decreased absorption of other medicine if taken within 1 to 2 hours of taking sodium bicarbonate.

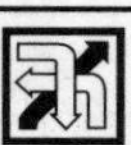

POSSIBLE INTERACTION WITH OTHER SUBSTANCES

INTERACTS WITH	COMBINED EFFECT
Alcohol:	Decreased effectiveness of sodium bicarbonate.
Beverages:	None expected.
Cocaine:	None expected.
Foods:	None expected.
Marijuana:	None expected.
Tobacco:	Decreased effectiveness of sodium bicarbonate.

***See Glossary**

SODIUM FLUORIDE

BRAND NAMES

Fluor-A-Day
Fluorident
Fluoritab
Fluorodex
Fluotic
Flura
Karidium
Listermint with Fluoride
Luride
Luride-SF
Pediaflor
Pedi-Dent
Solu-Flur

Numerous other multiple vitamin-mineral supplements. Check labels.

BASIC INFORMATION

Habit forming? No
Prescription needed? Yes, for some
Available as generic? Yes
Drug class: Mineral supplement (fluoride)

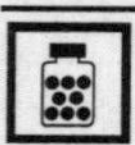

USES

- Reduces tooth cavities.
- Treats osteoporosis.

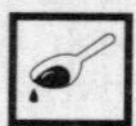

DOSAGE & USAGE INFORMATION

How to take:
- Tablet—Swallow with liquid or crumble tablet and take with liquid (not milk) or food.
- Liquid—Measure with dropper and take directly or with liquid.
- Chewable tablets—Chew slowly and thoroughly before swallowing.

When to take:
Usually at bedtime after teeth are thoroughly brushed.

Continued next column

OVERDOSE

SYMPTOMS:
Stomach cramps or pain, nausea, faintness, vomiting (possibly bloody), diarrhea, black stools, shallow breathing, muscle spasms, seizures, arrhythmias.
WHAT TO DO:
- **Dial 911 (emergency) or 0 (operator) for an ambulance or medical help. Then give first aid immediately.**
- **See emergency information on inside covers.**

If you forget a dose:
Take as soon as you remember. Don't double a forgotten dose. Return to schedule.

What drug does:
Provides supplemental fluoride to combat tooth decay.

Time lapse before drug works:
8 weeks to provide maximum effect.

Don't take with:
- Any other medicine simultaneously.
- See Interaction column.

POSSIBLE ADVERSE REACTIONS OR SIDE EFFECTS

SYMPTOMS	WHAT TO DO
Life-threatening: In case of overdose, see previous column.	
Common:	
Constipation, appetite loss.	Continue. Call doctor when convenient.
Infrequent:	
• Rash.	Discontinue. Call doctor right away.
• Tooth discoloration.	Continue. Call doctor when convenient.
Rare:	
• Severe upsets (digestive) only with overdose.	Discontinue. Seek emergency treatment.
• Sores in mouth and lips, aching bones, stiffness.	Discontinue. Call doctor right away.

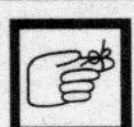

WARNINGS & PRECAUTIONS

Don't take if:
- Your water supply contains 0.7 parts fluoride per million. Too much fluoride stains teeth permanently.
- You are allergic to any fluoride-containing product.
- You have underactive thyroid.

Before you start, consult your doctor:
- If you have kidney disease.
- If you have ulcers.
- If you have joint pain.

Over age 60:
No problems expected.

Pregnancy:
Consult doctor. Risk category C (see page xxii).

Breast-feeding:
No problems expected. Consult doctor.

Infants & children:
No problems expected except accidental overdose. Keep vitamin-mineral supplements out of children's reach.

Prolonged use:
Excess may cause discolored teeth and decreased calcium in blood.

Skin & sunlight:
No problems expected.

Driving, piloting or hazardous work:
No problems expected.

Discontinuing:
No problems expected.

Others:
- Store in original plastic container. Fluoride decomposes glass.
- Some products contain tartrazine dye. Avoid, especially if you are allergic to aspirin.

POSSIBLE INTERACTION WITH OTHER DRUGS

GENERIC NAME OR DRUG CLASS	COMBINED EFFECT
Calcium supplements*	Decreased effect of calcium and fluoride.

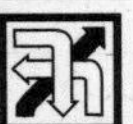

POSSIBLE INTERACTION WITH OTHER SUBSTANCES

INTERACTS WITH	COMBINED EFFECT
Alcohol:	None expected.
Beverages:	
Milk.	Prevents absorption of fluoride. Space dose 2 hours before or after milk.
Cocaine:	None expected.
Foods:	None expected.
Marijuana:	None expected.
Tobacco:	None expected.

SODIUM PHOSPHATE

BRAND NAMES

Fleet Enema
Fleet Phospho-Soda
Sal Hepatica

BASIC INFORMATION

Habit forming? No
Prescription needed? No
Available as generic? Yes
Drug class: Laxative (hyperosmotic)

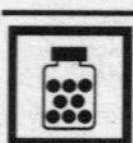

USES

Constipation relief.

DOSAGE & USAGE INFORMATION

How to take:

- Liquid, effervescent tablet or powder—Dilute dose in beverage before swallowing.
- Enema—Follow package instructions.

When to take:
Usually once a day, preferably in the morning.

If you forget a dose:
Take as soon as you remember up to 8 hours before bedtime. If later, wait for next scheduled dose (don't double this dose). Don't take at bedtime.

What drug does:
Draws water into bowel from other body tissues. Causes distention through fluid accumulation, which promotes soft stool and accelerates bowel motion.

Time lapse before drug works:
30 minutes to 3 hours.

Don't take with:
Any other medicine without consulting your doctor or pharmacist.

OVERDOSE

SYMPTOMS:
Fluid depletion, weakness, vomiting, fainting.
WHAT TO DO:
Overdose unlikely to threaten life. If person takes much larger amount than prescribed, call doctor, poison control center or hospital emergency room for instructions.

POSSIBLE ADVERSE REACTIONS OR SIDE EFFECTS

SYMPTOMS	WHAT TO DO
Life-threatening: In case of overdose, see previous column.	
Common:	
Weakness.	Continue. Call doctor when convenient.
Infrequent:	
• Irregular heartbeat.	Discontinue. Call doctor right away.
• Increased thirst, gaseousness, cramps, diarrhea, nausea.	Continue. Tell doctor at next visit.
Rare:	
Dizziness, confusion, tiredness or weakness.	Continue. Call doctor when convenient.

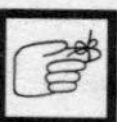

WARNINGS & PRECAUTIONS

Don't take if:
- You are allergic to any hyperosmotic laxative*.
- You have symptoms of appendicitis, inflamed bowel or intestinal blockage.
- You have missed a bowel movement for only 1 or 2 days.

Before you start, consult your doctor:
- If you have congestive heart disease.
- If you have diabetes.
- If you have high blood pressure.
- If you have a colostomy or ileostomy.
- If you have kidney disease.
- If you have a laxative habit.
- If you have rectal bleeding.
- If you take another laxative.

Over age 60:
Adverse reactions and side effects may be more frequent and severe than in younger persons.

Pregnancy:
Salt content may cause fluid retention and swelling. Avoid if possible. Consult doctor. Risk category C (see page xxii).

Breast-feeding:
No problems expected. Consult doctor.

Infants & children:
Use only under medical supervision.

Prolonged use:
Don't take for more than 1 week unless under a doctor's supervision. May cause laxative dependence.

Skin & sunlight:
No problems expected.

Driving, piloting or hazardous work:
No problems expected.

Discontinuing:
May be unnecessary to finish medicine. Follow doctor's instructions.

Others:
- Don't take to "flush out" your system or as a "tonic."
- Don't take within 2 hours of taking another medicine.

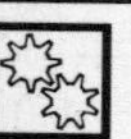

POSSIBLE INTERACTION WITH OTHER DRUGS

GENERIC NAME OR DRUG CLASS	COMBINED EFFECT
Chlordiazepoxide	Decreased chlordiazepoxide effect.
Chlorpromazine	Decreased chlorpromazine effect.
Dicumarol	Decreased dicumarol effect.
Digoxin	Decreased digoxin effect.
Diuretics, potassium-sparing*	Excessive potassium loss.
Isoniazid	Decreased isoniazid effect.
Mexiletine	May decrease effectiveness of mexiletine.
Potassium supplements*	Reduced potassium supplement effect.
Tetracyclines*	Possible intestinal blockage.

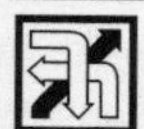

POSSIBLE INTERACTION WITH OTHER SUBSTANCES

INTERACTS WITH	COMBINED EFFECT
Alcohol:	None expected.
Beverages:	None expected.
Cocaine:	None expected.
Foods:	None expected.
Marijuana:	None expected.
Tobacco:	None expected.

*See Glossary

SPIRONOLACTONE

BRAND NAMES

Aldactone
Novospiroton

BASIC INFORMATION

Habit forming? No
Prescription needed? Yes
Available as generic? Yes
Drug class: Antihypertensive, diuretic

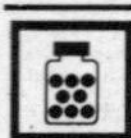

USES

- Reduces high blood pressure.
- Prevents fluid retention (edema).
- Treats hyperaldosteronism, hypokalemia, polycystic ovary syndrome, female hirsutism.

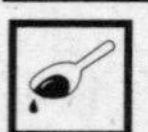

DOSAGE & USAGE INFORMATION

How to take:
Tablet—Swallow with liquid or food to lessen stomach irritation. If you can't swallow whole, crumble tablet and take with liquid or food.

When to take:
- 1 dose a day—Take after breakfast.
- More than 1 dose a day—Take last dose no later than 6 p.m.

If you forget a dose:
- 1 dose a day—Take as soon as you remember up to 12 hours late. If more than 12 hours, wait for next scheduled dose (don't double this dose).
- More than 1 dose a day—Take as soon as you remember. Wait 6 hours for next dose.

What drug does:
- Increases sodium and water excretion through increased urine production, decreasing body fluid and blood pressure.
- Retains potassium.

Continued next column

OVERDOSE

SYMPTOMS:
Thirst, drowsiness, confusion, fatigue, weakness, nausea, vomiting, irregular heartbeat, excessive blood pressure drop.
WHAT TO DO:
- **Dial 911 (emergency) or 0 (operator) for an ambulance or medical help. Then give first aid immediately.**
- **See emergency information on inside covers.**

Time lapse before drug works:
3 to 5 days.

Don't take with:
Any other medicine without consulting your doctor or pharmacist.

POSSIBLE ADVERSE REACTIONS OR SIDE EFFECTS

SYMPTOMS	WHAT TO DO
Life-threatening:	
In case of overdose, see previous column.	
Common:	
Drowsiness or headache, thirst, nausea, vomiting, diarrhea, abdominal cramping, muscle cramps.	Continue. Call doctor when convenient.
Infrequent:	
• Confusion, irregular heartbeat, shortness of breath, constipation, breast tenderness, unusual sweating.	Discontinue. Call doctor right away.
• Numbness, tingling in hands or feet; menstrual irregularities; change in sex drive; dizziness; energy loss.	Continue. Call doctor when convenient.
Rare:	
• Rash or itchy skin, fever.	Discontinue. Call doctor right away.
• Deep voice in women, excess hair growth, voice change, enlarged clitoris in women, enlarged breasts in males.	Continue. Tell doctor at next visit.

WARNINGS & PRECAUTIONS

Don't take if:
- You are allergic to spironolactone.
- You have impaired kidney function.
- Your serum potassium level is high.

Before you start, consult your doctor:
- If you have had kidney or liver disease.
- If you have diabetes.
- If you have menstrual abnormalities or breast enlargement.
- If you will have surgery within 2 months, including dental surgery, requiring general or spinal anesthesia.

Over age 60:
- Limit use to 2 to 3 weeks if possible.
- Adverse reactions and side effects may be more frequent and severe than in younger persons.
- Heat or fever can reduce blood pressure. May require dose adjustment.
- Overdose and extended use may cause blood clots.

Pregnancy:
Decide with your doctor if drug benefits justify risk to unborn child. Risk category C (see page xxii).

Breast-feeding:
Effect unknown. Consult doctor.

Infants & children:
Use only under medical supervision.

Prolonged use:
- Potassium retention with irregular heartbeat, unusual weakness and confusion.
- Talk to your doctor about the need for follow-up medical examinations or laboratory studies to check blood pressure, kidney function, ECG* and serum electrolytes.

Skin & sunlight:
Increased sensitivity to sunlight.

Driving, piloting or hazardous work:
Avoid if you feel drowsy. Otherwise, no problems expected.

Discontinuing:
Consult doctor about adjusting doses of other drugs.

Others:
No problems expected.

POSSIBLE INTERACTION WITH OTHER DRUGS

GENERIC NAME OR DRUG CLASS	COMBINED EFFECT
Amiloride	Dangerous potassium retention.
Angiotensin-converting enzyme (ACE) inhibitors*	Possible excessive potassium in blood.
Anticoagulants*, oral	Possible decreased anticoagulant effect.
Antihypertensives*, other	Increased anti-hypertensive effect.
Aspirin	Decreased spirono-lactone effect.
Carteolol	Increased anti-hypertensive effect.
Cyclosporine	Possible excessive potassium in blood.
Digitalis preparations*	Decreased digitalis effect.
Diuretics*, other	Increased effect of both drugs. Beneficial if needed and dose is correct.
Laxatives*	Reduced potassium levels.
Lithium	Likely lithium toxicity.
Nicardipine	Blood pressure drop. Dosages may require adjustment.
Nimodipine	Dangerous blood pressure drop.
Nitrates*	Excessive blood pressure drop.
Potassium iodide	May raise potassium level in blood to toxic levels.
Potassium supplements*	Dangerous potassium retention, causing possible heartbeat irregularity.
Salicylates*	May decrease spironolactone effect.
Sodium bicarbonate	Reduced high potassium levels.
Terazosin	Decreased effective-ness of terazosin.

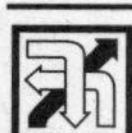

POSSIBLE INTERACTION WITH OTHER SUBSTANCES

INTERACTS WITH	COMBINED EFFECT
Alcohol:	None expected.
Beverages: Low-salt milk.	Possible potassium toxicity.
Cocaine:	Increased risk of heart block and high blood pressure.
Foods: Salt.	Don't restrict unless directed by doctor.
Salt substitutes.	Possible potassium toxicity.
Marijuana:	Increased thirst, fainting.
Tobacco:	None expected.

*See Glossary

SPIRONOLACTONE & HYDROCHLOROTHIAZIDE

BRAND NAMES

Aldactazide
Novospirozine
Spirozide

BASIC INFORMATION

Habit forming? Yes
Prescription needed? Yes
Available as generic? Yes
Drug class: Antihypertensive, diuretic (thiazide)

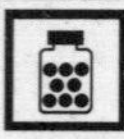

USES

- Controls, but doesn't cure, high blood pressure.
- Reduces fluid retention (edema).

DOSAGE & USAGE INFORMATION

How to take:
Tablet—Swallow with liquid. If you can't swallow whole, crumble tablet and take with liquid or food.

When to take:
- 1 dose a day—Take after breakfast.
- More than 1 dose a day—Take last dose no later than 6 p.m.

If you forget a dose:
- 1 dose a day—Take as soon as you remember up to 12 hours late. If more than12 hours, wait for next scheduled dose (don't double this dose).
- More than 1 dose a day—Take as soon as you remember. Wait 6 hours for next dose.

What drug does:
- Increases sodium and water excretion through increased urine production.
- Retains potassium.
- Relaxes muscle cells of small arteries.
- Reduces body fluid, and relaxed arteries lower blood pressure.

Time lapse before drug works:
4 to 6 hours. May require several weeks to lower blood pressure.

Don't take with:
Any other medicine without consulting your doctor or pharmacist.

OVERDOSE

SYMPTOMS:
Thirst, drowsiness, confusion, fatigue, weakness, nausea, vomiting, cramps, irregular heartbeat, weak pulse, excessive blood pressure drop, coma.
WHAT TO DO:
- **Dial 911 (emergency) or 0 (operator) for an ambulance or medical help. Then give first aid immediately.**
- **See emergency information on inside covers.**

POSSIBLE ADVERSE REACTIONS OR SIDE EFFECTS

SYMPTOMS	WHAT TO DO
Life-threatening:	
Irregular heartbeat, weak pulse, shortness of breath.	Discontinue. Seek emergency treatment.
Common:	
Drowsiness, headache, thirst, abdominal cramping, muscle cramps.	Continue. Call doctor when convenient.
Infrequent:	
• Blurred vision, abdominal pain, nausea, vomiting, constipation, breast tenderness.	Discontinue. Call doctor right away.
• Dizziness, mood change, headache, dry mouth, menstrual irregularities, diminished sex drive, increased sweating, weakness, tiredness, weight gain or loss, confusion, numbness or tingling in hands or feet, diarrhea.	Continue. Call doctor when convenient.
Rare:	
• Sore throat, fever, rash, jaundice.	Discontinue. Call doctor right away.
• Excess growth of hair, deep voice in in women, enlarged clitoris in women, enlarged breasts in males.	Continue. Call doctor when convenient.

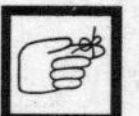

WARNINGS & PRECAUTIONS

Don't take if:
You are allergic to any thiazide diuretic drug.

Before you start, consult your doctor:
- If you are allergic to any sulfa drug*.
- If you have gout, liver, pancreas or kidney disorder.
- If you have had kidney or liver disease.

Continued next column

- If you will have surgery within 2 months, including dental surgery, requiring general or spinal anesthesia.

Over age 60:
- Adverse reactions and side effects may be more frequent and severe than in younger persons, especially dizziness and excessive potassium loss.
- Limit use to 2 to 3 weeks if possible.
- Heat or fever can reduce blood pressure. May require dose adjustment.
- Overdose and extended use may cause blood clots.

Pregnancy:
Decide with your doctor if drug benefits justify risk to unborn child. Risk category C (see page xxii).

Breast-feeding:
Drug passes into milk. Avoid drug or discontinue nursing until you finish medicine. Consult doctor.

Infants & children:
Use only under medical supervision.

Prolonged use:
- You may need medicine to treat high blood pressure for the rest of your life.
- Potassium retention with irregular heartbeat, unusual weakness and confusion.
- Talk to your doctor about the need for follow-up medical examinations or laboratory studies to check blood pressure, kidney function, ECG* and serum electrolytes.

Skin & sunlight:
May cause rash or intensify sunburn in areas exposed to sun or sunlamp.

Driving, piloting or hazardous work:
Don't drive or pilot aircraft until you learn how medicine affects you. Don't work around dangerous machinery. Don't climb ladders or work in high places. Danger increases if you drink alcohol or take medicine affecting alertness and reflexes.

Discontinuing:
- Don't discontinue without medical advice.
- Consult doctor about adjusting doses of other drugs.

Others:
- Hot weather and fever may cause dehydration and drop in blood pressure. Dose may require temporary adjustment. Weigh daily and report any unexpected weight decreases to your doctor.
- May cause rise in uric acid, leading to gout.
- May cause blood sugar rise in diabetics.

POSSIBLE INTERACTION WITH OTHER DRUGS

GENERIC NAME OR DRUG CLASS	COMBINED EFFECT
Allopurinol	Decreased allopurinol effect.
Angiotensin-converting enzyme (ACE) inhibitors*	Possible excessive potassium in blood.
Anticoagulants*, oral	Decreased anti-coagulant effect.
Antidepressants, tricyclic*	Dangerous drop in blood pressure. Avoid combination unless under medical supervision.
Antidiabetics*, oral	Increased blood sugar.
Antihypertensives*, other	Increased anti-hypertensive effect.
Aspirin	Decreased spironolactone effect.
Barbiturates*	Increased hydro-chlorothiazide effect.
Carteolol	Increased anti-hypertensive effect.

Continued on page 960

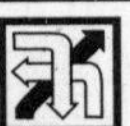

POSSIBLE INTERACTION WITH OTHER SUBSTANCES

INTERACTS WITH	COMBINED EFFECT
Alcohol:	Dangerous blood pressure drop.
Beverages:	
Low-salt milk.	Possible potassium toxicity.
Cocaine:	Decreased spironolactone effect.
Foods:	
Salt.	Don't restrict unless directed by doctor.
Salt substitutes.	Possible potassium toxicity.
Marijuana:	May increase blood pressure. Increased thirst, fainting.
Tobacco:	None expected.

*See Glossary

SUCRALFATE

BRAND NAMES

Carafate
Sulcrate

BASIC INFORMATION

Habit forming? No
Prescription needed? Yes
Available as generic? No
Drug class: Antiulcer

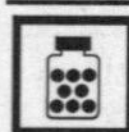

USES

- Treatment for duodenal and gastric ulcers.
- Used to relieve side effects of nonsteroidal anti-inflammatory therapy in rheumatoid arthritis.
- Treatment for gastroesophageal reflux disease (GERD).

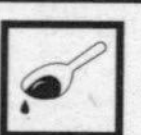

DOSAGE & USAGE INFORMATION

How to take:
Tablet—Take as directed on an empty stomach.

When to take:
1 hour before meals and at bedtime. Allow 2 hours to elapse before taking other prescription medicines.

If you forget a dose:
Take as soon as you remember up to 2 hours late. If more than 2 hours, wait for next scheduled dose (don't double this dose).

What drug does:
Covers ulcer site and protects from acid, enzymes and bile salts.

Time lapse before drug works:
Begins in 30 minutes. May require several days to relieve pain.

Don't take with:
Any other medicine without consulting your doctor or pharmacist.

OVERDOSE

SYMPTOMS:
None expected.
WHAT TO DO:
Overdose unlikely to threaten life. If person takes much larger amount than prescribed, call doctor, poison control center or hospital emergency room for instructions.

POSSIBLE ADVERSE REACTIONS OR SIDE EFFECTS

SYMPTOMS	WHAT TO DO
Life-threatening: None expected.	
Common: Constipation.	Continue. Call doctor when convenient.
Infrequent: Dizziness, sleepiness, rash, itchy skin, abdominal pain, indigestion, vomiting, nausea, dry mouth, diarrhea.	Continue. Call doctor when convenient.
Rare: Back pain.	Continue. Call doctor when convenient.

WARNINGS & PRECAUTIONS

Don't take if:
You are allergic to sucralfate.

Before you start, consult your doctor:
- If you will have surgery within 2 months, including dental surgery, requiring general or spinal anesthesia.
- If you have gastrointestinal or kidney disease.

Over age 60:
Adverse reactions and side effects may be more frequent and severe than in younger persons.

Pregnancy:
No proven harm to unborn child. Avoid if possible. Consult doctor. Risk category B (see page xxii).

Breast-feeding:
Unknown effects. Consult doctor.

Infants & children:
Safety not established.

Prolonged use:
Request blood counts if medicine needed longer than 8 weeks.

Skin & sunlight:
No problems expected.

Driving, piloting or hazardous work:
Don't drive or pilot aircraft until you learn how medicine affects you. Don't work around dangerous machinery. Don't climb ladders or work in high places. Danger increases if you drink alcohol or take medicine affecting alertness and reflexes, such as antihistamines, tranquilizers, sedatives, pain medicine, narcotics and mind-altering drugs.

Discontinuing:
Don't discontinue without consulting doctor. Dose may require gradual reduction if you have taken drug for a long time. Doses of other drugs may also require adjustment.

Others:
No problems expected.

POSSIBLE INTERACTION WITH OTHER DRUGS

GENERIC NAME OR DRUG CLASS	COMBINED EFFECT
Antacids*	Take 1/2 hour before or after sucralfate.
Cimetidine	Possible decreased absorption of cimetidine if taken simultaneously.
Ciprofloxacin	Decreased absorption of ciprofloxacin. Take 2 hours before sucralfate.
Digoxin	Decreased absorption of digoxin. Take 2 hours before sucralfate.
Norfloxacin	Decreased absorption of norfloxacin. Take 2 hours before sucralfate.
Ofloxacin	Decreased absorption of ofloxacin. Take 2 hours before sucralfate.
Phenytoin	Possible decreased absorption of phenytoin if taken simultaneously.
Tetracyclines*	Possible decreased absorption of tetracycline if taken simultaneously.
Theophylline	Decreased absorption of theophylline. Take 2 hours before sucralfate.
Vitamins A, D, E, K	Decreased vitamin absorption.

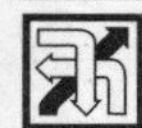

POSSIBLE INTERACTION WITH OTHER SUBSTANCES

INTERACTS WITH	COMBINED EFFECT
Alcohol:	Irritates ulcer. Avoid.
Beverages: Caffeine.	Irritates ulcer. Avoid.
Cocaine:	May make ulcer worse. Avoid.
Foods:	No problems expected.
Marijuana:	May make ulcer worse. Avoid.
Tobacco:	May make ulcer worse. Avoid.

*See Glossary

SULFACYTINE

BRAND NAMES

Renoquid

BASIC INFORMATION

Habit forming? No
Prescription needed? Yes
Available as generic? No
Drug class: Sulfa (sulfonamide)

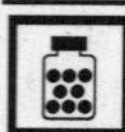

USES

Treatment for urinary tract infections responsive to this drug.

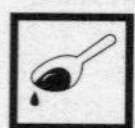

DOSAGE & USAGE INFORMATION

How to take:
Tablet—Swallow with liquid. Instructions to take on empty stomach mean 1 hour before or 2 hours after eating.

When to take:
At the same times each day, evenly spaced.

If you forget a dose:
Take as soon as you remember up to 2 hours late. If more than 2 hours, wait for next scheduled dose (don't double this dose).

What drug does:
Interferes with a nutrient (folic acid) necessary for growth and reproduction of bacteria. Will not attack viruses.

Time lapse before drug works:
2 to 5 days to affect infection.

Don't take with:
Any other medicine without consulting your doctor or pharmacist.

OVERDOSE

SYMPTOMS:
Less urine, bloody urine, coma.
WHAT TO DO:
- **Dial 911 (emergency) or 0 (operator) for an ambulance or medical help. Then give first aid immediately.**
- **See emergency information on inside covers.**

POSSIBLE ADVERSE REACTIONS OR SIDE EFFECTS

SYMPTOMS	WHAT TO DO
Life-threatening:	
In case of overdose, see previous column.	
Common:	
• Itchy skin, rash.	Discontinue. Call doctor right away.
• Headache, vomiting, nausea, diarrhea, appetite loss, skin sensitive to sun.	Continue. Call doctor when convenient.
Infrequent:	
• Red, peeling or blistering skin; sore throat; fever; swallowing difficulty; unusual bruising; aching joints or muscles; jaundice.	Discontinue. Call doctor right away.
• Dizziness, tiredness, weakness.	Continue. Call doctor when convenient.
Rare:	
Painful urination, low back pain, numbness or tingling in hands or feet, bloody urine, neck swelling.	Discontinue. Call doctor right away.

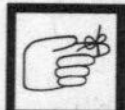

WARNINGS & PRECAUTIONS

Don't take if:
You are allergic to any sulfa drug.

Before you start, consult your doctor:
- If you are allergic to carbonic anhydrase inhibitors, oral antidiabetics, thiazide or loop diuretics.
- If you are allergic by nature.
- If you have liver or kidney disease.
- If you have porphyria.
- If you have developed anemia from use of any drug.

Over age 60:
Adverse reactions and side effects may be more frequent and severe than in younger persons.

Pregnancy:
Risk factor not designated. See category list on page xxii and consult doctor.

Breast-feeding:
Drug passes into milk. Avoid drug or discontinue nursing until you finish medicine. Consult doctor for advice on maintaining milk supply.

Infants & children:
Don't give to infants younger than 1 month.

Prolonged use:
- May enlarge thyroid gland.
- You may become more susceptible to infections caused by germs not responsive to this drug.
- Request frequent blood counts, liver and kidney function studies.

Skin & sunlight:
May cause rash or intensify sunburn in areas exposed to sun or sunlamp.

Driving, piloting or hazardous work:
Avoid if you feel dizzy. Otherwise, no problems expected.

Discontinuing:
Don't discontinue without doctor's advice until you complete prescribed dose, even though symptoms diminish or disappear.

Others:
- Drink 2 quarts of liquid each day to prevent adverse reactions.
- If you require surgery, tell anesthetist you take sulfa. Pentothal anesthesia should not be used.

POSSIBLE INTERACTION WITH OTHER DRUGS

GENERIC NAME OR DRUG CLASS	COMBINED EFFECT
Aminobenzoates	Possible decreased sulfa effect.
Anticoagulants*, oral	Increased anti-coagulant effect.
Anticonvulsants, hydantoin*	Toxic effect on brain.
Antidiabetics*	Toxic effect on brain.
Aspirin	Increased sulfa effect.
Calcium supplements*	Decreased sulfa effect.
Clozapine	Toxic effect on the central nervous system.
Hepatotoxic agents*	Increased liver toxicity.
Isoniazid	Possible anemia.
Mecamylamine	Decreased antibiotic effect.
Methenamine	Possible kidney blockage.
Methotrexate	Increased methotrexate effect.
Oxyphenbutazone	Increased sulfa effect.
Para-aminosalicylic acid	Decreased sulfa effect.
Penicillins*	Decreased penicillin effect.
Phenylbutazone	Increased sulfa effect.
Probenecid	Increased sulfa effect.
Sulfinpyrazone	Increased sulfa effect.
Sulfonureas*	May increase hypo-glycemic action.
Tiopronin	Increased risk of toxicity to kidneys.
Trimethoprim	Increased sulfa effect.
Zidovudine	Increased risk of toxic effects of zidovudine.

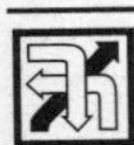

POSSIBLE INTERACTION WITH OTHER SUBSTANCES

INTERACTS WITH	COMBINED EFFECT
Alcohol:	Increased alcohol effect.
Beverages: Less than 2 quarts of fluid daily.	Kidney damage.
Cocaine:	None expected.
Foods:	None expected.
Marijuana:	None expected.
Tobacco:	None expected.

*See Glossary

SULFADOXINE AND PYRIMETHAMINE

BRAND NAMES

Fansidar

BASIC INFORMATION

Habit forming? No
Prescription needed? Yes
Available as generic? No
Drug class: Antiprotozoal

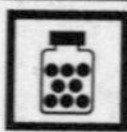

USES

- Treats malaria *(plasmodium faciparum).*
- Helps prevent malaria when traveling to areas where it exists.
- Also used to prevent isosporiasis in patients with acquired immunodeficiency disease.

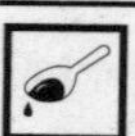

DOSAGE & USAGE INFORMATION

How to take:
Tablets—Swallow with liquid. If you can't swallow whole, crumble tablet and take with liquid or food. Instructions to take on empty stomach mean 1 hour before or 2 hours after eating.

When to take:
Follow doctor's instructions.

If you forget a dose:
Take as soon as you remember. If close to time for next dose, skip this one and wait for next scheduled dose. Don't double dose.

What drug does:
The sulfa component kills bacteria; the pyrimethamine works to kill malaria organisms in red blood cells or human tisue.

Time lapse before drug works:
2 to 6 hours.

Continued next column

OVERDOSE

SYMPTOMS:
Appetite loss, sore throat and fever, seizure, coma.
WHAT TO DO:
- **Dial 911 (emergency) or 0 (operator) for an ambulance or medical help. Then give first aid immediately.**
- **See emergency information on inside front covers.**

Don't take with:
- Any other medicines (including over-the-counter drugs such as cough and cold medicines, laxatives, antacids, diet pills, caffeine, nose drops or vitamins) without consulting your doctor.
- Mefloquine.

POSSIBLE ADVERSE REACTIONS OR SIDE EFFECTS

SYMPTOMS	WHAT TO DO
Life-threatening:	
In case of overdose, see previous column.	
Common:	
Loss or change of taste; diarrhea; skin rash; pale skin; sore throat; sore, red tongue; mouth ulcers; fever; excessive bleeding; tiredness, light sensitivity.	Discontinue. Call doctor right away.
Infrequent:	
Aching joints, fever, skin blisters or peeling, jaundice (yellow skin and eyes).	Discontinue. Call doctor right away.
Rare:	
Bloody urine, burning on urination, back pain, swollen neck.	Discontinue. Call doctor right away.

SULFADOXINE AND PYRIMETHAMINE

WARNINGS & PRECAUTIONS

Don't take if:
You know you are allergic to sulfa drugs, furosemide, thiazide diuretics, carbonase anhydrase inhibitors.

Before you start, consult your doctor:
- If you have AIDS.
- If you have anemia, seizures, G6PD* deficiency, liver disease, porphyria, kidney disease.
- If you can't tolerate sulfa drugs.

Over age 60:
Adverse reactions and side effects may be more frequent and severe than in younger persons. You may need smaller doses for shorter periods of time.

Pregnancy:
Use birth control so you won't get pregnant while in an endemic malaria area. Should not be taken during pregnancy if it can possibly be avoided. Consult doctor. Risk category C (see page xxii).

Breast-feeding:
Drug passes into milk. Avoid drug or discontinue nursing until you finish medicine. Consult doctor for advice on maintaining milk supply.

Infants & children:
Don't use in infants under 2 months old.

Prolonged use:
Talk to your doctor about the need for follow-up medical examinations or laboratory studies to check complete blood counts (white blood cell count, platelet count, red blood cell count, hemoglobin, hematocrit) and urinalyses.

Skin & sunlight:
Increased sensitivity to sunlight.

Driving, piloting or hazardous work:
Avoid if you feel confused, drowsy or dizzy.

Discontinuing:
Don't discontinue for 4 to 6 weeks after you leave endemic malaria areas.

Others:
- Advise any doctor or dentist whom you consult that you take this medicine.
- May affect results in some medical tests.
- Sleep under mosquito netting while in endemic areas. Wear long-sleeved shirts and long pants.
- Report to your doctor if you develop any symptoms of illness while you take this medicine—even if the symptoms seem minor.

POSSIBLE INTERACTION WITH OTHER DRUGS

GENERIC NAME OR DRUG CLASS	COMBINED EFFECT
Anticoagulants*	Increased risk of toxicity.
Anticonvulsants*	Increased risk of toxicity.
Antidiabetics*	Increased risk of toxicity.
Bone marrow depressants*	Increased risk of bleeding or other toxic symptoms.
Clozapine	Toxic effect on the central nervous system.
Contraceptives, oral*	Reduced reliability of the pill.
Hepatotoxic medicines*	Increased risk of liver toxicity.
Methenamine	Increased risk of kidney toxicity.
Methotrexate	Increased risk of toxicity.
Zidovudine	Increased risk of liver toxicity.

POSSIBLE INTERACTION WITH OTHER SUBSTANCES

INTERACTS WITH	COMBINED EFFECT
Alcohol:	Nausea and vomiting. Avoid.
Beverages:	No special problems expected.
Cocaine:	Increased likelihood of adverse reactions or seizures. Avoid.
Foods:	No special problems expected.
Marijuana:	Increased likelihood of adverse reactions. Avoid.
Tobacco:	No special problems expected.

***See Glossary**

SULFAMETHOXAZOLE

BRAND NAMES

See complete list of brand names in the *Brand Names Directory*, page 919.

BASIC INFORMATION

Habit forming? No
Prescription needed? Yes
Available as generic? Yes
Drug class: Sulfa (sulfonamide)

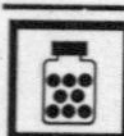

USES

Treatment for urinary tract infections responsive to this drug.

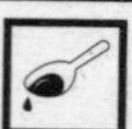

DOSAGE & USAGE INFORMATION

How to take:

- Tablet—Swallow with liquid. Instructions to take on empty stomach mean 1 hour before or 2 hours after eating.
- Liquid—Shake carefully before measuring.

When to take:
At the same times each day, evenly spaced.

If you forget a dose:
Take as soon as you remember up to 2 hours late. If more than 2 hours, wait for next scheduled dose (don't double this dose).

What drug does:
Interferes with a nutrient (folic acid) necessary for growth and reproduction of bacteria. Will not attack viruses.

Time lapse before drug works:
2 to 5 days to affect infection.

Don't take with:
Any other medicine without consulting your doctor or pharmacist.

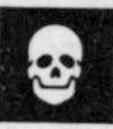

OVERDOSE

SYMPTOMS:
Less urine, bloody urine, coma.
WHAT TO DO:

- **Dial 911 (emergency) or 0 (operator) for an ambulance or medical help. Then give first aid immediately.**
- **See emergency information on inside covers.**

POSSIBLE ADVERSE REACTIONS OR SIDE EFFECTS

SYMPTOMS	WHAT TO DO
Life-threatening: In case of overdose, see previous column.	
Common:	
• Itchy skin, rash.	Discontinue. Call doctor right away.
• Headache, nausea, vomiting, diarrhea, appetite loss, skin sensitive to sun.	Continue. Call doctor when convenient.
Infrequent:	
• Red, peeling or blistering skin; sore throat; fever; swallowing difficulty; unusual bruising; aching joints or muscles; jaundice.	Discontinue. Call doctor right away.
• Dizziness, weakness, tiredness.	Continue. Call doctor when convenient.
Rare:	
Painful urination; low back pain; numbness, tingling, burning feeling in feet and hands, bloody urine, neck swelling.	Discontinue. Call doctor right away.

WARNINGS & PRECAUTIONS

Don't take if:
You are allergic to any sulfa drug.

Before you start, consult your doctor:

- If you are allergic to carbonic anhydrase inhibitors, oral antidiabetics or thiazide or loop diuretics.
- If you are allergic by nature.
- If you have liver or kidney disease.
- If you have porphyria.
- If you have developed anemia from use of any drug.

Over age 60:
Adverse reactions and side effects may be more frequent and severe than in younger persons.

Pregnancy:
Decide with your doctor if drug benefits justify risk to unborn child. Risk category C (see page xxii).

Breast-feeding:
Drug passes into milk. Avoid drug or discontinue nursing until you finish medicine. Consult doctor for advice on maintaining milk supply.

Infants & children:
Don't give to infants younger than 1 month.

Prolonged use:
- May enlarge thyroid gland.
- You may become more susceptible to infections caused by germs not responsive to this drug.
- Request frequent blood counts, liver and kidney function studies.

Skin & sunlight:
May cause rash or intensify sunburn in areas exposed to sun or sunlamp.

Driving, piloting or hazardous work:
Avoid if you feel dizzy. Otherwise, no problems expected.

Discontinuing:
Don't discontinue without doctor's advice until you complete prescribed dose, even though symptoms diminish or disappear.

Others:
- Drink 2 quarts of liquid each day to prevent adverse reactions.
- If you require surgery, tell anesthetist you take sulfa. Pentothal anesthesia should not be used.

POSSIBLE INTERACTION WITH OTHER DRUGS

GENERIC NAME OR DRUG CLASS	COMBINED EFFECT
Aminobenzoates	Possible decreased sulfa effect.
Anticoagulants*, oral	Increased anti-coagulant effect.
Anticonvulsants, hydantoin*	Toxic effect on brain.
Antidiabetics*	Toxic effect on brain.
Aspirin	Increased sulfa effect.
Calcium supplements*	Decreased sulfa effect.
Clozapine	Toxic effect on the central nervous system.
Hepatotoxic agents*	Increased liver toxicity.
Isoniazid	Possible anemia.
Mecamylamine	Decreased antibiotic effect.
Methenamine	Possible kidney blockage.
Methotrexate	Increased methotrexate effect.
Oxyphenbutazone	Increased sulfa effect.
Para-aminosalicylic acid	Decreased sulfa effect.
Penicillins*	Decreased penicillin effect.
Phenylbutazone	Increased sulfa effect.
Probenecid	Increased sulfa effect.
Sulfinpyrazone	Increased sulfa effect.
Sulfonureas*	May increase hypo-glycemic action.
Trimethoprim	Increased sulfa effect.
Zidovudine	Increased risk of toxic effects of zidovudine.

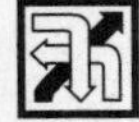

POSSIBLE INTERACTION WITH OTHER SUBSTANCES

INTERACTS WITH	COMBINED EFFECT
Alcohol:	Increased alcohol effect.
Beverages: Less than 2 quarts of fluid daily.	Kidney damage.
Cocaine:	None expected.
Foods:	None expected.
Marijuana:	None expected.
Tobacco:	None expected.

*See Glossary

SULFASALAZINE

BRAND NAMES

Azaline
Azulfidine
Azulfidine En-Tabs
PMS Sulfasalazine
PMS Sulfasalazine EC
Salazopyrin
Salazosulfapyridine
Salicylazosulfapyridine
S.A.S.-500
S.A.S. Enteric-500

BASIC INFORMATION

Habit forming? No
Prescription needed? Yes
Available as generic? Yes
Drug class: Sulfa (sulfonamide)

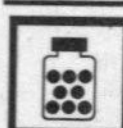

USES

Treatment for ulceration and bleeding during active phase of ulcerative colitis.

DOSAGE & USAGE INFORMATION

How to take:
- Tablet—Swallow with liquid. Instructions to take on empty stomach mean 1 hour before or 2 hours after eating.
- Liquid—Shake carefully before measuring.

When to take:
At the same times each day, evenly spaced.

If you forget a dose:
Take as soon as you remember up to 2 hours late. If more than 2 hours, wait for next scheduled dose (don't double this dose).

What drug does:
Anti-inflammatory action reduces tissue destruction in colon.

Time lapse before drug works:
2 to 5 days.

Don't take with:
Any other medicine without consulting your doctor or pharmacist.

OVERDOSE

SYMPTOMS:
Less urine, bloody urine, coma.
WHAT TO DO:
- **Dial 911 (emergency) or 0 (operator) for an ambulance or medical help. Then give first aid immediately.**
- **See emergency information on inside covers.**

POSSIBLE ADVERSE REACTIONS OR SIDE EFFECTS

SYMPTOMS	WHAT TO DO
Life-threatening: In case of overdose, see previous column.	
Common:	
• Itchy skin, rash.	Discontinue. Call doctor right away.
• Headache, nausea, vomiting, diarrhea, appetite loss, skin sensitive to sun.	Continue. Call doctor when convenient.
• Orange urine or skin.	Continue. Tell doctor at next visit.
Infrequent:	
• Red, peeling or blistering skin; sore throat; fever; swallowing difficulty; unusual bruising; aching joints or muscles; jaundice.	Discontinue. Call doctor right away.
• Dizziness, tiredness, weakness, impotence.	Continue. Call doctor when convenient.
Rare:	
Painful urination; low back pain; numbness, tingling, burning feeling in feet and hands, bloody urine, neck swelling.	Discontinue. Call doctor right away.

WARNINGS & PRECAUTIONS

Don't take if:
You are allergic to any sulfa drug*.

Before you start, consult your doctor:
- If you are allergic to carbonic anhydrase inhibitors, oral antidiabetics or thiazide or loop diuretics.
- If you are allergic by nature.
- If you have liver or kidney disease.
- If you have porphyria.
- If you have developed anemia from use of any drug.

Over age 60:
Adverse reactions and side effects may be more frequent and severe than in younger persons.

Pregnancy:
Consult doctor. Risk category B (see page xxii).

Breast-feeding:
Drug passes into milk. Avoid drug or discontinue nursing until you finish medicine. Consult doctor for advice on maintaining milk supply.

Infants & children:
Don't give to infants younger than 2 years.

Prolonged use:
- May enlarge thyroid gland.
- You may become more susceptible to infections caused by germs not responsive to this drug.
- Request frequent blood counts, liver and kidney function studies.

Skin & sunlight:
May cause rash or intensify sunburn in areas exposed to sun or sunlamp.

Driving, piloting or hazardous work:
Avoid if you feel dizzy. Otherwise, no problems expected.

Discontinuing:
Don't discontinue without doctor's advice until you complete prescribed dose, even though symptoms diminish or disappear.

Others:
- Drink 2 quarts of liquid each day to prevent adverse reactions.
- If you require surgery, tell anesthetist you take sulfa. Pentothal anesthesia should not be used.

POSSIBLE INTERACTION WITH OTHER DRUGS

GENERIC NAME OR DRUG CLASS	COMBINED EFFECT
Aminobenzoates	Possible decreased sulfa effect.
Antibiotics*	Decreased sulfa effect.
Anticoagulants*, oral	Increased anti-coagulant effect.
Anticonvulsants, hydantoin*	Toxic effect on brain.
Antidiabetics*	Toxic effect on brain.
Aspirin	Increased sulfa effect.
Calcium supplements*	Decreased sulfa effect.
Clozapine	Toxic effect on the central nervous system.
Digoxin	Decreased digoxin effect.
Hepatotoxic agents*	Increased liver toxicity.
Iron supplements*	Decreased sulfa effect.
Isoniazid	Possible anemia.
Mecamylamine	Decreased antibiotic effect.
Methenamine	Possible kidney blockage.
Methotrexate	Increased methotrexate effect.
Oxyphenbutazone	Increased sulfa effect.
Para-aminosalicylic acid	Decreased sulfa effect.
Penicillins*	Decreased penicillin effect.
Phenylbutazone	Increased sulfa effect.
Probenecid	Increased sulfa effect.
Sulfinpyrazone	Increased sulfa effect.
Sulfonureas*	May increase hypo-glycemic action.
Trimethoprim	Increased sulfa effect.
Vitamin C	Possible kidney damage. Avoid large doses of vitamin C.
Zidovudine	Increased risk of toxic effects of zidovudine.

POSSIBLE INTERACTION WITH OTHER SUBSTANCES

INTERACTS WITH	COMBINED EFFECT
Alcohol:	Increased alcohol effect.
Beverages: Less than 2 quarts of fluid daily.	Kidney damage.
Cocaine:	None expected.
Foods:	None expected.
Marijuana:	None expected.
Tobacco:	None expected.

*See Glossary

SULFINPYRAZONE

BRAND NAMES

Anturan
Anturane
Apo-Sulfinpyrazone
Novopyrazone

BASIC INFORMATION

Habit forming? No
Prescription needed? Yes
Available as generic? Yes
Drug class: Antigout

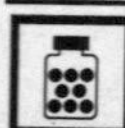

USES

- Treatment for chronic gout.
- Reduces severity of recurrent heart attack. (This use is experimental and not yet approved by the F.D.A.)

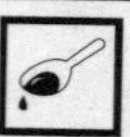

DOSAGE & USAGE INFORMATION

How to take:
Tablet or capsule—Swallow with liquid or food to lessen stomach irritation. If you can't swallow whole, crumble tablet or open capsule and take with liquid or food.

When to take:
At the same times each day.

If you forget a dose:
Take as soon as you remember up to 2 hours late. If more than 2 hours, wait for next scheduled dose (don't double this dose).

Continued next column

OVERDOSE

SYMPTOMS:
Breathing difficulty, vomiting, imbalance, seizures, convulsions, coma.
WHAT TO DO:

- **Dial 911 (emergency) or 0 (operator) for an ambulance or medical help. Then give first aid immediately.**
- **If patient is unconscious and not breathing, give mouth-to-mouth breathing. If there is no heartbeat, use cardiac massage and mouth-to-mouth breathing (CPR). Don't try to make patient vomit. If you can't get help quickly, take patient to nearest emergency facility.**
- **See emergency information on inside covers.**

What drug does:
Reduces uric acid level in blood and tissues by increasing amount of uric acid secreted in urine by kidneys.

Time lapse before drug works:
May require 6 months to prevent gout attacks.

Don't take with:
Any other medicine without consulting your doctor or pharmacist.

POSSIBLE ADVERSE REACTIONS OR SIDE EFFECTS

SYMPTOMS	WHAT TO DO
Life-threatening:	
In case of overdose, see previous column.	
Common:	
None expected.	
Infrequent:	
• Painful or difficult urination, worsening gout.	Discontinue. Call doctor right away.
• Rash, nausea, vomiting, abdominal pain, low back pain.	Continue. Call doctor when convenient.
Rare:	
• Black, bloody or tarry stools.	Discontinue. Seek emergency treatment.
• Sore throat; fever; unusual bleeding or bruising; red, painful joints; blood in urine; fatigue or weakness.	Discontinue. Call doctor right away.

WARNINGS & PRECAUTIONS

Don't take if:

- You are allergic to any uricosuric*.
- You have acute gout.
- You have active ulcers (stomach or duodenal), enteritis or ulcerative colitis.
- You have blood cell disorders.
- You are allergic to oxyphenbutazone or phenylbutazone.

Before you start, consult your doctor:
If you have kidney or blood disease.

Over age 60:
Adverse reactions and side effects may be more frequent and severe than in younger persons. You require lower dose because of decreased kidney function.

Pregnancy:
Decide with your doctor whether drug benefits justify risk to unborn child. Risk category C (see page xxii).

Breast-feeding:
Effect unknown. Consult doctor.

Infants & children:
Not recommended.

Prolonged use:
- Possible kidney damage.
- Talk to your doctor about the need for follow-up medical examinations or laboratory studies to check complete blood counts (white blood cell count, platelet count, red blood cell count, hemoglobin, hematocrit), kidney function, serum uric acid and urine uric acid.

Skin & sunlight:
No problems expected.

Driving, piloting or hazardous work:
No problems expected.

Discontinuing:
Don't discontinue without consulting doctor. Dose may require gradual reduction if you have taken drug for a long time. Doses of other drugs may also require adjustment.

Others:
- Drink 10 to 12 glasses of water each day you take this medicine.
- Periodic blood and urine laboratory tests recommended.

POSSIBLE INTERACTION WITH OTHER DRUGS

GENERIC NAME OR DRUG CLASS	COMBINED EFFECT
Allopurinol	Increased effect of each drug.
Anticoagulants*, oral	Increased anti-coagulant effect.
Antidiabetics*, oral	Increased anti-diabetic effect.
Aspirin	Bleeding tendency. Decreased sulfin-pyrazone effect.
Bismuth subsalicylate	Decreased sulfin-pyrazone effect.
Cephalosporins*	Increased risk of bleeding.
Cholestyramine	Decreased sulfin-pyrazone effect.
Contraceptives, oral*	Increased bleeding between menstrual periods.
Diuretics*	Decreased sulfin-pyrazone effect.
Nitrofurantoin	Increased risk of toxicity.
Penicillins*	Increased penicillin effect.
Salicylates*	Bleeding tendency. Decreased sulfin-pyrazone effect.
Sulfa drugs*	Increased effect of sulfa drugs.
Thioguanine	May need increased dosage of sulfinpyrazone.

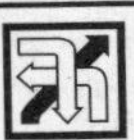

POSSIBLE INTERACTION WITH OTHER SUBSTANCES

INTERACTS WITH	COMBINED EFFECT
Alcohol:	Decreased sulfin-pyrazone effect.
Beverages: Caffeine drinks.	Decreased sulfin-pyrazone effect.
Cocaine:	None expected.
Foods:	None expected.
Marijuana:	Occasional use—None expected. Daily use—May increase blood level of uric acid.
Tobacco:	None expected.

*See Glossary

SULFISOXAZOLE

BRAND NAMES

Gantrisin
Novosoxazole
Sulfafurazole

BASIC INFORMATION

Habit forming? No
Prescription needed? Yes
Available as generic? Yes
Drug class: Sulfa (sulfonamide)

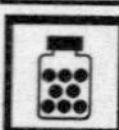

USES

Treatment for urinary tract infections responsive to this drug.

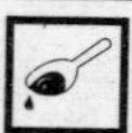

DOSAGE & USAGE INFORMATION

How to take:

- Tablet—Swallow with liquid. Instructions to take on empty stomach mean 1 hour before or 2 hours after eating.
- Liquid—Shake carefully before measuring.

When to take:
At the same times each day, evenly spaced.

If you forget a dose:
Take as soon as you remember up to 2 hours late. If more than 2 hours, wait for next scheduled dose (don't double this dose).

What drug does:
Interferes with a nutrient (folic acid) necessary for growth and reproduction of bacteria. Will not attack viruses.

Time lapse before drug works:
2 to 5 days to affect infection.

Don't take with:
Any other medicine without consulting your doctor or pharmacist.

OVERDOSE

SYMPTOMS:
Less urine, bloody urine, coma.
WHAT TO DO:

- **Dial 911 (emergency) or 0 (operator) for an ambulance or medical help. Then give first aid immediately.**
- **See emergency information on inside covers.**

POSSIBLE ADVERSE REACTIONS OR SIDE EFFECTS

SYMPTOMS	WHAT TO DO
Life-threatening: In case of overdose, see previous column.	
Common:	
• Itchy skin, rash.	Discontinue. Call doctor right away.
• Headache, nausea, vomiting, diarrhea, appetite loss, skin sensitive to sun.	Continue. Call doctor when convenient.
Infrequent:	
• Red, peeling or blistering skin; sore throat; fever; swallowing difficulty; unusual bruising; aching joints or muscles; jaundice.	Discontinue. Call doctor right away.
• Dizziness, tiredness, weakness.	Continue. Call doctor when convenient.
Rare:	
Painful urination; low back pain; numbness, tingling, burning feeling in feet and hands, bloody urine, neck swelling.	Discontinue. Call doctor right away.

WARNINGS & PRECAUTIONS

Don't take if:
You are allergic to any sulfa drug*.

Before you start, consult your doctor:

- If you are allergic to carbonic anhydrase inhibitors, oral antidiabetics or thiazide or loop diuretics.
- If you are allergic by nature.
- If you have liver or kidney disease.
- If you have porphyria.
- If you have developed anemia from use of any drug.

Over age 60:
Adverse reactions and side effects may be more frequent and severe than in younger persons.

SULFISOXAZOLE

Pregnancy:
Decide with your doctor whether drug benefits justify risk to unborn child. Risk category C (see page xxii).

Breast-feeding:
Drug passes into milk. Avoid drug or discontinue nursing until you finish medicine. Consult doctor for advice on maintaining milk supply.

Infants & children:
Don't give to infants younger than 1 month.

Prolonged use:
- May enlarge thyroid gland.
- You may become more susceptible to infections caused by germs not responsive to this drug.
- Request frequent blood counts, liver and kidney function studies.

Skin & sunlight:
May cause rash or intensify sunburn in areas exposed to sun or sunlamp.

Driving, piloting or hazardous work:
Avoid if you feel dizzy. Otherwise, no problems expected.

Discontinuing:
Don't discontinue without doctor's advice until you complete prescribed dose, even though symptoms diminish or disappear.

Others:
- Drink 2 quarts of liquid each day to prevent adverse reactions.
- If you require surgery, tell anesthetist you take sulfa.

POSSIBLE INTERACTION WITH OTHER DRUGS

GENERIC NAME OR DRUG CLASS	COMBINED EFFECT
Aminobenzoates	Possible decreased sulfisoxazole effect.
Anticoagulants*, oral	Increased anti-coagulant effect.
Anticonvulsants, hydantoin*	Toxic effect on brain.
Antidiabetics*	Toxic effect on brain.
Aspirin	Increased sulfa effect.
Calcium supplements*	Decreased sulfa effect.
Clozapine	Toxic effect on the central nervous system.
Flecainide	Possible decreased blood cell production in bone marrow.
Hepatotoxic agents*	Increased liver toxicity.
Isoniazid	Possible anemia.
Mecamylamine	Decreased antibiotic effect.
Methenamine	Possible kidney blockage.
Methotrexate	Increased possibility of toxic side effects from methotrexate.
Oxyphenbutazone	Increased sulfa effect.
Para-aminosalicylic acid	Decreased sulfa effect.
Penicillins*	Decreased penicillin effect.
Phenylbutazone	Increased sulfa effect.
Probenecid	Increased sulfa effect.
Sulfinpyrazone	Increased sulfa effect.
Sulfonureas*	May increase hypo-glycemic action.
Tocainide	Possible decreased blood cell production in bone marrow.
Trimethoprim	Increased sulfa effect.
Zidovudine	Increased risk of toxic effect of zidovudine.

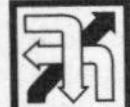

POSSIBLE INTERACTION WITH OTHER SUBSTANCES

INTERACTS WITH	COMBINED EFFECT
Alcohol:	Increased alcohol effect.
Beverages: Less than 2 quarts of fluid daily.	Kidney damage.
Cocaine:	None expected.
Foods:	None expected.
Marijuana:	None expected.
Tobacco:	None expected.

*See Glossary

SULFONAMIDES & PHENAZOPYRIDINE

BRAND AND GENERIC NAMES

Azo Gantanol
Azo Gantrisin
Azo-Sulfamethoxazole
Azo-Sulfisoxazole
Azo-Truxazole
Sul-Azo
Sulfafurazole & Phenazopyridine
SULFAMETHOXAZOLE & PHENAZOPYRIDINE
SULFISOXAZOLE & PHENAZOPYRIDINE

BASIC INFORMATION

Habit forming? No
Prescription needed? Yes
Available as generic? Yes
Drug class: Analgesic (urinary), sulfonamide

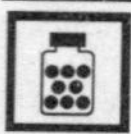

USES

- Treats infections responsive to this drug.
- Relieves pain of lower urinary tract irritation, as in cystitis, urethritis or prostatitis.

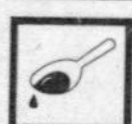

DOSAGE & USAGE INFORMATION

How to take:
Tablet—Swallow with liquid. Instructions to take on empty stomach mean 1 hour before or 2 hours after eating.

When to take:
At the same times each day, after meals.

If you forget a dose:
Take as soon as you remember up to 2 hours late. If more than 2 hours, wait for next scheduled dose (don't double this dose).

What drug does:
- Interferes with a nutrient (folic acid) necessary for growth and reproduction of bacteria. Will not attack viruses.
- Anesthetizes lower urinary tract. Relieves pain, burning, pressure and urgency to urinate.

Continued next column

OVERDOSE

SYMPTOMS:
Less urine, bloody urine, shortness of breath, weakness, coma.
WHAT TO DO:
- **Dial 911 (emergency) or 0 (operator) for an ambulance or medical help. Then give first aid immediately.**
- **See emergency information on inside covers.**

Time lapse before drug works:
2 to 5 days to affect infection.

Don't take with:
Any other medicine without consulting your doctor or pharmacist.

POSSIBLE ADVERSE REACTIONS OR SIDE EFFECTS

SYMPTOMS	WHAT TO DO
Life-threatening: In case of overdose, see previous column.	
Common:	
• Rash, itchy skin.	Discontinue. Call doctor right away.
• Dizziness, diarrhea, headache, appetite loss, nausea, vomiting, skin sensitive to sun.	Continue. Call doctor when convenient.
Infrequent:	
• Joint pain; swallowing difficulty; pale skin; blistering; peeling of skin; sore throat, fever, mouth sores; unexplained bleeding or bruising; jaundice.	Discontinue. Call doctor right away.
• Abdominal pain, indigestion, weakness, tiredness.	Continue. Call doctor when convenient.
Rare:	
Back pain; neck swelling; numbness, tingling, burning feeling in feet and hands; bloody urine; painful urination.	Discontinue. Call doctor right away.

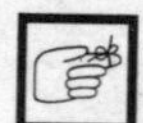

WARNINGS & PRECAUTIONS

Don't take if:
- You are allergic to any sulfa drug or urinary analgesic.
- You have hepatitis.

Before you start, consult your doctor:
- If you are allergic to carbonic anhydrase inhibitors, oral antidiabetics or thiazide or loop diuretics.
- If you are allergic by nature.
- If you have liver or kidney disease, porphyria.
- If you have developed anemia from use of any drug.
- If you have G6PD* deficiency.

SULFONAMIDES & PHENAZOPYRIDINE

Over age 60:
Adverse reactions and side effects may be more frequent and severe than in younger persons.

Pregnancy:
Risk factors vary for drugs in this group. See category list on page xxii and consult doctor.

Breast-feeding:
Drug passes into milk. Avoid drug or discontinue nursing until you finish medicine. Consult doctor for advice on maintaining milk supply.

Infants & children:
Don't give to infants younger than 1 month.

Prolonged use:
- May enlarge thyroid gland.
- You may become more susceptible to infections caused by germs not responsive to this drug.
- Request frequent blood counts, liver and kidney function studies.
- Orange or yellow skin.
- Anemia. Occasional blood studies recommended.

Skin & sunlight:
May cause rash or intensify sunburn in areas exposed to sun or sunlamp.

Driving, piloting or hazardous work:
Avoid if you feel dizzy. Otherwise, no problems expected.

Discontinuing:
Don't discontinue without doctor's advice until you complete prescribed dose, even though symptoms diminish or disappear.

Others:
- Drink 2 quarts of liquid each day to prevent adverse reactions.
- If you require surgery, tell anesthetist you take sulfa.
- Will probably cause urine to be reddish orange. Requires no action.
- May stain fabrics.

POSSIBLE INTERACTION WITH OTHER DRUGS

GENERIC NAME OR DRUG CLASS	COMBINED EFFECT
Aminobenzoates	Possible decreased sulfa effect.
Anticoagulants*, oral	Increased anti-coagulant effect.
Anticonvulsants, hydantoin*	Toxic effect on brain.
Antidiabetics*	Toxic effect on brain.
Aspirin	Increased sulfa effect.
Clozapine	Toxic effect on the central nervous system.
Didanosine	Increased risk of pancreatitis.
Hepatotoxic agents*	Increased liver toxicity.
Isoniazid	Possible anemia.
Mecamylamine	Decreased antibiotic effect.
Methenamine	Possible kidney blockage.
Methotrexate	Increased methotrexate effect.
Oxyphenbutazone	Increased sulfa effect.
Para-aminosalicylic acid	Decreased sulfa effect.
Penicillins*	Decreased penicillin effect.
Phenylbutazone	Increased sulfa effect.
Probenecid	Increased sulfa effect.
Sulfinpyrazone	Increased sulfa effect.
Sulfonureas*	May increase hypo-glycemic action.
Trimethoprim	Increased sulfa effect.
Zidovudine	Increased risk of toxic effects of zidovudine.

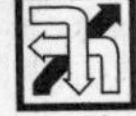

POSSIBLE INTERACTION WITH OTHER SUBSTANCES

INTERACTS WITH	COMBINED EFFECT
Alcohol:	Increased alcohol effect.
Beverages: Less than 2 quarts of fluid daily.	Kidney damage.
Cocaine:	None expected.
Foods:	None expected.
Marijuana:	None expected.
Tobacco:	None expected.

*See Glossary

SUMATRIPTAN

BRAND NAMES

Imitrex

BASIC INFORMATION

Habit forming? No
Prescription needed? Yes
Available as generic? No
Drug class: Antimigraine

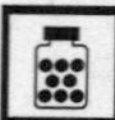

USES

- Treatment for acute migraine headaches not relieved by other medications (aspirin, acetaminophen and other nonsteroidal anti-inflammatory drugs). Does not prevent migraines.
- Treatment for cluster headaches.

DOSAGE & USAGE INFORMATION

How to take:

- Injection (self-administered)—Inject under the skin (subcutaneous) of the outer thigh or outer upper arm. Follow your doctor's instructions and written package instructions for proper injection technique and method for disposal of the cartridges.
- Tablets—Swallow whole with liquid. Do not crush, break or chew tablet.

When to take:

- At the first sign of a migraine (aura or pain). After you administer, lie down in a quiet, dark room to increase effectiveness of drug.
- An additional dose may be helpful if the migraine returns. Do not exceed the prescribed quantity or frequency. Do not use additional dose if first dose does not bring substantial relief.
- For cluster headache, follow doctor's directions.

Continued next column

OVERDOSE

SYMPTOMS:
Convulsions, tremor, swelling of arms and legs, breathing difficulty, chest pain, paralysis; skin and hair loss, scab formation at injection site .
WHAT TO DO:

- **Dial 911 (emergency) or 0 (operator) for an ambulance or medical help. Then give first aid immediately.**
- **See emergency information on inside covers.**

If you forget a dose:
Sumatriptan is not taken on a routine schedule. It can be taken any time during the course of a migraine.

What drug does:
Helps relieve headache pain and associated symptoms of migraine (nausea, vomiting, sensitivity to light and sound). It helps constrict dilated blood vessels that may contribute to development of migraines.

Time lapse before drug works:

- Oral dosage (tablet)—within 30 minutes.
- Injection—usually within 10 minutes for headache pain and within 20 minutes for associated nausea, vomiting, and sensitivity to light and sound.

Don't take with:

- Ergotamine-containing medicines. Delay 24 hours.
- Any other medication without consulting your doctor or pharmacist.

POSSIBLE ADVERSE REACTIONS OR SIDE EFFECTS

SYMPTOMS	WHAT TO DO
Life-threatening:	
In case of overdose, see previous column.	
Common:	
Burning, pain, or redness at injection site; nausea or vomiting (may be from migraine or from drug).	May readminister. Call doctor when convenient.
Infrequent:	
Sensation of burning, warmth, numbness, cold or tingling; discomfort of jaw, mouth, throat, nose or sinuses; dizziness; drowsiness; flushing; lightheadedness; muscle aches, cramps, stiffness or weakness; anxiety; tiredness; vision changes, general feeling of illness.	May readminister. Call doctor when convenient.
Rare:	
Pain, pressure or tightness in the chest; difficulty swallowing.	Discontinue. Seek emergency help.

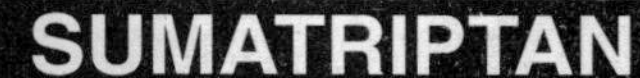

WARNINGS & PRECAUTIONS

Don't take if:
- You are allergic to sumatriptan.
- You have angina pectoris, a history of myocardial infarction or myocardial ischemia, Prinzmetal's angina, uncontrolled hypertension (high blood pressure).

Before you start, consult your doctor:
- If you have heart rhythm problems or coronary artery disease.
- If you have had a cerebrovascular accident (stroke).
- If you have liver or kidney disease.
- If you have controlled hypertension (high blood pressure).

Over age 60:
No problems expected.

Pregnancy:
Decide with your doctor whether drug benefits justify risk to unborn child. Risk category C (see page xxii).

Breast-feeding:
Unknown effects. Decide with your doctor whether drug benefits justify possible risk.

Infants & children:
Not recommended for patients under age 18.

Prolonged use:
Long-term effects unknown. As a precaution, do not use sumatriptan more often than every 5-7 days or as directed by your doctor.

Skin & sunlight:
No problems expected. Sensitivity to light is a symptom of migraine and is not drug-related.

Driving, piloting or hazardous work:
Avoid if you feel drowsy or dizzy. Otherwise no problems expected.

Discontinuing:
No problems expected. Talk to your doctor if you have plans to discontinue use of drug.

Others:
- Advise any doctor or dentist whom you consult that you take this medicine.
- May affect results in some medical tests (rare).
- Follow your doctor's recommendation of any additional treatment for prevention of migraines.

POSSIBLE INTERACTION WITH OTHER DRUGS

GENERIC NAME OR DRUG CLASS	COMBINED EFFECT
Antidepressants*	Adverse effects unknown. Avoid.
Ergotamine	Increased vasoconstriction. Delay 24 hours between drugs.
Furazolidone	Adverse effects unknown. Avoid.
Lithium	Adverse effects unknown. Avoid.
Monoamine oxidase (MAO) inhibitors*	Adverse effects unknown. Avoid.
Procarbazine	Adverse effects unknown. Avoid.
Selegiline	Adverse effects unknown. Avoid.

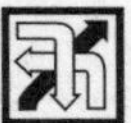

POSSIBLE INTERACTION WITH OTHER SUBSTANCES

INTERACTS WITH	COMBINED EFFECT
Alcohol:	No interaction known, but alcohol aggravates migraines. Avoid.
Beverages:	None expected.
Cocaine:	None expected.
Foods:	None expected.
Marijuana:	None expected.
Tobacco:	None expected.

***See Glossary**

TACRINE

BRAND NAMES

Cognex

BASIC INFORMATION

Habit forming? No
Prescription needed? Yes
Available as generic? No
Drug class: Cholinesterase inhibitor

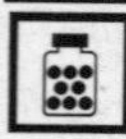

USES

Treatment for symptoms of mild to moderate Alzheimer's disease. May improve memory, reasoning and other cognitive functions slightly in some people.

DOSAGE & USAGE INFORMATION

How to take:
Capsule–Swallow with liquid.

When to take:
At the same times each day. Take 1 hour before or 2 hours after eating. Follow doctor's instructions.

If you forget a dose:
Take as soon as you remember up to 2 hours late. If more than 2 hours, wait for next scheduled dose (don't double this dose).

What drug does:
Slows breakdown of a brain chemical (acetycholine) that gradually disappears from the brains of people with Alzheimer's.

Continued next column

OVERDOSE

SYMPTOMS:
Severe nausea and vomiting, excessive saliva, sweating, blood pressure decrease, slow heartbeat, collapse, convulsions, muscle weakness (including respiratory muscles, which could lead to death).
WHAT TO DO:

- **Dial 911 (emergency) or 0 (operator) for an ambulance or medical help. Then give first aid immediately.**
- **If patient is unconscious and not breathing, use cardiac massage and mouth-to-mouth breathing (CPR). Don't try to make patient vomit. If you can't get help quickly, take patient to nearest emergency facility.**
- **See emergency information on inside covers.**

Time lapse before drug works:
May take several months before beneficial results are observed. Dosage is normally increased over a period of time to help prevent adverse reactions.

Don't take with:

- Any other prescription or nonprescription drug without consulting your doctor.
- See Interaction column and consult doctor.

POSSIBLE ADVERSE REACTIONS OR SIDE EFFECTS

SYMPTOMS	WHAT TO DO
Life-threatening: In case of overdose, see previous column.	
Common: Nausea, vomiting, diarrhea, lack of coordination.	Continue. Call doctor when convenient.
Infrequent: Rash, indigestion, headache, muscle aches, loss of appetite, stomach pain, nervousness, chills, dizziness, drowsiness, dry or itching eyes, increased sweating, joint pain, runny nose, sore throat, swelling of feet or legs, insomnia, weight loss, unusual tiredness or weakness, flushing of face.	Continue. Call doctor when convenient.
Rare: Changes in liver function (yellow skin or eyes; black, very dark or light stool color); lack of coordination, convulsions.	Continue. Call doctor right away.

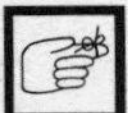

WARNINGS & PRECAUTIONS

Don't take if:
You are allergic to tacrine or acridine derivatives*.

Before you start, consult your doctor:
- If you have heart rhythm problems.
- If you have a history of ulcer disease or are at risk of developing ulcers.
- If you have a history of liver disease.
- If you have a history of asthma.
- If you have had previous treatment with tacrine that caused jaundice (yellow skin and eyes) or elevated bilirubin.

Over age 60:
No problems expected.

Pregnancy:
Unknown effect. Drug is usually not prescribed for women of childbearing age. Risk category C (see page xxii).

Breast-feeding:
Unknown effect. Not recommended for women of childbearing age.

Infants & children:
Not used in this age group.

Prolonged use:
- Drug may lose its effectiveness.
- Talk to your doctor about the need for follow-up medical examinations or laboratory studies to check blood chemistries and liver function.

Skin & sunlight:
No problems expected.

Driving, piloting or hazardous work:
Don't drive or pilot aircraft until you learn how medicine affects you. Don't work around dangerous machinery. Don't climb ladders or work in high places. Danger increases if you drink alcohol or take other medicines affecting alertness and reflexes such as antihistamines, tranquilizers, sedatives, pain medicine, narcotics and mind-altering drugs.

Discontinuing:
Do not discontinue drug unless advised by doctor. Abrupt decreases in dosage may cause a cognitive decline.

Others:
- Advise any doctor or dentist whom you consult that you take this medicine.
- May affect the results in some medical tests.
- Do not increase dosage without doctor's approval.
- Treatment with tacrine may need to be discontinued or the dosage lowered if weekly blood tests indicate a sensitivity to the drug or liver toxicity develops.

POSSIBLE INTERACTION WITH OTHER DRUGS

GENERIC NAME OR DRUG CLASS	COMBINED EFFECT
Anticholinergics*	Decreased anticholinergic effect.
Cimetidine	Increased tacrine effect.
Theophylline	Increased theophylline effect.

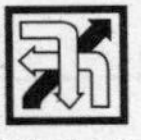

POSSIBLE INTERACTION WITH OTHER SUBSTANCES

INTERACTS WITH	COMBINED EFFECT
Alcohol:	None expected.
Beverages:	None expected.
Cocaine:	None expected.
Foods:	None expected.
Marijuana:	None expected.
Tobacco:	May decrease tacrine effect.

*See Glossary

TAMOXIFEN

BRAND NAMES

Alpha-Tamoxifen
Med Tamoxifen
Nolvadex
Nolvadex-D
Novo-Tamoxifen
Tamofen
Tamone
Tamoplex

BASIC INFORMATION

Habit forming? No
Prescription needed? Yes
Available as generic? No
Drug class: Antineoplastic

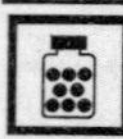

USES

Treats advanced breast cancer.

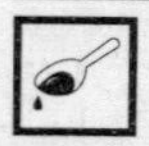

DOSAGE & USAGE INFORMATION

How to take:

- Tablets—Swallow with liquid. If you can't swallow whole, crumble tablet and take with liquid or food. Instructions to take on empty stomach mean 1 hour before or 2 hours after eating.
- Enteric-coated tablets—Swallow whole.

When to take:
Follow doctor's instructions.

If you forget a dose:
Skip the missed dose and return to regular schedule. Don't double dose.

What drug does:
Blocks uptake of estradiol and inhibits growth of cancer cells.

Time lapse before drug works:

- 4 to 10 weeks.
- With bone metastases—several months.

Don't take with:
Any other medicines (including over-the-counter drugs such as cough and cold medicines, laxatives, antacids, diet pills, caffeine, nose drops or vitamins) without consulting your doctor.

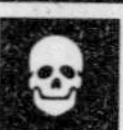

OVERDOSE

SYMPTOMS:
None expected.
WHAT TO DO:
Overdose unlikely to threaten life. If person takes much larger amount than prescribed, call doctor, poison control center or hospital emergency room for instructions.

POSSIBLE ADVERSE REACTIONS OR SIDE EFFECTS

SYMPTOMS	WHAT TO DO
Life-threatening:	
Leg pain, shortness of breath.	Seek emergency treatment immediately.
Common:	
Hot flashes, nausea and vomiting, weight gain.	Continue. Call doctor when convenient.
Infrequent:	
Headache, dry skin, menstrual irregularities, vaginal itching.	Continue. Call doctor when convenient.
Rare:	
Blurred vision, confusion, sleepiness.	Discontinue. Call doctor right away.

WARNINGS & PRECAUTIONS

Don't take if:
You are allergic to tamoxifen.

Before you start, consult your doctor:
- If you have cataracts.
- If you have blood disorders.

Over age 60:
Adverse reactions and side effects may be more frequent and severe than in younger persons. You may need smaller doses for shorter periods of time.

Pregnancy:
Consult doctor. Risk category D (see page xxii).

Breast-feeding:
Effect not documented. Consult your doctor.

Infants & children:
Not intended for use in children.

Prolonged use:
Talk to your doctor about the need for follow-up medical examinations (especially pelvic exams) or laboratory studies to check complete blood counts (white blood cell count, platelet count, red blood cell count, hemoglobin, hematocrit) and serum calcium.

Skin & sunlight:
No problems expected.

Driving, piloting or hazardous work:
Avoid if you feel confused, drowsy or dizzy.

Discontinuing:
No special problems expected.

Others:
- Advise any doctor or dentist whom you consult that you take this medicine.
- May affect results in some medical tests.
- Be sure you and your doctor discuss all aspects of using this drug, and read all instructional materials.

POSSIBLE INTERACTION WITH OTHER DRUGS

GENERIC NAME OR DRUG CLASS	COMBINED EFFECT
Antacids*	Decreased tamoxifen effect.
Cimetidine	Decreased tamoxifen effect.
Estrogens*	Decreased tamoxifen effect.
Famotidine	Decreased tamoxifen effect.
H_2 antagonist antihistamines*	Decreased tamoxifen effect.
Ranitidine	Decreased tamoxifen effect.

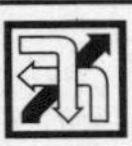

POSSIBLE INTERACTION WITH OTHER SUBSTANCES

INTERACTS WITH	COMBINED EFFECT
Alcohol:	No special problems expected.
Beverages:	No special problems expected.
Cocaine:	No special problems expected.
Foods:	No special problems expected.
Marijuana:	No special problems expected.
Tobacco:	No special problems expected.

***See Glossary**

TERAZOSIN

BRAND NAMES

Hytrin

BASIC INFORMATION

Habit forming? No
Prescription needed? Yes
Available as generic? No
Drug class: Antihypertensive

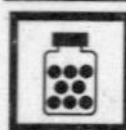

USES

- Treats high blood pressure.
- Treats symptoms of benign prostatic hyperplasia (BPH).

DOSAGE & USAGE INFORMATION

How to take:
Tablet—Swallow with liquid or food to lessen stomach irritation. If you can't swallow whole, crumble tablet and take with liquid or food.

When to take:
Once a day (usually) at bedtime.

If you forget a dose:
Take as soon as you remember. Don't ever double the dose.

What drug does:
Relaxes smooth muscle in arteries, reducing blood pressure. Terazosin doesn't cure hypertension, but controls it. Persons with hypertension may need lifelong treatment.

Continued next column

OVERDOSE

SYMPTOMS:
Difficult breathing, vomiting, fainting, slow heartbeat, coma, diminished reflexes.
WHAT TO DO:

- **Dial 911 (emergency) or 0 (operator) for an ambulance or medical help. Then give first aid immediately.**
- **If patient is unconscious and not breathing, give mouth-to-mouth breathing. If there is no heartbeat, use cardiac massage and mouth-to-mouth breathing (CPR). Don't try to make patient vomit. If you can't get help quickly, take patient to nearest emergency facility.**
- **See emergency information on inside covers.**

Time lapse before drug works:

- 15 minutes as an antihypertensive.
- For BPH may take 2 to 6 weeks for symptoms to improve.

Don't take with:
Any other drug (especially over-the-counter medicines containing alcohol) without consulting your doctor.

POSSIBLE ADVERSE REACTIONS OR SIDE EFFECTS

SYMPTOMS	WHAT TO DO
Life-threatening: In case of overdose, see previous column.	
Common: Headache, dizziness, tiredness or weakness.	Continue. Call doctor right away.
Infrequent: • Chest pain; lightheadedness on arising from bed or chair (more likely to occur with first dose); increased or rapid heartbeat, fainting, nausea and vomiting.	Discontinue. Call doctor right away.
• Fluid retention and weight gain.	Continue. Call doctor when convenient.
Rare: Back pain, joint pain, blurred vision, stuffy nose, drowsiness.	Continue. Call doctor when convenient.

WARNINGS & PRECAUTIONS

Don't take if:

- You are allergic to any alpha-adrenergic blocker*.
- You are under age 12.

Before you start, consult your doctor:

- If you will have surgery within 2 months, including dental surgery, requiring general or spinal anesthesia.
- If you have heart disease or chronic kidney disease.
- If you have a peripheral circulation disorder (intermittent claudication, Buerger's disease).
- If you have history of depression.
- If cancer of the prostate has not been ruled out.

Over age 60:
More sensitivity to drug, causing weakness, fainting episodes, low temperature.

Pregnancy:
Decide with your doctor whether drug benefits justify risk to unborn child. Risk category C (see page xxii).

Breast-feeding:
Effect unknown. Consult doctor.

Infants & children:
Not recommended for children. Adequate studies not complete.

Prolonged use:
Talk to your doctor about the need for follow-up medical examinations or laboratory studies.

Skin & sunlight:
No problems expected.

Driving, piloting or hazardous work:
Don't drive or pilot aircraft until you learn how medicine affects you. Don't work around dangerous machinery. Don't climb ladders or work in high places. Danger increases if you drink alcohol or take medicine affecting alertness and reflexes, such as antihistamines, tranquilizers, sedatives, pain medicine, narcotics and mind-altering drugs.

Discontinuing:
- Don't discontinue without consulting doctor. Dose may require gradual reduction if you have taken drug for a long time. Doses of other drugs may also require adjustment.
- Stopping abruptly may cause rebound high blood pressure, anxiety, chest pain, insomnia, headache, nausea, irregular heartbeat, flushed face, sweating.

Others:
- Avoid becoming overheated.
- Check blood pressure frequently.
- May affect results in some medical tests.

POSSIBLE INTERACTION WITH OTHER DRUGS

GENERIC NAME OR DRUG CLASS	COMBINED EFFECT
Anti-inflammatory drugs, nonsteroidal (NSAIDs)*	Decreases effectiveness of terazosin. Causes sodium and fluid retention.
Diclofenac	Decreases effectiveness of terazosin. Causes sodium and fluid retention.
Diuretics, loop*	Decreased effectiveness of terazosin.
Estrogens*	Decreases effectiveness of terazosin.
Lisinopril	Increases antihypertensive effect. Dosage of each may require adjustment.
Nicardipine	Blood pressure drop. Dosages may require adjustment.
Nimodipine	Dangerous blood pressure drop.
Other medicines to treat high blood pressure (antihypertensives*)	Decreases effectiveness of terazosin.
Sympathomimetics*	Decreases effectiveness of terazosin.

POSSIBLE INTERACTION WITH OTHER SUBSTANCES

INTERACTS WITH	COMBINED EFFECT
Alcohol:	Increased sensitivity to sedative effect of alcohol and very low blood pressure. Avoid.
Beverages: Caffeine drinks.	Decreased terazosin effect.
Cocaine:	Blood pressure rise. Avoid.
Foods:	No problems expected.
Marijuana:	Weakness on standing.
Tobacco:	No problems expected.

*See Glossary

TERFENADINE

BRAND NAMES

Seldane
Seldane D

BASIC INFORMATION

Habit forming? No
Prescription needed? Yes
U.S.: Yes
Canada: No
Available as generic? No
Drug class: Antihistamine, H_1 receptor antagonist

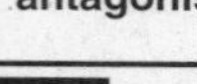

USES

Reduces allergic symptoms such as hay fever, hives, rash or itching. Less likely to cause drowsiness than most other antihistamines.

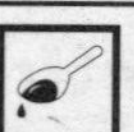

DOSAGE & USAGE INFORMATION

How to take:
- Tablet—Swallow with water or food to lessen stomach irritation.
- Oral suspension—Take as directed on package.

When to take:
Follow prescription instructions.

If you forget a dose:
Take as soon as you remember up to 2 hours late. If more than 2 hours, wait for next scheduled dose (don't double this dose).

What drug does:
Blocks effects of histamine, a chemical produced by the body as a result of contact with an allergen.

Time lapse before drug works:
1 to 2 hours; maximum effect at 3 to 4 hours.

Don't take with:
Any other medicine without consulting your doctor or pharmacist.

OVERDOSE

SYMPTOMS:
Headache, nausea, confusion, heart rhythm disturbance.
WHAT TO DO:
- **Dial 911 (emergency) or 0 (operator) for an ambulance or medical help. Then give first aid immediately.**
- **See emergency information on inside covers.**

POSSIBLE ADVERSE REACTIONS OR SIDE EFFECTS

SYMPTOMS	WHAT TO DO
Life-threatening: In case of overdose, see previous column.	
Common: None expected.	
Infrequent:	
• Nausea, vomiting sore throat, itching.	Discontinue. Call doctor right away.
• Fatigue, headache, dizziness, weakness.	Continue. Call doctor when convenient.
Rare:	
• Swollen lips, difficult breathing.	Discontinue. Seek emergency treatment.
• Irregular heartbeat, nightmares, frequent urination, wheezing.	Discontinue. Call doctor right away.
• Thinning hair.	Continue. Call doctor when convenient.

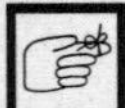

WARNINGS & PRECAUTIONS

Don't take if:
You are allergic to terfenadine.

Before you start, consult your doctor:
- If you have liver disease.
- If you are allergic to other antihistamines.
- If you have an enlarged prostrate or glaucoma.
- If you are under age 12.
- If you are allergic to any substance or any medicine.
- If you are pregnant or expect to become pregnant.
- If you have asthma.
- If you will have surgery within 2 months, including dental surgery, requiring general or spinal anesthesia.
- If you plan to have skin tests for allergies.

Over age 60:
Don't exceed recommended dose. Take only on advise of your doctor.

Pregnancy:
Decide with your doctor if drug benefits justify risk to unborn child. Risk category C (see page xxii).

Breast-feeding:
Drug may pass into milk although this has not been proven. Consult doctor for advice on using while breast feeding.

Infants & children:
Safety and effectiveness in children under age 12 have not been established.

Prolonged use:
Take only on advice of your doctor.

Skin & sunlight:
No problems expected.

Driving, piloting or hazardous work:
Don't drive or pilot aircraft until you learn how medicine affects you. Sedation and dizziness are less likely to occur with terfenadine than with other antihistamines.

Discontinuing:
No problems expected.

Others:
No problems expected.

POSSIBLE INTERACTION WITH OTHER DRUGS

GENERIC NAME OR DRUG CLASS	COMBINED EFFECT
Carteolol	Decreased antihistamine effect.
Erythromycins*	Life-threatening heartbeat irregularity. Avoid.
Itraconazole	Life-threatening heartbeat irregularity. Avoid.
Ketoconazole	Life-threatening heartbeat irregularity. Avoid.
Nabilone	Greater depression of central nervous system.

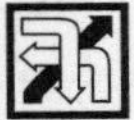

POSSIBLE INTERACTION WITH OTHER SUBSTANCES

INTERACTS WITH	COMBINED EFFECT
Alcohol:	Possible oversedation.
Beverages:	None expected.
Cocaine:	Decreased terfenadine effect.
Foods:	None expected.
Marijuana:	None expected.
Tobacco:	None expected.

***See Glossary**

TERPIN HYDRATE

BRAND AND GENERIC NAMES

Chexit
CODEINE AND TERPIN HYDRATE
DEXTROMETHORPHAN HYDROBROMIDE AND TERPIN HYDRATE
Prunicodeine
Terphan
Terpin-Dex
Terpin Hydrate and Codeine Syrup
Terpin Hydrate Elixir
Tricodene #1
Tricodene NN Cough and Cold Medication
Tussagesic

BASIC INFORMATION

Habit forming? Yes
Prescription needed? Yes
Available as generic? Yes
Drug class: Expectorant

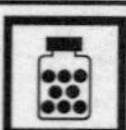

USES

Decreases cough due to simple bronchial irritation.

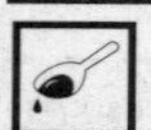

DOSAGE & USAGE INFORMATION

How to take:
Follow each dose with 8 oz. water or food to decrease gastric distress. Works better in combination with a cool-air vaporizer.

When to take:
3 to 4 times each day, spaced at least 4 hours apart.

If you forget a dose:
Take as soon as you remember. Wait 4 hours for next dose.

What drug does:
Loosens mucus in bronchial tubes to make mucus easier to cough up.

Time lapse before drug works:
10 to 15 minutes.

Don't take with:
Any other medicine without consulting your doctor or pharmacist.

OVERDOSE

SYMPTOMS:
Nausea, drowsiness.
WHAT TO DO:
Overdose unlikely to threaten life. If person takes much larger amount than prescribed, call doctor, poison control center or hospital emergency room for instructions.

POSSIBLE ADVERSE REACTIONS OR SIDE EFFECTS

SYMPTOMS	WHAT TO DO
Life-threatening:	
None expected.	
Common:	
None expected.	
Infrequent:	
Nausea, vomiting, abdominal pain.	Continue. Call doctor when convenient.
Rare:	
Symptoms of alcohol intoxication, especially in children.	Discontinue. Call doctor right away.

WARNINGS & PRECAUTIONS

Don't take if:
- You are allergic to terpin hydrate.
- You are a recovering or active alcoholic.

Before you start, consult your doctor:
If you plan to become pregnant within medication period.

Over age 60:
No problems expected.

Pregnancy:
Decide with your doctor if drug benefits justify risk to unborn child. Risk category C (see page xxii).

Breast-feeding:
Drug filters into milk. May harm child. Avoid.

Infants & children:
Use only under medical supervision.

Prolonged use:
Habit forming.

Skin & sunlight:
No problems expected.

Driving, piloting or hazardous work:
Don't drive or pilot aircraft until you learn how medicine affects you. Don't work around dangerous machinery. Don't climb ladders or work in high places. Danger increases if you drink alcohol or take medicine affecting alertness and reflexes, such as antihistamines, tranquilizers, sedatives, pain medicine, narcotics and mind-altering drugs.

Discontinuing:
May be unnecessary to finish medicine. Follow doctor's instructions.

Others:
- Exceeding recommended doses may cause intoxication; drug is 42.5% alcohol.
- Frequently combined with codeine, which increases hazards.

POSSIBLE INTERACTION WITH OTHER DRUGS

GENERIC NAME OR DRUG CLASS	COMBINED EFFECT
Antidepressants*	Increased sedation.
Antihistamines*	Increased sedation
Central nervous system (CNS) depressants*	Increased sedative effect of both.
Disulfiram	Possible disulfiram reaction*.
Muscle relaxants*	Increased sedation.
Narcotics*	Increased sedation.
Sedatives*	Increased sedation.
Sleep inducers*	Increased sedation.
Tranquilizers*	Increased sedation.

POSSIBLE INTERACTION WITH OTHER SUBSTANCES

INTERACTS WITH	COMBINED EFFECT
Alcohol:	Contains alcohol. Increased sedative effect of both drugs. Avoid.
Beverages:	None expected.
Cocaine:	Unpredictable effect on nervous system. Avoid.
Foods:	None expected.
Marijuana:	Unpredictable effect on nervous system. Avoid.
Tobacco:	None expected.

*See Glossary

TESTOLACTONE

BRAND NAMES

Teslac

BASIC INFORMATION

Habit forming? No
Prescription needed? Yes
Available as generic? No
Drug class: Antineoplastic

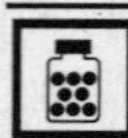

USES

Treats advanced breast cancer.

DOSAGE & USAGE INFORMATION

How to take:
Tablets—Swallow with liquid. If you can't swallow whole, crumble tablet and take with liquid or food. Instructions to take on empty stomach mean 1 hour before or 2 hours after eating.

When to take:
Follow doctor's instructions.

If you forget a dose:
Take as soon as you remember up to 2 hours late. If more than 2 hours, wait for next scheduled dose (don't double this dose).

What drug does:
Inhibits growth of cancer cells.

Time lapse before drug works:
6 to 12 weeks.

Don't take with:
Any other medicines (including over-the-counter drugs such as cough and cold medicines, laxatives, antacids, diet pills, caffeine, nose drops or vitamins) without consulting your doctor.

OVERDOSE

SYMPTOMS:
None expected.
WHAT TO DO:
Overdose unlikely to threaten life. If person takes much larger amount than prescribed, call doctor, poison control center or hospital emergency room for instructions.

POSSIBLE ADVERSE REACTIONS OR SIDE EFFECTS

SYMPTOMS	WHAT TO DO
Life-threatening: None expected.	
Common: Appetite loss.	Continue. Call doctor when convenient.
Infrequent: Diarrhea; swollen feet and legs; numb and tingling fingers, toes, face.	Continue. Call doctor when convenient.
Rare: Red tongue.	Continue. Call doctor when convenient.

WARNINGS & PRECAUTIONS

Don't take if:
You are allergic to testosterone.

Before you start, consult your doctor:
- If you have heart disease.
- If you have kidney disease.

Over age 60:
Adverse reactions and side effects may be more frequent and severe than in younger persons. You may need smaller doses for shorter periods of time.

Pregnancy:
Decide with your doctor if drug benefits justify risk to unborn child. Risk category C (see page xxii).

Breast-feeding:
Effect not documented. Consult your doctor.

Infants & children:
Not recommended.

Prolonged use:
Talk to your doctor about the need for follow-up medical examinations or laboratory studies to check serum calcium levels.

Skin & sunlight:
No problems expected.

Driving, piloting or hazardous work:
No problems expected.

Discontinuing:
No special problems expected.

Others:
- Advise any doctor or dentist whom you consult that you take this medicine.
- May affect results in some medical tests.

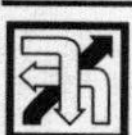

POSSIBLE INTERACTION WITH OTHER DRUGS

GENERIC NAME OR DRUG CLASS	COMBINED EFFECT
Anticoagulants*, oral	Increased anti-coagulant effect.

POSSIBLE INTERACTION WITH OTHER SUBSTANCES

INTERACTS WITH	COMBINED EFFECT
Alcohol:	No special problems expected.
Beverages:	No special problems expected.
Cocaine:	No special problems expected.
Foods:	No special problems expected.
Marijuana:	No special problems expected.
Tobacco:	No special problems expected.

***See Glossary**

TESTOSTERONE & ESTRADIOL

BRAND AND GENERIC NAMES

See complete list of brand and generic names in the *Brand Name Directory*, page 919.

BASIC INFORMATION

Habit forming? No
Prescription needed? Yes
Available as generic? Yes
Drug class: Androgens-estrogens

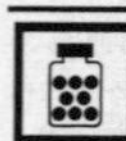

USES

- Prevents breast fullness in new mothers after childbirth.
- Relieves menopause symptoms such as unnecessary sweating, hot flashes, chills, faintness and dizziness.

DOSAGE & USAGE INFORMATION

How to take:
- Injection—Given deeply intramuscular.
- Tablets—Swallow with liquid or food to lessen stomach irritation.

When to take:
When directed.

If you forget a dose:
Check with your doctor.

What drug does:
- Restores normal estrogen level in tissues.
- Stimulates cells that produce male sex characteristics.
- Replaces hormones lost due to deficiencies.
- Stimulates red blood cell production.
- Suppresses production of estrogen.

Time lapse before drug works:
10 to 20 days.

Don't take with:
Any other medicine without consulting your doctor or pharmacist.

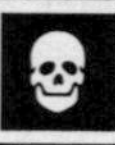

OVERDOSE

SYMPTOMS:
Headache (severe), coordination loss, vision changes, chest pain, shortness of breath (sudden), speech slurring.
WHAT TO DO:
Overdose unlikely to threaten life. If person takes much larger amount than prescribed, call doctor, poison control center or hospital emergency room for instructions.

POSSIBLE ADVERSE REACTIONS OR SIDE EFFECTS

SYMPTOMS	WHAT TO DO
Life-threatening:	
• In case of overdose, see previous column.	
• Hives, black stool, black or bloody vomit, intense itching, weakness, loss of consciousness.	Discontinue. Seek emergency treatment.
Common:	
• Red or flushed face; rash; swollen, tender breasts.	Discontinue. Call doctor right away.
• Depression, irritability, dizziness, confusion, acne or oily skin, enlarged clitoris, deepened voice, appetite loss, increased sex drive, unnatural hair growth, headache, constipation.	Continue. Call doctor when convenient.
Infrequent:	
• Nausea, vomiting, diarrhea, unusual vaginal bleeding or discharge, uncontrolled muscle movements.	Discontinue. Call doctor right away.
• Swollen feet and ankles, migraine headache.	Continue. Call doctor when convenient.
Rare:	
• Jaundice, abdominal pain.	Discontinue. Call doctor right away.
• Brown blotches on skin; hair loss; sore throat, fever, mouth sores.	Continue. Call doctor when convenient.

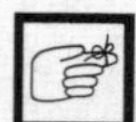

WARNINGS & PRECAUTIONS

Don't take if:
- You are allergic to any male hormone or any estrogen-containing drugs.
- You have impaired liver function.
- You have had blood clots, stroke or heart attack.
- You have unexplained vaginal bleeding.

Before you start, consult your doctor:
- If you might be pregnant or plan to become pregnant within 3 months.
- If you have heart disease, arteriosclerosis, diabetes, liver disease, high blood pressure, asthma, congestive heart failure, kidney disease or gallstones.

- If you have a high level of blood calcium.
- If you have had migraine headaches, epilepsy or porphyria.
- If you have had cancer of breast or reproductive organs, fibrocystic breast disease, fibroid tumors of the uterus or endometriosis.

Over age 60:
- May stimulate sexual activity.
- Can make high blood pressure or heart disease worse.
- Controversial. You and your doctor must decide if drug risks outweigh benefits.

Pregnancy:
Risk to unborn child outweighs drug benefits. Don't use. Risk category X (see page xxii).

Breast-feeding:
Drug passes into milk. Avoid drug or discontinue nursing until you finish medicine. Consult doctor for advice on maintaining milk supply.

Infants & children:
Not recommended.

Prolonged use:
- Increased growth of fibroid tumors of uterus.
- Possible kidney stones.
- Unnatural hair growth and deep voice in women.
- Talk to your doctor about the need for follow-up medical examinations or laboratory studies to check pap smear, liver function, mammogram, complete blood counts (white blood cell count, platelet count, red blood cell count, hemoglobin, hematocrit).
- Possible breast lumps, jaundice, sore throat, fever. If any of these occur, call your doctor.

Skin & sunlight:
May cause rash or intensify sunburn in areas exposed to sun or sunlamp.

Driving, piloting or hazardous work:
No problems expected.

Discontinuing:
You may need to discontinue estrogens periodically. Consult your doctor.

Others:
- In rare instances, may cause blood clot in lung, brain or leg. Symptoms are *sudden* severe headache, coordination loss, vision change, chest pain, breathing difficulty, slurred speech, pain in legs or groin. Seek emergency treatment immediately.
- Will not increase strength in athletes.
- Carefully read the paper delivered with your prescription called "Information for the Patient."
- Don't smoke.

POSSIBLE INTERACTION WITH OTHER DRUGS

GENERIC NAME OR DRUG CLASS	COMBINED EFFECT
Anticoagulants*, oral	Increased effect of anticoagulant.
Anticonvulsants*, hydantoin	Increased seizures.
Antidiabetics*, oral	Unpredictable increase or decrease in blood sugar.
Antifibrinolytic agents*	Increased possibility of blood clotting.
Carbamazepine	Increased seizures.
Chlorzoxazone	Decreased androgen effect.
Cholestyramine	Decreased cholestyramine effect.
Clofibrate	Decreased clofibrate effect.
Colestipol	Decreased colestipol effect.

Continued on page 961

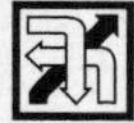

POSSIBLE INTERACTION WITH OTHER SUBSTANCES

INTERACTS WITH	COMBINED EFFECT
Alcohol:	None expected.
Beverages:	None expected.
Cocaine:	No proven problems.
Foods:	
Salt.	Excessive fluid retention (edema). Decrease salt intake while taking male hormones.
Marijuana:	Decreased blood levels of androgens. Possible menstrual irregularities and bleeding between periods.
Tobacco:	Increased risk of blood clots leading to stroke or heart attack.

***See Glossary**

TETRACYCLINES

BRAND AND GENERIC NAMES

See complete list of brand and generic names in the *Brand Name Directory*, page 919.

BASIC INFORMATION

Habit forming? No
Prescription needed? Yes
Available as generic? Yes
Drug class: Antibiotic (tetracycline), antiprotozoal

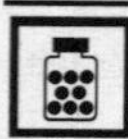

USES

- Treatment for infections susceptible to any tetracycline. Will not cure virus infections such as colds or flu.
- Treatment for acne.
- Used as diuretic.

DOSAGE & USAGE INFORMATION

How to take:
- Tablet or capsule—Take on empty stomach 1 hour before or 2 hours after eating. If you can't swallow whole, crumble tablet or open capsule and take with liquid or food.
- Liquid—Shake well. Take with measuring spoon.

When to take:
At the same times each day, evenly spaced.

If you forget a dose:
Take as soon as you remember up to 2 hours late. If more than 2 hours, wait for next scheduled dose (don't double this dose).

What drug does:
Prevents germ growth and reproduction.

Time lapse before drug works:
- Infections—May require 5 days to affect infection.
- Acne—May require 4 weeks to affect acne.

Don't take with:
Any other medicine without consulting your doctor or pharmacist.

OVERDOSE

SYMPTOMS:
Severe nausea, vomiting, diarrhea.
WHAT TO DO:
Overdose unlikely to threaten life. If person takes much larger amount than prescribed, call doctor, poison control center or hospital emergency room for instructions.

POSSIBLE ADVERSE REACTIONS OR SIDE EFFECTS

SYMPTOMS	WHAT TO DO
Life-threatening:	
Hives, rash, intense itching, faintness soon after a dose (anaphylaxis).	Seek emergency treatment immediately.
Common:	
• Sore mouth or tongue, nausea, vomiting, diarrhea.	Discontinue. Seek emergency treatment.
• Itching around rectum and genitals.	Discontinue. Call doctor right away.
• Vaginal discharge due to yeast, abdominal discomfort.	Continue. Call doctor when convenient.
• Dark tongue.	Continue. Tell doctor at next visit.
Infrequent:	
• Headache, rash.	Discontinue. Call doctor right away.
• Excessive thirst, increased urination, dizziness (with minocycline).	Continue. Call doctor when convenient.
Rare:	
Blurred vision, jaundice.	Discontinue. Call doctor right away.

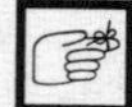

WARNINGS & PRECAUTIONS

Don't take if:
You are allergic to any tetracycline antibiotic.

Before you start, consult your doctor:
- If you have kidney or liver disease.
- If you have lupus.
- If you have myasthenia gravis.

Over age 60:
Dosage usually less than in younger adults. More likely to cause itching around rectum. Ask your doctor how to prevent it.

Pregnancy:
Risk to unborn child outweighs drug benefits. Don't use. Risk category D (see page xxii).

Breast-feeding:
Drug passes into milk. Avoid drug or discontinue nursing until you finish medicine. Consult doctor for advice on maintaining milk supply.

Infants & children:
May cause permanent teeth malformation or discoloration in children less than 8 years old. Don't use.

Prolonged use:
- You may become more susceptible to infections caused by germs not responsive to tetracycline.
- May cause rare problems in liver, kidney or bone marrow. Periodic laboratory blood studies, liver and kidney function tests recommended if you use drug a long time.

Skin & sunlight:
May cause rash or intensify sunburn in areas exposed to sun or sunlamp.

Driving, piloting or hazardous work:
No problems expected.

Discontinuing:
Don't discontinue without doctor's advice until you complete prescribed dose, even though symptoms diminish or disappear.

Others:
- Avoid using outdated drug.
- May affect results in some medical tests.

POSSIBLE INTERACTION WITH OTHER DRUGS

GENERIC NAME OR DRUG CLASS	COMBINED EFFECT
Antacids*	Decreased tetracycline effect.
Anticoagulants*, oral	Increased anti-coagulant effect.
Bismuth subsalicylate	Decreased tetra-cycline absorption .
Calcium supplements*	Decreased tetracycline effect.
Cefixime	Decreased antibiotic effect of cefixime.
Cholestyramine or colestipol	Decreased tetracycline effect.
Contraceptives, oral*	Decreased contra-ceptive effect.
Desmopressin	Possible decreased desmopressin effect.
Digitalis preparations*	Increased digitalis effect.
Etretinate	Increased chance of adverse reactions of etretinate.
Lithium	Increased lithium effect.
Mineral supplements* (iron, calcium, magnesium, zinc)	Decreased tetracycline absorption. Separate doses by 1 to 2 hours.
Penicillins*	Decreased penicillin effect.
Sodium bicarbonate	Greatly reduced tetracycline absorption.
Tiopronin	Increased risk of toxicity to kidneys (except with doxycycline and minocycline).
Zinc supplements	Decreased tetracycline absorption if taken within 2 hours of each other.

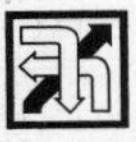

POSSIBLE INTERACTION WITH OTHER SUBSTANCES

INTERACTS WITH	COMBINED EFFECT
Alcohol:	Possible liver damage. Avoid.
Beverages: Milk.	Decreased tetracycline absorption. Take dose 2 hours after or 1 hour before drinking.
Cocaine:	No proven problems.
Foods: Dairy products.	Decreased tetracycline absorption. Take dose 2 hours after or 1 hour before eating.
Marijuana:	No interactions expected, but marijuana may slow body's recovery. Avoid.
Tobacco:	None expected.

*See Glossary

THEOPHYLLINE, EPHEDRINE & BARBITURATES

BRAND NAMES

Azma Aid	Tedrigen
Phedral-C.T.	T.E.P.
Primatene "P" Formula	Theodrine
Tedral	Theodrine Pediatric
Tedral SA	Theofed
	Theofedral

BASIC INFORMATION

Habit forming? Yes
Prescription needed? Some yes, others no
Available as generic? Some yes, others no
Drug class: Bronchodilator, barbiturate, sympathomimetic, sedative

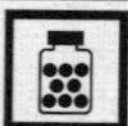

USES

- Treats bronchial asthma symptoms.
- Decreases congestion of breathing passages.
- Suppresses allergic reactions.
- Reduces anxiety or nervous tension (low dose).

DOSAGE & USAGE INFORMATION

How to take:
- Tablet or elixir—Swallow with liquid.
- Extended-release tablets—Swallow each dose whole. If you take regular tablets, you may chew or crush them.

When to take:
Most effective taken on empty stomach 1 hour before or 2 hours after eating. However, may take with food to lessen stomach upset.

Continued next column

If you forget a dose:
Take as soon as you remember up to 2 hours late. If more than 2 hours, wait for next scheduled dose (don't double this dose).

What drug does:
- Relaxes and expands bronchial tubes.
- Prevents cells from releasing allergy-causing chemicals (histamines).
- Decreases blood vessel size and blood flow, thus causing decongestion.
- May partially block nerve impulses at nerve cell connections.

Time lapse before drug works:
15 to 30 minutes.

Don't take with:
- Nonprescription drugs with ephedrine, pseudoephedrine or epinephrine.
- Nonprescription drugs for cough, cold, allergy or asthma without consulting doctor.
- Any other medicine without consulting your doctor or pharmacist.

OVERDOSE

SYMPTOMS:
Restlessness, irritability, anxiety, confusion, hallucinations, vomiting blood, delirium, muscle tremors, convulsions, rapid and irregular pulse, coma.

WHAT TO DO:
- **Dial 911 (emergency) or 0 (operator) for an ambulance or medical help. Then give first aid immediately.**
- **See emergency information on inside covers.**

POSSIBLE ADVERSE REACTIONS OR SIDE EFFECTS

SYMPTOMS	WHAT TO DO
Life-threatening:	
Difficult breathing, uncontrollable rapid heart rate, loss of consciousness.	Discontinue. Seek emergency treatment.
Common:	
• Headache, irritability, nervousness, restlessness, insomnia, nausea, vomiting, abdominal pain, irregular heartbeat, "hangover" effect.	Discontinue. Call doctor right away.
• Dizziness, light-headedness, paleness, heartburn.	Continue. Call doctor when convenient.
Infrequent:	
• Rash; hives; red or flushed face; appetite loss; diarrhea; cough; confusion; slurred speech; eyelid, face, lip swelling; joint pain.	Discontinue. Call doctor right away.
• Frequent urination.	Continue. Call doctor when convenient.
Rare:	
Agitation; sore throat, fever, mouth sores; jaundice.	Discontinue. Call doctor right away.

THEOPHYLLINE, EPHEDRINE & BARBITURATES

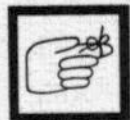

WARNINGS & PRECAUTIONS

Don't take if:
- You are allergic to any bronchodilator or barbiturate.
- You are allergic to ephedrine or any sympathomimetic drug*.
- You have an active peptic ulcer or porphyria.

Before you start, consult your doctor:
- If you have gastritis, peptic ulcer, high blood pressure or heart disease, diabetes, overactive thyroid gland, difficulty urinating, epilepsy, kidney or liver damage, asthma, anemia, chronic pain.
- If you have taken any MAO inhibitor in past 2 weeks, taken digitalis preparations in the last 7 days.
- If you have had impaired kidney or liver function.
- If you take medication for gout.
- If you will have surgery within 2 months, including dental surgery, requiring general or spinal anesthesia.

Over age 60:
- Adverse reactions and side effects may be more frequent and severe than in younger persons. Use small doses.
- More likely to develop high blood pressure, heart rhythm disturbances and angina and to feel drug's stimulant effects.

Pregnancy:
Risk to unborn child outweighs drug benefits. Don't use. Risk category D (see page xxii).

Breast-feeding:
Drug passes into milk. Avoid drug or discontinue nursing until you finish medicine.

Infants & children:
Use only under medical supervision.

Prolonged use:
- Stomach irritation.
- Excessive doses—Rare toxic psychosis.
- Men with enlarged prostate gland may have more urination difficulty.
- May cause addiction, anemia, chronic intoxication.
- May lower body temperature, making exposure to cold temperatures hazardous.

Skin & sunlight:
May cause rash or intensify sunburn in areas exposed to sun or sunlamp.

Driving, piloting or hazardous work:
Don't drive or pilot aircraft until you learn how medicine affects you. Don't work around dangerous machinery. Don't climb ladders or work in high places. Danger increases if you drink alcohol or take medicine affecting alertness and reflexes.

Discontinuing:
- May be unnecessary to finish medicine. Follow doctor's instructions.
- If you develop withdrawal symptoms of hallucinations, agitation or sleeplessness after discontinuing, call doctor right away.

Others:
Potential for abuse.

POSSIBLE INTERACTION WITH OTHER DRUGS

GENERIC NAME OR DRUG CLASS	COMBINED EFFECT
Allopurinol	Decreased allopurinol effect.
Anticoagulants*, oral	Decreased anticoagulant effect.
Anticonvulsants*, oral	Changed seizure patterns.
Antidepressants, tricyclic*	Decreased antidepressant effect. Possible dangerous oversedation.

Continued on page 961

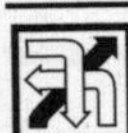

POSSIBLE INTERACTION WITH OTHER SUBSTANCES

INTERACTS WITH	COMBINED EFFECT
Alcohol:	Possible fatal oversedation. Avoid.
Beverages: Caffeine drinks.	Nervousness or insomnia.
Cocaine:	High risk of heartbeat irregularities and high blood pressure.
Foods:	None expected.
Marijuana:	Rapid heartbeat, possible heart rhythm disturbance.
Tobacco:	Decreased bronchodilator effect.

***See Glossary**

THEOPHYLLINE, EPHEDRINE, GUAIFENESIN & BARBITURATES

BRAND NAMES

Bronkolixir
Bronkotabs
Guaiphed
Mudrane GG

BASIC INFORMATION

Habit forming? Yes (barbiturates)
Prescription needed? Yes
Available as generic? Yes
Drug class: Bronchodilator (xanthine), cough/cold preparation, sympathomimetic, sedative

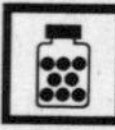

USES

- Treatment for symptoms of bronchial asthma, emphysema, chronic bronchitis.
- Relieves wheezing, coughing and shortness of breath.

DOSAGE & USAGE INFORMATION

How to take:
Tablet, capsule or elixir—Swallow with liquid.

When to take:
Most effective taken on empty stomach 1 hour before or 2 hours after eating. However, may take with food to lessen stomach upset.

If you forget a dose:
Take as soon as you remember up to 2 hours late. If more than 2 hours, wait for next scheduled dose (don't double this dose).

Continued next column

OVERDOSE

SYMPTOMS:
Restlessness, irritability, confusion, hallucinations, muscle tremors, severe anxiety, rapid and irregular pulse, mild weakness, nausea, vomiting blood, delirium, coma.
WHAT TO DO:

- **Overdose unlikely to threaten life. Depending on severity of symptoms and amount taken, call doctor, poison control center or hospital emergency room for instructions.**
- **Dial 911 (emergency) or 0 (operator) for an ambulance or medical help. Then give first aid immediately.**
- **See emergency information on inside covers.**

What drug does:

- Relaxes and expands bronchial tubes.
- Prevents cells from releasing allergy-causing chemicals (histamines).
- Relaxes muscles of bronchial tubes.
- Decreases blood vessel size and blood flow, thus causing decongestion.
- Increases production of watery fluids to thin mucus so it can be coughed out or absorbed.
- May partially block nerve impulses at nerve cell connections.

Time lapse before drug works:
30 to 60 minutes.

Don't take with:

- Nonprescription drugs with ephedrine, pseudoephedrine or epinephrine.
- Nonprescription drugs for cough, cold, allergy or asthma without consulting doctor.
- See Interaction column and consult doctor.

POSSIBLE ADVERSE REACTIONS OR SIDE EFFECTS

SYMPTOMS	WHAT TO DO
Life-threatening:	
Difficult breathing, uncontrollable rapid heart rate, loss of consciousness.	Discontinue. Seek emergency treatment.
Common:	
• Headache, irritability, nervousness, restlessness, insomnia, nausea, vomiting, abdominal pain, irregular heartbeat.	Discontinue. Call doctor right away.
• Dizziness, lightheadedness, paleness, heartburn.	Continue. Call doctor when convenient.
Infrequent:	
• Skin rash or hives, red or flushed face, appetite loss, diarrhea, abdominal pain.	Discontinue. Call doctor right away.
• Frequent urination.	Continue. Call doctor when convenient.
Rare:	
None expected.	

THEOPHYLLINE, EPHEDRINE, GUAIFENESIN & BARBITURATES

WARNINGS & PRECAUTIONS

Don't take if:
- You are allergic to any bronchodilator, ephedrine, any sympathomimetic drug*, cough or cold preparation containing guaifenesin.
- You have an active peptic ulcer.

Before you start, consult your doctor:
- If you have had impaired kidney or liver function.
- If you have gastritis, peptic ulcer, high blood pressure, heart disease, diabetes, overactive thyroid gland, difficulty urinating, epilepsy, anemia, chronic pain.
- If you take medication for gout or have taken any MAO inhibitor in past 2 weeks, or have taken digitalis preparations in the last 7 days.
- If you will have surgery within 2 months, including dental surgery, requiring general or spinal anesthesia.

Over age 60:
- Adverse reactions and side effects may be more frequent and severe than in younger persons. Use small doses. For drug to work, you must drink 8 to 10 glasses of fluid per day.
- More likely to develop high blood pressure, heart rhythm disturbances and angina and to feel drug's stimulant effects.

Pregnancy:
Risk to unborn child outweighs drug benefits. Don't use. Risk category D (see page xxii).

Breast-feeding:
Drug passes into milk. Avoid drug or discontinue nursing until you finish medicine. Consult doctor for advice on maintaining milk supply.

Infants & children:
Use only under medical supervision.

Prolonged use:
- Stomach irritation.
- Excessive doses—Rare toxic psychosis.
- Men with enlarged prostate gland may have more urination difficulty.
- May cause addiction, anemia, chronic intoxication.
- May lower body temperature, making exposure to cold temperature hazardous.

Skin & sunlight:
May cause rash or intensify sunburn in areas exposed to sun or sunlamp.

Driving, piloting or hazardous work:
Don't drive or pilot aircraft until you learn how medicine affects you. Don't work around dangerous machinery. Don't climb ladders or work in high places. Danger increases if you drink alcohol or take medicine affecting alertness and reflexes, such as antihistamines, tranquilizers, sedatives, pain medicine, narcotics and mind-altering drugs.

Discontinuing:
- May be unnecessary to finish medicine. Follow doctor's instructions.
- If you develop withdrawal symptoms of hallucinations, agitation or sleeplessness after discontinuing, call doctor right away.

Others:
Great potential for abuse.

POSSIBLE INTERACTION WITH OTHER DRUGS

GENERIC NAME OR DRUG CLASS	COMBINED EFFECT
Allopurinol	Decreased allopurinol effect.
Anticonvulsants*, oral	Changed seizure patterns.

Continued on page 962

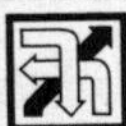

POSSIBLE INTERACTION WITH OTHER SUBSTANCES

INTERACTS WITH	COMBINED EFFECT
Alcohol:	Possible fatal oversedation. Avoid.
Beverages:	You must drink 8 to 10 glasses of fluid per day for drug to work.
Caffeine drinks.	Nervousness and insomnia.
Cocaine:	High risk of heartbeat irregularities and high blood pressure.
Foods:	None expected.
Marijuana:	Excessive sedation, rapid heartbeat, possible heart rhythm disturbance. Avoid.
Tobacco:	Decreased bronchodilator effect. Smoking is damaging to all problems this medicine treats. Avoid.

***See Glossary**

THEOPHYLLINE, EPHEDRINE & HYDROXYZINE

BRAND NAMES

Ami Rax
Hydrophed
Marax
Marax D.F.
T.E.H. Compound
Theomax DF

BASIC INFORMATION

Habit forming? No
Prescription needed? Yes
Available as generic? Yes
Drug class: Bronchodilator (xanthine), sympathomimetic, antihistamine

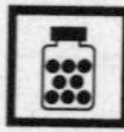

USES

- Treatment for symptoms of bronchial asthma, emphysema, chronic bronchitis.
- Relieves wheezing, coughing and shortness of breath.

DOSAGE & USAGE INFORMATION

How to take:
Tablet or syrup—Swallow with liquid.

When to take:
Most effective taken on empty stomach 1 hour before or 2 hours after eating. However, may take with food to lessen stomach upset.

If you forget a dose:
Take as soon as you remember up to 2 hours late. If more than 2 hours, wait for next scheduled dose (don't double this dose).

Continued next column

OVERDOSE

SYMPTOMS:
Restlessness, irritability, confusion, hallucinations, severe anxiety, muscle tremors, rapid and irregular pulse, agitation, purposeless movements, vomiting blood, delirium, convulsions, coma.
WHAT TO DO:

- **Dial 911 (emergency) or 0 (operator) for an ambulance or medical help. Then give first aid immediately.**
- **See emergency information on inside covers.**

What drug does:

- Relaxes and expands bronchial tubes.
- Prevents cells from releasing allergy-causing chemicals (histamines).
- Relaxes muscles of bronchial tubes.
- Decreases blood vessel size and blood flow, thus causing decongestion.
- May reduce activity in areas of the brain that influence emotional stability.

Time lapse before drug works:
15 to 60 minutes.

Don't take with:

- Nonprescription drugs with ephedrine, pseudoephedrine or epinephrine.
- Nonprescription drugs for cough, cold, allergy or asthma without consulting doctor.
- See Interaction column and consult doctor.

POSSIBLE ADVERSE REACTIONS OR SIDE EFFECTS

SYMPTOMS	WHAT TO DO
Life-threatening:	
Difficult breathing, uncontrollable rapid heart rate, loss of consciousness.	Discontinue. Seek emergency treatment.
Common:	
• Headache, irritability, nervousness, restlessness, insomnia, nausea, vomiting, abdominal pain, irregular heartbeat.	Discontinue. Call doctor right away.
• Dizziness, lightheadedness, paleness, heartburn.	Continue. Call doctor when convenient.
Infrequent:	
• Skin rash or hives, red or flushed face, appetite loss, diarrhea, abdominal pain.	Discontinue. Call doctor right away.
• Frequent urination.	Continue. Call doctor when convenient.
Rare:	
Tremor.	Discontinue. Call doctor right away.

THEOPHYLLINE, EPHEDRINE & HYDROXYZINE

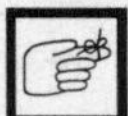

WARNINGS & PRECAUTIONS

Don't take if:
- You are allergic to any bronchodilator, ephedrine, any sympathomimetic drug*, or antihistamine.
- You have an active peptic ulcer.

Before you start, consult your doctor:
- If you have had impaired kidney or liver function.
- If you have gastritis, peptic ulcer, high blood pressure, heart disease, diabetes, overactive thyroid gland, difficulty urinating, epilepsy.
- If you take medication for gout or have taken any MAO inhibitor in past 2 weeks, taken digitalis preparations in the last 7 days.
- If you will have surgery within 2 months, including dental surgery, requiring general or spinal anesthesia.

Over age 60:
- Adverse reactions and side effects may be more frequent and severe than in younger persons.
- More likely to develop increased urination difficulty, high blood pressure, heart rhythm disturbances and angina and to feel drug's stimulant effects.

Pregnancy:
Risk factors vary for drugs in this group. See category list on page xxii and consult doctor.

Breast-feeding:
Drug passes into milk. Avoid drug or discontinue nursing until you finish medicine. Consult doctor for advice on maintaining milk supply.

Infants & children:
Use only under medical supervision.

Prolonged use:
- Stomach irritation.
- Excessive doses—Rare toxic psychosis.
- Men with enlarged prostate gland may have more urination difficulty.
- Tolerance develops and reduces effectiveness.

Skin & sunlight:
No problems expected.

Driving, piloting or hazardous work:
Don't drive or pilot aircraft until you learn how medicine affects you. Don't work around dangerous machinery. Don't climb ladders or work in high places. Danger increases if you drink alcohol or take medicine affecting alertness and reflexes, such as antihistamines, tranquilizers, sedatives, pain medicine, narcotics and mind-altering drugs.

Discontinuing:
Don't discontinue without consulting doctor. Dose may require gradual reduction if you have taken drug for a long time. Doses of other drugs may also require adjustment.

Others:
No problems expected.

POSSIBLE INTERACTION WITH OTHER DRUGS

GENERIC NAME OR DRUG CLASS	COMBINED EFFECT
Allopurinol	Decreased allopurinol effect.
Antidepressants, tricyclic*	Increased ephedrine effect. Excess stimulation of heart and blood pressure.
Antihistamines*	Increased hydroxyzine effect.
Antihypertensives*	Decreased anti-hypertensive effect.
Beta-adrenergic blocking agents*	Decreased effect of both drugs.

Continued on page 963

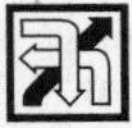

POSSIBLE INTERACTION WITH OTHER SUBSTANCES

INTERACTS WITH	COMBINED EFFECT
Alcohol:	Increased sedation and intoxication. Avoid.
Beverages: Caffeine drinks.	Nervousness and insomnia.
Cocaine:	High risk of heartbeat irregularities and high blood pressure.
Foods:	None expected.
Marijuana:	Slightly increased antiasthmatic effect of bronchodilator. Rapid heartbeat, possible heart rhythm disturbance.
Tobacco:	Decreased broncho-dilator effect. Smoking is damaging to all problems this medicine treats. Avoid.

***See Glossary**

THEOPHYLLINE & GUAIFENESIN

BRAND NAMES

Asbron G
Asbron G Inlay Tablets
Bronchial
Broncomar GG
Ed-Bron G
Elixophyllin-GG
Equibron G
Glyceryl T
Mudrane GG2
Quibron
Quibron 300
Slo-Phyllin GG
Syncophylate-GG
Theolate
Uni-Bronchial

BASIC INFORMATION

Habit forming? No
Prescription needed? Yes
Available as generic? Yes
Drug class: Bronchodilator, expectorant

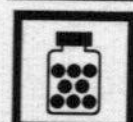

USES

- Treatment for bronchial asthma symptoms.
- Loosens mucus in respiratory passages.
- Relieves coughing, wheezing, shortness of breath.

DOSAGE & USAGE INFORMATION

How to take:
Tablet, capsule, elixir or syrup—Swallow with liquid.

When to take:
Most effective taken on empty stomach 1 hour before or 2 hours after eating. However, may take with food to lessen stomach upset.

If you forget a dose:
Take as soon as you remember up to 2 hours late. If more than 2 hours, wait for next scheduled dose (don't double this dose).

Continued next column

OVERDOSE

SYMPTOMS:
Restlessness, irritability, confusion, hallucinations, drowsiness, mild weakness, nausea, vomiting blood, delirium, convulsions, rapid pulse, coma.
WHAT TO DO:
- **Dial 911 (emergency) or 0 (operator) for an ambulance or medical help. Then give first aid immediately.**
- **See emergency information on inside covers.**

What drug does:
- Relaxes and expands bronchial tubes.
- Increases production of watery fluids to thin mucus so it can be coughed out or absorbed.

Time lapse before drug works:
15 to 30 minutes.

Don't take with:
Any other medicine without consulting your doctor or pharmacist.

POSSIBLE ADVERSE REACTIONS OR SIDE EFFECTS

SYMPTOMS	WHAT TO DO
Life-threatening:	
Difficult breathing, uncontrollable heart rate, loss of consciousness.	Discontinue. Seek emergency treatment.
Common:	
• Headache, irritability, nervousness, restlessness, insomnia, drowsiness, nausea, vomiting.	Discontinue. Call doctor right away.
• Dizziness, lightheadedness, diarrhea, abdominal pain, heartburn.	Continue. Call doctor when convenient.
Infrequent:	
Skin rash or hives, red or flushed face, appetite loss, diarrhea.	Discontinue. Call doctor right away.
Rare:	
None expected.	

WARNINGS & PRECAUTIONS

Don't take if:
- You are allergic to any bronchodilator or cough or cold preparation containing guaifenesin.
- You have an active peptic ulcer.

Before you start, consult your doctor:
- If you have had impaired kidney or liver function.
- If you have gastritis, peptic ulcer, high blood pressure or heart disease.
- If you take medication for gout.

Over age 60:
Adverse reactions and side effects may be more frequent and severe than in younger persons. For drug to work, you must drink 8 to 10 glasses of fluid per day.

Pregnancy:
Decide with your doctor if drug benefits justify risk to unborn child. Risk category C (see page xxii).

Breast-feeding:
Drug passes into milk. Avoid drug or discontinue nursing until you finish medicine. Consult doctor for advice on maintaining milk supply.

Infants & children:
Use only under medical supervision.

Prolonged use:
Stomach irritation.

Skin & sunlight:
No problems expected.

Driving, piloting or hazardous work:
Avoid if lightheaded, drowsy or dizzy. Otherwise, no problems expected.

Discontinuing:
May be unnecessary to finish medicine. Follow doctor's instructions.

Others:
No problems expected.

POSSIBLE INTERACTION WITH OTHER DRUGS

GENERIC NAME OR DRUG CLASS	COMBINED EFFECT
Allopurinol	Decreased allopurinol effect.
Anticoagulants*, oral	Possible risk of bleeding.
Ciprofloxacin	Increased possibility of central nervous system poisoning, such as nausea, vomiting, restlessness, palpitations.
Clarithromycin	Increased concentration of theophylline.
Ephedrine	Increased effect of both drugs.
Epinephrine	Increased effect of both drugs.
Erythromycins*	Increased bronchodilator effect.
Finasteride	Decreased theophylline effect.
Furosemide	Increased furosemide effect.
Lincomycins*	Increased bronchodilator effect.
Lithium	Decreased lithium effect.
Moricizine	Decreased bronchodilator effect.
Nicotine	Increased bronchodilator effect.
Probenecid	Decreased effect of both drugs.
Propranolol	Decreased bronchodilator effect.
Rauwolfia alkaloids*	Rapid heartbeat.
Sulfinpyrazone	Decreased sulfinpyrazone effect.
Ticlopidine	Increased theophylline effect.
Troleandomycin	Increased bronchodilator effect.

POSSIBLE INTERACTION WITH OTHER SUBSTANCES

INTERACTS WITH	COMBINED EFFECT
Alcohol:	No proven problems.
Beverages:	You must drink 8 to 10 glasses of fluid per day for drug to work.
Caffeine drinks.	Nervousness and insomnia.
Cocaine:	Excess stimulation. Avoid.
Foods:	None expected.
Marijuana:	Slightly increased antiasthmatic effect of bronchodilator.
Tobacco:	Decreased bronchodilator effect. Cigarette smoking worsens all problems that this medicine treats. Avoid.

*See Glossary

THIAMINE (Vitamin B-1)

BRAND NAMES

Betalin S
Betaxin
Bewon
Biamine

Numerous other multiple vitamin-mineral supplements. Check labels.

BASIC INFORMATION

Habit forming? No
Prescription needed? No
Available as generic? Yes
Drug class: Vitamin supplement

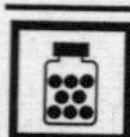

USES

- Dietary supplement to promote normal growth, development and health.
- Treatment for beri-beri (a thiamine-deficiency disease).
- Dietary supplement for alcoholism, cirrhosis, overactive thyroid, infection, breast-feeding, absorption diseases, pregnancy, prolonged diarrhea, burns.

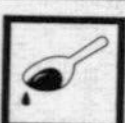

DOSAGE & USAGE INFORMATION

How to take:
Tablet or liquid—Swallow with beverage or food to lessen stomach irritation.

When to take:
At the same time each day.

If you forget a dose:
Take when remembered, then return to regular schedule.

What drug does:
- Promotes normal growth and development.
- Combines with an enzyme to metabolize carbohydrates.

Time lapse before drug works:
15 minutes.

Don't take with:
Any other medicine without consulting your doctor or pharmacist.

OVERDOSE

SYMPTOMS:
Increased severity of adverse reactions and side effects.
WHAT TO DO:
Overdose unlikely to threaten life. If person takes much larger amount than prescribed, call doctor, poison control center or hospital emergency room for instructions.

POSSIBLE ADVERSE REACTIONS OR SIDE EFFECTS

SYMPTOMS	WHAT TO DO
Life-threatening: Hives, rash, intense itching, faintness soon after a dose (anaphylaxis) (injection only).	Seek emergency treatment immediately.
Common: None expected.	
Infrequent: None expected.	
Rare:	
• Wheezing.	Discontinue. Seek emergency treatment.
• Rash or itchy skin.	Discontinue. Call doctor right away.

WARNINGS & PRECAUTIONS

Don't take if:
You are allergic to any B vitamin.

Before you start, consult your doctor:
If you have liver or kidney disease.

Over age 60:
No problems expected.

Pregnancy:
Consult doctor. Risk category A (see page xxii).

Breast-feeding:
No problems expected in meeting child's normal daily requirements. Consult doctor.

Infants & children:
No problems expected.

Prolonged use:
No problems expected.

Skin & sunlight:
No problems expected.

Driving, piloting or hazardous work:
No problems expected.

Discontinuing:
No problems expected.

Others:
A balanced diet should provide enough thiamine for healthy people to make a supplement unnecessary. Best dietary sources of thiamine are whole-grain cereals and meats.

POSSIBLE INTERACTION WITH OTHER DRUGS

GENERIC NAME OR DRUG CLASS	COMBINED EFFECT
Barbiturates*	Decreased thiamine effect.

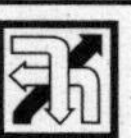

POSSIBLE INTERACTION WITH OTHER SUBSTANCES

INTERACTS WITH	COMBINED EFFECT
Alcohol:	None expected.
Beverages: Carbonates, citrates (additives listed on many beverage labels).	Decreased thiamine effect.
Cocaine:	None expected.
Foods: Carbonates, citrates (additives listed on many food labels).	Decreased thiamine effect.
Marijuana:	None expected.
Tobacco:	None expected.

*See Glossary

THIOGUANINE

BRAND NAMES

Lanvis

BASIC INFORMATION

Habit forming? No
Prescription needed? Yes
Available as generic? Yes
Drug class: Antineoplastic

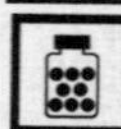

USES

Treats some forms of leukemia.

DOSAGE & USAGE INFORMATION

How to take:
Tablets—Swallow with liquid. If you can't swallow whole, crumble tablet and take with liquid or food. Instructions to take on empty stomach mean 1 hour before or 2 hours after eating.

When to take:
According to doctor's instructions.

If you forget a dose:
Skip the missed dose and return to regular schedule. Don't double dose.

What drug does:
Interferes with growth of cancer cells.

Time lapse before drug works:
Varies greatly among patients.

Don't take with:
Any other medicines (including over-the-counter drugs such as cough and cold medicines, laxatives, antacids, diet pills, caffeine, nose drops or vitamins) without consulting your doctor.

OVERDOSE

SYMPTOMS:
None expected.
WHAT TO DO:
Overdose unlikely to threaten life. If person takes much larger amount than prescribed, call doctor, poison control center or hospital emergency room for instructions.

POSSIBLE ADVERSE REACTIONS OR SIDE EFFECTS

SYMPTOMS	WHAT TO DO
Life-threatening:	
Black, tarry stools.	Discontinue. Seek emergency treatment.
Common:	
• Appetite loss, diarrhea, skin rash.	Continue. Call doctor when convenient.
• Nausea.	No action necessary.
Infrequent:	
Bloody urine; hoarseness or cough; fever or chills; lower back or side pain; painful or difficult urination; red spots on skin; unusual bleeding or bruising; joint pain; swollen feet and legs; unsteady gait.	Discontinue. Call doctor right away.
Rare:	
Mouth and lip sores; jaundice (yellow skin and eyes).	Discontinue. Call doctor right away.

WARNINGS & PRECAUTIONS

Don't take if:
- You are allergic to thioguanine.
- You have chicken pox or shingles.

Before you start, consult your doctor:
- If you have gout.
- If you have an infection.
- If you have kidney or liver disease.
- If you have had radiation or cancer chemotherapy within 6 weeks.

Over age 60:
Adverse reactions and side effects may be more frequent and severe than in younger persons. You may need smaller doses for shorter periods of time.

Pregnancy:
- Risk to unborn child outweighs drug benefits. Don't use.
- Don't use birth control pills for contraception.
- Risk category D (see page xxii).

Breast-feeding:
Drug may pass into milk. Avoid drug or discontinue nursing until you finish medicine. Consult doctor for advice on maintaining milk supply.

Infants & children:
No special problems expected.

Prolonged use:
- Increased likelihood of side effects.
- Talk to your doctor about the need for follow-up medical examinations or laboratory studies to check kidney and liver function, serum uric acid, and complete blood counts (white blood cell count, platelet count, red blood cell count, hemoglobin, hematocrit).

Skin & sunlight:
No problems expected.

Driving, piloting or hazardous work:
No problems expected.

Discontinuing:
Report to your doctor any of these symptoms that occur after discontinuing: black, tarry stools; bloody urine; hoarseness or cough; fever or chills; lower back or side pain; painful or difficult urination; red spots on skin; unusual bleeding or bruising.

Others:
- Advise any doctor or dentist whom you consult that you take this medicine.
- May affect results in some medical tests.
- Don't use birth control pills for contraception.

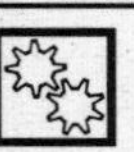

POSSIBLE INTERACTION WITH OTHER DRUGS

GENERIC NAME OR DRUG CLASS	COMBINED EFFECT
Antigout drugs*	May need increased antigout dosage.
Bone marrow depressants*, other	Increased risk of bone marrow depression.
Vaccines, live or killed	Increased risk of toxicity or reduced effectiveness of vaccine.
Zidovudine	More likelihood of toxicity of both drugs.

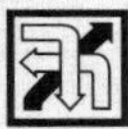

POSSIBLE INTERACTION WITH OTHER SUBSTANCES

INTERACTS WITH	COMBINED EFFECT
Alcohol:	Increased side effects.
Beverages:	None expected.
Cocaine:	Increased side effects.
Foods:	None expected.
Marijuana:	None expected.
Tobacco:	None expected.

THIOTHIXENE

BRAND NAMES

Navane
Thiothixene HCl Intensol

BASIC INFORMATION

Habit forming? No
Prescription needed? Yes
Available as generic? Yes
Drug class: Tranquilizer (thioxanthine), antiemetic

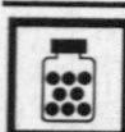

USES

- Reduces anxiety, agitation, psychosis.
- Stops vomiting, hiccups.

DOSAGE & USAGE INFORMATION

How to take:

- Capsule—Swallow with liquid. If you can't swallow whole, open capsule and take with liquid or food.
- Syrup—Dilute dose in beverage before swallowing.

When to take:
At the same time each day.

If you forget a dose:
Take as soon as you remember up to 2 hours late. If more than 2 hours, wait for next scheduled dose (don't double this dose).

What drug does:
Corrects imbalance of nerve impulses.

Continued next column

Time lapse before drug works:
3 weeks.

Don't take with:
Any other medicine without consulting your doctor or pharmacist.

OVERDOSE

SYMPTOMS:
Drowsiness, dizziness, weakness, muscle rigidity, twitching, tremors, confusion, dry mouth, blurred vision, rapid pulse, shallow breathing, low blood pressure, convulsions, coma.

WHAT TO DO:

- **Dial 911 (emergency) or 0 (operator) for an ambulance or medical help. Then give first aid immediately.**
- **If patient is unconscious and not breathing, give mouth-to-mouth breathing. If there is no heartbeat, use cardiac massage and mouth-to-mouth breathing (CPR). Don't try to make patient vomit. If you can't get help quickly, take patient to nearest emergency facility.**
- **See emergency information on inside covers.**

POSSIBLE ADVERSE REACTIONS OR SIDE EFFECTS

SYMPTOMS	WHAT TO DO
Life-threatening:	
Uncontrolled muscle movements of tongue, face and other muscles (neuroleptic malignant syndrome, rare).	Discontinue. Seek emergency treatment.
Common:	
• Fainting, jerky and involuntary movements, blurred vision, restlessness, rapid heartbeat.	Discontinue. Call doctor right away.
• Dizziness, drowsiness, constipation, muscle spasms, shuffling walk, decreased sweating, increased appetite, weight gain, sensitivity to light.	Continue. Call doctor when convenient.
• Dry mouth, nasal congestion.	Continue. Tell doctor at next visit.
Infrequent:	
• Rash, abdominal pain.	Discontinue. Call doctor right away.
• Less sexual ability, difficult urination.	Continue. Call doctor when convenient.
• Menstrual irregularities, swollen breasts, milk secretion by breasts.	Continue. Tell doctor at next visit.
Rare:	
Sore throat, fever, jaundice, lip smacking, cheek puffing, chewing movements of mouth, heatstroke, bleeding or bruising.	Discontinue. Call doctor right away.

WARNINGS & PRECAUTIONS

Don't take if:

- You are allergic to any thioxanthine or phenothiazine tranquilizer.
- You have serious blood disorder.
- You have Parkinson's disease.
- Patient is younger than 12.

Before you start, consult your doctor:

- If you have had liver or kidney disease.
- If you have epilepsy, glaucoma, prostate trouble.

- If you have high blood pressure or heart disease (especially angina).
- If you use alcohol daily.
- If you will have surgery within 2 months, including dental surgery, requiring general or spinal anesthesia.

Over age 60:
Adverse reactions and side effects may be more frequent and severe than in younger persons.

Pregnancy:
Decide with your doctor if drug benefits justify risk to unborn child. Risk category C (see page xxii).

Breast-feeding:
Studies inconclusive. Consult your doctor.

Infants & children:
Not recommended.

Prolonged use:
- Pigment deposits in lens and retina of eye.
- Involuntary movements of jaws, lips, tongue (tardive dyskinesia).
- Talk to your doctor about the need for follow-up medical examinations or laboratory studies to check complete blood counts (white blood cell count, platelet count, red blood cell count, hemoglobin, hematocrit), liver function, eyes.

Skin & sunlight:
May cause rash or intensify sunburn in areas exposed to sun or sunlamp.

Driving, piloting or hazardous work:
Don't drive or pilot aircraft until you learn how medicine affects you. Don't work around dangerous machinery. Don't climb ladders or work in high places. Danger increases if you drink alcohol or take medicine affecting alertness and reflexes.

Discontinuing:
Don't discontinue without consulting doctor. Dose may require gradual reduction if you have taken drug for a long time. Doses of other drugs may also require adjustment.

Others:
Hot temperatures increase chance of heat stroke.

POSSIBLE INTERACTION WITH OTHER DRUGS

GENERIC NAME OR DRUG CLASS	COMBINED EFFECT
Anticholinergics*	Increased anticholinergic effect.
Anticonvulsants*	Change in seizure pattern.
Antidepressants, tricyclic*	Increased thiothixene effect. Excessive sedation.
Antihistamines*	Increased thiothixene effect. Excessive sedation.
Antihypertensives*	Excessively low blood pressure.
Barbiturates*	Increased thiothixene effect. Excessive sedation.
Bethanechol	Decreased bethanechol effect.
Bupropion	Increased risk of major seizures.
Dronabinol	Increased effects of both drugs. Avoid.
Epinephrine	Excessively low blood pressure.
Guanethidine	Decreased guanethidine effect.
Levodopa	Decreased levodopa effect.
Mind-altering drugs*	Increased thiothixene effect. Excessive sedation.
Monoamine oxidase (MAO) inhibitors*	Excessive sedation.
Narcotics*	Increased thiothixene effect. Excessive sedation.
Pergolide	Decreased pergolide effect.
Procarbazine	Increased sedation.
Quinidine	Increased risk of heartbeat irregularities.

Continued on page 964

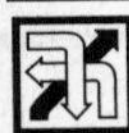

POSSIBLE INTERACTION WITH OTHER SUBSTANCES

INTERACTS WITH	COMBINED EFFECT
Alcohol:	Excessive brain depression. Avoid.
Beverages:	None expected.
Cocaine:	Decreased thiothixene effect. Avoid.
Foods:	None expected.
Marijuana:	Daily use—Fainting likely, possible psychosis.
Tobacco:	None expected.

***See Glossary**

THYROID HORMONES

BRAND AND GENERIC NAMES

Cytomel
Eltroxin
Euthroid
LEVOTHYROXINE
Levoid
Levothroid
Levoxyl
LIOTRIX
LIOTHYRONINE
Proloid
Synthroid
THYROGLOBULIN
THYROID
Thyrolar
THYROXINE

BASIC INFORMATION

Habit forming? No
Prescription needed? Yes
Available as generic? Yes, for some
Drug class: Thyroid hormone

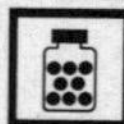

USES

Replacement for thyroid hormones lost due to deficiency.

DOSAGE & USAGE INFORMATION

How to take:
Tablet—Swallow with liquid.

When to take:
At the same time each day before a meal or on awakening.

If you forget a dose:
Take as soon as you remember up to 12 hours late. If more than 12 hours, wait for next scheduled dose (don't double this dose).

What drug does:
Increases cell metabolism rate.

Time lapse before drug works:
48 hours.

Continued next column

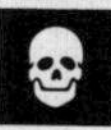

OVERDOSE

SYMPTOMS:
"Hot" feeling, heart palpitations, nervousness, sweating, hand tremors, insomnia, rapid and irregular pulse, headache, irritability, diarrhea, weight loss, muscle cramps, angina, congestive heart failure possible.
WHAT TO DO:
Overdose unlikely to threaten life. If person takes much larger amount than prescribed, call doctor, poison control center or hospital emergency room for instructions.

Don't take with:
Any other medicine without consulting your doctor or pharmacist.

POSSIBLE ADVERSE REACTIONS OR SIDE EFFECTS

SYMPTOMS	WHAT TO DO
Life-threatening: In case of overdose, see previous column.	
Common: Tremor, headache, irritability, insomnia, appetite change, diarrhea, leg cramps, menstrual irregularities, fever, heat sensitivity, unusual sweating, weight loss, nervousness.	Continue. Call doctor when convenient.
Infrequent: Hives, rash, vomiting, chest pain, rapid and irregular heartbeat, shortness of breath.	Discontinue. Call doctor right away.
Rare: None expected.	

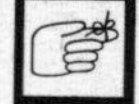

WARNINGS & PRECAUTIONS

Don't take if:
- You have had a heart attack within 6 weeks.
- You have no thyroid deficiency, but want to use this to lose weight.

Before you start, consult your doctor:
- If you have heart disease or high blood pressure.
- If you have diabetes.
- If you have Addison's disease, have had adrenal gland deficiency or use epinephrine, ephedrine or isoproterenol for asthma.

Over age 60:
More sensitive to thyroid hormone. May need smaller doses.

Pregnancy:
Considered safe if for thyroid deficiency only. Consult doctor. Risk category A (see page xxii).

Breast-feeding:
Present in milk. Consult doctor.

Infants & children:
Use only under medical supervision.

Prolonged use:

- No problems expected if dose is correct.
- Talk to your doctor about the need for follow-up medical examinations or laboratory studies to check thyroid, heart.

Skin & sunlight:
No problems expected.

Driving, piloting or hazardous work:
No problems expected.

Discontinuing:
Don't discontinue without consulting doctor. Dose may require gradual reduction if you have taken drug for a long time. Doses of other drugs may also require adjustment.

Others:

- Digestive upsets, tremors, cramps, nervousness, insomnia or diarrhea may indicate need for dose adjustment.
- Different brands can cause different results. Do not change brands without consulting doctor.
- Advise any doctor or dentist whom you consult that you take this medicine.

POSSIBLE INTERACTION WITH OTHER DRUGS

GENERIC NAME OR DRUG CLASS	COMBINED EFFECT
Amphetamines*	Increased amphetamine effect.
Anticoagulants*, oral	Increased anti-coagulant effect.
Antidepressants, tricyclic*	Increased anti-depressant effect. Irregular heartbeat.
Antidiabetics*, oral or insulin	Antidiabetic may require adjustment.
Aspirin (large doses, continuous use)	Increased effect of thyroid hormone.
Barbiturates*	Decreased barbiturate effect.
Beta-adrenergic blocking agents*	Possible decreased effect of beta blocker.
Cholestyramine	Decreased effect of thyroid hormone.
Colestipol	Decreased effect of thyroid hormone.
Contraceptives, oral*	Decreased effect of thyroid hormone.
Cortisone drugs*	Requires dose ad-justment to prevent cortisone deficiency.
Digitalis preparations*	Decreased digitalis effect.
Ephedrine	Increased ephedrine effect.
Epinephrine	Increased epinephrine effect.
Estrogens*	Decreased effect of thyroid hormone.
Methylphenidate	Increased methylphenidate effect.
Phenytoin	Possible decreased effect of thyroid hormone.
Sympathomimetics*	Increased risk of rapid or irregular heartbeat.

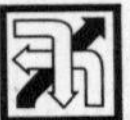

POSSIBLE INTERACTION WITH OTHER SUBSTANCES

INTERACTS WITH	COMBINED EFFECT
Alcohol:	None expected.
Beverages:	None expected.
Cocaine:	Excess stimulation. Avoid.
Foods:	None expected.
Marijuana:	None expected.
Tobacco:	None expected.

***See Glossary**

TICLOPIDINE

BRAND NAMES

Ticlid

BASIC INFORMATION

Habit forming? No
Prescription needed? Yes
Available as generic? No
Drug class: Platelet aggregation inhibitor

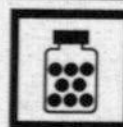

USES

Decreases the risk of stroke in patients who have warning signs of stroke or who have had strokes caused by blood clots.

DOSAGE & USAGE INFORMATION

How to take:
Tablets—Swallow with liquid. If you can't swallow whole, crumble tablet and take with liquid or food.

When to take:
Twice a day with food or as directed.

If you forget a dose:
Take as soon as you remember up to 2 hours late. If more than 2 hours, wait for next scheduled dose (don't double this dose).

What drug does:
Inhibits the clumping of platelets and thereby prevents blood clotting.

Time lapse before drug works:
2 hours.

Don't take with:
Any other drugs (particularly aspirin) without consulting doctor or pharmacist.

OVERDOSE

SYMPTOMS:
Bloody vomit or excessive bleeding from gums, nose or rectum.
WHAT TO DO:
Dial 911 (emergency) or 0 (operator) for an ambulance or medical help. Then give first aid immediately.

POSSIBLE ADVERSE REACTIONS OR SIDE EFFECTS

SYMPTOMS	WHAT TO DO
Life-threatening:	
None expected.	
Common:	
• Diarrhea, elevated level of cholesterol in blood.	Continue. Call doctor when convenient.
• Nausea, skin rash, abdominal pain.	Discontinue. Call doctor right away.
Infrequent:	
• Unusual bleeding or bruising.	Discontinue. Seek emergency treatment.
• Headache.	Continue. Call doctor when convenient.
Rare:	
• Sore throat, mouth ulcers, fever, chills.	Discontinue. Seek emergency treatment.
• Dizziness, loss of appetite, gaseousness.	Continue. Call doctor when convenient.

WARNINGS & PRECAUTIONS

Don't take if:
- You are allergic to ticlopidine.
- You have reduced white blood cells (neutropenia).

Before you start, consult your doctor:
- If you have liver disease, kidney disease, peptic ulcers or diverticulitis.
- If you have any bleeding disorder.

Over age 60:
No special problems expected.

Pregnancy:
Use during pregnancy only if clearly needed. Consult doctor. Risk category B (see page xxii).

Breast-feeding:
Safety not established. Consult doctor.

Infants & children:
Not recommended. Safety has not been established.

Prolonged use:
No special problems expected.

Skin & sunlight:
No special problems expected.

Driving, piloting or hazardous work:
Don't drive or pilot aircraft until you learn how the medicine affects you. Don't work around dangerous machinery. Don't climb ladders or work in high places.

Discontinuing:
No special problems expected.

Others:
- Advise any doctor or dentist whom you consult that you take this medicine. This is particularly important if any surgery is scheduled.
- May affect results of some medical tests.
- Report any unusual bleeding to your doctor.

POSSIBLE INTERACTION WITH OTHER DRUGS

GENERIC NAME OR DRUG CLASS	COMBINED EFFECT
Antacids*	Decreased ticlopidine effect.
Aspirin	Increased effects of both drugs.
Digoxin	Slightly decreased digoxin effect.
Theophylline	Increased theophylline effect.

POSSIBLE INTERACTION WITH OTHER SUBSTANCES

INTERACTS WITH	COMBINED EFFECT
Alcohol:	Increased alcohol in blood. Avoid.
Beverages:	No proven problems.
Cocaine:	No proven problems.
Foods:	Best to take with foods to prevent stomach upset.
Marijuana:	No proven problems.
Tobacco:	No proven problems.

*See Glossary

TIOPRONIN

BRAND NAMES

Capen
Captimer
Epatiol
Mucolysin
Sutilan
Thiola
Thiosol
Tioglis
Vincol

BASIC INFORMATION

Habit forming? No
Prescription needed? Yes
Available as generic? No
Drug class: Antiurolithic

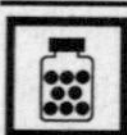

USES

Prevents the formation of kidney stones when there is too much cystine in the urine.

DOSAGE & USAGE INFORMATION

How to take:
Tablets—Swallow with liquid. If you can't swallow whole, crumble tablet and take with liquid or food. Instructions to take on empty stomach mean 1 hour before or 2 hours after eating.

When to take:
3 times daily (once approximately every 8 hours).

If you forget a dose:
Take as soon as you remember up to 2 hours late. If more than 2 hours, wait for next scheduled dose (don't double this dose).

What drug does:
Removes high levels of cystine from the body.

Time lapse before drug works:
Works immediately.

Continued next column

OVERDOSE

SYMPTOMS:
None expected. If massive overdose is suspected, follow instructions below.
WHAT TO DO:
- **Dial 911 (emergency) or 0 (operator) for an ambulance or medical help. Then give first aid immediately.**
- **See emergency information on inside covers.**

Don't take with:
- Medicines that are known to cause kidney damage or depress bone marrow.
- Any other medicine without consulting your doctor or pharmacist.

POSSIBLE ADVERSE REACTIONS OR SIDE EFFECTS

SYMPTOMS	WHAT TO DO
Life-threatening:	
In case of overdose, see previous column	
Common:	
• Skin rash, itching skin, mouth sores, mouth ulcers.	Discontinue. Call doctor right away.
• Abdominal pain, gaseousness, diarrhea, nausea or vomiting.	Continue. Call doctor when convenient.
Infrequent:	
• Cloudy urine, chills, breathing difficulty, joint pain.	Discontinue. Call doctor right away.
• Impaired smell or taste.	Continue. Call doctor when convenient.
Rare:	
Coughing up blood, fever, unusual tiredness or weakness, double vision, muscle weakness.	Discontinue. Call doctor right away.

WARNINGS & PRECAUTIONS

Don't take if:
You are allergic to tiopronin or penicillamine.

Before you start, consult your doctor:
If you have had any of the following in the past:
- Agranulocytosis*
- Aplastic anemia*
- Thrombocytopenia*
- Impaired kidney function

Over age 60:
May require dosage adjustment if kidney function is impaired due to normal aging.

Pregnancy:
Decide with your doctor if drug benefits justify risk to unborn child. Risk category C (see page xxii).

Breast-feeding:
Drug passes into milk. Avoid or discontinue nursing until you finish medicine. Consult doctor for advice on maintaining milk supply.

Infants & children:
Safety not established. Consult doctor.

Prolonged use:
No special problems expected.

Skin & sunlight:
No special problems expected.

Driving, piloting or hazardous work:
Don't drive or pilot aircraft until you learn how medicine affects you. Don't work around dangerous machinery. Don't climb ladders or work in high places. Danger increases if you drink alcohol or take medicine affecting alertness and reflexes.

Discontinuing:
No special problems expected.

Others:
- Advise any doctor or dentist whom you consult that you take this medicine.
- May affect results of some medical tests.

POSSIBLE INTERACTION WITH OTHER DRUGS

GENERIC NAME OR DRUG CLASS	COMBINED EFFECT
Bone marrow depressants*	May increase possibility of toxic effects of tiopronin.
Medications toxic to kidneys (nephrotoxins*)	May increase possibility of toxic effects of tiopronin.

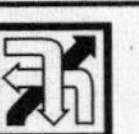

POSSIBLE INTERACTION WITH OTHER SUBSTANCES

INTERACTS WITH	COMBINED EFFECT
Alcohol:	None expected.
Beverages: Water.	Enhances effects of tiopronin. Drink 8 to 10 glasses daily.
Cocaine:	None expected.
Foods:	None expected.
Marijuana:	None expected.
Tobacco:	None expected.

*See Glossary

TOCAINIDE

BRAND NAMES

Tonocard

BASIC INFORMATION

Habit forming? No
Prescription needed? Yes
Available as generic? No
Drug class: Antiarrhythmic

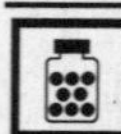

USES

Stabilizes irregular heartbeat, particularly irregular contractions of the ventricles of the heart or a too rapid heart rate.

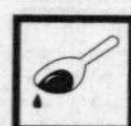

DOSAGE & USAGE INFORMATION

How to take:
Tablet—Swallow with food, water or milk. Dosage may need to be changed according to individual response.

When to take:
Take at regular times each day. For example, instructions to take 3 times a day means every 8 hours.

If you forget a dose:
Take as soon as you remember up to 4 hours late. If more than 4 hours, wait for next scheduled dose (don't double this dose).

What drug does:
Decreases excitability of cells of heart muscle.

Time lapse before drug works:
30 minutes to 2 hours.

Don't take with:
- Any other medicine without consulting your doctor or pharmacist.
- Wear identification information that states that you take this medicine so during an emergency a physician will know to avoid additional medicines that might be harmful or dangerous.

OVERDOSE

SYMPTOMS:
Convulsions, depressed breathing, cardiac arrest.
WHAT TO DO:
- **Dial 911 (emergency) or 0 (operator) for an ambulance or medical help. Then give first aid immediately.**
- **See emergency information on inside covers.**

POSSIBLE ADVERSE REACTIONS OR SIDE EFFECTS

SYMPTOMS	WHAT TO DO
Life-threatening:	
In case of overdose, see previous column.	
Common:	
• Nausea, vomiting, lightheadedness, dizziness.	Discontinue. Call doctor right away.
• Appetite loss.	Continue. Call doctor when convenient.
Infrequent:	
• Trembling, headache.	Discontinue. Call doctor right away.
• Numbness or tingling in hands or feet.	Continue. Call doctor when convenient.
Rare:	
• Sore throat, unexplained bleeding or bruising, fever, chills, blurred vision, accelerated heart rate or more irregular heartbeat, cough, difficult breathing, wheezing, double vision, disorientation, shakiness, seizures, blisters.	Discontinue. Call doctor right away.
• Rash, swollen feet and ankles, unusual sweating.	Continue. Call doctor when convenient.

WARNINGS & PRECAUTIONS

Don't take if:
- You are allergic to tocainide or anesthetics whose names end in "caine."
- You have myasthenia gravis.

Before you start, consult your doctor:
- If you have congestive heart failure.
- If you are pregnant or plan to become pregnant.
- If you take anticancer drugs, trimethoprim, pyrimethamine, primaquine, phenylbutazone, penicillamine or oxyphenbutazone. These may affect blood cell production in bone marrow.
- If you take any other heart medicine such as digitalis, flucystosine, colchicine, chloramphenicol, beta-adrenergic blockers or azathioprine. These can worsen heartbeat irregularity.

- If you will have surgery within 2 months, including dental surgery, requiring general, local or spinal anesthesia.
- If you have liver or kidney disease.

Over age 60:
Adverse reactions and side effects may be more frequent and severe than in younger persons.

Pregnancy:
Decide with your doctor whether drug benefits justify risk to unborn child. Risk category C (see page xxii).

Breast-feeding:
Avoid if possible. Consult doctor.

Infants & children:
Not recommended. Safety and dosage have not been established.

Prolonged use:
Request periodic lab studies on blood, liver function, potassium levels, x-ray, ECG*.

Skin & sunlight:
No problems expected.

Driving, piloting or hazardous work:
Use caution if medicine causes you to feel dizzy or weak. Otherwise, no problems expected.

Discontinuing:
Don't discontinue without consulting doctor, even though symptoms diminish or disappear.

Others:
No problems expected.

POSSIBLE INTERACTION WITH OTHER DRUGS

GENERIC NAME OR DRUG CLASS	COMBINED EFFECT
Antiarrhythmics*, others	Increased possibility of adverse reactions from either drug.
Beta-adrenergic blocking agents*	Irregular heartbeat. May worsen congestive heart failure.
Bone marrow depressants*	Decreased production of blood cells in bone marrow.

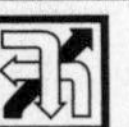

POSSIBLE INTERACTION WITH OTHER SUBSTANCES

INTERACTS WITH	COMBINED EFFECT
Alcohol:	Possible irregular heartbeat. Avoid.
Beverages: Caffeine drinks, iced drinks.	Possible irregular heartbeat.
Cocaine:	Possible light-headedness, dizziness, quivering, convulsions.
Foods:	None expected.
Marijuana:	None expected.
Tobacco:	Possible irregular heartbeat.

*See Glossary

TRAZODONE

BRAND NAMES

Desyrel
Trazon
Trialodine

BASIC INFORMATION

Habit forming? No
Prescription needed? Yes
Available as generic? Yes
Drug class: Antidepressant (nontricyclic)

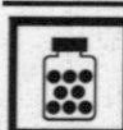

USES

- Treats mental depression.
- Treats anxiety.
- Treats some types of chronic pain.

DOSAGE & USAGE INFORMATION

How to take:
Tablet—Swallow with liquid or food to lessen stomach irritation. If you can't swallow whole, crumble tablet and take with liquid or food.

When to take:
According to prescription directions. Bedtime dose usually higher than other doses.

If you forget a dose:
Take as soon as you remember up to 2 hours late. If more than 2 hours, wait for next scheduled dose (don't double this dose).

What drug does:
Inhibits serotonin uptake in brain cells.

Continued next column

OVERDOSE

SYMPTOMS:
Fainting, irregular heartbeat, respiratory arrest, chest pain, seizures, coma.
WHAT TO DO:

- **Dial 911 (emergency) or 0 (operator) for an ambulance or medical help. Then give first aid immediately.**
- **If patient is unconscious and not breathing, give mouth-to-mouth breathing. If there is no heartbeat, use cardiac massage and mouth-to-mouth breathing (CPR). Don't try to make patient vomit. If you can't get help quickly, take patient to nearest emergency facility.**
- **See emergency information on inside covers.**

Time lapse before drug works:
2 to 4 weeks for full effect.

Don't take with:
Any other medicine without consulting your doctor or pharmacist.

POSSIBLE ADVERSE REACTIONS OR SIDE EFFECTS

SYMPTOMS	WHAT TO DO
Life-threatening: In case of overdose, see previous column.	
Common:	
Drowsiness.	Continue. Call doctor when convenient.
Infrequent:	
• Prolonged penile erections.	Seek emergency treatment immediately.
• Tremor, fainting, incoordination, blood pressue rise or drop, rapid heartbeat, shortness of breath.	Discontinue. Call doctor right away.
• Disorientation, confusion, fatigue, dizziness on standing, headache, nervousness, rash, itchy skin, blurred vision, ringing in ears, dry mouth, bad taste, diarrhea, nausea, vomiting, constipation, aching, menstrual changes, diminished sex drive, nightmares, vivid dreams.	Continue. Call doctor when convenient.
Rare:	
Unusual excitement	Discontinue. Call doctor right away.

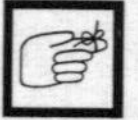

WARNINGS & PRECAUTIONS

Don't take if:

- You are allergic to trazodone.
- You are thinking about suicide.

Before you start, consult your doctor:

- If you have heart rhythm problem.
- If you have any heart disease.
- If you will have surgery within 2 months, including dental surgery, requiring general or spinal anesthesia.
- If you have liver or kidney disease.

Over age 60:
Adverse reactions and side effects may be more frequent and severe than in younger persons.

Pregnancy:
Decide with your doctor if drug benefits justify risk to unborn child. Risk category C (see page xxii).

Breast-feeding:
Drug passes into milk. Avoid drug or discontinue nursing until you finish medicine. Consult doctor for advice on maintaining milk supply.

Infants & children:
Not recommended.

Prolonged use:
Occasional blood counts, especially if you have fever and sore throat.

Skin & sunlight:
No problems expected.

Driving, piloting or hazardous work:
Don't drive or pilot aircraft until you learn how medicine affects you. Don't work around dangerous machinery. Don't climb ladders or work in high places. Danger increases if you drink alcohol or take medicine affecting alertness and reflexes, such as antihistamines, tranquilizers, sedatives, pain medicine, narcotics and mind-altering drugs.

Discontinuing:
Don't discontinue without consulting doctor. Dose may require gradual reduction if you have taken drug for a long time. Doses of other drugs may also require adjustment.

Others:
Electroshock therapy should be avoided.

POSSIBLE INTERACTION WITH OTHER DRUGS

GENERIC NAME OR DRUG CLASS	COMBINED EFFECT
Antidepressants*, other	Excess drowsiness.
Antihistamines*	Excess drowsiness.
Antihypertensives*	Possible too-low blood pressure. Avoid.
Barbiturates*	Too-low blood pressure. Avoid.
Central nervous system (CNS) depressants*	Increased sedation.
Digitalis preparations*	Possible increased digitalis level in blood.
Guanfacine	Increased effect of both medicines.
Monoamine oxidase (MAO) inhibitors*	May add to toxic effect of each.
Narcotics*	Excess drowsiness.
Phenytoin	Possible increased phenytoin level in blood.
Sedatives*	Excess drowsiness.
Sertraline	Increased depressive effects of both drugs.
Tranquilizers*	Excess drowsiness.

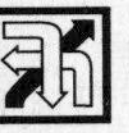

POSSIBLE INTERACTION WITH OTHER SUBSTANCES

INTERACTS WITH	COMBINED EFFECT
Alcohol:	Excess sedation. Avoid.
Beverages: Caffeine.	May add to heartbeat irregularity. Avoid.
Cocaine:	May add to heartbeat irregularity. Avoid.
Foods:	No problems expected.
Marijuana:	May add to heartbeat irregularity. Avoid.
Tobacco:	May add to heartbeat irregularity. Avoid.

*See Glossary

TRETINOIN (Topical)

BRAND NAMES

Retin-A Cream
Retin-A Cream Regimen Kit
Retin-A Gel
Retin-A Gel Regimen Kit
Retin-A Solution
Retinoic Acid
Stieva-A Cream
Stieva-A Cream Forte
Stieva-A Gel
Stieva-A Solution
Vitamin A Acid Cream
Vitamin A Acid Gel

BASIC INFORMATION

Habit forming? No
Prescription needed? Yes
Available as generic? Yes
Drug class: Anti-acne (topical), keratolytic

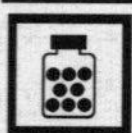

USES

- Treatment for acne, psoriasis, ichthyosis, keratosis, folliculitis, flat warts.
- Treatment for sun-damaged skin (wrinkles).

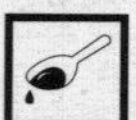

DOSAGE & USAGE INFORMATION

How to use:
Wash skin with nonmedicated soap, pat dry, wait 20 minutes before applying.
- Cream or gel—Apply to affected areas with fingertips and rub in gently.
- Solution—Apply to affected areas with gauze pad or cotton swab. Avoid getting too wet so medicine doesn't drip into eyes or mouth, onto lips or inside nose.
- Follow manufacturer's directions on container.

When to use:
At the same time each day.

If you forget an application:
Use as soon as you remember.

What drug does:
Increases skin cell turnover so skin layer peels off more easily.

Continued next column

OVERDOSE

SYMPTOMS:
None expected.
WHAT TO DO:
If person swallows drug, call doctor, poison control center or hospital emergency room for instructions.

Time lapse before drug works:
2 to 3 weeks. May require 6 weeks for maximum improvement.

Don't use with:
- Benzoyl peroxide. Apply 12 hours apart.
- Any other medicine without consulting your doctor or pharmacist.

POSSIBLE ADVERSE REACTIONS OR SIDE EFFECTS

SYMPTOMS	WHAT TO DO
Life-threatening:	
None expected.	
Common:	
• Pigment change in treated area, warmth or stinging, peeling.	Continue. Tell doctor at next visit.
• Sensitivity to wind or cold.	No action necessary.
Infrequent:	
Blistering, crusting, severe burning, swelling.	Discontinue. Call doctor right away.
Rare:	
None expected.	

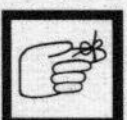

WARNINGS & PRECAUTIONS

Don't take if:
- You are allergic to tretinoin.
- You are sunburned, windburned or have an open skin wound.

Before you start, consult your doctor:
If you have eczema.

Over age 60:
Not recommended.

Pregnancy:
Discuss with your doctor if benefits outweigh risks to unborn child. Risk category C (see page xxii).

Breast-feeding:
Effect unknown. Consult doctor.

Infants & children:
Not recommended.

Prolonged use:
No problems expected.

Skin & sunlight:
- May cause rash or intensify sunburn in areas exposed to sun or sunlamp.
- In some animal studies, tretinoin caused skin tumors to develop faster when treated area was exposed to ultraviolet light (sunlight or sunlamp). No proven similar effects in humans.

Driving, piloting or hazardous work:
No problems expected.

Discontinuing:
Don't discontinue without doctor's advice until you complete prescribed dose, even though symptoms diminish or disappear.

Others:
Acne may get worse before improvement starts in 2 or 3 weeks. Don't wash face more than 2 or 3 times daily.

POSSIBLE INTERACTION WITH OTHER DRUGS

GENERIC NAME OR DRUG CLASS	COMBINED EFFECT
Antiacne topical preparations, other*	Severe skin irritation.
Cosmetics (medicated)	Severe skin irritation.
Etretinate	Increased chance of toxicity of each drug.
Skin preparations with alcohol	Severe skin irritation.
Soaps or cleansers (abrasive)	Severe skin irritation.

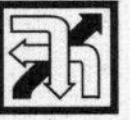

POSSIBLE INTERACTION WITH OTHER SUBSTANCES

INTERACTS WITH	COMBINED EFFECT
Alcohol:	None expected.
Beverages:	None expected.
Cocaine:	None expected.
Foods:	None expected.
Marijuana:	None expected.
Tobacco:	None expected.

*See Glossary

TRIAMCINOLONE

BRAND NAMES

See complete list of brand names in the *Brand Name Directory*, page 920.

BASIC INFORMATION

Habit forming? No
Prescription needed? Yes
Available as generic? Yes
Drug class: Cortisone drug (adrenal corticosteroid)

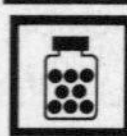

USES

- Reduces inflammation caused by many different medical problems.
- Treatment for some allergic diseases, blood disorders, kidney diseases, asthma and emphysema.
- Replaces corticosteroids lost due to deficiencies.

DOSAGE & USAGE INFORMATION

How to take:
- Tablet or syrup—Swallow with liquid or food to lessen stomach irritation. If you can't swallow whole, crumble tablet.
- Aerosol—Follow package instructions.

When to take:
At the same times each day. Take once-a-day or once-every-other-day doses in mornings.

If you forget a dose:
- Several-doses-per-day prescription—Take as soon as you remember up to 2 hours late. If more than 2 hours, wait for next scheduled dose (don't double this dose).
- Once-a-day dose or less—Wait for next dose. Double this dose.

What drug does:
Decreases inflammatory responses.

Time lapse before drug works:
2 to 4 days.

Continued next column

OVERDOSE

SYMPTOMS:
Headache, convulsions, heart failure.
WHAT TO DO:
- **Dial 911 (emergency) or 0 (operator) for an ambulance or medical help. Then give first aid immediately.**
- **See emergency information on inside covers.**

Don't take with:
Any other medicine without consulting your doctor or pharmacist.

POSSIBLE ADVERSE REACTIONS OR SIDE EFFECTS

SYMPTOMS	WHAT TO DO
Life-threatening:	
Hives, rash, intense itching, faintness soon after a dose (anaphylaxis).	Seek emergency treatment immediately.
Common:	
Acne, thirst, indigestion, nausea, vomiting, poor wound healing, decreased growth in children, constipation, gaseousness, unpleasant taste, diarrhea, headache, cough, dizziness, hoarseness, appetite gain or loss.	Continue. Call doctor when convenient.
Infrequent:	
• Black, bloody or tarry stool; various infections; swallowing difficulties.	Discontinue. Seek emergency treatment.
• Blurred vision, halos around lights, muscle cramps, swollen legs and feet, sore throat, fever.	Discontinue. Call doctor right away.
• Mood change, fatigue, weakness, insomnia, restlessness, frequent urination, weight gain, round face, menstrual irregularities, dry mouth, euphoria, nosebleeds.	Continue. Call doctor when convenient.
Rare:	
• Irregular heartbeat.	Discontinue. Seek emergency treatment.
• Rash, pancreatitis, numbness or tingling in hands or feet, thrombophlebitis, hallucinations, convulsions.	Discontinue. Call doctor right away.

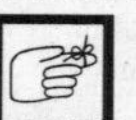

WARNINGS & PRECAUTIONS

Don't take if:
- You are allergic to any cortisone drug.
- You have tuberculosis or fungus infection.
- You have herpes infection of eyes, lips or genitals.

- You have bone disease, thyroid disease, colitis, peptic ulcer, diabetes, myasthenia gravis, liver or kidney disease, diverticulitis, glaucoma, heart disease.

Before you start, consult your doctor:
- If you have had tuberculosis.
- If you have congestive heart failure, diabetes, peptic ulcer, glaucoma, underactive thyroid, high blood pressure, myasthenia gravis, blood clots in legs or lungs.

Over age 60:
Adverse reactions and side effects may be more frequent and severe than in younger persons. Likely to aggravate edema, diabetes or ulcers. Likely to cause cataracts and osteoporosis (softening of the bones).

Pregnancy:
Decide with your doctor if drug benefits justify risk to unborn child. Risk category C (see page xxii).

Breast-feeding:
Drug passes into milk. Avoid drug or discontinue nursing until you finish medicine. Consult doctor for advice on maintaining milk supply.

Infants & children:
Use only under medical supervision.

Prolonged use:
- Retards growth in children.
- Possible glaucoma, cataracts, diabetes, fragile bones and thin skin.
- Functional dependence.
- Talk to your doctor about the need for follow-up medical examinations or laboratory studies to check blood pressure, serum electrolytes, stools for blood.

Skin & sunlight:
No problems expected.

Driving, piloting or hazardous work:
No problems expected.

Discontinuing:
- Don't discontinue without doctor's advice until you complete prescribed dose, even though symptoms diminish or disappear.
- Drug affects your response to surgery, illness, injury or stress for 2 years after discontinuing. Tell anyone who takes medical care of you within 2 years about drug.

Others:
- Avoid immunizations if possible.
- Your resistance to infection is less while taking this medicine.
- Advise any doctor or dentist whom you consult that you take this medicine.

POSSIBLE INTERACTION WITH OTHER DRUGS

GENERIC NAME OR DRUG CLASS	COMBINED EFFECT
Amphotericin B	Potassium depletion.
Anticholinergics*	Possible glaucoma.
Anticoagulants*, oral	Decreased anti-coagulant effect.
Anticonvulsants, hydantoin*	Decreased triamcinolone effect.
Antidiabetics*, oral	Decreased anti-diabetic effect.
Antihistamines*	Decreased triamcinolone effect.
Anti-inflammatory drugs nonsteroidal (NSAIDs)*	Increased risk of ulcers and triamcinolone effect.
Aspirin	Increased triamcinolone effect.
Attenuated virus vaccines*	Possible viral infection.
Barbiturates*	Decreased triamcinolone effect. Oversedation.
Chloral hydrate	Decreased triamcinolone effect.
Chlorthalidone	Potassium depletion.
Cholestyramine	Decreased triamci-nolone absorption.
Cholinergics*	Decreased cholinergic effect.

Continued on page 964

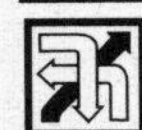

POSSIBLE INTERACTION WITH OTHER SUBSTANCES

INTERACTS WITH	COMBINED EFFECT
Alcohol:	Risk of stomach ulcers.
Beverages:	No proven problems.
Cocaine:	Overstimulation. Avoid.
Foods:	No proven problems.
Marijuana:	Decreased immunity.
Tobacco:	Increased triamcinolone effect Possible toxicity.

TRIAMTERENE

BRAND NAMES

Dyrenium

BASIC INFORMATION

Habit forming? No
Prescription needed? Yes
Available as generic? No
Drug class: Antihypertensive, diuretic

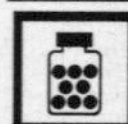

USES

- Reduces fluid retention (edema).
- Reduces potassium loss.

DOSAGE & USAGE INFORMATION

How to take:
Capsule—Swallow with liquid or food to lessen stomach irritation. If you can't swallow whole, open capsule and take with liquid or food.

When to take:
- 1 dose per day—Take after breakfast.
- More than 1 dose per day—Take last dose no later than 6 p.m.

If you forget a dose:
Take as soon as you remember up to 6 hours late. If more than 6 hours, wait for next scheduled dose (don't double this dose).

What drug does:
Increases urine production to eliminate sodium and water from body while conserving potassium.

Continued next column

OVERDOSE

SYMPTOMS:
Lethargy, nausea, vomiting, hypotension, irregular heartbeat, coma.
WHAT TO DO:
- **Dial 911 (emergency) or 0 (operator) for an ambulance or medical help. Then give first aid immediately.**
- **If patient is unconscious and not breathing, give mouth-to-mouth breathing. If there is no heartbeat, use cardiac massage and mouth-to-mouth breathing (CPR). Don't try to make patient vomit. If you can't get help quickly, take patient to nearest emergency facility.**
- **See emergency information on inside covers.**

Time lapse before drug works:
2 hours. May require 2 to 3 days for maximum benefit.

Don't take with:
Any other medicine without consulting your doctor or pharmacist.

POSSIBLE ADVERSE REACTIONS OR SIDE EFFECTS

SYMPTOMS	WHAT TO DO
Life-threatening:	
Hives, rash, intense itching, faintness soon after a dose (anaphylaxis).	Seek emergency treatment immediately.
Common:	
Constipation, decreased interest in sex.	Continue. Call doctor when convenient.
Infrequent:	
• Drowsiness, thirst, dry mouth, confusion, irregular heartbeat, shortness of breath, kidney stones, unusual tiredness, weakness, fever and chills, cracked mouth corners, black stools, dry mouth.	Discontinue. Call doctor right away.
• Diarrhea.	Continue. Call doctor when convenient.
• Anxiety.	Continue. Tell doctor at next visit.
Rare:	
• Rash, sore throat, red or inflamed tongue, unusual bleeding or bruising.	Discontinue. Call doctor right away.
• Headache.	Continue. Tell doctor at next visit.

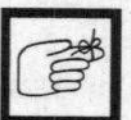

WARNINGS & PRECAUTIONS

Don't take if:
- You are allergic to triamterene.
- You have had severe liver or kidney disease.

Before you start, consult your doctor:
- If you have gout, diabetes, kidney stones.
- If you will have surgery within 2 months, including dental surgery, requiring general or spinal anesthesia.

Over age 60:
- Warm weather or fever can decrease blood pressure. Dose may require adjustment.
- Extended use can increase blood clots.

Pregnancy:
No proven harm to unborn child. Avoid if possible. Consult doctor. Risk category B (see page xxii).

Breast-feeding:
Safety not established. Consult doctor.

Infants & children:
Used infrequently. Use only under medical supervision.

Prolonged use:
- Potassium retention which may lead to heart rhythm problems.
- Talk to your doctor about the need for follow-up medical examinations or laboratory studies to check blood pressure, kidney function, ECG* and serum electrolytes.

Skin & sunlight:
May cause rash or intensify sunburn in areas exposed to sun or sunlamp.

Driving, piloting or hazardous work:
Avoid if you feel drowsy or confused. Otherwise, no problems expected.

Discontinuing:
Don't discontinue without consulting doctor. Dose may require gradual reduction if you have taken drug for a long time. Doses of other drugs may also require adjustment.

Others:
No problems expected.

POSSIBLE INTERACTION WITH OTHER DRUGS

GENERIC NAME OR DRUG CLASS	COMBINED EFFECT
Amantadine	Increased risk of amantadine toxicity.
Angiotensin-converting enzyme (ACE) inhibitors*	Possible excessive potassium in blood.
Antigout drugs*	Decreased antigout effect.
Antihypertensives*, other	Increased effect of other antihypertensives.
Anti-inflammatory drugs, nonsteroidal (NSAIDs)*	Possible excessive potassium in blood.
Carteolol	Increased anti-hypertensive effect.
Digitalis preparations*	Possible decreased digitalis effect.
Diuretics, potassium-sparing*, other	Possible excessive potassium levels.
Folic acid	Decreased folic acid effect.
Lithium	Increased lithium effect.
Nitrates*	Excessive blood pressure drop.
Potassium supplements*	Possible excessive potassium retention.
Potassium iodide	May raise potassium level in blood to toxic levels.

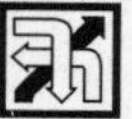

POSSIBLE INTERACTION WITH OTHER SUBSTANCES

INTERACTS WITH	COMBINED EFFECT
Alcohol:	None expected.
Beverages: Low-salt milk.	Possible potassium toxicity.
Cocaine:	Increased risk of heart block and high blood pressure.
Foods: Salt, substitutes.	Possible potassium toxicity.
Marijuana:	Daily use—Fainting likely.
Tobacco:	None expected.

*See Glossary

TRIAMTERENE & HYDROCHLOROTHIAZIDE

BRAND NAMES

Apo-Triazide
Dyazide
Maxzide
Novotriamzide

BASIC INFORMATION

Habit forming? No
Prescription needed? Yes
Available as generic? Yes
Drug class: Diuretic

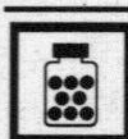

USES

- Reduces fluid retention (edema).
- Reduces potassium loss.
- Controls, but doesn't cure, high blood pressure.

DOSAGE & USAGE INFORMATION

How to take:
Tablet or capsule—Swallow with liquid. If you can't swallow whole, crumble tablet or open capsule and take with liquid or food.

When to take:
- 1 dose per day—Take after breakfast.
- More than 1 dose per day—Take last dose no later than 6 p.m.

If you forget a dose:
Take as soon as you remember up to 6 hours late. If more than 6 hours, wait for next scheduled dose (don't double this dose).

What drug does:
- Increases urine production to eliminate sodium and water from body while conserving potassium.
- Forces sodium and water excretion, reducing body fluid.
- Relaxes muscle cells of small arteries.
- Reduced body fluid and relaxed arteries lower blood pressure.

Continued next column

OVERDOSE

SYMPTOMS:
Lethargy, irregular heartbeat, cramps, nausea, vomiting, hypotension, weakness, drowsiness, weak pulse, coma.
WHAT TO DO:
- **Dial 911 (emergency) or 0 (operator) for an ambulance or medical help. Then give first aid immediately.**
- **See emergency information on inside covers.**

Time lapse before drug works:
4 to 6 hours. May require several weeks to lower blood pressure.

Don't take with:
Any prescription or nonprescription drugs without consulting your doctor.

POSSIBLE ADVERSE REACTIONS OR SIDE EFFECTS

SYMPTOMS	WHAT TO DO
Life-threatening:	
Irregular heartbeat, weak pulse, shortness of breath; hives, rash, intense itching, faintness soon after a dose (anaphylaxis).	Discontinue. Seek emergency treatment.
Common:	
• Mood change, muscle cramps.	Discontinue. Call doctor right away.
• Numbness or tingling in hands or feet, constipation, decreased interest in sex.	Continue. Call doctor when convenient.
Infrequent:	
• Blurred vision, abdominal pain, nausea, vomiting, kidney stones, fever and chills, red tongue, cracked mouth corners, black stools, dry mouth.	Discontinue. Call doctor right away.
• Dizziness, mood change, headache, weakness, tiredness, weight gain or loss.	Continue. Call doctor when convenient.
Rare:	
Sore throat, mouth sores, jaundice, rash, joint or muscle pain, hives, unexplained bleeding or bruising.	Discontinue. Call doctor right away.

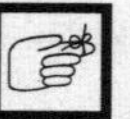

WARNINGS & PRECAUTIONS

Don't take if:
- If you are allergic to triamterene or any thiazide diuretic drug.
- If you have had severe liver or kidney disease.

Before you start, consult your doctor:
- If you have gout, diabetes, liver, pancreas or kidney disorder.
- You are allergic to any sulfa drug*.
- If you will have surgery within 2 months, including dental surgery, requiring general or spinal anesthesia.

TRIAMTERENE & HYDROCHLOROTHIAZIDE

Over age 60:

- Adverse reactions and side effects may be more frequent and severe than in younger persons, especially dizziness and excessive potassium loss.
- Warm weather or fever can decrease blood pressure. Dose may require adjustment.
- Extended use can increase blood clots.

Pregnancy:
Decide with your doctor if drug benefits justify risk to unborn child. Risk category C (see page xxii).

Breast-feeding:
Drug passes into milk. Avoid drug or discontinue nursing until you finish medicine. Consult doctor for advice on maintaining milk supply.

Infants & children:
Used infrequently. Use only under medical supervision.

Prolonged use:

- Potassium retention which may lead to heart rhythm problems.
- Talk to your doctor about the need for follow-up medical examinations or laboratory studies to check blood pressure, kidney function, ECG* and serum electrolytes.

Skin & sunlight:
May cause rash or intensify sunburn in areas exposed to sun or sunlamp.

Driving, piloting or hazardous work:
Don't drive or pilot aircraft until you learn how medicine affects you. Don't work around dangerous machinery. Don't climb ladders or work in high places. Danger increases if you drink alcohol or take medicine affecting alertness and reflexes, such as antihistamines, tranquilizers, sedatives, pain medicine, narcotics and mind-altering drugs.

Discontinuing:
Don't discontinue without consulting doctor. Dose may require gradual reduction if you have taken drug for a long time. Doses of other drugs may also require adjustment.

Others:

- Hot weather and fever may cause dehydration and drop in blood pressure. Dose may require temporary adjustment. Weigh daily and report any unexpected weight decreases to your doctor.
- May cause rise in uric acid, leading to gout.
- May cause blood sugar rise in diabetics.

POSSIBLE INTERACTION WITH OTHER DRUGS

GENERIC NAME OR DRUG CLASS	COMBINED EFFECT
Allopurinol	Decreased allopurinol effect.
Amantadine	Increased risk of amantadine toxicity.
Amphotericin B	Increased potassium.
Antidepressants*	Dangerous drop in blood pressure. Avoid combination unless under medical supervision.
Angiotensin-converting enzyme (ACE) inhibitors*	Possible excessive potassium in blood.
Antigout drugs*	Decreased antigout effect.
Antihypertensives*	Increased hypertensive effect.
Anti-inflammatory drugs, nonsteroidal (NSAIDs)*	Possible excessive potassium in blood.
Barbiturates*	Increased hydrochlorothiazide effect.
Beta-adrenergic blocking agents*	Increased antihypertensive effect. Dosages of both drugs may require adjustment.
Cholestyramine	Decreased hydrochlorothiazide effect.
Cortisone drugs*	Excessive potassium loss that causes dangerous heart rhythms.

Continued on page 965

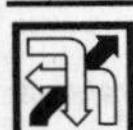

POSSIBLE INTERACTION WITH OTHER SUBSTANCES

INTERACTS WITH	COMBINED EFFECT
Alcohol:	Dangerous blood pressure drop.
Beverages: Low-salt milk.	Possible potassium toxicity.
Cocaine:	Decreased triamterene effect.
Foods: Salt, salt substitutes.	Possible potassium toxicity.
Marijuana:	Daily use—Fainting likely.
Tobacco:	Decreases drug's effectiveness.

***See Glossary**

TRIAZOLAM

BRAND NAMES

Apo-Triazo
Halcion
Novo-Triolam
Nu-Triazo

BASIC INFORMATION

Habit forming? Yes
Prescription needed? Yes
Available as generic? Yes
Drug class: Sedative (hypnotic)

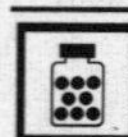

USES

- Treatment for insomnia.
- Prevention or treatment of transient insomnia associated with sudden sleep schedule changes such as travel across several time zones.

DOSAGE & USAGE INFORMATION

How to take:
Tablet—Swallow with liquid. If you can't swallow whole, crumble tablet and take with liquid or food.

When to take:
At the same time each day, according to instructions on prescription label.

If you forget a dose:
Take as soon as you remember up to 2 hours late. If more than 2 hours, wait for next scheduled dose (don't double this dose).

What drug does:
Affects limbic system of brain, the part that controls emotions.

Continued next column

OVERDOSE

SYMPTOMS:
Drowsiness, weakness, tremor, stupor, coma.
WHAT TO DO:

- **Dial 911 (emergency) or 0 (operator) for an ambulance or medical help. Then give first aid immediately.**
- **If patient is unconscious and not breathing, give mouth-to-mouth breathing. If there is no heartbeat, use cardiac massage and mouth-to-mouth breathing (CPR). Don't try to make patient vomit. If you can't get help quickly, take patient to nearest emergency facility.**
- **See emergency information on inside covers.**

Time lapse before drug works:
2 hours. May take 6 weeks for full benefit.

Don't take with:
Any prescription or nonprescription drugs without consulting your doctor.

POSSIBLE ADVERSE REACTIONS OR SIDE EFFECTS

SYMPTOMS	WHAT TO DO
Life-threatening: In case of overdose, see previous column.	
Common:	
Clumsiness, drowsiness, dizziness.	Continue. Call doctor when convenient.
Infrequent:	
• Amnesia, hallucinations, confusion, depression, irritability, rash, itch, vision changes, sore throat, fever, chills, dry mouth.	Discontinue. Call doctor right away.
• Constipation or diarrhea, nausea, vomiting, difficult urination, vivid dreams, behavior changes, abdominal pain, headache.	Continue. Call doctor when convenient.
Rare:	
• Slow heartbeat, breathing difficulty.	Discontinue. Seek emergency treatment.
• Mouth, throat ulcers; jaundice.	Discontinue. Call doctor right away.
• Decreased sex drive.	Continue. Call doctor when convenient.

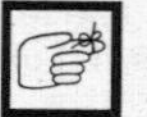

WARNINGS & PRECAUTIONS

Don't take if:

- You are allergic to any benzodiazepine.
- You have myasthenia gravis.
- You are an active or recovering alcoholic.
- Patient is younger than 6 months.

Before you start, consult your doctor:

- If you have liver, kidney or lung disease.
- If you have diabetes, epilepsy or porphyria.
- If you have glaucoma.

Over age 60:
Adverse reactions and side effects may be more frequent and severe than in younger persons. You may need smaller doses for shorter periods of time. You may develop agitation, rage or a "hangover" effect.

Pregnancy:
Risk to unborn child outweighs drug benefits. Don't use. Risk category X (see page xxii).

Breast-feeding:
Drug may pass into milk. Avoid drug or discontinue nursing until you finish medicine. Consult doctor for advice on maintaining milk supply.

Infants & children:
Use only under medical supervision for children older than 6 months.

Prolonged use:
May impair liver function.

Skin & sunlight:
No problems expected.

Driving, piloting or hazardous work:
Don't drive or pilot aircraft until you learn how medicine affects you. Don't work around dangerous machinery. Don't climb ladders or work in high places. Danger increases if you drink alcohol or take medicine affecting alertness and reflexes.

Discontinuing:
Don't discontinue without consulting doctor. Dose may require gradual reduction if you have taken drug for a long time. Doses of other drugs may also require adjustment.

Others:
- Hot weather, heavy exercise and profuse sweat may reduce excretion and cause overdose.
- Blood sugar may rise in diabetics, requiring insulin adjustment.
- Don't use for insomnia more than 4-7 days.
- Advise any doctor or dentist whom you consult that you take this medicine.
- Triazolam has a very short duration of action in the body.

POSSIBLE INTERACTION WITH OTHER DRUGS

GENERIC NAME OR DRUG CLASS	COMBINED EFFECT
Anticonvulsants*	Change in seizure frequency or severity.
Antidepressants*	Increased sedative effect of both drugs.
Antihistamines*	Increased sedative effect of both drugs.
Antihypertensives*	Excessively low blood pressure.
Central nervous system (CNS) depressants*, other	Increased central nervous system depression.
Cimetadine	Increased triazolam effect.
Clozapine	Toxic effect on the central nervous system.
Contraceptives, oral*	Increased triazolam effect.
Disulfiram	Increased triazolam effect.
Dronabinol	Increased effects of both drugs. Avoid.
Erythromycins*	Increased triazolam effect.
Isoniazid	Increased triazolam effect.
Ketoconazole	Increased triazolam effect.
Levodopa	Possible decreased levodopa effect.
Molindone	Increased tranquilizer effect.
Monoamine oxidase (MAO) inhibitors*	Convulsions, deep sedation, rage.
Nabilone	Greater depression of central nervous system.
Narcotics*	Increased sedative effect of both drugs.
Nizatidine	Increased effect and toxicity of triazolam.
Omeprazole	Delayed excretion of triazolam causing increased amount of triazolam in blood.

Continued on page 965

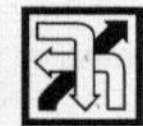

POSSIBLE INTERACTION WITH OTHER SUBSTANCES

INTERACTS WITH	COMBINED EFFECT
Alcohol:	Heavy sedation or amnesia. Avoid.
Beverages:	None expected.
Cocaine:	Decreased triazolam effect.
Foods:	None expected.
Marijuana:	Heavy sedation. Avoid.
Tobacco:	Decreased triazolam effect.

TRILOSTANE

BRAND NAMES

Modrastane

BASIC INFORMATION

Habit forming? No
Prescription needed? Yes
Available as generic? No
Drug class: Antiadrenal

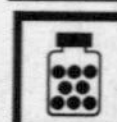

USES

Temporary treatment of Cushing's syndrome until surgery on adrenals or radiation to pituitary gland can be performed.

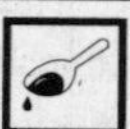

DOSAGE & USAGE INFORMATION

How to take:
Capsules—Swallow with liquid. If you can't swallow whole, open capsule and take with liquid or food. Instructions to take on empty stomach mean 1 hour before or 2 hours after eating.

When to take:
Follow doctor's instructions.

If you forget a dose:
Take as soon as you remember up to 2 hours late. If more than 2 hours, wait for next scheduled dose (don't double this dose).

What drug does:
Decreases function of the adrenal cortex.

Time lapse before drug works:
8 hours.

Don't take with:
Any other medicines (including over-the-counter drugs such as cough and cold medicines, laxatives, antacids, diet pills, caffeine, nose drops or vitamins) without consulting your doctor.

OVERDOSE

SYMPTOMS:
None expected.
WHAT TO DO:
Overdose unlikely to threaten life. If person takes much larger amount than prescribed, call doctor, poison control center or hospital emergency room for instructions.

POSSIBLE ADVERSE REACTIONS OR SIDE EFFECTS

SYMPTOMS	WHAT TO DO
Life-threatening: None expected.	
Common: Diarrhea, abdominal pain.	Discontinue. Call doctor right away.
Infrequent: Muscle ache, bloating, watery eyes, nausea, increased salivation, flushing, burning mouth or nose.	Continue. Call doctor when convenient.
Rare: Darkening skin, tiredness, appetite loss, depression, skin rash, vomiting.	Continue. Call doctor when convenient.

WARNINGS & PRECAUTIONS

Don't take if:
You know you are allergic to trilostane.

Before you start, consult your doctor:
- If you have an infection.
- If you will have surgery while taking.
- If you have a head injury.
- If you have kidney disease.

Over age 60:
Adverse reactions and side effects may be more frequent and severe than in younger persons. You may need smaller doses for shorter periods of time.

Pregnancy:
Risk to unborn child outweighs drug benefits. Don't use. Risk category X (see page xxii).

Breast-feeding:
Safety not established. Consult doctor.

Infants & children:
Effect not documented. Consult your pediatrician.

Prolonged use:
- Not intended for prolonged use.
- Talk to your doctor about the need for follow-up medical examinations or laboratory studies to check serum electrolytes and urinary 17 - hydroxycorticosteroid.

Skin & sunlight:
No problems expected.

Driving, piloting or hazardous work:
Avoid if you feel confused, drowsy or dizzy.

Discontinuing:
No special problems expected.

Others:
- Advise any doctor or dentist whom you consult that you take this medicine.
- May affect results in some medical tests.

POSSIBLE INTERACTION WITH OTHER DRUGS

GENERIC NAME OR DRUG CLASS	COMBINED EFFECT
Aminoglutethimide	Too much decrease in adrenal function.
Mitotane	Too much decrease in adrenal function.

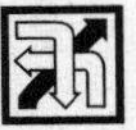

POSSIBLE INTERACTION WITH OTHER SUBSTANCES

INTERACTS WITH	COMBINED EFFECT
Alcohol:	No special problems expected.
Beverages:	No special problems expected.
Cocaine:	No special problems expected.
Foods:	No special problems expected.
Marijuana:	No special problems expected.
Tobacco:	No special problems expected.

TRIMETHOBENZAMIDE

BRAND NAMES

Arrestin	Tegamide
Benzacot	Ticon
Bio-Gan	Tigan
Stemetic	Tiject-20
T-Gen	Triban
Tebamide	Tribenzagan

BASIC INFORMATION

Habit forming? No
Prescription needed? Yes
Available as generic? Yes
Drug class: Antiemetic

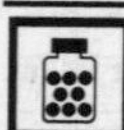

USES

Reduces nausea and vomiting.

DOSAGE & USAGE INFORMATION

How to take:

- Capsule—Swallow with liquid. If you can't swallow whole, open capsule and take with liquid or food.
- Suppositories—Remove wrapper and moisten suppository with water. Gently insert larger end into rectum. Push well into rectum with finger.

When to take:
When needed, no more often than label directs.

If you forget a dose:
Take when you remember. Wait as long as label directs for next dose.

Continued next column

OVERDOSE

SYMPTOMS:
Confusion, convulsions, coma.
WHAT TO DO:

- **Dial 911 (emergency) or 0 (operator) for an ambulance or medical help. Then give first aid immediately.**
- **If patient is unconscious and not breathing, give mouth-to-mouth breathing. If there is no heartbeat, use cardiac massage and mouth-to-mouth breathing (CPR). Don't try to make patient vomit. If you can't get help quickly, take patient to nearest emergency facility.**
- **See emergency information on inside covers.**

What drug does:
Possibly blocks nerve impulses to brain's vomiting centers.

Time lapse before drug works:
20 to 40 minutes.

Don't take with:
Any other prescription or nonprescription drugs without consulting doctor.

POSSIBLE ADVERSE REACTIONS OR SIDE EFFECTS

SYMPTOMS	WHAT TO DO
Life-threatening:	
In case of overdose, see previous column.	
Common:	
None expected.	
Infrequent:	
• Rash, blurred vision, low blood pressure.	Discontinue. Call doctor right away.
• Dizziness, headache, drowsiness, diarrhea, muscle cramps, unusual tiredness.	Continue. Call doctor when convenient.
Rare:	
• Convulsions.	Discontinue. Seek emergency treatment.
• Seizures, tremor, depression, sore throat, fever, repeated vomiting, back pain, jaundice, Parkinson symptoms, neck spasms.	Discontinue. Call doctor right away.

WARNINGS & PRECAUTIONS

Don't take if:

- You are allergic to trimethobenzamide.
- You are allergic to local anesthetics and have suppository form.

Before you start, consult your doctor:
If you have reacted badly to antihistamines.

Over age 60:
More susceptible to low blood pressure and sedative effects of this drug.

Pregnancy:
Decide with your doctor if drug benefits justify risk to unborn child. Risk category C (see page xxii).

Breast-feeding:
Effect unknown. Avoid if possible. Consult doctor.

Infants & children:
- Injectable form not recommended.
- Avoid during viral infections. Drug may contribute to Reye's syndrome.

Prolonged use:
- Damages blood cell production of bone marrow.
- Causes Parkinson's-like symptoms of tremors, rigidity.

Skin & sunlight:
Possible sun sensitivity. Use caution.

Driving, piloting or hazardous work:
- Use disqualifies you for piloting aircraft.
- Don't drive until you learn how medicine affects you. Don't work around dangerous machinery. Don't climb ladders or work in high places. Danger increases if you drink alcohol or take medicine affecting alertness and reflexes, such as antihistamines, tranquilizers, sedatives, pain medicine, narcotics and mind-altering drugs.

Discontinuing:
May be unnecessary to finish medicine. Follow doctor's instructions.

Others:
No problems expected.

POSSIBLE INTERACTION WITH OTHER DRUGS

GENERIC NAME OR DRUG CLASS	COMBINED EFFECT
Antidepressants*	Increased sedative effect.
Antihistamines*	Increased sedative effect.
Barbiturates*	Increased effect of both drugs.
Belladonna	Increased effect of both drugs.
Cholinergics*	Increased effect of both drugs.
Clozapine	Toxic effect on the central nervous system.
Ethinamate	Dangerous increased effects of ethinamate. Avoid combining.
Fluoxetine	Increased depressant effects of both drugs.
Guanfacine	May increase depressant effects of either medicine.
Leucovorin	High alcohol content of leucovorin may cause adverse effects.
Methyprylon	May increase sedative effect to dangerous level. Avoid.
Mind-altering drugs*	Increased effect of mind-altering drug.
Nabilone	Greater depression of central nervous system.
Narcotics*	Increased sedative effect.
Ototoxic medications*	May mask the symptoms of ototoxicity.
Phenothiazines*	Increased effect of both drugs.
Sedatives*	Increased sedative effect.
Sertraline	Increased depressive effects of both drugs.
Sleep inducers*	Increased effect of sleep inducer.
Tranquilizers*	Increased sedative effect.

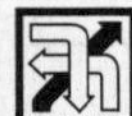

POSSIBLE INTERACTION WITH OTHER SUBSTANCES

INTERACTS WITH	COMBINED EFFECT
Alcohol:	Oversedation. Avoid.
Beverages:	None expected.
Cocaine:	None expected.
Foods:	None expected.
Marijuana:	Increased antinausea effect.
Tobacco:	None expected.

TRIMETHOPRIM

BRAND NAMES

Apo-Sulfatrim
Apo-Sulfatrim DS
Bactrim
Bactrim DS
Bethaprim
Cheragan with TMP
Cotrim
Cotrim DS
Novotrimel
Nu-Cotrimox
Nu-Cotrimox DS
Proloprim
Protrin
Roubac
Septra
Septra DS
SMZ-TMP
Sulfamethoprim
Sulfamethoprim DS
Sulfaprim
Sulfaprim DS
Sulfatrim
Sulfatrim DS
Sulfoxaprim
Sulfoxaprim DS
Sulmeprim
Triazole
Triazole DS
Trimeth-Sulfa
Trimpex
Trisulfam
Uroplus DS
Uroplus SS

BASIC INFORMATION

Habit forming? No
Prescription needed? Yes
Available as generic? Yes
Drug class: Antimicrobial (antibacterial)

USES

- Treats urinary tract infections susceptible to trimethoprim.
- Helps prevent recurrent urinary tract infections if taken once a day.
- Treats pneumocystis carinii pneumonia.

DOSAGE & USAGE INFORMATION

How to take:
Tablet—Swallow with liquid or food to lessen stomach irritation.

When to take:
Space doses evenly in 24 hours to keep constant amount in urine.

Continued next column

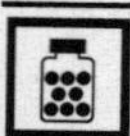

OVERDOSE

SYMPTOMS:
Nausea, vomiting, diarrhea.
WHAT TO DO:
Overdose unlikely to threaten life. If person takes much larger amount than prescribed, call doctor, poison control center or hospital emergency room for instructions.

If you forget a dose:
Take as soon as possible. Wait 5 to 6 hours before next dose. Then return to regular schedule.

What drug does:
Stops harmful bacterial germs from multiplying. Will not kill viruses.

Time lapse before drug works:
2 to 5 days.

Don't take with:
Any other medicine without consulting your doctor or pharmacist.

POSSIBLE ADVERSE REACTIONS OR SIDE EFFECTS

SYMPTOMS	WHAT TO DO
Life-threatening: None expected.	
Common:	
• Rash, itchy skin.	Discontinue. Seek emergency treatment.
• Unusual taste.	Continue. Call doctor when convenient.
Infrequent:	
• Diarrhea, nausea, vomiting, abdominal pain.	Discontinue. Call doctor right away.
• Headache, appetite loss, sore mouth or tongue.	Continue. Call doctor when convenient.
Rare:	
• Blue fingernails, lips and skin; difficult breathing.	Discontinue. Seek emergency treatment.
• Sore throat, fever, anemia, jaundice, unusual bleeding or bruising.	Discontinue. Call doctor right away.

WARNINGS & PRECAUTIONS

Don't take if:
- You are allergic to trimethoprim or any sulfa drug*.
- You are anemic due to folic acid deficiency.

Before you start, consult your doctor:
If you have had liver or kidney disease.

Over age 60:
- Reduced liver and kidney function may require reduced dose.
- More likely to have severe anal and genital itch.
- Increased susceptibility to anemia.

Pregnancy:
Decide with your doctor whether drug benefits justify risk to unborn child. Risk category C (see page xxii).

Breast-feeding:
No proven harm to unborn child. Avoid if possible. Consult doctor.

Infants & children:
Use under medical supervision only.

Prolonged use:
- Anemia.
- Talk to your doctor about the need for follow-up medical examinations or laboratory studies to check complete blood counts (white blood cell count, platelet count, red blood cell count, hemoglobin, hematocrit).

Skin & sunlight:
May cause rash or intensify sunburn in areas exposed to sun or sunlamp.

Driving, piloting or hazardous work:
No problems expected.

Discontinuing:
Don't discontinue without doctor's advice until you complete prescribed dose, even though symptoms diminish or disappear.

Others:
No problems expected.

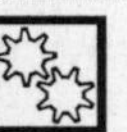

POSSIBLE INTERACTION WITH OTHER DRUGS

GENERIC NAME OR DRUG CLASS	COMBINED EFFECT
Bone marrow depressants*	Increased possibility of bone marrow supression.
Folate antagonists*, other	Increased risk of anemia.
Phenytoin	Increased phenytoin effect.

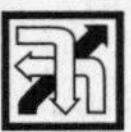

POSSIBLE INTERACTION WITH OTHER SUBSTANCES

INTERACTS WITH	COMBINED EFFECT
Alcohol:	Increased alcohol effect with Bactrim or Septra.
Beverages:	None expected.
Cocaine:	No proven problems.
Foods:	None expected.
Marijuana:	None expected.
Tobacco:	None expected.

***See Glossary**

URSODIOL

BRAND NAMES

Actigall
Ursofalk

BASIC INFORMATION

Habit forming? No
Prescription needed? Yes
Available as generic? No
Drug class: Anticholelithic

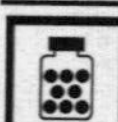

USES

Dissolves cholesterol gallstones in selected patients who either can't tolerate surgery or don't require surgery for other reasons. Not used when surgery is clearly indicated.

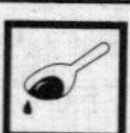

DOSAGE & USAGE INFORMATION

How to take:
Capsules—Swallow with liquid or food to lessen stomach irritation. If you can't swallow whole, open capsule and take with liquid or food.

When to take:
With meals, 2 or 3 times a day according to your doctor's instructions.

If you forget a dose:
Take as soon as you remember up to 2 hours late. If more than 2 hours, wait for next scheduled time. Don't double this dose.

What drug does:
Decreases secretion of cholesterol into bile by suppressing production and secretion of cholesterol by the liver. Ursodiol will not help gallstone problems unless the gallstones are made of cholesterol. It works best when the stones are small.

Time lapse before drug works:
Unpredictable. Varies among patients.

Don't take with:
Any other medicine without consulting your doctor or pharmacist.

OVERDOSE

SYMPTOMS:
Severe diarrhea.
WHAT TO DO:
Overdose not expected to threaten life. If person takes much larger amount than prescribed, call doctor, poison control center or hospital emergency room for instructions.

POSSIBLE ADVERSE REACTIONS OR SIDE EFFECTS

SYMPTOMS	WHAT TO DO
Life-threatening: None expected.	
Common: None expected.	
Infrequent: None expected.	
Rare: Diarrhea.	Continue. Call doctor when convenient.

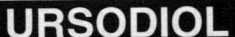

WARNINGS & PRECAUTIONS

Don't take if:
You can't tolerate other bile acids.

Before you start, consult your doctor:
- If you have complications of gallstones, such as infection or obstruction of the bile ducts.
- If you have had pancreatitis.
- If you have had chronically impaired liver function.
- If you take any other medicines for any reason.

Over age 60:
No special problems expected.

Pregnancy:
Consult doctor. Risk category B (see page xxii).

Breast-feeding:
Unknown, but no documented problems. Consult doctor.

Infants & children:
Not recommended. Adequate studies have not been performed.

Prolonged use:
- No special problems expected.
- Talk to your doctor about the need for follow-up medical examinations or laboratory studies to check kidney function.

Skin & sunlight:
No problems expected.

Driving, piloting or hazardous work:
Don't pilot aircraft until you learn how medicine affects you. Don't work around dangerous machinery. Don't climb ladders or work in high places. Danger increases if you drink alcohol or take medicine affecting alertness and reflexes, such as antihistamines, tranquilizers, sedatives, pain medicine, narcotics and mind-altering drugs.

Discontinuing:
Don't discontinue without consulting doctor.

Others:
Plan regular visits to your doctor while you take ursodiol. Have ultrasound and liver function studies done at appropriate intervals. Liver damage is unlikely, but theoretically could happen.

POSSIBLE INTERACTION WITH OTHER DRUGS

GENERIC NAME OR DRUG CLASS	COMBINED EFFECT
Antacids* (aluminum-containing)	Decreased absorption of ursodiol.
Cholestyramine	Decreased absorption of ursodiol.
Clofibrate	Decreased effect of ursodiol.
Colestipol	Decreased absorption of ursodiol.
Estrogens*	Decreased effect of ursodiol.
Progestins	Decreased effect of ursodiol.

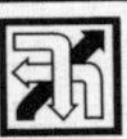

POSSIBLE INTERACTION WITH OTHER SUBSTANCES

INTERACTS WITH	COMBINED EFFECT
Alcohol:	None expected, unless you have impaired liver function from alcohol abuse.
Beverages:	None expected.
Cocaine:	None expected.
Foods:	None expected.
Marijuana:	None expected.
Tobacco:	None reported. However, tobacco may possibly impair intestinal absorption from the intestinal tract. Better to avoid.

*See Glossary

VALPROIC ACID (Dipropylacetic Acid)

BRAND NAMES

Depakene
Myproic Acid

BASIC INFORMATION

Habit forming? No
Prescription needed? Yes
Available as generic? Yes
Drug class: Anticonvulsant

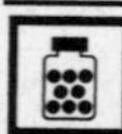

USES

- Controls petit mal (absence) seizures in treatment of epilepsy.
- Treatment for manic-depressive illness.

DOSAGE & USAGE INFORMATION

How to take:
Capsule or syrup—Swallow with liquid or food to lessen stomach irritation.

When to take:
Once a day.

If you forget a dose:
Take as soon as you remember. Don't ever double dose.

What drug does:
Increases concentration of gamma aminobutyric acid, which inhibits nerve transmission in parts of brain.

Time lapse before drug works:
1 to 4 hours.

Don't take with:
Any other medicine without consulting your doctor or pharmacist.

OVERDOSE

SYMPTOMS:
Coma
WHAT TO DO:

- **Dial 911 (emergency) or 0 (operator) for an ambulance or medical help. Then give first aid immediately.**
- **If patient is unconscious and not breathing, give mouth-to-mouth breathing. If there is no heartbeat, use cardiac massage and mouth-to-mouth breathing (CPR). Don't try to make patient vomit. If you can't get help quickly, take patient to nearest emergency facility.**
- **See emergency information on inside covers.**

POSSIBLE ADVERSE REACTIONS OR SIDE EFFECTS

SYMPTOMS	WHAT TO DO
Life-threatening: In case of overdose, see previous column.	
Common: Menstrual irregularities. nausea, vomiting, abdominal cramps, diarrhea, tremor, weight gain.	Continue. Call doctor when convenient.
Infrequent:	
• Rash, blood spots under skin, hair loss, bleeding (heart and lungs), easy bruising.	Discontinue. Call doctor right away.
• Sleepiness, weakness, easily upset emotionally, depression, psychic changes, headache, incoordination, appetite change, constipation.	Continue. Call doctor when convenient.
Rare:	
• Double vision, unusual movements of eyes (nystagmus), swelling of feet, ankles and abdomen; jaundice; increased bleeding tendency.	Discontinue. Call doctor right away.
• Anemia (paleness, fatigue).	Continue. Call doctor when convenient.

WARNINGS & PRECAUTIONS

Don't take if:
You are allergic to valproic acid.

Before you start, consult your doctor:

- If you have blood, kidney or liver disease.
- If you will have surgery within 2 months, including dental surgery, requiring general or spinal anesthesia.

Over age 60:
Adverse reactions and side effects may be more frequent and severe than in younger persons.

Pregnancy:
Risk to unborn child exists. Don't use. Risk category D (see page xxii).

Breast-feeding:
Drug passes into milk. Avoid drug or discontinue nursing until you finish medicine. Consult doctor for advice on maintaining milk supply.

Infants & children:
Under close medical supervision only.

VALPROIC ACID (Dipropylacetic Acid)

Prolonged use:
Request periodic blood tests, liver and kidney function tests.

Skin & sunlight:
No problems expected.

Driving, piloting or hazardous work:
Don't drive or pilot aircraft until you learn how medicine affects you. Don't work around dangerous machinery. Don't climb ladders or work in high places. Danger increases if you drink alcohol or take medicine affecting alertness and reflexes, such as antihistamines, tranquilizers, sedatives, pain medicine, narcotics and mind-altering drugs.

Discontinuing:
Don't discontinue without consulting doctor. Dose may require gradual reduction if you have taken drug for a long time. Doses of other drugs may also require adjustment.

Others:
No problems expected.

POSSIBLE INTERACTION WITH OTHER DRUGS

GENERIC NAME OR DRUG CLASS	COMBINED EFFECT
Anticoagulants*, oral	Increased chance of bleeding.
Aspirin	Increased chance of bleeding.
Carbamazepine	Decreased valproic acid effect.
Central nervous system (CNS) depressants*	Increased sedative effect.
Clonazepam	May prolong seizure.
Clozapine	Toxic effect on bone marrow.
Didanosine	Increased risk of pancreatitis.
Dipyridamole	Increased chance of bleeding.
Felbamate	Increased side effects and adverse reactions.
Flecainide	Possible decreased blood cell production in bone marrow.
Hepatotoxics*	Increased risk of liver toxicity.
Isoniazid	Increased risk of liver damage.
Levocarnitine	Decreased levocarnitine. Patients taking valproic acid may need to take the supplement levocarnitine.
Mefloquine	Decreased valproic acid effect.
Monoamine oxidase (MAO) inhibitors*	Increased sedative effect.
Nabilone	Greater depression of central nervous system.
Phenobarbital	Increased chance of toxicity.
Phenytoin	Unpredictable. Dose may require adjustment.
Primidone	Increased chance of toxicity.
Sertraline	Increased depressive effects of both drugs.
Sodium benzoate & sodium phenylacetate	May reduce effect of sodium benzoate & sodium phenylacetate.
Sulfinpyrazone	Increased chance of bleeding.
Tiopronin	Increased risk of toxicity to bone marrow.
Tocainide	Possible decreased blood cell production in bone marrow.

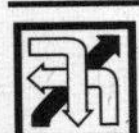

POSSIBLE INTERACTION WITH OTHER SUBSTANCES

INTERACTS WITH	COMBINED EFFECT
Alcohol:	Deep sedation. Avoid.
Beverages:	No problems expected.
Cocaine:	Increased brain sensitivity. Avoid.
Foods:	No problems expected.
Marijuana:	Increased brain sensitivity. Avoid.
Tobacco:	Decreased valproic acid effect.

*See Glossary

VANCOMYCIN

BRAND NAMES

Vancocin

BASIC INFORMATION

Habit forming? No
Prescription needed? Yes
Available as generic? Yes
Drug class: Antibiotic, antibacterial

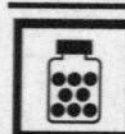

USES

- Treats colitis when caused by *clostridium* infections.
- Treats some forms of severe diarrhea.

DOSAGE & USAGE INFORMATION

How to take:

- Capsules—Swallow with liquid. If you can't swallow whole, open capsule and take with liquid or food. Instructions to take on empty stomach mean 1 hour before or 2 hours after eating.
- Oral solution—Use the calibrated measuring device. Swallow with other liquid to prevent nausea.
- There is also an injectable form. This information applies to the oral form only.

When to take:
According to doctor's instructions. Usually every 6 hours.

If you forget a dose:
Take as soon as you remember up to 2 hours late. If more than 2 hours, wait for next scheduled dose (don't double this dose).

What drug does:
Kills bacterial cells.

Time lapse before drug works:
None. Works right away. This medicine is not absorbed to a great extent through the intestinal tract.

Continued next column

OVERDOSE

SYMPTOMS:
None expected.
WHAT TO DO:
Overdose unlikely to threaten life. If person takes much larger amount than prescribed, call doctor, poison control center or hospital emergency room for instructions.

Don't take with:
Any other medicines (including over-the-counter drugs such as cough and cold medicines, laxatives, antacids, diet pills, caffeine, nose drops or vitamins) without consulting your doctor.

POSSIBLE ADVERSE REACTIONS OR SIDE EFFECTS

SYMPTOMS	WHAT TO DO
Life-threatening: None expected.	
Common: Bitter taste.	Continue. Tell doctor at next visit.
Infrequent: Nausea or vomiting.	Continue. Tell doctor at next visit.
Rare: Hearing loss, ears ringing or buzzing.	Discontinue. Call doctor right away.

WARNINGS & PRECAUTIONS

Don't take if:
You are allergic to vancomycin.

Before you start, consult your doctor:
- If you have hearing problems.
- If you have severe kidney disease.
- If you have intestinal obstruction.

Over age 60:
Adverse reactions and side effects may be more frequent and severe than in younger persons. You may need smaller doses for shorter periods of time.

Pregnancy:
Consult doctor. Risk category B (see page xxii).

Breast-feeding:
No special problems expected. Consult doctor.

Infants & children:
No special problems expected.

Prolonged use:
Talk to your doctor about the need for follow-up medical examinations or laboratory studies to check hearing acuity, kidney function, vancomycin serum concentration and urinalyses.

Skin & sunlight:
No problems expected.

Driving, piloting or hazardous work:
No problems expected.

Discontinuing:
No special problems expected.

Others:
- Advise any doctor or dentist whom you consult that you take this medicine.
- May affect results in some medical tests.

POSSIBLE INTERACTION WITH OTHER DRUGS

GENERIC NAME OR DRUG CLASS	COMBINED EFFECT
Cholestyramine	Decreased therapeutic effect of vancomycin.
Colestipol	Decreased therapeutic effect of vancomycin.
Nephrotoxics*	Increased risk of liver toxicity.

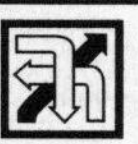

POSSIBLE INTERACTION WITH OTHER SUBSTANCES

INTERACTS WITH	COMBINED EFFECT
Alcohol:	No special problems expected.
Beverages:	No special problems expected.
Cocaine:	No special problems expected.
Foods:	No special problems expected.
Marijuana:	No special problems expected.
Tobacco:	No special problems expected.

***See Glossary**

VENLAFAXINE

BRAND NAMES

Effexor

BASIC INFORMATION

Habit forming? Not known
Prescription needed? Yes
Available as generic? No
Drug class: Bicyclic antidepressant

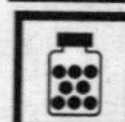

USES

Treats mental depression.

DOSAGE & USAGE INFORMATION

How to use:
Tablet—Swallow with liquid and take with food to lessen stomach irritation.

When to use:
At the same times each day (usually with meals or with a snack).

If you forget a dose:
Take as soon as you remember up to 2 hours late. If more than 2 hours, wait for the next scheduled dose (don't double this dose).

What drug does:
Increases the amount of certain chemicals in the brain that are required for the transmission of messages between nerve cells.

Time lapse before drug works:
Begins in 1 to 3 weeks, but may take 4 to 6 weeks for maximum benefit.

Don't take with:
Any other medication without consulting your doctor.

OVERDOSE

SYMPTOMS:
May cause no symptoms, or there may be extreme drowsiness, convulsions or rapid heartbeat.
WHAT TO DO:

- **Dial 911 (emergency) or 0 (operator) for an ambulance or medical help. Then give first aid immediately.**
- **See emergency information on inside covers.**

POSSIBLE ADVERSE REACTIONS OR SIDE EFFECTS

SYMPTOMS	WHAT TO DO
Life-threatening: In case of overdose, see previous column.	
Common:	
• Fast heartbeat, blurred vision, increased blood pressure.	Discontinue. Call doctor right away.
• Stomach pain, gas, insomnia or drowsiness, dizziness, decreased sexual drive, impotence, nausea or vomiting, headache, diarrhea or constipation, dryness of mouth, skin flushing, rash, loss of appetite, unusual tiredness, weakness, strange dreams, sweating, tremors, nervousness, headache.	Continue. Call doctor when convenient.
Infrequent:	
• Lightheadedness or faintness when arising from a sitting or lying position, mood or behavior changes, mental changes, difficulty in urinating.	Continue. Call doctor when convenient.
• Weight loss or gain, changes in taste, ringing in ears.	Continue. Tell doctor at next visit.
Rare:	
Seizures.	Discontinue. Seek emergency help.

WARNINGS & PRECAUTIONS

Don't take if:
You are allergic to venlafaxine.

Before you start, consult your doctor:
- If you have liver or kidney disease.
- If you have high blood pressure.
- If you have thoughts about suicide.
- If you are allergic to any other medications.
- If you have a history of seizures.

Over age 60:
Adverse reactions and side effects may be more severe than in younger persons.

Pregnancy:
Decide with your doctor if drug benefits justify any possible risk to unborn child. Risk category C (see page xxii).

Breast-feeding:
It is unknown if drug passes into milk. Avoid nursing until you finish medicine. Consult doctor for advice on maintaining milk supply.

Infants & children:
Safety in children under age 18 has not been established. Use only under close medical supervision.

Prolonged use:
Consult with your doctor on a regular basis while taking this drug to check your progress, to monitor your blood pressure and to determine the need for continued treatment.

Skin & sunlight:
No special problems expected.

Driving, piloting or hazardous work:
Don't drive or pilot aircraft until you learn how medicine affects you. Don't work around dangerous machinery. Don't climb ladders or work in high places. Danger increases if you drink alcohol or take medicine affecting alertness and reflexes.

Discontinuing:
Don't discontinue this drug without consulting doctor. Dosage may require a gradual reduction before stopping.

Others:
- Get up slowly from a sitting or lying position to avoid any dizziness, faintness or lightheadedness.
- Advise any doctor or dentist whom you consult that you take this medicine.
- Take medicine only as directed. Do not increase or reduce dosage without doctor's approval.

POSSIBLE INTERACTION WITH OTHER DRUGS

GENERIC NAME OR DRUG CLASS	COMBINED EFFECT
Antidepressants*, other	Increased sedative effect. Not recommended.
Central nervous system (CNS) depressants*, other	Increased sedative effect.
Cimetidine	Increased risk of adverse reactions.
Monoamine oxidase (MAO) inhibitors*	Increased risk and severity of adverse reactions. Allow 14 days between use of the two drugs.
Quinidine	Increased risk of venlafaxine toxicity.

POSSIBLE INTERACTION WITH OTHER SUBSTANCES

INTERACTS WITH	COMBINED EFFECT
Alcohol:	Increased sedative affect. Avoid.
Beverages:	None expected.
Cocaine:	Effect not known. Best to avoid.
Foods:	None expected.
Marijuana:	Effect not known. Best to avoid.
Tobacco:	None expected.

***See Glossary**

VITAMIN A

BRAND NAMES

Acon
Afaxin
Alphalin
Aquasol A
Dispatabs
Sust-A

Numerous multiple vitamin-mineral supplements. Check labels.

BASIC INFORMATION

Habit forming? No
Prescription needed? No
Available as generic? Yes
Drug class: Vitamin supplement

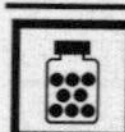

USES

- Dietary supplement to ensure normal growth and health, especially of eyes and skin.
- Beta carotene form decreases severity of sun exposure in patients with porphyria.

DOSAGE & USAGE INFORMATION

How to take:
- Drops or capsule—Swallow with liquid. If you can't swallow whole, open capsule and take with liquid or food.
- Oral solution—Swallow with liquid.
- Tablet—Swallow with liquid.

When to take:
At the same time each day.

If you forget a dose:
Take as soon as you remember, then resume regular schedule.

What drug does:
- Prevents night blindness.
- Promotes normal growth and health.

Continued next column

OVERDOSE

SYMPTOMS:
Increased adverse reactions and side effects. Jaundice (rare, but may occur with large doses), malaise, vomiting, irritability, bleeding gums, seizures, double vision, peeling skin.
WHAT TO DO:
If person takes much larger amount than prescribed, call doctor, poison control center or hospital emergency room for instructions.

Time lapse before drug works:
Requires continual intake.

Don't take with:
Any other medicine without consulting your doctor or pharmacist.

POSSIBLE ADVERSE REACTIONS OR SIDE EFFECTS

SYMPTOMS	WHAT TO DO
Life-threatening: In case of overdose, see previous column.	
Common: None expected.	
Infrequent: Confusion; dizziness; drowsiness; headache; irritability; dry, cracked lips; peeling skin; hair loss; sensitvity to light.	Continue. Call doctor when convenient.
Rare:	
• Bulging soft spot on baby's head, double vision, bone or joint pain, abdominal pain, frequent urination.	Discontinue. Call doctor right away.
• Diarrhea, appetite loss, nausea, vomiting.	Continue. Call doctor when convenient.

WARNINGS & PRECAUTIONS

Don't take if:
You have chronic kidney failure.

Before you start, consult your doctor:
If you have any kidney disorder.

Over age 60:
No problems expected.

Pregnancy:
Risk factor determined by length of pregnancy and dosage amount. See category list on page xxii and consult doctor.

Breast-feeding:
No problems expected. Consult doctor.

Infants & children:
- Avoid large doses.
- Keep vitamin-mineral supplements out of children's reach.

Prolonged use:
No problems expected.

Skin & sunlight:
Increased sensitivity to light.

Driving, piloting or hazardous work:
No problems expected.

Discontinuing:
Don't discontinue without doctor's advice until you complete prescribed dose, even though symptoms diminish or disappear.

Others:
- Don't exceed dose. Too much over a long time may be harmful.
- A balanced diet should provide all the vitamin A a healthy person needs and prevent need for supplements. Best sources are liver, yellow-orange fruits and vegetables, dark-green, leafy vegetables, milk, butter and margarine.

POSSIBLE INTERACTION WITH OTHER DRUGS

GENERIC NAME OR DRUG CLASS	COMBINED EFFECT
Anticoagulants*	Increased anticoagulant effect with large doses (over 10,000 I.U.) of vitamin A.
Calcium supplements*	Decreased vitamin effect.
Cholestyramine	Decreased vitamin A absorption.
Colestipol	Decreased vitamin absorption.
Contraceptives, oral*	Increased vitamin A levels.
Etretinate	Increased risk of toxic effects.
Isotretinoin	Increased risk of toxic effect of each.
Mineral oil (long-term)	Decreased vitamin A absorption.
Neomycin	Decreased vitamin absorption.
Vitamin A derivatives, other	Increased toxicity risk.
Vitamin E (excess dose)	Vitamin A depletion.

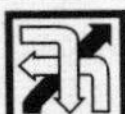

POSSIBLE INTERACTION WITH OTHER SUBSTANCES

INTERACTS WITH	COMBINED EFFECT
Alcohol:	None expected.
Beverages:	None expected.
Cocaine:	None expected.
Foods:	None expected.
Marijuana:	None expected.
Tobacco:	None expected.

*See Glossary

VITAMIN B-12 (Cyanocobalamin)

BRAND AND GENERIC NAMES

Acti-B-12
Alphamin
Alpha Redisol
Anocobin
Bedoz
Berubigen
Betalin 12
Codroxomin
Cyanabin
CYANOCOBALAMIN
Droxomin
HYDROXOCOBAL-AMIN
Kaybovite
Kaybovite-1000
Redisol
Rubion
Rubramin
Rubramin-PC

Numerous other multiple vitamin-mineral supplements.

BASIC INFORMATION

Habit forming? No
Prescription needed? No
Available as generic? Yes
Drug class: Vitamin supplement

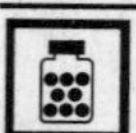

USES

- Dietary supplement for normal growth, development and health.
- Treatment for nerve damage.
- Treatment for pernicious anemia.
- Treatment and prevention of vitamin B-12 deficiencies in people who have had stomach or intestines surgically removed.
- Prevention of vitamin B-12 deficiency in strict vegetarians and persons with absorption diseases.

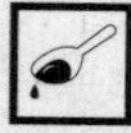

DOSAGE & USAGE INFORMATION

How to take:
- Tablets—Swallow with liquid.
- Injection—Follow doctor's directions.

When to take:
- Oral—At the same time each day.
- Injection—Follow doctor's directions.

Continued next column

OVERDOSE

SYMPTOMS:
Increased adverse reactions and side effects.
WHAT TO DO:
Overdose unlikely to threaten life. If person takes much larger amount than prescribed, call doctor, poison control center or hospital emergency room for instructions.

If you forget a dose:
Take when remembered. Don't double next dose. Resume regular schedule.

What drug does:
Acts as enzyme to promote normal fat and carbohydrate metabolism and protein synthesis.

Time lapse before drug works:
15 minutes.

Don't take with:
Any other medicine without consulting your doctor or pharmacist.

POSSIBLE ADVERSE REACTIONS OR SIDE EFFECTS

SYMPTOMS	WHAT TO DO
Life-threatening:	
Hives, rash, intense itching, faintness soon after a dose (anaphylaxis).	Seek emergency treatment immediately.
Common:	
None expected.	
Infrequent:	
None expected.	
Rare:	
• Itchy skin, wheezing.	Discontinue. Call doctor right away.
• Diarrhea.	Continue. Call doctor when convenient.

VITAMIN B-12 (Cyanocobalamin)

WARNINGS & PRECAUTIONS

Don't take if:
You have Leber's disease (optic nerve atrophy).

Before you start, consult your doctor:
- If you have gout.
- If you have heart disease.

Over age 60:
Don't take more than 100 mg per day unless prescribed by your doctor.

Pregnancy:
Risk factor determined by length of pregnancy and dosage amount. See category list on page xxii and consult doctor.

Breast-feeding:
Effect unknown. Consult doctor.

Infants & children:
No problems expected.

Prolonged use:
No problems expected.

Skin & sunlight:
No problems expected.

Driving, piloting or hazardous work:
No problems expected.

Discontinuing:
Don't discontinue without doctor's advice until you complete prescribed dose, even though symptoms diminish or disappear.

Others:
- A balanced diet should provide all the vitamin B-12 a healthy person needs and make supplements unnecessary. Best sources are meat, fish, egg yolk and cheese.
- Tablets should be used only for diet supplements. All other uses of vitamin B-12 require injections.
- Don't take large doses of vitamin C (1,000 mg or more per day) unless prescribed by your doctor.

POSSIBLE INTERACTION WITH OTHER DRUGS

GENERIC NAME OR DRUG CLASS	COMBINED EFFECT
Anticonvulsants*	Decreased absorption of vitamin B-12.
Chloramphenicol	Decreased vitamin B-12 effect.
Cholestyramine	Decreased absorption of vitamin B-12.
Cimetidine	Decreased absorption of vitamin B-12.
Colchicine	Decreased absorption of vitamin B-12.
Famotidine	Decreased absorption of vitamin B-12.
H_2 antagonists*	Decreased absorption of vitamin B-12.
Neomycin	Decreased absorption of vitamin B-12.
Para-aminosalicylic acid	Decreased effects of para-aminosalicyclic acid.
Potassium (extended-release forms)	Decreased absorption of vitamin B-12.
Ranitidine	Decreased absorption of vitamin B-12.
Vitamin C (ascorbic acid)	Destroys vitamin B-12 if taken at same time. Take 2 hours apart.

POSSIBLE INTERACTION WITH OTHER SUBSTANCES

INTERACTS WITH	COMBINED EFFECT
Alcohol:	Decreased absorption of vitamin B-12.
Beverages:	None expected.
Cocaine:	None expected.
Foods:	None expected.
Marijuana:	None expected.
Tobacco:	None expected.

*See Glossary

VITAMIN C (Ascorbic Acid)

BRAND NAMES

Ascorbicap	**Ce-Vi-Sol**
Cecon	**Cevita**
Cemill	**C-Span**
Cenolate	**Flavorcee**
Cetane	**Redoxon**
Cevalin	**Sunkist**
Cevi-Bid	

Numerous other multiple vitamin-mineral supplements.

BASIC INFORMATION

Habit forming? No
Prescription needed? No
Available as generic? Yes
Drug class: Vitamin supplement

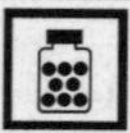

USES

- Prevention and treatment of scurvy and other vitamin C deficiencies.
- Treatment of anemia.
- Maintenance of acid urine.

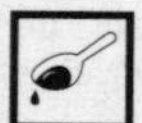

DOSAGE & USAGE INFORMATION

How to take:
- Tablets, capsules, liquid—Swallow with 8 oz. water.
- Extended-release tablets—Swallow whole.
- Drops—Squirt directly into mouth or mix with liquid or food.
- Chewable tablets—Chew well before swallowing.

When to take:
1, 2 or 3 times per day, as prescribed on label.

If you forget a dose:
Take as soon as you remember, then return to regular schedule.

Continued next column

OVERDOSE

SYMPTOMS:
Diarrhea, vomiting, dizziness.
WHAT TO DO:
Overdose unlikely to threaten life. If person takes much larger amount than prescribed, call doctor, poison control center or hospital emergency room for instructions.

What drug does:
- May help form collagen.
- Increases iron absorption from intestine.
- Contributes to hemoglobin and red blood cell production in bone marrow.

Time lapse before drug works:
1 week.

Don't take with:
Any other medicine without consulting your doctor or pharmacist.

POSSIBLE ADVERSE REACTIONS OR SIDE EFFECTS

SYMPTOMS	WHAT TO DO
Life-threatening: None expected.	
Common: None expected.	
Infrequent:	
• Mild diarrhea, nausea, vomiting.	Discontinue. Call doctor right away.
• Flushed face.	Continue. Call doctor when convenient.
Rare:	
• Kidney stones with high doses, anemia, abdominal pain.	Discontinue. Call doctor right away.
• Headache.	Continue. Tell doctor at next visit.

VITAMIN C (Ascorbic Acid)

WARNINGS & PRECAUTIONS

Don't take if:
You are allergic to vitamin C.

Before you start, consult your doctor:
- If you have sickle-cell or other anemia.
- If you have had kidney stones.
- If you have gout.

Over age 60:
Don't take more than 100 mg per day unless prescribed by your doctor.

Pregnancy:
Risk factor determined by length of pregnancy and dosage amount. See category list on page xxii and consult doctor.

Breast-feeding:
Avoid large doses. Consult doctor.

Infants & children:
- Avoid large doses.
- Keep vitamin-mineral supplements out of children's reach.

Prolonged use:
Large doses for longer than 2 months may cause kidney stones.

Skin & sunlight:
No problems expected.

Driving, piloting or hazardous work:
No problems expected.

Discontinuing:
No problems expected.

Others:
- Store in cool, dry place.
- May cause inaccurate tests for sugar in urine or blood in stool.
- May cause crisis in patients with sickle-cell anemia.
- A balanced diet should provide all the vitamin C a healthy person needs and make supplements unnecessary. Best sources are citrus, strawberries, cantaloupe and raw peppers.
- Don't take large doses of vitamin C (1,000 mg or more per day) unless prescribed by your doctor.
- Some products contain tartrazine dye. Avoid, if allergic (especially aspirin hypersensitivity).

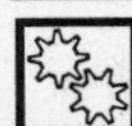

POSSIBLE INTERACTION WITH OTHER DRUGS

GENERIC NAME OR DRUG CLASS	COMBINED EFFECT
Amphetamines*	Possible decreased amphetamine effect.
Anticholinergics*	Possible decreased anticholinergic effect.
Anticoagulants*, oral	Possible decreased anticoagulant effect.
Antidepressants, tricyclic (TCA)*	Possible decreased antidepressant effect.
Aspirin	Decreased vitamin C effect and salicylate excretion.
Barbiturates*	Decreased vitamin C effect. Increased barbiturate effect.
Cellulose sodium phosphate	Decreased vitamin C effect.
Contraceptives, oral*	Decreased vitamin C effect.
Estrogens*	Increased likelihood of adverse effects from estrogen with 1 g or more of vitamin C per day.
Iron supplements*	Increased iron absorption.
Mexiletine	Possible decreased effectiveness of mexiletine.
Quinidine	Possible decreased quinidine effect.
Salicylates*	Decreased vitamin C effect and salicylate excretion. May lead to salicylate toxicity.
Tranquilizers* (phenothiazine)	May decrease phenothiazine effect if no vitamin C deficiency exists.

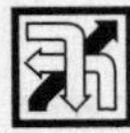

POSSIBLE INTERACTION WITH OTHER SUBSTANCES

INTERACTS WITH	COMBINED EFFECT
Alcohol:	None expected.
Beverages:	None expected.
Cocaine:	None expected.
Foods:	None expected.
Marijuana:	None expected.
Tobacco:	Increased requirement for vitamin C.

VITAMIN D

BRAND AND GENERIC NAMES

ALFACALCIDOL
Calciferol
CALCIFEDIOL
Calcijex
CALCITRIOL
Calderol
Deltalin
DHT
DHT Intensol
DIHYDROTA-CHYSTEROL
Drisdol
ERGOCALCIFEROL
Hytakerol
One-Alpha
Ostoforte
Radiostol
Radiostol Forte
Rocaltrol

Numerous other multiple vitamin-mineral supplements. Check labels.

BASIC INFORMATION

Habit forming? No
Prescription needed?
Low strength: No
High strength: Yes
Available as generic? Yes
Drug class: Vitamin supplement

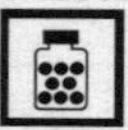

USES

- Dietary supplement.
- Prevention of rickets (bone disease).
- Treatment for hypocalcemia (low blood calcium) in kidney disease.
- Treatment for postoperative muscle contractions.
- Daily supplement for people who must use sunscreen daily.

DOSAGE & USAGE INFORMATION

How to take:
- Tablet, capsule or liquid—Swallow with liquid.
- Drops—Dilute dose in beverage.
- Injection—Take under doctor's supervision.

Continued next column

OVERDOSE

SYMPTOMS:
Severe stomach pain, nausea, vomiting, weight loss; bone and muscle pain; increased urination, cloudy urine; mood or mental changes (possible psychosis); high blood pressure, irregular heartbeat; eye irritation or light sensitivity; itchy skin.
WHAT TO DO:
Overdose unlikely to threaten life. If person takes much larger amount than prescribed, call doctor, poison control center or hospital emergency room for instructions.

When to take:
As directed, usually once a day at the same time each day.

If you forget a dose:
Take up to 12 hours late. If more than 12 hours, wait for next dose (don't double this dose).

What drug does:
- Maintains growth and health.
- Prevents rickets.
- Essential so body can use calcium and phosphate.

Time lapse before drug works:
2 hours. May require 2 to 3 weeks of continual use for maximum effect.

Don't take with:
Nonprescription drugs or drugs in Interaction column without consulting doctor.

POSSIBLE ADVERSE REACTIONS OR SIDE EFFECTS

SYMPTOMS	WHAT TO DO
Life-threatening: In case of overdose, see previous column.	
Common: None expected.	
Infrequent: Headache, metallic taste in mouth, thirst, dry mouth, constipation, appetite loss, nausea, vomiting, weakness, cloudy urine, sensitivity to light.	Continue. Call doctor when convenient.
Rare: • Increased urination, pink eye, psychosis, severe abdominal pain, fever.	Discontinue. Call doctor right away.
• Muscle pain, bone pain, diarrhea.	Continue. Tell doctor when convenient.

WARNINGS & PRECAUTIONS

Don't take if:
You are allergic to medicine containing vitamin D.

Before you start, consult your doctor:
- If you plan to become pregnant while taking vitamin D.
- If you have epilepsy.
- If you have heart or blood-vessel disease.
- If you have kidney disease.

Over age 60:
Adverse reactions and side effects may be more frequent and severe than in younger persons.

Pregnancy:
Risk factor determined by length of pregnancy and dosage amount. See category list on page xxii and consult doctor.

Breast-feeding:
No problems expected, but consult doctor.

Infants & children:
- Avoid large doses.
- Keep vitamins out of children's reach.

Prolonged use:
- No problems expected.
- Talk to your doctor about the need for follow-up medical examinations or laboratory studies to check kidney function, liver function, serum calcium.

Skin & sunlight:
Increased sensitivity to light.

Driving, piloting or hazardous work:
No problems expected.

Discontinuing:
Don't discontinue without doctor's advice until you complete prescribed dose, even though symptoms diminish or disappear.

Others:
- Don't exceed dose. Too much over a long time may be harmful.
- A balanced diet should provide all the vitamin D a healthy person needs and make supplements unnecessary. Best sources are fish and vitamin D-fortified milk and bread.
- Some products contain tartrazine dye. Avoid, if allergic (especially aspirin hypersensitivity).
- Sunscreen prevents the body from manufacturing vitamin D from sunshine. Take supplementary vitamin D if you use sunscreen daily. Ask doctor for dosage.

POSSIBLE INTERACTION WITH OTHER DRUGS

GENERIC NAME OR DRUG CLASS	COMBINED EFFECT
Antacids* (magnesium-containing)	Possible excess magnesium.
Anticonvulsants, hydantoin*	Decreased vitamin D effect.
Calcium (high doses)	Excess calcium in blood.
Calcium channel blockers*	Possible decreased effect of calcium channel blockers.
Calcium supplements*	Excessive absorption of vitamin D.
Cholestyramine	Decreased vitamin D effect.
Colestipol	Decreased vitamin D absorption.
Cortisone	Decreased vitamin D effect.
Digitalis preparations*	Heartbeat irregularities.
Diuretics, thiazide*	Possible increased calcium.
Mineral oil	Decreased vitamin D effect.
Neomycin	Decreased vitamin D absorption.
Nicardipine	Decreased nicardipine effect.
Phenobarbital	Decreased vitamin D effect.
Phosphorus preparations*	Accumulation of excess phosphorus.
Rifampin	Possible decreased vitamin D effect.
Vitamin D, other	Possible toxicity.

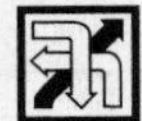

POSSIBLE INTERACTION WITH OTHER SUBSTANCES

INTERACTS WITH	COMBINED EFFECT
Alcohol:	None expected.
Beverages:	None expected.
Cocaine:	None expected.
Foods:	None expected.
Marijuana:	None expected.
Tobacco:	None expected.

*See Glossary

VITAMIN E

BRAND NAMES

Aquasol E
Chew-E
Eprolin
Epsilan-M
Pheryl-E
Viterra E

Numerous other multiple vitamin-mineral supplements. Check labels.

BASIC INFORMATION

Habit forming? No
Prescription needed? No
Available as generic? Yes
Drug class: Vitamin supplement

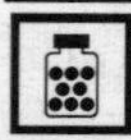

USES

- Dietary supplement to promote normal growth, development and health.
- Treatment and prevention of vitamin E deficiency, especially in premature or low-birth-weight infants.
- Treatment for fibrocystic disease of the breast.
- Treatment for circulatory problems to the lower extremities.
- Treatment for sickle-cell anemia.
- Treatment for lung toxicity from air pollution.

DOSAGE & USAGE INFORMATION

How to take:
- Tablet or capsule—Swallow with liquid or food to lessen stomach irritation.
- Drops—Dilute dose in beverage before swallowing or squirt directly into mouth.
- Injection—Take under doctor's supervision.

When to take:
At the same times each day.

If you forget a dose:
Take when you remember. Don't double next dose.

What drug does:
- Promotes normal growth and development.
- Prevents oxidation in body.

Continued next column

OVERDOSE

SYMPTOMS:
Nausea, vomiting, fatigue.
WHAT TO DO:
Overdose unlikely to threaten life. If person takes much larger amount than prescribed, call doctor, poison control center or hospital emergency room for instructions.

Time lapse before drug works:
Not determined.

Don't take with:
Any other medicine without consulting your doctor or pharmacist.

POSSIBLE ADVERSE REACTIONS OR SIDE EFFECTS

SYMPTOMS	WHAT TO DO
Life-threatening: None expected.	
Common: Breast enlargement, dizziness, headache.	Continue. Call doctor when convenient.
Infrequent: Nausea, abdominal pain, muscle aches, pain in lower legs, fever, tiredness, weakness.	Continue. Call doctor when convenient.
Rare: Blurred vision, diarrhea.	Discontinue. Call doctor right away.

WARNINGS & PRECAUTIONS

Don't take if:
You are allergic to vitamin E.

Before you start, consult your doctor:
- If you have had blood clots in leg veins (thrombophlebitis).
- If you have liver disease.

Over age 60:
No problems expected. Avoid excessive doses.

Pregnancy:
No problems expected with normal daily requirements. Don't exceed prescribed dose. Consult doctor.

Breast-feeding:
No problems expected. Consult doctor.

Infants & children:
Use only under medical supervision.

Prolonged use:
Toxic accumulation of vitamin E. Don't exceed recommended dose.

Skin & sunlight:
No problems expected.

Driving, piloting or hazardous work:
No problems expected.

Discontinuing:
No problems expected.

Others:
A balanced diet should provide all the vitamin E a healthy person needs and make supplements unnecessary. Best sources are vegetable oils, whole-grain cereals, liver.

POSSIBLE INTERACTION WITH OTHER DRUGS

GENERIC NAME OR DRUG CLASS	COMBINED EFFECT
Anticoagulants*, oral	Increased anti-coagulant effect.
Cholestyramine	Decreased vitamin E absorption.
Colestipol	Decreased vitamin E absorption.
Iron supplements*	Possible decreased effect of iron supplement in patients with iron-deficiency anemia. Decreased vitamin E effect in healthy persons.
Mineral oil	Decreased vitamin E effect.
Neomycin	Decreased vitamin E absorption.
Vitamin A	Recommended dose of vitamin E—Increased benefit and decreased toxicity of vitamin A. Excess dose of vitamin E—Vitamin A depletion.

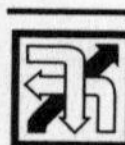

POSSIBLE INTERACTION WITH OTHER SUBSTANCES

INTERACTS WITH	COMBINED EFFECT
Alcohol:	None expected.
Beverages:	None expected.
Cocaine:	None expected.
Foods:	None expected.
Marijuana:	None expected.
Tobacco:	None expected.

*See Glossary

VITAMIN K

BRAND AND GENERIC NAMES

AquaMEPHYTON
Konakion
Menadione
MENADIOL
Mephyton
PHYTONADIONE
Synkayvite

BASIC INFORMATION

Habit forming? No
Prescription needed? No
Available as generic? Yes
Drug class: Vitamin supplement

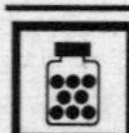

USES

- Dietary supplement.
- Treatment for bleeding disorders and malabsorption diseases due to vitamin K deficiency.
- Treatment for hemorrhagic disease of the newborn.
- Treatment for bleeding due to overdose of oral anticoagulants.

DOSAGE & USAGE INFORMATION

How to take:
- Usually given by injection in hospital or doctor's office.
- Tablet—Swallow with liquid. If you can't swallow whole, crumble tablet and take with liquid or food.

When to take:
At the same time each day.

If you forget a dose:
Take as soon as you remember up to 12 hours late. If more than 12 hours, wait for next scheduled dose (don't double this dose).

What drug does:
- Promotes growth, development and good health.
- Supplies a necessary ingredient for blood clotting.

Continued next column

OVERDOSE

SYMPTOMS:
Nausea, vomiting.
WHAT TO DO:
Overdose unlikely to threaten life. If person takes much larger amount than prescribed, call doctor, poison control center or hospital emergency room for instructions.

Time lapse before drug works:
15 to 30 minutes to support blood clotting.

Don't take with:
Any other medicine without consulting your doctor or pharmacist.

POSSIBLE ADVERSE REACTIONS OR SIDE EFFECTS

SYMPTOMS	WHAT TO DO
Life-threatening:	
None expected.	
Common:	
None expected.	
Infrequent:	
Unusual taste, face flushing.	Continue. Call doctor when convenient.
Rare:	
Rash, hives.	Discontinue. Call doctor right away.

WARNINGS & PRECAUTIONS

Don't take if:
- You are allergic to vitamin K.
- You have G6PD* deficiency.
- You have liver disease.

Before you start, consult your doctor:
If you are pregnant.

Over age 60:
No problems expected.

Pregnancy:
Risk factor determined by length of pregnancy and dosage amount. See category list on page xxii and consult doctor.

Breast-feeding:
No problems expected. Consult doctor.

Infants & children:
Phytonadione is the preferred form for hemorrhagic disease of the newborn.

Prolonged use:
Talk to your doctor about the need for follow-up medical examinations or laboratory studies to check prothrombin time.

Skin & sunlight:
No problems expected.

Driving, piloting or hazardous work:
No problems expected.

Discontinuing:
No problems expected.

Others:
- Tell all doctors and dentists you consult that you take this medicine.
- Don't exceed dose. Too much over a long time may be harmful.
- A balanced diet should provide all the vitamin K a healthy person needs and make supplements unnecessary. Best sources are green, leafy vegetables, meat or dairy products.

POSSIBLE INTERACTION WITH OTHER DRUGS

GENERIC NAME OR DRUG CLASS	COMBINED EFFECT
Anticoagulants*, oral	Decreased anti-coagulant effect.
Cholestyramine	Decreased vitamin K effect.
Colestipol	Decreased vitamin K absorption.
Dapsone	Increased risk of adverse effect on blood cells.
Mineral oil (long-term)	Vitamin K deficiency.
Neomycin	Decreased vitamin K absorption.
Sulfa drugs*	Vitamin K deficiency.

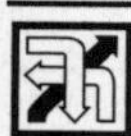

POSSIBLE INTERACTION WITH OTHER SUBSTANCES

INTERACTS WITH	COMBINED EFFECT
Alcohol:	None expected.
Beverages:	None expected.
Cocaine:	None expected.
Foods:	None expected.
Marijuana:	None expected.
Tobacco:	None expected.

*See Glossary

VITAMINS & FLUORIDE

BRAND AND GENERIC NAMES

Adeflor
Cari-Tab
Mulvidren-F
Poly-Vi-Flor
Tri-Vi-Flor
Vi-Daylin/F
Vi-Penta F
MULTIPLE VITAMINS & FLUORIDE
VITAMINS A, D & C & FLUORIDE

BASIC INFORMATION

Habit forming? No
Prescription needed? Yes
Available as generic? No
Drug class: Vitamins, minerals

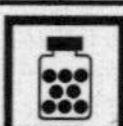

USES

- Reduces incidence of tooth cavities (fluoride). Children who need supplements should take until age 16.
- Prevents deficiencies of vitamin included in formula (some contain multiple vitamins whose content varies among products; others contain only vitamins A, D and C).

DOSAGE & USAGE INFORMATION

How to take:
- Chewable tablets—Chew or crush before swallowing.
- Oral liquid—Measure with specially marked dropper. May mix with food, fruit juice, cereal.

When to take:
- Bedtime or with or just after meals.
- If at bedtime, brush teeth first.

If you forget a dose:
Take as soon as you remember up to 2 hours late. If more than 2 hours, wait for next scheduled dose (don't double this dose).

Continued next column

OVERDOSE

SYMPTOMS:
Minor overdose—Black, brown or white spots on teeth.
Massive overdose—Shallow breathing, black or tarry stools, bloody vomit.
WHAT TO DO:
- **Dial 911 (emergency) or 0 (operator) for an ambulance or medical help. Then give first aid immediately.**
- **See emergency information on inside covers.**

What drug does:
Provides supplemental fluoride to combat tooth decay.

Time lapse before drug works:
8 weeks to provide maximum benefit.

Don't take with:
- Other medicine simultaneously.
- Any other medicine without consulting your doctor or pharmacist.

POSSIBLE ADVERSE REACTIONS OR SIDE EFFECTS

SYMPTOMS	WHAT TO DO
Life-threatening:	
Fainting, bloody vomit, bloody or black stool, breathing difficulty.	Discontinue. Seek emergency treatment.
Common:	
White, black or brown spots on teeth; nausea; vomiting.	Discontinue. Call doctor right away.
Infrequent:	
• Drowsiness; abdominal pain; increased salivation; watery eyes; weight loss; sore throat, fever, mouth sores; constipation; bone pain; rash; muscle stiffness; weakness; tremor; agitation.	Discontinue. Call doctor right away.
• Diarrhea.	Continue. Call doctor when convenient.
Rare:	
None expected.	

WARNINGS & PRECAUTIONS

Don't take if:
- Your water supply contains 0.7 parts fluoride per million. Too much fluoride stains teeth permanently.
- You are allergic to any fluoride-containing product.
- You have underactive thyroid.

Before you start, consult your doctor or dentist:
For proper dosage.

Over age 60:
No problems expected.

Pregnancy:
Risk factor determined by length of pregnancy and dosage amount. See category list on page xxii and consult doctor.

Breast-feeding:
No problems expected. Consult doctor.

Infants & children:
No problems expected in children over 3 years of age except in case of accidental overdose. Keep vitamin-mineral supplements out of children's reach.

Prolonged use:
Excess may cause discolored teeth and decreased calcium in blood.

Skin & sunlight:
No problems expected.

Driving, piloting or hazardous work:
No problems expected.

Discontinuing:
No problems expected.

Others:
- Store in original plastic container. Fluoride decomposes glass.
- Check with dentist once or twice a year to keep cavities at a minimum. Topical applications of fluoride may also be helpful.
- Fluoride probably not necessary if water contains about 1 part per million of fluoride or more. Check with health department.
- Don't freeze.
- Don't keep outdated medicine.

POSSIBLE INTERACTION WITH OTHER DRUGS

GENERIC NAME OR DRUG CLASS	COMBINED EFFECT
Anticoagulants*	Decreased effect of anticoagulant.
Iron supplements*	Decreased effect of any vitamin E if present in multivitamin product.
Vitamin A	May lead to vitamin A toxicity if vitamin A is in combination.
Vitamin D	May lead to vitamin D toxicity if vitamin D is in combination.

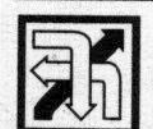

POSSIBLE INTERACTION WITH OTHER SUBSTANCES

INTERACTS WITH	COMBINED EFFECT
Alcohol:	None expected.
Beverages:	
Milk.	Prevents absorption of fluoride. Space dose 2 hours before or after milk.
Cocaine:	None expected.
Foods:	None expected.
Marijuana:	None expected.
Tobacco:	None expected.

***See Glossary**

XYLOMETAZOLINE

BRAND NAMES

See complete list of brand names in the *Brand Name Directory*, page 920.

BASIC INFORMATION

Habit forming? No
Prescription needed? No
Available as generic? Yes
Drug class: Sympathomimetic

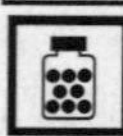

USES

Relieves congestion of nose, sinuses and throat from allergies and infections.

DOSAGE & USAGE INFORMATION

How to take:
Nasal solution, nasal spray—Use as directed on label. Avoid contamination. Don't use same container for more than 1 person.

When to take:
When needed, no more often than every 4 hours.

If you forget a dose:
Take as soon as you remember. Wait 4 hours for next dose.

What drug does:
Constricts walls of small arteries in nose, sinuses and eustachian tubes.

Time lapse before drug works:
5 to 30 minutes.

Continued next column

OVERDOSE

SYMPTOMS:
Headache, sweating, anxiety, agitation, rapid and irregular heartbeat (rare occurrence with systemic absorption).
WHAT TO DO:

- **Dial 911 (emergency) or 0 (operator) for an ambulance or medical help. Then give first aid immediately.**
- **If patient is unconscious and not breathing, give mouth-to-mouth breathing. If there is no heartbeat, use cardiac massage and mouth-to-mouth breathing (CPR). If you can't get help quickly, take patient to nearest emergency facility.**
- **See emergency information on inside covers.**

Don't take with:

- Nonprescription drugs for allergy, cough or cold without consulting doctor.
- Any other medicine without consulting your doctor or pharmacist.

POSSIBLE ADVERSE REACTIONS OR SIDE EFFECTS

SYMPTOMS	WHAT TO DO
Life-threatening:	
In case of overdose, see previous column.	
Common:	
None expected.	
Infrequent:	
Burning, dry or stinging nasal passages.	Continue. Call doctor when convenient.
Rare:	
Rebound congestion (increased runny or stuffy nose); headache, insomnia, nervousness (may occur with systemic absorption).	Discontinue. Call doctor right away.

WARNINGS & PRECAUTIONS

Don't take if:
You are allergic to any sympathomimetic nasal spray.

Before you start, consult your doctor:
- If you have heart disease or high blood pressure.
- If you have diabetes.
- If you have overactive thyroid.
- If you have taken a monoamine oxidase (MAO) inhibitor* in past 2 weeks.
- If you have glaucoma.

Over age 60:
Adverse reactions and side effects may be more frequent and severe than in younger persons.

Pregnancy:
Decide with your doctor if drug benefits justify risk to unborn child. Risk category C (see page xxii).

Breast-feeding:
No proven problems. Consult doctor.

Infants & children:
Don't give to children younger than 2.

Prolonged use:
Drug may lose effectiveness, cause increased congestion (rebound effect*) and irritate nasal membranes.

Skin & sunlight:
No problems expected.

Driving, piloting or hazardous work:
No problems expected.

Discontinuing:
May be unnecessary to finish medicine. Follow doctor's instructions.

Others:
No problems expected.

POSSIBLE INTERACTION WITH OTHER DRUGS

GENERIC NAME OR DRUG CLASS	COMBINED EFFECT
Antidepressants, tricyclic*	Possible rise in blood pressure.
Maprotiline	Possible increased blood pressure.

POSSIBLE INTERACTION WITH OTHER SUBSTANCES

INTERACTS WITH	COMBINED EFFECT
Alcohol:	None expected.
Beverages: Caffeine drinks.	Nervousness or insomnia.
Cocaine:	High risk of heartbeat irregularities and high blood pressure.
Foods:	None expected.
Marijuana:	Overstimulation. Avoid.
Tobacco:	None expected.

***See Glossary**

YOHIMBINE

BRAND NAMES

Actibine
Aphrodyne
Baron-X
Dayto Himbin
Prohim
Thybine
Yocon
Yohimar
Yohimex
Yoman
Yovital

BASIC INFORMATION

Habit forming? No
Prescription needed? Yes
Available as generic? Yes
Drug class: Impotence therapy agent

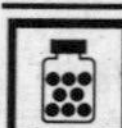

USES

Treatment for men who are unable to have sexual intercourse (impotent). It may be helpful for some, but not all, men who suffer sexual dysfunction.

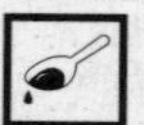

DOSAGE & USAGE INFORMATION

How to use:
Tablet—Swallow with liquid. May be taken with or without food.

When to use:
At the same times each day.

If you forget a dose:
Take as soon as you remember up to 4 hours late. If more than 4 hours, wait for next scheduled dose (don't double this dose).

What drug does:
It is unknown exactly how the drug works. It appears to increase the supply of certain body chemicals that can help produce erections.

Time lapse before drug works:
May take 2 to 3 weeks.

Don't take with:
Any other prescription or nonprescription drug without consulting your doctor or pharmacist.

OVERDOSE

SYMPTOMS:
None expected.
WHAT TO DO:
Overdose unlikely to threaten life. If person takes much larger amount than prescribed, call doctor, poison control center or hospital emergency room for instructions.

POSSIBLE ADVERSE REACTIONS OR SIDE EFFECTS

SYMPTOMS	WHAT TO DO
Life-threatening:	
None expected.	
Common:	
None expected.	
Infrequent:	
• Rapid heartbeat, increased blood pressure.	Discontinue. Call doctor right away.
• Headache, dizziness, restlessness, irritability, nervousness, anxiety, insomnia, muscle aches.	Continue. Call doctor when convenient.
Rare:	
Nausea, vomiting, flushed skin, sweating, tremor.	Continue. Call doctor when convenient.

WARNINGS & PRECAUTIONS

Don't take if:
- You have an allergy to yohimbine or any rauwolfia alkaloids*.
- You have angina pectoris.
- You have heart disease or high blood pressure.
- You have impaired kidney function.

Before you start, consult your doctor:
- If you suffer from depression.
- If you have any psychiatric disorder.
- If you have liver disease.
- If you have allergies to any medications, foods or other substances.

Over age 60:
Studies have not shown any specific problems. Discuss possible benefits and risk factors with your doctor.

Pregnancy:
Not used in females.

Breast-feeding:
Not used in females.

Infants & children:
Not used in this age group.

Prolonged use:
Effects of long-term use are unknown. Visit your doctor regularly while using this drug to check its effectiveness, as well as your blood pressure and heart rate.

Skin & sunlight:
No special problems expected.

Driving, piloting or hazardous work:
Avoid if you experience any side effects (especially dizziness).

Discontinuing:
No special problems expected.

Others:
Follow your doctor's instructions for using this drug. Don't take it more often or increase the dosage without your doctor's approval. It will increase the risk of high blood pressure and rapid heartbeat.

POSSIBLE INTERACTION WITH OTHER DRUGS

GENERIC NAME OR DRUG CLASS	COMBINED EFFECT
Antidepressants*	Decreased effect of antidepressant.
Antihypertensives*	Decreased effect of antihypertensive.

POSSIBLE INTERACTION WITH OTHER SUBSTANCES

INTERACTS WITH	COMBINED EFFECT
Alcohol:	Decreased yohimbine effect. Avoid.
Beverages:	None expected.
Cocaine	Effect unknown. Best to avoid.
Foods:	None expected.
Marijuana:	Effect unknown. Best to avoid.
Tobacco:	None expected.

*See Glossary

ZIDOVUDINE (AZT, Azidothymidine)

BRAND NAMES

Apo-Zidovudine
Novo-AZT
Retrovir

BASIC INFORMATION

Habit forming? No
Prescription needed? Yes
Available as generic? No
Drug class: Antiviral

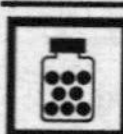

USES

Treatment of selected adult patients infected with HIV (human immunodeficiency virus), AIDS (acquired immune deficiency syndrome) and advanced ARC (AIDS-related complex). Does not cure the infection.

DOSAGE & USAGE INFORMATION

How to take:
- Capsule—Swallow with liquid.
- Syrup—Take with liquid.

When to take:
Every 4 hours around the clock unless instructed otherwise.

If you forget a dose:
Take as soon as you remember.

What drug does:
Inhibits reproduction of some viruses, including HIV virus (the virus that causes AIDS).

Time lapse before drug works:
May require several weeks of treatment for full effect. Absorption is rapid.

Don't take with:
- High-fat meals.
- Any other medicine without consulting your doctor or pharmacist.

OVERDOSE

SYMPTOMS:
Unusual bleeding or bruising, severe nausea and vomiting, seizures, unsteady gait.
WHAT TO DO:
- **Dial 911 (emergency) or 0 (operator) for an ambulance or medical help. Then give first aid immediately.**
- **See emergency information on inside covers.**

POSSIBLE ADVERSE REACTIONS OR SIDE EFFECTS

SYMPTOMS	WHAT TO DO
Life-threatening:	
Lip or tongue swelling.	Discontinue. Seek emergency treatment.
Common:	
• Pale skin (anemia), chills, diarrhea.	Discontinue. Call doctor right away.
• Severe headache, nausea, insomnia, diarrhea.	Continue. Call doctor when convenient.
Infrequent:	
Sweating, fever, appetite loss, abdominal pain, vomiting, aching muscles, dizziness, numbness in hands and feet, shortness of breath, skin rash, strange taste, nervousness, itching, mouth sores, discolored nails.	Continue. Call doctor when convenient.
Rare:	
Constipation, confusion, fainting, unexplained bleeding.	Discontinue. Call doctor right away.

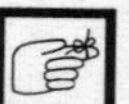

WARNINGS & PRECAUTIONS

Don't take if:
You are allergic to any component of this capsule.

Before you start, consult your doctor:
- If you know you have a low white blood cell count or severe anemia.
- If you have severe kidney or liver disease.

Over age 60:
Elimination may be slower.

Pregnancy:
Should not be used in pregnancy except when zidovudine is clearly indicated. Consult doctor. Risk category C (see page xxii).

Breast-feeding:
Not recommended for HIV-positive mothers.

Infants & children:
Use only under medical supervision.

Prolonged use:
Talk to your doctor about the need for follow-up medical examinations or laboratory studies to check complete blood counts (white blood cell count, platelet count, red blood cell count, hemoglobin, hematocrit).

Skin & sunlight:
No problems expected.

Driving, piloting, or hazardous work:
Don't drive or pilot aircraft until you learn how medicine affects you. Don't work around dangerous machinery. Don't climb ladders or work in high places. Danger increases if you drink alcohol or take medicine affecting alertness and reflexes, such as antihistamines, tranquilizers, sedatives, pain medicine, narcotics and mind-altering drugs.

Discontinuing:
Don't discontinue without consulting your doctor. Dose may require gradual reduction if you have taken drug for a long time. Doses of other drugs may also require adjustment.

Others:
- Zidovudine does not cure HIV virus infections. Transfusions or dose modification may be necessary if toxicity develops.
- Have blood counts followed closely during treatment to detect anemia or lowered white blood cell count.
- Zidovudine does not reduce risk of transmitting disease to others.
- Healing after dental procedures may be delayed.
- X-ray treatments may worsen anemia.
- Patients with AIDS or ARC may continue to develop complications, including opportunistic infections such as pneumocistis carnii pneumonia.

POSSIBLE INTERACTION WITH OTHER DRUGS

GENERIC NAME OR DRUG CLASS	COMBINED EFFECT
Acetaminophen	May increase toxic effects of zidovudine. Avoid.
Acyclovir	Lethargy, convulsions.
Aspirin	May increase toxic effects of zidovudine.
Benzodiazepines	May increase toxic effects of zidovudine. Avoid.
Bone marrow depressants*, other	Increased bone marrow toxicity.
Cimetidine	May increase toxic effects of zidovudine. Avoid.
Clarithromycin	Decreased zidovudine effect.
Clozapine	Toxic effect on bone marrow.
Ganciclovir	Increased toxicity of both drugs. Use combination with caution only when essential.
Morphine	May increase toxic effects of zidovudine. Avoid.
Probenecid	May increase toxic effects of zidovudine.
Ribavirin	Decreased zidovudine effect.
Sulfa drugs*	May increase toxic effects of zidovudine. Avoid.

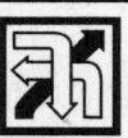

POSSIBLE INTERACTION WITH OTHER SUBSTANCES

INTERACTS WITH	COMBINED EFFECT
Alcohol:	Unknown. Best to avoid.
Beverages:	None expected.
Cocaine:	Unknown. Best to avoid.
Foods:	None expected.
Marijuana:	Unknown. Best to avoid.
Tobacco:	None expected.

***See Glossary**

ZINC SUPPLEMENTS

BRAND NAMES

Egozinc	ZINC GLUCONATE
Orazinc	ZINC SULFATE
PMS Egozinc	Zinc-220
Verazinc	Zincate
ZINC CHLORIDE	Zinkaps-220

Numerous multiple vitamin supplements. Check label.

BASIC INFORMATION

Habit forming? No
Prescription needed? No
Available as generic? Yes
Drug class: Nutritional supplement (mineral)

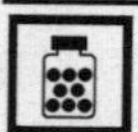

USES

- Treats zinc deficiency that may lead to growth retardation, appetite loss, changes in taste or smell, skin eruptions, slow wound healing, decreased immune function, diarrhea or impaired night vision.
- In absence of a deficiency, is used to treat burns, eating disorders, liver disorders, prematurity in infants, intestinal diseases, parasitism, kidney disorders, skin disorders and stress.
- May be useful as a supplement for those who are breast-feeding or pregnant (under a doctor's supervision).

DOSAGE & USAGE INFORMATION

How to take:
Tablet or capsule—Swallow with liquid. If you can't swallow whole, crumble tablet or open capsule and take with liquid or food.

When to take:
At the same time each day, according to a doctor's instructions or the package label.

Continued next column

OVERDOSE

SYMPTOMS:
Dizziness, yellow eyes and skin, shortness of breath, chest pain, vomiting.
WHAT TO DO:
- **Have patient drink lots of water.**
- **Dial 911 (emergency) or 0 (operator) for an ambulance or medical help. Then give first aid immediately.**

If you forget a dose:
Take as soon as you remember up to 2 hours late. If more than 2 hours, wait for next scheduled dose (don't double this dose).

What drug does:
Required by the body for the utilization of many enzymes, nucleic acids and proteins and for cell growth.

Time lapse before drug works:
2 hours.

Don't take with:
See Interaction column and consult doctor.

POSSIBLE ADVERSE REACTIONS OR SIDE EFFECTS

SYMPTOMS	WHAT TO DO
Life-threatening:	
In case of overdose, see previous column.	
Common:	
None expected.	
Infrequent:	
None expected.	
Rare:	
• Indigestion, heartburn, nausea and vomiting (only with large doses).	Continue. Call doctor when convenient.
• Fever, chills, sore throat, ulcers in throat or mouth, unusual tiredness or weakness (only with large doses).	Discontinue. Call doctor right away.

WARNINGS & PRECAUTIONS

Don't take if:
You have an upper respiratory infection (zinc makes this worse).

Before you start, consult your doctor:
If you are pregnant or breast-feeding.

Over age 60:
No special problems expected. Nutritional supplements may be helpful if the diet is restricted in any way.

Pregnancy:
Adequate zinc intake is important. Risk factor not designated. See category list on page xxii and consult doctor.

Breast-feeding:
Adequate zinc intake important. Consult a doctor.

Infants & children:
Normal daily requirements vary with age. Consult a doctor.

Prolonged use:
No special problems expected.

Skin & sunlight:
No special problems expected.

Driving, piloting or hazardous work:
No special problems expected.

Discontinuing:
No special problems expected.

Others:
The best natural sources of zinc are red meats, oysters, herring, peas and beans.

POSSIBLE INTERACTION WITH OTHER DRUGS

GENERIC NAME OR DRUG CLASS	COMBINED EFFECT
Copper supplements	Inhibited absorption of copper.
Diuretics, thiazide*	Increased need for zinc.
Folic acid	Increased need for zinc.
Iron supplements*	Increased need for zinc
Tetracyclines*	Decreased absorption of tetracycline if taken within 2 hours of each other.

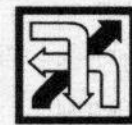

POSSIBLE INTERACTION WITH OTHER SUBSTANCES

INTERACTS WITH	COMBINED EFFECT
Alcohol:	May increase need for zinc.
Beverages:	No proven problems.
Cocaine:	No proven problems.
Foods:	
High-fiber.	May decrease zinc absorption.
Marijuana:	No proven problems.
Tobacco:	May increase need for zinc.

ZOLPIDEM

BRAND NAMES

Ambien

BASIC INFORMATION

Habit forming? Yes
Prescription needed? Yes
Available as generic? No
Drug class: Sedative (hypnotic)

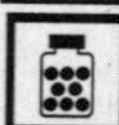

USES

Short-term (less than 2 weeks) treatment for insomnia.

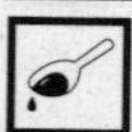

DOSAGE & USAGE INFORMATION

How to take:
Tablets—Swallow with liquid.

When to take:
Take immediately before bedtime. For best results, do not take with a meal or immediately after eating a meal.

If you forget a dose:
Take as soon as you remember. Take drug only when you are able to get 7 to 8 hours of sleep before your daily activity begins. Do not exceed prescribed dosage.

What drug does:
Acts as a central nervous system depressant, decreasing sleep problems such as trouble falling asleep, waking up too often during the night and waking up too early in the morning.

Time lapse before drug works:
Within 1 to 2 hours.

Don't take with:
Any other prescription or nonprescription drug without consulting your doctor.

OVERDOSE

SYMPTOMS:
Drowsiness, weakness, stupor, coma.
WHAT TO DO:

- **Dial 911 (emergency) or 0 (operator) for an ambulance or medical help. Then give first aid immediately.**
- **If patient is unconscious and not breathing, use cardiac massage and mouth-to-mouth breathing (CPR). Don't try to make patient vomit. If you can't get help quickly, take patient to nearest emergency facility.**
- **See emergency information on inside covers.**

POSSIBLE ADVERSE REACTIONS OR SIDE EFFECTS

SYMPTOMS	WHAT TO DO
Life-threatening: In case of overdose, see previous column.	
Common: Daytime drowsiness, lightheadedness, dizziness, clumsiness, headache, diarrhea, nausea.	Continue. Call doctor when convenient.
Infrequent: Dry mouth, muscle aches or pain, tiredness, indigestion, joint pain, memory problems.	Continue. Call doctor when convenient.
Rare: Behavioral changes, agitation, confusion, hallucinations, worsening of depression, bloody or cloudy urine, painful or difficult urination, increased urge to urinate, skin rash or hives, itching.	Discontinue. Call doctor right away.

WARNINGS & PRECAUTIONS

Don't take if:
You are allergic to zolpidem.

Before you start, consult your doctor:
- If you have respiratory problems.
- If you have kidney or liver disease.
- If you suffer from depression.
- If you are an active or recovering alcoholic.

Over age 60:
Adverse reactions and side effects may be more frequent and severe than in younger persons. You may need smaller doses for shorter periods of time.

Pregnancy:
Consult doctor. Risk category B (see page xxii).

Breast-feeding:
Drug passes into milk. Avoid drug or discontinue nursing until you finish medicine. Consult doctor for advice on maintaining milk supply.

Infants & children:
Not recommended for patients under age 18.

Prolonged use:
Not recommended for long-term usage. Don't take for longer than 1 to 2 weeks unless under doctor's supervision.

Skin & sunlight:
No special problems expected.

Driving, piloting or hazardous work:
Don't drive or pilot aircraft until you learn how medicine affects you. Don't work around dangerous machinery. Don't climb ladders or work in high places. Danger increases if you drink alcohol or take other medicines affecting alertness and reflexes.

Discontinuing:
- Don't discontinue without consulting doctor. Dose may require gradual reduction if you have taken drug for a long time.
- You may have sleeping problems for 1 or 2 nights after stopping drug.

Others:
- Advise any doctor or dentist whom you consult that you take this medicine.
- Don't take drug if you are traveling on an overnight airplane trip of less than 7 or 8 hours. A temporary memory loss may occur (traveler's amnesia).

POSSIBLE INTERACTION WITH OTHER DRUGS

GENERIC NAME OR DRUG CLASS	COMBINED EFFECT
Central nervous system (CNS) depressants*	Increased sedative effect. Avoid.
Chlorpromazine	Increased sedative effect. Avoid.
Imipramine	Increased sedative effect. Avoid.

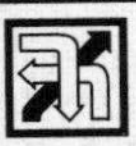

POSSIBLE INTERACTION WITH OTHER SUBSTANCES

INTERACTS WITH	COMBINED EFFECT
Alcohol:	Increased sedation. Avoid.
Beverages:	None expected.
Cocaine:	None expected.
Foods:	Decreased sedative effect if taken with a meal or right after a meal.
Marijuana:	None expected.
Tobacco:	None expected.

***See Glossary**

Brand and Generic Name Directory

The following drugs are alphabetized by generic name or drug class, shown in large capital letters. The brand and generic names that follow each title in this list are the complete list referred to on the drug charts. Generic names are in all capital letters on the lists.

ACETAMINOPHEN

4 Way Cold
Abenol
Acephen
Aceta
Acetaminophen Uniserts
Aclophen
Actamin
Actamin Extra
Actifed A
Actifed Plus
Actifed Plus capsules
Actimol
Advanced Formula Dristan
Advanced Formula Dristan Caplets
Alba-Temp 300
Allerest Headache Strength
Allerest No-Drowsiness
Allerest Sinus Pain Formula
Alumadrine
Amaphen
Aminofen
Aminofen Max
Anacin-3
Anatuss
Anatuss with Codeine
Anolor 300
Anoquan
Anuphen
Apacet
Apacet Extra Strength
Apacet Oral Solution
APAP
Apo-Acetaminophen
Arcet
Aspirin Free Anacin Maximum Strength Caplets
Aspirin Free Anacin Maximum Strength Tablets
Aspirin Free Bayer Select Maximum Strength Headache Plus Caplets
Aspirin-Free Excedrin Caplets
Aspirin Free Excedrin Dual Caplets
Atasol
Atasol Forte
Bayer Select Flu Relief Caplets
Bayer Select Head & Chest Cold Caplets
Bayer Select Head Cold Caplets
Bayer Select Maximum Strength Sinus Pain Relief Caplets
Bancap
Banesin
Benadryl Allergy/Sinus Headache Caplets
Benadryl Plus
Benadryl Plus Nighttime Liquid Oral Solution
Beta-Phed
BQ Cold
Bromo-Seltzer
Bucet
Butace
Calmylin Cough & Cold
Campain
Chexit
Children's Anacin 3
Children's Genapap
Children's Panadol
Children's Ty-Tab
Children's Tylenol
Children's Tylenol Cold
Children's Tylenol Suspension Liquid
Chlor-Trimeton Sinus Caplets
Co-Apap
Co-Tylenol
Codimal
Coldrine
Colrex Compound
Comtrex
Comtrex A/S Caplets
Comtrex Daytime Caplets
Comtrex Daytime Maximum Strength Cold and Flu Relief
Comtrex Daytime Maximum Strength Cold, Cough and Flu Relief
Comtrex Hot Flu Relief
Comtrex Multi-Symptom Cold Reliever
Comtrex Multi-Symptom Hot Flu Relief
Comtrex Multi-Symptom Non-Drowsy Caplets
Comtrex Nighttime
Comtrex Nighttime Maximum Strength Cold and Flu Relief
Comtrex Nighttime Maximum Strength Cold, Cough and Flu Relief
Conacetol
Conar-A
Conex Plus
Congespirin
Congespirin for Children Cold Tablets
Congespirin for Children Liquid Cold Medicine
Contac Allergy/Sinus Day Caplets
Contac Allergy/Sinus Night Caplets
Contac C Cold Care Formula Tablets
Contac Jr. Children's Cold Medicine
Contac Maximum Strength Sinus Caplets
Contac Night Caplets
Contac Severe Cold Formula
Contac Severe Cold Formula Night Strength
Coricidin D Decongestant
Coricidin D Medilets
Coricidin Demilets
Coricidin Maximum Strength Sinus Headache
CoTylenol Cold Medication
Covangesic
Dapa
Dapacin Cold
Datril Extra Strength
DayCare
DayQuil Liquicaps
DayQuil Non-Drowsy Cold/Flu
DayQuil Non-Drowsy Cold/Flu Liquicaps
DayQuil Non-Drowsy Sinus Pressure and Pain Relief Caplets
Dilotab
Dimetapp-A
Dimetapp-A Pediatric
Dimetapp Plus Caplets
Dolanex
Dolmar
Dorcol Children's Fever and Pain Reducer
Drinophen
Dristan
Dristan AF
Dristan AF Plus
Dristan Cold
Dristan Cold and Flu
Dristan Juice Mix-in Cold, Flu, and Cough
Dristan Maximum Strength Caplets
Drixoral Plus
Drixoral Sinus
Duadacin
Effervescent Tylenol Cold
Endolor
Esgic
Esgic Plus
Excedrin Caplets
Exdol
Exdol Strong
Extreme Cold Formula Caplets
Ezol
Febridyne
Femcet
Fendol
Feverall Sprinkle Caps
Fevernol Children's Strength
Fevernol Junior Strength
Fioricet
Genapap
Genapap Extra Strength
Genebs
Genebs Extra Strength
Genex
Halenol
Halenol Extra Strength
Histagestic Modified
Histosal
Hycomine Compound
Improved Sino-Tuss
Infants' Anacin-3
Infants Genapap

Infants' Tylenol Suspension Drops
Isopap
Kolephrin
Kolephrin/DM
Korigesic
Liquiprin Children's Elixir
Liquiprin Infants' Drops
Mapap Cold Formula
Maximum Strength Dristan Cold Multi-Symptom Caplets
Maximum Strength Tylenol Allergy Sinus Caplets
Maximum Strength Tylenol Flu Gelcaps
Meda Cap
Meda Tab
Medi-Flu
Medi-Flu Caplets
Medigesic
Myapap Elixir
Naldegesic
ND-Gesic
Neo Citran Sinus Medicine
Neopap
Nighttime Pamprin
Norel Plus
NyQuil Hot Therapy
NyQuil Liquicaps
NyQuil Nighttime Colds Medicine
Nytime Cold Medicine Liquid
Omnicol
Oraphen-PD
Ornex No Drowsiness Caplets
Pacaps
Panadol
Panadol Junior Strength
Panex
Panex 500
Paracetamol
Parafon Forte
Pedric
Pertussin PM
PhenAPAP No. 2
Phenapap Sinus Headache & Congestion
Phenaphen
Phentate T.D.
Phrenilin
Pyrroxate
Remcol-C
Remcol Cold
Repan
Rhinocaps
Rhinogesic
Robigesic
Robitussin Night Relief
Robitussin Night Relief Colds Formula Liquid
Rounox
Saleto-CF
Saleto D
Sedapap-10
Semcet
Sinapils
Sinarest
Sinarest Extra Strength
Sinarest No-Drowsiness
Sine-Aid
Sine-Aid Maximum Strength
Sine-Aid Maximum Strength Caplets
Sine-Off Maximum Strength Allergy
Sine-Off Maximum Strength Allergy/Sinus Formula Caplets
Sine-Off Maximum Strength-No Drowsiness
Singlet
Sinubid
Sinulin
Sinus Excedrin No Drowsiness
Sinus Excedrin No Drowsiness Caplets
Sinutab
Sinutab II Maximum Strength
Sinutab Extra Strength
Sinutab Maximum Strength without Drowsiness
Sinutab Maximum Strength without Drowsiness Caplets
Sinutab No Drowsiness
Sinutab No Drowsiness Extra Strength
Sinutab Regular
Sinutab SA
St. Joseph Aspirin Free
St. Joseph Cold Tablets for Children
Sudafed Severe Cold Formul
Sudafed Sinus Maximum Strength
Sudafed Sinus Maximum Strength Caplets
Summit
Super-Anahist
Suppap
Tapanol
Tapanol Extra Strength
Tapar
Tempra
Tempra Double Strength
Tencet
Tenol
TheraFlu/Flu & Cold
TheraFlu/Flu, Cold & Cough
TheraFlu Maximum Strength Non-Drowsy Formula Flu, Cold and Cough Medicine
TheraFlu Nighttime Maximum Strength
Thera-Hist
Triad
Triaminicin
Triaminicin w/Codeine
Triaprin
Tricom Tablets
Tussagesic
Two-Dyne
Ty-Cold Cold Formula
Ty Pap
Tylenol
Tylenol Allergy Sinus Gelcaps
Tylenol Allergy Sinus NightTime Maximum Strength Caplets
Tylenol Cold and Flu
Tylenol Cold Medication
Tylenol Cold Medication, Non-Drowsy
Tylenol Cold Night Time
Tylenol Cold No Drowsiness Formula Gelcaps
Tylenol Cough
Tylenol Cough with Decongestant
Tylenol Extra Strength
Tylenol Junior Strength
Tylenol Sinus Maximum Strength
Tylenol Sinus Maximum Strength Caplets
Tylenol Sinus Medication
Tylenol Sinus Medication Extra Strength
Valadol
Valadol Liquid
Valorin
Valorin Extra
Vicks 44 Cold, Flu and Cough Liqui-Caps
Vicks Formula 44M Multi-symptom Cough Mixture

ACETAMINOPHEN & SALICYLATES

ACETAMINOPHEN & ASPIRIN
ACETAMINOPHEN & SALICYLAMIDE
ACETAMINOPHEN & SODIUM SALICYLATE
ACETAMINOPHEN, ASPIRIN & SALICYLAMIDE
Arthralgin
Buffets II
Duoprin
Duradyne
Excedrin Extra Strength Caplets
Excedrin Extra Strength Tablets
Gelpirin
Gemnisyn
Goody's Extra Strength Tablet
Goody's Headache Powders
Presalin
Rid-A-Pain Compound
S-A-C
Salatin
Saleto
Salocol
Salphenyl
Supac
Tenol Plus
Tri-Pain
Trigesic
Vanquish

ADRENOCORTICOIDS (Topical)

9-1-1
Aclovate
Acticort-100
Adcortyl
Aeroseb-Dex
Aeroseb-HC
Ala-Cort
Ala-Scalp HP
ALCLOMETASONE (Topical)
Allercort
Alphaderm
Alphatrex
AMCINONIDE (Topical)
Anusol 2.5%, PD
Aristocort
Aristocort A
Aristocort C
Aristocort D
Aristocort R
Bactine
Barriere-HC
Beben

BECLOMETHASONE (Topical)
Beta HC
Betacort Scalp Lotion
Betaderm
Betaderm Scalp Lotion
Betamethacot
BETAMETHASONE (Topical)
Betatrex
Beta-Val
Betnovate
Betnovate 1/2
Bio-Syn
CaldeCORT Anti-Itch
CaldeCORT-Light
Carmol-HC
Celestoderm-V
Celestoderm-V/2
Cetacort
CLOBETASOL (Topical)
CLOBETASONE (Topical)
CLOCORTOLONE (Topical)
Cloderm
Cordran
Cordran SP
Cort-Dome
Cortacet
Cortaid
Cortate
Cortef
Cortef Feminine Itch
Corticaine
Corticreme
Cortifair
CORTISOL
Cortoderm
Cortril
Cultivate
Cyclocort
Decaderm
Decadron
Decaspray
Delacort
Delta-Tritex
Demarest DriCort
Dermabet
Dermacomb
Dermacort
DermAtop
DermiCort
Dermovate
Dermovate Scalp Application
Dermtex HC
DESONIDE (Topical)
DesOwen
DESOXIMETASONE (Topical)
DEXAMETHASONE (Topical)
DIFLORASONE (Topical)
DIFLUCORTOLONE (Topical)
Diprolene
Diprolene AF
Diprosone
Drenison
Drenison-1/4
Ectosone
Ectosone Regular
Ectosone Scalp Lotion
Efcortelan
Elcom
Elocon
Emo-Cort
Emo-Scalp Solution
Epifoam
Eumovate
Florene E
Florone
Florone E
Fludonid
Fludroxycortide
FLUMETHASONE (Topical)
Fluocet
Fluocin
FLUOCINOLONE (Topical)
FLUOCINONIDE (Topical)
Fluoderm
Fluolar
Fluonid
Fluonide
FLURANDRENOLIDE (Topical)
Flurosyn
Flutex
FLUTICASONE
Foille Cort
Gly-Cort
Gynecort
Gynecort 10
H2 Cort
Halciderm
HALCINONIDE (Topical)
HALOBETASOL
Halog
Halog E
Hi-Cor 1.0
Hi-Cor 2.5
Hyderm
Hydro-Tex
HYDROCORTISONE (Dental)
HYDROCORTISONE (Topical)
Hytone
Kenac
Kenalog
Kenalog-H
Kenalog in Orabase
Keronel
Lacticare-HC
Lanacort
Lanacort 10
Lemoderm
Licon
Lidemol
Lidex
Lidex-E
Locacorten
Locold
Lotrisone
Lyderm
Maxiflor
Maximum Strength Cortaid
Maxivate
Metaderm Mild
Metaderm Regular
METHYLPREDNISOLONE (Topical)
Metosyn
Metosyn FAPG
MOMETASONE (Topical)
My Cort
Nerisone
Nerisone Oily
Novobetamet
Novohydrocort
Nutracort
Orabase HCA
Oracort
Oralone
Pentacort
Pharma-Cort
PREDNICARBATE
Prevex B
Prevex HC
Propaderm
Psorcon
Rederm
Rhulicort
Sential
S-T Cort
Sarna HC
Synacort
Synalar
Synalar HP
Synamol
Synandone
Synemol
Teladar
Temovate
Temovate Scalp Application
Texacort
Topicort
Topicort LP
Topicort Mild
Topilene
Topisone
Topsyn
Triacet
Triaderm
TRIAMCINOLONE (Dental)
TRIAMCINOLONE (Topical)
Trianide Mild
Trianide Regular
Triderm
Tridesilon
Trymex
Ultravate
Unicort
Uticort
Valisone
Valisone Reduced Strength
Valisone Scalp Lotion
Valnac
Vioform-Hydrocortisone
Westcort
Some of these brands are available as oral medicine. Look under specific generic name for each brand.

ANDROGENS

Anabolin
Anabolin LA 100
Anadrol
Anapolon 50
Anavar
Andro 100
Andro-Cyp 100
Andro-LA 200
Android
Android-F
Android-T
Androlone
Andronaq-50
Andronaq-LA
Andronate
Andropository 100
Andryl 200
Deca-Durabolin
Delatest
Delatestryl
Dep Andro
Depo-Testosterone
Depotest
Durabolin
Duratest

Durathate 200
ETHYLESTRENOL
Everone
FLUOXYMESTERONE
Halotestin
Histerone
Hybolin Decanoate
Hybolin-Improved
Kabolin
Malogen
Malogex
Maxibolin
Metandren
METHYLTESTOSTERONE
Nancrobolic L.A.
Nandrobolic
NANDROLONE
Neo-Durabolic
Ora-Testryl
Oreton
OXANDROLONE
OXYMETHOLONE
STANOZOLOL
T-Cypionate
Testa-C
Testamone 100
Testaqua
Testex
Testoject-50
Testoject-LA
Testone L.A.
TESTOSTERONE
Testred
Testred-Cypionate 200
Testrin P.A.
Virilon
Virolon IM
Winstrol

ANESTHETICS (Topical)

Americaine
Aminobenzoate
BENZOCAINE
BENZOCAINE & MENTHOL
Benzocol
BUTACAINE
BUTAMBEN
Butesin Picrate
Butyl Aminobenzoate
Cinchocaine
Dermoplast
DIBUCAINE
EMLA
Ethyl Aminobenzoate
LIDOCAINE
LIDOCAINE AND PRILOCAINE
Lignocaine
Mercurochrome II
Nupercainal Cream
Nupercainal Ointment
Pontocaine Cream
Pontocaine Ointment
Pramegel
PRAMOXINE
Prax
TETRACAINE
TETRACAINE & MENTHOL
Tronothane
Unguentine
Unguentine Plus
Unguentine Spray
Xylocaine

ANGIOTENSIN-CONVERTING ENZYME (ACE) INHIBITORS

Accupril
Aceon
Altace
Apo-Capto
BENAZEPRIL
Capoten
CAPTOPRIL
ENALAPRIL
FOSINOPRIL
LISINOPRIL
Lotensin
Monopril
Novo-Captoril
PERINDOPRIL
Prinivil
QUINAPRIL
RAMIPRIL
Syn-Captopril
Vasotec
Zestril

ANGIOTENSIN-CONVERTING ENZYME (ACE) INHIBITORS & HYDROCHLOROTHIAZIDE

Capozide
CAPTOPRIL & HYDROCHLOROTHIAZIDE
ENALAPRIL & HYDROCHLOROTHIAZIDE
LISINOPRIL & HYDROCHLOROTHIAZIDE-
Prinzide
Vaseretic
Zestoretic

ANTACIDS

Advanced Formula Di-Gel
Alamag
Algenic Alka
Algenic Alka Improved
Algicon
Alka-Mints
Alkets
Alma-Mag Improved
Alma-Mag #4 Improved
Almacone
Almacone II
ALternaGEL
Alu-Cap
Alu-Tab
Aludrox
Alumid
Alumid Plus
Alumid Plus II
ALUMINA AND MAGNESIA
ALUMINA AND MAGNESIUM CARBONATE
ALUMINA AND MAGNESIUM TRISILICATE
ALUMINA, MAGNESIA, AND CALCIUM CARBONATE
ALUMINA, MAGNESIA, AND SIMETHICONE
ALUMINA, MAGNESIUM CARBONATE, AND CALCIUM CARBONATE
ALUMINA, MAGNESIUM TRISILICATE, AND SODIUM BICARBONATE
ALUMINUM CARBONATE, BASIC
ALUMINUM HYDROXIDE
Amitone
Amphojel
Amphojel Plus
Amphojel 500
AntaGel
AntaGel-II
Antiflux
Aspirin Free Excedrin Dual Caplets
Basaljel
Bisodol
Calcilac
Calcitrel
CALCIUM AND MAGNESIUM CARBONATES
CALCIUM AND MAGNESIUM CARBONATES AND MAGNESIUM OXIDE
CALCIUM CARBONATE
CALCIUM CARBONATE AND MAGNESIA
CALCIUM CARBONATE AND SIMETHICONE
CALCIUM CARBONATE, MAGNESIA, AND SIMETHICONE
Calglycine
Camalox
Chooz
Creamalin
Delcid
Di-Gel
Dialume
Dicarbosil
DIHYDROXYALUMINUM AMINOACETATE
DIHYDROXYALUMINUM AMINOACETATE, MAGNESIA, AND ALUMINA
DIHYDROXYALUMINUM SODIUM CARBONATE
Diovol Ex
Diovol Plus
Duracid
Equilet
Escot
Extra Strength Tylenol Headache Plus Caplets
Foamicon
Gas-is-gon
Gaviscon
Gaviscon Extra Strength Relief Formula
Gaviscon-2
Gelamal
Gelusil
Gelusil Extra-Strength
Gelusil-M
Gelusil-II
Genalac
Glycate
Gustalac
Kudrox Double Strength
Liquimint
Losotron Plus
Lowsium
Lowsium Plus
Maalox

Maalox No. 1
Maalox No. 2
Maalox Plus
Maalox Plus, Extra Strength
Maalox TC
Maalox Whip, Extra Strength
MAGALDRATE
MAGALDRATE AND SIMETHICONE
Magmalin
Magnagel
Magnatril
MAGNESIUM CARBONATE AND SODIUM BICARBONATE
MAGNESIUM HYDROXIDE
MAGNESIUM OXIDE
MAGNESIUM TRISILICATE, ALUMINA, AND MAGNESIUM CARBONATE
MAGNESIUM TRISILICATE, ALUMINA, AND MAGNESIA
Mag-Ox 400
Mallamint
Maox
Marblen
Mi-Acid
Mintox
Mintox Plus
Mygel
Mygel II
Mylanta
Mylanta-II
Mylanta-2 Extra Strength
Mylanta-2 Plain
Nephrox
Neutralca-S
Newtrogel II
Noralac
Pama No. 1
Par-Mag
Parviscon
Phillips' Milk of Magnesia
Riopan
Riopan Extra Strength
Riopan Plus
Riopan Plus 2
Riopan Plus Extra Strength
Robalate
Rolaids
Rolaids Calcium Rich
Rolaids Sodium Free
Rulox
Rulox No. 1
Rulox No. 2
Silain-Gel
Simaal Gel
Simaal 2 Gel
SIMETHICONE, ALUMINA, CALCIUM CARBONATE, AND MAGNESIA
SIMETHICONE, ALUMINA, MAGNESIUM CARBONATE, AND MAGNESIA
Spastosed
Tempo
Titracid
Titralac
Titralac Plus
Tralmag
Triconsil
Tums
Tums E-X
Tums Liquid Extra Strength
Tums Liquid Extra Strength w/Simethicone
Univol
Uro-Mag
WinGel

ANTIBACTERIALS (Ophthalmic)

Aerosporin
Achromycin
Ak-Chlor Ophthalmic Ointment
Ak-Chlor Ophthalmic Solution
Ak-Spore
Ak-Sulf
Aktob
Alcomicin
Aureomycin
Bio-Triple
Bleph-10
Cetamide
Chibroxin
Chloracol Ophthalmic Solution
CHLORAMPHENICOL (Ophthalmic)
Chlorofair Ophthalmic Ointment
Chlorofair Ophthalmic Solution
Chloromycetin Ophthalmic Ointment
Chloromycetin Ophthalmic Solution
Chloroptic Ophthalmic Solution
Chloroptic S.O.P.
CHLORTETRACYCLINE
Ciloxan
CIPROFLOXACIN
Cortisporin-Ophthalmic
Econochlor Ophthalmic Ointment
Econochlor Ophthalmic Solution
ERYTHROMYCIN (Ophthalmic)
Fenicol Ophthalmic Ointment
Gantrisin
Garamycin
Genoptic
Gentacidin
Gentafair
Gentak
GENTAMICIN
Gentrasul
I-Chlor Ophthalmic Solution
I-Sulfacet
Ilotycin
Isopto Cetamide
Isopto Fenicol
Liquifilm
Mycitracin
Neociden
NEOMYCIN
NEOMYCIN, POLYMIXIN B & BACITRACIN
NEOMYCIN, POLYMIXIN B & CORTISOL
NEOMYCIN, POLYMIXIN B & GRAMICIDIN
NEOMYCIN, POLYMIXIN B & HYDROCORTISONE
Neosporin
Neosporin Ophthalmic Solution
Neotal
Neotricin
NORFLOXACIN (Ophthalmic)
Ocu-Chlor Ophthalmic Ointment
Ocu-Chlor Ophthalmic Solution
Ocuflox
Ocu-Mycin
Ocu-Spor-B
Ocu-Spor-G
Ocusporin
Ocutricin
Ocu-Sul-10
Ocu-Sul-15
Ocu-Sul-30
Ocusulf-10
OFLOXACIN (Ophthalmic)
Ophthacet
Ophthalmic
Ophthochlor Ophthalmic Solution
Ophtho-Chloram Ophthalmic Solution
Pentamycetin
Pentamycetin Ophthalmic Ointment
Pentamycetin Ophthalmic Solution
P.N. Ophthalmic
POLYMYXIN B
Regasporin
Sodium Sulamyd
Sopamycetin Ophthalmic Ointment
Sopamycetin Ophthalmic Solution
Spectro-Chlor Ophthalmic Ointment
Spectro-Chlor Ophthalmic Solution
Spectro-Genta
Spectro-Sporin
Spectro-Sulf
Steri-Units Sulfacetamide
Sulf-10
SULFACETAMIDE (Ophthalmic)
Sulfair
Sulfair 10
Sulfair 15
Sulfair Forte
Sulfamide
Sulfex
SULFISOXAZOLE (Ophthalmic)
SULFONAMIDES (Ophthalmic)
Sulten-10
TOBRAMYCIN (Ophthalmic)
Tobrex
TETRACYCLINE (Ophthalmic)
Tribiotic
Tri-Ophthalmic
Tri-Thalmic

ANTICHOLINERGICS

AH-Chew
ANISTROPINE
Atrohist Plus
ATROPINE
Banthine
Baycodan
Cantil
Codan
D.A. Chewable
Dallergy
Dallergy Caplets
Darbid
Daricon
DuraVent/DA
Extendryl
Extendryl JR
Extendryl SR

Gastrozepin
Histor-D Timecelles
Homapin
HOMATROPINE
Hycodan
Hydromet
Hydropane
ISOPROPAMIDE
MEPENZOLATE
METHANTHELINE
METHSCOPOLAMINE
OMNIhist L.A.
OXYPHENCYCLIMINE
Pamine
Pathilon
Phenahist-TR
Phenchlor SHA
PIRENZEPINE
Prehist D
Rhinolar
Ru-Tuss
Stahist
TRIDIHEXETHYL
Tussigon
Valpin 50

ANTIDEPRESSANTS, TRICYCLIC

Adapin
AMITRYPTILINE
AMOXAPINE
Anafranil
Apo-Amitriptyline
Apo-Imipramine
Apo-Trimip
Asendin
Aventyl
CLOMIPRAMINE
DESIPRAMINE
DOXEPIN
Elavil
Emitrip
Endep
Enovil
IMIPRAMINE
Impril
Janimine
Levate
Limbitrol
Limbitrol DS
Norfranil
Norpramin
NORTRIPTYLINE
Novo-Doxepin
Novopramine
Novo-Tripramine
Novotriptyn
Pamelor
Pertofrane
PMS Amitriptyline
PMS Impramine
PROTRIPTYLINE
Rhotrimine
Sinequan
Surmontil
Tipramine
Tofranil
Tofranil-PM
Triadapin
TRIMIPRAMINE
Triptil
Vivactil

ANTIDIABETIC AGENTS

ACETOHEXAMIDE
Albert Glyburide
Alpha-Glibenclamide
Apo-Chlorpropamide
Apo-Glyburide
Apo-Tolbutamide
CHLORPROPAMIDE
DiaBeta
Diabinese
Dimelor
Dymelor
Euglucon
Gen-Glybe
GLIPIZIDE
Glucamide
Glucotrol
GLYBURIDE
Glynase PresTab
Micronase
Mobenol
Novo-Butamide
Novo-Glyburide
Novo-Propamide
Oramide
Orinase
Storzolamide
Tolamide
TOLAZAMIDE
TOLBUTAMIDE
Tolinase
Tol-Tab

ANTIDYSKINETICS

Akineton
Apo-Benztropine
Apo-Trihex
Artane
Artane Sequels
BENZTROPINE
BIPERIDEN
Cogentin
ETHOPROPAZINE
Kemadrin
Orap
Parsidol
Parsitan
PIMOZIDE
PMS Benztropine
PMS Procyclidine
PMS Trihexyphenidyl
Procyclid
PROCYCLIDINE
Trihexane
Trihexy
TRIHEXYPHENIDYL

ANTIFUNGALS (Topical)

Aftate for Athlete's Foot Aerosol Spray Liquid
Aftate for Athlete's Foot Aerosol Spray Powder
Aftate for Athlete's Foot Gel
Aftate for Athlete's Foot Sprinkle Powder
Aftate for Jock Itch Aerosol Spray Powder
Aftate for Jock Itch Gel
Aftate for Jock Itch Sprinkle Powder
AMPHOTERICIN B
Caldesene Medicated Powder
Canesten Cream
Canesten Solution
CICLOPIROX
Ciloxam
CLOTRIMAZOLE
Cruex Aerosol Powder
Cruex Antifungal Cream
Cruex Antifungal Powder
Cruex Antifungal Spray Powder
Cruex Cream
Cruex Powder
Decylenes
Decylenes Powder
Desenex Aerosol Powder
Desenex Antifungal Cream
Desenex Antifungal Liquid
Desenex Antifungal Ointment
Desenex Antifungal Penetrating Foam
Desenex Antifungal Powder
Desenex Antifungal Spray Powder
Desenex Ointment
Desenex Powder
Desenex Solution
ECONAZOLE
Ecostatin
Exelderm
Fungizone
Genaspore Cream
Gordochom Solution
HALOPROGIN
Halotex
KETOCONAZOLE (Topical)
Lamisil
Loprox
Lotriderm
Lotrimin Cream
Lotrimin Lotion
Lotrimin Ointment
Lotrisone
Micatin
MICONAZOLE
Monistat-Derm
Mycelex Cream
Mycelex Solution
Myclo Cream
Myclo Solution
Miclo Spray
Mycostatin
Nadostine
NAFTIFINE
Naftin
Nilstat
Nizoral Shampoo
NP-27 Cream
NP-27 Powder
NP-27 Solution
NP-27 Spray Powder
Nyaderm
NYSTATIN
Nystex
OXICONAZOLE (Topical)
Oxistat
Pitrex Cream
Spectazole
SULCONAZOLE
TERBINAFINE
Tinactin Aerosol Liquid
Tinactin Aerosol Powder
Tinactin Antifungal Deodorant Powder Aerosol
Tinactin Cream

Tinactin Jock Itch Aerosol Powder
Tinactin Jock Itch Cream
Tinactin Jock Itch Spray Powder
Tinactin Plus Powder
Tinactin Powder
Tinactin Solution
Ting Antifungal Cream
Ting Antifungal Powder
Ting Antifungal Spray Liquid
Ting Antifungal Spray Powder
TOLNAFTATE
UNDECYLENIC ACID
Zeasorb-AF Powder

ANTIFUNGALS (Vaginal)

BUTOCONAZOLE
Canesten
Canesten 1
Canesten 3
Canesten 10%
CLOTRIMAZOLE
ECONAZOLE
Ecostatin
FemCare
Femstat
Genapax
GENTIAN VIOLET
Gyne-Lotrimin
Gyno-Trosyd
MICONAZOLE
Monistat
Monistat 3
Monistat 5
Monistat 7
Mycelex-7
Mycelex-G
Myclo
Mycostatin
Nadostine
Nilstat
Nyaderm
NYSTATIN
Terazol 3
Terazol 7
TERCONAZOLE
TIOCONAZOLE
Vagistat

ANTIHISTAMINES

4 Way Cold
12-Hour Cold
Aclophen
Actacin
Actagen-C Cough
ACRIVASTINE
Actidil
Actifed
Actifed 12-Hour
Actifed A
Actifed Allergy Nighttime Caplets
Actifed DM
Actifed Plus
Actifed w/Codeine Cough
Advanced Formula Dristan
AH-Chew
Alamine
Alamine-C Liquid
Alersule
Alka-Selzer Plus Cold
Alka-Seltzer Plus Maximum Strength Sinus Allergy
Alka-Selzer Plus Nighttime Cold
Allent
Aller-Chlor
Alleract
Allerdryl
Allerest
Allerest 12 Hour
Allerest 12 Hour Caplets
Allerest Headache Strength
Allerest Sinus Pain Formula
Allerfrin
Allerfrin w/Codeine
Allergy Formula Sinutab
Allergy Relief Medicine
AllerMax
Allerphed
Allert
Amaril D
Amaril D Spantab
Ambay Cough
Ambenyl Cough
Ambophen Expectorant
Anamine
Anamine HD
Anamine TD
Anaplex
Anatuss
Anatuss w/Codeine
Apo-Dimenhydrinate
Aprodrine
A.R.M. Maximum Strength Caplets
ASTEMIZOLE
Atrofed
Atrohist Plus
Atrohist Sprinkle
AZATADINE
Banophen
Bayaminicol
Baydec DM Drops
Bayhistine DH
BC Cold Powder
Beldin Cough
Belix
Bena-D
Bena-D 50
Benadryl
Benadryl Allergy/Sinus Headache Caplets
Benadryl Complete Allergy
Benadryl Decongestant
Benadryl Plus
Benadryl Plus Nighttime Liquid
Benahist 10
Benahist 50
Ben-Allergin 50
Benaphen
Benoject-10
Benoject-50
Benylin Cold
Benylin Cough
Benylin Decongestant
Benylin w/Codeine
Benylin-DM
Biphetane DC Cough
BQ Cold
Brexin
Brexin-L.A.
Bromanate DC Cough
Bromatap
Bromatapp
Brombay
Bromfed
Bromfed-AT
Bromfed-DM
Bromfed-PD
BROMODIPHENHYDRAMINE
Bromophen T.D.
Bromphen
Bromphen DC
BROMPHENIRAMINE
Brompheril
Bronkotuss Expectorant
Brotane DX Cough
Bydramine Cough
Caldomine-DH Forte
Caldomine-DH Pediatric
Calm X
Calmylin #4
Calmylin w/Codeine
CARBINOXAMINE
Carbinoxamine Compound
Carbiset
Carbodec
Carbodec DM Drops
Carbodec TR
Cardec-S
Cenafed Plus
Cerose-DM
Cheracol Plus
Cheracol Sinus
Children's Dramamine
Children's Nyquil Nighttime Cold Medicine
Children's Tylenol Cold
Chexit
Chlo-Amine
Chlor-100
Chlorafed
Chlorafed H.S. Timecelles
Chlorafed Timecelles
Chlorate
Chlorgest-HD
Chlor-Niramine
Chlorphed
CHLORPHENIRAMINE
Chlor-Pro
Chlor-Pro 10
Chlor-Rest
Chlorspan-12
Chlortab-4
Chlortab-8
Chlor-Trimeton
Chlor-Trimeton Allergy
Chlor-Trimeton Decongestant
Chlor-Trimeton Repetabs
Chlor-Trimeton Sinus Caplets
Chlor-Tripolon
Chlor-Tripolon Decongestant
Chlor-Tripolon Decongestant Extra Strength
Chlor-Tripolon Decongestant Repetabs
Citra Forte
Claritin
Claritin Extra
CLEMASTINE FUMARATE
Clistin
CoActifed
CoActifed Expectorant
Co-Apap
Codehist DH
Codimal
Codimal-A
Codimal DH
Codimal DM
Codimal L.A.

Codimal-LA Half
Codimal PH
Colrex Compound
Colrex Cough
Coltab Children's
Comhist
Comhist LA
Compoz
Comtrex A/S
Comtrex Hot Flu Relief
Comtrex Multi-Symptom Cold Reliever
Comtrex Multi-Symptom Hot Flu Relief
Comtrex Nighttime
Comtrex Nighttime Maximum Strength Cold and Flu Relief
Comtrex Nighttime Maximum Strength Cold, Cough and Flu Relief
Condrin LA
Conex D.A.
Conex Plus
Conjec-B
Contac 12-Hour
Contac 12-Hour Allergy
Contac Allergy/Sinus Night Caplets
Contac C Cold Care Formula Caplets
Contac Day Caplets
Contac Maximum Strength 12-Hour Caplets
Contac Night Caplets
Contac Severe Cold Formula
Contac Severe Cold Formula Night Strength
Cophene No. 2
Cophene-B
Cophene-S
Cophene-X
Cophene-XP
Co-Pyronil 2
Coricidin D
Coricidin Demilets
Coricidin Maximum Strength Sinus Headache
Coricidin w/Codeine
Coristex-DH
Coristine-DH
Corsym
Cotridin
Cotridin Expectorant
CoTylenol Cold Medication
Covangesic
Cremacoat 4 Throat Coating Cough Medicine
CYPROHEPTADINE
D.A. Chewable
Dallergy
Dallergy Caplets
Dallergy Jr.
Dallergy-D
Dapacin Cold
Decohist
Deconamine
Deconamine SR
Decongestabs
Dehist
Demazin
Demazin Repetabs
Dexaphen SA
DEXBROMPHENIRAMINE

Dexchlor
DEXCHLORPHENIRAMINE
Dexbrompheniramine
Dexophed
Diahist
Diamine T.D.
Dihistine
Dihistine DH
Dihydrex
Dimaphen S.A.
DIMENHYDRINATE
Dimentabs
Dimetane
Dimetane-DC Cough
Dimetane Decongestant
Dimetane Decongestant Caplets
Dimetane-DX Cough
Dimetane Expectorant
Dimetane Expectorant-C
Dimetane Expectorant-DC
Dimetane Extentabs
Dimetane-Ten
Dimetapp
Dimetapp 4-Hour Liqui-Gels Maximum Strength
Dimetapp-A
Dimetapp-DM
Dimetapp Extentabs
Dimetapp Maximum Strength Liquigels
Dimetapp Oral Infant Drops
Dimetapp Plus Caplets
Dimetapp w/Codeine
Dinate
Diphen Cough
Diphenacen-10
Diphenacen-50
Diphenadryl
DIPHENHYDRAMINE
DIPHENYLPYRALINE
Disobrom
Disophrol
Disophrol Chronotabs
Dommanate
Donatussin
Donatussin Drops
Dondril
Dorcol Children's Cold Formula
Dormarex 2
Dormin
DOXYLAMINE
Dramamine
Dramamine Chewable
Dramamine Liquid
Dramanate
Dramilin
Dramocen
Dramoject
Dristan
Dristan AF
Dristan Cold
Dristan Cold and Flu
Dristan Formula P
Drixoral
Drixoral Plus
Drixtab
Drize
Duadacin
Duralex
Dura-Tap PD
DuraVent/A
DuraVent/DA
Dymenate

EDA-Hist
Effervescent Tylenol Cold
Efficol Cough Whip (Cough Suppressant/Decongestant/ Antihistamine)
Efricon Expectorant Liquid
Endafed
Endal HD
Endal-HD Plus
Extendryl
Extendryl JR
Extendryl SR
Extreme Cold Formula Caplets
Father John's Medicine Plus
Fedahist
Fedahist Decongestant
Fedahist Gyrocaps
Fedahist Timecaps
Fenylhist
Fiogesic
Fynex
Genac
Genallerate
Genamin
Genatap
Gencold
Gen-D-phen
Gentab LA
Gravol
Gravol L/A
Guistrey Fortis
Hismanal
Hispril
Histabid Duracaps
Histadyl E.C.
Histafed C
Histagesic Modified
Histaject Modified
Histalet
Histalet DM
Histalet Forte
Histamic
Histatab Plus
Histatan
Histatuss Pediatric
Hista-Vadrin
Histor-D
Histor-D Timecelles
Histosal
Histussin HC
Hycomine
Hycomine Compound
Hycomine-S Pediatric
Hydramine
Hydramine Cough
Hydrate
Hydril
Hyrexin-50
Improved Sino-Tuss
Insomnal
Isoclor
Isoclor Timesules
Klerist
Kolephrin
Kolephrin/DM
Kolephrin NN Liquid
Kophane
Kophane Cough and Cold Formula
Korigesic
Kronofed-A
Kronofed-A Jr.
Lanatuss Expectorant

LORATADINE
Mapap Cold Formula
Marmine
Maximum Strength Dristan Cold Multi-Symptom Caplets
Maximum Strength Tylenol Allergy Sinus Caplets
Medatussin Plus
Meda Syrup Forte
Medi-Flu
Medi-Flu Caplets
Midahist DH
Motion-Aid
Myfed
Myfedrine Plus
Myhistine
Myhistine DH
Myidil
Myminic
Myphetane DC Cough
Myphetapp
Naldecon
Naldecon Pediatric
Naldelate
Naldelate Pediatric Syrup
Nalgest
Napril
Nasahist
Nasahist B
Nauseatol
ND Clear T.D.
ND-Gesic
ND Stat Revised
NeoCitran DM Coughs & Cold
Nervine Night-time Sleep-Aid
New-Decongest
New-Decongest Pediatric Syrup
Nico-Vert
Nidryl
Nighttime Pamprin
Nisaval
Nolahist
Nolamine
Noradryl
Norafed
Noraminic
Nordryl
Nordryl Cough
Norel Plus
Normatane
Normatane DC
Novafed A
Novahistex
Novahistex C
Novahistex DH
Novahistex DH Expectorant
Novahistex DM
Novahistine
Novahistine DH
Novahistine DH Expectorant
Novahistine DH Liquid
Novodimenate
Novopheniram
NyQuil Liquicaps
NyQuil Nighttime Colds Medicine
Nytime Cold Medicine Liquid
Nytol Maximum Strength
Nytol w/DPH
Omni-Tuss
Omnicol
OMNIhist L.A.
Optimine
Oragest S.R.
Oraminic II
Oraminic Spancaps
Ornade
Ornade A.F.
Ornade Expectorant
Ornade Spansules
Ornade-DM 10
Ornade-DM 15
Ornade-DM 30
Orthoxicol Cough
Panadyl
Par Decon
PBZ
PBZ-SR
PediaCare Allergy
Pediacare Children's Cold Relief Night Rest Cough-Cold Formula
PediaCare Children's Cough Cold Formula
Pediacare Cold Formula
Pediacof Cough
Pelamine
Penntuss
Periactin
Pertussin PM
Pfeiffer's Allergy
Phanadex
Phenahist-TR
Phenapap Sinus Headache & Congestion
Phenchlor SHA
Phenetron
Phenetron Lanacaps
PHENINDAMINE
PHENIRAMINE
Phentate T.D.
Phentox Compound
PHENYLTOLOXAMINE
PMS-Dimenhydrinate
Poladex T.D.
Polaramine
Polaramine Expectorant
Polaramine Repetabs
Polargen
Poly-Histine-CS
Poly-Histine-D
Poly-Histine-D Ped
Poly-Histine-DM
Prehist D
Prominicol Cough
Promist HD Liquid
Pseudo-Car DM
Pseudo-Chlor
Pseudodine C Cough
Pseudo-gest Plus
P-V-Tussin
Pyribenzamine
PYRILAMINE
Pyrilamine Maleate Tablets
Pyrroxate
Quelidrine Cough
Reactine
Remcol Cold
Reidamine
Remcol-C
Rentamine
Resaid S.R.
Resporal TR
Rhinogesic
Rhinolar
Rhinolar-EX
Rhinolar-EX 12
Rhinosyn-DM
Rinade B.I.D.
Robitussin A-C
Robitussin Night Relief
Robitussin Night Relief Colds Formula Liquid
Robitussin w/Codeine
Rondec
Rondec Drops
Rondec-DM
Rondec-DM Drops
Rondec-TR
R-Tannate
Ru-Tuss
Ru-Tuss II
Ru-Tuss w/Hydrocodone Liquid
Ryna
Ryna-C Liquid
Rynatan
Rynatuss
Rynatuss Pediatric
Salphenyl
Scot-tussin Original 5-Action Cold Medicine
Semprex-D
Silphen
Sinapils
Sinarest
Sinarest Extra Strength
Sine-Off Maximum Strength Allergy/Sinus Formula
Sine-Off Sinus Medicine
Singlet
Sinubid
Sinucon Pediatric Drops
Sinulin
Sinusol-B
Sinutab
Sinutab Extra Strength
Sinutab Maximum Strength
Sinutab Regular
Sinutab SA
Sleep-Eze 3
Snaplets Multi
Snaplets-D
Sominex Liquid
Stahist
Statuss Expectorant
Statuss Green
Sudafed Plus
Tamine S.R.
Tavist
Tavist-1
Tavist-D
T-Dry
T-Dry Junior
Tega-Vert
Telachlor
Teldrin
TheraFlu/Flu & Cold
TheraFlu/Flu, Cold & Cough
TheraFlu Nighttime Maximum Strength
Thera-Hist
T-Koff
Touro A&H
Travamine
Triacin C Cough
Triaminic
Triaminic Allergy
Triaminic Chewables
Triaminic Cold
Triaminic DM Nighttime For Children
Triaminic Expectorant
Triaminic Expectorant DH

Triaminic Nite Light
Triaminic Oral Infant Drops
Triaminic TR
Triaminic-12
Triaminic-DM Expectorant
Triaminicin
Triaminicin w/Codeine
Triaminicol DM
Triaminicol Multi-Symptom Relief
Tricodene Forte
Tricodene NN
Tricom Tablets
Trifed
Trifed-C Cough
Trimedine Liquid
Trinalin Repetabs
Trind
Trind DM Liquid
Tri-Nefrin Extra Strength
Trinex
Triofed
Triotann
Tripalgin Cold
Trip-Tone
TRIPELENNAMINE
Tri-Phen-Chlor
Tri-Phen-Chlor T.D.
Triphenyl
Triphenyl T.D.
Tripodrine
Triposed
TRIPROLIDINE
Tritann Pediatric
Trymegen
Tusquelin
Tuss-Ornade Spansules
Tussafed
Tussagesic
Tussaminic DH Forte
Tussaminic DH Pediatric
Tussanil DH
Tussanil Plain
Tussar DM
Tussar SF
Tussar-2
Tussionex
Tussirex w/Codeine Liquid
Tusstat
Twilite
Ty-Cold Cold Formula
Tylenol Allergy Sinus Gelcaps
Tylenol Allergy Sinus Night Time Maximum Strength Caplets
Tylenol Cold and Flu
Tylenol Cold Medication
Tylenol Cold Night Time
Unisom Nighttime Sleep Aid
Unisom SleepGels Maximum Strength
Valdrene
Vanex-HD
Vasominic T.D.
Veltane
Veltap
Vertab
Vicks 44 Cold, Flu and Cough Liquid-Caps
Vicks DayQuil 4 Hour Allergy Relief
Vicks DayQuil 12 Hour Allergy Relief
Vicks Formula 44 Cough Mixture
Viro-Med
Wehamine
Wehdryl
Wehdryl-10
Wehdryl-50

ANTIHISTAMINES, PHENOTHIAZINE-DERIVATIVE

Anergan 25
Anergan 50
Histantil
Mallergan-VC with Codeine
METHDILAZINE
Panectyl
Pentazine
Phenameth
Phenameth VC with Codeine
Phenazine 25
Phenazine 50
Phencen-50
Phenergan
Phenergan Fortis
Phenergan Plain
Phenergan VC
Phenergan VC with Codeine
Phenergan with Codeine
Phenergan with Dextromethorphan
Phenoject-50
Pherazine VC
Pherazine VC with Codeine
PMS Promethazine
Pro-50
Promerhegan
Prometh VC Plain
Prometh VC with Codeine
Prometh-25
Prometh-50
Prometharazine VC
PROMETHAZINE
Prorex-25
Prorex-50
Prothazine
Prothazine Plain
TRIMEPRAZINE
V-Gan-25
V-Gan-50

ANTI-INFLAMMATORY DRUGS, NON-STEROIDAL (NSAIDs)

Aches-N-Pain
Advil
Advil Caplets
Advil First
Albert Tiafen
Aleve
Alka-Butazolidin
Alka-Phenylbutazone
Alkabutazone
Alrheumat
Amersol
Anaprox
Anaprox DS
Ansaid
Apo-Diclo
Apo-Flurbiprofen
Apo-Ibuprofen
Apo-Indomethacin
Apo-Keto
Apo-Keto-E
Apo-Naproxen
Apo-Piroxicam
Apsifen
Apsifen-F
Bayer Select Pain Relief Formula Caplets
Brufen
Butacote
Butazone
Cataflam
Children's Advil
Clinoril
CoAdvil
Cotybutazone
Cramp End
Daypro
DICLOFENAC
DIFLUNISAL
Dolgesic
Dolobid
ETODOLAC
Excedrin-IB Caplets
Excedrin-IB Tablets
Feldene
FENOPROFEN
Fenopron
FLOCTAFENINE
FLURBIPROFEN
Froben
Genpril
Haltran
Ibifon-600 Caplets
Ibren
Ibu
Ibu-4
Ibu-6
Ibu-8
Ibu-200
Ibumed
Ibuprin
Ibupro-600
IBUPROFEN
Ibutex
Idarac
Ifen
Imbrilon
Indameth
Indocid
Indocid SR
Indocin
Indocin SR
Indolar SR
INDOMETHACIN
Intrabutazone
KETOPROFEN
KETOROLAC
Lidifen
Lodine
Meclofen
MECLOFENAMATE
Meclomen
Medipren
MEFENAMIC ACID
Midol 200
Midol-IB
Mobiflex
Motrin
Motrin-IB
Motrin-IB Caplets
Motrin-IB Sinus
Motrin-IB Sinus Caplets
Motrin, Children's
NABUMETONE
Nalfon
Nalfon 200

Naprosyn
NAPROXEN
Naxen
Novo-Keto-EC
Novo-Sundac
Novobutazone
Novomethacin
Novonaprox
Novopirocam
Novoprofen
Nu-Indo
Nu-Pirox
Nuprin
Nuprin Caplets
Orudis
Orudis-E
Oruvail
OXAPROZIN
Pamprin-IB
Paxofen
Pedia
PHENYLBUTAZONE
Phenylone Plus
Ponstan
Ponstel
PIROXICAM
Profen
Progesic
Relafen
Rhodis-EC
Ro-Profen
Rufen
Saleto-200
Saleto-400
Saleto-600
Saleto-800
Sine-Aid IB
SULINDAC
Surgam
Synflex
Telectin DS
TENOXICAM
TIAPROFENIC ACID
TOLMETIN
Toradol
Trendar
Voltaren
Voltaren Rapide
Voltaren SR
Voltarol
Voltarol Retard

ANTI-INFLAMMATORY DRUGS, STEROIDAL (Ophthalmic)

Ak-Dex
Ak-Pred
Ak-Tate
Baldex
BETAMETHASONE
Betnesol
Cortamed
Cortisol
Decadron
Dexair
DEXAMETHASONE
Dexotic
Econopred
Econopred Plus
Flarex
FLUOROMETHOLONE
Fluor-Op
FML Forte
FML Liquifilm
FML S.O.P.
HMS Liquifilm
HYDROCORTISONE
I-Methasone
I-Pred
Inflamase Forte
Inflamase-Mild
Life-Pred
Maxidex
MEDRYSONE
Ocu-Dex
Ocu-Pred
Ocu-Pred-A
Ocu-Pred Forte
Pred Forte
Pred Mild
Predair
Predair-A
Predair Forte
PREDNISOLONE
Storz-Dexa
Ultra Pred

ANTISEBORRHEICS (Topical)

Buf-Bar
Capitrol
CHLOROXINE
DHS Zinc
Danex
Dan-Gard
Episel
Exsel
Glo-Sel
Head & Shoulders
Head & Shoulders Antidandruff Cream Shampoo Normal to Dry Formula
Head & Shoulders Antidandruff Cream Shampoo Normal to Oily Formula
Head & Shoulders Antidandruff Lotion Shampoo Normal to Dry Formula
Head & Shoulders Antidandruff Lotion Shampoo Normal to Oily Formula
Head & Shoulders Antidandruff Lotion Shampoo 2 in 1 Formula
Head & Shoulders Dry Scalp Conditioning Formula Lotion Shampoo
Head & Shoulders Dry Scalp Regular Formula Lotion Shampoo
Head & Shoulders Dry Scalp 2 in 1 Formula Lotion Shampoo
Head & Shoulders Intensive Treatment Conditioning Formula Dandruff Lotion Shampoo
Head & Shoulders Intensive Treatment Regular Formula Dandruff Lotion Shampoo
Head & Shoulders Intensive Treatment 2 in 1 Formula Dandruff Lotion Shampoo
Meted Maximum Strength Anti-Dandruff Shampoo with Conditioners
PYRITHIONE
SALICYLIC ACID, SULFUR AND COAL TAR
Sebex-T Tar Shampoo
Sebulex Conditioning Suspension Shampoo
Sebulex Lotion Shampoo
Sebulon
Sebutone
SELENIUM SULFIDE
Selsun
Selsun Blue
Selsun Blue Regular Formula
Theraplex Z
Vanseb-T
Vanseb Cream Dandruff Shampoo
Vanseb Lotion Dandruff Shampoo
Zincon
ZNP

APPETITE SUPPRESSANTS

Adipex-P
Adipost
Adphen
Anorex
Anoxine-AM
Appecon
Bacarate
BENZPHETAMINE
Bontril PDM
Bontril Slow Release
Dapex-37.5
Didrex
DIETHYLPROPION
Dital
Dyrexan-OD
Fastin
FENFLURAMINE
Ionamin
M-Orexic
Marlibar A
MAZINDOL
Mazanor
Melfiat-105 Unicelles
Metra
Nobesine
Obalan
Obe-Del
Obe-Mar
Obe-Nix
Obephen
Obermine
Obestin-30
Obeval
Obezine
Oby-Trim
Panrexin M
Panrexin MTP
Panshape
Parmine
Parzine
Phendiet
Phendimet
PHENDIMETRAZINE
Phentercot
PHENTERMINE
Phenterxene
Phentra
Phentride
Phentrol

Phenzine
Plegine
Ponderal
Ponderal Pacaps
Pondimin
Pondimin Extentabs
Prelu-2
Preludin-Endurets
PT 105
Rexigen
Rexigen Forte
Sanorex
Slynn-LL
Span-RD
Statobex
T-Diet
Tega-Nil
Tenuate
Tenuate Dospan
Tepanil
Tepanil Ten-Tab
Teramin
Trimcaps
Trimstat
Trimtabs
Uni Trim
Wehless
Wehless Timecelles
Weightrol
Wescoid
Wilpowr
X-Trozine
X-Trozine LA
Zantryl

ASPIRIN

217
217 Strong
8-Hour Bayer Timed Release
A.S.A.
A.S.A. Enseals
Acetylsalicylic Acid
Alka-Seltzer Effervescent Pain Reliever & Antacid
Alka-Seltzer Plus
Alka-Seltzer Plus Cold
Alka-Seltzer Plus Maximum Strength Sinus Allergy
Alka-Seltzer Plus Nighttime Cold
Alpha-Phed
Anacin
APAC Improved
APF Arthritic Pain Formula
Arthinol
Arthritis Pain Formula
Artria S.R.
Ascriptin
Ascriptin A/D
Aspergum
Astrin
Bayer
Bayer Enteric
Bayer Timed-Release Arthritic Pain Formula
BC Cold Powder
Bexophene
Buffaprin
Bufferin
Buffinol
Cama Arthritis Reliever
Coricidin D
Coricidin w/Codeine
Coryphen
Dristan
Dristan Formula P
Easprin
Ecotrin
Empirin
Entrophen
Fiogesic
Halfprin
Magnaprin
Magnaprin Arthritis Strength
Maprin
Maprin I-B
Measurin
Norwich Aspirin
Novasen
P-A-C Revised Formula
Robaxisal
Rhinocaps
Riphen
St. Joseph Adult Chewable Aspirin
Sal-Adult
Salatin
Saleto
Sal-Infant
Salocol
Sine-Off Sinus Medicine
Supasa
Synalgos
Therapy Bayer
Triaphen
Ursinus Inlay
Vanquish
Viro-Med
Zorprin

BARBITURATES

Alurate
Amaphen
AMOBARBITAL
Amytal
Ancalixir
Anolor-300
Anoquan
APROBARBITAL
Arcet
Bancap
Barbita
Bucet
Busodium
BUTABARBITAL
Butace
Butalan
BUTALBITAL
Butisol
Dolmar
Endolor
Esgic
Esgic-Plus
Ezol
Femcet
Fioricet
G-1
Gemonil
Isocet
Isopap
Lotusate Caplets
Luminal
Mebaral
Medigesic
MEPHOBARBITAL
METHARBITAL
Nembutal
Nova Rectal
Novopentobarb
Novosecobarb
Pacaps
PENTOBARBITAL
PHENOBARBITAL
Repan
Sarisol No. 2
SECOBARBITAL
SECOBARBITAL AND AMOBARBITAL
Seconal
Sedapap
Solfoton
TALBUTAL
Tencet
Triad
Triaprin
Tuinal
Two-Dyne

BARBITURATES & ASPIRIN (Also contains caffeine)

Axotal
B-A-C
Butalbital A-C
BUTALBITAL, ASPIRIN & CAFFEINE
Butalbital Compound
Butalgen
Farbital
Fiorex
Fiorgen PF
Fiorinal
Fiormor
Florital
Fortabs
Idenal
Isobutal
Isobutyl
Isolin
Isollyl (Improved)
Laniroif
Lanorinal
Marnal
Salipral
Tecnal
Vibutal

BARBITURATES, ASPIRIN & CODEINE

ABC Compound with Codeine
Ascomp with Codeine No. 3
B-A-C with Codeine
BUTALBITAL, ASPIRIN & CODEINE
Butalbital Compound with Codeine
Butinal with Codeine No. 3
Fiomor with Codeine
Fiorgen with Codeine
Fiorinal-C1/4
Fiorinal-C1/2
Fiorinal with Codeine
Fiorinal with Codeine No. 3
Idenal with Codeine
Isollyl with Codeine
Phenaphen with Codeine No. 2
Phenaphen with Codeine No. 3
Phenaphen with Codeine No. 4
PHENOBARBITAL, ASPIRIN & CODEINE

BELLADONNA ALKALOIDS & BARBITURATES

Antrocol
ATROPINE & PHENOBARBITAL
ATROPINE, HYOSCYAMINE, SCOPOLAMINE & BUTABARBITAL
ATROPINE, HYOSCYAMINE, SCOPOLAMINE & PHENOBARBITAL
Barbidonna
Barbidonna 2
Barophen
Belladenal
Belladenal-S
Belladenal Spacetabs
BELLADONNA & AMOBARBITAL
BELLADONNA & BUTABARBITAL
Bellalphen
Butibel
Chardonna-2
Donnamor
Donnapine
Donna-Sed
Donnatal
Donnatal Extentabs
Donnatal No. 2
Donphen
HYOSCYAMINE & PHENOBARBITAL
Hyosophen
Kinesed
Levsin-PB
Levsin with Phenobarbital
Levsinex with Phenobarbital Timecaps
Malatal
Pheno-Bella
Relaxadon
Spaslin
Spasmolin
Spasmophen
Spasquid
Susano

BENZODIAZEPINES

ALPRAZOLAM
Alzapam
Apo-Alpraz
Apo-Chlorax
Apo-Chlordiazepoxide
Apo-Clorazepate
Apo-Diazepam
Apo-Flurazepam
Apo-Lorazepam
Apo-Oxazepam
Ativan
BROMAZEPAM
Centrax
CHLORDIAZEPOXIDE
Clindex
Clinoxide
Clipoxide
CLONAZEPAM
CLORAZEPATE
Corium
Dalmane
Diazemuls
DIAZEPAM
Diazepam Intensol
Doral
Durapam
ESTAZOLAM
FLURAZEPAM
Gen-XENE
HALAZEPAM
KETAZOLAM
Klonopin
Lectopam
Librax
Libritabs
Librium
Lidox
Limbitrol
Limbitrol DS
Lipoxide
Lodoxide
Loftran
LORAZEPAM
Lorazepam Intensol
Medilium
Meval
MIDAZOLAM
Mogadon
NITRAZEPAM
Novo-Alprazol
Novoclopate
Novodipam
Novoflupam
Novolorazem
Novopoxide
Novoxapam
Nu-Alpraz
Nu-Loraz
OXAZEPAM
Paxipam
PMS Diazepam
PRAZEPAM
ProSom
QUAZEPAM
Razepam
Restoril
Rivotril
Serax
Solium
Somnol
TEMAZEPAM
T-Quil
Tranxene
Tranxene-SD
Tranxene T-Tab
Valium
Valrelease
Vasepam
Vivol
Xanax
Zapex
Zebrax
Zetran

BENZOYL PEROXIDE

Acetoxyl 2.5 Gel
Acetoxyl 5 Gel
Acetoxyl 10 Gel
Acetoxyl 20 Gel
Acne Aid 10 Cream
Acne-5 Lotion
Acne-10 Lotion
Acne-Mask
Acnomel B.P. 5 Lotion
Ben-Aqua 2½ Gel
Ben-Aqua 2½ Lotion
Ben-Aqua 5 Gel
Ben-Aqua 5 Lotion
Ben-Aqua 10 Gel
Ben-Aqua 10 Lotion
Ben-Aqua Masque 5
Benoxyl 5 Lotion
Benoxyl 10 Lotion
Benoxyl 20 Lotion
Benzac Ac 2½ Gel
Benzac Ac 5 Gel
Benzac Ac 10 Gel
Benzac W 2½ Gel
Benzac W 5 Gel
Benzac W 10 Gel
Benzagel 5 Acne Lotion
Benzagel 5 Acne Wash
Benzagel 5 Gel
Benzagel 10 Gel
Benzamycin
BenzaShave 5 Cream
BenzaShave 10 Cream
Brevoxyl 4 Gel
Buf-Oxal 10
Clear By Design 2.5 Gel
Clearasil BP Plus 5 Cream
Clearasil BP Plus 5 Lotion
Clearasil Maximum Strength Medicated Anti-Acne 10 Tinted Cream
Clearasil Maximum Strength Medicated Anti-Acne 10 Vanishing Cream
Clearasil Medicated Anti-Acne 10 Vanishing Lotion
Cuticura Acne 5 Cream
Del-Aqua-5 Gel
Del-Aqua-10 Gel
Del-Ray
Dermoxyl 2.5 Gel
Dermoxyl 5 Gel
Dermoxyl 10 Gel
Dermoxyl 20 Gel
Dermoxyl Aqua
Desquam-E 2.5 Gel
Desquam-E 5 Gel
Desquam-E 10 Gel
Desquam-X 2.5 Gel
Desquam-X 5 Gel
Desquam-X 5 Wash
Desquam-X 10 Gel
Desquam-X 10 Wash
Dry and Clear 5 Lotion
Dry and Clear Double Strength 10 Cream
Fostex 5 Gel
Fostex 10 Bar
Fostex 10 Cream
Fostex 10 Gel
Fostex 10 Wash
H_2Oxyl 2.5 Gel
H_2Oxyl 5 Gel
H_2Oxyl 10 Gel
H_2Oxyl 20 Gel
Loroxide 5 Lotion with Flesh Tinted Base
Loroxide 5.5 Lotion
Neutrogena Acne Mask 5
Noxzema Clear-Ups Maximum Strength 10
Noxzema Clear-Ups On-the-Spot 10 Lotion
Oxy 5 Tinted Lotion
Oxy 5 Vanishing Formula Lotion
Oxy 5 Vanishing Lotion

Oxy 10
Oxy 10 Daily Face Wash
Oxy 10 Tinted Lotion
Oxy 10 Vanishing Lotion
Oxyderm 5 Lotion
Oxyderm 10 Lotion
Oxyderm 20 Lotion
PanOxyl 5 Bar
PanOxyl 5 Gel
PanOxyl 10 Bar
PanOxyl 10 Gel
PanOxyl 15 Gel
PanOxyl 20 Gel
PanOxyl AQ 2½ Gel
PanOxyl AQ 5 Gel
Persa-Gel 5
Persa-Gel 10
Persa-Gel W 5
Persa-Gel W 10
pHisoAc BP 10
Propa P.H. 10 Acne Cover Stick
Propa P.H. 10 Liquid Acne Soap
Stri-Dex Maximum Strength
Treatment 10 Cream
Theroxide 5 Lotion
Theroxide 10 Lotion
Theroxide 10 Wash
Topex 5 Lotion
Topex 10 Lotion
Vanoxide 5 Lotion
Xerac BP 5 Gel
Xerac BP 10 Gel
Zeroxin-5 Gel
Zeroxin-10 Gel

BETA-ADRENERGIC BLOCKING AGENTS

ACEBUTOLOL
Apo-Atenolol
Apo-Metoprolol
Apo-Metoprolol (Type L)
Apo-Propranolol
Apo-Timol
ATENOLOL
Betaloc
Betaloc Durules
Betapace
BETAXOLOL
BISOPROLOL
Blocadren
CARTEOLOL
Cartrol
Corgard
Detensol
Inderal
Inderal LA
Kerlone
LABETALOL
Levatol
Lopresor
Lopressor SR
Lopressor
METOPROLOL
Monitan
NADOLOL
Normodyne
Novo-Atenol
Novometoprol
Novo-Pindol
Novopranol
Novo-Timol
Nu-Atenol
NuMetop
OXPRENOLOL
PENBUTOLOL
PINDOLOL
pms Propranolol
PROPRANOLOL
Sectral
Slow-Trasicor
Sotacor
SOTALOL
Syn-Nadolol
Syn-Pindolol
Tenormin
TIMOLOL
Toprol XL
Trandate
Trasicor
Visken
Zebeta

BETA-ADRENERGIC BLOCKING AGENTS & THIAZIDE DIURETICS

ATENOLOL & CHLORTHALIDONE
BETAXOLOL & CHLORTHALIDONE
BISOPROLOL & HYDROCHLOROTHIAZIDE
Co-Betaloc
Corzide
Inderide
Inderide LA
Kerledex
LABETALOL & HYDROCHLOROTHIAZIDE
Lopressor HCT
METOPROLOL & HYDROCHLOROTHIAZIDE
NADOLOL & BENDROFLUMETHIAZIDE
Normozide
PINDOLOL & HYDROCHLOROTHIAZIDE
PROPRANOLOL & HYDROCHLOROTHIAZIDE
Tenoretic
Timolide
TIMOLOL & HYDROCHLOROTHIAZIDE
Trandate HCT
Viskazide
Ziac

BETAMETHASONE

Betnelan
Betnesol
Celestone
Celestone Phosphate
Celestone Soluspan
Selestoject

BRONCHODILATORS, ADRENERGIC

Adrenalin
Aerolone
ALBUTEROL
Alupent
Arm-a-Med Isoetharine
Arm-a-Med Metaproterenol
AsthmaHaler
AsthmaNefrin
Berotec
BITOLTEROL
Brethaire
Brethine
Bricanyl
Bronitin Mist
Bronkaid Mist
Bronkaid Mist Suspension
Bronkaid Mistometer
Bronkephrine
Bronkometer
Bronkosol
Dey-Dose Isoetharine
Dey-Dose Isoetharine S/F
Dey-Dose Isoproterenol
Dey-Dose Metaproterenol
Dey-Dose Racepinephrine
Dey-Lute Isoetharine
Dey-Lute Isoetharine S/F
Dey-Lute Metaproterenol
Dispos-a-Med Isoetharine
Dispos-a-Med Isoptroterenol
Ephed II
EPHEDRINE SULFATE
EPINEPHRINE
EpiPen Auto-Injector
EpiPen Jr. Auto-Injector
ETHYLNOREPINEPHRINE
FENOTEROL
ISOETHARINE
ISOPROTERENOL
Isuprel
Isuprel Glossets
Isuprel Mistometer
Maxair
Medihaler-Epi
Medihaler-Iso
Metaprel
METAPROTERENOL
microNEFRIN
Norisodrine Aerotrol
Novosalmol
PIRBUTEROL
Primatene Mist
Primatene Mist Suspension
Pro-Air
PROCATEROL
Prometa
Proventil
Proventil Repetabs
SALMETEROL
Serevent
Sus-Phrine
TERBUTALINE
Tornalate
Vapo-Iso
Vaponefrin
Ventolin
Ventolin Rotocaps

BRONCHODILATORS, XANTHINE

Accurbron
Aerolate
Aerolate III
Aerolate Jr.
Aerolate Sr.
Aerophyllin
Aminophyllin
AMINOPHYLLINE
Apo-Oxtriphylline
Aquaphyllin
Asbron

Asmalix
Bronkodyl
Choledyl
Choledyl Delayed-Release
Choledyl SA
Constant-T
Corophyllin
Dilor
Dilor-400
Duraphyl
Dyflex
Dyflex 400
DYPHILLINE
Elixicon
Elixomin
Elixophyllin
Elixophyllin SR
Lanophyllin
Lixolin
Lufyllin
Lufyllin-400
Neothylline
Novotriphyl
OXTRIPHYLLINE
Palaron
Phyllocontin
Phyllocontin-350
PMS Theophylline
Primatene, P Formula
Protophylline
Pulmophylline
Quibron-T
Quibron-T Dividose
Quibron-T/SR Dividose
Respbid
Slo-Bid
Slo-bid Gyrocaps
Slophyllin
Slo-Phyllin
Slo-Phyllin Gyrocaps
Solu-Phyllin
Somophyllin
Somophyllin-12
Somophyllin-CRT
Somophyllin-DF
Somophyllin-T
Sustaire
Synophylate
T.E.H.
T.E.P.
Theo-24
Theo-250
Theobid Duracaps
Theobid Jr. Duracaps
Theochron
Theoclear-80
Theoclear L.A. 130 Cenules
Theoclear L.A. 260 Cenules
Theocot
Theo-Dur
Theo-Dur Sprinkle
Theolair
Theolair-SR
Theomar
Theon
THEOPHYLLINE
Theophylline SR
Theo-Sav
Theospan SR
Theo-SR
Theostat
Theostat 80
Theo-Time
Theox
Theovent Long-acting
Thylline
T-Phyl
Truphylline
Truxophyllin
Uniphyl

CAFFEINE

Amaphen
Anacin
Anoquan
A.P.C.
Aspirin Free Bayer Select Maximum Strength Headache Pain Relief Caplets
Aspirin-Free Excedrin Caplets
Cafetrate
Caffedrine
Caffefrine Caplets
Citrated Caffeine
Dexitac
Dristan
Dristan AF
Dristan AF Plus
Esgic
Esgic-Plus
Excedrin Caplets
Excedrin Extra Strength Caplets
Excedrin Extra Strength Tablets
Fendol
Florinal
Histosal
Kolephrin
Korigesic
Lanorinal
NoDoz
Pacaps
P-A-C Compound
Propoxyphene Compound
Quick Pep
S-A-C
Salatin
Saleto-D
Salocol
Scot-tussin Original 5-Action Cold Medicine
Sinapils
Supac
Synalgos-DC
Tirend
Triaminicin with Codeine
Trigesic
Two-Dyne
Vanquish
Vivarin

CALCIUM CHANNEL BLOCKERS

Adalat
Adalat CC
Adalat FT
Adalat P.A.
AMLODIPINE
Apo-Diltiaz
Apo-Nifed
Apo-Verap
Bepadin
BEPRIDIL
Calan
Calan SR
Cardene
Cardizem
Cardizem CD
Cardizem SR
Chase
Dilacor-XR
DILTIAZEM
Dyna Circ
FELODIPINE
FLUNARIZINE
Isoptin
Isoptin SR
ISRADIPINE
NICARDIPINE
NIFEDIPINE
Norvasc
Novo-Diltazem
Novo-Nifedin
Novo-Veramil
Nu-Diltiaz
Nu-Nifed
Nu-Verap
Plendil
Procardia
Procardia XL
Renedil
Sibelium
Syn-Diltiazem
Vascor
VERAPAMIL
Verelan

CALCIUM SUPPLEMENTS

Apo-Cal
BioCal
Calbarb 600
Calci-Chew
Calciday
Calciject
Calcilac
Calcite
Calcium-500
Calcium-600
CALCIUM CARBONATE (also used as an antacid)
CALCIUM CITRATE
CALCIUM GLUBIONATE
CALCIUM GLUCONATE
CALCIUM GLYCEROPHOSPHATE & CALCIUM LACTATE
CALCIUM LACTATE
Calcium-Sandoz
Calcium-Sandoz Forte
Calcium Stanley
Calglycine
Calphosan
Calsan
Caltrate
Caltrate-300
Caltrate-600
Caltrate Chewable
Chooz
Citracal
Citracal Liquitabs
DIBASIC CALCIUM PHOSPHATE
Dicarbosil
Gencalc
Gramcal
Kalcinate
Mallimint
Mega-Cal
Neo-Calglucon
Nephro-Calci
Os-Cal
Os-Cal Chewable

Os-Cal 500
Oysco
Oysco 500 Chewable
Oyst-Cal
Oyst-Cal 500 Chewable
Oystercal 500
Posture
Rolaids-Calcium Rich
Super Calcium 1200
Titralac
TRIBASIC CALCIUM PHOSPHATE
Tums
Tums E-X

COAL TAR (Topical)

Alphosyl
Aquatar
Balnetar
Balnetar Therapeutic Tar Bath
Cutar Water Dispersible Emollient Tar
Denorex
Denorex Extra Strength Medicated Shampoo
Denorex Extra Strength Medicated Shampoo with Conditioners
Denorex Medicated Shampoo
Denorex Medicated Shampoo and Conditioner
Denorex Mountain Fresh Herbal Scent Medicated Shampoo
DHS Tar Gel Shampoo
DHS Tar Shampoo
Doak Oil
Doak Oil Forte
Doak Oil Forte Therapeutic Bath Treatment
Doak Oil Therapeutic Bath Treatment For All-Over Body Care
Doak Tar Lotion
Doak Tar Shampoo
Doctar
Doctar Hair & Scalp Shampoo and Conditioner
Estar
Fototar
Ionil-T Plus
LAVATAR
Liquor Carbonis Detergens
Medotar
Pentrax Extra-Strength Therapeutic Tar Shampoo
Pentrax Tar Shampoo
psoriGel
PsoriNail
Taraphilic
Tarbonis
Tar Doak
TARPASTE
Tarpaste Doak
T/Derm Tar Emollient
Tegrin Lotion for Psoriasis
Tegrin Medicated Cream Shampoo
Tegrin Medicated Shampoo Concentrated Gel
Tegrin Medicated Shampoo Extra Conditioning Formula
Tegrin Medicated Shampoo Herbal Formula
Tegrin Medicated Shampoo Original Formula
Tegrin Medicated Soap for Psoriasis
Tegrin Skin Cream for Psoriasis
Tersa-Tar Mild Therapeutic Shampoo with Protein and Conditioner
Tersa-Tar Soapless Tar Shampoo
Tersa-Tar Therapeutic Shampoo
T-Gel
T/Gel Therapeutic Conditioner
T/Gel Therapeutic Shampoo
Theraplex T Shampoo
Zetar
Zetar Emulsion
Zetar Medicated Antiseborrheic Shampoo

CONTRACEPTIVES, ORAL

Brevicon
Brevicon 0.5/35
Brevicon 1/35
Cyclen
Demulen 1/35
Demulen 1/50
Demulen 30
Demulen 50
Desogen 28
Desogen Ortho-Cept
DESOGESTREL & ETHINYL ESTRADIOL
ETHYNODIOL DIACETATE & ETHINYL ESTRADIOL
GenCept 0.5/35
GenCept 1/35
GenCept 10/11
Genora 0.5/35
Genora 1/35
Genora 1/50
Jenest-28
Levlen
LEVONORGESTREL & ETHINYL ESTRADIOL
Levora
Lo/Ovral
Loestrin 1/20
Loestrin 1.5/30
Marvelon
Minestrin 1/20
Min-Ovral
ModiCon
N.E.E. 1/35
N.E.E. 1/50
Nelova 0.5/35E
Nelova 1/35E
Nelova 1/50M
Nelova 10/11
Nelulen 1/35E
Nelulen 1/50E
Norcept-E 1/35
Nordette
Norethin 1/35E
Norethin 1/50M
NORETHINDRONE & ETHINYL ESTRADIOL
NORETHINDRONE & MESTRANOL
NORETHINDRONE ACETATE & ETHINYL ESTRADIOL
NORGESTIMATE & ETHINYL ESTRADIOL
NORGESTREL & ETHINYL ESTRADIOL
Norinyl 1+35
Norinyl 1+50
Norinyl 1/50
Norlestrin 1/50
Norlestrin 2.5/50
Orth-Novum 0.5
Ortho 0.5/35
Ortho 1/35
Ortho 7/7/7
Ortho 10/11
Ortho-Cept
Ortho-Cyclen
Ortho-Novum 0.5
Ortho-Novum 1/35
Ortho-Novum 1/50
Ortho-Novum 1/80
Ortho-Novum 2
Ortho-Novum 7/7/7
Ortho-Novum 10/11
Ortho-Tri-Cyclen 21
Ortho-Tri-Cyclen 28
Ovcon-35
Ovcon-50
Ovral
Symphasic
Tri-Cyclen
Tri-Levlen
Tri-Norinyl
Triphasil
Triquilar

CONTRACEPTIVES, VAGINAL (Spermicides)

BENZALKONIUM CHLORIDE
Because
Conceptrol-Contraceptive Inserts
Conceptrol Gel
Delfen
Emko
Encare
Gynol II Extra Strength
Gynol II Original Formula
Intercept
Koromex Cream
Koromex Crystal Gel
Koromex Foam
Koromex Jelly
NONOXYNAL 9
OCTOXYNOL 9
Ortho-Creme
Ortho-Gynol
Pharmatex
Pre-Fil
Ramses Contraceptive Foam
Ramses Contraceptive Vaginal Jelly
Ramses Crystal Clear Gel
Semicid
Shur-Seal
Today
VCF

DEXAMETHASONE

Ak-Dex
Dalalone
Dalalone D.P.
Dalalone L.A.
Decadrol
Decadron
Decadron L.A.

Decadron Phosphate
Decaject
Decaject-L.A.
Deronil
Desasone L.A.
Dexacen
Dexacen L.A.
Dexasone
Dexone
Dexone LA
Hexadrol
Hexadrol Phosphate
Mymethasone
Oradexon
Solurex
Solurex LA

DEXTROMETHORPHAN

2/G-DM Cough
Actifed DM
Ambenyl-D Decongestant Cough Formula
Anatuss
Anatuss DM
Anti-Tuss DM Expectorant
Balminil DM
Bayaminicol
Baydec DM Drops
Bayer Cough Syrup for Children
Bayer Select Flu Relief Caplets
Bayer Select Head and Chest Cold Caplets
Baytussin DM
Benylin-DM
Benylin DM-D
Benylin DM-D-E
Benylin DM-D-E Expectorant
Benylin DM-E
Benylin Expectorant Cough Formula
Bromfed-AT
Bromfed-DM
Broncho-Grippol-DM
Brotane DX Cough
Calmylin
Calmylin Cough & Cold
Calmylin #1
Calmylin #2
Calmylin #4
Calmylin Pediatric
Carbinoxamine Compound
Carbodec DM Drops
Cerose-DM
Cheracol D Cough
Cheracol Plus
Chexit
Children's Benylin
Children's Nyquil Nighttime Cold Medicine
Co-Apap
Codimal DM
Codistan No. 1
Colrex Cough
Comtrex Daytime Caplets
Comtrex Hot Flu Relief
Comtrex Multi-Symptom Cold Reliever
Comtrex Multi-Symptom Hot Flu Relief
Comtrex Multi-Symptom Non-Drowsy Caplets
Comtrex Nighttime
Comtrex Nighttime Maximum Strength Cold and Flu Relief
Comtrex Nighttime Maximum Strength Cold, Cough and Flu Relief
Conar
Conar-A
Conar Expectorant
Concentrin
Congespirin
Contac Day Caplets
Contac Jr. Children's Cold Medicine
Contac Night Caplets
Contac Severe Cold Formula
Contac Severe Cold Formula Night Strength
Coricidin Cough
CoTylenol Cold Medication
Cough X
Cremacoat 1
Cremacoat 3 Throat Coating Cough Medicine
Cremacoat 4 Throat Coating Cough Medicine
Creo-Terpin
DayCare
DayQuil Liquicaps
DayQuil Non-Drowsy Cold/Flu
DayQuil Non-Drowsy Cold/Flu LiquiCaps
Delsym
DEXTROMETHORPHAN HYDROBROMIDE AND TERPIN HYDRATE
Dimacol
Dimetane-DX Cough
Dimetapp DM Cough and Cold
Dimetapp-DM
DM Cough
DM Syrup
Donatussin
Dondril
Dorcol Children's Cough
Dorcol DM
Dristan Cold and Flu
Dristan Juice Mix-in
Efficol Cough Whip (Cough Suppressant/Decongestant)
Efficol Cough Whip (Cough Suppressant/Decongestant/ Antihistamine)
Efficol Cough Whip (Cough Suppressant/Expectorant)
Extra Action Cough
Father John's Medicine Plus
Glycotuss-dM
Guiamid D.M. Liquid
Guiatuss-DM
Halls Mentho-Lyptus Decongestant Cough Formula
Halotussin-DM Expectorant
Histalet-DM
Hold
Hold (Children's Formula)
Improved Sino-Tuss
Iotuss-DM
Ipsatol Cough Formula for Children
Kiddy Koff
Koffex
Kolephrin/DM
Kolephrin GG/DM
Kolephrin NN Liquid
Kophane
Kophane Cough and Cold Formula
Mapap Cold Formula
Maximum Strength Tylenol Flu Gelcaps
Meda Syrup Forte
Medatussin
Medatussin Plus
Medi-Flu
Medi-Flu Caplets
Mediquell
Mediquell Decongestant Formula
Mytussin DM
Naldecon-DX
Naldecon-DX Adult Liquid
Naldecon-DX Children's Syrup
Naldecon-DX Pediatric Drops
Naldecon Senior DX
NeoCitran Coughs & Colds
Neo-DM
Niquil Hot Therapy
Noratuss II Liquid
Novahistex DM
Novahistine Cough & Cold Formula Liquid
Novahistine DMX Liquid
NyQuil Liquicaps
NyQuil Nighttime Colds Medicine
Nytime Cold Medicine Liquid
Omnicol
Ornade-DM 10
Ornade-DM 15
Ornade-DM 30
Orthoxicol Cough
PediaCare 1
PediaCare Children's Cold Relief Night Rest Cough-Cold Formula
PediaCare Children's Cough-Cold Formula
Par Glycerol-DM
Pertussin AM
Pertussin CS
Pertussin PM
Phanadex
Phanatuss
Phenergan w/Dextromethorphan
Poly-Histine-DM
Prominicol Cough
Pseudo-Car DM
Quelidrine Cough
Queltuss
Remcol-C
Rhinosyn-DM
Rhinosyn-DMX Expectorant
Rhinosyn-X
Robidex
Robitussin Cold and Cough Liqui-Gels
Robitussin-CF
Robitussin-DM
Robitussin Maximum Strength Cough
Robitussin Night Relief
Robitussin Night Relief Colds Formula Liquid
Robitussin-Pediatric
Rondec-DM
Rondec-DM Drops
Ru-Tuss Expectorant
Safe Tussin 30
Saleto-CF
Sedatuss

Silexin Cough
Snaplets-DM
Snaplets-Multi
St. Joseph for Children
Sucrets Cough Control
Sudafed Cough
Sudafed DM
Sudafed Severe Cold Formula
Syracol Liquid
Terphan
Terpin-Dex
TheraFlu/Flu, Cold & Cough
TheraFlu Maximum Strength Non-Drowsy Formula Flu, Cold and Cough Medicine
TheraFlu Nighttime Maximum Strength
Tolu-Sed DM Cough
Triaminic DM Cough Formula
Triaminic DM Daytime
Triaminic DM Expectorant
Triaminic DM Nighttime for Children
Triaminic Nite Light
Triaminicol DM
Triaminicol Multi-Symptom Relief
Tricodene Forte
Tricodene NN
Tricodene Pediatric
Trimedine Liquid
Trind DM Liquid
Trocal
Tusquelin
Tussafed
Tussagesic
Tussar DM
Tuss-DM
Tussi-Organidin DM Liquid
Tusso-DM
Ty-Cold Cold Formula
Tylenol Cold and Flu
Tylenol Cold Medication
Tylenol Cold Medication, Non-Drowsy
Tylenol Cold Night Time
Tylenol Cold No Drowsiness Formula Gelcaps
Tylenol Cough
Tylenol Cough with Decongestant
Unproco
Vicks 44 Cold, Flu and Cough Liqui-Caps
Vicks 44 Non-Drowsy Cold and Cough LiquiCaps
Vicks Children's Cough
Vicks Formula 44 Cough Mixture
Vicks Formula 44D Decongestant Cough Mixture
Vicks Formula 44M Multi-symptom Cough Mixture
Viro-Med

DICYCLOMINE

A-Spas
Antispas
Bentyl
Bentylol
Byclomine
Dibent
Di-Cyclonex
Dilomine
Di-Spaz
Forulex
Lomine
Neoquess
Or-Tyl
Protylol
Spasmoban
Spasmoject
Viscerol

DIURETICS, THIAZIDE

Anhydron
Apo-Chlorthalidone
Apo-Hydro
Aquatensen
BENDROFLUMETHIAZIDE
BENZTHIAZIDE
CHLOROTHIAZIDE
CHLORTHALIDONE
CYCLOTHIAZIDE
Diucardin
Diuchlor H
Diulo
Diuril
Duretic
Enduron
Esidrix
Fluidil
HYDROCHLOROTHIAZIDE
HydroDIURIL
HYDROFLUMETHIAZIDE
Hydromox
Hygroton
Metahydrin
METHYCLOTHIAZIDE
METOLAZONE
Mykrox
Naqua
Naturetin
Neo-Codema
Novo-Hydrazide
Novo-Thalidone
Oretic
POLYTHIAZIDE
QUINETHAZONE
Renese
Saluron
Thalitone
TRICHLORMETHIAZIDE
Uridon
Urozide
Zaroxolyn

DOCUSATES

Afko-Lube
Afko-Lube Lax
Bilax
Colace
Colax
Correctol
Correctol Extra Gentle
Dialose
Dialose Plus
Diocto
Diocto-C
Diocto-K
Diocto-K Plus
Dioeze
Diosuccin
Dio-Sul
Diothron
Disanthrol
Disolan
Disolan Forte
Disonate
Disoplex
Di-Sosul
Di-Sosul Forte
Docucal-P
Docu-K Plus
DOCUSATE CALCIUM
DOCUSATE POTASSIUM
DOCUSATE SODIUM
Doss
Doxidan
Doxinate
DSMC Plus
D-S-S
D-S-S plus
Dulcodos
Duosol
Feen-a-Mint
Feen-a-Mint Pills
Gentlax-S
Kasof
Laxinate 100
Modane Soft
Molatoc
Molatoc-CST
Neolax
Peri-Colase
Phillip's Gelcaps
Phillip's LaxCaps
Pro-Cal-Sof
Pro-Sof
Pro-Sof Liquid Concentrate
Pro-Sof Plus
Regulace
Regulax SS
Regulex
Regulex-D
Regutol
Senokot-S
Stulex
Surfak
Therevac Plus
Therevac-SB
Trilax

EPHEDRINE

Broncholate
Bronkotuss Expectorant
Histatuss Pediatric
KIE
Omni-Tuss
Quelidrine Cough
Rentamine Pediatric
Rynatuss
Rynatuss Pediatric

ERYTHROMYCINS

Apo-Erythro-S
E-Base
E.E.S.
E/Gel
Emgel
E-Mycin
Eryc
EryPed
Ery-Tab
Erythro
Erythrocin
Erythrocot
Erythromid
ERYTHROMYCIN-BASE

ERYTHROMYCIN ESTOLATE
ERYTHROMYCIN ETHYLSUCCINATE
ERYTHROMYCIN GLUCEPTATE
ERYTHROMYCIN LACTOBIONATE
ERYTHROMYCIN STEARATE
Erythrozone
Ethril
Ilosone
Ilotycin
Kenmycin
My-E
Mythromycin
Novorythro
PCE Dispersatabs
Pediamycin
Robimycin
Ro-Mycin
Staticin
Stiefel
Theramycinz
T-Stat
Wintrocin
Wyamycin E
Wyamycin S

ESTROGENS

Aquest
C.E.S.
CHLOROTRIANISENE
Clinagen LA 40
Congest
CONJUGATED ESTROGENS
Deladiol-40
Delestrogen
depGynogen
Depo Estradiol
Depogen
DES
DIETHYLSTILBESTROL
Dioval
Dioval XX
Duragen
Dura-Estrin
Duragen-20
Duragen-40
E-Cypionate
Estragen 5
Estragen LA 5
ESTERIFIED ESTROGENS
Estinyl
Estrace
Estraderm
ESTRADIOL
Estra-L
Estratab
Estro-A
Estro-Cyp
Estro-L.A.
Estrofem
ESTROGEN
Estroject-L.A.
ESTRONE
Estrone 5
ESTROPIPATE
Estro-Span
Estrovis
ETHINYL ESTRADIOL
Femogex
Gynogen
Gynogen L.A. 40
Honvol
Kestrane-5
Mannest
Menaval-20
Menest
Neo-Estrone
Ogen
Ogen 1.25
Ogen 2.5
Ogen 6.25
Ortho-Est
Piperazine
Premarin
QUINESTROL
Stilphostrol
TACE
Valergen-10
Valergen-20
Valergen-40
Wehgen

GUAIFENESIN

2/G-DM Cough
Adatuss D.C. Expectorant
Alamine Expectorant
Ambenyl-D Decongestant Cough Formula
Ami-Tex LA
Amonidrin
Anatuss
Anatuss with Codeine
Anti-Tuss
Anti-Tuss DM Expectorant
Balminil
Banex
Banex-LA
Bayaminic Expectorant
Bayer Select Head and Chest Cold Caplets
Bayhistine Expectorant
Baytussin AC
Baytussin DM
Benylin DM-D-E
Benylin DM-D-E Expectorant
Benylin DM-E
Benylin Expectorant Cough Formula
Breonesin
Brexin
Broncholate
Bronkotuss Expectorant
Brontex
Calmylin Codeine
Calmylin Cough & Cold
Calmylin Expectorant
Cheracol
Cheracol D Cough
CoActifed Expectorant
Codegest-Expectorant
Codiclear DH
Codimal Expectorant
Codistan No. 1
Colrex Expectorant
Conar-A
Conar Expectorant
Concentrin
Conex
Conex w/Codeine Liquid
Congess JR
Congess SR
Coricidin Cough
Cotridin Expectorant
Cremacoat 2
Cremacoat 3 Throat Coating Cough Medicine
C-Tussin Expectorant
DayCare
DayQuil Liquicaps
DayQuil Non-Drowsy Cold/Flu
DayQuil Non-Drowsy Cold/Flu LiquiCaps
DayQuil Non-Drowsy Sinus Pressure and Congestion Relief Caplets
Despec
Deproist Expectorant w/Codeine
Detussin Expectorant
Diabetic Tussin EX
Dilaudid Cough
Dimacol
Dimetane Expectorant
Dimetane Expectorant-C
Dimetane Expectorant-DC
Donatussin
Donatussin DC
Donatussin Drops
Dorcol Children's Cough
Dorcol DM
Duratuss
Duratuss HD
Dura-Vent
Efficol Cough Whip (Cough Suppressant/Expectorant)
Entex
Entex LA
Entex Liquid
Entex PSE
Entuss Expectorant
Entuss Pediatric Expectorant
Entuss-D
Extra Action Cough
Father John's Medicine Plus
Fedahist Expectorant
Fedahist Expectorant Pediatric Drops
Fendol
Gee-Gee
GG-CEN
Genatuss
Gentab LA
Glyate
Glycotuss
Glycotuss-dM
Glydeine Cough
Guaifed
Guaifed-PD
GuaiMAX-D
Guaipax
Guaitab
Guiamid D.M. Liquid
Guiatuss A.C.
Guiatuss-DM
Guiatussin w/Codeine Liquid
Guistrey Fortis
Gulatuss
Halotussin
Halotussin-DM Expectorant
Head & Chest
Histalet X
Humibid L.A.
Humibid Sprinkle
Hycotuss Expectorant
Hytuss
Hytuss-2X
Ipsatol Cough Formula for Children
Isoclor Expectorant

Kiddy Koff
Kolephrin GG/DM
Kwelcof Liquid
Lanatuss Expectorant
Malotuss
Meda Syrup Forte
Medatussin
Medatussin Plus
Myhistine Expectorant
Mytussin AC
Mytussin DAC
Mytussin DM
Naldecon
Naldecon-CX Adult Liquid
Naldecon-DX Adult Liquid
Naldecon-DX Children's Syrup
Naldecon-DX Pediatric Drops
Naldecon-EX
Naldecon Senior DX
Nolex LA
Noratuss II Liquid
Nortussin
Nortussin w/Codeine
Novahistex DH Expectorant
Novahistine DH Expectorant
Novahistine DMX Liquid
Novahistine Expectorant
Nucochem Expectorant
Nucochem Pediatric Expectorant
Nucofed Expectorant
Nucofed Pediatric Expectorant
Organidin
Ornade Expectorant
Pertussin AM
Pertussin CS
Phanadex
Phanatuss
Phenhist Expectorant
Phenylfenesin L.A.
Pneumomist
Polaramine Expectorant
Poly-Histine Expectorant Plain
Prominic Expectorant
Pseudo-Bid
Pseudo-Hist Expectorant
P-V-Tussin Tablets
Queltuss
Respaire-60 SR
Respaire-120 SR
Respinol-G
Respinol LA
Resyl
Rhinosyn-DMX Expectorant
Rhinosyn-X
Robafen
Robitussin
Robitussin with Codeine
Robitussin A-C
Robitussin-CF
Robitussin-DAC
Robitussin-DM
Robitussin-PE
Robitussin Severe Congestion Liqui-Gels
Ru-Tuss Expectorant
Rymed
Rymed Liquid
Rymed-TR
Ryna-CX Liquid
Safe Tussin 30
Silexin Cough
Sinufed Timecelles
Snaplets-EX
Stamoist E
Stamoist LA
SRC Expectorant
Sudafed Cough
Sudafed Expectorant
T-Moist
Tolu-Sed Cough
Tolu-Sed DM Cough
Touro Ex
Triaminic DM Daytime
Triaminic DM Expectorant
Triaminic Expectorant
Triaminic Expectorant DH
Triaminic Expectorant w/Codeine
Trinex
Triphenyl Expectorant
Trocal
Tussanil DH Tablets
Tussar SF
Tussar-2
Tuss-DM
Tuss-LA
ULR-LA
Unproco
Utex-S.R.
Vicks Children's Cough
Vicks Formula 44D Decongestant Cough Mixture
Vicks Formula 44M Multi-symptom Cough Mixture
Vicodin-Tuss
Viro-Med
Zephrex
Zephrex-LA

HYDROCORTISONE (Cortisol)

A-hydroCort
Cortef
Cortenema
Cortifoam
Hydrocortone
Hydrocortone Acetate
Hydrocortone Phosphate
Solu-Cortef

HYDROXYZINE

Anxanil
Apo-Hydroxyzine
Atarax
Multipax
Novo-Hydroxyzin
Vistaril

INSULIN

Humulin BR
Humulin L
Humulin N
Humulin R
Humulin U
Insulatard NPH
Insulatard NPH Human
Lente
Lente Iletin I
Lente Iletin II
Lente Insulin
Mixtard
Mixtard Human
Novolin 70/30
Novolin L
Novolin N
Novolin R
NPH
NPH Iletin I
NPH Iletin II
NPH Insulin
Protamine Zinc & Iletin
Protamine Zinc & Iletin I
Protamine Zinc & Iletin II
PZI
Regular
Regular (Concentrated) Iletin
Regular (Concentrated) Iletin II, U-500
Regular Iletin I
Regular Iletin II
Regular Insulin
Semilente
Semilente Iletin
Semilente Iletin I
Ultralente
Ultralente Iletin I
Velosulin
Velosulin Human

IRON SUPPLEMENTS

Apo-Ferrous Gluconate
Apo-Ferrous Sulfate
Femiron
Feosol
Feostat
Fergon
Fer-In-Sol
Fer-Iron
Fero-folic 500
Fero-Grad
Fero-Gradumet
Ferralet
Ferralyn
Ferra-TD
Ferrospace
FERROUS FUMARATE
FERROUS GLUCONATE
FERROUS SULFATE
Fertinic
Fumasorb
Fumerin
Geritol Tablets
Hemocyte
Hytinic
Iberet
Ircon
IRON POLYSACCHARIDE
Mol-Iron
Neo-Fer
Niferex
Niferex-150
Novoferrogluc
Novoferrosulfa
Novofumar
Nu-Iron
Nu-Iron 150
Palafer
Palmiron
PMS Ferrous Sulfate
Simiron
Slow Fe
Span-FF

KERATOLYTICS

Acne-Aid Gel
Acno
Acnomel-Acne Cream

Acnomel Cake
Acnomel Cream
Acnomel Vanishing Cream
Acnotex
Anti-acne
Antinea
Aveeno Acne Bar
Aveeno Cleansing Bar
Bensulfoid Cream
Buf-Puf Acne Cleansing Bar with Vitamin E
Buf-Puf Medicated Maximum Strength Pads
Buf-Puf Medicated Regular Strength Pads
Calicylic
Clear Away
Clear by Design Medicated Cleansing Pads
Clearasil Adult Care Medicated Blemish Cream
Clearasil Adult Care Medicated Blemish Stick
Clearasil Clearstick Maximum Strength Topical Solution
Clearasil Clearstick Regular Strength Topical Solution
Clearasil Double Textured Pads Maximum Strength
Clearasil Double Textured Pads Regular Strength
Clearasil Medicated Deep Cleanser Topical Solution
Compound W Gel
Compound W Liquid
Creamy SS Shampoo
Cuplex Gel
Cuticura Ointment
Derma & Soft Creme
Diasporal Cream
Duofilm
Duoplant
Duoplant Topical Solution
Finac
Fostex CM
Fostex Medicated Cleansing Bar
Fostex Medicated Cleansing
Fostex Medicated Cleansing Liquid
Fostex Regular Strength Medicated Cleansing Bar
Fostex Regular Strength Medicated Cleansing Cream
Fostex Regular Strength Medicated Cover-Up
Fostril Cream
Fostril Lotion
Freezone
Gordofilm
Hydrisalic
Ionax Astringent Skin Cleanser Topical Solution
Ionil Plus Shampoo
Ionil Shampoo
Keralyt
Keratex Gel
Lactisol
Listerex Golden Scrub Lotion
Listerex Herbal Scrub Lotion
Lotio Asulfa
Mediplast
Meted Maximum Strength Anti-Dandruff Shampoo with Conditioners
Night Cast R
Night Cast Regular Formula Mask-Lotion
Night Cast Special Formula Mask-Lotion
Noxzema Anti-Acne Gel
Noxzema Anti-Acne Pads Maximum Strength
Noxzema Anti-Acne Pads Regular Strength
Occlusal Topical Solution
Occlusal-HP Topical Solution
Off-Ezy Topical Solution Corn & Callus Removal Kit
Off-Ezy Topical Solution Wart Removal Kit
Oxy Clean Medicated Cleanser
Oxy Clean Medicated Pads Maximum Strength
Oxy Clean Medicated Pads Sensitive Skin
Oxy Clean Regular Strength
Oxy Clean Regular Strength Medicated Cleanser Topical Solution
Oxy Clean Regular Strength Medicated Pads
Oxy Clean Sensitive Skin Cleanser Topical Solution
Oxy Clean Sensitive Skin Pads
Oxy Night Watch Maximum Strength Lotion
Oxy Night Watch Night Time Acne Medication Extra Strength Lotion
Oxy Night Watch Night Time Acne Medication Regular Strength Lotion
Oxy Night Watch Sensitive Skin Lotion
Oxy Sensitive Skin Vanishing Formula Lotion
P&S
Paplex
Paplex Ultra
Pernox Lemon Medicated Scrub Cleanser
Pernox Lotion Lathering Abradant Scrub Cleanser
Pernox Lotion Lathering Scrub Cleanser
Pernox Regular Medicated Scrub Cleanser
Propa pH Medicated Acne Cream Maximum Strength
Propa pH Medicated Cleansing Pads Maximum Strength
Propa pH Medicated Cleansing Pads Sensitive Skin
Propa pH Perfectly Clear Skin Cleanser Topical Solution Oily Skin
Propa pH Perfectly Clear Skin Cleanser Topical Solution Sensitive Skin Formula
R.A.
RESORCINOL
RESORCINOL & SULFUR
Rezamid Lotion
Salac
Salacid
Sal-Acid Plaster
Salactic Film Topical Solution
Sal-Clens Plus Shampoo
Sal-Clens Shampoo
SALICYLIC ACID
SALICYLIC ACID & SULFUR
Saligel
Salonil
Sal-Plant Gel Topical Solution
Sastid (AL) Scrub
Sastid Plain
Sastid Plain Shampoo and Acne Wash
Sastid Soap
Sebasorb Liquid
Sebex
Sebucare
Sebulex Antiseborrheic Treatment and Conditioning Shampoo
Sebulex Antiseborrheic Treatment Shampoo
Sebulex Conditioning Shampoo
Sebulex Cream Medicated Shampoo
Sebulex Medcicated Dandruff Shampoo with Conditioners
Sebulex Medicated Shampoo
Sebulex Regular Medicated Dandruff Shampoo
Sebulex Shampoo
Stri-Dex
Stri-Dex Dual Textured Pads Maximum Strength
Stri-Dex Dual Textured Pads Regular Strength
Stri-Dex Dual Textured Pads Sensitive Skin
Stri-Dex Maximum Strength Pads
Stri-Dex Regular Strength Pads
Stri-Dex Super Scrub Pads
Sulfo-Lac
Sulforcin
SULFUR (Topical)
Sulsal Soap
Tersac Cleansing Gel
Therac Lotion
Trans-Plantar
Trans-Ver-Sal
Vanseb Cream Dandruff Shampoo
Vanseb Lotion Dandruff Shampoo
Verukan Topical Solution
Verukan-HP Topical Solution
Viranol
Viranol Ultra
Wart-Off Topical Solution
X-Seb

MEPROBAMATE

Acabamate
Apo-Meprobamate
Equanil
Equanil Wyseals
Medi-Tran
Meprospan
Miltown
Neuramate
Novomepro
Novo-Mepro
Pax 400

Probate
Sedabamate
Trancot
Tranmep

METHYLPREDNISOLONE

A-methaPred
dep Medalone
Depo-Medrol
Depo-Pred-40
Depo-Pred-80
Depo-Predate
Depoject-40
Depoject-80
Duralone
Duralone-40
Duralone-80
Medralone-40
Medralone-80
Medrol
Meprolone
Rep-Pred
Solu-Medrol

NARCOTIC & ACETAMINOPHEN

Aceta with Codeine
Acetaco
ACETAMINOPHEN & CODEINE
Allay
Amacodone
Anexsia
Anodynos DHC
Anolor-DH5
APAP with Codeine
Atasol with Codeine
Bancap-HC
Capital with Codeine
Codalan
Codamin
Codaminophen
Co-gesic
Compal
Darvocet-N 100
Darvocet-N 50
Demerol-APAP
Dolacet
Dolene-AP 65
Doxapap
D-Rex
Duocet
Duradyne DHC
E-Lor
Empracet 30
Empracet 60
Emtec
Endocet
Exdol with Codeine
Genagesic
Hy-5
Hycomed
Hycopap
Hydrocet
HYDROCODONE & ACETAMINOPHEN
Hydrocodone with APAP
Hydrogesic
HY-PHEN
Lenoltec
Lorcet
Lorcet 10/650
Lorcet-HD
Lortab
Lortab 5
Lortab 7
Megagesic
MEPERIDINE & ACETAMINOPHEN
M-Gesic
Myapap with Codeine
Norcet
Novogesic
Oxycocet
OXYCODONE & ACETAMINOPHEN
PENTAZOCINE & ACETAMINOPHEN
Percocet
Percocet-Demi
Phenaphen with Codeine
Polygesic
Pro Pox with APAP
Propacet
Propain-HC
PROPOXYPHENE & ACETAMINOPHEN
Proval
Proxy 65
Pyregesic-C
Rogesic
Rounox with Codeine
Roxicet
Senefen III
Talacen
Tylaprin with Codeine
Tylenol with Codeine
Tylox
Ty-Pap with Codeine
Ty-Tab with Codeine No. 2
Ty-Tab with Codeine No. 3
Ty-Tab with Codeine No. 4
Ultragesic
Veganin
Vicodin
Wygesic
Zydone

NARCOTIC ANALGESICS

642
Actagen-C Cough
Actifed w/Codeine
Actifed w/Codeine Cough
Adatuss D.C.
Adatuss D.C. Expectorant
Alamine-C Liquid
Alamine Expectorant
Allerfrin w/Codeine
Ambay Cough
Ambenyl Cough
Ambophen Expectorant
Anamine HD
Anatuss with Codeine
Astramorph
Astramorph-PF
Baycodan
Baycomine
Baycomine Pediatric
BayCotussend Liquid
Bayhistine DH
Bayhistine Expectorant
Baytussin AC
Benylin with Codeine
Biphetane DC Cough
Bromanate DC Cough
Bromphen DC w/Codeine Cough
Brontex
Buprenex
BUPRENORPHINE
Calcidrine
Caldomine-DH Forte
Caldomine-DH Pediatric
Calmylin with Codeine
Cheracol
Chlorgest-HD
Citra Forte
CoActifed
CoActifed Expectorant
Codamine
Codamine Pediatric
Codan
Codegest Expectorant
Codehist DH
CODEINE
CODEINE AND TERPIN HYDRATE
Codeine Sulfate
Codiclear DH
Codimal DH
Codimal PH
Colrex Compound
Conex w/Codeine Liquid
Cophene-S
Coricidin w/Codeine
Coristex-DH
Coristine-DH
Cotridin
Cotridin Expectorant
C-Tussin Expectorant
Darvon
Darvon-N
De-Tuss
Demerol
Deproist Expectorant w/Codeine
Detussin Expectorant
Detussin Liquid
Dihistine DH
DIHYDROCODEINE
Dihydromorphinone
Dilaudid
Dilaudid Cough
Dilaudid-HP
Dimetane Expectorant-C
Dimetane Expectorant-DC
Dimetane-DC Cough
Dimetapp with Codeine
Dolene
Dolophine
Doloxene
Donatussin DC
Doraphen
Doxaphene
Dromoran
Duragesic
Duramorph
Duratuss HD
Efricon Expectorant Liquid
Endal-HD
Endal-HD Plus
Entuss-D
Entuss Expectorant
Entuss Pediatric Expectorant
Epimorph
FENTANYL
Fortral
Glydeine Cough
Guiatuss A.C.
Guiatussin w/Codeine Liquid
Histafed C

Histussin HC
Hycodan
Hycomine
Hycomine Compound
Hycomine Pediatric
Hycomine-S Pediatric
Hycotuss Expectorant
HYDROCODONE
HYDROCODONE AND HOMATROPINE
Hydromet
Hydromine
Hydromine Pediatric
HYDROMORPHONE
Hydropane
Hydrophen
Hystadyl E.C.
Iophen-C Liquid
Iotuss
Isoclor Expectorant
Kwelcof Liquid
Laudanum
Levo-Dromoran
Levorphan
LEVORPHANOL
Mallergan-VC w/Codeine
MEPERIDINE
METHADONE
Methadose
Midahist DH
MORPHINE
Morphitec
M.O.S.
M.O.S.-SR
MS Contin
MSIR
MST Continus
Mycotussin
Myhistine DH
Myhistine Expectorant
Myhydromine
Myhydromine Pediatric
Myphetane DC Cough
Mytussin AC
Mytussin DAC
NALBUPHINE
Naldecon-CX
Normatane DC
Nortussin w/Codeine
Novahistex C
Novahistex DH
Novahistex DH Expectorant
Novahistine DH
Novahistine DH Expectorant
Novahistine DH Liquid
Novahistine Expectorant
Novopropoxyn
Nubain
Nucochem
Nucochem Expectorant
Nucochem Pediatric Expectorant
Nucofed
Nucofed Expectorant
Nucofed Pediatric Expectorant
Numorphan
Omni-Tuss
OPIUM
Oramorph
Oramorph-SR
OXYCODONE
OXYMORPHONE
P-V-Tussin
Pantapon
Par Glycerol C
Paveral
Pediacof Cough
Penntuss
PENTAZOCINE
Pethidine
Phenameth VC w/Codeine
Phenergan w/Codeine
Phenergan VC with Codeine
Phenhist Expectorant
Pherazine VC w/Codeine
Physeptone
Poly-Histine w/Codeine
Poly-Histine-CS
Profene
Prometh VC w/Codeine
PROMETHAZINE AND CODEINE
Promist HD Liquid
Pro Pox
Propoxycon
PROPOXYPHENE
Prunicodeine
Pseudo-Hist Expectorant
Pseudodine C Cough
RMS Uniserts
Robidone
Robitussin with Codeine
Robitussin A-C
Robitussin-DAC
Roxanol
Roxanol SR
Roxicodone
Ru-Tuss w/Hydrocodone Liquid
Ryna-C Liquid
Ryna-CX Liquid
Soma Compound w/Codeine
SRC Expectorant
Statex
Statuss Expectorant
Statuss Green
Supeudol
Talwin
Talwin-NX
Temgesic
T-Koff
Tolu-Sed Cough
Triacin C Cough
Triaminic w/Codeine
Triaminic Expectorant w/Codeine
Triaminic Expectorant DH
Triaminicin w/Codeine
Tricodene #1
Trifed-C Cough
Tussaminic DH Forte
Tussaminic DH Pediatric
Tussanil DH
Tussar-2
Tussar SF
Tussi-Organidin Liquid
Tussigon
Tussionex
Tussirex w/Codeine Liquid
Vanex-HD
Vicodin-Tuss

NARCOTIC & ASPIRIN

222
282
292
293
692
A.C.&C.
Anacin with Codeine
Ancasal
ASPIRIN & CODEINE
Azdone
Bexophrene
BUFFERED ASPIRIN & CODEINE
Coryphen with Codeine
Cotanal 65
Damason-P
Darvon Compound
Darvon with A.S.A.
Darvon-N with A.S.A.
Darvon-N Compound
Doraphen Compound 65
Doxaphene Compound
Drocade and Aspirin
DROCODE & ASPIRIN
Emcodeine
Empirin with Codeine
Endodan
HYDROCODONE & ASPIRIN
Lortab ASA
Margesic A-C
Novopropoxyn Compound
Oxycodan
OXYCODONE & ASPIRIN
PENTAZOCINE & ASPIRIN
Percodan
Percodan-Demi
Pro Pox Plus
PROPOXYPHENE & ASPIRIN
Roxiprin
Synalgos-DC
Talwin Compound
Talwin Compound-50

NITRATES

Apo-ISDN
Cardilate
Cedocard-SR
Coradur
Coronex
Deponit
Dilatrate-SR
Duotrate
ERYTHRITYL TETRANITRATE
Glyceryl Trinitrate
IMDUR
ISMO
Iso-Bid
Isonate
Isorbid
Isordil
ISOSORBIDE DINITRATE
ISOSORBIDE MONONITRATE
Isotrate
Klavikordal
Minitran
Monoket
Naptrate
Niong
Nitro-Bid
Nitrocap
Nitrocap T.D.
Nitrocine
Nitrodisc
Nitro-Dur
Nitro-Dur II
Nitrogard-SR
NITROGLYCERIN (GLYCERYL TRINITRATE)
Nitroglyn
Nitrol
Nitrolin
Nitrolingual

Nitronet
Nitrong
Nitrong SR
Nitrospan
Nitrostat
Novosorbide
NTS
PENTAERYTHRITOL
TETRANITRATE
Pentritol
Pentylan
Peritrate
Peritrate Forte
Peritrate SA
P.E.T.N.
Sorbitrate
Sorbitrate SA
Transderm-Nitro
Tridil

OXYMETAZOLINE (Nasal)

4-Way Long Acting Nasal Spray
Afrin 12 Hour Nasal Spray
Afrin 12 Hour Nose Drops
Afrin Cherry Scented Nasal Spray
Afrin Children's Strength 12 Hour Nose Drops
Afrin Children's Strength Nose Drops
Afrin Extra Moisturizing Nasal Decongestant Spray
Afrin Menthol Nasal Spray
Afrin Nasal Spray
Afrin Nasal Spray Pump
Afrin Nose Drops
Afrin Sinus
Allerest 12 Hour Nasal Spray
Cheracol Nasal Spray
Cheracol Nasal Spray Pump Cherry Scented
Coricidin Nasal Mist
Dristan 12-Hr Nasal Spray
Dristan Long Lasting Menthol Nasal Spray
Dristan Long Lasting Nasal Pump Spray
Dristan Long Lasting Nasal Spray
Dristan Long Lasting Nasal Spray 12 Hour Metered Dose Pump
Duramist Plus Up To 12 Hours Decongestant Nasal Spray
Duration 12 Hour Nasal Spray Pump
Nafrine Decongestant Nasal Drops
Nafrine Decongestant Nasal Spray
Nafrine Decongestant Pediatric Nasal Spray/Drops
Neo-Synephrine 12 Hour Nasal Spray
Neo-Synephrine 12 Hour Nasal Spray Pump
Neo-Synephrine 12 Nose Drops
Neo-Synephrine 12 Hour Vapor Nasal Spray
Nostrilla 12 Hour Nasal Decongestant
Nostril Nasal Decongestant Mild
Nostril Nasal Decongestant Regular
NTZ Long Acting Decongestant Nasal Spray
NTZ Long Acting Decongestant Nose Drops
Sinarest 12 Hour Nasal Spray
Vicks Sinex 12-Hour Formula Decongestant Nasal Spray
Vicks Sinex 12-Hour Formula Decongestant Ultra Fine Mist
Vicks Sinex Long-Acting 12 Hour Nasal Spray

PENICILLINS

AMOXICILLIN
Amoxil
AMPICILLIN
Apo-Amoxi
Apo-Ampi
Apo-Cloxi
Apo-Ven VK
BACAMPICILLIN
Bactocill
Beepen-VK
Betapen-VK
CARBENICILLIN
CLOXACILLIN
Cloxapen
DICLOXACILLIN
Dycill
Dynapen
Fluclox
FLUCOXACILLIN
Geocillin
Geopen Oral
Ledercillin-VK
Megacillin
Nadopen-V
Nadopen-V 200
Nadopen-V 400
NAFCILLIN
Novamoxin
Novo-Ampicillin
Novo-Cloxin
Novo-Pen VK
Nu-Amoxi
Nu-Ampi
Nu-Cloxi
Nu-Pen-VK
Omnipen
Orbenin
OXACILLIN
Pathocil
Pen Vee
Pen Vee K
Penbritin
Penglobe
PENICILLIN G
PENICILLIN V
Pentids
PIVAMPICILLIN
PIVMECILLINAM
Polycillin
Polymox
Pondocillin
Principen
Prostaphlin
PVF
PVF K
Selexid
Spectrobid
Tegopen
Totacillin
Trimox
Unipen
V-Cillin K
Veetids
Wymox

PHENOTHIAZINES

ACETOPHENAZINE
Apo-Fluphenazine
Apo-Perphenazine
Apo-Thioridazine
Apo-Trifluoperazine
Chlorpromanyl-20
Chlorpromanyl-40
CHLORPROMAZINE
Compazine
Compazine Spansule
Dartal
FLUPHENAZINE
Largactil
Largactil Liquid
Largactil Oral Drops
Levoprome
Majeptil
Mellaril
Mellaril Concentrate
Mellaril-S
MESORIDAZINE
METHOTRIMEPRAZINE
Modecate
Moditen Enanthate
Moditen HCl
Moditen HCl-H.P
Neuleptil
Novo-Chlorpromazine
Novo-Flurazine
Novo-Ridazine
Nozinan
Nozinan Liquid
Nozinan Oral Drops
PERICYAZINE
Permitil
Permitil Concentrate
PERPHENAZINE
Piportil L_4
PIPOTIAZINE
PMS Thioridazine
PROCHLORPERAZINE
Prolixin
Prolixin Concentrate
Prolixin Decanoate
Prolixin Enanthate
PROMAZINE
Prozine
Serentil
Serentil Concentrate
Solazine
Stelazine
Stelazine Concentrate
Stemetil
Stemetil Liquid
Suprazine
Terfluzine Concentrate
THIOPROPAZATE
THIOPROPERAZINE
THIORIDAZINE
Thorazine
Thorazine Concentrate
Thorazine Spansule
Thor-Prom
Tindal
TRIFLUOPERAZINE
TRIFLUPROMAZINE
Trilafon
Trilafon Concentrate
Vesprin

PHENYLEPHRINE

Aclophen
Advanced Formula Dristan
Advanced Formula Dristan Caplets
AH-Chew
Alersule
Amaril D
Amaril D Spantab
Anamine HD
Anatuss
Atrohist Plus
Atrohist Sprinkle
Banex
Banex Liquid
Bromophen T.D.
Cerose-DM
Citra Forte
Chlorgest-HD
Codimal DH
Codimal DM
Codimal PH
Colrex Compound
Colrex Cough
Coltab Children's
Comhist
Comhist LA
Conar
Conar Expectorant
Conar-A
Congespirin for Children Cold Tablets
Cophene-S
Cophene-X
Cophene-XP
Coristex-DH
Coristine-DH
Covangesic
D.A. Chewable
Dallergy
Dallergy Caplets
Dallergy-D Syrup
Decohist
Decongestabs
Despec
Dihistine
Dimaphen S.A.
Dimetane Decongestant Caplets
Dimetane Expectorant
Dimetane Expectorant-C
Dimetane Expectorant-DC
Dimetapp-A
Dimetapp-A Pediatric
Dimetapp Elixir
Dimetapp Oral Infant Drops
Dimetapp with Codeine
Dimetapp-DM
Donatussin
Donatussin DC
Donatussin Drops
Dondril
Dristan-AF
Dristan-AF Plus
Dristan Cold
Dristan Formula P
DuraVent/DA
EDA-HIST
Efricon Expectorant Liquid
Endal-HD
Endal-HD Plus
Entex
Entex Liquid
Extendryl
Extendryl JR
Extendryl SR
Father John's Medicine Plus
Fendol
Guistrey Fortis
Histagesic Modified
Histalet Forte
Histamic
Histatab
Histatan
Histatuss Pediatric
Hista-Vadrin
Histor-D
Histor-D Timecelles
Histussin HC
Hycomine
Hycomine Compound
Hycomine-S Pediatric
Improved Sino-Tuss
Kolephrin
Korigesic
Mallergan-VC w/Codeine
Meda Syrup Forte
Myhistine
Naldecon
Naldecon Pediatric
Naldelate
Nalgest
Nasahist
ND-Gesic
NeoCitran DM Coughs & Colds
NeoCitran Sinus Medicine
New-Decongest
New-Decongest Pediatric Syrup
Normatane
Novahistex C
Novahistex DH
Novahistex DH Expectorant
Novahistex DM
Novahistine
Novahistine DH
Novahistine DH Expectorant
Omnicol
OMNIhist L.A.
P-V-Tussin
Par Decon
Pediacof Cough
Phenahist-TR
Phenameth VC
Phenameth VC w/Codeine
Phenchlor SHA
Phenergan VC
Phenergan VC w/Codeine
Phentox Compound
Prehist D
Pherazine VC
Pherazine VC w/Codeine
Prometh VC Plain
Prometh VC w/Codeine
Promethazine VC
Quelidrine Cough
Respinol G
Respinol LA
Rhinogesic
Robitussin Night Relief
Robitussin Night Relief Colds Formula Liquid
R-Tannate
Ru-Tuss
Ru-Tuss w/Hydrocodone
Ru-Tuss Expectorant
Ru-Tuss w/Hydrocodone Liquid
Rymed
Rymed Liquid
Rynatan
Salphenyl
Scot-Tussin
Sinucon Pediatric Drops
Stahist
Statuss Expectorant
Statuss Green
Tamine S.R.
T-Koff
Trimedine Liquid
Triotann
Tri-Phen-Chlor
Tri-Phen-Chlor T.D.
Tritann Pediatric
Tusquelin
Tussanil DH
Tussanil Plain
Tussirex w/Codeine
Tussirex w/Codeine Liquid
Vanex-HD
Vasominic T.D.
Veltap

PHENYL-PROPANOLAMINE

12-Hour Cold
Acutrim II Maximum Strength
Acutrim 16 Hour
Acutrim Late Day
Alamine
Alka-Seltzer Plus Cold
Alka-Seltzer Plus Maximum Strength Sinus Allergy
Alka-Seltzer Plus Maximum Strength Sinus Allergy Medicine
Alka-Seltzer Plus Nighttime Cold
Allerest
Allerest 12 Hour Allergy Relief Medicine
Allerest Headache Strength
Allerest Sinus Pain Formula
Alumadrine
Amaril D
Ami-Tex LA
Anatuss
Anatuss with Codeine
A.R.M. Maximum Strength Caplets
Atrohist Plus
BC Cold Powder
BC Cold Powder Non-Drowsy Formula
Banex
Banex Liquid
Banex-LA
Bayaminic Expectorant
Bayaminicol
Baycomine
Baycomine Pediatric
Bayer Cough Syrup
Bayer Cough Syrup for Children
Biphetane DC Cough Syrup
BQ Cold
Bromanate DC Cough Syrup
Bromatap
Bromatapp
Bromophen T.D.
Bromphen DC w/Codeine Cough
Caldomine-DH Forte
Caldomine-DH Pediatric
Cheracol Plus
Chexit

Chlor-Rest
Chlor-Trimeton Sinus Caplets
Chlor-Tripolon Decongestant
Codamine
Codamine Pediatric
Codegest Expectorant
Codimal Expectorant
Comtrex Multi-Symptom Cold Reliever
Condrin-LA
Conex
Conex D.A.
Conex Plus
Conex w/Codeine Liquid
Congespirin for Children Liquid Cold Medicine
Contac C Cold Care Formula Caplets
Contac Jr. Children's Cold Medicine
Contac 12-Hour
Contac Maximum Strength 12-Hour
Contac Maximum Strength 12-Hour Caplets
Control
Cophene-S
Cophene-X
Cophene-XP
Coricidin Cough
Coricidin D
Coricidin D Decongestant
Coricidin D Medilets
Coricidin Demilets
Coricidin Maximum Strength Sinus Headache
Corsym
Dapacin Cold
DayQuil Non-Drowsy Sinus Pressure and Congestion Relief Caplets
Decongestabs
Dehist
Demazin
Demazin Repetabs
Despec
Dexatrim Maximum Strength Caplets
Dexatrim Maximum Strength Capsules
Dexatrim Maximum Strength Tablets
Diet-Aide Maximum Strength
Dilotab
Dimaphen S.A.
Dimetane Expectorant
Dimetane Expectorant-C
Dimetane Expectorant-DC
Dimetane-DC Cough
Dimetapp
Dimetapp 4-Hour Liqui-Gels Maximum Strength
Dimetapp-A
Dimetapp-A Pediatric
Dimetapp-DM
Dimetapp with Codeine
Dimetapp Extentabs
Dimetapp Maximum Strength Liquigels
Dimetapp Oral Infant Drops
Dimetapp Plus Caplets
Dorcol DM
Drinophen
Dristan
Drize
Duadacin
Dura-Vent
Dura-Vent/A
Efed II Yellow
Effervescent Tylenol Cold
Efficol Cough Whip (Cough Suppressant/Decongestant)
Efficol Cough Whip (Cough Suppressant/Decongestant/ Antihistamine)
Efficol Whip
Entex
Entex LA
Entex Liquid
Extreme Cold Formula Caplets
Fiogesic
Genamin
Genatap
Gencold
Genex
Gentab-LA
Guaipax
Halls Mentho-Lyptus
Halls Mentho-Lyptus Decongestant Cough Formula
Head & Chest
Histabid Duracaps
Histalet Forte
Histamic
Hista-Vadrin
Histosal
Hold (Children's Formula)
Hycomine
Hycomine Pediatric
Hydromine
Hydromine Pediatric
Hydrophen
Ipsatol Cough Formula for Children
Kiddy Koff
Kolephrin/DM
Kolephrin NN Liquid
Kophane
Kophane Cough and Cold Formula
Lanatuss Expectorant
Medatussin Plus
Myhydromine
Myhydromine Pediatric
Myminic
Myphetane DC Cough
Myphetapp
Naldecon
Naldecon Pediatric
Naldecon-CX Adult Liquid
Naldecon-DX Adult Liquid
Naldecon-DX Children's Syrup
Naldecon-DX Pediatric Drops
Naldecon-EX
Naldelate
Naldelate Pediatric Syrup
Nalgest
Nasahist
New-Decongest
New-Decongest Pediatric Syrup
Nolamine
Nolex LA
Noraminic
Norel Plus
Normatane
Normatane DC
Oragest S.R.
Oraminic Spancaps
Ornade
Ornade A.F.
Ornade-DM
Ornade-DM 10
Ornade-DM 15
Ornade-DM 30
Ornade Expectorant
Orthoxicol Cough
Panadyl
Par Decon
Pertussin AM
Phanadex
PhenAPAP No. 2
Phenate T.D.
Phena-TR
Phenchlor SHA
Phentox Compound
Phenyldrine
Phenylfenesin L.A.
Poly-Histine-CS
Poly-Histine-D
Poly-Histine-D Ped
Poly-Histine-DM
Prolamine
Prominic Expectorant
Prominicol Cough
Propagest
Pyrroxate
Remcol Cold
Rentamine
Resaid S.R.
Rescaps-D S.R.
Respinol-G
Respinol LA
Rhinocaps
Rhinolar
Rhinolar-EX
Rhinolar-EX 12
Robitussin-CF
Ru-Tuss
Ru-Tuss II
Ru-Tuss w/Hydrocodone Liquid
Saleto-CF
Saleto-D
Sinapils
Sinarest
Sinarest Extra Strength
Sine-Off Sinus Medicine
Sinubid
Sinucon Pediatric Drops
Sinulin
Sinutab SA
Snaplets-D
Snaplets-DM
Snaplets-EX
Snaplets-Multi
St. Joseph Cold Tablets for Children
Stahist
Stamoist LA
Statuss Green
Syracol Liquid
Tamine S.R.
Tavist-D
T-Koff
Triaminic
Triaminic Allergy
Triaminic Chewables
Triaminic Cold
Triaminic DM Daytime
Triaminic Expectorant
Triaminic Expectorant DH

Triaminic Expectorant w/Codeine
Triaminic Oral Infant Drops
Triaminic TR
Triaminic-DM Cough Formula
Triaminic-DM Expectorant
Triamincin
Triaminicin w/Codeine
Triaminicol DM
Triaminicol Multi-Symptom Relief
Tricodene Forte
Tricodene NN
Tricodene NN Pediatric Medication
Tricodene Pediatric
Trind
Trind DM Liquid
Tri-Nefrin Extra Strength
Tripalgen Cold
Tri-Phen-Chlor
Tri-Phen-Chlor T.D.
Triphenyl
Triphenyl Expectorant
Triphenyl T.D.
Tusquelin
Tuss-Ade
Tuss Allergine Modified T.D.
Tussagesic
Tussaminic C Forte
Tussaminic C Pediatric
Tussaminic DH Forte
Tussaminic DH Pediatric
Tussanil DH Tablets
Tussogest
Tuss-Ornade Liquid
Tuss-Ornade Spansules
Tylenol Cold Medicine
ULR-LA
Utex-S.R.
Vasominic T.D.
Veltap
Vicks DayQuil 4 Hour Allergy Relief
Vicks DayQuil 12 Hour Allergy Relief

POTASSIUM SUPPLEMENTS

Apo-K
Cena-K
K-10
Kallum Durules
Kaochlor
Kaochlor-Eff
Kaochlor S-F
Kaon
Kaon-Cl
Kaon-Cl 10
Kaon-Cl 20
Kato
Kay Ciel
Kay Ciel Elixir
Kaylixir
K+Care ET
KCL
K-Dur
K-G Elixir
K-Lease
K-Long
K-Lor
Klor-Con
Klor-Con/25
Klor-Con/EF
Klorvess
Klorvess 10% Liquid
Klotrix
K-Lyte
K-Lyte DS
K-Lyte/Cl
K-Lyte/Cl 50
K-Lyte/CL Powder
K-Norm
Kolyum
K-Tab
Micro-K
Micro-K 10
Micro-K LS
Neo-K
Novo-Lente-K
Potachlor 10%
Potachlor 20%
Potage
Potasalan
POTASSIUM ACETATE
POTASSIUM BICARBONATE
POTASSIUM BICARBONATE & POTASSIUM CHLORIDE
POTASSIUM BICARBONATE & POTASSIUM CITRATE
POTASSIUM CHLORIDE
POTASSIUM CHLORIDE, POTASSIUM BICARBONATE & POTASSIUM CITRATE
POTASSIUM GLUCONATE
POTASSIUM GLUCONATE & POTASSIUM CHLORIDE
POTASSIUM GLUCONATE & POTASSIUM CITRATE
POTASSIUM GLUCONATE, POTASSIUM CITRATE & AMMONIUM
Potassium-Rougier
Potassium-Sandoz
Potassium Triplex
Roychlor 10%
Roychlor 20%
Royonate
Rum-K
Slo-Pot 600
Slow-K
Ten K
Tri-K
Trikates
Twin-K
Twin-K-Cl

PREDNISOLONE

Articulose
Delta-Cortef
Hydeltrasol
Hydeltra-TBA
Key-Pred
Key-Pred-SP
Nor-Pred-TBA
Pediapred
Predaject
Predalone
Predate-50
Predate-S
Predate-TBA
Predcor 25
Predcor 50
Predicort-50
Prelone

PROGESTINS

Amen
Aygestin
Curretab
Cycrin
Depo-Provera
Duralutin
Femotrone
Gesterol
Gesterol L.A.
HYDROXYPROGESTERONE
Hylutin
Hyprogest
Hyproval P.A.
MEDROXYPROGESTERONE
Megace
Megace Oral Suspension
MEGESTROL
Micronor
Nor-Q.D.
NORETHINDRONE
NORGESTREL
Norlutate
Norlutin
Ovrette
Pro-Depo
Prodrox
Progestaject
PROGESTERONE
Progestilin
Provera

PSEUDOEPHEDRINE

Actacin
Actagen
Actagen-C Cough
Actifed
Actifed A
Actifed Allergy Nighttime Caplets
Actifed Plus
Actifed Plus Caplets
Actifed w/Codeine Cough
Actifed DM
Actifed 12-Hour
Afrinol Repetabs
Alamine-C Liquid
Alamine Expectorant
Allent
Allerest No-Drowsiness
Allerfrin Allergy Formula Sinutab
Allerfrin w/Codeine
AlleRid
Allerphed
Alpha-Phed
Ambenyl-D Decongestant Cough
Anamine
Anamine T.D.
Anaplex
Anatuss DM
Aprodrine
Atrofed Formula
Balminil Decongestant
Banophen
BayCotussend Liquid
Baydec DM Drops
Bayer Select Flu Relief Caplets
Bayer Select Head Cold Caplets
Bayer Select Maximum Strength Sinus Pain Relief Caplets
Bayhistine DH
Bayhistine Expectorant
Benadryl Allergy/Sinus Headache Caplets

Benadryl Decongestant
Benadryl Plus
Benadryl Plus Nighttime Liquid Oral Suspension
Benylin Cold
Benylin Decongestant
Benylin DM-D
Benylin DM-D-E
Benylin DM-D-E Extra Strength
Beta-Phed
Brexin
Brexin-L.A.
Bromfed
Bromfed-AT
Bromfed-DM
Bromphed-PD
Brompheril
Brotane DX Cough
Calmylin
Calmylin Codeine
Calmylin Pediatric
Carbinoxamine Compound
Carbiset
Carbodec
Carbodec DM Drops
Carbodec TR
Cardec-S
Cenafed
Cenafed Plus
Cheracol Sinus
Children's Benylin DM-D
Children's NyQuil Nighttime Cold Medicine
Children's Sudafed Liquid
Children's Tylenol Cold
Chlorafed
Chlorafed H.S. Timecelles
Chlorafed Timecelles
Chlor-Trimeton Decongestant
Chlor-Trimeton Decongestant Repetabs
Chlor-Trimeton Non-Drowsy Decongestant 4 Hour
Chlor-Tripolon Decongestant Extra Strength
Chlor-Tripolon Decongestant Repetabs
Chlor-Tripolon Decongestant Tablets
Claritin Extra
CoActifed
CoActifed Expectorant
CoAdvil
CoAdvil Caplets
Co-Apap
Codehist DH
Codimal
Codimal-LA
Coldrine
Comtrex A/S
Comtrex Daytime Caplets
Comtrex Daytime Maximum Strength Cold and Flu Relief
Comtrex Daytime Maximum Strength Cold, Cough and Flu Relief
Comtrex Hot Flu Relief
Comtrex Multi-Symptom Hot Flu Relief
Comtrex Multi-Symptom Non-Drowsy Caplets
Comtrex Nighttime
Comtrex Nighttime Maximum Strength Cold and Flu Relief
Comtrex Nighttime Maximum Strength Cold, Cough and Flu Relief
Concentrin
Congess JR
Congess SR
Congestac N.D. Caplets
Contac Allergy/Sinus Day Caplets
Contac Allergy/Sinus Night Caplets
Contac Day Caplets
Contac Maximum Strength Sinus Caplets
Contac Night Caplets
Contac Severe Cold Formula
Contac Severe Cold Formula Night Strength
Cophene No. 2
Co-Pyronil 2
Cotridin
Cotridin Expectorant
CoTylenol Cold Medication
Cremacoat 3 Throat Coating Cough Medicine
Cremacoat 4 Throat Coating Cough Medicine
C-Tussin Expectorant
Dallergy-D
Dallergy Jr.
DayCare
DayQuil Liquicaps
DayQuil Non-Drowsy Cold/Flu
DayQuil Non-Drowsy Cold/Flu LiquiCaps
DayQuil Non-Drowsy Sinus Pressure and Pain Relief Caplets
Decofed
Deconamine
Deconamine SR
DeFed-60
Deproist Expectorant w/Codeine
De-Tuss
Detussin Expectorant
Detussin Liquid
Dexaphen SA
Dexophed
Dihistine DH
Dimacol
Dimetane-DX Cough
Dimetapp Sinus Caplets
Disobrom
Disophrol
Disophrol Chronotabs
Dorcol Children's Cold Formula
Dorcol Children's Cough
Dorcol Children's Decongestant
Dristan Cold and Flu
Dristan Juice Mix-in Cold, Flu, and Cough
Dristan Maximum Strength Caplets
Dristan Sinus Caplets
Drixoral
Drixoral Non-Drowsy Formula
Drixoral Plus
Drixoral Sinus
Drixtab
Duralex
Dura-Tap PD
Duratuss
Duratuss HD
Efidec/24
Eltor-120
Endafed
Entuss-D
Entuss Pediatric Expectorant
Fedahist
Fedahist Decongestant
Fedahist Expectorant
Fedahist Expectorant Pediatric Drops
Fedahist Gyrocaps
Fedahist Timecaps
Genac
Genaphed
Guaifed
Guaifed-PD
Guaimax-D
Guaitab
Halofed
Halofed Adult Strength
Head & Chest
Histadyl E.C.
Histafed C
Histalet
Histalet-DM
Histalet X
Isoclor
Isoclor Expectorant
Isoclor Timesules
Klerist-D
Kronofed-A
Kronofed-A Jr.
Maxenal
Maximum Strength Dristan Cold Multi-Symptom Caplets
Maximum Strength Tylenol Allergy Sinus Caplets
Maximum Strength Tylenol Flu Gelcaps
Medi-Flu
Medi-Flu Caplets
Mediquell Decongestant Formula
Midahist DH
Motrin IB Sinus
Motrin IB Sinus Caplets
Mycotussin
Myfed
Myfedrine
Myfedrine Plus
Myhistine DH
Myhistine Expectorant
Mytussin DAC
Naldegesic
Napril
ND Clear T.D.
Neofed
Noratuss II Liquid
Novafed
Novafed A
Novahistex
Novahistine Cough & Cold Formula Liquid
Novahistine DH Liquid
Novahistine DMX Liquid
Novahistine Expectorant
Nucochem
Nucochem Expectorant
Nucochem Pediatric Expectorant
Nucofed
Nucofed Expectorant

Nucofed Pediatric Expectorant
NyQuil Hot Therapy
NyQuil Liquicaps
NyQuil Nighttime Colds Medicine
Nytime Cold Medicine Liquid
Ornex Cold
Ornex No Drowsiness Caplets
Otrivin
PediaCare Children's Cough-Cold Formula
PediaCare Children's Cold Relief Night Rest Cough-Cold Formula
PediaCare Cold Formula
PediaCare Infants' Oral Decongestant Drops
Pertussin AM
Pertussin PM
Phenapap Sinus Headache & Congestion
Phenergan-D
Phenhist Expectorant
Polaramine Expectorant
Promist HD Liquid
Pseudo
Pseudo-Bid
Pseudo-Car DM
Pseudo-Chlor
Pseudodine C Cough
Pseudofrin
Pseudogest
Pseudogest Plus
Pseudo-Hist Expectorant
Respaire-60 SR
Respaire-120 SR
Resporal TR
Rhinosyn-DM
Rhinosyn-X
Rinade B.I.D.
Robidrine
Robitussin Cold and Cough Liqui-Gels
Robitussin-DAC
Robitussin Night Relief
Robitussin-PE
Robitussin Severe Congestion Liqui-Gels
Rondec
Rondec Drops
Rondec-DM
Rondec-DM Drops
Ru-Tuss Expectorant
Rymed-TR
Ryna
Ryna-C Liquid
Ryna-CX Liquid
Seldane D
Semprex-D
Sinarest No-Drowsiness
Sine-Aid
Sine-Aid IB
Sine-Aid Maximum Strength
Sine-Off Maximum Strength Allergy/Sinus Formula
Sine-Aid Maximum Strength Caplets
Sine-Off Maximum Strength No Drowsiness Formula Caplets
Singlet
Sinufed Timecelles
Sinus Excedrin No Drowsiness
Sinus Excedrin No Drowsiness Caplets
SinuStat
Sinutab
Sinutab II Maximum Strength
Sinutab Extra Strength
Sinutab Maximum Strength
Sinutab Maximum Strength Without Drowsiness
Sinutab Maximum Strength Without Drowsiness Caplets
Sinutab No Drowsiness
Sinutab No Drowsiness Extra Strength
Sinutab Regular
SRC Expectorant
Stamoist E
Sudafed
Sudafed 12 Hour
Sudafed 60
Sudafed Cough
Sudafed DM
Sudafed Expectorant
Sudafed Plus
Sudafed Severe Cold Formula Caplets
Sudafed Sinus Maximum Strength
Sudafed Sinus Maximum Strength Caplets
Sudrin
Sufedrin
Super-Anahist
TheraFlu/Flu & Cold
TheraFlu/Flu, Cold & Cough
TheraFlu Nighttime Maximum Strength
Thera-Hist
T-Dry
T-Dry Junior
TheraFlu Maximum Strength Non-Drowsy Formula Flu, Cold and Cough Medicine
T-Moist
Touro A&H
Triacin C Cough
Triaminic DM Nighttime for Children
Triaminic Nite Light
Tricom Caplets
Trifed
Trifed-C Cough
Trinalin Repetabs
Trinex
Triofed
Tripodrine
Triposed
Tussafed
Tussar DM
Tussend
Tussend Expectorant
Tussend Liquid
Tuss-LA
Ty-Cold Cold Formula
Tylenol Allergy Sinus Gelcaps
Tylenol Allergy Sinus Night Time Maximum Strength Caplets
Tylenol Cold Medication
Tylenol Cold Night Time
Tylenol Cold No Drowsiness Gelcaps
Tylenol Cold Medication, Non-Drowsy
Tylenol Cold Night Time
Tylenol Cold and Flu
Tylenol Cough
Tylenol Cough with Decongestant
Tylenol Sinus Maximum Strength
Tylenol Sinus Maximum Strength Caplets
Tylenol Sinus Maximum Strength Gelcaps
Tylenol Sinus Medication
Tylenol Sinus Medication Extra Strength
Ursinus Inlay
Vicks 44 Non-Drowsy Cold and Cough Liqui-Caps
Vicks Formula 44D Decongestant Cough Mixture
Vicks Formula 44M Multi-symptom Cough Mixture
Viro-Med
Zephrex
Zephrex-LA

PSYLLIUM

Cillium
Effersyllium
Fiberall
Hydrocil
Hydrocil Instant
Karacil
Konsyl
Konsyl-D
Konsyl-Orange
Metamucil
Metamucil Instant Mix
Metamucil Instant Mix, Orange Flavor
Metamucil Orange Flavor
Metamucil Strawberry Flavor
Metamucil Sugar Free
Modane Bulk
Naturacil
Perdiem
Perdiem Plain
Pro-Lax
Prodiem
Prodiem Plain
Prompt
Reguloid Natural
Reguloid Orange
Serutan
Serutan Toasted Granules
Siblin
Syllact
V-Lax
Versabran

RADIO-PHARMACEUTICALS

Cyanocobalamin Co 57
Cyanocobalamin Co 60
Ferrous Citrate Fe 59
Gallium Citrate Ga 67
Indium In 111 Pentetate
Iodinated I 131 Albumin
Iodohippurate Sodium I 123
Iodohippurate Sodium I 131
Iothalamate Sodium I 125
Krypton KR 81m
Selenomethionine Se 75
Sodium Chromate Cr 51
Sodium Iodide I 123
Sodium Iodide I 131

Sodium Pertechnetate Tc 99m
Sodium Phosphate P 32
Technetium Tc 99m Albumin Aggregated
Technetium Tc 99m Disofenin
Technetium Tc 99m Gluceptate
Technetium Tc 99m Human Serum Albumin
Technetium Tc 99m Medronate
Technetium Tc 99m Oxidronate
Technetium Tc 99m Pentetate
Technetium Tc 99m Pyrophosphate
Technetium Tc 99m Succimer
Technetium Tc 99m Sulfur Colloid
Thallous Chloride Tl 201
Xenon Xe 127
Xenon Xe 133

RAUWOLFIA ALKALOIDS

DESERPIDINE
Harmonyl
Novoreserpine
Raudixin
Rauval
Rauverid
RAUWOLFIA SERPENTINA
Reserfia
RESERPINE
Serpalan
Serpasil
Wolfina

RAUWOLFIA & THIAZIDE DIURETICS

Demi-Regroton
DESERPIDINE & HYDROCHLOROTHIAZIDE
DESERPIDINE & METHYCLOTHIAZIDE
Diupres
Diurese R
Diurigen with Reserpine
Diutensen-R
Dureticyl
Enduronyl
Enduronyl Forte
Hydropine
Hydropres
Hydrosine
Hydrotensin
Mallopres
Metatensin
Naquival
Oreticyl
Oreticyl Forte
RAUWOLFIA SERPENTINA & BENDROFLUMETHIAZIDE
Rauzide
Regroton
Renese-R
RESERPINE & CHLOROTHIAZIDE
RESERPINE & CHLORTHALIDONE
RESERPINE & HYDROCHLOROTHIAZIDE
RESERPINE & HYDROFLUMETHIAZIDE
RESERPINE & METHYLCLOTHIAZIDE
RESERPINE & POLYTHIAZIDE
RESERPINE & QUINETHAZONE
RESERPINE & TRICHLORMETHIAZIDE
Salazide
Salutensin
Salutensin-Demi

SALICYLATES

Amigesic
Arthropan
Back-Ese
CHOLINE MAGNESIUM SALICYLATES
Choline Magnesium Trisalicylate
CHOLINE SALICYLATE
Citra Forte
Diagen
Disalcid
Doan's Pills
Dodd's Pills
Fendol
Improved SinoTuss
Kolephrin
Kolephrin NN Liquid
Magan
MAGNESIUM SALICYLATE
Mobidin
Mono-Gesic
Omnicol
Rhinogesic
Salcylic Acid
Salflex
Salgesic
SALICYLAMIDE
SALSALATE
Salsitab
Scot-tussin Original 5-Action Cold Medicine
SODIUM SALICYLATE
Tricosal
Trilisate
Tussanil DH Tablets
Tussirex w/Codeine Liquid
Uracel

SCOPOLAMINE (Hyoscine)

Atrohist Plus
Barbidonna
Barbidonna 2
Buscopan
Kinesed
Phenahist TR
Phenchlor SHA
Ru-Tuss
Stahist
Transderm-Scop
Transderm-V

SULFAMETHOXAZOLE

Apo-Sulfamethoxazole
Apo-Sulfatrim
Apo-Sulfatrim DS
Bactrim
Bactrim DS
Bethaprim
Cheragan w/TMP
Cotrim
Cotrim DS
Co-trimoxazole
Gantanol
Gantanol DS
Novotrimel
Nu-Cotrimox
Nu-Cotrimox DS
Protrin
Roubac
Septra
Septra DS
SMZ-TMP
Sulfamethoprim
Sulfamethoprim DS
Sulfaprim
Sulfaprim DS
Sulfatrim
Sulfatrim DS
Sulfoxaprim
Sulfoxaprim DS
Sulmeprim
Triazole
Triazole DS
Trimeth-Sulfa
Trisulfam
Uroplus DS
Uroplus SS

TESTOSTERONE & ESTRADIOL

Andrest
Andro-Estro
Andro/Fem
Androgyn L.A.
De-Comberol
Deladumone
Delatestadiol
depAndrogyn
Depo-Testadiol
Depotestogen
Ditate DS
Duo-Cyp
Duo-Gen L.A.
Duogex LA
Duoval PA
Duratestrin
Estrand
Estra-Testrin
Menoject-L.A.
Neo-Pause
Teev
T.E.-Ionate P.A.
Testadiate-Depo
Test-Estra-C
Test-Estro Cypionates
TESTOSTERONE CYPIONATE & ESTRADIOL CYPIONATE
TESTOSTERONE ENANTHATE & ESTRADIOL VALERATE
Testradiol
Testradiol L.A.
Valertest

TETRACYCLINES

Achromycin
Achromycin V
Apo-Doxy
Apo-Tetra
Declomycin
DEMECLOCYCLINE
Doryx
Doxy-Caps
Doxy-Tabs
Doxycin
DOXYCYCLINE

E.P. Mycin
Minocin
MINOCYCLINE
Monodox
Novodoxlin
Novotetra
Nu-Tetra
OXYTETRACYCLINE
Panmycin
Robitet
Sumycin
Terramycin
TETRACYCLINE
Tetracyn
Tija
Vibramycin
Vibra-Tabs

TRIAMCINOLONE

Amcort
Aristocort Forte
Aristocort Intralesional
Aristospan
Articulose-L.A.
Cenocort A 40
Cenocort Forte
Cinalone 40
Cinonide 40
Kanacort
Kenaject-40
Kenalog 10
Kenalog 40
Myco II
Myco-Triacet II
Mycobiotic II
Mycogen II
Mycolog II
Mykacet
Mykacet II
Mytrex
Tac-3
Triam A
Triam-Forte
Triamolone
Triamonide 40
Tri-Kort
Trilog
Trilone
Tristatin II
Tristoject
Some of these brands are avaiable as topical medicines (ointments, creams or lotions).
See ADRENOCORTICOIDS (Topical) in this section.

XYLOMETAZOLINE

Chlorohist-LA
Neo-Synephrine II Long Acting Nasal Spray Adult Strength
Neo-Synephrine II Long Acting Nose Drops Adult Strength
Otrivin Decongestant Nose Drops
Otrivin Nasal Drops
Otrivin Nasal Spray
Otrivin Pediatric Decongestant Nose Drops
Otrivin Pediatric Nasal Drops
Otrivin Pediatric Nasal Spray
Otrivin With M-D Pump

Additional Drug Interactions

The following lists of drugs and their interactions with other drugs are continuations of lists found in the alphabetized drug charts beginning on page 2. These lists are alphabetized by generic name or drug class name, shown in large capital letters. Only those lists too long for the drug charts are included in this section. For complete information about any generic drug, see the alphabetized charts.

ACETAMINOPHEN & SALICYLATES

GENERIC NAME OR DRUG CLASS	COMBINED EFFECT
Cortisone drugs*	Increased cortisone effect. Risk of ulcers and stomach bleeding.
Furosemide	Possible salicylate toxicity, decreased furosemide effect.
Hepatotoxic drugs*	Increased liver toxicity.
Indomethacin	Risk of stomach bleeding and ulcers.
Lisinopril	Decreased lisinopril effect.
Methotrexate	Increased methotrexate effect.
Para-aminosalicylic acid (PAS)	Possible salicylate toxicity.
Phenobarbital	Decreased effect of acetaminophen and salicylates because of quicker elimination.
Phenytoin	Increased phenytoin effect.
Primidone	Increased liver toxicity.
Probenecid	Decreased probenecid effect.
Propranolol	Decreased aspirin effect.
Rauwolfia alkaloids*	Decreased aspirin effect.
Rifampin	Increased liver toxicity.
Sotalol	Decreased antihypertensive effect of sotalol.
Spironolactone	Decreased spironolactone effect.
Sulfinpyrazone	Decreased sulfinpyrazone effect.
Terazosin	Decreased effectiveness of terazosin. Causes sodium and fluid retention.
Tetracyclines* (effervescent granules or tablets)	May slow tetracycline absorption. Space doses 2 hours apart.
Vancomycin	Hearing loss.
Verapamil	Increased risk of toxicity.
Vitamin C (large doses)	Possible aspirin toxicity.
Urinary alkalizers*	Increased risk of toxicity.
Zidovudine	Increased toxicity of both.

AMILORIDE & HYDROCHLOROTHIAZIDE

GENERIC NAME OR DRUG CLASS	COMBINED EFFECT
Cyclosporine	Increased potassium levels.
Digitalis preparations*	Excessive potassium loss that causes dangerous heart rhythms.
Diuretics, thiazide*	Increased diuretic effect.
Diuretics, other*	Increased effect of both drugs.
Indapamide	Increased diuretic effect.
Lisinopril	Increased antihypertensive effect. Dosage of each may require adjustment.

***See Glossary**

GENERIC NAME OR DRUG CLASS	COMBINED EFFECT	GENERIC NAME OR DRUG CLASS	COMBINED EFFECT

AMILORIDE & HYDROCHLOROTHIAZIDE continued

GENERIC NAME OR DRUG CLASS	COMBINED EFFECT
Lithium	Possible lithium toxicity.
Monoamine oxidase (MAO) inhibitors*	Increased hydrochlorothiazide effect.
Nicardipine	Dangerous blood pressure drop. Dosages may require adjustment.
Nimodipine	Dangerous blood pressure drop.
Nitrates*	Excessive blood pressure drop.
Oxprenolol	Increased antihypertensive effect. Dosages may require adjustment.
Probenecid	Decreased phenytoin effect.
Potassium supplements*	Increased potassium levels.
Sodium bicarbonate	Decreased potassium levels.
Sotalol	Increased antihypertensive effect.
Terazosin	Decreased effectiveness of terazosin
Zinc supplements	Increased need for zinc.

ANGIOTENSIN-CONVERTING ENZYME (ACE) INHIBITORS

GENERIC NAME OR DRUG CLASS	COMBINED EFFECT
Sotalol	Increased antihypertensive effects of both drugs. Dosages may require adjustment.
Spironolactone	Possible excessive potassium in blood
Terazosin	Decreased effectiveness of terazosin.
Tiopronin	Increased risk of toxicity to kidneys.
Triamterene	Possible excessive potassium in blood.

ANGIOTENSIN-CONVERTING ENZYME (ACE) INHIBITORS & HYDROCHLOROTHIAZIDE

GENERIC NAME OR DRUG CLASS	COMBINED EFFECT
Digitalis preparations*	Excessive potassium loss that causes dangerous heart rhythms
Diuretics*	Decreased blood pressure.
Lisinopril	Increased antihypertensive effect. Dosage of each may require adjustment.
Lithium	Increased lithium effect.
Monoamine oxidase (MAO) inhibitors*	Increased hydrochlorothiazide effect.
Nicardipine	Blood pressure drop. Dosages may require adjustment.
Nimodipine	Possible irregular heartbeat. May worsen congestive heart failure.
Nitrates*	Excessive blood pressure drop.
Potassium supplements*	Excessive potassium in blood.
Probenecid	Decreased probenecid effect.
Sotalol	Increased antihypertensive effects of both drugs. Dosages may require adjustment.
Spironolactone	Possible excessive potassium in blood.
Triamterene	Possible excessive potassium in blood.

***See Glossary**

GENERIC NAME OR DRUG CLASS	COMBINED EFFECT	GENERIC NAME OR DRUG CLASS	COMBINED EFFECT

ANTICOAGULANTS (Oral)

GENERIC NAME OR DRUG CLASS	COMBINED EFFECT
Clofibrate	Increased effect of anticoagulant.
Colestipol	Decreased effect of anticoagulant.
Contraceptives, oral*	Decreased effect of anticoagulant.
Danazol	Increased effect of anticoagulant.
Dextrothyroxine	Increased effect of anticoagulant.
Diclofenac	Increased risk of bleeding.
Diflunisal	Increased effect of anticoagulant.
Dipyridamole	Increased risk of hemorrhage.
Disulfiram	Increased effect of anticoagulant.
Erythromycins*	Increased effect of anticoagulant.
Estramustine	Decreased effect of anticoagulant.
Estrogens	Decreased effect of anticoagulant.
Fenoprofen	Increased effect of anticoagulant.
Fluconazole	Increased effect of anticoagulant.
Fluoxetine	May cause confusion, agitation, convulsions and high blood pressure. Avoid combining.
Gemfibrozil	Increased effect of anticoagulant.
Glutethimide	Decreased effect of anticoagulant.
Griseofulvin	Decreased effect of anticoagulant.
Indomethacin	Increased effect of anticoagulant.
Itraconazole	Increased effect of anticoagulant.
Levamisole	Increased risk of bleeding.
Methimazole	Increased effect of anticoagulant.
Metronidazole	Increased effect of anticoagulant.
Mineral Oil	Decreased absorption of anticoagulant.
Nalidixic acid	Increased effect of anticoagulant.
Nicardipine	Possible increased effect of anticoagulant.
Nimodipine	Possible increased effect of anticoagulant.
Nizatidine	Increased effect of anticoagulant.
Omeprazole	Increased effect of anticoagulant
Paroxetine	Increased effect of anticoagulant.
Phenylbutazone	Increased effect of anticoagulant.
Phenytoin	Decreased levels of phenytoin.
Plicamycin	Increased effect of anticoagulant.
Propafenone	May require adjustment of anticoagulant dosage.
Primadone	Decreased effect of anticoagulant.
Rifampin	Decreased effect of anticoagulant.
Quinidine	Increased effect of anticoagulant.
Salicylates	Increased effect of anticoagulant.
Sulfadoxine and pyrimethamine	Increased risk of toxicity.
Sulindac	Increased effect of anticoagulant.
Suprofen	Increased risk of bleeding.
Testolactone	Increased effect of anticoagulant.
Thyroid hormones*	Increased effect of anticoagulant.
Vitamin E	Increased risk of bleeding.
Vitamin K	Decreased effect of anticoagulant.
Note: Any medicine	Unpredictable absorption.

***See Glossary**

ADDITIONAL DRUG INTERACTIONS

ANTICONVULSANTS, HYDANTOIN

GENERIC NAME OR DRUG CLASS	COMBINED EFFECT
Furosemide	Decreased furosemide effect.
Gold compounds*	Increased anti-convulsant blood levels Hydantoin dose may require adjustment.
Glutethimide	Decreased anti-convulsant effect.
Griseofulvin	Increased griseofulvin effect.
Hypoglycemics, oral*	Possible decreased hypoglycemic effect.
Hypoglycemics, other*	Possible decreased hypoglycemic effect.
Isoniazid	Increased anti-convulsant effect.
Itraconazole	Decreased itra-conazole effect.
Leucovorin	May counteract the effect of phenytoin or any hydantoin anti-convulsant.
Loxapine	Decreased anti-convulsant effect of phenytoin or any hydantoin anticonvulsant.
Methadone	Decreased methadone effect.
Methotrexate	Increased methotrexate effect.
Methylphenidate	Increased anti-convulsant effect.
Molindone	Increased phenytoin effect.
Monoamine oxidase (MAO) inhibitors*	Increased polythiazide effect.
Nicardipine	Increased anticonvulsant effect.
Nimodipine	Increased anticonvulsant effect.
Nitrates*	Excessive blood pressure drop.
Nizatidine	Increased effect and toxicity of phenytoin.
Omeprazole	Delayed excretion of phenytoin causing increased amount of phenytoin in blood.
Oxyphenbutazone	Increased anti-convulsant effect.
Para-aminosalicylic acid (PAS)	Increased anti-convulsant effect.
Paroxetine	Decreased anti-convulsant effect.
Phenacemide	Increased risk of paranoid symptoms.
Phenothiazines*	Increased anti-convulsant effect.
Phenylbutazone	Increased anti-convulsant effect.
Potassium supplements*	Decreased potassium effect.
Probenecid	Decreased probenecid effect.
Propafenone	Increased effect of both drugs and increased risk of toxicity.
Propranolol	Increased propranolol effect.
Quinidine	Increased quinidine effect.
Rifampin	Decreased anti-convulsant effect.
Sedatives*	Increased sedative effect.
Sotalol	Decreased sotalol effect.
Sucralfate	Decreased anti-convulsant effect.
Sulfa drugs*	Increased anti-convulsant effect.
Theophylline	Reduced anticonvulsant effect.
Trimethoprim	Increased phenytoin effect.
Valproic acid	Breakthrough seizures.
Xanthines*	Decreased effects of both drugs.

***See Glossary**

GENERIC NAME OR DRUG CLASS	COMBINED EFFECT	GENERIC NAME OR DRUG CLASS	COMBINED EFFECT

ANTIDEPRESSANTS TRICYCLIC

GENERIC NAME OR DRUG CLASS	COMBINED EFFECT
Antihistamines*	Increased antihistamine effect.
Barbiturates*	Decreased antidepressant effect. Increased sedation.
Benzodiazepines*	Increased sedation.
Bupropion	Increased risk of major seizures.
Central nervous system (CNS) depressants*	Excessive sedation.
Cimetidine	Possible increased tricyclic anti-depressant effect and toxicity.
Clonidine	Possible decreased clonidine effect.
Clozapine	Toxic effect on the central nervous system.
Dextrothyroxine	Increased antidepressant effect. Irregular heartbeat.
Disulfiram	Delirium.
Ethchlorvynol	Delirium.
Ethinamate	Dangerous increased effects of ethinamate. Avoid combining.
Fluoxetine	Increased depressant effects of both drugs.
Furazolidine	Sudden, severe increase in blood pressure.
Guanabenz	Decreased guanabenz effect.
Guanadrel	Decreased guanadrel effect.
Guanethidine	Decreased guanethidine effect.
Leucovorin	High alcohol content of leucovorin may cause adverse effects.
Levodopa	May increase blood pressure.
Lithium	Possible decreased seizure threshold.
Methyldopa	Possible decreased methyldopa effect.
Methylphenidate	Possible increased tricyclic anti-depressant effect and toxicity.
Methyprylon	Increased sedative effect, perhaps to dangerous level. Avoid.
Metyrosine	Increased sedative effect.
Molindone	Increased molindone effect.
Monoamine oxidase (MAO) inhibitors*	Fever, delirium, convulsions.
Nabilone	Greater depression of central nervous system.
Narcotics*	Oversedation.
Nicotine	Increased effect of antidepressant (with imipramine).
Contraceptives*, oral	Increased depression.
Phenothiazines*	Possible increased tricyclic antidepressant effect and toxicity.
Phenytoin	Decreased phenytoin effect.
Procainamide	Possible irregular heartbeat.
Quinidine	Possible irregular heartbeat.
Sedatives*	Dangerous oversedation.
Sertraline	Increased depressive effects of both drugs.
Sympathomimetics*	Increased sympathomimetic effect.
Thyroid hormones*	Irregular heartbeat.
Zolpidem	Increased sedative effect. Avoid.

***See Glossary**

GENERIC NAME OR DRUG CLASS	COMBINED EFFECT	GENERIC NAME OR DRUG CLASS	COMBINED EFFECT

ANTIDIABETIC AGENTS

GENERIC NAME OR DRUG CLASS	COMBINED EFFECT
Insulin	Increased blood sugar lowering.
Isoniazid	Decreased blood sugar lowering.
Labetalol	Increased blood sugar lowering, may mask hypoglycemia.
MAO inhibitors*	Increased blood-sugar lowering.
Nicotinic acid	Decreased blood-sugar lowering.
Oxyphenbutazone	Increased blood-sugar lowering.
Phenothiazines*	Decreased blood-sugar lowering.
Phenylbutazone	Increased blood-sugar lowering.
Phenyramidol	Increased blood-sugar lowering.
Phenytoin	Decreased blood-sugar lowering.
Probenecid	Increased blood-sugar lowering.
Pyrazinamide	Decreased blood-sugar lowering.
Ranitidine	Increased blood-sugar lowering.
Rifampin	Decreased blood-sugar lowering.
Sulfa drugs*	Increased blood-sugar lowering.
Sulfadoxine and pyrimethamine	Increased risk of toxicity.
Sulfaphenazole	Increased blood-sugar lowering.
Thyroid hormones*	Decreased blood-sugar lowering.

ANTIHISTAMINES, PHENOTHIAZINE-DERIVATIVE

GENERIC NAME OR DRUG CLASS	COMBINED EFFECT
Guanfacine	May increase depressant effects of either medicine.
Leucovorin	High alcohol content of leucovorin may cause adverse effects.
Levodopa	Decreased levodopa effect.
Methyprylon	May increase sedative effect to dangerous level. Avoid.
Metyrosine	Increased likelihood of toxic symptoms of each.
Mind-altering drugs*	Increased effect of mind-altering drugs.
Molindone	Increased sedative and antihistamine effect.
Monoamine oxidase (MAO) inhibitors*	Increased antihistamine effect.
Nabilone	Greater depression of central nervous system.
Narcotics*	Increased narcotic effect.
Sedatives*	Increased sedative effect.
Sertraline	Increased depressive effects of both drugs.
Sotalol	Increased antihistamine effect.
Tranquilizers*	Increased tranquilizer effect. Avoid.

ANTI-INFLAMMATORY DRUGS, NONSTEROIDAL (NSAIDs)

GENERIC NAME OR DRUG CLASS	COMBINED EFFECT
Diuretics*	May decrease diuretic effect.
Gold compounds*	Increased risk of kidney toxicity.
Lithium	Increased lithium effect.
Methotrexate	Increased risk of methotrexate.

***See Glossary**

GENERIC NAME OR DRUG CLASS	COMBINED EFFECT	GENERIC NAME OR DRUG CLASS	COMBINED EFFECT

ANTI-INFLAMMATORY DRUGS, NONSTEROIDAL (NSAIDs) continued

GENERIC NAME OR DRUG CLASS	COMBINED EFFECT
Minoxidil	Decreased minoxidil effect.
Probenecid	Increased pain relief.
Terazosin	Decreased effectiveness of terazosin. Causes sodium and fluid retention.
Thyroid hormones*	Rapid heartbeat, blood pressure rise.
Tiopronin	Increased risk of toxicity to kidneys.
Triamterene	Reduced triamterene effect.

ASPIRIN

GENERIC NAME OR DRUG CLASS	COMBINED EFFECT
Indomethacin	Risk of stomach bleeding and ulcers.
Ketoprofen	Increased risk of stomach ulcer.
Levamisole	Increased risk of bleeding.
Methotrexate	Increased methotrexate effect.
Minoxidil	Decreased minoxidil effect.
Oxprenolol	Decreased anti-hypertensive effect of oxprenolol.
Para-aminosalicylic acid	Possible aspirin toxicity.
Penicillins*	Increased effect of both drugs.
Phenobarbital	Decreased aspirin effect.
Phenytoin	Increased phenytoin effect.
Probenecid	Decreased probenecid effect.
Propranolol	Decreased aspirin effect.
Rauwolfia alkaloids*	Decreased aspirin effect.
Salicylates*	Likely aspirin toxicity.
Sotalol	Decreased anti-hypertensive effect of sotalol.
Spironolactone	Decreased spironolactone effect.
Sulfinpyrazone	Decreased sulfinpyrazone effect.
Terazosin	Decreased effectiveness of terazosin. Causes sodium and fluid retention.
Terfenadine	May conceal symptons of aspirin overdose, such as ringing in ears.
Ticlopidine	Increased effect of both drugs.
Vitamin C (large doses)	Possible aspirin toxicity.
Valproic acid	May increase valproic acid effect.

ATROPINE, HYOSCYAMINE, METHENAMINE, METHYLENE BLUE, PHENYLSALICYLATE & BENZOIC ACID

GENERIC NAME OR DRUG CLASS	COMBINED EFFECT
Indomethacin	Risk of stomach bleeding and ulcers.
Ketoconazole	Reduced ketoconazole effect.
Meperidine	Increased atropine and hyoscyamine effect.
Methylphenidate	Increased atropine and hyoscyamine effect.
Minoxidil	Decreased minoxidil effect.
Monoamine oxidase (MAO) inhibitors*	Increased belladonna and atropine effect.

*See Glossary

ATROPINE, HYOSCYAMINE, METHENAMINE, METHYLENE BLUE, PHENYLSALICYLATE & BENZOIC ACID continued

GENERIC NAME OR DRUG CLASS	COMBINED EFFECT
Orphenadrine	Increased atropine and hyoscyamine effect.
Oxprenolol	Decreased anti-hypertensive effect of oxprenolol.
Para-aminosalicylic acid (PAS)	Possible salicylate toxicity.
Penicillins*	Increased effect of both drugs.
Phenobarbital	Decreased salicylate effect.
Phenothiazines*	Increased atropine and hyoscyamine effect.
Phenytoin	Increased phenytoin effect.
Pilocarpine	Loss of pilocarpine effect in glaucoma treatment.
Potassium supplements*	Possible intestinal ulcers with oral potassium tablets.
Probenecid	Decreased probenecid effect.
Propranolol	Decreased salicylate effect.
Rauwolfia alkaloids*	Decreased salicylate effect.
Salicylates*	Likely salicylate toxicity.
Sedatives* or central nervous system (CNS) depressants*	Increased sedative effect of both drugs.
Sodium bicarbonate	Decreased methenamine effect.
Spironolactone	Decreased spironolactone effect.
Sulfa drugs*	Possible kidney damage.
Sulfinpyrazone	Decreased sulfinpyrazone effect.
Terfenadine	May conceal symptoms of salicylate overdose, such as ringing in ears.
Vitamin C (1 to 4 grams per day)	Increased effect of methenamine, contributing to urine acidity; decreased atropine effect; possible salicylate toxicity.

BARBITURATES

GENERIC NAME OR DRUG CLASS	COMBINED EFFECT
Narcotics*	Dangerous sedation. Avoid.
Pain relievers*	Dangerous sedation. Avoid.
Sedatives*	Dangerous sedation. Avoid.
Sertraline	Increased depressive effects of both drugs.
Sleep inducers*	Dangerous sedation. Avoid.
Sotalol	Increased barbiturate effect. Dangerous sedation.
Tranquilizers*	Dangerous sedation. Avoid.
Valproic acid	Increased barbiturate effect.

BARBITURATES & ASPIRIN (Also contains caffeine)

GENERIC NAME OR DRUG CLASS	COMBINED EFFECT
Anti-inflammatory drugs, nonsteroidal (NSAIDs)*	Risk of stomach bleeding and ulcers.
Aspirin, other	Likely aspirin toxicity.
Beta-adrenergic blocking agents*	Decreased effect of beta-adrenergic blocker.
Contraceptives, oral*	Decreased contraceptive effect.
Cortisone drugs*	Increased cortisone effect. Risk of ulcer and stomach bleeding.

***See Glossary**

GENERIC NAME OR DRUG CLASS	COMBINED EFFECT	GENERIC NAME OR DRUG CLASS	COMBINED EFFECT

BARBITURATES & ASPIRIN (Also contains caffeine) continued

GENERIC NAME OR DRUG CLASS	COMBINED EFFECT
Digitoxin	Decreased digitoxin effect.
Doxycycline	Decreased doxycycline effect.
Dronabinol	Increased effect of both drugs.
Furosemide	Possible aspirin toxicity.
Gold compounds*	Increased likelihood of kidney damage.
Griseofulvin	Decreased griseofulvin effect.
Indapamide	Increased indapamide effect.
Indomethacin	Risk of stomach bleeding and ulcers.
Methotrexate	Increased methotrexate effect.
Mind-altering drugs*	Dangerous sedation. Avoid.
Minoxidil	Decreased minoxidil effect.
Monoamine oxidase (MAO) inhibitors*	Increased butalbital effect.
Naltrexone	Decreased analgesic effect.
Narcotics*	Dangerous sedation. Avoid.
Pain relievers*	Dangerous sedation. Avoid.
Rifampin	May decrease butalbital effect.
Salicylates*	Likely aspirin toxicity.
Sedatives*	Dangerous sedation. Avoid.
Sleep inducers*	Dangerous sedation. Avoid.
Spironolactone	Decreased spirono-lactone effect.
Sulfinpyrazone	Decreased sulfin-pyrazone effect.
Terfenadine	May conceal symptoms of aspirin overdose, such as ringing in ears.
Tranquilizers*	Dangerous sedation. Avoid.
Valproic acid	Increased butalbital effect.
Vitamin C (large doses)	Possible aspirin toxicity.
Zidovudine	Increased toxicity of both.

BARBITURATES, ASPIRIN & CODEINE (Also contains caffeine)

GENERIC NAME OR DRUG CLASS	COMBINED EFFECT
Antidepressants*	Decreased anti-depressant effect. Possible dangerous oversedation.
Antidiabetics, oral*	Increased butalbital effect. Low blood sugar.
Antihistamines*	Dangerous sedation. Avoid.
Anti-inflammatory drugs, nonsteroidal (NSAIDs)*	Risk of stomach bleeding and ulcers.
Aspirin, other	Likely aspirin toxicity.
Beta-adrenergic blocking agents*	Decreased effect of beta-adrenergic blocker.
Carteolol	Increased narcotic effect. Dangerous sedation.
Contraceptives, oral*	Decreased contra-ceptive effect.
Cortisone drugs*	Increased cortisone effect. Risk of ulcer and stomach bleeding.
Digitoxin	Decreased digitoxin effect.
Doxycycline	Decreased doxycycline effect.
Dronabinol	Increased effect of drugs.
Furosemide	Possible aspirin toxicity.

ADDITIONAL DRUG INTERACTIONS

***See Glossary**

GENERIC NAME OR DRUG CLASS	COMBINED EFFECT	GENERIC NAME OR DRUG CLASS	COMBINED EFFECT

BARBITURATES, ASPIRIN & CODEINE (Also contains caffeine) continued

GENERIC NAME OR DRUG CLASS	COMBINED EFFECT
Gold compounds*	Increased likelihood of kidney damage.
Griseofulvin	Decreased griseofulvin effect.
Indapamide	Increased indapamide effect.
Indomethacin	Risk of stomach bleeding and ulcers.
Methotrexate	Increased methotrexate effect.
Mind-altering drugs*	Dangerous sedation. Avoid.
Minoxidil	Decreased minoxidil effect.
Monoamine oxidase (MAO) inhibitors*	Increased butalbital effect.
Naltrexone	Decreased analgesic effect.
Narcotics*	Dangerous sedation. Avoid.
Nitrates*	Excessive blood pressure drop.
Pain relievers*	Dangerous sedation. Avoid.
Para-aminosalicylic acid	Possible aspirin toxicity.
Penicillins*	Increased effect of drugs.
Phenobarbital	Decreased aspirin effect.
Phenothiazines*	Increased phenothiazine effect.
Phenytoin	Increased phenytoin effect.
Probenecid	Decreased probenecid effect.
Propranolol	Decreased aspirin effect.
Rauwolfia alkaloids*	Decreased aspirin effect.
Salicylates*	Likely aspirin toxicity.
Sedatives*	Dangerous sedation. Avoid.
Sleep inducers*	Dangerous sedation. Avoid.
Sotalol	Increased narcotic effect. Dangerous sedation.
Spironolactone	Decreased spirono-lactone effect.
Sulfinpyrazone	Decreased sulfin-pyrazone effect.
Terfenadine	May conceal symptoms of aspirin overdose, such as ringing in ears.
Tranquilizers*	Dangerous sedation. Avoid.
Valproic acid	Increased phenobarbital effect.
Vitamin C (large doses)	Possible aspirin toxicity.
Zidovudine	Increased toxicity of both.

BELLADONNA ALKALOIDS & BARBITURATES

GENERIC NAME OR DRUG CLASS	COMBINED EFFECT
Attapulgite	Decreased belladonna effect.
Beta-adrenergic blocking agents*	Decreased effects of beta-adrenergic blocker.
Carteolol	Increased barbiturate effect. Dangerous sedation.
Central nervous system (CNS) depressants*	Dangerous sedation. Avoid.
Contraceptives, oral*	Decreased contra-ceptive effect.
Cortisone drugs*	Increased internal eye pressure. Decreased cortisone effect.
Digitoxin	Decreased digitoxin effect.
Doxycycline	Decreased doxycycline effect.
Dronabinol	Increased effects of both drugs. Avoid.
Furosemide	Possible orthostatic hypotension.

*See Glossary

GENERIC NAME OR DRUG CLASS	COMBINED EFFECT	GENERIC NAME OR DRUG CLASS	COMBINED EFFECT

BELLADONNA ALKALOIDS & BARBITURATES continued

GENERIC NAME OR DRUG CLASS	COMBINED EFFECT
Griseofulvin	Decreased griseofulvin effect.
Haloperidol	Increased internal eye pressure.
Indapamide	Increased indapamide effect.
Ketoconazole	Decreased ketoconazole effect.
Meperidine	Increased belladonna effect.
Methylphenidate	Increased belladonna effect.
Metronidazole	Decreased metronidazole effect.
Mind-altering drugs*	Dangerous sedation. Avoid.
Monoamine oxidase (MAO) inhibitors*	Increased belladona and barbiturate effect.
Narcotics*	Dangerous sedation. Avoid.
Nitrates*	Increased internal eye pressure.
Nizatidine	Increased nizatidine effect.
Orphenadrine	Increased belladonna effect.
Pain relievers*	Dangerous sedation. Avoid.
Phenothiazines*	Increased belladonna effect. Danger of oversedation.
Pilocarpine	Loss of pilocarpine effect in glaucoma treatment.
Potassium supplements*	Possible intestinal ulcers with oral potassium tablets.
Quinidine	Increased belladonna effect.
Sedatives*	Dangerous sedation. Avoid.
Sleep inducers*	Dangerous sedation. Avoid.
Sotalol	Increased barbiturate effect. Dangerous sedation.
Tranquilizers*	Dangerous sedation. Avoid.
Valproic acid	Increased barbiturate effect.
Vitamin C	Decreased belladonna effect. Avoid large doses of vitamin C.

BENZODIAZEPINES

GENERIC NAME OR DRUG CLASS	COMBINED EFFECT
Tranquilizers*	Increased sedative effect of both drugs.
Zidovudine	Increased toxicity of zidovudine.

BETA-ADRENERGIC BLOCKING AGENTS

GENERIC NAME OR DRUG CLASS	COMBINED EFFECT
Diazoxide	Additional blood pressure drop.
Dextrothyroxine	Possible decreased beta blocker effect.
Digitalis preparations*	Can either increase or decrease heartrate. Improves irregular heart beat.
Encainide	Increased effect of toxicity on heart muscle.
Guanabenz	Additional blood pressure drop.
Indomethacin	Decreased effect of beta blocker.
Insulin	Hypoglycemic effects may be prolonged.
Levobunolol eyedrops	Possible increased beta blocker effect.
Molindone	Increased tranquilizer effect.
Monoamine oxidase (MAO) inhibitors*	High blood pressure following MAO discontinuation.
Narcotics*	Increased narcotic effect. Dangerous sedation.

ADDITIONAL DRUG INTERACTIONS

*See Glossary

GENERIC NAME OR DRUG CLASS	COMBINED EFFECT	GENERIC NAME OR DRUG CLASS	COMBINED EFFECT

BETA-ADRENERGIC BLOCKING AGENTS continued

GENERIC NAME OR DRUG CLASS	COMBINED EFFECT
Nicardipine	Possible irregular heartbeat and congestive heart failure.
Nicotine	Increased beta blocker effect.
Nimodipine	Possible irregular heartbeat. May worsen congestive heart failure.
Nitrates*	Possible excessive blood pressure drop.
Phentoin	Decreased beta blocker effect.
Propafenone	Increased beta blocker effect.
Quinidine	Slows heart excessively.
Reserpine	Increased reserpine effect. Excessive sedation and depression. Additional blood pressure drop.
Sympathomimetics*	Decreased effect of both drugs.
Timolol eyedrops	Possible increased beta blocker effect.
Tocainide	May worsen congestive heart failure.
Verapamil	Increased effect of both drugs.
Xanthines (aminophylline, theophylline)	Decreased effects of both drugs.

BETA-ADRENERGIC BLOCKING AGENTS & THIAZIDE DIURETICS

GENERIC NAME OR DRUG CLASS	COMBINED EFFECT
Antidiabetics*	Increased antidiabetic effect.
Antihistamines*	Decreased antihistamine effect.
Antihypertensives*	Increased antihypertensive effect.
Anti-inflammatory drugs, nonsteroidal (NSAIDs)*	Decreased anti-inflammatory effect.
Barbiturates*	Increased barbiturate effect. Dangerous sedation.
Bumetanide	Increased diuretic effect.
Calcium channel blockers*	Increased antihypertensive effect. Dosages of both drugs may require adjustments.
Cholestyramine	Decreased hydrochlorthiazide effect.
Cortisone drugs*	Excessive potassium loss that causes dangerous heart rhythms.
Diclofenac	Decreased antihypertensive effect.
Digitalis preparations*	Excessive potassium loss that causes dangerous heart rhythms. Can either increase or decrease heart rate. Improves irregular heartbeat.
Diuretics, thiazide*	Increased effect of other thiazide diuretics.
Ethacrynic acid	Increased diuretic effect.
Furosemide	Increased diuretic effect.
Guanfacine	Increased effect of both drugs.
Hypoglycemics, oral*	Decreased ability to lower blood glucose.
Indapamide	Increased diuretic effect.
Insulin	Decreased ability to lower blood glucose.
Lisinopril	Increased antihypertensive effect. Dosage of each may require adjustment.
Metolazone	Increased diuretic effect.

***See Glossary**

GENERIC NAME OR DRUG CLASS	COMBINED EFFECT	GENERIC NAME OR DRUG CLASS	COMBINED EFFECT

BETA-ADRENERGIC BLOCKING AGENTS & THIAZIDE DIURETICS continued

GENERIC NAME OR DRUG CLASS	COMBINED EFFECT	GENERIC NAME OR DRUG CLASS	COMBINED EFFECT
Monoamine oxidase (MAO) inhibitors*	Increased hydro chlorothiazide effect.	**Propafenone**	Increased beta blocker effect.
Narcotics*	Increased narcotic effect. Dangerous sedation.	**Quinidine**	Slows heart excessively.
Nicardipine	Possible irregular heartbeat and congestive heart failure.	**Reserpine**	Increased reserpine effect. Excessive sedation and depression.
Nicotine	Increased beta blocker effect.	**Sympathomimetics***	Decreased effectiveness of both.
Nitrates*	Excessive blood pressure drop.	**Theophylline**	Decreased effectiveness of both.
Phenytoin	Increased beta adrenergic effect.	**Tocainide**	May worsen congestive heart failure.
Potassium supplements*	Decreased potassium effect.	**Zinc supplements**	Increased need for zinc.
Probenecid	Decreased probenecid effect.		

BETAMETHASONE

GENERIC NAME OR DRUG CLASS	COMBINED EFFECT	GENERIC NAME OR DRUG CLASS	COMBINED EFFECT
Ephedrine	Decreased betamethasone effect.	**Insulin**	Decreased insulin effect.
Estrogens*	Increased betamethasone effect.	**Isoniazid**	Decreased isoniazid effect.
Ethacrynic acid	Potassium depletion.	**Oxyphenbutazone**	Possible ulcers.
Furosemide	Potassium depletion.	**Phenylbutazone**	Possible ulcers.
Glutethimide	Decreased betamethasone effect.	**Phenytoin**	Decreased betamethasone effect.
Indapamide	Possible excessive potassium loss, causing dangerous heartbeat irregularity.	**Potassium supplements***	Decreased potassium effect.
		Rifampin	Decreased betamethasone effect.
Indomethacin	Increased betamethasone effect.	**Sympathomimetics***	Possible glaucoma.

CALCIUM CHANNEL BLOCKERS

GENERIC NAME OR DRUG CLASS	COMBINED EFFECT	GENERIC NAME OR DRUG CLASS	COMBINED EFFECT
Rifampin	Decreased effect of calcium channel blocker.	**Vitamin D**	Decreased effect of calcium channel blockers.
Theophylline	May increase effect and toxicity of theophylline.		

CALCIUM SUPPLEMENTS

GENERIC NAME OR DRUG CLASS	COMBINED EFFECT	GENERIC NAME OR DRUG CLASS	COMBINED EFFECT
Vitamin A	Decreased vitamin effect.	**Vitamin D**	Increased vitamin absorption, sometimes excessively.

*See Glossary

GENERIC NAME OR DRUG CLASS	COMBINED EFFECT	GENERIC NAME OR DRUG CLASS	COMBINED EFFECT

CARBAMAZEPINE

GENERIC NAME OR DRUG CLASS	COMBINED EFFECT
Doxycycline	Decreased doxycycline effect.
Estrogens	Decreased estrogen effect.
Erythromycins*	Increased carbamazepine effect.
Ethinamate	Dangerous increased effects of ethinamate. Avoid combining.
Felbamate	Increased side effects and adverse reactions.
Fluoxetine	Increased depressant effects of both drugs.
Guanfacine	May increase depressant effects of either drug.
Isoniazid	Increased risk of liver damage.
Itraconazole	Decreased itraconazole effect.
Leucovorin	High alcohol content of leucovorin may cause adverse effects.
Mebendazole	Decreased effect of mebendazole.
Methyprylon	Increased sedative effect, perhaps to dangerous level. Avoid.
Monoamine oxidase (MAO) Inhibitors*	Dangerous overstimulation. Avoid.
Nabilone	Greater depression of central nervous system.
Nicardipine	May increase carbamazepine effect and toxicity.
Nimodipine	May increase carbamazepine effect and toxicity.
Nizatidine	Increased carbamazepine effect and toxicity.
Phenytoin	Decreased carbamazepine effect.
Phenobarbital	Decreased carbamazepine effect.
Primidone	Decreased carbamazepine effect.
Propoxyphene (Darvon)	Increased toxicity of both. Avoid.
Sertraline	Increased depressive effects of both drugs.
Tiopronin	Increased risk of toxicity to bone marrow.
Tranquilizers* (benzodiazepine)	Increased carbamazepine effect.
Verapamil	Possible increased carbamazepine effect.

CHLORPROTHIXENE

GENERIC NAME OR DRUG CLASS	COMBINED EFFECT
Sleep inducers*	Increased chlorprothixene effect Excessive sedation.
Tranquilizers*	Increased chlorprothixene effect. Excessive sedation.

CHLORZOXAZONE & ACETAMINOPHEN

GENERIC NAME OR DRUG CLASS	COMBINED EFFECT
Tranquilizers*	Increased sedation.
Zidovudine	Increased toxicity of zidovudine.

CLONIDINE

GENERIC NAME OR DRUG CLASS	COMBINED EFFECT
Methyprylon	Increased sedative effect, perhaps to dangerous level. Avoid.
Nabilone	Greater depression of central nervous system.

***See Glossary**

GENERIC NAME OR DRUG CLASS	COMBINED EFFECT	GENERIC NAME OR DRUG CLASS	COMBINED EFFECT

CLONIDINE continued

GENERIC NAME OR DRUG CLASS	COMBINED EFFECT	GENERIC NAME OR DRUG CLASS	COMBINED EFFECT
Nicardipine	Blood pressure drop. Dosages may require adjustment.	**Sertraline**	Increased depressive effects of both drugs.
Nimodipine	Dangerous blood pressure drop	**Sotalol**	Increased anti-hypertensive effect.
Nitrates*	Possible excessive blood pressure drop	**Terazosin**	Decreased effective-ness of terazosin.

CLONIDINE & CHLORTHALIDONE

GENERIC NAME OR DRUG CLASS	COMBINED EFFECT	GENERIC NAME OR DRUG CLASS	COMBINED EFFECT
Central nervous system (CNS) depressants*	Increased sedative effect.	**Monoamine oxidase (MAO) inhibitors***	Increased chlor-thalidone effect.
Cholestyramine	Decreased chlor-thalidone effect.	**Nabilone**	Greater depression of central nervous system.
Cortisone drugs*	Excessive potassium loss that causes dangerous heart rhythms.	**Nicardipine**	Blood pressure drop. Dosage may require adjustment.
Digitalis preparations*	Excessive potassium loss that causes dangerous heart rhythms.	**Nitrates***	Possible excessive blood pressure drop.
Diuretics*	Excessive blood pressure drop.	**Potassium supplements***	Decreased potassium effect.
Fenfluramine	Possible increased clonidine effect.	**Probenecid**	Decreased probenecid effect.
Guanfacine	Impaired blood pressure control.	**Sedatives* or central nervous system (CNS) depressants***	Increased sedative effect of both drugs.
Indapamide	Increased diuretic effect.	**Sotalol**	Decreased anti-hypertensive effect.
Lithium	Increased lithium effect.	**Terazosin**	Decreased terazosin effect.

CONTRACEPTIVES, ORAL

GENERIC NAME OR DRUG CLASS	COMBINED EFFECT	GENERIC NAME OR DRUG CLASS	COMBINED EFFECT
Meprobamate	Decreased contraceptive effect.	**Terazosin**	Decreases terazosin effect.
Mineral oil	Decreased contraceptive effect.	**Tetracyclines***	Decreased contra-ceptive effect.
Phenothiazines*	Increased pheno-thiazine effect.	**Ursodiol**	Decreased ursodiol effect.
Rifampin	Decreased contra-ceptive effect.	**Vitamin A**	Vitamin A excess.
Sulfadoxine and pyrimethamine	Reduced reliability of the pill.	**Vitamin C**	Possible increased contraceptive effect.

*See Glossary

GENERIC NAME OR DRUG CLASS	COMBINED EFFECT	GENERIC NAME OR DRUG CLASS	COMBINED EFFECT

CORTISONE

GENERIC NAME OR DRUG CLASS	COMBINED EFFECT
Digitalis preparations*	Dangerous potassium depletion. Possible digitalis toxicity.
Diuretics, thiazide*	Potassium depletion.
Ephedrine	Decreased cortisone effect.
Estrogens*	Increased cortisone effect.
Ethacrynic acid	Potassium depletion.
Furosemide	Potassium depletion.
Glutethimide	Decreased cortisone effect.
Indapamide	Possible excessive potassium loss, causing dangerous heatbeat irregularity.
Indomethacin	Increased cortisone effect.
Insulin	Decreased insulin effect.
Isoniazid	Decreased isoniazid effect.
Ketoprofen	Increased risk of stomach ulcer and bleeding.
Mitotane	Decreased cortisone effect.
Oxyphenbutazone	Possible ulcers.
Phenobarbital	Decreased cortisone effect.
Phenylbutazone	Possible ulcers.
Potassium supplements*	Decreased potassium effect.
Rifampin	Decreased cortisone effect.
Salicylates*	Decreased salicylate effect.
Sodium bicarbonate	Sodium overload.
Sympathomimetics*	Possible glaucoma.
Theophylline	Possible increased theophylline effect.
Vaccines, other immunizations	Increased risk of developing disease vaccine is for or decreased vaccine effect.

DEXAMETHASONE

GENERIC NAME OR DRUG CLASS	COMBINED EFFECT
Digitalis preparations*	Dangerous potassium depletion. Possible digitalis toxicity.
Diuretics, thiazide*	Potassium depletion.
Ephedrine	Decreased dexamethasone effect.
Estrogens*	Increased dexamethasone effect.
Ethacrynic acid	Potassium depletion.
Furosemide	Potassium depletion.
Glutethimide	Decreased dexamethasone effect.
Indapamide	Possible excessive potassium loss, causing dangerous heartbeat irregularity.
Indomethacin	Increased dexamethasone effect.
Insulin	Decreased insulin effect.
Isoniazid	Decreased isoniazid effect.
Mitotane	Decreased dexamethasone effect.
Oxyphenbutazone	Possible ulcers.
Phenobarbital	Decreased dexamethasone effect.
Phenylbutazone	Possible ulcers.
Potassium supplements*	Decreased potassium effect.
Rifampin	Decreased dexamethasone effect.
Salicylates*	Decreased salicylate effect.
Sympathomimetics*	Possible glaucoma.
Theophylline	Possible increased theophylline effect.

***See Glossary**

GENERIC NAME OR DRUG CLASS	COMBINED EFFECT

DIDANOSINE

GENERIC NAME OR DRUG CLASS	COMBINED EFFECT
Tetracyclines	Decreased antibiotic effect.
Valproic acid	Increased risk of pancreatitis.
Vincristine	Increased risk of peripheral neuropathy.

DIFENOXIN & ATROPINE

GENERIC NAME OR DRUG CLASS	COMBINED EFFECT
Nitrates*	Increased internal eye pressure.
Orphenadrine	Increased atropine effect.
Phenothiazines*	Increased atropine effect.
Pilocarpine	Loss of pilocarpine effect in glaucoma treatment.
Potassium supplements*	Possible intestinal ulcers with oral potassium tablets.
Procainamide	Increased atropine effect.
Sertraline	Increased depressive effects of both drugs.
Vitamin C	Decreased atropine effect. Avoid large doses of vitamin C.

DIGITALIS PREPARATIONS (Digitalis Glycosides)

GENERIC NAME OR DRUG CLASS	COMBINED EFFECT
Mineral Oil	Decreased digitalis effect.
Nicardipine	Increased digitalis effect. May need to reduce dose.
Nizatidine	Increased digitalis effect.
Oxyphenbutazone	Decreased digitalis effect.
Paroxetine	Increased levels of paroxetine in blood.
Phenobarbital	Decreased digitalis effect.
Phenylbutazone	Decreased digitalis effect.
Potassium supplements*	Overdose of either drug may cause severe heartbeat irregularity.
Propafenone	Increased digitalis absorption. May require decreased digitalis dosage.
PTU/Metronidazole	Decreased digitalis effect.
Quinidine	Increased digitalis effect.
Rauwolfia alkaloids*	Increased digitalis effect.
Rifampin	Possible decreased digitalis effect.
Sotalol	Can either increase or decrease heart rate. Improves irregular heartbeat.
Spironolactone	Increased digitalis effect. May require digitalis dosage reduction.
Sulfasalazine	Decreased digitalis absorption.
Sympathomimetics*	Increased risk of heartbeat irregularities.
Tetracycline	May increase digitalis absorption.
Thyroid hormones*	Digitalis toxicity.
Ticlopidine	Slightly decreased digitalis effect (digoxin only).
Trazodone	Possible increased digitalis toxicity.
Triamterene	Possible decreased digitalis effect.
Verapamil	Increased digitalis effect.

*See Glossary

GENERIC NAME OR DRUG CLASS	COMBINED EFFECT	GENERIC NAME OR DRUG CLASS	COMBINED EFFECT

DIURETICS, LOOP

GENERIC NAME OR DRUG CLASS	COMBINED EFFECT
Probenecid	Decreased probenecid effect.
Salicylates* **(including aspirin)**	Dangerous salicylate retention.
Sedatives*	Increased diuretic effect.

DIURETICS, THIAZIDE

GENERIC NAME OR DRUG CLASS	COMBINED EFFECT
Indapamide	Increased diuretic effect.
Indomethacin	Decreased anti-hypertensive effect.
Lithium	Increased effect of lithium.
Monoamine oxidase (MAO) inhibitors*	Increased anti-hypertensive effect.
Nicardipine	Blood pressure drop. Dosages may require adjustment.
Nimodipine	Dangerous blood pressure drop.
Nitrates*	Excessive blood pressure drop.
Opiates*	Dizziness or weakness when standing up after sitting or lying down.
Pentoxifylline	Increased anti-hypertensive effect.
Potassium supplements*	Decreased potassium effect.
Probenecid	Decreased probenecid effect.
Sotalol	Increased anti-hypertensive effect.
Terazosin	Decreased terazosin effect.
Zinc supplements	Increased need for zinc.

ERGOTAMINE, BELLADONNA & PHENOBARBITAL

GENERIC NAME OR DRUG CLASS	COMBINED EFFECT
Ephedrine	Dangerous blood pressure rise.
Epinephrine	Dangerous blood pressure rise.
Erythromycin	Decreased ergotamine effect.
Griseofulvin	Decreased griseofulvin effect.
Guanethidine	Decreased belladonna effect.
Haloperidol	Increased internal eye pressure.
Indapamide	Increased indapamide effect.
Meperidine	Increased belladonna effect.
Methylphenidate	Increased belladonna effect.
Metoclopramide	May decrease metoclopramide effect.
Mind-altering drugs*	Dangerous sedation. Avoid.
Monoamine oxidase (MAO) inhibitors*	Increased belladonna and phenobarbital effect.
Narcotics*	Dangerous sedation. Avoid.
Nitrates*	Increased internal eye pressure.
Nitroglycerin	Decreased nitroglycerin effect.
Orphenadrine	Increased belladonna effect.
Pain relievers*	Dangerous sedation. Avoid.
Phenothiazines*	Increased belladonna effect.
Pilocarpine	Loss of pilocarpine effect in glaucoma treatment.
Potassium supplements*	Possible intestinal ulcers with oral potassium tablets.
Quinidine	Increased belladonna effect.

***See Glossary**

GENERIC NAME OR DRUG CLASS	COMBINED EFFECT	GENERIC NAME OR DRUG CLASS	COMBINED EFFECT

ERGOTAMINE, BELLADONNA & PHENOBARBITAL continued

GENERIC NAME OR DRUG CLASS	COMBINED EFFECT
Reserpine	Decreased belladonna effect.
Sedatives*	Dangerous sedation. Avoid.
Sleep inducers*	Dangerous sedation. Avoid.
Sumatriptan	Increased vasoconstriction. Delay 24 hours between drugs.
Tranquilizers*	Dangerous sedation. Avoid.
Troleandomycin	Increased adverse reactions of ergotamine.
Valproic acid	Increased phenobarbital effect.
Vitamin C	Decreased belladonna effect. Avoid large doses of vitamin C.

ERGOTAMINE & CAFFEINE

GENERIC NAME OR DRUG CLASS	COMBINED EFFECT
Tranquilizers*	Decreased tranquilizer effect.
Troleandomycin	Decreased ergotamine effect.

ERGOTAMINE, CAFFEINE, BELLADONNA & PENTOBARBITAL

GENERIC NAME OR DRUG CLASS	COMBINED EFFECT
Anticonvulsants*	Changed seizure patterns.
Antidepressants, tricyclic*	Decreased antidepressant effect. Possible dangerous oversedation.
Antidiabetics, oral*	Increased pentobarbital effect.
Antihistamines*	Dangerous sedation. Avoid.
Aspirin	Decreased aspirin effect.
Anti-inflammatory drugs, nonsteroidal (NSAIDs)*	Decreased anti-inflammatory effect.
Beta-adrenergic blocking agents*	Decreased effect of beta-adrenergic blocker.
Cimetidine	Increased caffeine effect.
Contraceptives, oral*	Decreased contraceptive effect.
Cortisone drugs*	Decreased cortisone effect. Increased internal eye pressure.
Digitoxin	Decreased digitoxin effect.
Disulfiram	Possible increased pentobarbital effect.
Doxycycline	Decreased doxycycline effect.
Dronabinol	Increased effect of drugs.
Ephedrine	Dangerous blood pressure rise.
Epinephrine	Dangerous blood pressure rise.
Erythromycin	Decreased ergotamine effect.
Estrogens*	Decreased estrogen effect.
Griseofulvin	Possible decreased griseofulvin effect.
Guanethidine	Decreased belladonna effect.
Haloperidol	Increased internal eye pressure.
Indapamide	Increased indapamide effect.
Isoniazid	Increased caffeine effect.
Meperidine	Increased belladonna effect.
Methylphenidate	Increased belladonna effect.
Metoclopramide	May decrease metoclopramide effect.
Metronidazole	Possible decreased metronidazole effect.

*See Glossary

ERGOTAMINE, CAFFEINE, BELLADONNA & PENTOBARBITAL continued

GENERIC NAME OR DRUG CLASS	COMBINED EFFECT
Mind-altering drugs*	Dangerous sedation. Avoid.
Monoamine oxidase (MAO) inhibitors*	Increased belladona effect, dangerous blood pressure rise.
Narcotics*	Dangerous sedation. Avoid.
Nitrates*	Increased internal eye pressure.
Nitroglycerin	Decreased nitroglycerin effect.
Orphenadrine	Increased belladonna effect.
Pain relievers*	Dangerous sedation. Avoid.
Phenothiazines*	Increased belladonna effect.
Pilocarpine	Loss of pilocarpine effect in glaucoma treatment.
Potassium supplements*	Possible intestinal ulcers with oral potassium tablets.
Quinidine	Increased belladonna effect.
Reserpine	Decreased belladonna effect.
Rifampin	Possible decreased pentobarbital effect.
Sedatives*	Dangerous sedation. Avoid.
Sleep inducers*	Dangerous sedation. Avoid.
Sumatriptan	Increased vasoconstriction. Delay 24 hours between drugs.
Sympathomimetics*	Overstimulation, blood pressure rise.
Thyroid hormones*	Increased thyroid effect.
Terazosin	Decreased effectiveness of terazosin.
Thyroid hormones*	Decreased thyroid effect.
Ursodiol	Decreased effect of ursodiol.
Vitamin C	Possible increased estrogen effect.

ESTROGENS

GENERIC NAME OR DRUG CLASS	COMBINED EFFECT
Terazosin	Decreased effectiveness of terazosin.
Thyroid hormones*	Decreased thyroid effect.
Ursodiol	Decreased effect of ursodiol.
Vitamin C	Possible increased estrogen effect.

GUANETHIDINE

GENERIC NAME OR DRUG CLASS	COMBINED EFFECT
Rauwolfia alkaloids*	Excessively slow heartbeat. Weakness and faintness upon rising from chair or bed.
Sotalol	Increased antihypertensive effect.
Terazosin	Decreased effectiveness of terazosin.
Thioxanthenes*	Decreased guanethidine effect.
Trimeprazine	Decreased guanethidine effect.

GUANETHIDINE & HYDROCHLOROTHIAZIDE

GENERIC NAME OR DRUG CLASS	COMBINED EFFECT
Cortisone drugs*	Excessive potassium loss that causes dangerous heart rhythms.
Digitalis preparations*	Excessive potassium loss that causes dangerous heart rhythms.

*See Glossary

GENERIC NAME OR DRUG CLASS	COMBINED EFFECT	GENERIC NAME OR DRUG CLASS	COMBINED EFFECT

GUANETHIDINE & HYDROCHLOROTHIAZIDE continued

GENERIC NAME OR DRUG CLASS	COMBINED EFFECT
Diuretics, thiazide*	Increased thiazide and guanethidine effects.
Haloperidol	Decreased guanethidine effect.
Indapamide	Possible increased effects of both drugs. When monitored carefully, combination may be beneficial in controlling hypertension.
Insulin	Increased insulin effect.
Lithium	Increased lithium effect.
Minoxidil	Dosage adjustments may be necessary to keep blood pressure at proper level.
Monoamine oxidase (MAO) inhibitors*	Increased hydrochlorothiazide effect.
Nicardipine	Blood pressure drop. Dosages may require adjustment.
Nimodipine	Dangerous blood pressure drop.
Nitrates*	Excessive blood pressure drop.
Oxprenolol	Increased antihypertensive effects. Dosages of both drugs may require adjustments.
Phenothiazines*	Decreased guanethidine effect.
Potassium supplements*	Decreased potassium effect.
Probenecid	Decreased probenecid effect.
Sotalol	Increased antihypertensive effect.
Terazosin	Decreased effectiveness of terazosin.

GUANFACINE

GENERIC NAME OR DRUG CLASS	COMBINED EFFECT
Sympathomimetics*	May decrease antihypertensive effects of guanfacine.
Terazosin	Decreased effectiveness of terazosin.

HALOPERIDOL

GENERIC NAME OR DRUG CLASS	COMBINED EFFECT
Levodopa	Decreased levodopa effect.
Lithium	Increased toxicity.
Loxapine	May increase toxic effects of both drugs.
Methyldopa	Possible psychosis.
Methyprylon	Increased sedative effect, perhaps to dangerous level. Avoid.
Nabilone	Greater depression of central nervous system.
Narcotics*	Excessive sedation.
Pergolide	Decreased pergolide effect.
Phenindione	Decreased anticoagulant effect.
Procarbazine	Increased sedation.
Sedatives*	Excessive sedation.
Sertraline	Increased depressive effects of both drugs.
Tranquilizers*	Excessive sedation.

HISTAMINE H_2 RECEPTOR ANTAGONISTS

GENERIC NAME OR DRUG CLASS	COMBINED EFFECT
Metoclopramide	Decreased absorption of histamine H_2 receptor antagonist.
Methadone	Increased effect and toxicity of methadone.

*See Glossary

GENERIC NAME OR DRUG CLASS	COMBINED EFFECT

HISTAMINE H_2 RECEPTOR ANTAGONISTS continued

GENERIC NAME OR DRUG CLASS	COMBINED EFFECT
Metoclopramide	Decreased absorption of histamine H_2 receptor antagonist.
Methadone	Increased effect and toxicity of methadone.
Metoprolol	Increased effect and toxicity of metoprolol.
Metronidazole	Increased effect and toxicity of metronidazole.
Moricizine	Increased concentration of H_2 receptor antagonist in the blood.
Morphine	Increased effect and toxicity of morphine.
Nicardipine	Possible increased effect and toxicity of nicardipine.
Nimodipine	Possible increased effect and toxicity of nimodipine.
Paroxetine	Increased levels of paroxetine in blood.
Phenytoin	Increased effect and toxicity of phenytoin
Propafenone	Increased effect of both drugs and increased risk of toxicity.
Propranolol	Possible increased propranolol effect.
Quinidine	Increased quinidine effect.
Tacrine	Increased tacrine effect.
Tamoxifen	Decreased tamoxifen effect.
Theophylline	Increases theophylline effect.
Triazolam	Increased effect and toxicity of triazolam.
Venlafaxine	With cimetidine—Increased risk of adverse reactions.
Verapamil	Increased effect and toxicity of verapamil.

HYDRALAZINE

GENERIC NAME OR DRUG CLASS	COMBINED EFFECT
Sotalol	Increased anti-hypertensive effect.
Terazosin	Decreased effectiveness of terazosin.

HYDRALAZINE & HYDROCHLOROTHIAZIDE

GENERIC NAME OR DRUG CLASS	COMBINED EFFECT
Antihypertensives, other*	Increased anti-hypertensive effect.
Barbiturates*	Increased hydrochlorothiazide effect.
Carteolol	Decreased anti-hypertensive effect.
Cholestyramine	Decreased hydrochlorothiazide effect.
Cortisone drugs*	Excessive potassium loss that causes dangerous heart rhythms.
Diazoxide	Increased anti-hypertensive effect.
Didanosine	Increased risk of peripheral neuropathy.
Digitalis preparations*	Excessive potassium loss that causes dangerous heart rhythms.
Diuretics, oral*	Increased effect of both drugs. When monitored carefully, combination may be beneficial in controlling hypertension.
Indapamide	Increased diuretic effect.
Lithium	Increased lithium effect.
Monoamine oxidase (MAO) inhibitors*	Increased effect of drugs.

*See Glossary

GENERIC NAME OR DRUG CLASS	COMBINED EFFECT	GENERIC NAME OR DRUG CLASS	COMBINED EFFECT

HYDRALAZINE & HYDROCHLOROTHIAZIDE continued

GENERIC NAME OR DRUG CLASS	COMBINED EFFECT
Nimodipine	Dangerous blood pressure drop.
Nitrates*	Excessive blood pressure drop.
Potassium supplements*	Decreased potassium effect.
Probenecid	Decreased probenecid effect.

HYDROCORTISONE (Cortisol)

GENERIC NAME OR DRUG CLASS	COMBINED EFFECT
Cyclosporine	Increased risk of infection.
Digitalis preparations*	Dangerous potassium depletion. Possible digitalis toxicity.
Diuretics, thiazide*	Potassium depletion.
Ephedrine	Decreased hydro-cortisone effect.
Estrogens*	Increased hydro-cortisone effect
Ethacrynic acid	Potassium depletion.
Furosemide	Potassium depletion.
Glutethimide	Decreased hydro-cortisone effect
Indapamide	Possible excessive potassium loss, causing dangerous heartbeat irregularity.
Indomethacin	Increased hydro-cortisone effect
Insulin	Decreased insulin effect.
Isoniazid	Decreased isoniazid effect.
Mitotane	Decreased hydro-cortisone effect.
Oxyphenbutazone	Possible ulcers.
Phenobarbital	Decreased hydro-cortisone effect.
Phenylbutazone	Possible ulcers.
Potassium supplements*	Decreased potassium effect.
Rifampin	Decreased hydro-cortisone effect.
Salicylates*	Decreased salicylate effect.
Sympathomimetics*	Possible glaucoma.
Theophylline	Possible increased theophylline effect.

INDAPAMIDE

GENERIC NAME OR DRUG CLASS	COMBINED EFFECT
Opiates*	Weakness and faint-ness when arising from bed or chair.
Probenecid	Decreased probenecid effect.
Sotalol	Increased anti-hypertensive effect.
Terazosin	Decreased effective-ness of terazosin.

KAOLIN, PECTIN, BELLADONNA & OPIUM

GENERIC NAME OR DRUG CLASS	COMBINED EFFECT
Ketoconazole	Decreased ketoconazole effect.
Lincomycins*	Decreased absorp-tion of lincomycin. Separate doses by at least 2 hours.
MAO inhibitors*	Increased belladonna effect.
Meperidine	Increased belladonna effect.
Methylphenidate	Increased belladonna effect.
Mind-altering drugs*	Increased sedative effect.
Narcotics, other*	Increased narcotic effect.
Nitrates*	Increased internal eye pressure.
Orphenadrine	Increased belladonna effect.

*See Glossary

GENERIC NAME OR DRUG CLASS	COMBINED EFFECT	GENERIC NAME OR DRUG CLASS	COMBINED EFFECT

KAOLIN, PECTIN, BELLADONNA & OPIUM continued

GENERIC NAME OR DRUG CLASS	COMBINED EFFECT
Phenothiazines*	Increased sedative effect of paregoric.
Pilocarpine	Loss of pilocarpine effect in glaucoma treatment.
Potassium supplements*	Possible intestinal ulcers with oral potassium tablets.
Sedatives*	Excessive sedation.
Sleep inducers*	Increased effect of sleep inducers.
Sotalol	Increased narcotic effect. Dangerous sedation.
Tranquilizers*	Increased tranquilizer effect.
Vitamin C	Decreased belladon-na effect. Avoid large doses of vitamin C.
All other oral medicines	Decreased absorption of other medicines. Separate doses by at least 2 hours.

LITHIUM

GENERIC NAME OR DRUG CLASS	COMBINED EFFECT
Ketoprofen	May increase lithiumin blood.
Methyldopa	Increased lithium effect.
Molindone	Brain changes.
Muscle relaxants, skeletal*	Increased skeletal muscle relaxation.
Nicardipine	Possible decreased lithium effect.
Nimodipine	Possible decreased lithium effect.
Oxyphenbutazone	Increased lithium effect.
Phenothiazines*	Decreased lithium effect.
Phenylbutazone	Increased lithium effect.
Phenytoin	Increased lithium effect.
Potassium iodide	Increased potassium iodide effect.
Sodium bicarbonate	Decreased lithium effect.
Sumatriptan	Adverse effects unknown. Avoid.
Tetracyclines*	Increased lithium effect.
Theophylline	Decreased lithium effect.
Tiopronin	Increased risk of toxicity to kidneys.
Verapamil	Decreased lithium effect.

LOXAPINE

GENERIC NAME OR DRUG CLASS	COMBINED EFFECT
Pergolide	Decreased pergolide effect.
Phenothiazines*	May increase toxic effects of both drugs.
Pimozide	May increase toxic effects of both drugs.
Rauwolfia	May increase toxic effects of both drugs.
Sertraline	Increased depressive effects of both drugs.
Thioxanthenes*	May increase toxic effects of both drugs

MAPROTILINE

GENERIC NAME OR DRUG CLASS	COMBINED EFFECT
Fluoxetine	Increased depressant effects of both drugs.
Guanabenz	Possible decreased clonidine effect.
Guanethidine	Decreased guanethidine effect.
Guanfacine	May increase depressant effects of either drug.

*See Glossary

GENERIC NAME OR DRUG CLASS	COMBINED EFFECT

MAPROTILINE continued

GENERIC NAME OR DRUG CLASS	COMBINED EFFECT
Leucovorin	High alcohol content of leucovorin may cause adverse effects.
Levodopa	May increase blood pressure.
Lithium	Possible decreased seizure threshold.
Methyldopa	Decreased methyldopa effect.
Methylphenidate	Possible increased antidepressant effect and toxicity.
Methyprylon	Increased sedative effect, perhaps to dangerous level. Avoid.
Molindone	Increased tranquilizer effect.
Monoamine oxidase (MAO) inhibitors*	Fever, delirium, convulsions.
Nabilone	Greater depression of central nervous system.
Narcotics*	Dangerous oversedation.
Phenothiazine	Possible increased antidepressant effect and toxicity.
Phenytoin	Decreased phenytoin effect.
Procainamide	Possible irregular heartbeat.
Quinidine	Irregular heartbeat.
Sedatives*	Dangerous oversedation.
Sertraline	Increased depressive effects of both drugs.
Sympathomimetics*	Increased sympathomimetic effect.
Thyroid hormones*	Irregular heartbeat.

MEPROBAMATE & ASPIRIN

GENERIC NAME OR DRUG CLASS	COMBINED EFFECT
Ethacrynic acid	Possible aspirin toxicity.
Furosemide	Possible aspirin toxicity. May decrease furosemide effect.
Gold compounds*	Increased likelihood of kidney damage.
Indomethacin	Risk of stomach bleeding and ulcers.
Methotrexate	Increased methotrexate effect.
Minoxidil	Decreased minoxidil effect.
Monoamine oxidase (MAO) inhibitors*	Increased meprobamate effect.
Narcotics*	Increased narcotic effect.
Oxprenolol	Decreased antihypertensive effect of oxprenolol.
Para-aminosalicylic acid (PAS)	Possible aspirin toxicity.
Penicillins*	Increased effect of both drugs.
Phenobarbital	Decreased aspirin effect.
Phenytoin	Increased phenytoin effect.
Probenecid	Decreased probenecid effect
Propranolol	Decreased aspirin effect.
Rauwolfia alkaloids*	Decreased aspirin effect.
Salicylates, other*	Likely aspirin toxicity.
Sedatives*	Increased sedative effect.
Sleep inducers*	Increased effect of sleep inducer.
Spironolactone	Decreased spironolactone effect.
Sulfinpyrazone	Decreased sulfinpyrazone effect.
Terfenadine	Possible excessive sedation. May conceal symptoms of aspirin overdose, such as ringing in ears.

*See Glossary

MEPROBAMATE & ASPIRIN continued

GENERIC NAME OR DRUG CLASS	COMBINED EFFECT
Tranquilizers*	Increased tranquilizer effect.
Vancomycin	Increased chance of hearing loss.
Vitamin C (large doses)	Possible aspirin toxicity.

METHOTREXATE

GENERIC NAME OR DRUG CLASS	COMBINED EFFECT
Sulfadoxine and pyrimethamine	Increased risk of toxicity.
Sulfa drugs*	Possible methotrexate toxicity.
Tetracyclines*	Possible methotrexate toxicity.
Tiopronin	Increased risk of toxicity to bone marrow and kidneys.
Vaccines, live or killed	Increased risk of toxicity or reduced effectiveness of vaccine.

METHYLDOPA

GENERIC NAME OR DRUG CLASS	COMBINED EFFECT
Monoamine oxidase (MAO) inhibitors*	Dangerous blood pressure rise.
Nabilone	Greater depression of central nervous system.
Nicardipine	Blood pressure drop. Dosages may require adjustment.
Nimodipine	Dangerous blood pressure drop.
Norepinephrine	Decreased methyldopa effect.
Pergolide	Decreased pergolide effect.
Phenytoin	Possible increased methotrexate toxicity.
Probenecid	Possible methotrexate toxicity.
Pyrimethamine	Increased toxic effect of methotrexate.
Salicylates* (including aspirin)	Possible methotrexate toxicity.
Phenoxybenzamine	Urinary retention.
Phenylephrine	Decreased methyldopa effect.
Phenylpropanolamine	Decreased methyldopa effect.
Propranolol	Increased blood pressure (rarely).
Sertraline	Increased depressive effects of both drugs.
Sotalol	Increased antihypertensive effect.
Sympathomimetic drugs*	Increased risk of heart block and high blood pressure.
Terazosin	Decreased effectiveness of terazosin.
Tolbutamide	Increased tolbutamide effect.

METHYLDOPA & THIAZIDE DIURETICS

GENERIC NAME OR DRUG CLASS	COMBINED EFFECT
Antihypertensives*	Increased antihypertensive effect.
Barbiturates*	Increased hydrochlorothiazide effect.
Carteolol	Increased antihypertensive effect.
Cholestyramine	Decreased hydrochlorothiazide effect
Cortisone drugs*	Excessive potassium loss that causes dangerous heart rhythms.
Dapsone	Increased risk of adverse effect on blood cells.
Didanosine	Increased risk of pancreatitis.

*See Glossary

GENERIC NAME OR DRUG CLASS	COMBINED EFFECT	GENERIC NAME OR DRUG CLASS	COMBINED EFFECT

METHYLDOPA & THIAZIDE DIURETICS continued

GENERIC NAME OR DRUG CLASS	COMBINED EFFECT
Digitalis preparations*	Excessive potassium loss that causes dangerous heart rhythms.
Diuretics, thiazide*	Increased effect of both drugs.
Haloperidol	Increased sedation, possibly dementia.
Indapamide	Increased diuretic effect.
Levodopa	Increased effect of both drugs.
Lithium	Increased lithium effect.
Monoamine oxidase (MAO) inhibitors*	Dangerous blood pressure changes.
Nabilone	Greater depression of central nervous system.
Nicardipine	Blood pressure drop. Dosages may require adjustment.
Nimodipine	Dangerous blood pressure drop.
Nitrates*	Excessive blood pressure drop.
Norepinephrine	Decreased methyldopa effect.
Phenoxybenzanine	Urinary retention.
Phenylephrine	Decreased methyldopa effect.
Phenylpropanolamine	Decreased methyldopa effect.
Potassium supplements*	Decreased potassium effect.
Propranolol	Increased blood pressure (rarely).
Sertraline	Increased depressive effects of both drugs.
Sotalol	Increased antihypertensive effect.
Terazosin	Decreased terazosin effect.
Tolbutamide	Increased tolbutamide effect.
Zinc supplements	Increased need for zinc.

METHYLPREDNISOLONE

GENERIC NAME OR DRUG CLASS	COMBINED EFFECT
Barbiturates*	Decreased methylprednisolone effect. Oversedation.
Chloral hydrate	Decreased methylprednisolone effect.
Chlorthalidone	Potassium depletion.
Cholestyramine	Decreased methylprednisolone absorption.
Cholinergics*	Decreased cholinergic effect.
Colestipol	Decreased methyprednisolone absorption.
Contraceptives, oral*	Increased methylprednisolone effect.
Digitalis preparations*	Dangerous potassium depletion Possible digitalis toxicity.
Diuretics, thiazide*	Potassium depletion.
Ephedrine	Decreased methylprednisolone effect.
Estrogens*	Increased methylprednisolone effect.
Ethacrynic acid	Potassium depletion.
Furosemide	Potassium depletion.
Glutethimide	Decreased methylprednisolone effect.
Indapamide	Possible excessive potassium loss, causing dangerous heartbeat irregularity.
Indomethacin	Increased methylprednisolone effect.
Insulin	Decreased insulin effect.
Isoniazid	Increased isoniazid effect.
Mitotane	Decreased methylprednisolone effect.
Oxyphenbutazone	Possible ulcers.
Phenobarbital	Decreased methylprednisolone effect.

*See Glossary

ADDITIONAL DRUG INTERACTIONS

METHYLPREDNISOLONE continued

GENERIC NAME OR DRUG CLASS	COMBINED EFFECT
Phenylbutazone	Possible ulcers.
Potassium supplements*	Decreased potassium effect.
Rifampin	Decreased methyl-prednisolone effect.
Salicylates*	Decreased salicylates effect.
Sympathomimetics*	Possible glaucoma.
Theophylline	Possible increased theophylline effect.

METOCLOPRAMIDE

GENERIC NAME OR DRUG CLASS	COMBINED EFFECT
Narcotics*	Decreased metoclo-pramide effect.
Nizatidine	Decreased nizatidine absorption.
Pergolide	Decreased pergolide effect.
Phenothiazines*	Increased chance of muscle spasm and trembling.
Sertraline	Increased depressive effects of both drugs.
Tetracyclines*	Slow stomach emptying.
Thiothixines*	Increased chance of muscle spasm and trembling.

MOLINDONE

GENERIC NAME OR DRUG CLASS	COMBINED EFFECT
Nabilone	Greater depression of central nervous system.
Narcotics*	Increased narcotic effect.
Pergolide	Decreased pergolide effect.
Phenytoin	Increased phenytoin effect.
Procarbazine	Increased sedation.
Quinidine	Impaired heart function. Dangerous mixture.
Sedatives*	Increased sedative effect.
Sertraline	Increased depressive effects of both drugs.
Sotalol	Increased tranquilizer effect.
Tetracyclines*	May decrease absorption of both drugs.
Tranquilizers, other*	Increased tranquilizer effect.

MONOAMINE OXIDASE (MAO) INHIBITORS

GENERIC NAME OR DRUG CLASS	COMBINED EFFECT
Clozapine	Toxic effect on the central nervous system.
Cyclobenzaprine	Fever, seizures. Avoid.
Dextromethorphan	Very high blood pressure.
Diuretics*	Excessively low blood pressure.
Ephedrine	Increased blood pressure.
Ethinamate	Dangerous increased effects of ethinamate. Avoid combining.
Fluoxetine	Increased depressant effects of both drugs.
Furazolidine	Sudden, severe increase in blood pressure.
Guanadrel	High blood pressure.
Guanethidine	Blood pressure rise to life-threatening level.
Guanfacine	May increase depressant effects of either drug.
Hypoglycemics, oral*	Increased hypo-glycemic effect.

***See Glossary**

GENERIC NAME OR DRUG CLASS	COMBINED EFFECT	GENERIC NAME OR DRUG CLASS	COMBINED EFFECT

MONOAMINE OXIDASE (MAO) INHIBITORS continued

GENERIC NAME OR DRUG CLASS	COMBINED EFFECT	GENERIC NAME OR DRUG CLASS	COMBINED EFFECT
Indapamide	Increased indapamide effect.	**Narcotic analgesics***	Severe high blood pressure.
Insulin	Increased hypoglycemic effect.	**Paroxetine**	Can cause a life-threatening reaction. Avoid.
Leucovorin	High alcohol content of leucovorin may cause adverse effects.	**Phenothiazines***	Possible increased phenothiazine toxicity.
Levodopa	Sudden, severe blood pressure rise.	**Phenylpropanolamine**	Increased blood pressure.
Maprotiline	Dangerous blood pressure rise.	**Pseudoephedrine**	Increased blood pressure.
Methyldopa	Sudden, severe blood pressure rise.	**Sertraline**	Increased depressive effects of both drugs.
Methylphenidate	Increased blood pressure.	**Sympathomimetics***	Blood pressure rise to life-threatening level.
Methyprylon	Increased sedative effect, perhaps to dangerous level. Avoid.	**Trazodone**	Increased risk of mental status changes.
Monoamine oxidase (MAO) inhibitors* (others, when taken together)	High fever, convulsions, death	**Tryptophan**	Increased blood pressure.
Nabilone	Greater depression of central nervous system.	**Venlafaxine**	Increased risk and severity of side effects. Allow 14 days between use of the 2 drugs.

NARCOTIC & ACETAMINOPHEN

GENERIC NAME OR DRUG CLASS	COMBINED EFFECT	GENERIC NAME OR DRUG CLASS	COMBINED EFFECT
Phenothiazines*	Increased phenothiazine effect.	**Sotalol**	Increased narcotic effect. Dangerous sedation.
Sedatives*	Increased sedative effect.	**Terfenadine**	Possible oversedation.
Selegiline	Severe toxicity characterized by breathing difficulty, seizures, coma.	**Tetracyclines***	May slow tetracycline absorption. Space doses 2 hours apart.
Sertraline	Increased depressive effects of both drugs.	**Tranquilizers***	Increased sedative effect.
Sleep inducers*	Increased sedative effect.	**Zidovudine**	Increased toxicity of zidovudine.

NARCOTIC ANALGESICS

GENERIC NAME OR DRUG CLASS	COMBINED EFFECT	GENERIC NAME OR DRUG CLASS	COMBINED EFFECT
Mind-altering drugs*	Increased sedative effect.	**Molindone**	Increased narcotic effect.

*See Glossary

GENERIC NAME OR DRUG CLASS	COMBINED EFFECT	GENERIC NAME OR DRUG CLASS	COMBINED EFFECT

NARCOTIC ANALGESICS continued

GENERIC NAME OR DRUG CLASS	COMBINED EFFECT
Monoamine oxidase (MAO) inhibitors*	Serious toxicity (including death).
Nabilone	Greater depression of central nervous system.
Nalbuphine	Possibly precipitates withdrawal with chronic narcotic use.
Naltrexone	Precipitates withdrawal symptoms. May lead to respiratory arrest, coma and death.
Narcotics, other*	Increased narcotic effect.
Nicotine	Increased narcotic effect.
Nitrates*	Excessive blood pressure drop.
Pentazocine	Possibly precipitates withdrawal with chronic narcotic use.
Phenothiazines*	Increased sedative effect.
Phenytoin	Possible decreased narcotic effect.
Rifampin	Possible decreased narcotic effect.
Sedatives*	Increased sedative effect.
Selegiline	Severe toxicity characterized by breathing difficulties, seizures, coma.
Sertraline	Increased depressive effects of both drugs.
Sleep inducers*	Increased sedative effect.
Sotalol	Increased narcotic effect. Dangerous sedation.
Tranquilizers*	Increased sedative effect.

NARCOTIC & ASPIRIN

GENERIC NAME OR DRUG CLASS	COMBINED EFFECT
Cortisone drugs*	Increased cortisone effect. Risk of ulcers and stomach bleeding.
Ethacrynic acid	Possible aspirin toxicity.
Furosemide	Possible aspirin toxicity. May decrease furosemide effect.
Gold compounds*	Increased likelihood of kidney damage.
Indomethacin	Risk of stomach bleeding and ulcers.
Methotrexate	Increased methotrexate effect.
Minoxidil	Decreased minoxidil effect.
Narcotics*, other	Increased narcotic effect.
Nitrates*	Excessive blood pressure drop.
Propranolol	Decreased aspirin effect.
Rauwolfia alkaloids*	Decreased aspirin effect.
Salicylates, other*	Likely aspirin toxicity.
Sedatives*	Increased sedative effect.
Selegiline	Severe toxicity characterized by breathing difficulties, seizures, coma.
Sleep inducers*	Increased sedative effect.
Sotalol	Increased narcotic effect. Dangerous sedation.
Spironolactone	Decreased spironolactone effect.
Sulfinpyrazone	Decreased sulfinpyrazone effect.
Terfenadine	Possible excessive sedation. May conceal symptoms of aspirin overdose, such as ringing in ears.
Ticlopidine	Decreased effects of both drugs.

*See Glossary

NARCOTIC & ASPIRIN continued

GENERIC NAME OR DRUG CLASS	COMBINED EFFECT
Tranquilizers*	Increased sedative effect.
Valproic acid	May increase valproic acid effect.
Vitamin C (large doses)	Possible aspirin toxicity.

NIMODIPINE

GENERIC NAME OR DRUG CLASS	COMBINED EFFECT
Theophylline	May increase theophylline effect and toxicity.
Timolol eye drops	May cause increased effect of nimodipine on heart function.
Tocainide	Increased likelihood of adverse reactions from either drug.
Vitamin D (large doses)	Decreased nimodipine effect.

ORPHENADRINE, ASPIRIN & CAFFEINE

GENERIC NAME OR DRUG CLASS	COMBINED EFFECT
Allopurinol	Decreased allopurinol effect.
Antacids*	Decreased aspirin effect.
Anticholinergics*	Increased anticholinergic effect.
Anticoagulants*	Increased anticoagulant effect. Abnormal bleeding.
Antidepressants, tricyclic*	Increased sedation.
Antidiabetics, oral*	Low blood sugar.
Anti-inflammatory drugs, nonsteroidal (NSAIDs)*	Risk of stomach bleeding and ulcers.
Aspirin, other	Likely aspirin toxicity.
Chlorpromazine	Hypoglycemia (low blood sugar).
Contraceptives, oral*	Increased caffeine effect.
Cortisone drugs*	Increased cortisone effect. Risk of ulcers and stomach bleeding.
Furosemide	Possible aspirin toxicity.
Gold compounds*	Increased likelihood of kidney damage.
Griseofulvin	Decreased griseofulvin effect.
Indomethacin	Risk of stomach bleeding and ulcers.
Isoniazid	Increased caffeine effect.
Levodopa	Increased levodopa effect. (Improves effectiveness in treating Parkinson's disease.)
Methotrexate	Increased methotrexate effect.
Minoxidil	Decreased minoxidil effect.
Monoamine oxidase (MAO) inhibitors*	Dangerous blood pressure rise.
Nitrates*	Increased internal eye pressure.
Para-aminosalicylic acid (PAS)	Possible aspirin toxicity.
Penicillins*	Increased effect of drugs.
Phenobarbital	Decreased aspirin effect.
Potassium supplements*	Increased possibility of intestinal ulcers with oral potassium tablets.
Probenecid	Decreased probenecid effect.
Propoxyphene	Possible confusion, nervousness, tremors.
Propranolol	Decreased aspirin effect.
Rauwolfia alkaloids*	Decreased aspirin effect.

*See Glossary

GENERIC NAME OR DRUG CLASS	COMBINED EFFECT

ORPHENADRINE, ASPIRIN & CAFFEINE continued

GENERIC NAME OR DRUG CLASS	COMBINED EFFECT
Salicylates, other*	Likely aspirin toxicity.
Sedatives*	Decreased sedative effect.
Sleep inducers*	Decreased sedative effect.
Spironolactone	Decreased spironolactone effect.
Sulfinpyrazone	Decreased sulfinpyrazone effect.
Sympathomimetics*	Overstimulation.
Terfenadine	May conceal symptoms of aspirin overdose, such as ringing in ears.
Thyroid hormones*	Increased thyroid effect.
Tranquilizers*	Decreased tranquilizer effect.
Valproic acid	May increase valproic acid effect.
Vitamin C (large doses)	Possible aspirin toxicity.

PANCREATIN, PEPSIN, BILE SALTS, HYOSCYAMINE, ATROPINE, SCOPOLAMINE & PHENOBARBITAL

GENERIC NAME OR DRUG CLASS	COMBINED EFFECT
Attapulgite	Decreased anticholinergic effect.
Beta-adrenergic blocking agents*	Decreased effect of beta-adrenergic blocker.
Buclizine	Increased scopolamine effect.
Central nervous system (CNS) depressants*	Increased CNS depression.
Contraceptives, oral*	Decreased contraceptive effect.
Cortisone drugs*	Decreased cortisone effect.
Digitalis	Possible decreased absorption of digitalis.
Disopyramide	Increased atropine effect.
Dronabinol	Increased phenobarbital effect.
Griseofulvin	Decreased griseofulvin effect.
Haloperidol	Increased internal eye pressure.
Indapamide	Increased indapamide effect.
Ketoconazole	Decreased ketoconazole effect.
Meperidine	Increased atropine effect.
Methylphenidate	Increased atropine effect.
Mind-altering drugs*	Dangerous sedation. Avoid.
Monoamine oxidase (MAO) inhibitors*	Increased atropine effect.
Narcotics*	Dangerous sedation. Avoid.
Nitrates*	Increased internal eye pressure.
Nizatidine	Increased nizatidine effect.
Orphenadrine	Increased atropine effect.
Phenothiazines*	Increased atropine effect.
Pilocarpine	Loss of pilocarpine effect in glaucoma treatment.
Potassium supplements*	Possible intestinal ulcers with oral potassium tablets.
Quinidine	Increased quinidine and scopolamine effect.
Sedatives*	Dangerous sedation. Avoid.
Sleep inducers*	Dangerous sedation. Avoid.
Tranquilizers*	Dangerous sedation. Avoid.
Valproic acid	Increased phenobarbital effect.
Vitamin C	Decreased atropine effect. Avoid large doses of vitamin C.

***See Glossary**

GENERIC NAME OR DRUG CLASS	COMBINED EFFECT	GENERIC NAME OR DRUG CLASS	COMBINED EFFECT

PARAMETHASONE

GENERIC NAME OR DRUG CLASS	COMBINED EFFECT
Colestipol	Decreased paramethasone absorption.
Contraceptives, oral*	Increased paramethasone effect.
Digitalis preparations*	Dangerous potassium depletion Possible digitalis toxicity.
Diuretics, thiazide*	Potassium depletion.
Ephedrine	Decreased paramethasone effect.
Estrogens*	Increased paramethasone effect.
Ethacrynic acid	Potassium depletion.
Furosemide	Potassium depletion.
Glutethimide	Decreased paramethasone effect.
Indapamide	Possible excessive potassium loss, causing dangerous heartbeat irregularity.
Indomethacin	Increased paramethasone effect.
Insulin	Decreased insulin effect.
Isoniazid	Increased isoniazid effect.
Mitotane	Decreased paramethasone effect.
Oxyphenbutazone	Possible ulcers.
Phenobarbital	Decreased paramethasone effect.
Phenylbutazone	Possible ulcers.
Potassium supplements*	Decreased potassium effect.
Rifampin	Decreased paramethasone effect.
Salicylates*	Decreased salicylate effect.
Sympathomimetics*	Possible glaucoma.
Theophylline	Possible increased theophylline effect.

PERPHENAZINE & AMITRIPTYLINE

GENERIC NAME OR DRUG CLASS	COMBINED EFFECT
Dronabinol	Increased effect of both drugs.
Ethchlorvynol	Delirium.
Guanabenz	Possible decreased guanabenz effect.
Guanethidine	Decreased guanethidine effect.
Guanfacine	Possible decreased guanfacine effect.
Levodopa	Decreased levodopa effect.
Lithium	Possible decreased seizure threshold.
Methyldopa	Possible decreased methyldopa effect.
Methylphenidate	Possible increased antidepressant effect.
Mind-altering drugs*	Increased effect of mind-altering drugs.
Monoamine oxidase (MAO) inhibitors*	Fever, delirium, convulsions.
Nabilone	Greater depression of central nervous system.
Narcotics*	Increased narcotic effect and dangerous sedation.
Phenothiazines*	Possible increased antidepressant effect.
Procainamide	Possible irregular heartbeat.
Procarbazine	Increased sedation.
Quinidine	Impaired heart function. Dangerous mixture.
Sedatives*	Dangerous oversedation.
Sympathomimetics*	Increased sympathomimetics effect.
Thyroid hormones*	Irregular heartbeat.
Tranquilizers*, other	Increased tranquilizer effect.

*See Glossary

PHENOTHIAZINES

GENERIC NAME OR DRUG CLASS	COMBINED EFFECT
Molindone	Increased tranquilizer effect.
Nabilone	Greater depression of central nervous system.
Narcotics*	Increased narcotic effect.
Procarbazine	Increased sedation.
Quinidine	Impaired heart function. Dangerous mixture.
Sedatives*	Increased sedation.
Tranquilizers*, other	Increased tranquilizer effect.
Zolpidem	Increased sedation effect. Avoid.

PRAZOSIN & POLYTHIAZIDE

GENERIC NAME OR DRUG CLASS	COMBINED EFFECT
Antidepressants, tricyclic*	Dangerous drop in blood pressure. Avoid combination unless under medical supervision.
Antidiabetics, other*	Increased blood sugar.
Antihypertensives*	Increased anti-hypertensive effect. dosages may require adjustments.
Anti-inflammatory drugs, nonsteroidal (NSAIDs)*	Decreased prazosin effect.
Barbiturates*	Increased polythiazide effect.
Carteolol	Increased anti-hypertensive effect.
Cholestyramine	Decreased polythiazide effect.
Chlorpromazine	Acute agitation.
Cortisone drugs*	Excessive potassium loss that causes dangerous heart rhythms.
Digitalis preparations*	Excessive potassium loss that causes dangerous heart rhythms.
Diuretics, other*	Increased effect of other thiazide diuretics.
Estrogens*	Decreased prazosin effect.
Indapamide	Increased diuretic effect.
Indomethacin	Decreased polythiazide effect.
Lithium	Increased lithium effect.
Monoamine oxidase (MAO) inhibitors*	Blood pressure drop. Increased polythiazide effect.
Nicardipine	Blood pressure drop. Dosages may require adjustment.
Nifedipine	Weakness and faintness when arising from bed or chair.
Nimodipine	Dangerous blood pressure drop.
Nitrates*	Possible excessive blood pressure drop.
Opiates*	Weakness and faintness when arising from bed or chair.
Potassium	Decreased potassium effect.
Probenecid	Decreased probenecid effect.
Sotalol	Decreased anti-hypertensive effect.
Sympathomimetics*	Decreased prazosin effect.
Terazosin	Decreased terazosin effect.
Verapamil	Weakness and faintness when arising from bed or chair.

*See Glossary

PREDNISOLONE

GENERIC NAME OR DRUG CLASS	COMBINED EFFECT
Chlorthalidone	Potassium depletion.
Cholestyramine	Decreased prednisolone absorption effect.
Cholinergics*	Decreased cholinergic effect.
Colestipol	Decreased prednisolone absorption effect.
Contraceptives, oral*	Increased prednisolone effect.
Digitalis preparations*	Dangerous potassium depletion. Possible digitalis toxicity.
Diuretics, thiazide*	Potassium depletion.
Ephedrine	Decreased prednisolone effect.
Estrogens*	Increased prednisolone effect.
Ethacrynic acid	Potassium depletion.
Furosemide	Potassium depletion.
Glutethimide	Decreased prednisolone effect.
Indapamide	Possible excessive potassium loss, causing dangerous heartbeat irregularity.
Beta-adrenergic blocking agents*	Decreased prednisolone effect.
Chloral hydrate	Decreased prednisolone effect.
Indomethacin	Increased prednisolone effect.
Insulin	Decreased insulin effect.
Isoniazid	Decreased isoniazid effect.
Mitotane	Decreased prednisolone effect.
Oxyphenbutazone	Possible ulcers.
Phenobarbital	Decreased prednisolone effect.
Phenylbutazone	Possible ulcers.
Potassium supplements*	Decreased potassium effect.
Rifampin	Decreased prednisolone effect.
Salicylates*	Decreased salicylate effect.
Sympathomimetics*	Possible glaucoma.
Theophylline	Possible increased theophylline effect.

PREDNISONE

GENERIC NAME OR DRUG CLASS	COMBINED EFFECT
Barbiturates*	Decreased prednisone effect. Oversedation.
Chloral hydrate	Decreased prednisone effect.
Chlorthalidone	Potassium depletion.
Cholestyramine	Decreased prednisone absorption.
Cholinergics*	Decreased cholinergic effect.
Colestipol	Decreased prednisone absorption.
Contraceptives, oral*	Increased prednisone effect.
Digitalis preparations*	Dangerous potassium depletion. Possible digitalis toxicity.
Diuretics, thiazide*	Potassium depletion.
Ephedrine	Decreased prednisone effect.
Estrogens*	Increased prednisone effect.
Ethacrynic acid	Potassium depletion.
Furosemide	Potassium depletion.
Glutethimide	Decreased prednisone effect.
Indapamide	Possible excessive potassium loss, causing dangerous heartbeat irregularity
Indomethacin	Increased prednisone effect.
Insulin	Increased insulin effect.
Isoniazid	Decreased isoniazid effect.

*See Glossary

GENERIC NAME OR DRUG CLASS	COMBINED EFFECT	GENERIC NAME OR DRUG CLASS	COMBINED EFFECT

PREDNISONE continued

GENERIC NAME OR DRUG CLASS	COMBINED EFFECT
Mitotane	Decreased prednisone effect.
Oxyphenbutazone	Possible ulcers.
Phenobarbital	Decreased prednisone effect.
Phenylbutazone	Possible ulcers.
Potassium supplements*	Decreased potassium effect.
Rifampin	Decreased prednisone effect.
Salicylates*	Decreased salicylate effect.
Sympathomimetics*	Possible glaucoma.
Theophylline	Possible increased theophylline effect.

PRIMIDONE

GENERIC NAME OR DRUG CLASS	COMBINED EFFECT
Narcotics*	Increased narcotic effect.
Oxyphenbutazone	Decreased oxyphenbutazone effect.
Phenylbutazone	Decreased phenylbutazone effect.
Phenytoin	Possible increased primidone toxicity.
Rifampin	Possible decreased primidone effect.
Sedatives*	Increased sedative effect.
Sertraline	Increased depressive effects of both drugs.
Sleep inducers*	Increased effect of sleep inducer.
Tranquilizers*	Increased tranquilizer effect.

PROBENECID & COLCHICINE

GENERIC NAME OR DRUG CLASS	COMBINED EFFECT
Ketoprofen	Increased effect of ketoprofen toxicity.
Methotrexate	Increased methotrexate effect.
Mind-altering drugs*	Oversedation.
Narcotics*	Oversedation.
Nitrofurantoin	Increased nitrofurantoin effect.
Para-aminosalicylic acid (PAS)	Increased effect of para-aminosalicylic acid.
Penicillins*	Enhanced penicillin effect.
Phenylbutazone	Decreased antigout effect of colchicine.
Pyrazinamide	Decreased probenecid effect.
Salicylates*	Decreased probenecid effect.
Sedatives*	Oversedation.
Sleep inducers*	Oversedation.
Sulfa drugs*	Slows elimination. May cause harmful accumulation of sulfa.
Thioguanine	More likelihood of toxicity of both drugs.
Tranquilizers*	Oversedation.
Vitamin B-12	Decreased absorption of vitamin B-12.
Zidovudine	Increased risk of zidovudine toxicity.

PROCARBAZINE

GENERIC NAME OR DRUG CLASS	COMBINED EFFECT
Diuretics*	Excessively low blood pressure.
Doxapam	Increased blood pressure.
Ethinamate	Dangerous increased effects of ethinamate. Avoid combining.

*See Glossary

PROCARBAZINE continued

GENERIC NAME OR DRUG CLASS	COMBINED EFFECT
Fluoxetine	Increased depressant effects of both drugs.
Guanethidine	Blood pressure rise to life-threatening level.
Guanfacine	May increase depressant effects of either medicine.
Leucovorin	High alcohol content of leucovorin may cause adverse effects.
Levamisole	Increased risk of bone marrow depression.
Levodopa	Sudden, severe blood pressure rise.
Methyldopa	Severe high blood pressure.
Methylphenidate	Excessive high blood pressure.
Methyprylon	May increase sedative effect to dangerous level. Avoid.
Monoamine oxidase (MAO) inhibitors, other*	High fever, convulsions, death.
Nabilone	Greater depression of central nervous system.
Narcotics*	Increased sedation.
Phenothiazines*	Increased sedation.
Rauwolfia alkaloids*	Very high blood pressure.
Reserpine	Increased blood pressure, excitation.
Sertraline	Increased depressive effects of both drugs.
Sumatriptan	Adverse effects unknown. Avoid.
Sympathomimetics*	Heartbeat abnormalities, severe high blood pressure.
Tiopronin	Increased risk of toxicity to bone marrow.

QUINIDINE

GENERIC NAME OR DRUG CLASS	COMBINED EFFECT
Rauwolfia alkaloids*	Possibly disturbs heart rhythms.
Rifampin	Decreased quinidine effect.
Tocainide	Increased possibility of adverse reactions from either drug.
Venlafaxine	Increased risk of venlafaxine toxicity.
Verapamil	Hypotension.

RAUWOLFIA ALKALOIDS

GENERIC NAME OR DRUG CLASS	COMBINED EFFECT
Lisinopril	Increased antihypertensive effect. Dosage of each may require adjustment.
Loxapine	May increase toxic effects of both drugs.
Methyprylon	May increase sedative effect to dangerous level. Avoid.
Mind-altering drugs*	Excessive sedation.
Monoamine oxidase (MAO) inhibitors*	Severe depression.
Nabilone	Greater depression of central nervous system.
Nicardipine	Blood pressure drop. Dosages may require adjustment.
Nimodipine	Dangerous blood pressure drop.
Pergolide	Decreased pergolide effect.
Sertraline	Increased depressive effects of both drugs.
Sotalol	Decreased antihypertensive effect.
Terazosin	Decreased effectiveness of terazosin.

*See Glossary

GENERIC NAME OR DRUG CLASS	COMBINED EFFECT	GENERIC NAME OR DRUG CLASS	COMBINED EFFECT

RAUWOLFIA & THIAZIDE DIURETICS

GENERIC NAME OR DRUG CLASS	COMBINED EFFECT
Barbiturates*	Increased hydrochlorothiazide effect.
Beta-adrenergic blocking agents*	Increased effect of rauwolfia alkaloids. Excessive sedation.
Carteolol	Increased anti-hypertensive effect.
Cholestyramine	Decreased hydro-cholorothiazide effect.
Cortisone drugs*	Excessive potassium loss that causes dangerous heart rhythms.
Digitalis preparations*	Excessive potassium loss that causes dangerous heart rhythms.
Diuretics, thiazide*	Increased effect of other thiazide diuretics.
Dronabinol	Increased effect of both drugs. Avoid.
Indapamide	Increased diuretic effect.
Levodopa	Decreased levodopa effect.
Lisinopril	Increased anti-hypertensive effect. Dosage of each may require adjustment.
Lithium	Increased effect of lithium.
Mind-altering drugs*	Excessive sedation.
Monoamine oxidase (MAO) inhibitors*	Increased hydrochlorothiazide effect. Severe depression.
Nicardipine	Blood pressure drop. Dosages may require adjustment.
Nitrates*	Excessive blood pressure drop.
Oxprenolol	Increased anti-hypertensive effect. Dosages of both drugs may require adjustments.
Pergolide	Decreased pergolide effect.
Potassium supplements*	Decreased potassium effect.
Probenecid	Decreased probenecid effect.
Sotalol	Decreased anti-hypertensive effect.
Terazosin	Decreased effectiveness of terazosin.

RESERPINE, HYDRALAZINE & HYDROCHLOROTHIAZIDE

GENERIC NAME OR DRUG CLASS	COMBINED EFFECT
Allopurinol	Decreased allopurinol effect.
Amphetamines*	Decreased hydralazine effect.
Anticoagulants*, oral	Unpredictable increased or decreased effect of anticoagulant.
Anticonvulsants*	Serious change in seizure pattern.
Antidepressants, tricyclic*	Dangerous drop in blood pressure. Avoid combination unless under medical supervision.
Antihistamines*	Increased antihistamine effect.
Antihypertensives, other*	Increased anti-hypertensive effect.
Anti-inflammatory drugs, nonsteroidal (NSAIDs)*	Decreased hydralazine effect.
Aspirin	Decreased aspirin effect.
Barbiturates*	Increased hydrochlorothiazide effect.
Beta-adrenergic blocking agents*	Increased effect of rauwolfia alkaloids. Excessive sedation.
Carteolol	Increased anti-hypertensive effect.
Cholestyramine	Decreased hydrochlorothiazide effect.

*See Glossary

GENERIC NAME OR DRUG CLASS	COMBINED EFFECT	GENERIC NAME OR DRUG CLASS	COMBINED EFFECT

RESERPINE, HYDRALAZINE & HYDROCHLOROTHIAZIDE continued

GENERIC NAME OR DRUG CLASS	COMBINED EFFECT
Cortisone drugs*	Excessive potassium loss that causes dangerous heart rhythms.
Diazoxide	Increased anti-hypertensive effect.
Digitalis preparations*	Excessive potassium loss that causes dangerous heart rhythms.
Diuretics, oral*	Increased effects of drugs. When monitored carefully, combination may be beneficial in controlling hypertension.
Dronabinol	Increased effects of drugs.
Indapamide	Increased diuretic effect.
Levodopa	Decreased levodopa effect.
Lisinopril	Increased anti-hypertensive effect. Dosage of each may require adjustment.
Lithium	Increased lithium effect.
Mind-altering drugs*	Excessive sedation.
Monoamine oxidase (MAO) inhibitors*	Increased effects of both drugs. Severe depression.
Nicardipine	Blood pressure drop. Dosages may require adjustment.
Nimodipine	Dangerous blood pressure drop.
Nitrates*	Excessive blood pressure drop.
Oxprenolol	Increased anti-hypertensive effect. Dosages of drugs may require adjustments.
Pergolide	Decreased pergolide effect.
Potassium supplements*	Decreased potassium effect.
Probenecid	Decreased probenecid effect.
Sotalol	Decreased anti-hypertensive effect.
Terazosin	Decreased effectiveness of terazosin.

SALICYLATES

GENERIC NAME OR DRUG CLASS	COMBINED EFFECT
Insulin	Decreased blood sugar.
Ketocanazole	With buffered salicylates—Decreased ketoconazole effect.
Methotrexate	Increased methotrexate effect and toxicity.
Para-aminosalicylic acid	Possible salicylate toxicity.
Penicillins*	Increased effect of both drugs.
Phenobarbital	Decreased salicylate effect.
Phenytoin	Increased phenytoin effect.
Probenecid	Decreased probenecid effect.
Rauwolfia alkaloids*	Decreased salicylate effect.
Salicylates*, other	Likely salicylate toxicity.
Sotalol	Decreased anti-hypertensive effect of sotalol.
Spironolactone	Decreased spironolactone effect.
Sulfinpyrazone	Decreased sulfinpyrazone effect.
Terazosin	Decreased effectiveness of terazosin. Causes sodium and fluid retention.
Urinary acidifiers*	Decreased excretion, increased salicylate effect.
Urinary alkalizers*	Increased excretion, decreased salicylate effect.

*See Glossary

GENERIC NAME OR DRUG CLASS	COMBINED EFFECT	GENERIC NAME OR DRUG CLASS	COMBINED EFFECT

SALICYLATES continued

Valproic acid	Possible increased valproic acid toxicity.	**Zidovudine**	increased zidovudine effect.
Vitamin C (large doses)	Possible salicylate toxicity.		

SCOPOLAMINE (Hyoscine)

Nizatidine	Increased nizatidine effect.	**Quinidine**	Increased scopolamine effect.
Orphenadrine	Increased scopolamine effect.	**Sedatives* or central nervous system (CNS) depressants***	Increased sedative effect of both drugs.
Phenothiazines*	Increased scopolamine effect.	**Sertraline**	Increased depressive effects of both drugs.
Pilocarpine	Loss of pilocarpine effect in glaucoma treatment.	**Vitamin C**	Decreased scopolamine effect. Avoid large doses of vitamin C.
Potassium supplements*	Possible intestinal ulcers with oral potassium tablets.		

SELEGILINE

Sertraline	Increased depressive effects of both drugs.	**Sumatriptan**	Adverse effects unknown. Avoid.

SPIRONOLACTONE & HYDROCHLOROTHIAZIDE

Cholestyramine	Decreased hydro-chlorothiazide effect.	**Nicardipine**	Blood pressure drop. Dosages may require adjustment.
Cortisone drugs*	Excessive potassium loss that causes dangerous heart rhythms.	**Nimodipine**	Dangerous blood pressure drop.
Cyclosporine	Possible excessive potassium in blood.	**Nitrates***	Excessive blood pressure drop.
Diuretics, other*	Increased effect of both drugs. Beneficial if needed and dose is correct.	**Opiates***	Weakness and faintness when arising from bed or chair.
Indapamide	Increased diuretic effect.	**Potassium supplements***	Decreased potassium effect. Dangerous potassium retention, causing possible heartbeat irregularity.
Indomethacin	Decreased hydro-chlorothiazide effect.		
Laxatives*	Reduced potassium levels.	**Potassium iodide**	May raise potassium level in blood to toxic levels.
Lithium	Increased lithium effect. Likely lithium toxicity.	**Probenecid**	Decreased probenecid effect.
Monoamine oxidase (MAO) inhibitors*	Increased hydro-chlorothiazide effect.	**Salicylates***	May decrease spironolactone effect.

*See Glossary

SPIRONOLACTONE & HYDROCHLOROTHIAZIDE continued

GENERIC NAME OR DRUG CLASS	COMBINED EFFECT
Sodium bicarbonate	Reduces high potassium levels.
Sotalol	Decreased anti-hypertensive effect.
Terazosin	Decreased effectiveness of terazosin.
Triamterene	Dangerous potassium retention.
Zinc supplements	Increased need for zinc.

TESTOSTERONE & ESTRADIOL

GENERIC NAME OR DRUG CLASS	COMBINED EFFECT
Insulin	Unpredictable increase or decrease in blood sugar.
Nicotinic acid	Decreased nicotinic acid.
Oxyphenbutazone	Decreased androgen and estrogen effect.
Phenobarbital	Decreased androgen and estrogen effect.
Phenylbutazone	Decreased androgen and testosterone effect.
Primidone	Decreased estrogen and testosterone effect.
Rifampin	Decreased estrogen and testosterone effect.
Terazosin	Decreased effectiveness of terazosin.
Thyroid hormones*	Decreased thyroid effect.
Ursodiol	Decreased ursodiol effect.

THEOPHYLLINE, EPHEDRINE & BARBITURATES

GENERIC NAME OR DRUG CLASS	COMBINED EFFECT
Antidiabetics*, oral	Increased phenobarbital effect.
Antihistamines*	Dangerous sedation. Avoid.
Antihypertensives*	Decreased anti-hypertensive effect.
Anti-inflammatory drugs, nonsteroidal (NSAIDs)*	Decreased anti-inflammatory effect.
Aspirin	Decreased aspirin effect.
Beta-adrenergic blocking agents*	Decreased effect of drugs.
Carteolol	Increased barbiturate effect. Dangerous sedation.
Ciprofloxacin	Increased possibility of central nervous system poisoning, such as nausea, vomiting, restlessness, palpitations.
Clarithromycin	Increased concentration of theophylline.
Contraceptives, oral*	Decreased contraceptive effect.
Cortisone drugs*	Decreased cortisone effect.
Digitalis preparations*	Serious heart rhythm disturbances.
Doxycycline	Decreased doxycycline effect.
Dronabinol	Increased effect of drugs. Avoid.
Ephedrine	Increased effect of drugs.
Epinephrine	Increased effect of drugs.
Ergot preparations*	Serious blood pressure rise.
Erythromycins*	Increased bronchodilator effect.
Finasteride	Decreased theophylline effect.
Furosemide	Increased furosemide effect.
Griseofulvin	Decreased griseofulvin effect.
Guanethidine	Decreased effect of drugs.

*See Glossary

ADDITIONAL DRUG INTERACTIONS

GENERIC NAME OR DRUG CLASS	COMBINED EFFECT	GENERIC NAME OR DRUG CLASS	COMBINED EFFECT

THEOPHYLLINE, EPHEDRINE & BARBITURATES continued

GENERIC NAME OR DRUG CLASS	COMBINED EFFECT
Indapamide	Increased indapamide effect.
Lincomycins*	Increased bronchodilator effect.
Lithium	Decreased lithium effect.
Mind-altering drugs*	Dangerous sedation. Avoid.
Monoamine oxidase (MAO) inhibitors*	Increased ephedrine effect. Dangerous blood pressure rise.
Narcotics*	Dangerous sedation. Avoid.
Nicardipine	May increase theophylline effect and toxicity.
Nicotine	Increased bronchodilator effect.
Nitrates*	Possible decreased effect of drugs.
Probenecid	Decreased effect of drugs.
Propranolol	Decreased bronchodilator effect.
Pseudoephedrine	Increased pseudoephedrine effect.
Rauwolfia alkaloids*	Rapid heartbeat.
Sotalol	Increased barbiturate effect. Dangerous sedation.
Sulfinpyrazone	Decreased sulfinpyrazone effect.
Terazosin	Decreased terazosin effect.
Ticlopidine	Increased theophylline effect.
Troleandomycin	Increased bronchodilator effect.
Valproic acid	Increased barbiturate effect.

THEOPHYLLINE, EPHEDRINE, GUAIFENESIN & BARBITURATES

GENERIC NAME OR DRUG CLASS	COMBINED EFFECT
Antidepressants, tricyclic*	Decreased antidepressant effect.
Antidiabetics, oral*	Increased phenobarbital effect.
Antihistamines*	Dangerous sedation. Avoid.
Anti-inflammatory drugs, nonsteroidal (NSAIDs)*	Decreased anti-inflammatory effect.
Aspirin, other	Decreased aspirin effect.
Beta-adrenergic blocking agents*	Decreased effect of drugs.
Carteolol	Increased barbiturate effect. Dangerous sedation.
Clarithromycin	Increased concentration of theophylline.
Ciprofloxacin	Increased possibility of central nervous system poisoning, such as nausea, vomiting, restlessness, palpitations.
Contraceptives, oral*	Decreased contraceptive effect
Cortisone drugs*	Increased cortisone effect.
Digitalis preparations*	Serious heart rhythm disturbances.
Digitoxin	Decreased digitoxin effect.
Doxycycline	Decreased doxycycline effect.
Dronabinol	Increased effect of drugs.
Ephedrine	Increased effect of drugs.
Ergot preparations*	Serious blood pressure rise.
Erythromycins*	Increased bronchodilator effect.
Finasteride	Decreased theophylline effect.
Furosemide	Increased furosemide effect.

*See Glossary

THEOPHYLLINE, EPHEDRINE, GUAIFENESIN & BARBITURATES continued

GENERIC NAME OR DRUG CLASS	COMBINED EFFECT
Griseofulvin	Decreased griseofulvin effect.
Guanethidine	Decreased effect of drugs.
Indapamide	Increased indapamide effect.
Lincomycins*	Increased bronchodilator effect.
Lithium	Decreased lithium effect.
Mind-altering drugs*	Dangerous sedation. Avoid.
Monoamine oxidase (MAO) inhibitors*	Increased phenobarbital effect.
Narcotics*	Dangerous sedation. Avoid.
Nicardipine	May increase theophylline effect and toxicity.
Nicotine	Increased bronchodilator effect.
Nitrates*	Possible decreased effect of drugs.
Pain relievers*	Dangerous sedation. Avoid.
Probenecid	Decreased effect of drugs.
Propranolol	Decreased bronchodilator effect.
Pseudoephedrine	Increased pseudo-ephedrine effect.
Rauwolfia alkaloids*	Rapid heartbeat.
Sedatives*	Dangerous sedation. Avoid.
Sleep inducers*	Dangerous sedation. Avoid.
Sulfinpyrazone	Decreased sulfin-pyrazone effect.
Terazosin	Decreased terazosin effect.
Ticlopidine	Increased theophylline effect.
Tranquilizers*	Dangerous sedation. Avoid.
Troleandomycin	Increased bronchodilator effect.
Valproic acid	Increased phenobarbital effect.

THEOPHYLLINE, EPHEDRINE & HYDROXYZINE

GENERIC NAME OR DRUG CLASS	COMBINED EFFECT
Carteolol	Decreased anti-histamine effect.
Ciprofloxacin	May cause kidney dysfunction.
Clarithromycin	Increased concentra-tion of theophylline.
Digitalis preparations*	Serious heart rhythm disturbances.
Dronabinol	Increased effect of drugs.
Ephedrine	Increased effect of drugs.
Epinephrine	Increased effect of drugs.
Ergot preparations*	Serious blood pressure rise.
Erythromycins*	Increased bronchodilator effect.
Finasteride	Decreased theophylline effect.
Furosemide	Increased furosemide effect.
Guanethidine	Decreased effect of drugs.
Lincomycins*	Increased bronchodilator effect.
Lithium	Decreased lithium effect.
Monoamine oxidase (MAO) inhibitors*	Increased ephedrine effect. Dangerous blood pressure rise.
Moricizine	Decreased antihistamine effect.
Nabilone	Greater depression of central nervous system.
Nicardipine	May increase theophylline effect and toxicity.
Nicotine	Increased bronchodilator effect.

***See Glossary**

GENERIC NAME OR DRUG CLASS	COMBINED EFFECT	GENERIC NAME OR DRUG CLASS	COMBINED EFFECT

THEOPHYLLINE, EPHEDRINE & HYDROXYZINE continued

GENERIC NAME OR DRUG CLASS	COMBINED EFFECT
Nitrates*	Possible decreased effect of drugs.
Pain relievers*	Increased effect of drugs.
Probenecid	Decreased effect of drugs.
Propranolol	Decreased bronchodilator effect.
Pseudoephedrine	Increased pseudo-ephedrine effect.
Rauwolfia alkaloids*	Rapid heartbeat.
Sotalol	Decreased antihistamine effect.
Sulfinpyrazone	Decreased sulfin-pyrazone effect.
Terazosin	Decreased effect of terazosin.
Ticlopidine	Increased theophylline effect.
Tranquilizers*	Increased effect of drugs.
Troleandomycin	Increased bronchodilator effect.

THIOTHIXENE

GENERIC NAME OR DRUG CLASS	COMBINED EFFECT
Sedatives*	Increased thiothixene effect. Excessive sedation.
Sertraline	Increased depressive effects of both drugs.
Sleep inducers*	Increased thiothixene effect. Excessive sedation.
Tranquilizers*	Increased thiothixene effect. Excessive sedation.

TRIAMCINOLONE

GENERIC NAME OR DRUG CLASS	COMBINED EFFECT
Colestipol	Decreased triamci-nolone absorption.
Contraceptives, oral*	Increased triamcinolone effect.
Digitalis preparations*	Dangerous potassium depletion. Possible digitalis toxicity.
Diuretics, thiazide*	Potassium depletion.
Ephedrine	Decreased triamcinolone effect.
Estrogens*	Increased triamcinolone effect.
Ethacrynic acid	Potassium depletion.
Furosemide	Potassium depletion.
Glutethimide	Decreased triamcin-olone effect.
Indapamide	Possible excessive potassium loss, causing dangerous heartbeat irregularity.
Indomethacin	Increased triamcinolone effect.
Insulin	Decreased insulin effect.
Isoniazid	Decreased isoniazid effect.
Mitotane	Decreased triamcin-olone effect.
Oxyphenbutazone	Possible ulcers.
Phenobarbital	Decreased triamcin-olone effect.
Phenylbutazone	Possible ulcers.
Potassium supplements*	Decreased potassium effect.
Rifampin	Decreased triamcin-olone effect.
Salicylates*	Decreased salicylate effect.
Sympathomimetics*	Possible glaucoma.
Theophylline	Possible increased theophylline effect.

*See Glossary

GENERIC NAME OR DRUG CLASS	COMBINED EFFECT	GENERIC NAME OR DRUG CLASS	COMBINED EFFECT

TRIAMTERENE & HYDROCHLOROTHIAZIDE

GENERIC NAME OR DRUG CLASS	COMBINED EFFECT
Digitalis preparations*	Excessive potassium loss that causes dangerous heart rhythms.
Diuretics, potassium-sparing*, other	Possible excessive potassium levels.
Diuretics, thiazide*	Increased effect of other thiazide diuretics.
Folic acid	Decreased folic acid effect.
Indapamide	Increased diuretic effect.
Lisinopril	Possible severe blood pressure drop with first dose.
Lithium	Increased lithium effect.
Monoamine oxidase (MAO) inhibitors*	Increased hydro-chlorothiazide effect.
Nitrates*	Excessive blood pressure drop.
Opiates*	Weakness and faintness when arising from bed or chair.
Potassium supplements*	Possible excessive potassium retention. Decreased potassium effect.
Probenecid	Decreased probenecid effect.

TRIAZOLAM

GENERIC NAME OR DRUG CLASS	COMBINED EFFECT
Probenecid	Increased triazolam effect.
Sedatives*	Increased sedative effect of both drugs.
Sleep inducers*	Increased sedative effect of both drugs.
Tranquilizers*	Increased sedative effect of both drugs.
Zidovudine	Increased toxicity of zidovudine.

***See Glossary**

Glossary

The following medical terms are found in the drug charts. Where drug names are listed, the generic or drug class is first, with brand names following in parentheses.

A

Angiotensin-Converting Enzyme (ACE) Inhibitors—A family of drugs used to treat hypertension and congestive heart failure. Inhibitors decrease the rate of conversion of angiotensin I into angiotensin II, which is the normal process for the angiotensin-converting enzyme. These drugs include benazepril, captopril, enalapril, fosinopril, lisinopril, ramipril.

Acne Preparations—Creams, lotions and liquids applied to the skin to treat acne. These include alcohol and acetone; alcohol and sulfur; benzoyl peroxide; clindamycin; erythromycin; erythromycin and benzoyl peroxide; isotretinoin; meclocycline; resorcinol; resorcinol and sulfur; salicylic acid gel USP; salicylic acid lotion; salicylic acid ointment; salicylic acid pads; salicylic acid soap; salicylic acid and sulfur bar soap; salicylic acid and sulfur cleansing lotion; salicylic acid and sulfur cleansing suspension; salicylic acid and sulfur lotion; sulfurated lime; sulfur bar soap; sulfur cream; sulfur lotion; tetracycline, oral; tetracycline hydrochloride for topical solution; tretinoin.

Acridine Derivatives—Dyes or stains (usually yellow or orange) used for some medical tests and as antiseptic agents.

Acute—Having a short and relatively severe course.

Addiction—Psychological or physiological dependence upon a drug.

Addictive drugs—Any drug that can lead to physiological dependence on the drug. These include alcohol, cocaine, marijuana, nicotine, opium, morphine, codeine, heroin (and other narcotics) and others.

Addison's Disease—Changes in the body caused by a deficiency of hormones manufactured by the adrenal gland. Usually fatal if untreated.

Adrenal Cortex—Center of the adrenal gland.

Adrenal Gland—Gland next to the kidney that produces cortisone and epinephrine (adrenalin).

Agranulocytosis—A symptom complex characterized by (1) a sharply decreased number of granulocytes (one of the types of white blood cells), (2) lesions of the throat and other mucous membranes, (3) lesions of the gastrointestinal tract and (4) lesions of the skin. Sometimes also called granulocytopenia.

Alkalizers—These drugs neutralize acidic properties of the blood and urine by making them more alkaline (or basic). Systemic alkalizers include potassium citrate and citric acid, sodium bicarbonate, sodium citrate and citric acid, and tricitrates. Urinary alkalizers include potassium citrate, potassium citrate and citric acid, potassium citrate and sodium citrate, sodium citrate and citric acid.

Alkylating Agent—Chemical used to treat malignant diseases.

Allergy—Excessive sensitivity to a substance.

Alpha-Adrenergic Blocking Agents—A group of drugs used to treat hypertension. These drugs include prazosin, terazosin, doxazosin and labetalol (an alpha-adrenergic and beta-adrenergic combination drug). Also included are other drugs that produce an alpha-adrenergic blocking action such as haloperidol, loxapine, phenothiazines, thioxanthenes.

Amebiasis—Infection with amoebas, one-celled organisms. Causes diarrhea, fever and abdominal cramps.

Aminoglycosides—A family of antibiotics used for serious infections. Their usefulness is limited because of relative toxicity compared to some other antibiotics. These drugs include amikacin, gentamicin, kanamycin, neomycin, netilmicin, streptomycin, tobramycin.

Amphetamines—A family of drugs that stimulates the central nervous system, prescribed to treat attention-deficit disorders in children and also for narcolepsy. They are habit-forming, are controlled under U.S. law and are no longer prescribed as appetite suppressants. These drugs include amphetamine, dextroamphetamine, methamphetamine. They may be ingredients of several combination drugs.

ANA Titers—A test to evaluate the immune system and to detect antinuclear antibodies (ANAs), substances which appear in the blood of some patients with autoimmune disease.

Analgesics—Agents that reduce pain without reducing consciousness.

Anaphylaxis—Severe allergic response to a substance. Symptoms are wheezing, itching, hives, nasal congestion, intense burning of hands and feet, collapse, loss of consciousness and cardiac arrest. Symptoms appear within a few seconds or minutes after exposure. Anaphylaxis is a severe medical emergency. Without appropriate treatment, it can cause death.

Instructions for home treatment for anaphylaxis are on the front inside cover.
Androgens—Male hormones, including fluoxymesterone, methyltestosterone, testosterone.
Anemia—Not enough healthy red blood cells in the bloodstream or too little hemoglobin in the red blood cells. Anemia is caused by an imbalance between blood loss and blood production.
Anemia, Aplastic—A form of anemia in which the bone marrow is unable to manufacture adequate numbers of blood cells of all types—red cells, white cells, and platelets.
Anemia, Hemolytic—Anemia caused by a shortened lifespan of red blood cells. The body can't manufacture new cells fast enough to replace old cells.
Anemia, Iron-Deficiency—Anemia caused when iron necessary to manufacture red blood cells is not available.
Anemia, Pernicious—Anemia caused by a vitamin B-12 deficiency. Symptoms include weakness, fatigue, numbness and tingling of the hands or feet and degeneration of the central nervous system.
Anemia, Sickle-Cell—Anemia caused by defective hemoglobin that deprives red blood cells of oxygen, making them sickle-shaped.
Anesthesias, General—Gases that are used in surgery to render patients unconscious and able to withstand the pain of surgical cutting and manipulation. They include enflurane, etomidate, fentanyl, halothane, isoflurane, ketamine, methohexital, methoxyflurane, nitrous oxide, propofol, thiamylal, thiopental, alfentanil, amobarbital, butabarbital, butorphanol, chloral hydrate, etomidate, fentanyl, tentanyl, hydroxyzine, ketamine, levorphanol, meperidine, midazolam, morphine parenteral, nalbuphine, oxymorphone, pentazocine, pentobarbital, phenobarbital, promethazine, propiomazine, scopolamine, secobarbital, sufentanil.
Anesthetics—Drugs that eliminate the sensation of pain.
Angina (Angina Pectoris)—Chest pain with a sensation of suffocation and impending death. Caused by a temporary reduction in the amount of oxygen to the heart muscle through diseased coronary arteries.
Antacids—A large family of drugs prescribed to treat hyperacidity, peptic ulcer, esophageal reflux and other conditions. These drugs include alumina and magnesia; alumina, magnesia and calcium carbonate; alumina, magnesia and simethicone; alumina and magnesium carbonate; alumina and magnesium trisilicate; alumina, magnesium trisilicate and sodium bicarbonate; aluminum carbonate; aluminum hydroxide; bismuth subsalicylate; calcium carbonate; calcium carbonate and magnesia; calcium carbonate, magnesia and simethicone; calcium and magnesium carbonates; calcium and magnesium carbonates and magnesium oxide; calcium carbonate and simethicone; dihydroxyaluminum aminoacetate; dihydroxyaluminum sodium carbonate; magaldrate; magaldrate and simethicone; magnesium carbonate and sodium bicarbonate; magnesium hydroxide; magnesium oxide; magnesium trisilicate, alumina and magnesia; simethicone, alumina, calcium carbonate and magnesia; simethicone, alumina, magnesium carbonate and magnesia; sodium bicarbonate.
Antacids, Calcium Carbonate—These antacids include calcium carbonate and magnesium, calcium carbonate and simethicone, calcium carbonate and magnesium carbonates.
Antacids, Magnesium-Containing—These antacids include magnesium carbonate, magnesium hydroxide, magnesium oxide and magnesium trisilicate. All these medicines are designed to treat excess stomach acidity. In addition to being an effective antacid, magnesium can sometimes cause unpleasant side effects and drug interactions. Look for the presence of magnesium in nonprescription drugs.
Anthelmintics—A family of drugs used to treat intestinal parasites. Names of these drugs include niclosamide, piperazine, pyrantel, pyrvinium, quinacrine, mebendazole, metronidazole, oxamniquine, praziquantel, thiabendazole.
Antiacne Topical Preparations—See Acne Preparations.
Antiadrenals—Medicines or drugs that prevent the effects of the hormones liberated by the adrenal glands.
Antianginals—A group of drugs used to treat angina pectoris (chest pain that comes and goes, caused by coronary artery disease). These drugs include acebutolol, amlodipine, amyl nitrite, atenolol, bepridril, carteolol, diltiazem, erythrityl, felodipine, isosorbide dinitrate, labetalol, metoprolol, nadolol, nicardipine, nifedipine, nitroglycerin, oxprenolol, penbutolol, pentaerythritol, pindolol, propranolol, sotalol, tetranitrate, timolol, verapamil.
Antianxiety Drugs—A group of drugs prescribed to treat anxiety. These drugs include alprazolam, bromazepam, buspirone, chlordiazepoxide, chlorpromazine, clomipramine, clorazepate, diazepam, halazepam, hydroxyzine, imipramine, ketazolam, lorazepam, meprobamate, oxazepam, prazepam, prochlorperazine, thioridazine, trifluoperazine.

Antiarrhythmics—A group of drugs used to treat heartbeat irregularities (arrhythmias). These drugs include acebutolol, amiodarone, atenolol, atropine, bretylium, deslanoside, digitalis, digitoxin, diltiazem, disopyramide, edrophonium, encainide, esmolol, flecainide, glycopyrrolate, hyoscyamine, lidocaine, methoxamine, metoprolol, mexiletine, moricizine, nadolol, oxprenolol, phenytoin, procainamide, propafenone, propranolol, quinidine, scopolamine, sotalol, timolol, tocainide, verapamil.

Antiasthmatics—Medicines used to treat asthma, which may be tablets, liquids or aerosols (to be inhaled to get directly to the bronchial tubes rather than through the bloodstream). These medicines include adrenocorticoids, glucocorticoid; albuterol; aminophylline; beclomethasone; bitolterol; corticotropin; cromolyn; dexamethasone; dyphylline; ephedrine; epinephrine; ethylnorepinephrine; fenoterol; flunisolide; ipratropium, isoetharine; isoproterenol; isoproterenol and phenylephrine; metaproterenol; oxtriphylline; oxtriphylline and guaifenesin; pirbuterol; racepinephrine; terbutaline; theophylline; theophylline and guaifenesin; triamcinolone.

Antibacterials (Antibiotics)—A group of drugs prescribed to treat infections. These drugs include aminocillin, amikacin, amoxicillin, amoxicillin and clavulanate, ampicillin, azlocillin, aztreonam, bacampicillin, carbenicillin, cefaclor, cefadroxil, cefamandole, cefazolin, cefonicid, cefoperazone, ceforanide, cefotaxime, cefotetan, cefoxitin, ceftazidime, ceftizoxime, ceftriaxone, cefuroxime, cephalexin, cephalothin, cephapirin, cephradine, chloramphenicol, cinoxacine, clindamycin, cloxacillin, cyclacillin, cycloserine, demeclocycline, dicloxacillin, doxycycline, erythromycin, erythromycin and sulfisoxazole, flucloxacillin, fusidic acid, gentamicin, imipenem and cilastatin, kanamycin, lincomycin, methacycline, methenamine, methicillin, metronidazole, mezlocillin, minocycline, moxalactam, nafcillin, nalidixic acid, netilmicin, nitrofurantoin, norfloxacin, oxacillin, oxytetracycline, penicillin G, penicillin V, piperacillin, pivampicillin, rifampin, spectinomycin, streptomycin, sulfacytine, sulfadiazine and trimethoprim, sulfamethoxazole, sulfamethoxazole and trimethoprim, sulfisoxazole, tetracycline, ticarcillin, ticarcillin and clavulanate, tobramycin, trimethoprim, vancomycin.

Antibiotics—Chemicals that inhibit the growth of or kill germs. See Antibacterials.

Anticholinergics—Drugs that work against acetylcholine, a chemical found in many locations in the body, including connections between nerve cells and connections between muscle and nerve cells. Anticholinergic drugs include anisotropine, atropine, belladonna, clidinium, dicyclomine, glycopyrrolate, hyoscyamine, ipratropium, isopropamide, mepenzolate, methantheline, methscopolamine, oxyphencyclimine, pirenzepine, propantheline, scopolamine, tridihexethyl.

Anticoagulants—A family of drugs prescribed to slow the rate of blood clotting. These drugs include acenocoumarol, anisindione, dicumarol, dihydroergotamine and heparin, heparin, warfarin.

Anticonvulsants—A group of drugs prescribed to treat or prevent seizures (convulsions). These drugs include these families: barbiturates, carbonic anhydrase ingibitors, diones, hydantoins and succinamides. These are the names of the generic drugs in these families: acetazolamide, amobarbital, carbamazepine, carbonic anhydrase inhibitors, clonazepam, clorazepate, diazepam, dichlorphenamide, divalproex, ethosuximide, ethotoin, lorazepam, magnesium sulfate, mephenytoin, mephobarbital, metharbital, methazolamide, methsuximide, metocurine, nitrazepam, paraldehyde, paramethadione, pentobarbital, phenobarbital, phensuximide, phenytoin, primidone, secobarbital, trimethadione, tubocurarine, valproic acid.

Antidepressants—A group of medicines prescribed to treat mental depression. These drugs include amitriptyline, amoxapine, clomipramine, desipramine, doxepin, fluoxetine, imipramine, isocarboxazid, maprotiline, nortriptyline, paroxetine, phenelzine, protriptyline, tranylcypromine, trazodone, trimipramine.

Antidepressants, MAO (Monamine Oxidase Inhibitors)—A special group of drugs prescribed for mental depression. These are not as popular as in years past because of a relatively high incidence of adverse effects. These drugs include isocarboxazid (Marplan), phenelzine (Nardil), tranylcypromine (Parnate).

Antidepressants, Tricyclic —A group of medicines with similar chemical structure and pharmacologic activity used to treat mental depression. These drugs include amitriptyline (Amitril, Apo-Amitriptyline, Elavil, Emitrip, Endep, Levate, Meravil, Novotriptyn); amoxapine (Asendin); clomipramine (Anafranil); desipramine (Pertofrane, Norpramin); doxepin (Adapin, Sinequan, Triadapin); imipramine (Apo-Imipramine, Impril, Janimine, Novopramine, Tipramine, Tofranil, Tofranil-PM); nortriptyline (Aventyl, Pamelor); protriptyline (Triptil, Vivactil); trimipramine (Surmontil).

Antidiabetic Agents—A group of drugs used in the treatment of diabetes mellitus. These medicines all reduce blood sugar. These drugs include acetohexamide, chlorpropamide, glipizide, glyburide, insulin, metformin, tolazamide, tolbutamide.

Antidiarrheal Preparations—Medicines that treat diarrhea symptoms. Most do not cure the cause. Oral medicines include aluminum hydroxide; charcoal, activated; kaolin and pectin; loperamide; polycarbophil; psyllium hydrophilic mucilloid. Systemic medicines include carbohydrates, codeine; difenoxin and atropine; diphenoxylate and atropine; and electrolytes; glycopyrrolate; kaolin, pectin, belladonna alkaloids and opium; kaolin, pectin and paregoric; opium tincture; paregoric.

Antidyskinetics—A group of drugs used for treatment of Parkinsonism (paralysis agitans) and drug-induced extrapyramidal reactions (see elsewhere in Glossary). These drugs include amantadine, benztropine, biperiden, bromocriptine, carbidopa and levodopa, diphenhydramine, ethopropazine, levodopa, levodopa and benserazide, procyclidine, trihexyphenidyl.

Antiemetics—A group of drugs used to treat nausea and vomiting. These drugs include buclizine, cyclizine, chlorpromazine, dimenhydrinate, diphenhydramine, diphenidol, domperidone, dronabinol, haloperidol, hydroxyzine, meclizine, metoclopramide, nabilone, perphenazine, prochlorperazine, promethazine, scopolamine, thiethylperazine, triflupromazine, trimethobenzamide.

Antifibronyltic Drugs—Drugs that are used to treat serious bleeding. These drugs include aminocaproic acid and tranexamic acid.

Antifungals—A group of drugs used to treat fungus infections. Those listed as systemic are taken orally or given by injection. Those listed as topical are applied directly to the skin and include liquids, powders, creams, ointments and liniments. Those listed as vaginal are used topically inside the vagina and sometimes on the vaginal lips. These drugs include: Systemic—amphotericin B, miconazole, fluconazole, flucytosine, griseofulvin, itraconazole, ketoconazole, potassium iodide. Topical—carbol-fuchsin; ciclopirox; clioquinol; clotrimazole; econazole; haloprogin; ketoconzaole; miconazole; nystatin; salicylic acid, sulfur and coal; tolnaftate. Vaginal—butoconazole, clotrimazole, gentian violet, miconazole, nystatin.

Antiglaucoma Drugs—Medicines used to treat glaucoma. Those listed as systemic are taken orally or given by injection. Those listed as ophthalmic are used as eye drops. These drugs include: Systemic—acetazolamide, dichlorphenamide, glycerin, mannitol, methazolamide, timolol, urea. Ophthalmic—betaxolol, carbachol ophthalmic solution, demecarium, dipivefrin, echothiophate, epinephrine, epinephrine bitartrate, epinephryl borate, isoflurophate, levobunolol, physostigmine, pilocarpine, timolol.

Antigout Drugs—Drugs to treat the metabolic disease called gout. Gout causes recurrent attacks of joint pain caused by deposits of uric acid in the joints. Antigout drugs include allopurinol, carprofen, colchicine, fenoprofen, ibuprofen, indomethacin, ketoprofen, naproxen, phenylbutazone, piroxicam, probenecid, probenecid and colchicine, sulfinpyrazone, sulindac.

Antihistamines—A family of drugs used to treat allergic conditions, such as hay fever, allergic conjunctivitis, itching, sneezing, runny nose, motion sickness, dizziness, sedation, insomnia and others. These drugs include astemizole (Hismanal), azatadine (Optimine); brompheniramine (Bromphen, Chlorphed, Dehist, Dimetane, Dimetane Extentabs, Dimetane-Ten, Histaject Modified, Nasahist B, ND-Stat Revised, Oraminic II, Veltane); carbinoxamine (Clistin); chlorpheniramine (Aller-Chlor, Allerid-O.D., Chlo-Amine, Chlor-100, Chlor-Mal, Chlor-Niramine, Chlorphen, Chlor-Pro, Chlorspan, Chlortab, Chlor-Trimeton, Chlor-Trimeton Repetabs, Chlor-Tripolon, Hal-Chlor, Histrey, Novopheniram, Phenetron, Phenetron Lanacaps, T.D. Alermine, Teldrin, Trymegen); clemastine (Tavist); cyproheptadine (Periactin); dexchlorpheniramine (Polaramine, Polaramine Repetabs); dimenhydrinate (Apo-Dimenhydrinate, Calm X, Dimentabs, Dinate, Dommanate, Dramamine, Dramilin, Dramocen, Dramoject, Dymenate, Gravol, Hydrate, Marmine, Motion-Aid, Nauseatol, Novodimenate, PMS-Dimenhydrinate, Reidamine, Travamine, Wehamine); diphenhydramine (Beldin, Benadryl, Benadryl Children's Allergy, Benadryl Complete Allergy, Bendylate, Benylin, Compoz, Diahist, Diphen, Diphenadril, Fenylhist, Fynex, Hydramine, Hydril, Insomnal, Nervine Nighttime Sleep-Aid, Noradryl, Nordryl, Nytol with DPH, Robalyn, Sleep-Eze 3, Sominex Formula 2, Tusstate, Twilite, Valdrene); diphenylpyraline (Hispril); doxylamine (Unisom Nighttime Sleep-Aid); phenindamine (Nolahist); pyrilamine (Dormarex, Somnicaps, Sominex); terfenadine (Seldane); tripelennamine (PBZ, PBZ-SR); triprolidine (Actidil, Bayidyl).

Antihyperammonemias—Medications that decrease the amount of ammonia in the blood. The ones with this pharmacological property that are available in the United States are lactulose, sodium benzoate and sodium phenylacetate.

Antihypertensives—Drugs used to treat high blood pressure. These medicines can be used singly or in combination with other drugs. They work best if accompanied by a low-salt, low-fat diet plus an active exercise program. These drugs include acebutolol, amiloride, amiloride and hydrochlorothiazide, amlodipine, atenolol, atenolol and chlorthalidone, benazepril, bendroflumethiazide, benzthiazide, betaxolol, bisoprolol, bumetanide, captopril, captopril and hydrochlorothiazide, carteolol, chlorothiazide, chlorthalidone, clonidine, clonidine and chlorthalidone, cyclothiazide, debrisoquine, deserpidine, deserpidine and hydrochlorothiazide, deserpidine and methyclothiazide, diazoxide, diltiazem, doxazosin, enalapril, enalapril and hydrochlorothiazide, ethacrynic acid, felodipine, fosinopril, furosemide, guanabenz, guanadrel, guanethidine, guanethidine and hydrochlorothiazide, guanfacine, hydralazine, hydralazine and hydrochlorothiazide, hydrochlorothiazide, hydroflumethiazide, indapamide, isradipine, labetalol, labetalol and hydrochlorothiazide, lisinopril, lisinopril and hydrochlorothiazide, mecamylamine, methyclothiazide, methyldopa, methyldopa and chlorothiazide, methyldopa and hydrochlorothiazide, metolazone, metoprolol, metoprolol and hydrochlorothiazide, minoxidil, nadolol, nadolol and bendroflumethiazide, nicardipine, nifedipine, nitroglycerin, nitroprusside, oxprenolol, penbutolol, pindolol, pindolol and hydrochlorothiazide, polythiazide, prazosin, prazosin and polythiazide, propranolol, propranolol and hydrochlorothiazide, quinapril, quinethazone, ramipril, rauwolfia serpentina, rauwolfia serpentina and bendroflumethazide, reserpine, reserpine and chlorothiazide, reserpine and chlorthalidone, reserpine and hydralazine, reserpine, hydralazine and hydrochlorothiazide, reserpine and hydrochlorothiazide, reserpine and hydroflumethiazide, reserpine and methyclothiazide, reserpine and polythiazide, reserpine and quinethazone, reserpine and trichlormethiazide, sotalol, spironolactone, spironolactone and hydrochlorothiazide, terazosin, timolol, timolol and hydrochlorothiazide, triamterene, triamterene and hydrochlorothiazide, trichlormethiazide, trimethaphan, verapamil.

Anti-Inflammatory Drugs, Nonsteroidal (NSAIDs)—A family of drugs not related to cortisone or other steroids that decrease inflammation wherever it occurs in the body. Used for treatment of pain, fever, arthritis, gout, menstrual cramps and vascular headaches. These drugs include aspirin; aspirin, alumina and magnesia tablets; buffered aspirin; bufexamac; choline salicylate; choline and magnesium salicylates; diclofenac, diflunisal; fenoprofen; flurbiprofen, ibuprofen; indomethacin; ketoprofen; magnesium salicylate; meclofenamate; naproxen; piroxicam; salsalate; sodium salicylate; sulindac; tolmetin.

Anti-Inflammatory Drugs, Steroidal—A family of drugs with pharmacologic characteristics similar to those of cortisone and cortisone-like drugs. They are used for many purposes to help the body deal with inflammation no matter what the cause. Steroidal drugs may be taken orally or by injection (systemic) or applied locally for the skin, eyes, ears, bronchial tubes (topical) and others. These drugs include: Nasal—beclomethasone, dexamethasone, flunisolide. Ophthalmic (eyes)—betamethasone, dexamethasone, fluorometholone, hydrocortisone, medrysone, prednisolone. Otic (ears)—betamethasone, desonide and acetic acid, dexamethasone, hydrocortisone, hydrocortisone and acetic acid, prednisolone. Systemic—betamethasone, corticotroprin, cortisone, dexamethasone, hydrocortisone, methylprednisolone, paramethasone, prednisolone, prednisone, triamcinolone. Topical—alclometasone; amcinonide; beclomethasone; betamethasone; clobetasol; clobetasone; clocortolone; desonide; desoximetasone;
dexamethasone; diflorasone; diflucortolone; flumethasone; fluocinolone; fluocinonide; fluocinonide, procinonide and ciprocinonide; flurandrenolid; halcinonide; hydrocortisone; methylprednisolone; mometasone; triamcinolone.

Antimalarials (also called Antiprotozoals)—A group of drugs used to treat malaria. The choice depends on the precise type of malaria organism and its developmental state. These drugs include amphotericin B, chloroquine, dapsone, demeclocycline, doxycycline, hydroxychloroquine, iodoquinol, methacycline, mefloquine, metronidazole, minocycline, oxytetracycline, pentamidine, primaquine, pyrimethamine, quinacrine, quinidine, quinine, sulfadoxine and pyrimethamine, sulfamethoxazole, sulfamethoxazole and trimethoprim, sulfisoxazole, tetracycline.

Antimuscarines—Drugs that block the muscarinic action of acetylcholine and therefore decrease spasms of the smooth muscles. They are prescribed for peptic ulcers, dysmenorrhea, dizziness, seasickness, bedwetting, slow heart rate, treatment of toxicity from pesticides made from organophosphates and other medical problems. These drugs include anisotropine, atropine, belladonna, clidinium dicyclomine, glycopyrrolate, homatropine, hyoscyamine, hyoscyamine and scopolamine, isopropamide, mepenzolate, methantheline, methscopolamine, oxyphencyclimine, pirenzepine, propantheline, scopolamine, tridihexethyl.

Antimyasthenics—Medicines to treat myasthenia gravis, a muscle disorder (especially of the face and head) with increasing fatigue and weakness as muscles tire from use. These medicines include ambenonium, azathioprine, neostigmine, pyridostigmine.

Antineoplastics—Potent drugs used for malignant disease, they are listed here for completeness. Some of these are not described in this book. These drugs include: Systemic—aminoglutethimide, amsacrine, antithyroid agents, asparaginase, azathioprine, bleomycin, busulfan, carboplatin, carmustine, chlorambucil, chloramphenicol, chlorotrianisene, chromic phosphate, cisplatin, colchicine, cyclophosphamide, cyclosporine, cyproterone, cytarabine, dacarbazine, dactinomycin, daunorubicin, deferoxamine, diethylstilbestrol, doxorubicin, dromostanolone, epirubicin, estradiol, estradiol valerate, estramustine, estrogens (conjugated and esterified), estrone, ethinyl estradiol, etoposide, floxuridine, flucytosine, fluorouracil, flutamide, fluoxymesterone, gold compounds, hexamethylmelamine, hydroxyprogesterone, hydroxyurea, interferon alfa-2a and alfa-2b (recombinant), ketoconazole, leuprolide, levamisole, levothyroxine, liothyronine, liotrix, lithium, lomustine, masoprocol, mechlorethamine, medroxyprogesterone, megestrol, melphalan, methyltestosterone, mercaptopurine, methotrexate, mitomycin, mitotane, mitoxantrone, nandrolone, paclitaxel, phenpropionate, penicillamine, plicamycin, procarbazine, sodium iodide I 131, sodium phosphate P 32, streptozocin, tamoxifen, teniposide, testolactone, testosterone, thioguanine, thiotepa, thyroglobulin, thyroid, thyrotropin, uracil mustard, vinblastine, vincristine, vindesine, zidovudine. Topical—fluorouracil, mechlorethamine.

Antiparkisonism Drugs—Drugs used to treat Parkinson's disease. A disease of the central nervous system in older adults, it is characterized by gradual progressive muscle rigidity, tremors and clumsiness. These drugs include amantadine, benztropine, biperiden, bromocriptine, carbidopa and levodopa, diphenhydramine, ethopropazine, levodopa, levodopa and benserazide, orphenadrine, pergolide, procyclidine, seligiline, trihexyphenidyl.

Antipsychotic Drugs—A group of drugs used to treat the mental disease of psychosis, including such variants as schizophrenia, manic-depressive illness, anxiety states, severe behavior problems and others. These drugs include acetophenazine, carbamazepine, chlorpromazine, chlorprothixene, fluphenazine, flupenthixol, fluspirilene, haloperidol, loxapine, mesoridazine, methotrimeprazine, molindone, pericyazine, perphenazine, pimozide, pipotiazine, prochlorperazine, promazine, thioproperazine, thioridazine, thiothixene, trifluoperazine, triflupromazine.

Antithyroid Drugs—These drugs decrease the amount of thyroid hormone produced by the thyroid gland.

Antitussives—A group of drugs used to suppress cough. These drugs include chlophedianol, codeine (oral), dextromethorphan, diphenhydramine syrup, hydrocodone, hydromorphone, methadone, morphine.

Antiulcer Drugs—A group of medicines used to treat peptic ulcer in the stomach, duodenum or the lower end of the esophagus. These drugs include antacids, anticholinergics, antispasmotics, cimetidine, doxepin, famotidine, omeprazole, ranitidine, rimantadine, sucralfate, trimipramine.

Antiurolithics—Medicines that prevent the formation of kidney stones.

Antiviral Drugs—A group of drugs to treat viral infection. These drugs include Ophthalmic (eye) idoxuridine, trifluridine, vidarabine. Systemic acyclovir, amantadine, ribavirin, rimantadine, zidovudine. Topical acyclovir.

Appendicitis—Inflammation or infection of the appendix. Symptoms include loss of appetite, nausea, low-grade fever and tenderness in the lower right of the abdomen.

Appetite Suppressants—A group of drugs used to decrease the appetite as part of an overall treatment for obesity. These drugs include benzphetamine, diethylpropion, fenfluramine, mazindol, phendimetrazine, phenmetrazine, phentermine, phenylpropanolamine.

Artery—Blood vessel carrying blood away from the heart.

Asthma—Recurrent attacks of breathing difficulty due to spasms and contractions of the bronchial tubes.

Attentuated Virus Vaccines—Liquid products of killed germs used for injections to prevent certain diseases.

B

Bacteria—Microscopic organisms. Some bacteria contribute to health; others (germs) cause disease.

Barbiturates—Powerful drugs used for sedation, to help induce sleep and sometimes to prevent seizures. Except for use in seizures (phenobarbital), barbiturates are being used less and less because there are better, less hazardous drugs that produce the same or better effects. These drugs include amobarbital, aprobarbital, butabarbital, mephobarbital, metharbital, pentobarbital, phenobarbital, secobarbital, secobarbital and amobarbital, talbutal.

Basal Area of Brain—Part of the brain that regulates muscle control and tone.

Benzethonium Chloride—A compound used as a preservative in some drug preparations. It is also used in various concentrations for cleaning cooking and eating utensils and as a disinfectant.

Benzodiazepines—A family of drugs prescribed to treat anxiety and alcohol withdrawal and sometimes prescribed for sedation. These drugs include alprazolam, bromazepam, chlordiazepoxide, clonazepam, clorazepate, diazepam, estazolam, flurazepam, halazepam, ketazolam, lorazepam, nitrazepam, oxazepam, prazepam, quazepam, triazolam.

Beta Agonists—A group of drugs that act directly on cells in the body (beta-adrenergic receptors) to relieve spasms of the bronchial tubes and other organs consisting of smooth muscles. These drugs include albuterol, bitolerol, isoetharine, isoproterenol, methproterenol, terbutaline.

Beta-Adrenergic Blocking Agents—A family of drugs with similar pharmacological actions with some variations. These drugs are prescribed for angina, heartbeat irregularities (arrhythmias), high blood pressure, hypertrophic subaortic stenosis, vascular headaches (as a preventative, not to treat once the pain begins) and others. Timolol is prescribed for treatment of open-angle glaucoma. These drugs include acebutolol (Monitan, Sectral); atenolol (Esmolol); betaxolol (Kerlone); bisoprolol (Zebeta); carteolol (Cartrol); labetalol (Normodyne, Trandate); metoprolol (Apo-Metoprolol, Betaloc, Betaloc Durules, Lopresor, Lopresor SR, Lopressor, Novometoprol); nadolol (Corgard); oxprenolol (Trasicor, Slow-Trasicor); pindolol (Visken); propranolol (Apo-Propranolol, Detensol, Inderal, Inderal LA, Novopranol, pms-Propranolol); sotalol (Sotacor); timolol (Blocadren).

Bile Acids—Components of bile that are derived from cholesterol and formed in the liver. Bile acids aid the digestion of fat.

Blood Count—Laboratory studies to count white blood cells, red blood cells, platelets and other elements of the blood.

Blood Dyscrasia-Causing Medicines—Drugs which cause unpredictable damaging effects to human bone marrow. These effects occur in a small minority of patients and are not dependent upon dosage. These medicines include the following (some of which are ot described in this book): ACE inhibitors, anticonvulsants (dione, hydantoin, succinimide), antidepressants (tricyclic), antidiabetic agents (oral), anti-inflammatory analgesics, antithyroid agents, carbamazepine, chloramphenicol, clozapine, dapsone, divalproex, flecainide acetate, foscarnet, gold compounds, levamisole, loxapine, maprotiline, mephenytoin, methsuximide, penicillins (some), penicillamine, pentamidine, phenacemide, phenothiazines, phensuximide, phenytoin, pimozide, primaquine, primidone, procainamide, propafenone, pyrimethamine (large doses), rifampin, sulfasalazine, thioxanthenes, ticlopidine, tocainide, trimethoprim, valproic acid.

Blood Pressure, Diastolic—Pressure (usually recorded in millimeters of mercury) in the large arteries of the body when the heart muscle is relaxed and filling for the next contraction.

Blood Pressure, Systolic—Pressure (usually recorded in millimeters of mercury) in the large arteries of the body at the instant the heart muscle contracts.

Blood Sugar (Blood Glucose)—Necessary element in the blood to sustain life.

Bone Marrow Depressants—Medicines that affect the bone marrow to depress its normal function of forming blood cells. These medicines include the following (some of which are not described in this book): aldesleukin, altretamine, amophotericin B (systemic), anticancer drugs, anthithyroid drugs, azathioprine, busulfan, carboplatin, carmustine, chlorambucil, chloramphenicol, chromic phosphate, cisplatin, clozapine, colchicine, cyclophosphamide, cytarabine, dacarbazine, dactinomycin, daunorubicin, didanosine, doxorubicin, eflornithine, etoposide, felbamate, floxuridine, flucytosine, fludarabine, fluorouracil, ganciclovir, hydroxyurea, idarubicin, ifosfamide, interferon, lomustine, mechlorethamine, melphalan, mercaptopurine, methotrexate, mitomycin, mitoxantrone, paclitaxel, pentostatin, plicamycin, procarbazine, streptozocin, sulfa drugs, thioguanine, uracil mustard, vidarabine (large doses), vinblastine, vincristine, zidovudine.

Bone Marrow Depression—Many drugs taken for long periods of time in high doses can cause toxicity to the blood-producing capacity of human bone marrow.

Brain Depressants—Any drug that depresses brain function, such as tranquilizers, narcotics, alcohol, barbiturates.

Bronchodilators—A group of drugs used to dilate the bronchial tubes to treat such problems as asthma, emphysema, bronchitis, bronchiectasis, allergies and others. These drugs include albuterol, aminophylline, bitolterol, dyphylline, ephedrine, epinephrine, ethylnorepinephrine, fenoterol, ipratropium, isoetharine, isoproterenol, metaproterenol, oxtriphylline, oxtriphylline and guaifenesin, pirbuterol, terbutaline, theophylline, guaifenesin.

Bronchodilators, Xanthine-Derivative—Drugs of similar chemical structure and pharmacological activity that are prescribed to dilate bronchial tubes in disorders such as asthma, bronchitis, emphysema and other chronic lung diseases. These drugs include aminophylline, dyphylline, oxtriphylline, theophylline.

BUN—Abbreviation for blood urea nitrogen. A test often used as a measurement of kidney function.

C

Calcium Channel Blockers—A group of drugs used to treat angina and heartbeat irregularities. These drugs include bepridril, diltiazem, felodipine, flunarizine, isradipine, nicardipine, nifedipine, nimodipine, verapamil.

Calcium Supplements—Supplements used to increase calcium concentration in the blood in an attempt to make bones denser (as in osteoporosis). These supplements include calcium citrate, calcium glubionate, calcium gluconate, calcium glycerophosphate and calcium lactate, calcium lactate, dibasic calcium phosphate, tribasic calcium phosphate.

Carbamates—A group of drugs derived from carbamic acid and used for anxiety or as sedatives. They include meprobamate and ethinamate.

Carbonic Anhydrase Inhibitors—Drugs used to treat glaucoma and seizures and to prevent high altitude sickness\ They include acetazolamide, dichlorphenamide, methazolamid.

Cataract—Loss of transparency in the lens of the eye.

Catecholamines—A group of drugs used to treat excess catecholamine production (often a cause of hypertension). These drugs include dopamine, norepinephrine and epinephrine.

Cell—Unit of protoplasm, the essential living matter of all plants and animals.

Central Nervous System (CNS) Depressants—These drugs cause sedation or otherwise diminish brain activity and other parts of the nervous system. These drugs include alcohol, aminoglutethimide, anesthetics (general and injection-local), anticonvulsants, antidepressants (MAO inhibitors, tricyclic), antidyskinetics (except amantadine), antihistamines, apomorphine, baclofen, barbiturates, benzodiazepines, beta-adrenergic blocking agents, buclizine, carbamazepine, chlophedianol, chloral hydrate, chlorzoxazone, clonidine, clozapine, cyclizine, difenoxin and atropine, diphenoxylate and atropine, disulfiram, dronabinol, ethchlorvynol, ethinamate, etomidate, fenfluramine, fluoxetine, glutethimide, guanabenz, guanfacine, haloperidol, hydroxyzine, interferon, loxapine, magnesium sulfate (injection), maprotiline, meclizine, meprobamate, methyldopa, methyprylon, metoclopramide, metyrosine, mitotane, molindone, nabilone, opioid (narcotic) analgesics, oxybutynin, paraldehyde, paregoric, pargyline, paroxetine, phenothiazines, pimozide, procarbazine, promethazine, propiomazine, rauwolfia alkaloids, risperidone, scopolamine, sertraline, skeletal muscle relaxants (centrally acting), thioxanthenes, trazodone, trimeprazine, trimethobenzamide, zolpidem.

Central Nervous System (CNS) Stimulants—Drugs that cause excitation, anxiety and nervousness or otherwise stimulate the brain and other parts of the central nervous system. These drugs include amantadine, amphetamines, anesthetics (local), appetite suppressants (except fenfluramine), bronchodilators (xanthine-derivative), bupropion, caffeine, caffeine and sodium benzoate, chlophedianol, cocaine, dextroamphetamine, doxapram, dronabinol, ephedrine (oral), fluoxetine, methamphetamine, methylphenidate, nabilone, pemoline, selegiline, sertraline, sympathomimetics, tranylcpromine.

Cephalosporins—Antibiotics that kill many bacterial germs that penicillin and sulfa drugs can't destroy.

Cholinergics (Parasympathomimetics)—Chemicals that facilitates passage of nerve impulses through the parasympathetic nervous system.

Cholinesterase Inhibitors—Drugs that prevent the action of cholinesterase (an enzyme that breaks down acetylcholine in the body).

Chronic—Long-term, continuing. Chronic illnesses may not be curable, but they can often be prevented from becoming worse. Symptoms usually can be alleviated or controlled.

Cirrhosis—Disease that scars and destroys liver tissue.

Citrates—Medicines taken orally to make urine more acid. Citrates include potassium citrate, potassium citrate and citric acid, potassium citrate and sodium citrate, sodium citrate and acid, tricitrates.

Coal Tar Preparations—Creams, ointments and lotions used on the skin for various skin ailments.

Cold Urticaria—Hives that appear in areas of the body exposed to the cold.

Colitis, Ulcerative—Chronic, recurring ulcers of the colon for unknown reasons.

Collagen—Support tissue of skin, tendon, bone, cartilage and connective tissue.

Colostomy—Surgical opening from the colon, the large intestine, to the outside of the body.

Congestive—Characterized by excess accumulation of blood. In congestive heart failure, congestion occurs in the lungs, liver, kidney and other parts of the body to cause shortness of breath, swelling of the ankles and feet, rapid heartbeat and other symptoms.

Constriction—Tightness or pressure.

Contraceptives, Oral (Birth Control Pills)—A group of hormones used to prevent ovulation, therefore preventing pregnancy. These hormones include ethynodiol diacetate and ethinyl estradiol, ethynodiol diacetate and mestranol, levonorgestrel and ethinyl estradiol, medroxyprogesterone, norethindrone tablets, norethindrone acetate and ethinyl estradiol, norethindrone and ethinyl estradiol, norethindrone and mestranol, norethynodrel and mestranol, norgestrel, norgestrel, ethinyl estradiol.

Contraceptives, Vaginal—Topical medications or devices applied inside the vagina to prevent pregnancy.

Convulsions—Violent, uncontrollable contractions of the voluntary muscles.

Corticosteroids (Adrenocorticosteroids)—Steroid hormones produced by the body's adrenal cortex or their synthetic equivalents.

Cortisone (Adrenocorticoids, Glucocorticoids) and Other Adrenal Steroids—Medicines that mimic the action of the steroid hormone cortisone, manufactured in the cortex of the adrenal gland. These drugs decrease the effects of inflammation within the body. They are available for injection, oral use, topical use for the skin and nose and inhalation for the bronchial tubes. These drugs include alclometasone; amcinonide; beclomethasone; benzyl benzoate; betamethasone; bismuth; clobetasol; clobetasone 17-butyrate; clocortolone; cortisone; desonide; desoximetasone; desoxycorticosterone; dexamethasone; diflorasone; diflucortolone; fludrocortisone; flumethasone; flunisolide; fluocinonide; fluocinonide, procinonide and ciprocinonide; fluorometholone; fluprednisolone, flurandrenolide; halcinonide; hydrocortisone; medrysone; methylprednisolone; mometasone; paramethasone; peruvian balsam; prednisolone; prednisone; triamcinolone; zinc oxide.

Cyclopegics—Eye drops that prevent the pupils from accommodating to varying degrees of light.

Cystitis—Inflammation of the urinary bladder.

D

Decongestants—Drugs used to open nasal passages by shrinking swollen membranes lining the nose. These drugs include: Cough-suppressing—phenylephrine and dextromethorphan, phenylpropanolamine and caramiphen, phenylpropanolamine and dextromethorphan, phenylpropanolamine and hydrocodone, pseudoephedrine and codeine, pseudoephedrine and dextromethorphan, pseudoephedrine and hydrocodone. Cough-suppressing and pain-relieving—phenylpropanolamine, dextromethorphan and acetaminophen. Cough-suppressing and sputum-thinning—phenylephrine, dextromethorphan and guaifenesin; phenylephrine, hydrocodone and guaifenesin; phenylpropanolamine, codeine and guaifenesin; phenylpropanolamine, dextromethorphan and guaifenesin; pseudoephedrine, codeine and guaifenesin; pseudoephedrine, dextromethorphan and guaifenesin; pseudoephedrine, hydrocodone and guaifenesin; phenylephrine, dextromethorphan, guaifenesin and acetaminophen; pseudoephedrine, dextromethorphan, guaifenesin and acetaminophen. Sputum-thinning—ephedrine and guaifenesin; ephedrine and potassium iodide; phenylephrine, phenylpropanolamine and guaifenesin; phenylpropanolamine and guaifenesin; pseudoephedrine and guaifenesin. Nasal—ephedrine (oral), phenylpropanolamine, pseudoephedrine. Ophthalmic (eye)—naphazoline, oxymetazoline, phenylephrine. Topical—oxymetazoline, phenylephrine, xylometazoline.

Delirium—Temporary mental disturbance characterized by hallucinations, agitation and incoherence.

Diabetes —Metabolic disorder in which the body can't use carbohydrates efficiently. This leads to a dangerously high level of glucose (a carbohydrate) in the blood.

Dialysis—Procedure to filter waste products from the bloodstream of patients with kidney failure.

Digitalis Preparations (Digitalis Glycosides)—Important drugs to treat heart disease, such as congestive heart failure, heartbeat irregularities and cardiogenic shock. These drugs include digitoxin, digoxin.

Digoxin—One of the digitalis drugs used to treat heart disease. All digitalis products were originally derived from the foxglove plant.

Dilation—Enlargement.

Disulfiram Reaction—Disulfiram (Antabuse) is a drug to treat alcoholism. When alcohol in the bloodstream interacts with disulfiram, it causes a flushed face, severe headache, chest pains, shortness of breath, nausea, vomiting, sweating and weakness. Severe reactions may cause death. A disulfiram reaction is the interaction of any drug with alcohol or another drug to produce these symptoms.

Diuretics—Drugs that act on the kidneys to prevent reabsorption of electrolytes, especially chlorides. They are used to treat edema, high blood pressure, congestive heart failure, kidney and liver failure and others. These drugs include amiloride, amiloride and hydrochlorothiazide, bendroflumethiazide, benzthiazide, bumetanide, chlorothiazide, chlorthalidone, cyclothiazide, ethacrynic acid, furosemide, glycerin, hydrochlorothiazide, hydroflumethiazide, indapamide, mannitol, methyclothiazide, metolazone, polythiazide, quinethazone, spironolactone, sprionolactone and hydrochlorothiazide, triamterene, triamterene and hydrochlorothiazide, trichlormethiazide, urea.

Diuretics, Loop—Drugs that act on the kidneys to prevent reabsorption of electrolytes, especially chlorides. They are used to treat edema, high blood pressure, congestive heart failure, kidney and liver failure and others. These drugs include bumetanide, ethacrynic acid, furosemide.

Diuretics, Potassium-Sparing—Drugs that act on the kidneys to prevent reabsorption of electrolytes, especially chlorides. They are used to treat edema, high blood pressure, congestive heart failure, kidney and liver failure and others. This particular group of diuretics does not allow the unwanted side effect of low potassium in the blood to occur. These drugs include amiloride, spironolactone, triamterene.

Diuretics, Thiazide—Drugs that act on the kidneys to prevent reabsorption of electrolytes, especially chlorides. They are used to treat edema, high blood pressure, congestive heart failure, kidney and liver failure and others. These drugs include bendroflumethiazide (Naturetin); benzthiazide (Aquatag, Exna, Hydrex); chlorothiazide (Diuril); chlorthalidone (Apo-Chlorthalidone, Hygroton, Novothalidone, Thalitone, Uridon); cyclothiazide (Anhydron, Fluidil); hydrochlorothiazide (Apo-Hydro, Diuchlor H, Esidrix, Hydrochlorothiazide Intensol, HydroDIURIL, Mictrin, Natrimax, Neo-Codema, Novohydrazide, Oretic, Thiuretic, Urozide); hydroflumethiazide (Diucardin, Saluron); methyclothiazide (Aquatensen, Duretic, Enduron); metolazone (Diulo, Zaroxolyn); polythiazide (Renese); quinethazone (Aquamox, Hydromox); trichlormethiazide (Metahydrin, Naqua).

Duodenum—The first 12 inches of the small intestine.

E

ECG (or EKG)—Abbreviation for electrocardiogram or electrocardiograph. An ECG is a graphic tracing representing the electrical current produced by impulses passing through the heart muscle. This is a useful test in the diagnosis of heart disease, but used alone it usually can't make a complete diagnosis. An ECG is most useful in two areas: (1) demonstrating heart rhythm disturbances and (2) demonstrating changes when there is a myocardial infarction (heart attack). It will detect enlargement of either heart chamber, but will not establish a diagnosis of heart failure or disease of the heart valves.

Eczema—Disorder of the skin with redness, itching, blisters, weeping and abnormal pigmentation.

EEG—Electroencephalogram or electroencephalograph. An EEG is a graphic recording of electrical activity generated spontaneously from nerve cells in the brain. This test is useful in the diagnosis of brain dysfunction, particularly in studying seizure disorders.

Electrolytes—Substances that can transmit electrical impulses when dissolved in body fluids.

Embolism—Sudden blockage of an artery by a clot or foreign material in the blood.

Emphysema—Disease in which the lung's air sacs lose elasticity and air accumulates in the lungs.

Endometriosis—Condition in which uterus tissue is found outside the uterus. Can cause pain, abnormal menstruation and infertility.

Enzymes—Protein chemicals that can accelerate chemical reactions in the body.

Epilepsy—Episodes of brain disturbance that cause convulsions and loss of consciousness.

Ergot Preparations—Medicines used to treat migraine and other types of throbbing headaches. Also used after delivery of babies to make the uterus clamp down and reduce excessive bleeding.

Erythromycins—A group of drugs with similar structure used to treat infections. These drugs include erythromycin (Eryc, Eryc Sprinkle, Erythromid, Novorythro, E-Mycin, Ery-Tab, Ilotycin, PCE Dispersatabs, Robimycin, RP-Mycin); erythromycin estolate (Ilosone, Novorythro); erythromycin ethylsuccinate (E.E.S., E-Mycin E, Pediamycin, Wyamycin E, EryPed); erthromycin gluceptate (Ilotycin); erythromycin lactobionate (Erythrocin); erythromycin stearate (ApoErythro-S).

Esophagitis—Inflammation of the lower part of the esophagus, the tube connecting the throat and the stomach.

Estrogens—Female hormones used to replenish the body's stores after the ovaries have been removed or become nonfunctional after menopause. Also used with progesterone in some birth control pills and for other purposes. These drugs include: Systemic—chlorotrianisene, diethylstilbestrol, estradiol, estrogens (conjugated and esterified), estrone, estropipate, ethinyl estradiol, quinestrol. Vaginal—dienestrol, estradiol, estrogens (conjugated), estrone, estropipate.

Eustachian Tube—Small passage from the middle ear to the sinuses and nasal passages.
Extrapyramidal Reactions—Abnormal reactions in the power and coordination of posture and muscular movements. Movements are not under voluntary control. Some drugs associated with producing extrapyramidal reactions include amoxapine, antidepressants (tricyclic), droperidol, haloperidol, loxapine, metoclopramide, metyrosine, molindone, phenothiazines, pimozide, rauwolfia alkaloids, tacrine, thioxanthenes.
Extremity—Arm, leg, hand or foot.

F

Fecal Impaction—Condition in which feces become firmly wedged in the rectum.
Fibrocystic Breast Disease—Overgrowth of fibrous tissue in the breast, producing non-malignant cysts.
Fibroid Tumors—Non-malignant tumors of the muscular layer of the uterus.
Flu (Influenza)—A virus infection of the respiratory tract that lasts three to ten days. Symptoms include headache, fever, runny nose, cough, tiredness and muscle aches.
Fluoroquinolones—A class of drugs used to treat bacterial infections, such as urinary tract infections and some types of bronchitis. These drugs include ciprofloxacin, enoxacin, lomefloxacin, norfloxacin and ofloxacin.
Folliculitis—Inflammation of a follicle.

G

G6PD—Deficiency of glucose 6-phosphate, necessary for glucose metabolism.
Ganglionic Blockers—Medicines that block the passage of nerve impulses through a part of the nerve cell called a ganglion. Ganglionic blockers are used to treat urinary retention and other medical problems. Bethanechol is one of the best ganglionic blockers.
Gastritis—Inflammation of the stomach.
Gastrointestinal—Of the stomach and intestinal tract.
Gland—Organ that manufactures and excretes materials not required for its own metabolic needs.
Glaucoma—Eye disease in which increased pressure inside the eye damages the optic nerve, causes pain and changes vision.
Glucagon—Injectable drug that immediately elevates blood sugar by mobilizing glycogen from the liver.
Gold Compounds—Medicines which use gold as their base and are usually used to treat joint or arthritic disorders. These medicines include auranofin, aurothioglucose, gold sodium thiomalate.

H

H_2 Antagonists—Antihistamines that work against H_2 histamine. H_2 histamine may be liberated at any point in the body, but most often in the skin, bronchial tubes and gastrointestinal tract.
Hangover Effect—The same feelings as a "hangover" after too much alcohol consumption. Symptoms include headache, irritability and nausea.
Hemochromatosis—Disorder of iron metabolism in which excessive iron is deposited in and damages body tissues, particularly of the liver and pancreas.
Hemoglobin—Pigment that carries oxygen in red blood cells.
Hemolytics—Drugs that separate hemoglobin from the blood cells. These include acetohydroxamic acid, antidiabetic agents (oral), doxapram, furazolidone, mefenamic acid, methyldopa, nitrofurans, primaquine, procainamide, quinidine, quinine, sulfonamides (systemic), sulfones, vitamin K.
Hemorrhage—Heavy bleeding.
Hemorrheologic Agents—Medicines to help control bleeding.
Hemosiderosis—Increase of iron deposits in body tissues without tissue damage.
Hepatitis—Inflammation of liver cells, usually accompanied by jaundice.
Hepatotoxics—Medications that can possibly cause toxicity or decreased normal function of the liver. These drugs include the following (some of which are not described in this book): acetaminophen (with long-term use); alcohol; amiodarone; anabolic steroids; androgens; angiotensin-converting enzyme (ACE) inhibitors; anti-inflammatory drugs, nonsteroidal (NSAIDs); antithyroid agents; asparaginase; azlocillin; carbamazepine; carmustine;
dantrolene; dapsone; daunorubicin; disulfiram; divalproex; erythromycins; estrogens; ethionamide; etretinate; fluconazole; flutamide; gold compounds; halothane; HMG-CoA reductase inhibitors; isoniazid; itraconazole; ketoconazole (oral); labetalol; lovastatin; mercaptopurine; methotrexate; methyldopa; mezlocillin; naltrexone; niacin (high doses); nitrofurans; phenothiazines; phenytoin; piperacillin; plicamycin; pravastatin; rifampin; simvastatin; sulfonamides; tacrine; testosterone; valproic acid; zidovudine.
Hiatal Hernia—Section of stomach that protrudes into the chest cavity.
Histamine—Chemical in body tissues that dilates the smallest blood vessels, constricts the smooth muscle surrounding the bronchial tubes and stimulates stomach secretions.
History—Past medical events in a patient's life.

Hives—Elevated patches on the skin that are redder or paler than surrounding skin and often itch severely.

Hormones—Chemical substances produced in the body to regulate other body functions.

Hypercalcemia—Too much calcium in the blood. This happens with some malignancies and in calcium overdose.

Hyperkalemia-Causing Medications—Medicines that cause too much potassium in the bloodstream. These include ACE inhibitors; anti-inflammatory drugs, nonsteroidal (NSAIDs); cyclosporine; digitalis glycosides; diuretics (potassium-sparing); pentamidine; succinylcholine chloride; possibly any medicine that is combined with potassium.

Hypersensitivity—Serious reactions to many medications. The effects of hypersensitivity may be characterized by wheezing, shortness of breath, rapid heart rate, severe itching, faintness, unconsciousness and severe drop in blood pressure.

Hypertension—High blood pressure.

Hypervitaminosis—A condition due to an excess of one or more vitamins. Symptoms may include weakness, fatigue, loss of hair and changes in the skin.

Hypnotics—Drugs used to induce a sleeping state. See Barbiturates.

Hypocalcemia—Abnormally low level of calcium in the blood.

Hypoglycemia—Low blood sugar (blood glucose). A critically low blood sugar level will interfere with normal brain function and can damage the brain permanently.

Hypoglycemics—Drugs that reduce blood sugar. These include acetohexamide, chlorpropamide, glipizide, glyburide, insulin, metformin, tolazamide, tolbutamide.

Hypokalemia-Causing Medications—Medicines that cause a depletion of potassium in the bloodstream. These include adrenocorticoids (systemic), alcohol, amphotericin B (systemic), bronchodilators (adrenergic), carbonic anhydrase inhibitors, diuretics (loop and thiazide), foscarnet, indapamide, insulin, laxatives (if dependent on), penicillins (some), salicylates, sodium bicarbonate, urea, vitamin D (overdose of).

Hypotension—Blood pressure decreased below normal. Symptoms may include weakness, lightheadedness and dizziness.

Hypotension-causing drugs—Medications that might cause hypotension. These include alcohol, alprostadil, amantadine, anesthetics (general), angiotensin-converting enzyme inhibitors (ACE inhibitors), anti-depressants (MAO inhibitors, tricyclic), anti-hypertensives, benzodiazepines used as preanesthetics, beta-adrenergic blocking agents, bromocriptine, calcium channel-blocking agents, captopril, carbidopa and levodopa, clozapine, diuretics, edetate calcium disodium, edetate disodium, enalapril, encainide, haloperidol, hydralazine, levodopa, lidocaine (systemic), loxapine, maprotiline, molindone, nabilone (high doses), nitrates, opioid analgesics (including fentanil, fentanyl and sufentanil), paclitaxel, pentamidine, phenothiazines, pimozide, prazosin, procainamide, quinidine, radiopaques (materials used in x-ray studies), thioxanthenes, tocainide, trazodone. If you take any of these medications, be sure to tell a dentist, anesthesiologist or anyone else who intends to give you an anesthetic to put you to sleep.

Hypothermia-Causing Medications—Medicines that can cause a significant lowering of body temperature. These drugs include alcohol, alpha-adrenergic blocking agents (dihydroergotamine, ergotamine, labetol, phenoxybenzamine, phentolamine, prazosin, tolazoline), barbiturates (large amounts), beta-adrenergic blocking agents, clonidine, insulin, minoxidil, narcotic analgesics (with overdose), vasodilators.

I

Ichthyosis—Skin disorder with dryness, scaling and roughness.

Ileitis—Inflammation of the ileum, the last section of the small intestine.

Ileostomy—Surgical opening from the ileum, the end of the small intestine, to the outside of the body.

Immunosuppressants—Powerful drugs that suppress the immune system. Immunosuppressants are used in patients who have had organ transplants or severe disease associated with the immune system. These drugs include the following (some of which are not described in this book): azathioprine, betamethasone, chlorambucil, corticotropin, cortisone, cyclophosphamide, cyclosporine, dexamethasone, hydrocortisone, mercaptopurine, methylprednisolone, muromonab, muromonab-CD3, paramethasone, prednisolone, prednisone, triamcinolone.

Impotence—Male's inability to achieve or sustain erection of the penis for sexual intercourse.

Insomnia—Sleeplessness.

Interaction—Change in the body's response to one drug when another is taken. Interaction may decrease the effect of one or both drugs, increase the effect of one or both drugs or cause toxicity.

Iron Supplements—Products that contain iron in a form that can be absorbed from the intestinal tract. Supplements include ferrous fumarate, ferrous gluconate, ferrous sulfate, iron dextran, iron-polysaccharide.

J

Jaundice—Symptoms of liver damage, bile obstruction or destruction of red blood cells. Symptoms include yellowed whites of the eyes, yellow skin, dark urine and light stool.

K

Keratosis—Growth that is an accumulation of cells from the outer skin layers.

Kidney Stones—Small, solid stones made from calcium, cholesterol, cysteine and other body chemicals.

L

Laxatives—Medicines prescribed to treat constipation. These medicines include bisacodyl; bisacodyl and docusate; casanthranol; casanthranol and docusate; cascara sagrada; cascara sagrada and aloe; cascara sagrada and phenolphthalein; castor oil; danthron; danthron and docusate; danthron and poloxamer 188; dehydrocholic acid; dehydrocholic acid and docusate; docusate; docusate and phenolphthalein; docusate and mineral oil; docusate and phenolphthalein; docusate, carboxymethylcellulose and casanthranol; glycerin; lactulose; magnesium citrate; magnesium hydroxide; magnesium hydroxide and mineral oil; magnesium oxide; magnesium sulfate; malt soup extract; malt soup extract and psyllium; methylcellulose; mineral oil; mineral oil and cascara sagrada; mineral oil and phenolphthalein; mineral oil, glycerin and phenolphthalein; phenolphthalein; poloxamer; polycarbophil; potassium bitartrate and sodium bicarbonate; psyllium; psyllium and senna; psyllium hydrophilic mucilloid; psyllium hydrophilic mucilloid and carboxymethylcellulose; psyllium hydrophilic mucilloid and sennosides; psyllium hydrophilic musilloid and senna; senna; senna and docusate; sennosides; sodium phosphate.

LDH—Abbreviation for lactate dehydrogenase. It is a measurement of cardiac enzymes used to confirm some heart conditions.

Lincomycins—A family of antibiotics used to treat certain infections.

Low-Purine Diet—A diet that avoids high-purine foods, such as liver, sweetbreads, kidneys, sardines, oysters and others. If you need a low-purine diet, request instructions from your doctor.

Lupus—Serious disorder of connective tissue that primarily affects women. Varies in severity with skin eruptions, joint inflammation, low white blood cell count and damage to internal organs, especially the kidney.

Lymph Glands—Glands in the lymph vessels throughout the body that trap foreign and infectious matter and protect the bloodstream from infection.

M

Macrolides—A class of antibiotic (antibacterial) drugs. They include erythromycin, lincomycin and vancomycin.

Male Hormones—Chemical substances secreted by the testicles, ovaries and adrenal glands in humans. Some male hormones used by humans are derived synthetically. Male hormones include testosterone cypionate and estradiol cypionate, testosterone enanthate and estradiol valerate.

Manic-Depressive Illness—Psychosis with alternating cycles of excessive enthusiasm and depression.

MAO Inhibitors—See Monoamine Oxidase (MAO) Inhibitors.

Mast Cell—Connective tissue cell.

Menopause—The end of menstruation in the female, often accompanied by irritability, hot flashes, changes in the skin and bones and vaginal dryness.

Metabolism—Process of using nutrients and energy to build and break down wastes.

Migraine—Periodic headaches caused by constriction of arteries to the skull. Symptoms include severe pain, vision disturbances, nausea, vomiting and sensitivity to light.

Mind-Altering Drugs—Any drugs that decrease alertness, perception, concentration, contact with reality or muscular coordination.

Mineral Supplements—Mineral substances added to the diet to treat or prevent mineral deficiencies. They include iron, copper, magnesium, calcium, etc.

Monoamine Oxidase (MAO) Inhibitors—Drugs that prevent the activity of the enzyme monoamine oxidase (MAO) in brain tissue, thus affecting mood. MAO inhibitors include anti-depressants, the use of which is frequently restricted because of severe side effects. These side effects may be interactions with other drugs (such as ephedrine or amphetamine) or foods containing tyramine (such as cheese) and may produce a sudden increase in blood pressure. MAOs include isocarboxazid, phenelzine, tranylcypromine.

Muscle Blockers—Same as muscle relaxants or skeletal muscle relaxants.

Muscle Relaxants—Medicines to lessen painful contractions and spasms of muscles. These include atracurium, carisoprodol, chlorphenesin, chlorzoxazone, cyclobenzaprine, metaxalone, methcarbamol, metocurine, orphenadrine citrate, orphenadrine hydrochloride, pancuronium, succinylcholine, tubocurarine, vecuronium.

Myasthenia Gravis—Disease of the muscles characterized by fatigue and progressive paralysis. It is usually confined to muscles of the face, lips, tongue and neck.

Mydriatics—Eye drops that cause the pupils to dilate to a marked degree.

N

Narcotics—A group of habit-forming, addicting drugs used for treatment of pain, diarrhea, cough, acute pulmonary edema and others. They are all dervied from opium, a milky exudate in capsules of *papaver somniferum*. Law requires licensed physicians to dispense by prescription. These drugs include alfentanil, buprenorphine, butorphanol, codeine, fentanyl, hydrocodone, hydromorphone, levorphanol, meperidine, methadone, morphine, nalbuphine, opium, oxycodone, oxymorphone, paregoric, pentazocine, propoxyphene, sufetanil.

Nephrotoxic (Kidney-Poisoning) Medications—Under some circumstances, these medicines can be toxic to the kidneys. These medicines include acetaminophen (in high doses); acyclovir (given internally); aminoglycosides; amphotericin B (given internally); analgesic combinations containing acetaminophen and aspirin or other salicylates (with chronic high-dose use); anti-inflammatory analgesics (nonsteroidal); bacitracin (given internally); capreomycin; carmustine; ciprofloxacin; cisplatin; cyclosporine; demeclocycline (nephrogenic diabetes insipidus); edetate calcium disodium (with high doses); edetate disodium (with high dose); enalapril; foscarnet; gold compounds; lithium; methotrexate (with high dose therapy); methoxyflurane; neomycin (oral); penicillamine; pentamidine; plicamycin; polymyxins (given internally); radiopaques (materials used for special x-ray examinations); rifampin; streptozocin; sulfonamides; tetracyclines (except doxycycline and minocycline); tiopronin; vancomycin (given internally).

Neuroleptic Malignant Syndrome—Ceaseless, involuntary, jerky movements of the tongue, facial muscles and hands.

Neuromuscular Blocking Agents—A group of drugs prescribed to relax skeletal muscles. They are all given by injection, and descriptions are not included in this book. These drugs include atracurium, edrohponium, gallamine, neostigmine, metocurine, pancuronium, pyridostigmine, succinylcholine, tubocurarine, vecuronium.

Neurotoxic Medications—Medicines that cause toxicity to the nerve tissues in the body. These drugs include anticonvulsants (hydantoin), carbamazepine, chloramphenicol (oral), chloroquine, ciprofloxacin, cisplatin, cycloserine, didanosine, disulfiram, ethambutol, ethionamide, hydroxychloroquine, isoniazid, lincomycins, lindane (topical), lithium, metronidazole, mexiletine, nitrofurantoin, pemoline, pyridoxine (large amounts), quinacrine, quinidine, quinine, stavudine, tetracyclines, vincristine, zalcitabine.

Nitrates—Medicines made from a chemical with a nitrogen base. Nitrates include erythrityl tetranitrate, isosorbide dinitrate, nitroglycerin, pentaerythritol tetranitrate.

Nonsteroidal Anti-Inflammatory Drugs (NSAIDs)—See Anti-Inflammatory Drugs, Nonsteroidal.

Nutritional Supplements—Substances used to treat and prevent deficiencies when the body is unable to absorb them by eating a well-balanced, nutritional diet. These supplements include: Vitamins—ascorbic acid, ascorbic acid and sodium ascorbate, calcifediol, calcitriol, calcium pantothenate, cyanocobalamin, dihydrotachysterol, ergocalciferol, folate sodium, folic acid, hydroxocobalamin, niacin, niacinamide, pantothenic, pyridoxine, riboflavin, sodium ascorbate, thiamine, vitamin A, vitamin E. Minerals—calcium carbonate, calcium citrate, calcium glubionate, calcium gluconate, calcium lactate, calcium phosphate (dibasic and tribasic), sodium fluoride. Other—levocarnitine, omega-3 polyunsaturated fatty acids.

O

Opiates—Pain-killing medicines derived from opium that have a high index of addiction. Some of these include butorphanol, codeine, hydrocodone, hydromorphone, levorphanol, meperidine, methadone, morphine, nalbuphine, opium, oxycodone, oxymorphone, paregoric, pentazocine, propoxyphene.

Osteoporosis—Softening of bones caused by a loss of chemicals usually found in bone.

Ototoxic Medications—These medicines may possibly cause hearing damage. They include aminoglycosides, 4-aminoquinolines, anti-inflammatory analgesics (nonsteroidal), bumetanide (injected), capreomyucin, chloroquine, cisplatin, deferoxamine, erythromycins, ethacrynic acid, furosemide, hydroxychloroquine, minocycline, quinidine, quinine, salicylates, vancomycin (injected).

Ovary—Female sexual gland where eggs mature and ripen for fertilization.

P

Pain Relievers—Non-narcotic medicines to treat pain.

Palpitations—Rapid heartbeat noticeable to the patient.

Pancreatitis—Serious inflammation or infection of the pancreas that causes upper abdominal pain.

Parkinson's Disease or Parkinson's Syn-

drome—Disease of the central nervous system. Characteristics are a fixed, emotionless expression of the face, tremor, slower muscle movements, weakness, changed gait and a peculiar posture.

Pellagra—Disease caused by a deficiency of the water-soluble vitamin thiamine (vitamin B-1). Symptoms include brain disturbance, diarrhea and skin inflammation.

Penicillin—Chemical substance (antibiotic) originally discovered as a product of mold, which can kill some bacterial germs.

Phenothiazines—Drugs used to treat mental, nervous and emotional conditions. These drugs include acetophenazine, chlorpromazine, fluphenazine, mesoridazine, methotrimeprazine, pericyazine, perphenazine, prochlorperazine, promazine, thiopropazate, thioproperazine, thioridazine, trifluoperazine, triflupromazine.

Pheochromocytoma—A tumor of the adrenal gland which produces chemicals that cause high blood pressure, headache, nervousness and other symptoms.

Phlegm—Thick mucus secreted by glands in the respiratory tract.

Photophobia—Increased sensitivity to light as perceived by the human eye. Drugs that can cause photophobia include antidiabetic drugs*, atropine, belladonna, bromides, chloraquine, ciprofloxacin, chlordiazepoxide, clidinium, clomiphene, dicyclomine, digitalis drugs, doxepin, ethambutol, ethionamide, ethosuximide, etretinate, glycopyrrolate, hydroxychloroquine, hydroxyzine, hyoscyamine, mephenytoin, methenamine, methsuximide, monoamine oxidase (MAO) inhibitors, nalidixic acid, norfloxacin, oral contraceptives, orphenadrine, paramethadione, phenothiazines, propantheline, quinidine, quinine, scopolamine, sopropamide, tetracyclines, tridihexethyl, trimethadione.

Photosensitizing Medications—Medicines that can cause abnormally heightened skin reactions to the effects of sunlight. These medicines include acetohexamide, amiodarone, amitriptyline, amoxapine, anthralin, antidiabetic agents (oral), antihistamines, barbiturates, bendroflumethiazide, benzocaine, carbamazepine, chlordiazepoxide, chloroquine, chlorothiazide, chlorpromazine, chlorpropamide, chlortetracycline, chlorthalidone, clindamycin, coal tar, contraceptives (estrogen-containing, oral), cyproheptadine, demeclocycline, desipramine, diethylstilbestrol, diltiazem, diphenhydramine, diuretics (thiazide), doxepin, doxycycline, estrogens, ethionamide, etretinate, fluorouracil, fluphenazine, furosemide, griseofulvin, glyburide, gold preparations, hydrocholothiazide, hydroflumethiazide, imipramine, isotretinoin, ketoprofen, lincomycin, maprotiline, mesoridazine, methacycline, methotrexate, methoxsalen, nalidixic acid, naproxen, nortriptyline, oral contraceptives, oxyphenbutazone, oxytetracycline, perphenazine, phenobarbital, phenothiazines, phenylbutazone, phenytoin, piroxicam, prochlorperazine, promazine, promethazine, protriptyline, pyrazinamide, sulfonamides, sulindac, tetracyclines, thioridazine, thioxanthenes, tolazamide, tolbutamide, tranylcypromine, tretinoin, triamterene, trifluoperazine, trioxsalen, trimeprazine, trimipramine, triproldine.

Pinworms—Common intestinal parasites that cause rectal itching and irritation.

Pituitary Gland—Gland at the base of the brain that secretes hormones to stimulate growth and other glands to produce hormones.

Platelet—Disc-shaped element of the blood, smaller than a red or white blood cell, necessary for blood clotting.

Polymixins—A family of antibiotics that kill bacteria.

Polyp—Growth on a mucous membrane.

Porphyria—Inherited metabolic disorder characterized by changes in the nervous system and kidney.

Post-Partum—Following delivery of a baby.

Potassium—Important chemical found in body cells.

Potassium Foods—Foods high in potassium content, including dried apricots and peaches, lentils, raisins, citrus and whole-grain cereals.

Potassium Supplements—Medicines needed by people who don't have enough potassium in their diets or by those who develop a deficiency due to illness or taking diuretics and other medicines. These supplements include chloride; potassium acetate; potassium bicarbonate; potassium bicarbonate and potassium chloride; potassium bicarbonate and potassium citrate; potassium chloride; potassium chloride, potassium bicarbonate and potassium citrate; potassium gluconate; potassium gluconate and potassium chloride; potassium gluconate and potassium citrate; potassium gluconate, potassium citrate and ammonium; trikates.

Prostaglandins—A group of drugs used for a variety of therapeutic purposes. These drugs include alprostadil (treats newborns with congenital heart disease), carboprost and dinoprost (both used to induce labor) and dinoprostone (used to induce labor or to induce a late abortion).

Prostate—Gland in the male that surrounds the neck of the bladder and the urethra.

Prothrombin—Blood substance essential in clotting.

Prothrombin Time (Pro Time)—Laboratory study used to follow prothrombin activity and keep coagulation safe.

Psoriasis—Chronic, inherited skin disease. Symptoms are lesions with silvery scales on the edges.

Psychosis—Mental disorder characterized by deranged personality, loss of contact with reality and possible delusions, hallucinations or illusions.

Purine Foods—Foods that are metabolized into uric acid. Foods high in purines include anchovies, liver, brains, sweetbreads, sardines, kidney, oysters, gravy and meat extracts.

R

Rauwolfia Alkaloids—Drugs that belong to the family of antihypertensives (drugs that lower blood pressure). Rauwolfia alkaloids are not used as extensively as in years past. They include alseroxylon, deserpidine, rauwolfia serpentina, reserpine.

RDA—Recommended daily allowance of a vitamin or mineral.

Rebound Effect—Return of a condition, often with increased severity, once the prescribed drug is withdrawn.

Renal—Pertaining to the kidney.

Retina—Innermost covering of the eyeball on which the image is formed.

Retinoids—A group of drugs that are synthetic vitamin A-like compounds used to treat skin conditions. These drugs include etretinate, isotretinoin and retinoic acid.

Retroperitoneal Imaging—Special x-rays or CT scans of the organs attached to the abdominal wall, behind the peritoneum (the covering of the intestinal tract and lining of the walls of the abdominal and pelvic cavities).

Reye's Syndrome—Rare, sometimes fatal, disease of children that causes brain and liver damage.

Rickets—Bone disease caused by vitamin D deficiency. Bones become bent and distorted during infancy or childhood.

S

Salicylates—Medicines to relieve pain and reduce fever. These include aspirin, aspirin and caffeine, buffered aspirin, choline salicylate, choline and magnesium salicylates, magnesium salicylate, salicylamide, salsalate, sodium salicylate.

Sedatives—Drugs that reduce excitement or anxiety.

Seizure—Brain disorder causing changes of consciousness or convulsions.

SGOT—Abbreviation for serum glutamic-oxaloacetic transaminase. Measuring the level in the blood helps demonstrate liver disorders and diagnose recent heart damage.

SGPT—Abbreviation for a laboratory study measuring the blood level of serum glutamic-pyruvic transaminase. Deviations from a normal level may indicate liver disease.

Sick Sinus Syndrome—A complicated, serious heartbeat rhythm disturbance characterized by a slow heart rate alternating with a fast or slow heart rate with heart block.

Sinusitis—Inflammation or infection of the sinus cavities in the skull.

Skeletal Muscle Relaxants (Same as Skeletal Muscle Blockers)—A group of drugs prescribed to treat spasms of the skeletal muscles. These drugs include carisoprodol, chlorphenesin, chlorzoxazone, cyclobenzaprine, diazepam, lorazepam, metaxalone, methocarbamol, orphenadrine, phenytoin.

Sleep Inducers—Night-time sedatives to aid in falling asleep. See Benzodiazepines.

Streptococci—Bacteria that cause infections in the throat, respiratory system and skin. Improperly treated, can lead to disease in the heart, joints and kidneys.

Stroke—Sudden, severe attack. Usually sudden paralysis from injury to the brain or spinal cord caused by a blood clot or hemorrhage in the brain.

Stupor—Near unconsciousness.

Sublingual—Under the tongue. Some drugs are absorbed almost as quickly this way as by injection.

Sulfa Drugs—Shorthand for sulfonamide drugs, which are used to treat infections.

Sulfonamides—Sulfa drugs prescribed to treat infections. They include sulfacytine, sulfamethoxazole, sulfamethoxazole and trimethoprin, sulfasalazine, sulfisoxazole.

Sulfonureas—A family of drugs that lower blood sugar (hypoglycemic agents). Used in the treatment of some forms of diabetes.

Sympathomimetics—A large group of drugs that mimic the effects of stimulation of the sympathetic part of the autonomic nervous system. These drugs include adrenalin (epinephrine); appetite suppressants (such as benzphetamine, diethylpropion, fenfluramine, mazindol, phendimetrazine, phenmetrazine, phentermine, phenylpropanolamine); aramine; cocaine; dobutamine; ephedrine; epinephrine; mephentermine; methoxamine; norepinephrine; phenylephrine; phenylpropanolamine; metaraminol; isoproterenol.

T

Tardive Dyskinesia—Involuntary movements of the jaw, lips and tongue caused by an unpredictable drug reaction.

Tartrazine Dye—A dye used in foods and medicine preparations that may cause an allergic reaction in some people.

Tetracyclines—A group of medicines with similar chemical structure used to treat infections. These drugs include demeclocycline, doxycycline, methacycline, minocycline, oxytetracycline, tetracycline.

Thiazides—A group of chemicals that cause diuresis (loss of water through the kidney). Frequently used to treat high blood pressure and congestive heart failure. Thiazides include bendroflumethiazide, benzthiazide, chlorothiazide, chlorthalidone, cyclothiazide, hydrochlorothiazide, hydroflumethiazide, methyclothiazide, metolazone, polythiazide, quinethazone, trichlormethiazide.

Thiothixines—See Thioxanthenes.

Thioxanthenes—Drugs used to treat emotional, mental and nervous conditions. These drugs include chlorprothixene, fluphenthixol, thiothixene.

Thrombocytopenias—Diseases characterized by inadequate numbers of blood platelets circulating in the bloodstream.

Thrombolytic Agents—Drugs that help to dissolve blood clots. They include alteplase, streptokinase, urokinase.

Thrombophlebitis—Inflammation of a vein caused by a blood clot in the vein.

Thyroid—Gland in the neck that manufactures and secretes several hormones.

Thyroid Hormones—Medications that mimic the action of the thyroid hormone made in the thyroid gland. They include dextrothyroxine, levothyroxine, liothyronine, liotrix, thyroglobulin, thyroid.

Tic Douloureux—Painful condition caused by inflammation of a nerve in the face.

Tolerance–A decreasing response to repeated constant doses of a drug or a need to increase doses to produce the same physical or mental response.

Toxicity—Poisonous reaction to a drug that impairs body functions or damages cells.

Transdermal Patches—There are more and more medications in a form known as transdermal (stick-on) patches. If you are using this form, follow these instructions: Choose an area of skin without cuts, scars or hair, such as the upper arm, chest or behind the ear. Thoroughly clean the area where patch is to be applied. If patch gets wet and loose, cover with an additional piece of plastic. Apply a fresh patch if the first one falls off. Apply each dose to a different area of skin if possible.

Tranquilizers—Drugs that calm a person without clouding consciousness.

Tremor—Involuntary trembling.

Trichomoniasis—Infestation of the vagina by *trichomonas*, an infectious organism. The infection causes itching, vaginal discharge and irritation.

Triglyceride—Fatty chemical manufactured from carbohydrates for storage in fat cells.

Tyramine—Normal chemical component of the body that helps sustain blood pressure. Can rise to fatal levels in combination with some drugs.

Tyramine is found in many foods:

Beverages—Alcohol beverages, especially Chianti or robust red wines, vermouth, ale, beer.

Breads—Homemade bread with a lot of yeast and breads or crackers containing cheese.

Fats—Sour cream.

Fruits—Bananas, red plums, avocados, figs, raisins, raspberries.

Meats and meat substitutes—Aged game, liver (if not fresh), canned meats, salami, sausage, aged cheese, salted dried fish, pickled herring, meat tenderizers.

Vegetables—Italian broad beans, green bean pods, eggplant.

Miscellaneous—Yeast concentrates or extracts, marmite, soup cubes, commercial gravy, soy sauce, any protein food that has been stored improperly or is spoiled.

U

Ulcer, Peptic—Open sore on the mucous membrane of the esophagus, stomach or duodenum caused by stomach acid.

Urethra—Hollow tube through which urine (and semen in men) is discharged.

Urethritis—Inflammation or infection of the urethra.

Uricosurics—A group of drugs that promotes excretion of uric acid in the urine. These drugs include probenecid and sulfinpyrazone.

Urinary Acidifiers—Medications that cause urine to become acid. These include ascorbic acid, potassium phosphate, potassium and sodium phosphates.

Urinary Alkalizers—Medications that cause urine to become alkaline. These include potassium citrate, potassium citrate and citric acid, potassium citrate and sodium citrate, sodium bicarbonate, sodium citrate and citric acid, tricitrate.

Uterus—Also called womb. A hollow muscular organ in the female in which the embryo develops into a fetus.

V

Vascular—Pertaining to blood vessels.

Vascular Headache Preventatives—Medicines prescribed to prevent the occurrence of or reduce the frequency and severity of vascular headache such as migraine. These drugs include atenolol;

clonidine; ergotamine, belladonna alkaloids and phenobarbital; fenoprofen; ibuprofen; indomethacin; isocarboxazid, lithium; mefenamic acid; methysergide; metoprolol; nadolol; naproxen; phenelzine; pizotyline; propranolol; timolol, tranylcypromine, verapamil.

Vascular Headache Treatment—Medicine prescribed to treat vascular headaches such as migraine. These drugs include butalbital (combined with acetaminophen, aspirin, caffeine or codeine); cyproheptadine; diclofenac; diflunisal; dihydroergotamine; ergotamine; ergotamine and caffeine; ergotamine, caffeine, belladonna alkaloids and pentobarbital; etodolac; fenoprofen; ibuprofen; indomethacin (capsules, oral suspension, rectal); isometheptene, dichloralphenazone and acetaminophen; ketoprofen; meclofenamate; mefenamic acid; metoclopramide; naproxen; phenobarbital; sumatriptan.

Virus—Infectious organism that reproduces in the cells of the infected host.

X

Xanthines—Substances that stimulate muscle tissue, especially that of the heart. Types of xanthines include aminophylline, caffeine, dyphylline, oxtriphylline, theophylline.

Y

Yeast—A single-cell organism that can cause infections of the mouth, vagina, skin and parts of the gastrointestinal system.

GUIDE TO INDEX

Alphabetical entries in the index include three categories—generic names, brand names and drug-class names.

1. Generic names appear in capital letters, followed by their chart page number:

   ASPIRIN 120

2. Brand names appear in *italic*, followed by their generic ingredient and chart page number:

   Bayer - See ASPIRIN 120

   Some brand names contain two or more generic ingredients. These generic ingredients are listed in capital letters, following the brand name:

   Anacin - See
   ASPIRIN 120
   CAFFEINE 180

3. Drug-class names appear in regular type, capital and lower-case letters. All generic drug names in this book that fall into a drug class are listed after the class name:

   Anticonvulsant - See
   CARBAMAZEPINE 190
   DIVALPROEX 328
   FELBAMATE 372
   GABAPENTIN 394
   PARALDEHYDE 644
   PRIMIDONE 708
   VALPROIC ACID (Dipropylacetic Acid) 860

B

E

F

H

INDEX

I

J

K

L

M

N

O

Q

R

T

INDEX

V

EMERGENCY GUIDE FOR OVERDOSE VICTIMS

This section lists *basic* steps in recognizing and treating immediate effects of drug overdose.

Study the information before you need it. If possible, take a course in first aid and learn external cardiac massage and mouth-to-mouth breathing techniques, called *cardiopulmonary resuscitation* (CPR).

For quick reference, list emergency telephone numbers in the spaces provided on the inside front cover for fire department paramedics, ambulance, poison control center and your doctor. These numbers, except for that of a doctor, are usually listed on the inside cover of your telephone directory.

IF VICTIM IS UNCONSCIOUS, NOT *BREATHING:*

1. Yell for help. Don't leave victim.
2. Dial 911 (emergency) or 0 (operator) for an ambulance or medical help. If the victim is a child, give mouth-to-mouth breathing for one minute, then dial 911 or 0.
3. Begin mouth-to-mouth breathing immediately.
4. If there is no heartbeat, give external cardiac massage.
5. Don't stop CPR until help arrives.
6. Don't try to make victim vomit.
7. If vomiting occurs, save vomit to take to emergency room for analysis.
8. Take medicine or empty bottles with you to emergency room.

IF VICTIM IS UNCONSCIOUS AND *BREATHING:*

1. Dial 911 (emergency) or 0 (operator) for an ambulance or medical help.
2. If you can't get help immediately, take victim to the nearest emergency room.
3. Don't try to make victim vomit.
4. If vomiting occurs, save vomit to take to emergency room for analysis.
5. Watch victim carefully on the way to the emergency room. If heart or breathing stops, use cardiac massage and mouth-to-mouth breathing (CPR).
6. Take medicine or empty bottles with you to emergency room.